Mastering the BDS II
(Last 25 Years Solved Questions)

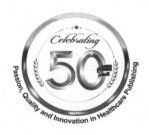

Celebrating 50

Passion, Quality and Innovation in Healthcare Publishing

Mastering the BDS IIIrd Year
(Last 25 Years Solved Questions)

Thoroughly Revised and Updated According to the Latest Syllabus of DCI

Eighth Edition

Hemant Gupta MDS
(Oral and Maxillofacial Pathology, Microbiology and Forensic Odontology)
General Practitioner and Consultant
Shivom Multispeciality Dental Clinic
Indore, Madhya Pradesh, India

JAYPEE BROTHERS MEDICAL PUBLISHERS
The Health Sciences Publisher
New Delhi | London

Jaypee Brothers Medical Publishers (P) Ltd

Headquarters

Jaypee Brothers Medical Publishers (P) Ltd
4838/24, Ansari Road, Daryaganj
New Delhi 110 002, India
Phone: +91-11-43574357
Fax: +91-11-43574314
Email: jaypee@jaypeebrothers.com

Overseas Office

J.P. Medical Ltd
83 Victoria Street, London
SW1H 0HW (UK)
Phone: +44 20 3170 8910
Fax: +44 (0)20 3008 6180
Email: info@jpmedpub.com

Website: www.jaypeebrothers.com
Website: www.jaypeedigital.com

Inquiries for bulk sales may be solicited at: jaypee@jaypeebrothers.com

Mastering the BDS IIIrd Year (Last 25 Years Solved Questions)

Eighth Edition: **2020**

ISBN 978-81-947090-9-1

Printed at Sanat Printers

Dedicated to

Almighty SAI BABA
My grandparents Shri HD Gupta and Smt Vijaylakshmi Gupta
In loving memory of my parents
Late Shri VK Gupta and Late Smt Anju Gupta

To my wife Smita Sharma Gupta
for being so much understanding and
Last but not least my lovely angel son Meetaan Gupta
for making life worthwhile

PREFACE TO THE EIGHTH EDITION

It is a matter of great pride and pleasure to introduce the eighth edition of *Mastering the BDS IIIrd Year (Last 25 Years Solved Questions)*. The aim of this book is to enable the student of dentistry to learn fundamentals. All the sections are updated and the answers of each and every section are revised as per the latest syllabus. This new edition is updated and expanded, bringing forth new information gained since production of last edition. The text has been made more clinically oriented so as to better correlate the text with clinical aspects. The text consists of a large number of illustrations, which enhances the understanding of written description. In this edition, additional matter along with image-based questions is added, which will help students to know the basic pattern of competitive examinations, such as AIIMS, NEET, PGI, etc. I, as an author, wish to express my hope that material presented is clear and understandable. The book is never meant to replace any of the textbook. All the respective textbooks of all subjects should be read thoroughly to gain the deep knowledge of subject. This book provides an idea of questions and answers in BDS examinations and MDS basic science examination and multiple choice questions (MCQs) and image-based questions (IBQs) in pre-PG examinations. I hope that the content will be enough to stimulate the insight and new trends of thoughts in all the subjects of 3rd Year.

Any of the suggestions and criticism are welcomed at *macrocyte@gmail.com*.

Hemant Gupta

PREFACE TO THE FIRST EDITION

It is a matter of great pride and pleasure to introduce the first edition of *Mastering the BDS IIIrd Year*. As our previous books have got continued support and good response, we have kept the same basic pattern, but the sequence of chapters has been arranged in a simpler way for a wider and systematic coverage of the topics.

The subjects of IIIrd year still ring fear in the minds of students—baseless fear that rest on silent assumptions and those that distort thinking. However, self-study, dedication, motivation and hard work are the virtues that go a long way in the making of a genius—a success. Listen, think, read and analyze with an open mind and you definitely cannot go wrong. I would like to clarify that this book is not meant to replace your standard textbooks, but yet coupled with your effort and sincerity, it will definitely make you clinch and help you put your best foot forward to reach great heights of success.

And last but not least, I thank our publisher, Shri Jitendar P Vij (Group Chairman) of M/s Jaypee Brothers Medical Publishers (P) Ltd, New Delhi, India, for his whole-hearted support and help to make this book a reality.

Hemant Gupta

ACKNOWLEDGMENTS

Achievement of this book was possible by the help and support of Almighty *SAI BABA,* my grandparents, parents, my wife, teachers and friends.

Special thanks to those who remain behind the curtain and help in arrangement of study material for the book.

Heartily thanks to Dr Deepak Aggarwal (MDS), and Mrs Kriti Gorkhe, for helping in arranging the appropriate question papers.

Thanks to Mr Jai Singh Bundela from M/s Jaypee Brothers Medical Publishers (P) Ltd, Indore, Madhya Pradesh, India, for his whole-hearted support.

I am very grateful to the whole team of M/s Jaypee Brothers Medical Publishers (P) Ltd, New Delhi, India, who helped and guided me, especially Shri Jitendar P Vij (Group Chairman), Mr Ankit Vij (Managing Director), Mr MS Mani (Group President), Dr Madhu Choudhary (Publishing Head–Education), Ms Pooja Bhandari (Production Head), Ms Sunita Katla (Executive Assistant to Group Chairman and Publishing Manager), Dr Astha Sawhney (Development Editor), Ms Samina Khan (Executive Assistant to Publishing Head–Education), Mr Rajesh Sharma (Production Coordinator), Ms Seema Dogra (Cover Visualizer), Mr Ajeet Rathor (Typesetter), Mr Vakil Khan (Proofreader), Mr Manoj Pahuja (Graphic Designer) and his team members, for all their support to work in this project and make it a success. Without their cooperation, I could not have completed this project.

CONTENTS

Plate 1

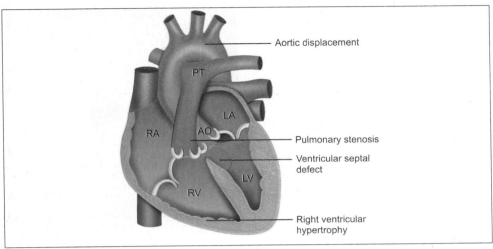

Page 46, Q. 13: Tetralogy of Fallot.

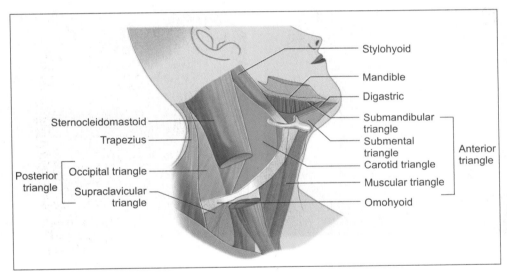

Page 412, Q. 6: Triangles of neck.

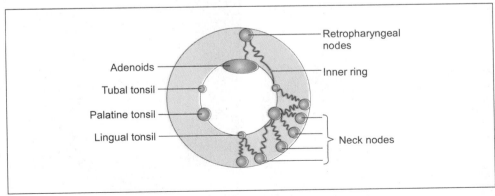

Page 414, Q. 8: Inner and outer Waldeyer ring anatomy.

Plate 2

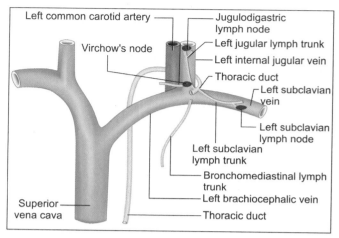

Page 443, Q. 2: Virchow's node.

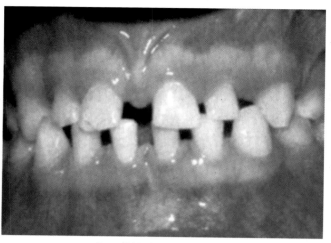

Page 515, Q. 2: Microdontia.

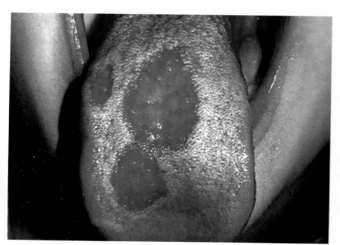

Page 516, Q. 3: Geographic tongue.

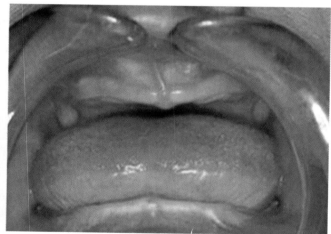

Page 517, Q. 6: Anodontia.

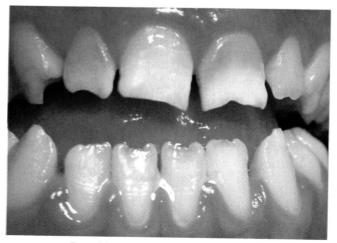

Page 518, Q. 7: Amelogenesis imperfecta.

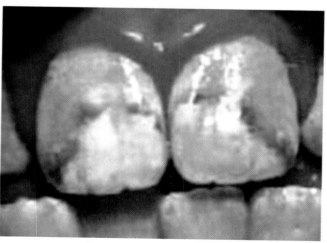

Page 518, Q. 8: Mottled enamel.

Plate 3

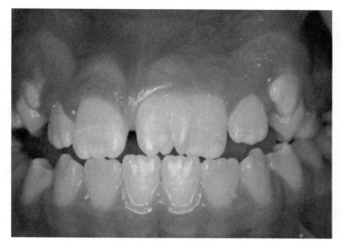

Page 520, Q. 11: Fusion.

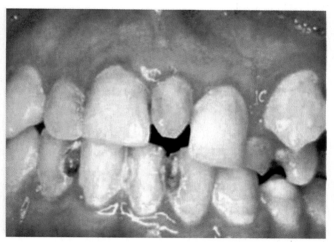

Page 521, Q. 13: Supernumerary teeth.

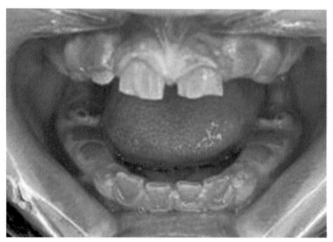

Page 521, Q. 14: Dentinogenesis imperfecta.

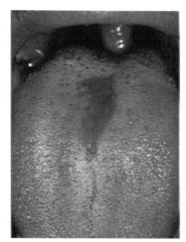

Page 522, Q. 15: Median rhomboid glossitis.

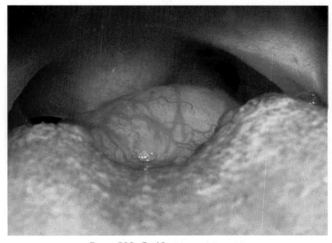

Page 522, Q. 16: Lingual thyroid.

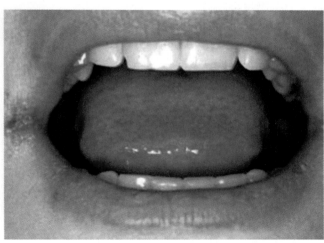

Page 522, Q. 17: Perleche.

Plate 4

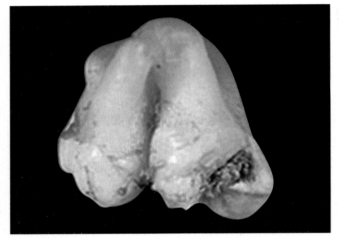

Page 523, Q. 19: Concrescence.

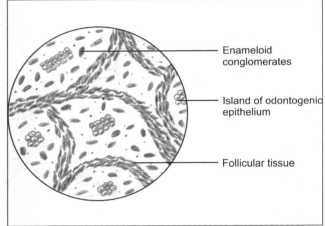

- Enameloid conglomerates
- Island of odontogenic epithelium
- Follicular tissue

Page 528, Q. 26: Ghost teeth.

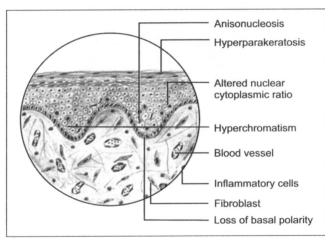

- Anisonucleosis
- Hyperparakeratosis
- Altered nuclear cytoplasmic ratio
- Hyperchromatism
- Blood vessel
- Inflammatory cells
- Fibroblast
- Loss of basal polarity

A. Mild dysplasia

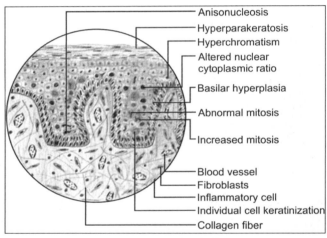

- Anisonucleosis
- Hyperparakeratosis
- Hyperchromatism
- Altered nuclear cytoplasmic ratio
- Basilar hyperplasia
- Abnormal mitosis
- Increased mitosis
- Blood vessel
- Fibroblasts
- Inflammatory cell
- Individual cell keratinization
- Collagen fiber

B. Moderate dysplasia

Page 535 Q. 1: Leukoplakia.

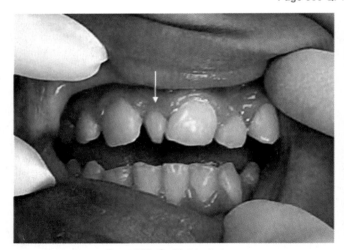

Page 532, Q. 41: Mesiodens.

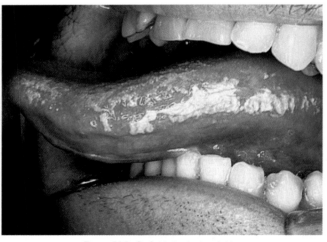

Page 536, Q. 3: Hairy leukoplakia.

Plate 5

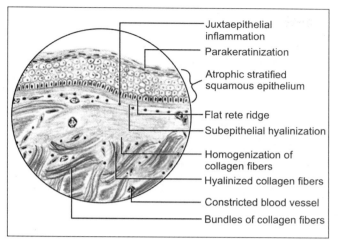

Juxtaepithelial inflammation
Parakeratinization
Atrophic stratified squamous epithelium
Flat rete ridge
Subepithelial hyalinization
Homogenization of collagen fibers
Hyalinized collagen fibers
Constricted blood vessel
Bundles of collagen fibers

Page 537, Q. 4: Oral Submucous fibrosis.

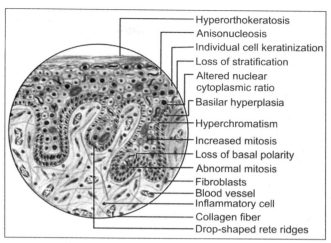

Hyperorthokeratosis
Anisonucleosis
Individual cell keratinization
Loss of stratification
Altered nuclear cytoplasmic ratio
Basilar hyperplasia
Hyperchromatism
Increased mitosis
Loss of basal polarity
Abnormal mitosis
Fibroblasts
Blood vessel
Inflammatory cell
Collagen fiber
Drop-shaped rete ridges

Page 537, Q. 5: Intraepithelial carcinoma.

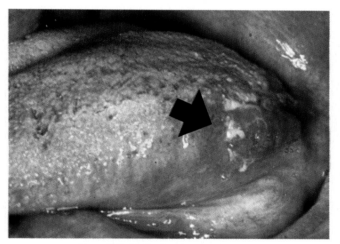

Page 538, Q. 6: Carcinoma of tongue.

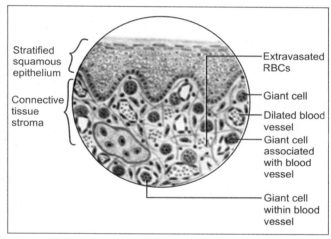

Stratified squamous epithelium
Connective tissue stroma
Extravasated RBCs
Giant cell
Dilated blood vessel
Giant cell associated with blood vessel
Giant cell within blood vessel

Page 538, Q. 7: Peripheral giant cell granuloma.

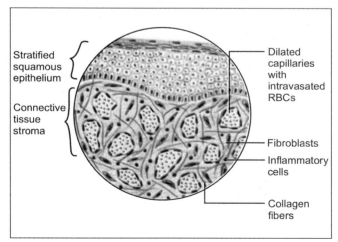

Stratified squamous epithelium
Connective tissue stroma
Dilated capillaries with intravasated RBCs
Fibroblasts
Inflammatory cells
Collagen fibers

Page 539, Q. 8: Capillary hemangioma.

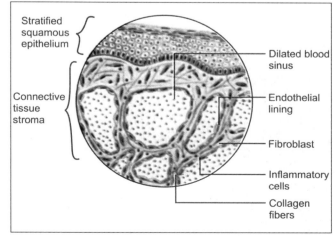

Stratified squamous epithelium
Connective tissue stroma
Dilated blood sinus
Endothelial lining
Fibroblast
Inflammatory cells
Collagen fibers

Page 539, Q. 8: Cavernous hemangioma.

Plate 6

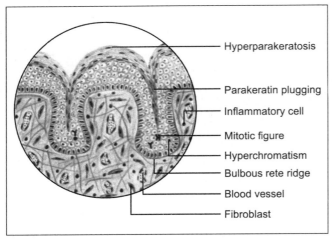

Page 540, Q. 11: Verrucous carcinoma.

- Hyperparakeratosis
- Parakeratin plugging
- Inflammatory cell
- Mitotic figure
- Hyperchromatism
- Bulbous rete ridge
- Blood vessel
- Fibroblast

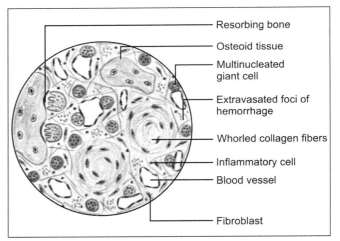

Page 540, Q. 13: Central giant cell granuloma.

- Resorbing bone
- Osteoid tissue
- Multinucleated giant cell
- Extravasated foci of hemorrhage
- Whorled collagen fibers
- Inflammatory cell
- Blood vessel
- Fibroblast

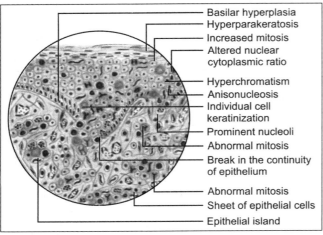

Page 541, Q. 15: Moderately differentiated squamous cell carcinoma.

- Basilar hyperplasia
- Hyperparakeratosis
- Increased mitosis
- Altered nuclear cytoplasmic ratio
- Hyperchromatism
- Anisonucleosis
- Individual cell keratinization
- Prominent nucleoli
- Abnormal mitosis
- Break in the continuity of epithelium
- Abnormal mitosis
- Sheet of epithelial cells
- Epithelial island

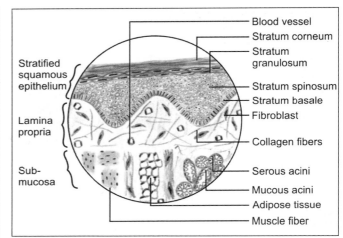

Page 542, Q. 17: van Gieson's stain.

- Stratified squamous epithelium
- Lamina propria
- Sub-mucosa
- Blood vessel
- Stratum corneum
- Stratum granulosum
- Stratum spinosum
- Stratum basale
- Fibroblast
- Collagen fibers
- Serous acini
- Mucous acini
- Adipose tissue
- Muscle fiber

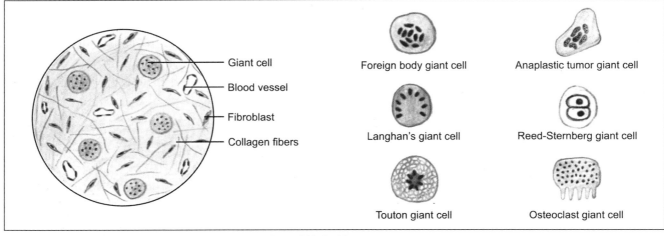

- Giant cell
- Blood vessel
- Fibroblast
- Collagen fibers

Foreign body giant cell

Anaplastic tumor giant cell

Langhan's giant cell

Reed-Sternberg giant cell

Touton giant cell

Osteoclast giant cell

Page 542, Q. 16: Giant cell.

Plate 7

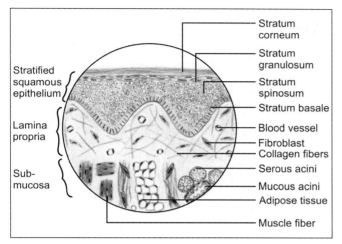

Stratified squamous epithelium
- Stratum corneum
- Stratum granulosum
- Stratum spinosum
- Stratum basale

Lamina propria
- Blood vessel
- Fibroblast
- Collagen fibers

Sub-mucosa
- Serous acini
- Mucous acini
- Adipose tissue
- Muscle fiber

Page 543, Q. 17: Mallory stain.

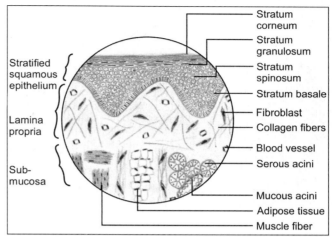

Stratified squamous epithelium
- Stratum corneum
- Stratum granulosum
- Stratum spinosum
- Stratum basale

Lamina propria
- Fibroblast
- Collagen fibers

Sub-mucosa
- Blood vessel
- Serous acini
- Mucous acini
- Adipose tissue
- Muscle fiber

Page 543, Q. 17: PAS stain.

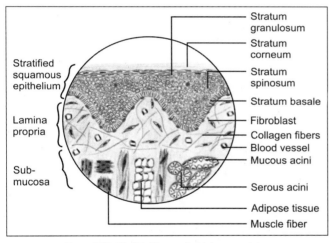

Stratified squamous epithelium
- Stratum granulosum
- Stratum corneum
- Stratum spinosum
- Stratum basale

Lamina propria
- Fibroblast
- Collagen fibers
- Blood vessel
- Mucous acini

Sub-mucosa
- Serous acini
- Adipose tissue
- Muscle fiber

Page 543, Q. 17: Masson's trichrome stain.

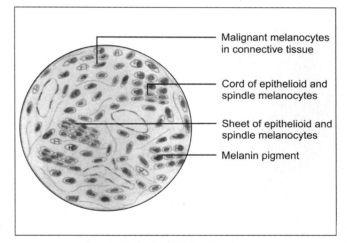

- Malignant melanocytes in connective tissue
- Cord of epithelioid and spindle melanocytes
- Sheet of epithelioid and spindle melanocytes
- Melanin pigment

Page 546, Q. 20: Malignant melanoma.

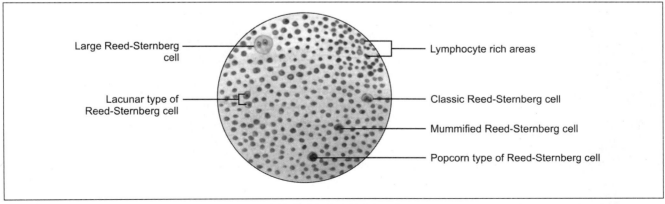

- Large Reed-Sternberg cell
- Lacunar type of Reed-Sternberg cell
- Lymphocyte rich areas
- Classic Reed-Sternberg cell
- Mummified Reed-Sternberg cell
- Popcorn type of Reed-Sternberg cell

Page 547, Q. 22: Hodgkin's lymphoma.

Plate 8

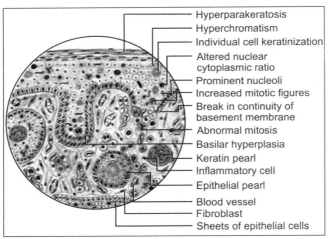

Hyperparakeratosis
Hyperchromatism
Individual cell keratinization
Altered nuclear cytoplasmic ratio
Prominent nucleoli
Increased mitotic figures
Break in continuity of basement membrane
Abnormal mitosis
Basilar hyperplasia
Keratin pearl
Inflammatory cell
Epithelial pearl
Blood vessel
Fibroblast
Sheets of epithelial cells

Page 548, Q. 23: Well-differentiated squamous cell carcinoma.

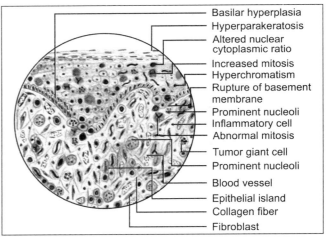

Basilar hyperplasia
Hyperparakeratosis
Altered nuclear cytoplasmic ratio
Increased mitosis
Hyperchromatism
Rupture of basement membrane
Prominent nucleoli
Inflammatory cell
Abnormal mitosis
Tumor giant cell
Prominent nucleoli
Blood vessel
Epithelial island
Collagen fiber
Fibroblast

Page 548, Q. 23: Poorly-differentiated squamous cell carcinoma.

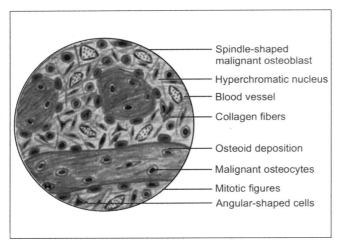

Spindle-shaped malignant osteoblast
Hyperchromatic nucleus
Blood vessel
Collagen fibers
Osteoid deposition
Malignant osteocytes
Mitotic figures
Angular-shaped cells

Page 549, Q. 25: Osteosarcoma.

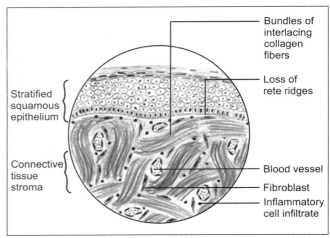

Bundles of interlacing collagen fibers
Loss of rete ridges
Stratified squamous epithelium
Connective tissue stroma
Blood vessel
Fibroblast
Inflammatory cell infiltrate

Page 550, Q. 29: Fibroma.

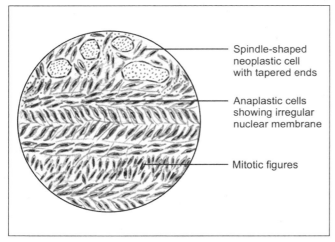

Spindle-shaped neoplastic cell with tapered ends
Anaplastic cells showing irregular nuclear membrane
Mitotic figures

Page 551, Q. 31: Fibrosarcoma.

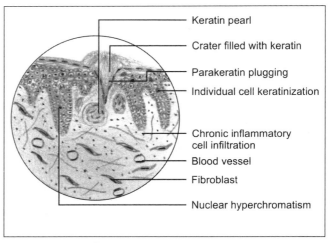

Keratin pearl
Crater filled with keratin
Parakeratin plugging
Individual cell keratinization
Chronic inflammatory cell infiltration
Blood vessel
Fibroblast
Nuclear hyperchromatism

Page 552, Q. 32: Keratoacanthoma.

Plate 9

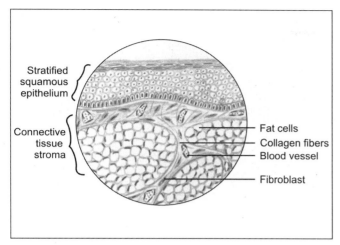

Stratified squamous epithelium

Connective tissue stroma

Fat cells
Collagen fibers
Blood vessel
Fibroblast

Page 554, Q. 38: Lipoma.

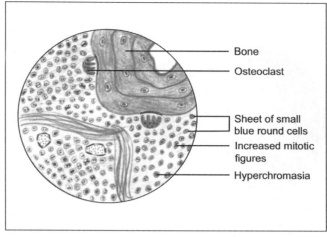

Bone
Osteoclast

Sheet of small blue round cells
Increased mitotic figures
Hyperchromasia

Page 555, Q. 39: Ewing's sarcoma.

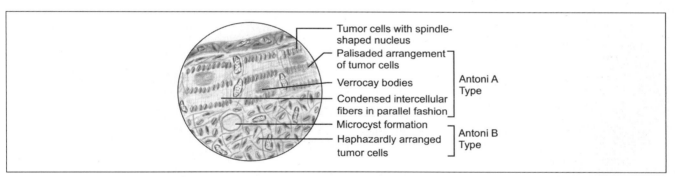

Tumor cells with spindle-shaped nucleus
Palisaded arrangement of tumor cells — Antoni A Type
Verrocay bodies
Condensed intercellular fibers in parallel fashion
Microcyst formation — Antoni B Type
Haphazardly arranged tumor cells

Page 556, Q. 41: Neurilemmoma.

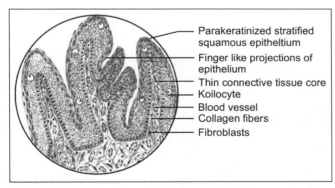

Parakeratinized stratified squameltium
Finger like projections of epithelium
Thin connective tissue core
Koilocyte
Blood vessel
Collagen fibers
Fibroblasts

Page 557, Q. 44: Papilloma (H and E stain).

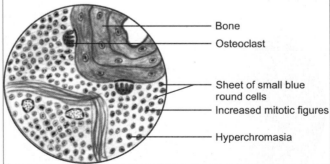

Bone
Osteoclast

Sheet of small blue round cells
Increased mitotic figures
Hyperchromasia

Page 558, Q. 45: Ewing's sarcoma (H and E Stain).

Plate 10

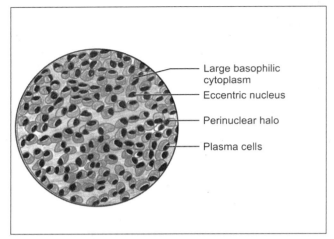

Large basophilic cytoplasm
Eccentric nucleus
Perinuclear halo
Plasma cells

Page 559, Q. 47: Multiple myeloma.

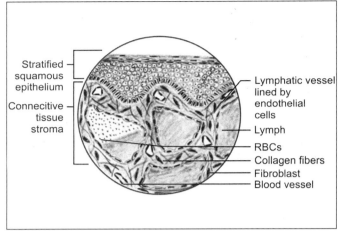

Stratified squamous epithelium
Connecitive tissue stroma
Lymphatic vessel lined by endothelial cells
Lymph
RBCs
Collagen fibers
Fibroblast
Blood vessel

Page 561, Q.50: Lymphangioma.

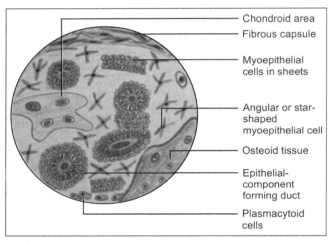

Chondroid area
Fibrous capsule
Myoepithelial cells in sheets
Angular or star-shaped myoepithelial cell
Osteoid tissue
Epithelial-component forming duct
Plasmacytoid cells

Page 563, Q. 1: Pleomorphic adenoma.

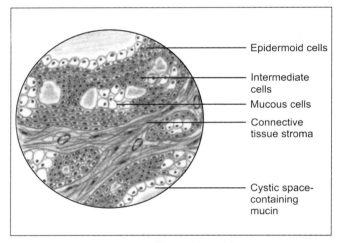

Epidermoid cells
Intermediate cells
Mucous cells
Connective tissue stroma
Cystic space-containing mucin

Page 565, Q. 3: Mucoepidermoid tumor.

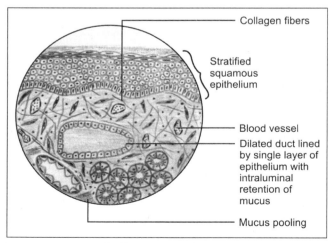

Collagen fibers
Stratified squamous epithelium
Blood vessel
Dilated duct lined by single layer of epithelium with intraluminal retention of mucus
Mucus pooling

A. Mucous retention cyst

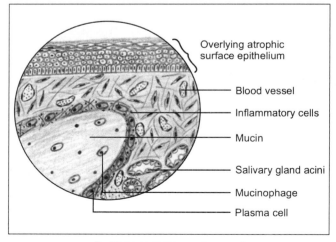

Overlying atrophic surface epithelium
Blood vessel
Inflammatory cells
Mucin
Salivary gland acini
Mucinophage
Plasma cell

B. Mucous extravasation cyst

Page 567, Q. 7: Mucocele

Plate 11

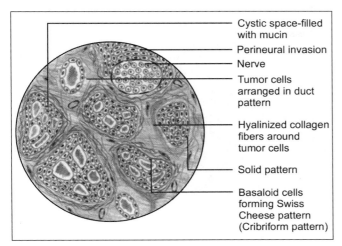

Cystic space-filled with mucin
Perineural invasion
Nerve
Tumor cells arranged in duct pattern
Hyalinized collagen fibers around tumor cells
Solid pattern
Basaloid cells forming Swiss Cheese pattern (Cribriform pattern)

Page 566, Q. 4: Adenoid cystic carcinoma.

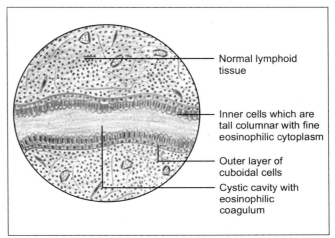

Normal lymphoid tissue
Inner cells which are tall columnar with fine eosinophilic cytoplasm
Outer layer of cuboidal cells
Cystic cavity with eosinophilic coagulum

Page 568, Q. 13: Warthin's tumor.

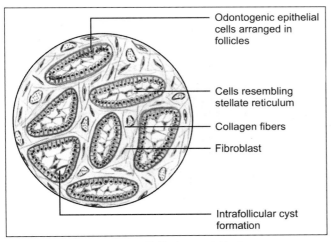

Odontogenic epithelial cells arranged in follicles
Cells resembling stellate reticulum
Collagen fibers
Fibroblast
Intrafollicular cyst formation

Page 571, Q. 1: Follicular ameloblastoma.

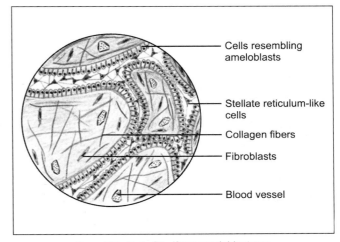

Cells resembling ameloblasts
Stellate reticulum-like cells
Collagen fibers
Fibroblasts
Blood vessel

Page 571, Q. 1: Plexiform ameloblastoma.

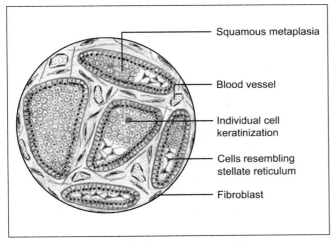

Squamous metaplasia
Blood vessel
Individual cell keratinization
Cells resembling stellate reticulum
Fibroblast

Page 571, Q. 1: Acanthomatous ameloblastoma.

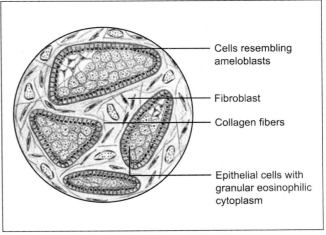

Cells resembling ameloblasts
Fibroblast
Collagen fibers
Epithelial cells with granular eosinophilic cytoplasm

Page 571, Q. 1: Granular cell ameloblastoma.

Plate 12

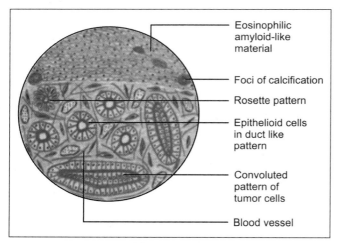

Eosinophilic amyloid-like material

Foci of calcification

Rosette pattern

Epithelioid cells in duct like pattern

Convoluted pattern of tumor cells

Blood vessel

Page 572, Q. 4: Adenomatoid odontogenic tumor.

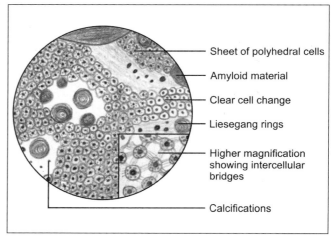

Sheet of polyhedral cells

Amyloid material

Clear cell change

Liesegang rings

Higher magnification showing intercellular bridges

Calcifications

Page 573, Q. 5: Pindborg's tumor.

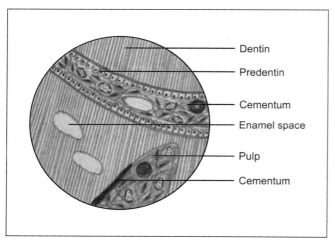

Dentin

Predentin

Cementum

Enamel space

Pulp

Cementum

Page 573, Q. 6: Complex composite odontome.

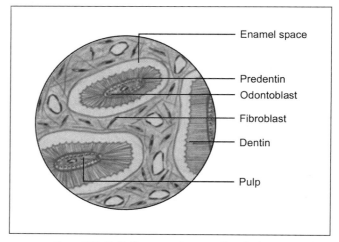

Enamel space

Predentin

Odontoblast

Fibroblast

Dentin

Pulp

Page 574, Q. 6: Compound composite odontome.

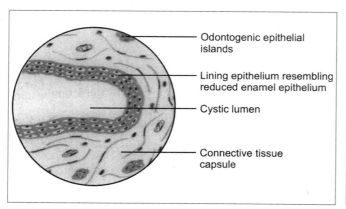

Odontogenic epithelial islands

Lining epithelium resembling reduced enamel epithelium

Cystic lumen

Connective tissue capsule

Page 577, Q. 1: Dentigerous cyst.

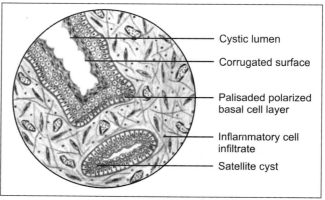

Cystic lumen

Corrugated surface

Palisaded polarized basal cell layer

Inflammatory cell infiltrate

Satellite cyst

Page 578, Q. 4: Odontogenic keratocyst.

Plate 13

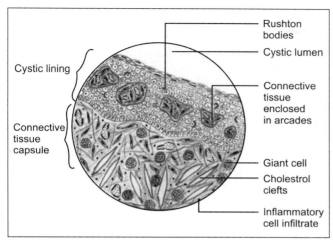

Page 579, Q. 5: Radicular cyst.

Labels: Rushton bodies, Cystic lumen, Connective tissue enclosed in arcades, Giant cell, Cholestrol clefts, Inflammatory cell infiltrate, Cystic lining, Connective tissue capsule

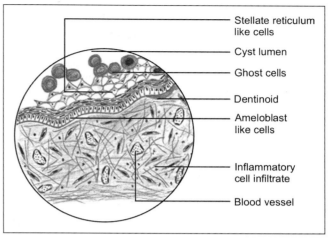

Page 582, Q. 20: Calcifying odontogenic cyst.

Labels: Stellate reticulum like cells, Cyst lumen, Ghost cells, Dentinoid, Ameloblast like cells, Inflammatory cell infiltrate, Blood vessel

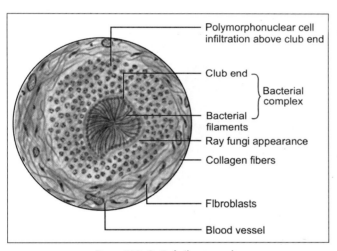

Page 586, Q. 5: Actinomycosis.

Labels: Polymorphonuclear cell infiltration above club end, Club end, Bacterial complex, Bacterial filaments, Ray fungi appearance, Collagen fibers, Fibroblasts, Blood vessel

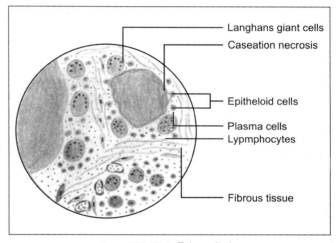

Page 586, Q. 6: Tuberculosis.

Labels: Langhans giant cells, Caseation necrosis, Epitheloid cells, Plasma cells, Lypmphocytes, Fibrous tissue

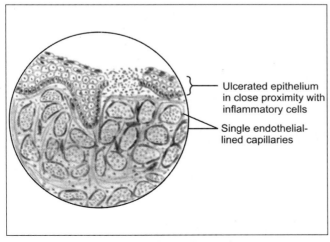

Page 588, Q. 9: Pyogenic granuloma.

Labels: Ulcerated epithelium in close proximity with inflammatory cells, Single endothelial-lined capillaries

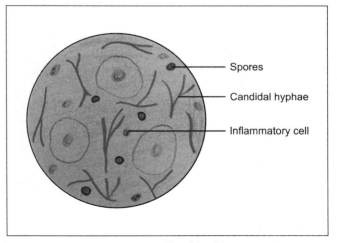

Page 599, Q. 1: Candida albicans.

Labels: Spores, Candidal hyphae, Inflammatory cell

Plate 14

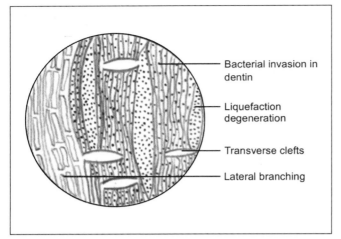

Bacterial invasion in dentin

Liquefaction degeneration

Transverse clefts

Lateral branching

Page 608, Q. 3: Dentinal caries H and E (DS).

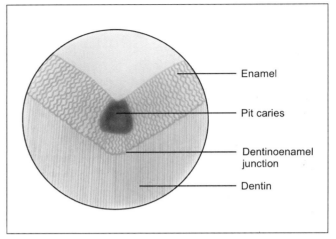

Enamel

Pit caries

Dentinoenamel junction

Dentin

Page 611, Q. 14: Pit and fissure caries (GS).

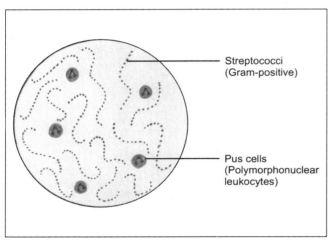

Streptococci (Gram-positive)

Pus cells (Polymorphonuclear leukocytes)

Page 612, Q. 15: *Streptococcus mutans*.

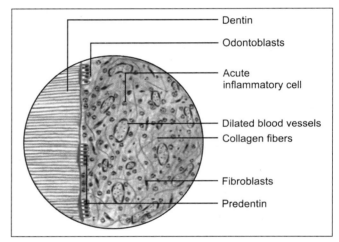

Dentin

Odontoblasts

Acute inflammatory cell

Dilated blood vessels

Collagen fibers

Fibroblasts

Predentin

Page 615, Q. 1: Acute pulpitis.

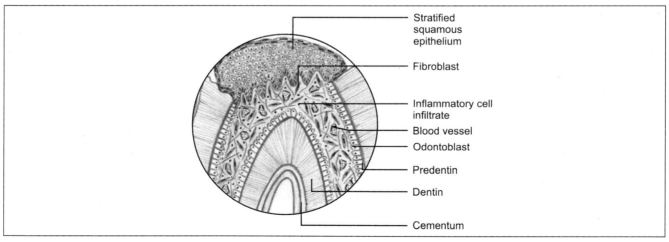

Stratified squamous epithelium

Fibroblast

Inflammatory cell infiltrate

Blood vessel

Odontoblast

Predentin

Dentin

Cementum

Page 616, Q. 2: Pulp polyp/chronic hyperplastic pulpitis.

Plate 15

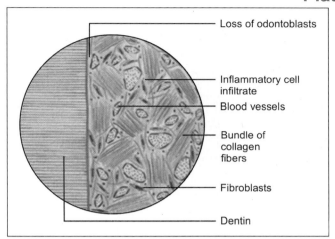

Loss of odontoblasts

Inflammatory cell infiltrate

Blood vessels

Bundle of collagen fibers

Fibroblasts

Dentin

Page 617, Q. 3: Chronic pulpitis.

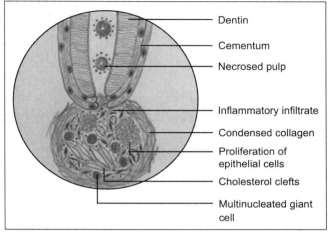

Dentin

Cementum

Necrosed pulp

Inflammatory infiltrate

Condensed collagen

Proliferation of epithelial cells

Cholesterol clefts

Multinucleated giant cell

Page 618, Q. 5: Periapical granuloma.

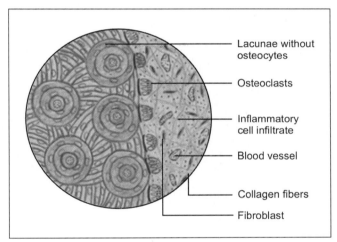

Lacunae without osteocytes

Osteoclasts

Inflammatory cell infiltrate

Blood vessel

Collagen fibers

Fibroblast

Page 619, Q. 8: Osteomyelitis.

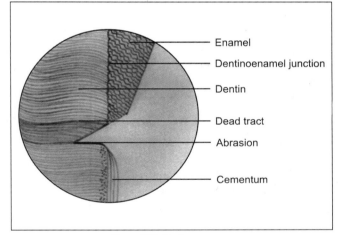

Enamel

Dentinoenamel junction

Dentin

Dead tract

Abrasion

Cementum

Page 628, Q. 1: Abrasion.

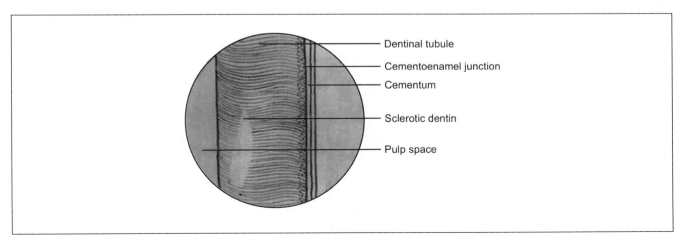

Dentinal tubule

Cementoenamel junction

Cementum

Sclerotic dentin

Pulp space

Page 628, Q. 2: Sclerotic dentin.

Plate 16

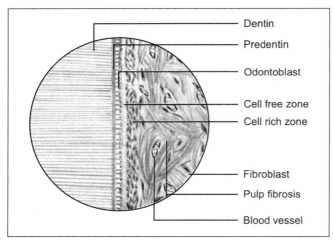

Dentin
Predentin
Odontoblast
Cell free zone
Cell rich zone
Fibroblast
Pulp fibrosis
Blood vessel

Page 629, Q. 3: Pulp fibrosis.

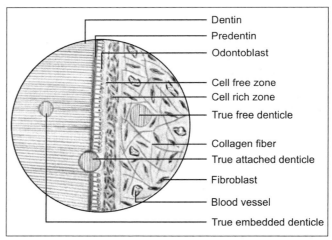

Dentin
Predentin
Odontoblast
Cell free zone
Cell rich zone
True free denticle
Collagen fiber
True attached denticle
Fibroblast
Blood vessel
True embedded denticle

Page 629, Q. 3; Page 633, Q. 12: True pulp stones.

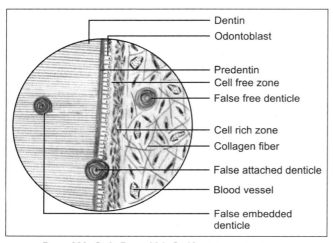

Dentin
Odontoblast
Predentin
Cell free zone
False free denticle
Cell rich zone
Collagen fiber
False attached denticle
Blood vessel
False embedded denticle

Page 629, Q. 3; Page 634, Q. 12: False pulp stones.

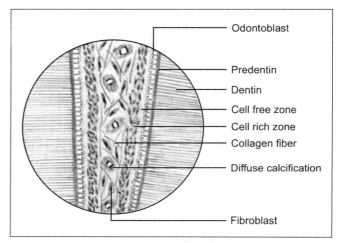

Odontoblast
Predentin
Dentin
Cell free zone
Cell rich zone
Collagen fiber
Diffuse calcification
Fibroblast

Page 630, Q. 3: Diffuse calcification.

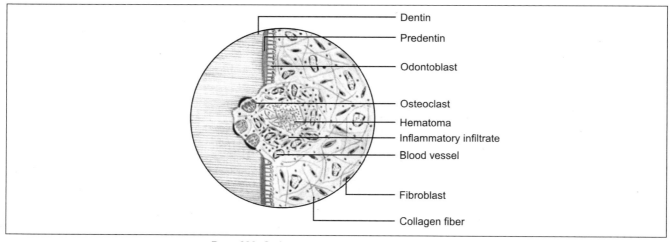

Dentin
Predentin
Odontoblast
Osteoclast
Hematoma
Inflammatory infiltrate
Blood vessel
Fibroblast
Collagen fiber

Page 630, Q. 4: Internal resorption of teeth or pink tooth.

Plate 17

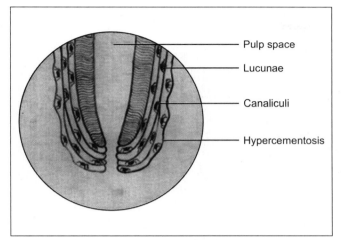

- Pulp space
- Lucunae
- Canaliculi
- Hypercementosis

Page 631, Q. 5: Hypercementosis.

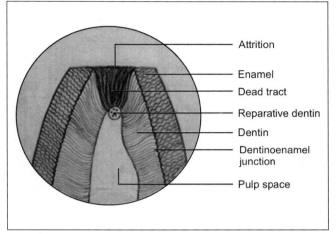

- Attrition
- Enamel
- Dead tract
- Reparative dentin
- Dentin
- Dentinoenamel junction
- Pulp space

Page 631, Q. 6: Attrition.

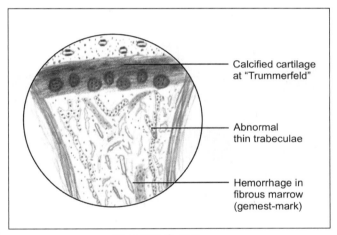

- Calcified cartilage at "Trummerfeld"
- Abnormal thin trabeculae
- Hemorrhage in fibrous marrow (gemest-mark)

Page 640, Q. 5: Scurvy.

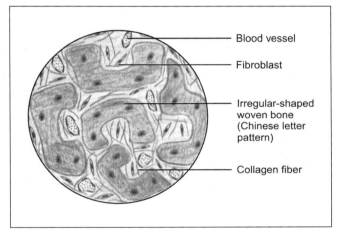

- Blood vessel
- Fibroblast
- Irregular-shaped woven bone (Chinese letter pattern)
- Collagen fiber

Page 643, Q. 5: Fibrous dysplasia.

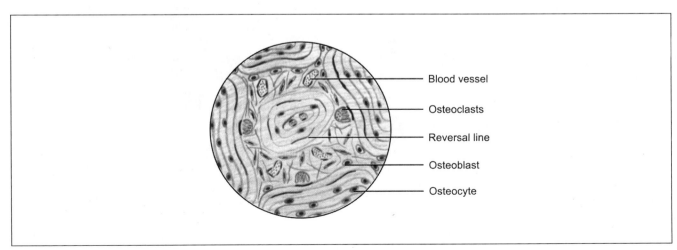

- Blood vessel
- Osteoclasts
- Reversal line
- Osteoblast
- Osteocyte

Page 644, Q. 6: Paget's disease of bone.

Plate 18

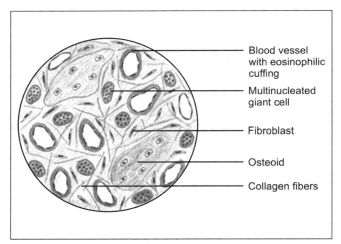

Blood vessel with eosinophilic cuffing

Multinucleated giant cell

Fibroblast

Osteoid

Collagen fibers

Page 645, Q. 10: Cherubism.

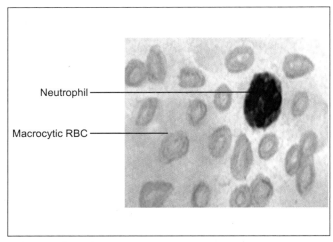

Neutrophil

Macrocytic RBC

Page 649, Q. 1: Peripheral smear showing pernicious anemia.

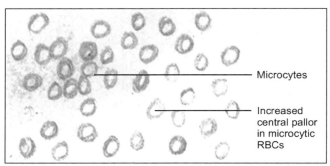

Microcytes

Increased central pallor in microcytic RBCs

Page 652, Q. 8: Peripheral smear showing iron deficiency anemia.

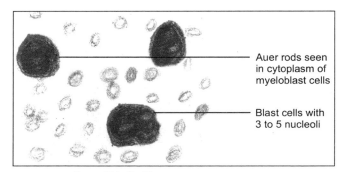

Auer rods seen in cytoplasm of myeloblast cells

Blast cells with 3 to 5 nucleoli

Page 654, Q. 10: Acute myeloid leukemia.

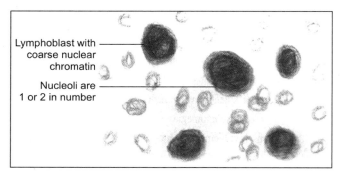

Lymphoblast with coarse nuclear chromatin

Nucleoli are 1 or 2 in number

Page 654, Q. 10: Acute lymphoblastic leukemia.

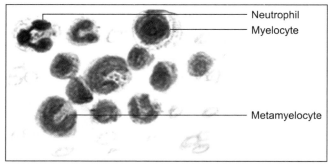

Neutrophil

Myelocyte

Metamyelocyte

Page 654, Q. 10: Chronic myeloid leukemia.

Plate 19

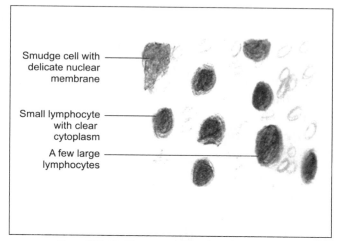

Smudge cell with delicate nuclear membrane

Small lymphocyte with clear cytoplasm

A few large lymphocytes

Page 654, Q. 10: Chronic lymphocytic leukemia.

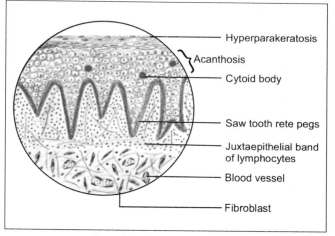

Hyperparakeratosis

Acanthosis

Cytoid body

Saw tooth rete pegs

Juxtaepithelial band of lymphocytes

Blood vessel

Fibroblast

Page 657, Q. 1: Lichen planus.

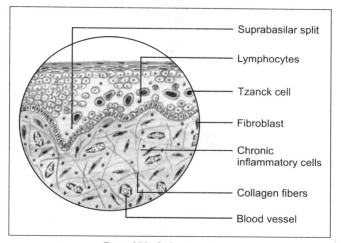

Suprabasilar split

Lymphocytes

Tzanck cell

Fibroblast

Chronic inflammatory cells

Collagen fibers

Blood vessel

Page 658, Q. 3: Pemphigus.

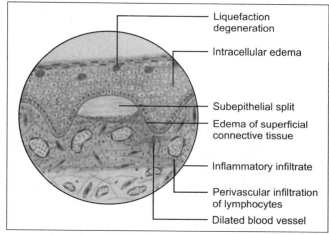

Liquefaction degeneration

Intracellular edema

Subepithelial split

Edema of superficial connective tissue

Inflammatory infiltrate

Perivascular infiltration of lymphocytes

Dilated blood vessel

Page 658, Q. 5: Erythema multiforme.

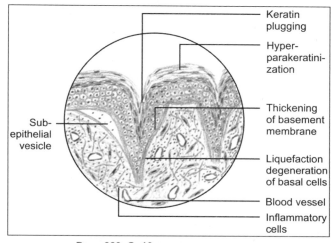

Keratin plugging

Hyper-parakeratini-zation

Sub-epithelial vesicle

Thickening of basement membrane

Liquefaction degeneration of basal cells

Blood vessel

Inflammatory cells

Page 660, Q. 13: Lupus erythematosus.

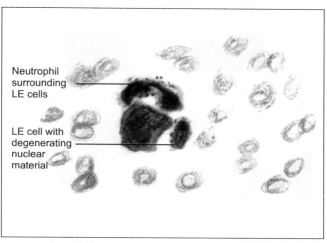

Neutrophil surrounding LE cells

LE cell with degenerating nuclear material

Page 665, Q. 22: LE Cell inclusion phenomenon.

Plate 20

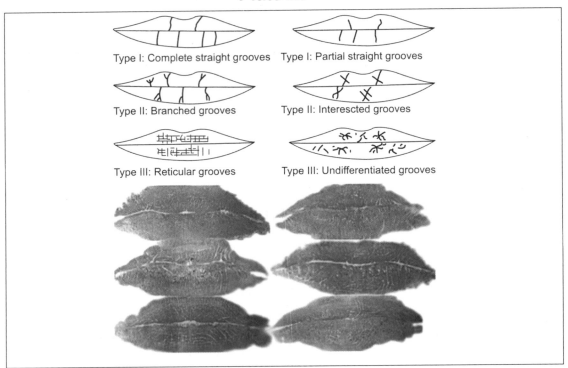

Type I: Complete straight grooves   Type I: Partial straight grooves

Type II: Branched grooves   Type II: Interescted grooves

Type III: Reticular grooves   Type III: Undifferentiated grooves

Page 668, Q. 2: Lip patterns.

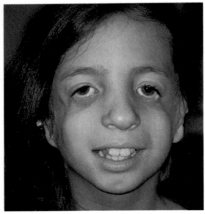

Page 715, Q. 1

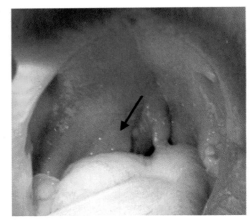

Page 716, Q. 1

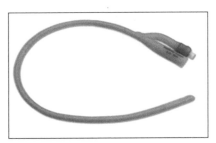

Page 716, Q. 2

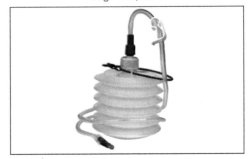

Page 716, Q. 3

1. INTRODUCTION

Q.1. Write important causes of digital clubbing.

(Mar 2011, 2 Marks)

Ans. Clubbing is a bulbous enlargement of soft part of terminal phalanges with both transverse and longitudinal curving of nails.

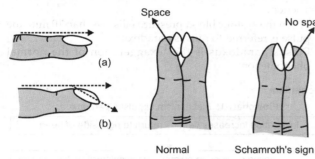

(a) Normal nail bed; Profile angle = 180°
(b) Severe clubbing; Profile angle = >180°

Fig. 1: Clubbing.

Causes of Clubbing

♦ **Pulmonary disorders**
   • *Suppuration of lung*
     – Bronchiectasis
     – Lung abscess
     – Suppurative pneumonia
   • *Tumors of lung*
     – Mesothelioma
     – Primary lung cancer
     – Metastatic lung cancer
♦ **Cardiac disorders**
   • Cyanotic congenital heart diseases
   • Subacute bacterial endocarditis
   • Atrial myxoma
♦ **Disorders of gastrointestinal system and liver**
   • Inflammatory bowel disease
     – Regional ileitis
     – Ulcerative colitis
     – Malabsorption syndrome
   • Cirrhosis of liver
   • Malignancy of liver
♦ **Disorders of endocrine system**
   • Myxedema
   • Thyroid acropachy
   • Acromegaly
♦ **Miscellaneous**
   • Hereditary
   • Idiopathic
   • *Unilateral:* Pancoast tumor, subclavian and innominate artery aneurysm
   • *Unidigital:* Traumatic or tophi deposit in gout
   • Only in upper limbs in heroin addicts due to chronic obstructive phlebitis.

Grades of Clubbing

♦ **Grade I:** Softening of nail bed because of hypertrophy of tissue at that site.
♦ **Grade II:** In addition to grade I changes, there is obliteration of angle between nail base and adjacent skin of the finger.
♦ **Grade III:** In addition to grade II changes, nail itself loses its longitudinal ridges, becomes convex from above downwards and from side to side. The nails assume shape of "parrot's beak" or terminal segment may become bulbous like a "drum stick".
♦ **Grade IV:** Finger changes are associated with hypertrophic pulmonary osteoarthropathy.

Q.2. Write short note on cyanosis.

(Feb 2013, 5 Marks) (Apr 2015, 3 Marks)

Or

Write short answer on cyanosis. *(Apr 2018, 3 Marks)*

Ans. Cyanosis is a bluish discoloration of the skin and mucus membrane due to reduced hemoglobin (more than 5 mg%) in blood.

Type of Cyanosis

Generally, there are four types of cyanosis:
   i. Central cyanosis
   ii. Peripheral cyanosis
   iii. Cyanosis due to abnormal pigments
   iv. Mixed cyanosis.

Central Cyanosis

♦ It occur because of poor oxygenation of blood in lungs due to interference of exchange of gases, i.e., oxygen and carbon dioxide in respiratory failure or pulmonary edema.
♦ Central cyanosis is also visible in some congenital heart diseases where deoxygenated blood from right side mixes to the oxygenated blood from left side. This brings down oxygen saturation of blood.
♦ Central cyanosis is visible at under surface of tongue and mucous membrane of oral cavity and palate.

Peripheral Cyanosis

♦ It occurs because of removal of oxygen from the blood when circulation is slow due to congestive cardiac failure or due to shock causing vasoconstriction.
♦ This can also occur in healthy people when extremities are very cold.
♦ It is visible in lip, nail, tip of nose, lobule of ear.

Cyanosis due to Abnormal Pigments

♦ Normal hemoglobin has iron in ferrous form. In methemoglobinemia, iron is in the ferric form designated as methemoglobin. Several substances, such as nitrite ingestion, sulfonamide or aniline dyes oxidize hemoglobin to methemoglobin, but this is immediately reduced back to hemoglobin by methemoglobin reductase I or diaphorase I. If there is deficiency of diaphorase I, methemoglobin circulates in blood, causing cyanosis.

♦ Sulfhemoglobin is an abnormal sulfur containing substance, which is not normally present, but is formed by toxic action of drugs and chemicals like sulfonamides, phenacetin and acetanilide. Sulfhemoglobin forms an irreversible change in the hemoglobin pigment that has no capacity to carry oxygen and causes cyanosis.

Mixed Cyanosis

Due to combination of both the factors, e.g., cor pulmonale due to pulmonary emphysema.

Causes of Cyanosis

♦ **Central cyanosis**
  • *Pulmonary causes*
    – Lobar pneumonia
    – High altitudes
    – Pneumothorax
    – Multiple small pulmonary thromboembolism
    – Chronic obstructive pulmonary disease
    – Respiratory failure
    – Severe acute asthma
  • *Cardiovascular causes*
    – Cyanotic heart disease
    – Acute pulmonary edema
    – Cor pulmonale
    – Arterio venous fistula
  • *Abnormal hepatopulmonary syndrome*
♦ **Peripheral cyanosis**
  • Congestive heart failure
  • Exposure to cold
  • Due to arterial obstruction
  • Due to venous obstruction
♦ **Cyanosis due to abnormal pigments**
  • Methemoglobin formation due to ingestion sulfonamide and aniline dye
  • Sulfhemoglobin formation due to sulfonamide, phenacetin
♦ **Mixed cyanosis**
  • Acute left ventricular failure
  • Mitral stenosis

Q.3. Write important causes of central cyanosis.

(Mar 2011, 2 Marks)

Ans. Following are the causes of central cyanosis:
♦ *Pulmonary causes*
  • Lobar pneumonia
  • High altitudes
  • Pneumothorax
  • Multiple small pulmonary thromboembolism
  • Chronic obstructive pulmonary disease
  • Respiratory failure
  • Severe acute asthma
♦ *Cardiovascular causes*
  • Cyanotic heart disease
  • Acute pulmonary edema

  • Cor pulmonale
  • Arteriovenous fistula
♦ *Abnormal hepatopulmonary syndrome*

Q.4. Describe briefly pulsus paradoxus.

(Feb 1999, 3 Marks)

Ans. The term pulsus paradoxus is used to describe dramatically fall in blood pressure during inspiration, i.e., characteristic of *tamponade, pericardial constriction and severe airway obstruction.
♦ When the systolic blood pressure falls less than 10 mm, the pulse is referred to pulsus paradoxus.
♦ Pulsus paradoxus is the *exaggeration of the normal phenomenon.

Mechanism

Flowchart 1: Mechanism of pulsus paradoxus.

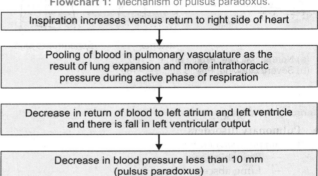

Causes

♦ Superior vena cava obstruction
♦ Lung conditions
  • Asthma
  • Emphysema
  • Airway obstruction
♦ Cardiac condition
  • Pericardial effusion
  • Constrictive pericarditis
  • Severe congestive cardiac failure

Q.5. Describe briefly water hammer pulse.

(Sep 2009, 4 Marks)

Ans. It is also called as Corrigan pulse.
♦ Water hammer pulse is a large bounding pulse with increased stroke volume of left ventricle and decrease in the peripheral resistance, leading to wide pulse pressure.
♦ The pulse strikes palpating finger with rapid, forceful jerk and quickly disappears.
♦ It is best felt in radial artery with patient's arm elevated.
♦ It is described as having a water hammer quality because of its sudden impact and collapsing quality because it falls away so rapidly.
♦ The collapsing pulse caused by artery suddenly emptying as some of the blood flow from aorta to ventricle.

Q 4.   *Tamponade = Compression of the heart by an accumulation of fluid in the pericardial sac.
      *Exaggeration = Greater than it really is

Causes

- Physiological
  - Fever
  - Chronic alcoholism
  - Pregnancy
- High output states or syndrome
  - Anemia
  - Beri beri
  - Cor pulmonale
  - Liver cirrhosis
  - Paget's disease
  - Arteriovenous fistula
  - Thyrotoxicosis
- Cardiac lesions
  - Aortic regurgitation
  - Rupture of sinus of valsalva into heart chamber
  - Patent ductus arteriosus
  - Aortopulmonary window
  - Bradycardia
  - Systolic hypertension

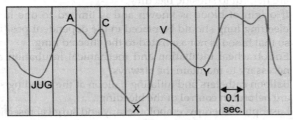

Fig. 2: Water hammer pulse.

Q.6. How will you differentiate arterial and venous pulse?

(Mar 2008, 2 Marks)

Ans.

Arterial pulse	Venous pulse
• Normal pulse has a small *anacrotic wave on upstroke, which is not felt. This is followed by percussion wave which is felt by palpating finger	• Normal venous pulse consists of three positive waves and two negative waves
• Arterial pulse is better felt than seen in appearance	• Venous pulse is better seen than felt
• Pressure below the angle of mandible has no change on the wave	• Pressure below the angle of mandible obliterates the wave
• Changes with respiration and changes on position are absent	• Changes with the respiration and position are present
• It has no effect of posture	• It disappears when patient sits up on bed
• There is no effect of abdominal compression	• Pressure over the liver distends the vein

Q.7. Enumerate the causes of hematemesis.

(Sep 1999, 4 Marks)

Ans. Rapid loss of blood from a lesion in esophagus, stomach or duodenum above the level of ampulla of Vater will result in vomiting of blood.

Causes

- Common causes
  - Duodenal ulcer
  - Esophagitis
  - Gastric erosion
  - Varices
  - Gastric ulcer.
- Less common
  - Carcinoma stomach
  - Bleeding diathesis
  - Aortic aneurysm
- Rare cases
  - Acute pancreatitis
  - Angiomas
  - Telangiectasia
  - COPD
  - Polycythemia vera
  - Hypoparathyroidism.

Q.8. Write short note on hematemesis. *(Mar 2009, 5 Marks)*

Ans. *For definition and causes refer to Ans. 7 of same chapter.*

Clinical Features

- Patient presents with vomiting of blood or complaint of passing the *tarry stools.
- Many patients with coffee ground vomiting are present.
- In cases of severe hemorrhage, there may be fresh rectal bleeding or *giddiness and *syncope due to sudden hypo-volemia.
- Hematemesis is mixed with food particles.

Management

General

- Put the patient to the bed.
- Arrange fresh blood transfusion.
- Maintain nutrition and hydration.
- Pass a Ryle's tube and do constant suction. In cases of suspected peptic ulcer an antacid in gel form is given too early.

Specific

- Treat underlying condition appropriately.
- Once the crisis is over and bleeding subsides, than treatment is to be planned according to the basic disease. Drug-induced hematemesis shall require symptomatic relief.

Q.9. Enumerate the causes of hemoptysis.

(Feb 2006, 2.5 Marks)

Ans. Hemoptysis is defined as coughing out of the blood which includes stained sputum.

Q 6. *Anacrotic wave = A secondary wave on the ascending limb of the main wave.

Q 8. *Tarry = Smeared with tar
     *Giddiness = Dizziness
     *Syncope = Transient loss of consciousness, accompanied by inability to maintain an upright posture

Causes

♦ **Causes for true hemoptysis**
- *Cardiac*
  - Mitral stenosis
  - Aneurysm of aorta
  - Left ventricular failure and primary pulmonary hypertension.
- *Respiratory*
  - Pneumonia
  - Tuberculosis
  - Bronchogenic carcinoma and adenoma
  - Pulmonary embolism
  - Lung abscess
  - Bronchiectasis and other infections of lung and bronchi
  - Trauma to the airways and lung
  - AV malformations.
- *Immunological*
  - Goodpasture's syndrome
  - Wegener's granulomatosis
  - Polyarteritis nodosa.
- *Bleeding disorders*
  - Thrombocytopenia
  - Purpura
  - Agranulocytosis
  - Leukemia
  - Hemophilia and anticoagulant therapy.
- *Iatrogenic*
  - Following bronchoscopy
  - Lung biopsy
  - Endotracheal intubation
  - Anticoagulant therapy

♦ **Causes for pseudohemoptysis**
- Trauma of mouth, pharynx and larynx
- Tuberculosis, syphilis or pyogenic infection of mouth, pharynx and larynx.
- Malignancy of mouth, pharynx and larynx
- Bleeding spongy gums in scurvy.

Q.10. How will you differentiate hemoptysis from hematemesis? *(Apr 1999, 5 Marks)*

Ans.

Hemoptysis	Hematemesis
• Symptoms and sign are of pulmonary and cardiac disease	• Symptoms and signs are of gastric or abdominal disease
• Blood is coughed up	• Blood is vomited
• Blood is bright red, frothy and mixed with the sputum	• Blood is coffee ground, mixed with food particles
• Blood is relatively in small amount	• Blood is in large amount
• Reaction is alkaline	• Reaction is acidic
• Stool become rusty next day	• Stool is tarry next day

Q.11. Outline the investigation and management of hemoptysis. *(Mar 2000, 5 Marks)*

Ans. Hemoptysis is defined as expectoration of blood from respiratory tract, spectrum varies from blood streak of sputum to cough up or large amount of pure blood.

Investigation

- Hemodynamic resuscitation and bronchoscopy is done.
- Chest radiograph for TB, pneumonia, tumor, pulmonary infarction.
- Full blood count and hematological tests.
- Bronchoscopy to exclude central bronchial carcinoma and to provide tissue diagnosis for the suspected.
- *CT scan:* For peripheral lesion investigation which are seen on chest radiograph.

Management

- Establishing a diagnosis is a first priority.
- When hemoptysis is maintained, adequate gas exchange preventing blood from spleen into unaffected area of lung and avoiding asphyxiation are the highest priority.
- Keeping the patient at rest and partially suppressing cough are helpful to subside bleeding.
- If origin of blood is known and is limited to one lung, bleeding lung should be placed in the dependent position so that blood is not aspirated to the affected lung.
- Endotracheal intubation and mechanical intubation are necessary to maintain the airways.
- Balloon catheters and inflating balloon at the bleeding site are helpful in control of the bleeding.
- Laser phototherapy, embolotherapy and surgical resection of involved area of lung are the other methods. Surgical resection is done in life-threatening hemoptysis.

Q.12. Enumerate the causes of malena.
(Mar 1998, 5 Marks)

Ans. Malena is defined as the passage of dark colored blood in stool.

Causes

- Peptic ulcer
- Portal hypertension
- Typhoid fever
- Malignant GI tract
- Ulcerative colitis
- Bleeding diathesis, i.e., purpura, hemophilia, leukemia.

Q.13. Enumerate common causes of fever.
(Sep 2008, 2.5 Marks)

Ans.

Causes of Fever

- *Infections:* Bacterial, viral, rickettsial, fungal, parasitic, etc.
- *Neoplasms:* Fever may be present with any neoplasm but commonly with hypernephroma, lymphoproliferative malignancies, carcinoma of pancreas, lung and bone and hepatoma.
- *Vascular:* Acute myocardial infarction, pulmonary embolism, pontine hemorrhage, etc.
- *Traumatic:* Crush injury.

♦ *Immunological:*
  • Collagen disease, SLE, rheumatoid arthritis.
  • Drug fever
  • Serum sickness
♦ *Endocrine:* Thyrotoxicosis, Addison's disease.
♦ *Metabolic:* Gout, porphyria, acidosis, dehydration
♦ *Hematological:* Acute hemolytic crisis
♦ *Physical agents:* Heat stroke, radiation sickness.
♦ *Miscellaneous:* Factitious fever, habitual hyperpyrexia, cyclic neutropenia

Q.14. How will you investigate a case of prolong fever?
(Sep 2009, 5 Marks) (Feb/Mar 2004, 5 Marks)
Ans.

Important Investigation in Case of a Prolong Fever

♦ **ESR platelet correlation:** If ESR is more than 100 mm/h with thrombocytosis, following diseases can be think off, i.e.
  • Tuberculosis
  • Malignancy
  • Connective tissue diseases.
    If ESR is <100 mm/h with thrombocytosis, viral infection can be suspected.
♦ **Assessment of alkaline phosphatase levels:** If alkaline phosphatase levels are higher following infections are suspected, i.e., biliary tract infections, alcoholic hepatitis, primary and secondaries of liver, hypernephroma, lymphoma, military tuberculosis, cytomegalovirus infection.
♦ **Serological tests:** They are helpful in assessing enteric fever, hepatitis, CMV infection, tularemia, secondary syphilis, brucellosis, Q fever, amoebiasis, HIV.
♦ **Imaging techniques:**
  • *X-ray chest:* In cases with prolonged fever when initial X-ray is normal, a second X-ray must be taken after three weeks to rule out military tuberculosis.
  • *Ultrasound:* Excellent imaging is done in thin individuals and poor imaging in obese individuals, SOL in hepatobiliary tree of more than 1 cm and endocarditis vegetation of more than 2 mm can be detected.
  • *CT scan:* Provide excellent imaging in obese patient. SOL in liver is more than 1 cm and CNS lesion is more than 0.2 cm.
  • *Radionuclide scans:* ^{99m}Tc-sulfur colloid is used for scanning liver and spleen. ^{111}Indium labeled leukocytes are used for detection of intra-abdominal mass.

Q.15. Write short note on pedal edema. *(Sep 2005, 3 Marks)*
Ans. Pedal edema is defined as swelling of feet and ankle caused by collection of fluid in the tissues and is a possible sign of congestive heart failure.

Causes

Trauma.

Clinical Features

♦ Swelling appears on the feet and ankle.
♦ Pitting type of edema is present.
♦ Obstruction of inferior vena cava.

Treatment

♦ Sodium restriction is done.
♦ Diuretics should be used, i.e., spironolactone.
♦ Management of underlying disorder.
♦ ACE inhibitors are given.
♦ Leg elevation of patient.

Q.16. Enumerate the causes of hematuria.
(Sep 2008, 2.5 Marks)
Ans. Hematuria is defined as presence of blood in urine.

Causes

♦ Renal
  • Glomerulonephritis
    – Primary
      » Mesangial proliferative
      » Mesangiocapillary
      » Berger's disease
    – Secondary
      » Systemic lupus erythematosus
      » Polyarthritis nodosa
      » Infective endocarditis
    – Others
      » Alport's syndrome
      » Fabry's disease
      » Benign familial hematuria
  • Interstitial disease
    – Acute pyelonephritis
    – Papillary necrosis
    – Neoplasms
  • Cystic disease
    – Adult polycystic disease
    – Medullary cystic disease
  • Renal stones
  • Trauma to kidneys
♦ Ureter
  • Stone
  • Neoplasm
♦ Urinary bladder
  • Neoplasm
  • Cystitis
  • Stone
  • Trauma or catheter induced
  • Schistosomiasis
♦ Prostate
  • Prostatitis
  • Benign enlargement of prostate
  • Neoplasm
♦ Urethra
  • Injury
  • Urethritis
♦ Disorders of hemostasis
  • Bleeding or coagulation disorders
  • Anticoagulants
♦ Systemic diseases
  • Diabetes
  • Amyloidosis
  • Collagen disease
  • Disseminated intravascular coagulation

Q.17. Write short note on bronchial breathing.

(Sep 2009, 4 Marks)

Ans. Bronchial breathing is blowing or hollow in character, inspiratory phase equals expiratory phase and there is pause between the two.

♦ Bronchial breathing may be low pitched (Cavernous) medium pitched or high pitched (tubular). Low pitched bronchial breathing is heard over moderately large cavities in the lung and in a case of open pneumothorax.

♦ High pitched or tubular breathing is heard where consolidation of lung has occurred round small sized bronchial tubes as in consolidation of lung, lobar pneumonia, malignant disease, pulmonary infarction and pleural effusion.

♦ Another variety of bronchial breathing is amphoric which is like blowing across a bottle and has a distinct 'echo like' quality. It is heard over a large cavity with smooth wall or in a case of pneumothorax in direct contact with a bronchus.

Q.18. Write short note on clubbing.

(Dec 2010, 5 Marks) (Dec 2015, 3 Marks)

Or

Write short answer on clubbing. *(Sep 2018, 3 Marks)*

Ans. Clubbing is an enlargement of distal segment of fingers and toes due to increase in soft tissue.

Causes of Clubbing

♦ **Pulmonary disorders**
  • *Suppuration of lung*
    – Bronchiectasis
    – Lung abscess
    – Suppurative pneumonia
  • *Tumors of lung*
    – Mesothelioma
    – Primary lung cancer
    – Metastatic lung cancer
♦ **Cardiac disorders**
  • Cyanotic congenital heart diseases
  • Subacute bacterial endocarditis
  • Atrial myxoma
♦ **Disorders of gastrointestinal system and liver**
  • Inflammatory bowel disease
    – Regional ileitis
    – Ulcerative colitis
    – Malabsorption syndrome
  • Cirrhosis of liver
  • Malignancy of liver
♦ **Disorders of endocrine system**
  • Myxedema
  • Thyroid acropachy
  • Acromegaly
♦ **Miscellaneous**
  • Hereditary
  • Idiopathic
  • *Unilateral:* Pancoast tumor, subclavian and innominate artery aneurysm
  • *Unidigital:* Traumatic or tophi deposit in gout
  • Only in upper limbs in heroin addicts due to chronic obstructive phlebitis.

Grading

♦ **Grade I:** Softening of nail bed due to the hypertrophy of tissue at that particular site.

♦ **Grade II:** In addition to grade I changes, there is obliteration of the angle of nail bed

♦ **Grade III:** In addition to grade II changes, there is swelling of the subcutaneous tissues over the base of the nail causing the overlying skin to become tense, shiny and wet and increasing the curvature of the nail, resulting in parrot beak or drumstick appearance.

♦ **Grade IV:** Swelling of the fingers in all dimensions associated with hypertrophic pulmonary osteoarthropathy causing pain and swelling of the hand, wrist, etc., and radiographic evidence of subperiosteal new bone formation.

Q.19. Write short note on drug fever. *(Dec 2010, 5 Marks)*

Ans. Drug fever is a prolonged fever and any belong to any febrile pattern.

♦ In drug fever, there is relative bradycardia and hypotension.

♦ Pruritus, skin rash and arthralgia may occur.

♦ It begins 1 to 3 weeks after the drug is started and persists of 2 to 3 days after drug is withdrawn.

♦ Eosinophilia may be present.

♦ Almost all the drugs may lead to drug fever.

♦ Drugs which commonly leads to drug fever are sulfonamide, penicillin, iodide, antitubercular drugs, methyldopa, anti-convulsants, propylthiouracil.

Q.20. Write important causes of pitting edema.

(Mar 2011, 2 Marks)

Ans.

Causes of Pitting Edema

♦ Ingestion of excessive salt

♦ Due to steroids

♦ Premenstrual

♦ Due to portal obstruction

♦ Due to obstruction of inferior vena cava

♦ In beri beri

♦ Anemia and hypoproteinemia

♦ Epidemic dropsy

♦ Pregnancy

♦ *Miscellaneous:* Dermatomyositis, Raynaud's phenomenon and old age

♦ If pitting remains for more than a minute most likely cause is congestion

♦ If pitting remains for 40 seconds it is caused by hypoalbuminemia

Q.21. Write short note on causes and investigations of dysphagia. *(Mar 2013, 3 Marks)*

Ans. Dysphagia is difficulty in swallowing.

Causes

♦ **Due to narrowing of esophagus**
  • Intrinsic, i.e., obstruction inside esophagus
    – Esophageal stricture
    – Esophageal ulceration
    – Congenital atresia of esophagus
    – Plummer-Vinson syndrome
    – Tumors either benign or malignant

- Tonsillitis
- Stomatitis
- Glossitis
- Esophagitis
- Pharyngitis
- Extrinsic, i.e., obstruction outside esophagus
  - Aortic aneurysm
  - Retropharyngeal mass
  - Mitral stenosis which lead to left atrial enlargement
  - Thyroid gland enlargement which compresses esophagus.
- **Motor Dysphagia:**
  - Paralysis of esophageal sphincter
    - Esophageal spasm
    - Cardiac achalasia.
  - Paralysis of 9th and 10th cranial nerve nuclei
    - Systemic sclerosis
    - Polymyelitis.
  - Esophageal muscle weakness
    - Myopathy.
  - Neuromuscular paralysis
    - Myasthenia gravis.

Investigations

- Complete hemogram is done to check for the anemia
- Chest X-ray should be done to check for the tuberculosis, cardiomegaly, mediastinal enlargement
- Endoscopy of esophagus helps in detection of lesion and finding its cause
- Barium meal examination is carried out purely for localization of lesion in esophagus
- Esophageal manometry is carried out for assessing motility disorders of esophagus.

2. DISEASES OF GASTROINTESTINAL TRACT

Q.1. Write short note on stomatitis.

(Sep 2007, 2 Marks) (Apr 2010, 5 Marks)
(June 2010, 5 Marks) (Aug 2012, 5 Marks)

Or

Write notes on stomatitis.   *(Aug 2011, 10 Marks)*

Ans. Stomatitis is the inflammation of mouth and is caused by bacterial, viral and fungal infections in persons with poor oral hygiene or in blood dyscrasias.

Causes of Stomatitis

Local Causes

- Poor oral hygiene
- Excessive use of tobacco
- Alcohol and spices
- Use of broad spectrum antibiotics
- Drugs, such as iodine or gold.

General causes

The main general causes are the infectious diseases. There are various types of infective stomatitis:

- Bacterial, e.g., streptococcal stomatitis and Vincent's stomatitis
- Viral, e.g., herpes simplex and herpes zoster
- Fungal, e.g., candidiasis and actinomycosis
- Recurrent aphthous stomatitis
- Mucocutaneous diseases, e.g., Lichen planus, pemphigus vulgaris, lupus erythematous, etc.
- Miscellaneous, e.g., diabetes, uremia and drug toxicity.

Clinical Features

- Lip, tongue and gums are inflamed, swollen and painful.
- Tongue is furred and foul smell is present.
- Sometimes ulceration of mucus membrane is present when person is suffering from infectious stomatitis.
- Patient feels pain and difficulty in opening the mouth.
- There was an *excoriation and redness of mucus membrane of oral cavity.

Treatment

- If drug is the causative factor discontinuation of the drug is done.
- If allergen is the causative factor remove allergen.
- Antihistaminic drugs, such as cetirizine to be given to the patient.
- Topical corticosteroid application should be done. Triamcinolone acetate is effective.
- Tetracycline mouthwash should be given which should be used four times a day for 5 to 7 days.
- Nutritional supplements to be given, such as vitamin B12, iron, folic acid.

Q.2. Write short note on chronic gastritis.

(Sep 1999, 5 Marks)

Ans. When the acute gastritis remain for the longer time and is not treated, it becomes chronic and is known as chronic gastritis.

Etiology

- Repeated injury to gastric mucosa by tea, coffee, alcohol, spices
- Infection from throat, teeth, gums and sinuses
- NSAIDs
- Autoimmune pathology
- Very hot beverage
- Gastrectomy.

Types of Gastritis

- Superficial
- Atrophic
- Hypertrophic
- Infectious
- Eosinophilic.

Q 1.   *Excoriation = An abrasion of skin or the surface of other organs by scratching, traumatic injury, burn or other causes.

There are mainly two types of chronic gastritis:

A. Type A gastritis
B. Type B gastritis.

Type A Gastritis (Less Common)

♦ It involves body of stomach and spars antrum.
♦ It is caused during autoimmune disorders like type I diabetes mellitus, Sjögrens syndrome, Graves' disease, Hashimoto disease, myasthenia gravis, etc.
♦ It is caused due to autoimmune activity against parietal cells.
♦ Parietal cell antibodies can be detected in serum.
♦ In severe cases, parietal cell atrophy leads to deficiency of intrinsic factor which leads to pernicious anemia.
♦ Disease is asymptomatic and long-term complication is gastric carcinoma.

Treatment

♦ In severe cases, corticosteroids are administered.
♦ In mild cases, parenteral iron should be administered.

Type B Gastritis

♦ This is more common form of gastritis and involves antrum of stomach.
♦ Usual cause is gram-negative bacteria *H. pylori*.
♦ The condition is precursor of peptic ulcer.
♦ There is possibility of gastric carcinoma.

Diagnosis

♦ Gastric acid study, i.e., achlorhydria
♦ Hemoglobin decreases
♦ Serum gastrin increases.

Management

♦ *Anti-H. pylori* treatment
   • *Triple drug therapy:* Proton pump inhibitor or ranitidine 400 mg BD + Bismuth subcitrate + Amoxicillin 1 g or clarithromycin 500 mg or metronidazole 500 mg BD
   • *Quadruple therapy:* Omeprazole 10 mg BD + Tetracycline 500 mg QID + Bismuth subcitrate QID + Metronidazole 500 mg TDS.
     In both the cases 14 days course is preferred.
♦ Parenteral vitamin B12 is administered.

Q.3. Write short note on amoebiasis.

(Mar 2006, 5 Marks) (Feb 2006, 2.5 Marks)

Ans.

♦ Amoebic dysentery is caused by a protozoan called *Entamoeba histolytica*.
♦ *Entamoeba histolytica* exist in two forms, i.e., trophozoite and cystic stage.
♦ Trophozoites are responsible for production for disease and cysts are responsible for transmission of disease.
♦ *Reservoir of infection:* Man is the only known reservoir.
♦ *Mode of transmission:* Fecal-oral route, i.e., through contaminated food and water.
♦ Incubation period is two to four months or longer.

Clinical Features

Symptoms

♦ Patient has diarrhea and pass 10–15 stools per day.
♦ Presence of abdominal pain.
♦ Stools consist of blood and mucus.
♦ Flatulence is present.
♦ Fever is present between 38 and 40 degrees with rigors.

Signs

♦ Palpation of abdomen show diffuse tenderness.
♦ Chronic cases show thickened tender sigmoid colon.
♦ Amoeba is felt as a sausage shaped mass in right iliac fossa.
♦ Tender hepatomegaly is present.

Management

Investigations

♦ *Stool examination:* Show various forms of *E. histolytica*
♦ Serological test
♦ Sigmoidoscopy for ulcer.
♦ Immunofluorescence test for autoantibodies

Treatment

♦ Nitroimidazole classes of antimicrobial agents are main drugs of treatment.
   • Metronidazole 400 to 800 mg TDS 5 to 7 days.
   • Tinidazole 2 g as single or divided three days dose.
   • Secnidazole 2 g as single dose.
   • Diloxanide furoate: It should be added because it has effect on cyst. It is given 500 mg TDS for 10 days. Metronidazole has no effect on cyst.
♦ General supportive measures, fluid and electrolyte imbalance correction is there.
♦ Diet given should be soft, liquid or semi-liquid.

Q.4. Outline the management of Amoebic liver abscess.

(Sep 1999, 4 Marks)

Ans.

Investigation

♦ *TLC and DLC:* Leukocytosis is present.
♦ Stool study shows cyst.
♦ *Sigmoidoscopy:* Ulcers are seen.
♦ USG.
♦ Aspiration study.
♦ Immunofluorescence test for autoantibodies

Management of Amoebic Liver Abscess/Hepatic Amoebiasis

♦ Early cases are responding well with metronidazole 800 mg TID for 5 days or tinidazole 2 g daily for three days.
♦ *Luminal amoebicide:* Diloxanide furoate 500 mg 8 hourly for 10 days should be given to determine luminal cyst.
♦ If abscess is large and not respond to chemotherapy repeated aspiration under ultrasonic guidance is required.
♦ Rupture of abscess into peritoneal cavity requires immediate aspiration or surgical drainage.

Q.5. Write short note on malabsorption syndrome.
(May/June 2009, 5 Marks) (Mar 2009, 5 Marks)

Or

What is malabsorption syndrome, causes of malabsorption, clinical features and its management.
(Nov 2011, 8 Marks)

Ans. Malabsorption syndrome comprises a large number of pathological condition in which there is disturbance of processes by which nutrients are transferred from lumen of intestine into circulation.

Etiology

♦ *Stomach:*
  • Precipitate emptying after postgastrectomy dumping.
  • Lack of intrinsic factor.
  • Excess acid secretion in Zollinger-Ellison syndrome.
♦ *Pancreatic:* Inadequate enzyme and bicarbonate secretion.
♦ *Biliary:* Due to defective micelle formation.
♦ Endocrine diseases
♦ Parasitic or drug.

Various diseases along with their etiologies can cause malabsorption as:

♦ **Disorders of intraluminal digestion**
  • Pancreatic enzyme deficiency in chronic pancreatitis, cystic fibrosis and pancreatic carcinoma
  • Disturbances of gastric function after gastroenterostomy and partial gastrectomy
  • Deficiency of bile acids in Crohn's disease, resection of terminal ileum, stagnant loop syndrome or blind loop syndrome.
♦ **Disorders of transport in the intestinal mucosal cell**
  • With histologically abnormal mucosa (infiltration, inflammation or infection of mucosa) in celiac disease, tropical sprue, lymphoma, Whipple's disease, giardiasis and radiation enteritis
  • With histologically normal mucosa (genetic diseases) in lactase deficiency, pernicious anemia
  • Disorders of transport from mucosal cell in abdominal lymphoma, tuberculosis, telangiectasia of mesenteric lymphatics, A beta lipoproteinemia,
  • Impaired nutrient uptake in lymphatic obstruction, cardiac heart failure, and pericarditis
  • Miscellaneous: Diabetes mellitus, hyperthyroidism, hyperparathyroidism

Clinical Features

♦ *Steatorrhea is presenting symptom.
♦ Diarrhea or abdominal discomfort.
♦ Nutritional deficiencies, i.e., deficiency of vitamin A, D, B12 and K
♦ General features, such as anemia, sore mouth, loss of weight, fatigue and lethargy.
♦ Bone pain may be present.
♦ Skin changes, such as pellagra are present

_____

Q 5.   *Steatorrhea = Defective absorption of fat

♦ Patient also suffers from peripheral neuropathy, irritability and lack of confidence.

Investigations

Tests are carried out to detect the nutritional deficiency. These tests indicate the malabsorption of particular nutrient and not its cause.

♦ *Fecal fat stimulation:* It confirms steatorrhea and fat malabsorption. Sudan III stain may show an increase in the stool fat. Quantitative estimation of fat in the stool is more reliable and sensitive. A 72-hour stool collection while the patient is on a defined diet is used for fat estimation. Excretion of more than 10 g fat per day suggests fat malabsorption.
♦ *Schilling test:* This is useful in the diagnosis of cobalamin (B12) malabsorption and its causes, such as pernicious anemia, chronic pancreatitis, achlorhydria and bacterial overgrowth. In this test, radiolabeled cobalamin (1 mg 68°C) should be given orally and its excretion in urine is measured. 1 mg cobalamin is administered intramuscularly to saturate hepatic binding sites so that all radiolabeled cobalamin is excreted in the urine. The test is abnormal, if <10% of the radiolabeled cobalamin is excreted in the urine in 24 hours. This will help in differentiating the various defects responsible for malabsorption of cobalamin.
♦ *D-xylose test:* It detects carbohydrate malabsorption. 25 g of D-xylose is given orally and its excretion is measured in urine. Excretion of <4.5 g in 5 hours is suggestive of malabsorption.
♦ *Upper gastrointestinal endoscopy and biopsy of small intestinal mucosa:* It is essential for the diagnosis of conditions, such as tropical sprue, celiac sprue, Whipple's disease, and Crohn's disease.
♦ *Barium meal contrast radiography:* Radiological assessment of the small intestine with barium contrast is helpful in evaluation of structural abnormalities in Crohn's disease, diverticulae and strictures.
♦ *Pancreatic exocrine functions:* They should be carried out in patients with steatorrhea.
♦ *Serological studies:* In some of the conditions, such as celiac sprue and pernicious anemia autoantibodies are detected.
♦ *Small intestinal biopsy (duodenal or jejunal):* It is carried out for conformational diagnosis.

Management

♦ *Diet:* High protein and low fat diet is taken.
♦ *Digestants:* Pancreatic enzyme preparations are administered after meals.
♦ *Treatment of anemia:* All three hematinics vitamin B12, folic acid and iron is given.
♦ *Vitamin supplements:* Vitamin B complex and vitamin D are given.
♦ *Treatment of diarrhea:* Codeine and loperamide are administered.
♦ *Steroids:* Prolong therapy with prednisolone is given.

♦ *Elimination of bacterial overgrowth:* Tetracycline 250 mg TDS for one week.

Q.6. Enumerate causes of acute diarrhea.

(Feb 2006, 2.5 Marks)

Or

Enumerate causes of diarrhea. *(Jan 2012, 5 Marks)*

Ans.

I. Acute Diarrhea

♦ *Infective diarrhea*
- *Bacterial:* The bacteria which causes acute diarrhea are *Shigella, Salmonella, E.coli*, etc.
- *Viral:* Viruses which results in diarrhea are parvovirus, Hawaii, etc.
- *Protozoal:* The protozoans are *E. histolytica*, giardia, etc.
- Toxic and systemic causes
- Some drugs result in acute diarrhea, i.e., broad spectrum antibiotics.

♦ Non-infective diarrhea
- Crohn's disease
- Irritable bowel syndrome
- Acute psychological stress
- Drugs, such as amoxicillin, antacids, cholinergics, etc.

II. Chronic Diarrhea

♦ Ulcerative colitis
♦ HIV associated enteritis
♦ Whipple's disease
♦ Pancreatic insufficiency
♦ Zollinger-Ellison syndrome
♦ Medullary carcinoma of thyroid
♦ Irritable bowel syndrome.

Q.7. Write short note on bacillary dysentery.

(Mar 2000, 5 Marks)

Ans. Bacillary dysentery is mainly caused by *Shigella*.

Etiology

♦ It occurs by contaminated food or flies.
♦ It is caused by unwashed hands after defecation.
♦ It is also caused due to wars and natural calamities which causes poor sanitation and crowding.

Clinical Features

♦ Diarrhea, colicky abdominal pain and tenesmus, i.e., spasmodic contraction of anal or bladder sphincter with pain.
♦ Fever, dehydration and weakness with tenderness over colon.
♦ Arthritis may be seen.

Management

♦ Oral rehydration therapy is given.
♦ IV replacement of water and electrolyte loss is necessary.
♦ Ciprofloxacin 500 mg 12 hourly for two days is given.
♦ Antidiarrheal medication is given.

Q.8. Differentiate between gastric ulcer and duodenal ulcer.

(Feb 2006, 3 Marks)

Ans.

Characteristic	Gastric ulcer	Duodenal ulcer
Age	It occur in individuals more than 40 years	It occur in individuals from age range of 20 to 50 years
Sex	It is equal in both sexes	It is more in females
Course of illness	It is less remittent	It is more remittent
Duration of episode of pain	Duration is long	Duration is short
Nature of pain	Diffuse	Sharp pointing pain present in epigastrium
Occurrence of pain	Pain occur after meal	Pain occur on fastening
Hemorrhage	More common	Less common
Malena	Less common	More common
Anorexia and nausea	Present	Less often
Hematemesis	Present	Less common
Heart burn	Less common	More common

Q.9. Discuss causes of acute gastritis.

(Feb/Mar 2004, 5 Marks)

Ans. The causes of acute gastritis are:

♦ *NSAIDs and analgesics:* They not only cause gastric erosion by predisposing to peptic ulcer.
♦ Antimitotic drugs
♦ Renal failure
♦ *H. pylori* initial infection
♦ Other infections, i.e., streptococcal, viral, fungal, etc.
♦ Iron therapy
♦ Stress and burns
♦ Postoperative.

Q.10. Enumerate the causes of upper GI hemorrhage.

(Sep 2010, 5 Marks)

Ans.

The Causes for Upper GI Hemorrhage

Esophageal Causes

♦ Esophageal varices
♦ Esophagitis
♦ Esophageal ulcers
♦ Esophageal cancers.

Gastric Causes

♦ Gastric ulcer
♦ Gastric cancer
♦ Gastritis
♦ Gastric varices.

Duodenal Causes

♦ Duodenal ulcer
♦ Vascular malformations

- *Hematobilia
- Bleeding from the pancreatic duct.

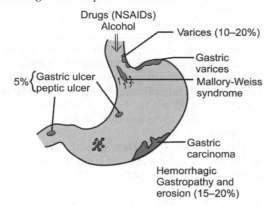

Fig. 3: Upper GI hemorrhage.

Q.11. Outline the treatment of acute gastroenteritis.
(Sep 2008, 2.5 Marks)

Ans. Inflammation of stomach and intestinal tract that causes vomiting, diarrhea or both.

Treatment

- Rehydration with liquid is keyword to avoid dehydration and electrolytic imbalance.
- Antidiarrheal treatment is given, i.e.
  - Antimicrobial agent
    - Ciprofloxacin 500 mg BD for three days or nalidixic acid 1 g 6 hourly for 5 to 7 days. It may be combined with the tinidazole 300 mg BD for 6 days.
  - Antimotility agent
    This should be used in children before 5 years of age.
    - Loperamide or diphenoxylate atropine.
    - Codeine could be used.
    - Sodium and water conserving agent, i.e., Racecadotril is the newer drug safely given in the children and adult. It reduces the loss of sodium and water in the stool.

General Management

- Rest, maintenance of fluid and electrolyte balance.
- ORS should be given in all children as early as possible.
- Patient with constant vomiting or moderate to severe dehydration require IV fluid.
- Ringer lactate is ideal, normal saline may be given.

Q.12. Write short note on peptic ulcer. *(Sep 2006, 5 Marks)*

Or

Write short note on diagnosis and treatment of peptic ulcer. *(Nov 2014, 3 Marks)*

Or

Write in detail about peptic ulcer and its management.
(Mar 2007, 5 Marks)

Q 10. *Hematobilia = Blood in the bile

Ans. Peptic ulcer is defined as mucosal ulceration near the acid bearing regions of gastrointestinal tract. It is the ulcer in duodenum and stomach.

Etiology

- *Hereditary:* Patient with blood group O has much incidence.
- *H. pylori:* Gram-negative bacteria are supposed to be main cause accounting for 70% of gastric ulcer.
- *NSAIDs:* They lead to 30% of gastric ulcers. By depleting mucosal prostaglandin levels aspirin and NSAIDs impairs cytoprotection resulting in mucosal injury, erosion and ulceration
- *Smoking:* It does not cause ulcer but more likely to cause complication and is responsible for nonhealing or delayed healing.
- *Corticosteroids:* They are responsible for silent perforation of ulcer.
- *Acid-pepsin versus mucosal resistance:* Cause of peptic ulceration is digestion of the mucosa with acid and pepsin of gastric juice. Normal stomach is capable of resisting this digestion. So, the concept of peptic ulceration is acid plus pepsin versus mucosal resistance. Factors which tilt this balance leads to the production of ulcers. The factors are:
  - Gastric hypersecretion.
  - Severe ulceration occurs in Zollinger-Ellison syndrome, which is characterized by very high acid secretion.
  - Acid secretion is more important in the etiology of duodenal ulcer than in gastric ulcer.
- *Factors reducing mucosal resistance:*
  - Several drugs, particularly those used in rheumatoid arthritis.
  - Aspirin is an important etiological factor in gastric ulcer.
  - The organism *Helicobacter pylori*
  - Reflux of bile and intestinal contents into stomach due to poorly functioning pyloric sphincter.
- Other risk factors are smoking and alcohol consumption.

Clinical Features

- Patient presents with the recurrent abdominal pain which consists of three characters, i.e., localization of epigastrium, relationship to food and periodicity.
- Patient has epigastric pain. Pain is very sharply localized in the manner that the patient localize the site with one finger only. This is also known as pointing sign. In its character, the pain is burning.
- *Hunger pain:* As person remain empty stomach pain gets started which is relieved only by taking the foods.
- *Night pain:* Patient wakes from the sleep due to the pain at around 3 AM. This is relieved by taking the food, milk or antacid.
- *Periodicity of pain*
  - Pain usually occur in episodes and last for 1 to 3 weeks every time for 3 to 4 times a year. In between the episodes patients become asymptomatic.

- Initially episodes are short in duration and are less frequent. With the time episodes get longer in duration and their frequency increases.
- In winter and spring seasons, patients remain more symptomatic.
- In smokers, relapse is more common as compared to non-smokers.

Management

Investigations/Diagnosis

- **Endoscopy:** It is the ideal method of diagnosing. Ulcer appears as severe aphthous ulcer with the creamy base.
- **Barium meal:** Peptic ulcer is seen in the form of crater along the lesser curvature.
- **Gastric acid secretion tests:** Fractional test meal is done in which gruel meal is given for stimulating gastric secretion. Both free and total acidity are estimated. Augmented histamine test is more specific and is used.
- **Test for *H. pylori*:** It consists of invasive and non-invasive tests:
  - Invasive tests
    - Rapid urease test
    - Histology
    - Culture
  - Non-invasive tests
    - Serology
    - Urea breath test

Treatment

Treatment of peptic ulcer is mainly medical.
- **General measure:**
  - Stop smoking
  - Stop NSAIDs, corticosteroids and alcohols
  - Avoid stress.
- **Pharmacotherapy:**
  - *Short-term treatment*
    - *Antacid and alginates:* These are the antacids which are the combination of aluminum and magnesium compounds, i.e., aluminum hydroxide, magnesium trisilicate and alginic acid. These drugs form protective mucosal raft. Sodium bicarbonate is the quickest acting antacid. Its dose is 15 to 30 mL liquid antacid 1 to 3 hours after the food and at bed time for 4 to 6 weeks.
    - *H2 receptor antagonists:*, i.e., ranitidine 150 mg BD or 300 mg at night; Famotidine can be given 20 mg BD or 40 mg at night. In gastric ulcers dose should be given for 6 weeks followed by endoscopy.
    - Proton pump inhibitors are given, i.e., omeprazole or rabeprazole 20 to 40 mg/day; pantoprazole 40 mg/day and lansoprazole 15 to 30 mg/day is given. These should be given for 4 to 8 weeks. Drugs omeprazole and lansoprazole should be given 30 minutes before taking a meal.
    - *Prostaglandin analogue:* Misoprostol 200 mg QDS helps to prevent NSAID induced mucosal injury.
    - *Colloidal bismuth compounds:* Here drugs, such as bismuth subsalicylate and colloidal bismuth subcitrate are given.

- *Complex salts:* Sucralfate forms the protective covering for the ulcers.

H. pylori eradication
- Here triple drug therapy is used. Regimen includes two antibiotics and a proton pump inhibitor
- Commonly given regimen consists of amoxicillin l g twice daily along with clarithromycin 500 mg twice daily with twice a day proton pump inhibitor, i.e., omeprazole or rabeprazole 20 mg, lansoprazole 30 mg, pantoprazole 40 mg for 14 days. If person is allergic from penicillin, metronidazole may be used in place of amoxicillin.
- If infection persists after giving triple therapy, quadruple therapy, i.e., proton pump inhibitor, bismuth, tetracycline, metronidazole is given.
- *Long-term treatment*
- Intermittent treatment
  - This should be given in cases where symptomatic relapses are <4 times a year.
  - Four weeks course of one of the ulcer healing agents is given.
- Maintenance treatment
  - Continuous maintenance treatment is not needed after successful *H. pylori* eradication.
  - In minority who do require it, the lowest effective dose should be given.
  - Long-term maintenance is with H2 receptor antagonists, i.e., cimetidine 400 mg at night, ranitidine 150 mg at night, famotidine 20 mg at night or nizatidine 150 mg at night.
- Surgical treatment
  - In cases with gastric ulcer, partial gastrectomy with a Billroth I anastomosis is procedure of choice, in which ulcer itself and ulcer bearing area of the stomach are resected.
  - Duodenal ulcer treatment could be truncal vagotomy along with pyloroplasty or gastroenterostomy.
  - In the emergency condition, 'under-running' the ulcer for bleeding or 'over sewing', i.e., patch repair for perforation is all that is required, in addition to taking a biopsy.
  - In patients with giant duodenal ulcers, partial gastrectomy using a 'Polya' or Billroth II reconstruction may be required.
  - Elective surgery is done in gastric outflow obstruction and recurrent ulcer despite the medical treatment.

Q.13. Write short note on dysphagia.
(Mar 2007, 2 Marks) (Sep 2008, 2.5 Marks)

Or

Write short answer on dysphagia. *(May 2018, 3 Marks)*

Ans. Dysphagia is defined as difficulty in swallowing.

Causes

- Disease pertaining to esophagus and its surrounding structures.
  - Stomatitis
  - Pharyngitis

- Glossitis
- Plummer-Vinson syndrome
- Esophagitis
- Carcinoma of esophagus
- Pressure by mediastinal tumor on esophagus
- Achalasia (Failure of reflex) of lower end of esophagus.
- Dysphagia in neurological disorders
  - Post-diphtheric paralysis
  - Myasthenia gravis
  - Motor neuron disease
  - Scleroderma or other related collagen disorders
  - Acute bulbar paralysis.

Clinical Features

- Presence of anemia
- Koilonychia
- Glaze tongue
- Malnutrition
- Nasal regurgitation
- Bulbar palsy
- Severe weight loss
- Malignancy
- Chest pain
- Hoarseness of voice.

Treatment

Dysphagia is a symptom complex of number of disease hence treatment has to be planned depending on the etiological factors.

Q.14.   Write short note on gastroesophageal reflux disease.
(Apr 2007, 10 Marks)

Ans. A chronic condition in which the lower esophageal sphincter allows gastric acids to reflux into the esophagus, causing heartburn, acid indigestion, and possible injury to the esophageal lining.

Mechanism

Flowchart 2: Mechanism of gastroesophageal reflux disease.

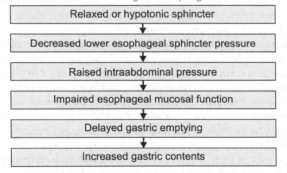

```
Relaxed or hypotonic sphincter
          ↓
Decreased lower esophageal sphincter pressure
          ↓
Raised intraabdominal pressure
          ↓
Impaired esophageal mucosal function
          ↓
Delayed gastric emptying
          ↓
Increased gastric contents
```

Etiology

- *Relaxed or hypotonic sphincter:* It is due to diabetes mellitus, hiatus hernia, fatty meal.
- *Decreased lower esophageal sphincter pressure:* It is due to prolonged gastric tube intubation, scleroderma and use of certain drugs, such as calcium channel blockers, nitrates.
- *Raised intra-abdominal pressure:* It is due to ascites, obesity and pregnancy.
- *Impaired esophageal mucosal function:* It is due to usage of alcohol and smoking.
- *Delayed gastric emptying:* It is due to pyloric obstruction, fatty foods and gastroparesis.
- *Increased gastric contents:* It is due to large meals and Zollinger-Ellison syndrome.
- *Sliding hiatus hernia:* Where the esophagogastric junction slides up through the diaphragm resulting in:
  - Loss of the obliquity of entry of esophagus into stomach.
  - Loss of the reinforcing effect of intra-abdominal pressure on the lower esophageal sphincter.

  These two above mentioned factors of hiatus hernia facilitate gastroesophageal reflux, but do not directly cause it.
- *Cardiomyotomy and vagotomy:* They decrease the efficiency of the lower esophageal sphincter.
- *Increased intra-abdominal pressure:* Pregnancy, obesity, ascites, weight-lifting and straining increases the intra-abdominal pressure.
- *Reduced tone of lower esophageal sphincter:* Cigarette smoking, alcohol, fatty foods and caffeine act by reducing the lower esophageal sphincter tone.
- *Impaired gastric emptying:* Impaired gastric emptying due to obstruction of gastric outlet or use of anticholinergic drugs, fatty foods and large volume meals act by increasing the gastric content available for reflux.
- Systemic sclerosis.
- Drugs which reduce the lower esophageal sphincter tone, e.g., aminophylline, beta-agonists, nitrates, calcium channel blockers, etc.

Clinical Features

- *Typical symptoms:* Heart burn and acid regurgitation
- *Atypical symptoms:* Dysphagia, globus sensation, non-cardiac chest pain, dyspepsia or abdominal pain.
- *Extra-esophageal symptoms:* Hoarseness, sore throat, sinusitis, otitis media, chronic cough, laryngitis, dental erosion and recurrent aspiration.
- *Malignancy:* Head and neck cancer, esophageal adeno-carcinoma

Complications

- Esophagitis
- Esophageal strictures
- Esophageal ulcers
- Aspiration pneumonia
- Iron deficiency anemia
- Barrett's esophagus
- Carcinoma of esophagus

Investigations

- *Endoscopy:* Enables visualization of esophagitis, strictures and Barrett's mucosa which all can be confirmed by biopsy.
- Barium meal can reveal hiatus hernia.
- Bernstein test is done in patients with high clinical suspicion but negative endoscopy.
- Resting ECG and stress ECG to rule out ischemic heart disease.
- Esophageal motility studies.

Management

1. **Conservative measures:**

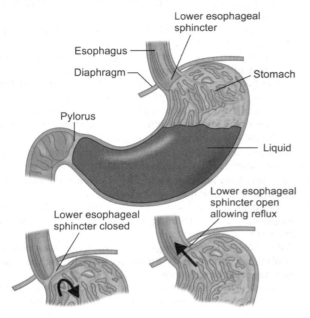

Fig. 4: Gastroesophageal reflux disease.

- Abstain from eating within 2 hours of bed time
- Elevate head of bed by 6 inches
- Sleep in left lateral decubitus position
- *Avoid:* Caffeine, nicotine, alcohol, chocolate, mints, carbonated beverages, high-fat foods, tomato or citrus-based products
- Avoid if possible medications that can worsen GERD - anticholinergic, theophylline, prostaglandin, calcium channel blockers, alendronate
- Weight loss if patient is obese
- Rabeprazole, esomeprazole provide superior gastric acid suppression.

2. **Medical treatment**
- In mild cases liquid antacid is used, i.e., 10 to 15 mL, one to three hours after the meal it provide relief in heart burn.
- In moderate cases, H_2 receptor antagonist, i.e., ranitidine 150 mg BD or QID with meals and before bed time for 6 weeks.
- In severe cases, proton pump inhibitors are given, i.e., omeprazole 20 to 40 mg/day, pantoprazole 40 mg/day and rabeprazole 10 to 20 mg/day is given. These should be given for 6 to 8 weeks. For maintenance therapy treatment should be given for 6 to 8 months.
- Metaclopramide or domperidone 10 mg TID increases lower esophageal sphincter tone and promote gastric emptying.
- Repeated dilatations are used to treat esophageal strictures.
- In anemics oral iron or blood transfusion is given.

3. **Surgical treatment**
- Surgical resection of strictures should be carried out.
- Surgical return of lower esophageal sphincter to abdomen in patient with sliding hiatus hernia, construction of an additional valve mechanism is done.

Q.15. Write in brief signs, symptoms and treatment of amoebiasis. *(Apr 2008, 5 Marks)*

Or

Write short note on treatment of amoebiasis.
(Feb 2013, 5 Marks)

Ans. Amoebiasis is the infection of gastrointestinal tract by protozoan parasite *Entamoeba histolytica*.

Symptoms
- Patient has diarrhea and pass 10–15 stools per day.
- Presence of abdominal pain.
- Stools consist of blood and mucus.
- Flatulence is present.
- Fever is present between 38 and 40° with rigors.

Signs
- Palpation of abdomen show diffuse tenderness.
- Chronic cases show thickened tender sigmoid colon.
- Amoeba is felt as a sausage shaped mass in right iliac fossa.
- Tender hepatomegaly is present.

Treatment
- Diloxanide furoate is given 500 mg TDS × 10 days.
- Metronidazole Or Ornidazole 500 mg TDS × 5 days
- Secnidazole plus 2 g single dose is given
- Nitazoxanide 500 mg BD is given
- Dehydroemetine 1.5 mg/kg/day × 5 days IM

Q.16. Write short note on hepatic amoebiasis.
(May/Jun 2009, 5 Marks)

Ans. It is the most common complication of amoebiasis.

Pathophysiology

Amoeba after reaching the liver multiply and block small intrahepatic portal radicles, producing thrombosis and infarction resulting in necrosed areas surrounded by areas of congestion. Necrotic area consists of degenerated liver cells, leukocytes, connective tissue strands and enmeshed in between *Entamoeba histolytica*. Cytolytic enzyme liberated from amoebae destroy the liver parenchyma and fusion of these small necrosed areas results in abscess formation. An abscess generally is single but may be multiple. Its walls are lined by a shaggy necrotic zone in whose center there is thick reddish brown pus containing fragments of liver tissue, necrotic material and erythrocytes. The pus typically is called "Anchovy sauce" like and is sterile on culture.

Clinical Features

- Onset of Amoebic hepatitis is insidious and patient may come with irregular or intermittent fever

- There is stretching sensation in the liver area. Gradually with the progression of disease, anorexia hepatic pain and epigastric discomfort appear
- Examination shows a uniform tender hepatomegaly
- There are signs of toxemia
- Jaundice is not very common
- When hepatitis progresses on to a liver abscess, pain in the liver area becomes a constant feature
- Intermittent fever, loss of weight, lassitude, peculiar sallowness of skin, irritability, sleeplessness are common features.

Investigations

- TLC and DLC shows leukocytosis with increase in polymorphs.
- Stool examination is done and cysts and trophozoites of E. histolytica should be look over.
- Amoebic fluorescent antibody titer is positive.

Management of Amoebic Liver Abscess/Hepatic Amoebiasis

- Early cases are responding well with metronidazole 800 mg TID for 5 days or tinidazole 2 g daily for three days.
- Luminal amoebicide: Diloxamide furoate 500 mg 8 hourly for 10 days should be given to determine luminal cyst.
- If abscess is large and not respond to chemotherapy repeated aspiration under ultrasonic guidance is required.
- Rupture of abscess into peritoneal cavity requires immediate aspiration or surgical drainage.

Q.17. Describe etiology, clinical features and management of intestinal amoebiasis. *(Jan 2012, 15 Marks)*

Ans.

Etiology

- Amoebiasis is caused by infection by protozoan parasite known as *Entamoeba histolytica*.
- Common source of transmission is water especially when it is contaminated by fecal matter or sanitary conditions of water supply being defective.
- Flies spread infection by feeding on fecal matter or contaminated food.
- Auto-spread in a patient when cysts embedded underneath the nails and person may get infected if he had not properly washed his hands.

Clinical Features

Symptoms

- Patient has diarrhea and pass 10–15 stools per day.
- Presence of abdominal pain.
- Stools consist of blood and mucus.
- Flatulence is present.
- Fever is present between 38 and 40° with rigors.

Signs

- Palpation of abdomen show diffuse tenderness.
- Chronic cases show thickened tender sigmoid colon.

- Amoeba is felt as a sausage shaped mass in right iliac fossa.
- Tender hepatomegaly is present.

Management

- Diloxanide furoate is given 500 mg TDS × 10 days.
- Metronidazole Or Ornidazole 500 mg TDS × 5 days
- Secnidazole plus 2 g single dose is given
- Nitazoxanide 500 mg BD is given.
- Dehydroemetine 1.5 mg/kg/day × 5 days IM

Q.18. Write sign and symptoms of malabsorption syndrome. *(Aug 2012, 5 Marks)*

Ans.

Sign and Symptoms of Malabsorption Syndrome

Symptoms

- Presence of lassitude and laziness
- Mood fluctuation
- Fatigue and weakness is present
- Pain in bone is present
- Weight loss is present.

Signs

- **Skin:** edema over legs and purpuras
- **Eyes:** Xerophthalmia and night blindness
- **Hematopoietic:** Hemorrhagic tendencies are present, anemia
- **Gastrointestinal system:** Malnutrition is generalized, angular stomatitis, glossitis and diarrhea
- **Genitourinary system:** Hypotension, amenorrhea, loss of libido, Nocturia
- **Skeletal:** Muscle wasting, tetany and presence of paresthesia.
- **Nervous system:** Peripheral neuropathy.

Q.19. Write acid peptic disease under the following headings: *(Feb 2014, 2 Marks Each)*
   a. Etiology
   b. Clinical features
   c. Investigations
   d. Treatment

Or

Write short answer on acid peptic disorder.
(Feb 2019, 3 Marks)

Ans. Excessive secretion of acid and pepsin or a weakened stomach mucosal defense is responsible for damage to the delicate mucosa and the lining of the stomach, esophagus and duodenum resulting in ulceration which is known as "Acid Peptic Disease".

"Acid peptic disease" is a collective term used to include many conditions, such as gastroesophageal reflux disease (GERD), gastritis, gastric ulcer, duodenal ulcer, esophageal ulcer, Zollinger-Ellison Syndrome (ZES) and Meckel's diverticular ulcer.

Etiology

- *Helicobacter pylori*: H. pylori is responsible for around 60–90% of all gastric and duodenal ulcers.

- **NSAIDs:** Prostaglandins protect the mucus lining of the stomach. Nonsteroidal anti-inflammatory drugs (NSAIDs), such as aspirin, diclofenac and naproxen prevent the production of these prostaglandins by blocking cyclo-oxygenase enzyme leading to ulceration and bleeding.
- **Smoking, alcohol and tobacco:** Cigarettes, alcohol and tobacco cause an instant and intense acid production which acts as though gasoline is poured over a raging fire.
- **Blood group O:** People with blood group "O" are reported to have higher risks for the development of stomach ulcers as there is an increased formation of antibodies against the *Helicobacter bacteria*, which causes an inflammatory reaction and ulceration.
- **Heredity:** Patients suffering from peptic ulcer diseases usually have a family history of the disease, particularly the development of duodenal ulcer which may occur below the age of 20.
- **Steroids/other medicines:** Drugs, such as corticosteroids, anticoagulants like warfarin (Coumarin), niacin, some chemotherapy drugs, and spironolactone can aggravate or cause ulcers.
- **Diet:** Low fiber diet, caffeinated drinks and fatty foods are linked to peptic ulcer.
- **Other diseases:** Chronic liver, lung and kidney diseases especially tumors of the acid producing cells all predispose to peptic ulcers. Zollinger-Ellison syndrome (ZES) is a rare pre-cancerous condition which causes peptic ulcer disease. Endocrine disorders, such as hyperparathyroidism are also implicated in the development of peptic ulcers.
- **Stress:** Stress and neurological problems can also be associated with the Cushing's ulcer and peptic ulcer.

Clinical Features

- *Abdominal Pain:* A burning pain in the upper part of the abdomen usually related to mealtimes together with fullness, distension of the abdomen, bloating, with/without nausea and generalized discomfort also known as "dyspepsia". The pain is usually so sharply localized that the patient can often indicate the exact place with two or three fingers called the "pointing sign". Gastric ulcer pain is more after the ingestion of meals while duodenal ulcer pain occurs more due to hunger.
- Nausea, heart burn, vomiting, loss of appetite and weight loss.
- *Gastric outlet obstruction:* The ulcer could heal with scarring and result in narrowing of the gastric or intestinal lumen. This could cause an obstruction to food being passed forward.
- *Vomiting or passing blood in stool:* Signs of bleeding as vomiting of blood or black tarry color of the stool.
- *Bleeding and perforation from the ulcer:* Bleeding from the site of the ulcer with thinning of the wall may result in perforation.

Investigations

- **Blood tests:** Blood tests, such as ELISA help in the measurement of antibodies to *H. pylori*. Serum gastrin levels should be measured in patients with multiple ulcers to consider gastrin secreting tumors or Zollinger-Ellison syndrome. Tests for gastric secretion include the "pentagastrin test", the "chew and spit test" and the "Hollander insulin test".
- **Stool Test:** Stool test detects the presence of *H. pylori* in the feces and also establishes whether there is any recurrence after antibiotic therapy.
- **Breath test:** The urea breath test (UBT) is helpful in the detection of *H. pylori*. The patient is made to drink a liquid containing carbon-labeled urea, which is broken down by the bacteria. The patient is subsequently asked to breathe into a sealed bag, which is tested for the presence of labeled carbon. A positive test indicates the presence of *H. pylori* infection.
- **Endoscopy:** Endoscopy is considered a more accurate test for the diagnosis of "peptic ulcer diseases" and also helps in taking biopsy of the affected area. Gastroscopy or esophagogastroduodenoscopy (EGD) is a kind of endoscopy which is carried out on patients to detect peptic ulcer.
- **Barium radiography:** X-rays are taken of the stomach, esophagus and duodenum after swallowing barium and the retention of contrast in the ulcer is monitored.

Treatment

- *Eradication of H. pylori:* The standard protocol to eradicate *H. pylori* involves the use of two or three antibiotics, i.e., amoxicillin, tetracycline, clarithromycin, metronidazole and the use of a proton pump inhibitor, i.e., esomeprazole, omeprazole, lansoprazole, rabeprazole, pantoprazole with or without a bismuth compound for around 2–3 weeks and repeated if there is recurrence.
- Avoid NSAIDs or the concurrent use of a prostaglandin analogue (misoprostol) may be prescribed to prevent peptic ulceration due to NSAIDs.
- The use of antacids or H_2 receptor antagonist (H_2RAs), such as cimetidine, ranitidine, famotidine, and nizatidine which help in the reduction of gastric acid secretion and in turn increase the gastric pH and reduce the secretion of pepsin.
- Treatment of peptic ulcer complications include a blood transfusion for hematemesis and malena, the use of antacids and H_2 receptor antagonists for pain, the treatment of peritonitis in case of perforation of peptic ulcer disease.

Q.20. Write short answer on inflammatory bowel disease.

(Apr 2019, 3 Marks)

Ans. Inflammatory bowel disease constitutes Crohn's disease and ulcerative colitis which are nonspecific inflammatory disorders of bowel.

Both disorders are less common in blacks and more common in American Jews.

Both the diseases can occur at any age but I more frequent during 15 to 20 years of age.

Ulcerative colitis is a chronic recurrent inflammatory disorder of rectum and colonic mucosa which leads to ulceration and bleeding.

Crohn's disease is a chronic granulomatous inflammation of terminal ileum and adjoining colon resulting in ulceration, stricture formation, fistulation and abscess formation.

Etiology

♦ Basically, the exact cause in both of the diseases is unknown, but few factors are implicated in pathogenesis:

♦ **Familial and genetic disorders:** In both of the diseases, 10 to 15% of patients have inflammatory bowel disease. In Crohn's disease, monozygotic twins are mainly affected. So genetic predisposition is to be considered.

♦ **Infective disorders:** Colonization of gut with bacterial overgrowth is hypothesized and there is an exaggerated immune response to the luminal bacterial antigens and their products due to genetic predisposition. Bacterial antigens produce an inflammatory response by producing receptor ligands which interact with luminal mucosa and produces ulceration.

♦ **Immunological disorders:** Due to the histopathological evidence of the inflammation of bowel and the non-isolation of infective agent, immunological basis of disease has been proposed which causes infiltration of lamina propria along with inflammatory cells. Till now no antigen has been detected. So autoimmunity is considered as strong possibility in pathogenesis due to presence of extraintestinal manifestations and its response to corticosteroids and azathioprine.

♦ **Smoking:** It is strongly associated with Crohn's disease and not with ulcerative colitis.

Clinical Features

Clinical manifestation	Ulcerative colitis	Crohn's disease
Symptoms	Presence of diarrhea along with blood, mucus and the pus There is tenderness over left side of abdomen or in the left iliac fossa	Presence of diarrhea and pain in abdomen in right lower quadrant
Palpation	No mass is palpable	While palpating on abdomen and rectum a mass is felt
Colics/Diffuse pain	There is no colicky pain. Megacolon can produce diffuse pain which is associated with distention of abdomen and stoppage of the loose motions	Abdomen colics are common because of obstruction
Features of malabsorption	• Diarrhea with tenesmus • Anemia and weight loss • Dehydration	• Moderate diarrhea and fever • Loose or well formed stools • Features of malabsorption of fat, carbohydrate, protein, vitamin D and vitamin B12 • Anemia • Weight loss • Growth retardation in children
Extraintestinal features		
Eye, i.e., conjunctivitis, uveitis, episcleritis	It is common	It is less common
Skin, i.e., erythema nodosum, pyoderma gangrenosa	It is less common	It is common
Joints, i.e., arthritis, arthralgia and ankylosing spondylitis	It is common	It is less common
Heart, i.e., aortic regurgitation, mitral valve prolapse	It is common	It is less common
Liver, i.e., sclerosing cholangitis, hepatitis, fatty liver	It is uncommon	It is common

Investigations

1. **General tests**
   • Presence of mild-to-moderate normocytic normochromic iron deficiency anemia.
   • Leukocytosis
   • Hypoproteinemia
   Above features are seen in both the diseases.
2. **Stool and blood cultures:** They are performed to exclude other causes of septicemia and also to rule out amoebic dysentery or amoebic colitis.
3. **Special tests for Crohn's disease:**
   • *Barium meal study:* Barium meal follows through barium enema as diagnostic for Crohn's disease. It can show disturbed mucosal pattern, malabsorption pattern and pathognomic string sign due to marked narrowing of segment of thee affected bowel. In chronic cases strictures are seen.
   • *Endoscopy:* Ulcers are seen in stomach and duodenum.
   • *Sigmoidoscopy and colonoscopy:* They detect rectal and colonic lesions. These are seen less common in Crohn's disease
   • *Radioactive labeled white cell counting:* It is done to detect all cases of active involvement.
4. **Special tests for ulcerative colitis:**
   • *Sigmoidocopy:* It shows hyperemic rectal mucosa and normal vascular pattern is lost. In mild cases mucosa

bleeds on touch while in severe cases spontaneous bleeding is seen.

- *Plain X-ray abdomen:* It shows dilated gases filled colon with diameter >5 cm. It is essential if sign and symptoms of toxic megacolon are seen.
- *Barium enema:* It is the double contrast study which in severe cases show ulceration and pseudopolyposis and in long standing cases, narrowing of lumen and loss of haustrations leading to pipe stem appearance.
- *Colonoscopy:* It demonstrates severity and extent of disease. Colon biopsy is done to differentiate it from Crohn's disease and amoebic colitis.

Management

Treatment of Crohn's Disease

Medical Treatment

- High protein and high energy diet should be given to the patient by orally or by parenteral route depending on the severity of disease.
- Plasma and blood transfusion should be done to improve moderate anemia and hypoproteinemia.
- Low fat diet or milk free diet should be given to the patient which improve symptoms o lactate deficiency or malabsorption. This reduces the colics and obstruction of intestine.
- For infection broad spectrum antibiotics and metronidazole should be given in the presence of infection. In Crohn's disease, infection is common.
- Supplementation of iron, folic acid, calcium, vitamin D, electrolytes whenever there I deficiency.

Drug Treatment

- For treatment of diarrhea oral doses of diphenoxylate 5 mg TID or loperamide 2 mg TID and codeine phosphate 30 mg TID can be given
- Oral prednisolone 40 to 60 mg daily should be given in active disease for 2 to 4 weeks, this leads to remission and improvement of symptoms, it is withdrawn for the period of 4 to 6 weeks to prevent the early relapse.
- Azathioprine 2.5 mg/k/day is given in patients who relapse on steroidal therapy and in whom surgery cannot be done.

Surgical Treatment

Resection of bowel is done in following situations:

- Frequent intestinal obstruction not relieved by dietary and drug therapy.
- Presence of fistula, stricture or abscess
- Emergency surgery during perforation
- Extensive involvement of ileum and colon

Treatment of ulcerative colitis

Medical Treatment

- Admit the patient to hospital.
- Provide supportive treatment in form of parenteral fluid, nutrition, electrolyte and blood to correct dehydration, electrolyte imbalance, anemia and hypoproteinemia in the severe cases. If disease is mild to moderate it need high protein and low residual diet.

- Corticosteroids given in form of suppositories and or enema and orally for systemic effects. Prednisolone-21-phosphate or betamethasone suppositories are helpful for treating proctitis once or twice a day. This provides relief in mild form.
- If disease is severe administer systemic corticosteroids, i.e., prednisolone 40 to 60 mg/day orally in divided doses or single dose for 4 to 6 weeks. In severe cases, IV hydrocortisone 100 to 200 mg 6 hourly or methylprednisolone 48 to 60 mg in four divided doses is given. Administration of potassium is must with corticosteroid therapy. Steroids give remission in 4 to 6 weeks and now dose is reduced to 5 to 10 mg at weekly intervals for next 4 to 6 weeks.
- Sulfasalazine is given in mild to moderate disease and it is less effective as compared to steroidal therapy. Its oral dose is 2 to 4 g/day. This decreases risk of relapse. As remission is induced by steroidal therapy patient is maintained on oral dose of sulfasalazine 0.5 g 6 hourly for around 1 to 2 years.
- Immunomodulatory drug, such as mercaptopurine or azathioprine or methotrexate in steroidal dependant patients to withdraw corticosteroid and maintain the remission.
- Biological agents, such as anti – TNF therapy with monoclonal antibodies and anti-integrins are highly effective against corticosteroid dependent or refractory disease.

Surgical Treatment

Proctocolectomy with ileostomy is done when:

- Acute ulcerative colitis is resistant to medical treatment or relapse frequently occur after giving proper treatment.
- In chronic disease along with stricture formation and duration of disease is more than 10 years.
- If disease gets localized to rectum, then ileorectal or ileoanal anastomosis with formation of ileal pouch should be preferred.

3. DISEASES OF LIVER

Q.1. Write short note on tender hepatomegaly.

(Jan 2012, 5 Marks) (May/June 2009, 5 Marks)

Ans. The term tender hepatomegaly itself means there is enlargement of liver with tenderness present in it.

Causes

- Infections
  - Viral hepatitis
  - Amoebic abscess
  - Acute alcoholic hepatitis
  - Autoimmune hepatitis
  - Actinomycosis of liver
  - Weil's disease
  - Malaria

- Circulatory disturbances
  - Congestive heart failure
  - Hepatic vein occlusion
- Tumors
  - Hepatocellular carcinoma
  - Angiosarcoma
- Budd-Chiari syndrome

Hepatitis

- *Viral hepatitis:* Inflammation of liver due to viral hepatitis is common cause of producing tender hepatomegaly. There is moderate enlargement of liver which is smooth with consistency varying from soft to firm.
- *Amoebic liver abscess:* In this, liver is enlarged and is tender and tenderness present on lower costal cartilages on right side.
- *Bacterial liver abscess:* Multiple small pyogenic abscesses or a single large abscess involves liver mainly the right lobe producing an enlarged tender liver.
- *Acute alcoholic hepatitis:* This follows the period of heavy drinking. There is presence of right upper abdominal pain, anorexia, nausea and vomiting, profound weakness. Liver become enlarged and tender.
- *Autoimmune hepatitis:* Prevalence is in young females. Presence of enlarged and tender liver, spider nevi and enlarged spleen.
- *Actinomycosis of liver:* Here liver becomes enlarged and tender.
- *Weil's disease:* Spirochetes causes Weil's disease. There is presence of enlarged and tender liver.
- *Malaria:* In malignant form of malaria, there is hepatomegaly and tenderness over the liver. Liver is palpable in half of the cases. Spleen is always palpable.

Circulatory Disturbances

- *Congestive heart failure:* Congestive heart failure is an important cause of hepatomegaly moderate to massive. The liver is firm and tender.
- *Hepatic vein occlusion:* It is uncommon condition and there is presence of enlarged and tender liver.

Tumors

- *Hepatocellular carcinoma:* Liver becomes enlarged but sometimes it is tender.
- *Angiosarcoma:* In patients with exposure to gaseous chemical, liver becomes enlarged and tender.

Budd-Chiari syndrome

Here liver is enlarged and tender. There is failure of jugular vein to fill when liver is pressed.

Q.2. Write short note on ascites. *(Mar 2006, 5 Marks)*
(Mar 2007, 2 Marks) (June 2010, 5 Marks)
(Mar 2011, 2 Marks) (Jan 2012, 5 Marks)

Or

Enumerate causes of ascites. *(Sep 2007, 2 Marks)*
Ans. Collection of the fluid in peritoneal cavity is called ascites.

At least 1500 mL of fluid must collect in peritoneal cavity before physical examination.

Pathogenesis of Ascites

Flowchart 3: Pathogenesis of ascites.

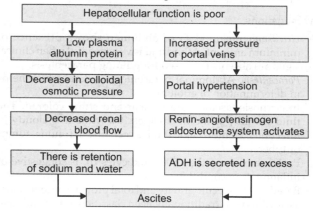

Causes of Ascites

- Disease of peritoneum
  - Infections:
    - Tuberculous peritonitis.
    - Spontaneous bacterial peritonitis.
    - Fungal—Candida, histoplasma.
    - Parasitic—Schistosoma, enterobius.
    - Viral—Acute severe hepatitis.
  - Neoplasms:
    - Primary mesothelioma.
    - Secondary carcinomatosis, e.g., adenocarcinoma, sarcoma, teratoma, leukemia, Hodgkin's disease, lymphocytic lymphoma, myeloid metaplasia.
    - Pseudomyxoma peritonei
  - Familial paroxysmal peritonitis
  - Miscellaneous
    - Vasculitis — SLE and other collagen vascular diseases, allergic vasculitis (Henoch-Schonlein purpura).
    - Eosinophilic gastroenteritis.
    - Whipple's disease.
    - Granulomatous peritonitis — Sarcoidosis, Crohn's disease, starch peritonitis.
    - Peritoneal loose bodies.
    - Peritoneal encapsulation.
- Portal hypertension
- Congestive heart failure
- Hypoalbuminemia
  - Nephrosis
  - Malnutrition
  - Protein-losing enteropathy
- Beri-beri
- Myxedema
- *Ovarian disease:*
  - Meigs syndrome
  - Struma ovari
  - Ovarian overstimulation syndrome

♦ Pancreatic ascites due to retroperitoneal leakage of pancreatic enzymes from a ruptured cyst or pancreatic duct.
♦ Bile ascites
♦ Chylous ascites
♦ Epidemic dropsy

Investigations

♦ *Ultrasonography:* USG of abdomen shows presence of minimum amount of fluid and is very needful when clinical signs are absent. This used for guiding paracentesis.
♦ *Paracentesis:* Abdominal paracentesis is done which helps in determination of etiology.
♦ In cirrhosis, ascitic fluid is clear and straw colored. The fluid is milky white in chyle ascites while it is cloudy in infections. Hemorrhagic fluid is seen due to trauma, tumor or tuberculosis.
♦ Presence of more than 500 leukocytes/μL is suggestive of inflammatory conditions.
♦ Based on the specific gravity and total protein concentration, ascitic fluid has traditionally been classified as transudative and exudative.

Management of Ascites

♦ In every case of ascites oral diuretics, i.e., furosemide 40 to 80 mg + spironolactone 25 to 100 mg is administered.
♦ Sodium intake is restricted and diet which is low in sodium is given.
♦ In case of massive ascites which produce cardiorespiratory enlargement, abdominal paracentesis is done and fluid is drained slowly. Fluid should not be drained quickly because it causes vasovagal attack.
♦ Portacaval shunt surgery or implantation of peritoneovenous shunt can be done in refractory ascites.

Q.3. Describe causes, clinical features, diagnosis and management of jaundice. *(Apr 2017, 12 Marks)*

Ans. Jaundice is a condition where there is yellow pigmentation of skin or sclera due to excess bilirubin in the blood.

Causes

The causes are based on the type of jaundice.

♦ **Hemolytic jaundice:** In hemolytic jaundice, there is excessive break down of RBC due to which bilirubin is produced in excess from hemoglobin. The causes of hemolytic jaundice are:
• Jaundice of prematurity, physiological jaundice
• Defect in shape of erythrocytes, i.e., spherocytes and sickle cell anemia
• There is parasitic destruction of erythrocyte
• Toxic agents, i.e., metal like lead, poison like snake venom
• Incompatible blood transfusion
• ABO and Rh-incompatibility
• Excessive burns of body
• Bacterial toxins, septicemia.
♦ **Obstructive jaundice:** In obstructive jaundice bilirubin conjugation takes place normally in the liver, but it does not reach into the intestine and goes into the blood stream,

the result is rise in bilirubin level. The causes of obstructive jaundice are:
• *Extrahepatic:*
  – Obstruction within the bile ducts: The common cause is gallstone.
  – Obstruction due to change in wall of ducts: Congenital obliteration of ducts during operation procedure, sclerosing cholangitis, etc.
  – Due to pressure on bile ducts: Pressure on the bile duct occur in number of disease, e.g., carcinoma of liver, hydatid cyst or fever, etc.
• *Intrahepatic:* In it, there is no mechanical obstruction in bile ducts and it is due to intake of drugs, such as oral contraceptives, antitubercular drugs and chlorpromazine.
• *Hepatocellular jaundice:* In this liver cells fall to conjugate and excrete all the bile pigments. The causes of hepatocellular jaundice are:
  – Infection, such as viral hepatitis, yellow fever, malaria, typhoid, etc.
  – Chemical poisons, such as chloroform, halothane, CCl4, etc.
  – Alcoholic hepatitis, postnecrotic cirrhosis, etc.

Clinical Features

Symptoms

♦ Symptoms of a case of jaundice shall vary with the type of jaundice the patient is suffering from and the underlying condition.
♦ Commonest form of jaundice is due to hepatitis where the patient may start with malaise, low grade fever, vomiting and loss of appetite.
♦ Person may take his/her morning breakfast normally and as the day passes, appetite for food almost disappears.
♦ In smokers, urge to smoke is the earliest to go. Yellowness appears first in the conjunctiva and then the mucous membrane of the lips and palate became pale.
♦ Urine is high colored while in early stage, the stools may remain of normal color.
♦ When a person has got features of obstructive jaundice, color of conjunctiva is yellowish green. Stools become clay colored and there is severe degree of itching.
♦ Pulse becomes slow.
♦ Patient may suffer from bruises and bleeding from mucous surfaces due to lack of fat soluble vitamin K.
♦ If jaundice remains for prolonged periods as in case of malignancy patient suffers from marked asthenia and wasting.

Signs

♦ Patient may show signs of anemia, malnutrition suggestive of malignancy or cirrhosis.
♦ In cirrhotics look for spider nevi, white nails, enlargement of parotid glands, testicular atrophy, palmar erythema, gynecomastia, edema over legs and feet, and ascites.
♦ There may be scratch marks on skin suggestive of cholestasis due to obstructive jaundice, bruising and petechial spots indicating prothrombin deficiency in alcoholic or Laennec's cirrhosis may be observed.

- Liver may be palpable, smooth and tender in infective hepatitis, hard and nodular in malignancy.
- Gallbladder becomes palpable when obstruction at the level of common bile duct is incomplete. A hard, small nodular gallbladder may be palpated in carcinoma.
- In chronic cholecystitis, gallbladder may be palapable and tender (Murphy's sign). In addition to looking for signs of disease in general examination, look specifically in abdomen for ascites, liver, spleen and any lymphadenopathy.
- Rectal examination may be carried out for any primary growth in rectum.

Diagnosis

- **Biochemical test:**
  - *White cell count*: Leukopenia is present in the hepatocellular jaundice. Eosinophilia is present in drug hepatitis.
  - *Urine*: Urobilinogen is absent in the obstructive jaundice and is in excess in hemolytic jaundice. Bilirubin is in excess in urine in obstructive jaundice.
  - *Liver function test*: Serum bilirubin estimation is done to asses level of jaundice. The flocculation test is positive for hepatocellular and is negative for hemolytic and obstructive jaundice. Serum albumin levels are low and globulin levels are high in chronic hepatocellular jaundice.
  - *Hematology*: In hemolytic jaundice, blood film shows immature cells and spherocytosis, erythrocyte fragility is increased and Coombs test is positive.
- **Radiology:**
  - Imaging of liver by ultrasound technique should be initial technique for all the jaundiced patients.
  - Imaging of liver through CT scan is done. The dilated bile ducts are seen during obstructive jaundice while imaging through CT scan.
- **Aspiration needle biopsy of liver:**
  - It is done cautiously in jaundice. Menghini needle is used. The histological appearance of hemolytic, hepatocellular and obstructive jaundice is distinctive.

Management

Treatment is directed towards the underlying cause

- Patient should be given small feeds of fat free, low protein and high carbohydrate diet which can be easily assimilated.
- Additionally vitamin B and C are given orally in high dosages.
- In obstructive jaundice, vitamin K should be given 10 mg parentrally.

Q.4. Write in detail about viral hepatitis.
(Sep 2007, 5 Marks)

Or

Write in brief the clinical features and treatment of viral hepatitis. *(June 2010, 5 Marks)*

Or

Describe clinical features, investigations and treatment of viral hepatitis. *(Sep 2010, 15 Marks)*

Ans. Viral hepatitis is a clinical entity where systemic infection causes inflammation and hepatic cell necrosis.

Viruses causing viral hepatitis are:

- Hepatitis A virus
- Hepatitis B virus
- Hepatitis C virus
- Hepatitis D virus
- Hepatitis E virus

Other viruses are:

- Cytomegalovirus
- Epstein-Barr virus
- Herpes simplex virus, etc.

Clinical Manifestations

Prodromal symptoms proceed the development of jaundice in sclera and behind the tongue from few days to two weeks and common symptoms are:

- Mild fever with or without chills
- Headache
- Malaise
- Arthralgia and skin rashes particularly in HBV infection
- Prominent gastroenteritis symptoms like anorexia, nausea and vomiting
- Steady upper mild abdominal pain in right hypochondrium
- Liver is not palpable.

Physical Signs

- Liver is usually tender but is not palpable initially.
- Enlarged cervical nodes may be found.
- Splenomegaly is present, particularly in children.
- Dark urine and a yellow tint of sclera held the onset of jaundice.

Features of Jaundice

- It is first observed in sclera in bulbar conjunctivitis
- Jaundice deepens following obstruction of bile canaliculi.
- Stool become pallor
- Urine is dark
- Liver is tender and is easily palpable
- At this time appetite often improves
- Gastrointestinal symptoms diminished intensity.

Thereafter jaundice recedes and all features comes to normal in 3 to 6 weeks of time which can be revealed by:

- Normal skin, sclera and urine color
- Normal stool color
- Appetite improves
- Liver enlargement regresses.

Diagnosis

Diagnosis of viral hepatitis is done in a patient with history of severe anorexia, nausea, vomiting and fever for a few days, elevated serum bilirubin and value of SGPT over 500 indicates viral hepatitis. The etiological agent is detected by serological markers.

- **Hepatitis A:**
  - Nonspecific lab tests
    - Raised serum bilirubin within few days and remain high up to 12 weeks.
    - Serum AST and ALT levels remain high for 1 to 3 weeks.
    - Alkaline phosphatase level is mildly elevated, though it remains persistently high, it suggest hepatitis associated cholestasis.
  - Specific test
    - Hepatitis A specific IgM antibody can be detected at the onset of symptoms and at first rise in serum ALT. It peaks within first month and remain positive for 3 to 6 months.
    - IgG and hepatitis A virus become positive at onset of illness and is detectable for many years
    - Nucleic acid based test like PCR.
- **Hepatitis B:**
  In a patient with history of severe anorexia, nausea, vomiting, fever for few days, elevated serum bilirubin and value of SGPT over 500 indicates HBV. The etiological agent is identified by serological markers.

Serological diagnosis of hepatitis B:

Stage of infection	HBsAg	Anti-HBc		Anti-HBs
		IgM	IgG	
Incubation	Positive	Positive	Negative	Negative
Acute hepatitis B				
Early	Positive	Positive	Negative	Negative
Late or established	Positive	Positive	Positive	Negative
Convalescence				
3 to 6 months	Negative	Positive or Negative	Positive	Positive or Negative
6 to 9 months	Negative	Negative	Positive	Positive
Post-infection				
More than 1 year	Negative	Negative	Positive	Positive
Chronic infection	Positive	--------	Positive	Negative
Immunization without exposure to infection	Negative	Negative	Negative	Positive

Markers of hepatitis B infection

Markers	Interpretation
HBsAg	Indicates presence of virus in body
HBeAg	Indicates active replication of virus
HBe antibody	Indicates seroconversion and non-replicative stage
IgM anti-HBc	Indicate recent infection or acute flare of chronic infection. Low levels in chronic infection
HBs antibody	Indicates immunity against the infection either manual or following the vaccine
HBV DNA quantitative	Indicates viral load

Viral Blood

HBV-DNA is measured by polymerase chain reaction in blood. Viral loads are in excess of 105 copies/mL in presence of active viral replication.

Other Investigations

- During early phase of hepatitis there is an increase in more than 400 units/L increase in plasma alanine aminotransferase and aspartate aminotransferase.
- High levels of alkaline phosphatase is suggestive of cholestasis.
- Prothrombin time is increased which indicates severe liver damage.
- **Hepatitis C**
  - Antibodies to HCV (anti-HCV)
    - Detection of antibodies to recombinant HCV polypeptides. Enzyme immunoassay measures antibodies against two antigens NS4 and NS3.
    - These assays can detect antibodies within 6 to 8 weeks of exposure.
    - Average time for seroconversion is 2 to 3 weeks
  - Recombinant immunoassay
  - Hepatitis C virus RNA testing qualitative test
  - Hepatitis C virus RNA testing quantitative test
  - HCV genotyping is helpful in predicting response to therapy.
- **Hepatitis D**
  - During Hepatitis D viral infection both IgM and IgG antibodies can be detected in serum in acute phase.
  - HDV infection can also be detected using reverse transcriptase polymerase chain reaction (RT-PCR)
- **Hepatitis E**
  - Identification of IgM antibodies to HEV from acute plasma serum samples. Antibodies detected are against ORF-2 and ORF-3

Management

- Only the more severely affected patients require care in hospital.
- Posthepatic syndrome is treated by reassurance.

Diet

- Nutritious diet containing 2000–3000 kcal daily is given.
- Light diet supplemented with glucose and food debris is acceptable.
- A good protein diet should be encouraged.
- In case of severe vomiting, IV fluids and glucose may be required.
- Highly fatty diet should be avoided however complete restriction of fatty diet is not required.

Drugs

- Drugs should be avoided, especially in severe hepatitis.
- Sedative and hypotonic drugs, alcohol, oral contraceptives should be especially avoided.

Surgery

During acute viral hepatitis surgery carries a significant role of postoperative liver failure. Only life saving operation should be carried.

Liver Transplantation

This may be required in acute or chronic liver failure due to hepatitis virus.

Prevention of Viral Hepatitis

Prophylaxis of only hepatitis A virus and hepatitis B virus is present, i.e., active immunization.

In active immunization recombinant hepatitis B vaccine which consists of HBsAg is available and produce active immunization in 95% of individuals.

Q.5. Mention the complication of viral hepatitis.

(Apr 2007, 5 Marks)

Ans.

Complications of Viral Hepatitis

- Acute hepatic failure: Fatalities are rare and usually occur in this case.
- Relapsing hepatitis: There is return of signs and symptom during recovery. It can be detected by clinical signs and biochemical tests. It resolves jaundice.
- Cholestasis: It can develop at any stage of illness and gives features of obstructive jaundice.
- Gillbert's syndrome: It may come into picture during viral hepatitis.
- Connective tissue disease, such as polyarteritis nodosa is observed in HBV and HCV infection.
- Renal failure, i.e., glomerulonephritis can occur also in relation to HBV and HCV infection.
- Henoch-Schönlein purpura and papular *acrodermatitis is repeated in children.
- Chronic hepatitis is observed with HBV infection with or without HDV and HCV viruses.
- Cirrhosis is also the complication of HBV and HCV and follows chronic hepatitis.
- *Hepatocellular carcinoma:* It is also the complication of HBV and HCV following cirrhosis of liver.

Q.6. Write short note on viral hepatitis.

(Aug 2012, 5 Marks)

Or

Discuss clinical features diagnosis, management and complications of viral hepatitis.

(Jan 2017, 12 Marks)

Ans. *Refer to Ans. 4 and Ans. 5 of same chapter.*

Q.7. Describe briefly viral hepatitis B.

(Dec 2015, 3 Marks) (Feb 2013, 5 Marks)

Or

Discuss mode of transmission and clinical features of hepatitis B infection. *(May 2018, 5 Marks)*

Ans. Hepatitis B is a virus which results in causing of disease known as hepatitis in man.

Route of Transmission or Etiology

- *Horizontal transmission*
  - By use of drug injection
  - By infected unscreened blood products
  - By tattooing and acupuncture needles
  - In sexually active individuals, i.e., either homosexuals or heterosexuals
- *Vertical transmission*
  - By HBsAg positive mother
  - High risk groups of HBV infection are patients of hemodialysis, physician, dentists, surgeons, paramedical staff and persons in laboratory and blood bank.

Clinical Features

The cases of hepatitis pass through three phases:

1. **Preicteric phase:**
   - Prodromal period of 4 to 7 days
   - Mild fatigue fever for 2 to 5 days
   - Anorexia, nausea and vomiting
   - Distaste for smoking
   - Abdominal distress
2. **Icteric phase:**
   - Jaundice on third or fourth days deepens or rapidly increases
   - Tea colored urine is present
   - Loss of weight
   - Stool becomes light in color
   - Spleen is palpable
3. **Posticteric phase:**
   - Jaundice recedes and all features come back to normal in 3 to 6 weeks
   - Appetite is good.
   - Stool and urine regain their natural color.

Investigations

Serology

- HBV consists of number of antigens. The three important antigens are hepatitis B surface antigen (HBsAg), core antigen (HBeAg) and hepatitis e antigen (HBeAg).
- Appearance of hepatitis B surface antigen (HBsAg) in serum is the first evidence of infection. It normally persists for 3–4 weeks but can persist up to 6 months. After disappearance of HBsAg, antibody against HBsAg (Anti-HBs) appears and persists for years and confers immunity. Presence of Anti-HBs antibody means either previous infection or vaccination.
- HBeAg is not seen in the blood. However, antibody to it (anti-HBc) appears early during the illness. Presence of IgM anti-HBc indicates acute infection and IgG anti-HBc suggests chronic infection (when HBsAg positive) or recovery (when anti-HBs positive).
- Presence of HBeAg indicates active viral replication and high degree of infectivity. Anti-HBe appears as HBeAg disappears and its presence suggests low level of viral replication and decreased infectivity.
- Above mentioned serological tests are done to identify the cause of hepatitis.

Viral Blood

HBV-DNA is measured by polymerase chain reaction in blood. Viral loads are in excess of 105 copies/mL in presence of active viral replication.

Q 5. *Acrodermatitis = Dermatitis of extremities

Other Investigations

- During early phase of hepatitis, there is an increase in more than 400 units/L increase in plasma alanine aminotransferase and aspartate aminotransferase.
- High levels of alkaline phosphatase is suggestive of cholestasis.
- Prothrombin time is increased which indicates severe liver damage.

Management

- **Supportive treatment:**
  This is given in acute hepatitis
  - Restrict the physical activity and bed rest is strictly recommended.
  - High calorie diet is given. Good protein intake should be there. Hospitalization and intravenous fluid (10% glucose) are indicated, if oral intake is not proper or there is marked nausea and vomiting.
  - Avoid the drugs which are hepatotoxic or those that are metabolized in the liver.
  - Bile salt sequestering agent (cholestyramine) decreases pruritus in cases with cholestasis.
  - Patients having features of severe hepatic failure, such as alteration in mental status (hepatic encephalopathy) and prolonged prothrombin time or bleeding time should be hospitalized.
  - No specific therapy is recommended for acute viral hepatitis except in acute HCV infection. Subcutaneous interferon alpha has been shown to reduce the rate of chronicity in acute HCV hepatitis.

- **Specific management:**
  It is done in case of chronic hepatitis B
  - Interferon inhibits the division of virus and antiviral drug lamivudine 100 mg OD is given.
  - Interferon is given in dose of 5 MU daily or 10 MU three times per week for 16 days.
  - Lamivudine is anti-DNA polymerase agent. It has shown significant improvement but when the drug is stopped HBV replication recurs and resistance to lamivudine is another problem.

Complication/Fate of HBV

Flowchart 4: Complication/Fate of HBV.

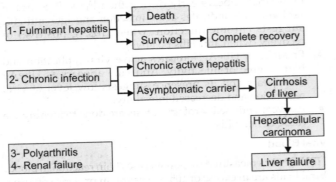

Q.8. Describe the causes, clinical features, complications and management in cases of cirrhosis of liver.
(Apr 2010, 15 Marks)

Or

Describe clinical features, etiology and management of cirrhosis of liver. *(Dec 2009, 15 Marks)*

Or

Write short note on clinical features and complications of cirrhosis of liver. *(Dec 2012, Marks)*

Or

Write short note on cirrhosis of liver.
(Dec 2015, 3 Marks) (Mar 2016, 3 Marks)

Or

Write etiology, clinical features, investigations and management of cirrhosis. *(July 2016, 12 Marks)*

Or

Write etiology, clinical features, diagnosis and management of liver cirrhosis. *(Aug 2018, 12 Marks)*

Or

Write in detail about cirrhosis of liver.
(Apr 2019, 5 Marks)

Ans. The term cirrhosis is applied to chronic diffuse liver disease of varied etiology and is characterized by hepatic cell necrosis, proliferation of connective tissue and nodular regeneration.

Causes of Cirrhosis of Liver

- *Common causes*
  Alcohol
  Viruses: Hepatitis B virus, hepatitis C virus.
- *Other causes*
  - Hepatic venous congestion
  - Veno-occlusive disease
  - Budd-Chairi syndrome
  - Wilson's disease
  - Galactosemia
  - Glycogen storage diseases
  - *Hemochromatosis
  - Drugs, such as isoniazid, oral contraceptives, etc.
  - Biliary cirrhosis (primary or secondary)
  - Autoimmune chronic active hepatitis

Clinical Features

- Hepatomegaly
- Jaundice
- Ascites
- Circulatory changes
- Spider angioma
- Palmar erythema
- Cyanosis
- Endocrine changes.
  - Loss of libido
  - Hair loss of chest.
    Men: Gynecomastia, testicular atrophy, impotence

Q 8. *Hemochromatosis = A hereditary disorder in which iron salts are deposited in the tissues, leading to liver damage, diabetes mellitus, and bronze discoloration of the skin.

Women: Breast atrophy, irregular menstrual cycle, amenorrhea
- *Hemorrhage tendency:* Bruises, purpura, epistaxis, menorrhagia
- *Portal hypertension:* Splenomegaly, collateral vessels, variceal bleeding
- Hepatic encephalopathy
- *Miscellaneous:* Pigmentation, clubbing, low grade fever.

Complications

- Posthepatic vein obstruction "Budd-Chiari syndrome" or extrahepatic and postsinusoidal.
- Intrahepatic postsinusoidal/cirrhosis
- Esophageal varices causes severe hemorrhage
- Development of hepatocellular failure due to hepatocellular carcinoma.
- Renal failure
- Hypersplenism
- Due to infection, spontaneous bacterial peritonitis and secondary bacterial peritonitis occur.

Investigations/Diagnosis

- Blood examination:
  - Anemia can be present secondary to bleeding, folate deficiency, marrow suppression or hypersplenism. Leukopenia and thrombocytopenia.
  - Aminotransferases (ALT, AST) get frequently elevated whereas a rise in the serum bilirubin and ALP may occur later. Serum albumin is low and Prothrombin time is frequently prolonged.
- Imaging: Ultrasonography is done to assess the liver size and texture, ascites, portal hypertension and splenomegaly.
- Endoscopy: Upper gastrointestinal endoscopy is being carried out to detect esophageal varices and to exclude other causes of upper gastrointestinal bleeding in the stomach and duodenum.
- *Liver biopsy:* It is done for the assessment of severity of the cirrhotic changes and also confirms the specific cause of the cirrhosis.

Management

No treatment can reverse cirrhosis or even ensure that no further progression occurs, but medical therapy can improve general health and treat the symptom of disease effectively.

The main objectives are:

- Detect treatable causes
- Prevent and correct malnutrition
- Manage chronic cholestasis
- Treat the complication.
  - *Treatable causes:* The treatable causes are alcohol abuse, drug ingestion, hemochromatosis and Wilson's disease, relief of biliary obstruction will prevent secondary biliary cirrhosis.
  - *Nutrition:* In absence of ascites, a high energy 3000 kcal/day, protein rich (80–100 g/day) diet should

be advised. Salt restriction is required if ascites are present. Fat intake is not restricted unless cholestasis is a feature. Complete absence of alcohol. Vitamin and other supplements are not required when good diet is taken.
- *Drug treatment:* Any drug should be avoided because as most of the drugs are metabolized in the liver which are liable to develop toxic reaction because they will unable to get metabolize.
- *Liver transplantation:* It is considered in all patients with chronic liver disease who develop liver failure.

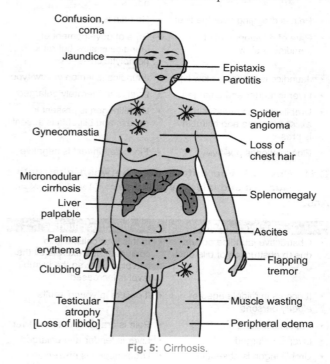

Fig. 5: Cirrhosis.

Q.9. Discuss management and etiopathogenesis of cirrhosis. *(Oct 2003, 16 Marks)*

Ans. *For management refers to Ans. 10 of same chapter.*

Etiopathogenesis

Hepatic cirrhosis can occur at any age and often causes prolong morbidity. Any condition leading to persistent or recurrent hepatocyte death may lead to hepatic cirrhosis, e.g., viral hepatitis and alcohol, prolonged biliary damage and obstruction as occur in primary biliary cirrhosis, sclerosing cholangitis and postsurgical biliary structures will also result in cirrhosis. Persistent blockages of venous return from liver, e.g., veno-occlusive disease and Budd-Chiari syndrome, will eventually result in liver cirrhosis.

Common to all cause of liver cirrhosis is activation of hepatic stellate cells. These cells are widely distributed throughout the liver in the space of disse. Following activation the fat storing stellate cells become transformed into multifunctional cells, and cytokine synthesis.

Q.10. Differentiate between hepatocellular jaundice and hemolytic jaundice. *(Feb 2006, 3 Marks)*

Ans.

Hepatocellular jaundice	Hemolytic jaundice
• In this liver cells fails to conjugate and excrete all the bile pigments, so the bilirubin level is increased	• There is excessive brake down of RBC due to which excess bilirubin is produced
• It occurs in young adults	• It occurs in infants and young adults
• Pain is dragging over the liver	• No pain is present
• Rate of development of jaundice is slow	• Rate of development of jaundice is slow but rapid in hemolytic crisis
• Jaundice is orange yellow type	• Jaundice is lemon yellow type
• Liver is tender and enlarged	• Liver is moderately enlarged
• Urobilinogen is present in excess in urine and bilirubin is present	• Urobilinogen is present in excess and bilirubin is absent
• Flocculation is positive	• Flocculation test is negative

Q.11. How will you differentiate between obstructive jaundice and infective jaundice? *(Apr 1999, 5 Marks)*

Ans.

Obstructive jaundice	Infective jaundice
• Obstructive jaundice occurs due to obstruction of bile duct	• In this liver cells fails to conjugate and excrete all the bile pigments, so the bilirubin level is increased
• It occurs in middle aged or elderly persons	• It occurs in young adults
• Pain is colicky	• Pain is dragging over the liver
• Liver is enlarged	• Liver is tender and enlarged
• Urobilinogen is absent in urine examination but bilirubin is present	• Urobilinogen is present in excess in urine and bilirubin is present
• Type of jaundice is greenish yellow	• Type of jaundice is orange yellow type
• Flocculation test is negative	• Flocculation test is positive

Q.12. Enumerate the causes of hepatomegaly.

(Dec 2010, 5 Marks) (Feb 2006, 2.5 Marks)

Ans.

Causes of Hepatomegaly

♦ Infections
  • Viral
    – Viral hepatitis
    – Yellow fever
    – Infectious mononucleosis
    – Lassa fever
  • Bacterial
    – Typhoid
    – Pneumonia
    – Brucellosis
    – Tuberculosis

  • Protozoal
    – Amoebiasis
    – Malaria
    – kala-azar
  • Spirochetal
    – Weil's disease
    – Syphilis
    – Relapsing fever
  • Parasitic
    – Schistosomiasis
    – *Echinococcus*
    – Clonorchiasis
  • Fungal
    – Actinomycosis
    – Histoplasmosis
♦ Metabolic
  • Fatty liver
  • Amyloid
  • Glycogen storage disease
♦ Congestive
  • General
    – Congestive heart failure
    – Tricuspid regurgitation
    – Constrictive pericarditis
  • Local
    – Portal hypertension (cirrhosis)
    – Hepatic vein thrombosis
♦ Tumors
  • Primary
    – Benign and malignant hepatoma
    – Benign and malignant cholangioma
    – Fibroma
    – Sarcoma
    – Hemangioma
  • *Secondary:* Direct due to spread by contiguity, or embolic metastatic
♦ Cysts
  • Hydatid
  • Polycystic
♦ Biliary obstruction
  • Gallstones
  • Strictures of bile ducts
♦ Hematological
  • Leukemias
  • Lymphoma
  • Myeloproliferative disorders
♦ Storage disorders
  • Gaucher's disease
  • Niemann-Pick's disease
  • Amyloidosis
  • Glycogen storage disease
  • Gargoylism,
  • Hemochromatosis
♦ Myeloid metaplasia
  • Secondary carcinoma of bone
  • Myelofibrosis
  • Myelosclerosis

- Multiple myeloma
- Marble-bone disease
♦ Genetic abnormalities: Sickle cell disease
♦ Congenital: Riedel's lobe

Q.13. Write short note on soft tender liver.

(Sep 2005, 5 Marks)

Ans. Soft tender liver is the clinical condition of the liver in which on palpitation the liver assumes to be soft and palpable.

Etiology

♦ Hydatid cyst
♦ Calcinosis cutis
♦ Nephritis and cerebellar ataxia
♦ Hypersensitivity reaction
♦ Oral contraceptives
♦ HIV
♦ Acute renal failure
♦ Obstructive jaundice
♦ Hepatocellular carcinoma
♦ Pleural and pericardial effusion
♦ Gallbladder injury.

Clinical Features

♦ Fever is present
♦ Hepatomegaly is present
♦ Muscle cramp/fatigue due to lactic acid accumulation
♦ Jaundice is seen
♦ Non-pitting edema is present
♦ Anorexia, ascites and anemia is present
♦ Amyloidosis is present.

Diagnosis

♦ MRI should be done
♦ USG is done
♦ X-ray of lower abdomen shows moderate enlargement of liver
♦ Lipid profile shows increase in lipid value.
♦ Blood picture reveals microcytic hypochromic anemia.

Treatment

♦ Treatment of cause is done
♦ No drug is given, only conservative treatment is done.
♦ Fluid diet is given, restriction of salt and fatty acids and spicy foods is done.
♦ Electrolyte balance is maintained with digestive enzymes.

Q.14. How history taking and investigation will help in finding the cause of the jaundice?

(Sep 2005, 18 Marks)

Ans. History taking of person mainly concerned with its illness, present past and family history which he describe to the doctor. Its basic aim is to arrive a diagnosis of disease and outline the treatment.

♦ History taking is an important clinical presentation which helps in the diagnosis and finding the etiology/cause of jaundice.

♦ In history taking, we are mainly concerned with the abdominal pain which patient undergoes like in hepatocellular jaundice patient will not feel abdominal colic while in obstructive and hemolytic jaundice patient feels sharp pain.

♦ The second point concerned in history taking with patient is pruritis, i.e., discoloration of skin. Pruritis is transient in hepatocellular jaundice. It is well, marked and is present in obstructive jaundice while it is fully absent in hemolytic jaundice.

♦ Last and most important point in history taking is past history of patient, such as patient can develop hepatocellular jaundice if he/she is in contact with jaundice patient before as well as certain drug can cause hepatocellular jaundice.

♦ A patient of obstructive jaundice will explain about pain, weight loss or any abdominal surgery before, which can give rise to the obstructive jaundice.

♦ A patient of hemolytic jaundice has a blood transfusion or certain drugs which can cause hemolytic jaundice which patient had taken in past.

Investigations

Investigation means laboratory diagnosis.

Investigation	Hepatocellular	Obstructive	Hemolytic
• Urine Bilirubin Urobilinogen	• Present • Present	• Present • Absent	• Absent • Present
• Stools Stercobilinogen	• Present	• Absent	Present
• Peripheral smear	• Leukopenia in infective hepatitis	• Normal	Reticulocytosis and spherocytosis
• Laboratory finding test - Bilirubin - Alkaline phosphate - SGOT	• + + • Raised • Markedly raised	• + + • Markedly raised • Raised	• + + • Normal • Normal
• Barium meal and cholangiography	Normal	May reveal pancreatic growth	Normal
• RBC survival	Normal	Normal	Decreased

Q.15. Write short note on liver function test.

(Mar 2007, 2 Marks)

Ans.

Liver Function Test

Serum Bilirubin

♦ The normal level is 1 mg/100 mL.
♦ It increases in:
  • Hepatocellular injury
  • Posthepatic biliary obstruction.

Thymol Turbidity Test

♦ Demonstrating hepatic cellular dysfunction
♦ Gamma globulins are mainly responsible for positivity in this test.

Enzyme in Liver Disease

♦ Alkaline phosphate:
  • Elevation occurs in obstructive jaundice.
  • Mild elevation in xanthomatous cirrhosis, hepatocellular injury, liver abscess.
♦ SGOT (serum glutamine oxalate transferase):
  • Normal level is 5 to 40 unit
  • It increases in all conditions leading to hepatic necrosis and in alcoholic liver damage.
♦ SGPT (serum glutamine pyruvic transferase)
  • It is more specific for liver disease.
  • It is raised in sever parenchymal damage to liver. For example, chronic acute hepatitis, alcoholic liver disease, biliary obstruction.
♦ GGT (gamma glutamyl transpeptidase): Sensitivity test for alcoholic liver disease and for hepatobiliary disease.
♦ Leucine aminopeptidase: It increases in primary liver diseases.
♦ Serum pseudocholinesterase:
  • It has limited value.
  • Value decreases in subacute and chronic parenchymal diseases of liver (Cirrhosis).

Q.16. Write short note on hepatitis B importance in dental practice.   *(Mar 2007, 2 Marks)*

Ans. Hepatitis may be defined as an infection of the liver caused by the hepatitis virus B.

The prevention for hepatitis will be:

♦ Prevention of mode of transmission:
  • Avoid infected blood transfusion, body organs, sperms and other tissues. Blood should be screened before transfusion.
  • Strict sterilization process should be ensured in clinics.
  • Presterilized needles and syringe should be used.
  • Avoid injections unless they are absolutely necessary.
  • Carrier should be told not to share razors or tooth brushes, use barrier methods of contraceptions, avoid blood donation.
♦ Hepatitis B vaccination should be given.

Q.17. Differentiate between hepatitis A and hepatitis B viral infection.   *(Mar 2008, 2 Marks)*

Ans.

Hepatitis A viral infection	Hepatitis B viral infection
• It spreads by feco-oral route	• It spreads by parental route
• Incubation period ranges from 15 days to 45 days	• Incubation period ranges from 6 weeks to 6 months
• Chronic infection is not present	• Chronic infection is present
• It is caused by enterovirus which is RNA virus	• It is caused by hepadna which is DNA virus
• For prevention passive immunity is given by immune serum globulin	• For prevention passive immunity is given by hyperimmune serum globulin

Q.18. Write short note on jaundice.
                    (Mar 2011, 4 Marks) (Sep 2009, 4 Marks)
                              Or
Write briefly on signs and symptoms and treatment of jaundice.   *(May/June 2009, 5 Marks)*
                              Or
Write short answer on jaundice.   *(Apr 2018, 3 Marks)*

Ans. Jaundice is a condition where there is yellow pigmentation of the skin or sclera by excess of bilirubin in the blood. When levels of bilirubin exceed 2 mg or above clinical jaundice become apparent.

Classification

♦ **Hemolytic:**
  • *Physiological*: Jaundice of prematurity
  • *Congenital*: Spherocytosis, sickle cell anemia
  • Parasitic destruction of erythocytes—malaria
  • Toxins—heavy metals
  • Poisons—snake venom
  • Drugs—sulfonamides, nitrofurantoin
  • Bacterial toxins— septicemia
  • Incompatible blood transfusions—ABO and Rh blood group incompatibility
  • Extensive burns.
♦ **Obstructive:**
  • *Extrahepatic:*
    – Obstruction within the bile ducts—gallstones, neoplasm, roundworm.
    – Obstruction due to changes in the wall of the ducts—congenital obstruction (biliary atresia), traumatic (following surgery), sclerosing cholangitis.
    – *Pressure from without:* Carcinoma of liver (primary/secondary) gumma, hydatid cyst, enlarged glands in porta hepatis (Hodgkin's, leukemia, tuberculosis) carcinoma head of pancreas, cancer stomach.
  • *Intrahepatic* (obstruction without mechanical cause):
    – Drugs, such as chlorpromazine, antitubercular drugs, methyl testosterone, oral contraceptives.
    – Viral hepatitis with prolonged cholestasis.
    – Jaundice of pregnancy
    – Primary biliary cirrhosis
    – *Hepatocellular:*
      » Viral hepatitis
      » Infectious mononucleosis
      » Yellow fever
      » Bacterial diseases with fever, typhoid
      » Malaria
      » Weil's disease
      » Chemicals, such as chloroform, halothane, trinitrotoluene, carbon tetrachloride.
      » Post-necrotic cirrhosis
      » Alcoholic hepatitis
      » Hemochromatosis.
    – Congenital hyperbilirubinemia
      » *Without liver pigment:*
        ▪ Gilbert's disease
        ▪ Crigler-Najjar syndrome.

» *With liver pigment:*
  ▪ Dubin-Johnson syndrome
  ▪ Rotor syndrome.

Symptoms

♦ Symptoms of a case of jaundice shall vary with the type of jaundice the patient is suffering from and the underlying condition.

♦ Most common form of jaundice is due to hepatitis where the patient may start with malaise, low grade fever, vomiting and loss of appetite.

♦ Person may take his/her morning breakfast normally and as the day passes, appetite for food almost disappears.

♦ In smokers, urge to smoke is the earliest to go. Yellowness appears first in the conjunctiva and then the mucous membrane of the lips and palate became pale.

♦ Urine is high colored while in early stage, the stools may remain of normal color.

♦ When a person has got features of obstructive jaundice, color of conjunctiva is yellowish green. Stools become clay colored and there is severe degree of itching.

♦ Pulse becomes slow.

♦ Patient may suffer from bruises and bleeding from mucous surfaces due to lack of fat soluble vitamin-K.

♦ If jaundice remains for prolonged periods as in case of malignancy patient suffers from marked asthenia and wasting.

Signs

♦ Patient may show signs of anemia, malnutrition suggestive of malignancy or cirrhosis.

♦ In cirrhotics look for spider naevi, white nails, enlargement of parotid glands, testicular atrophy, palmar erythema, gynecomastia, edema over legs and feet, and ascites.

♦ There may be scratch marks on skin suggestive of cholestasis due to obstructive jaundice, bruising and petechial spots indicating prothrombin deficiency in alcoholic or Laennec's cirrhosis may be observed.

♦ Liver may be palpable, smooth and tender in infective hepatitis, hard and nodular in malignancy.

♦ Gallbladder becomes palpable when obstruction at the level of common bile duct is incomplete. A hard, small nodular gall bladder may be palpated in carcinoma.

♦ In chronic cholecystitis, gallbladder may be palapable and tender (Murphy's sign). In addition to looking for signs of disease in general examination, look specifically in abdomen for ascites, liver, spleen and any lymphadenopathy.

♦ Rectal examination may be carried out for any primary growth in rectum.

Treatment

Treatment is directed towards the underlying cause:

♦ Patient should given small feeds of fat free, low protein and high carbohydrate diet which can be easily assimilated.

♦ Additionally Vitamin B and C are given orally in high dosages.

♦ In obstructive jaundice, vitamin K should be given 10 mg parentrally.

Q.19. Describe causes, clinical features and management of portal cirrhosis. *(Sep 2009, 4.5 Marks)*

Ans. It is characterized by the diffuse involvement of the liver in form of necrosis of liver cells, collapse of hepatic lobules, reticulin framework followed by diffuse fibrosis and formation of structurally abnormal nodules. This interferes not only with liver blood flow, but also its function. This results in portal cirrhosis which is due to inadequacy of liver cells and portal hypertension.

Causes

♦ Hepatitis B and D
♦ Consumption of excessive alcohol
♦ Hemochromatosis
♦ Alpha-1 antitrypsin deficiency
♦ Autoimmune chronic active hepatitis
♦ Wilson's disease
♦ Malaria
♦ Schistosomiasis
♦ Veno-occlusive disease
♦ Hepatic venous congestion to drugs, such as methyldopa, etc.

Clinical Features

Case of cirrhosis may present either in compensated or decompensated forms.

Compensated Form

♦ A compensated case of cirrhosis has features of dyspepsia in the form of morning anorexia, nausea, vomiting and vague ill-health. This is more so when it is early stage of alcoholic cirrhosis.

♦ There is palmar erythema, spider naevi, splenomegaly and hepatomegaly with a nontender liver.

♦ There is loss of weight, ill-health and edema of the ankles.

♦ There may be no firm signs of cirrhosis and diagnosis is made on clinical suspicion to be confirmed by biochemical investigations and liver biopsy.

♦ This stage of compensated form of cirrhosis may continue for a variable period of time ranging from months to years and bleed from esophageal varices may draw attention to the disease or some precipitating cause like severe bacteremia may produce hepatocellular decompensation.

Decompensated Form

♦ A decompensated cirrhosis is characterized by a downhill course, abdominal distension, ascites, weight loss, edema over the dependent parts, cirrhotic facies (sunken eyes, hollow cheeks, pinched nose), skin dry and sallow.

♦ Jaundice may appear indicating progressive liver cell destruction.

♦ Liver may be palpable with irregular surface or it may not be palpable when it is shrunken.

♦ Splenomegaly is present in 80% of patients. Nails are white and clubbed.

◆ Endocrinal changes in the form of spider nevi, palmar erythema, gynecomastia, loss of axillary and pubic hair, and testicular atrophy are seen. There may be bleeding spots or bruising due to prothrombin deficiency.

◆ Ascites may be massive and is disproportionate to the edema of feet.

◆ Hepatocellular failure may supervene as liver cell necrosis proceeds.

◆ Breath becomes foul smelling often giving a mousy smell (Fetor hepaticus).

◆ Flapping tremors and encephalopathy appear.

◆ Appearance of jaundice, rapid accumulation of ascites and development of hepatic encephalopathy are poor signs in cirrhosis.

Management

It is palliative:

◆ *Rest in bed:* To maximize treatment of any reversible element of underlying liver disease and to improve renal perfusion.

◆ *Correction of any etiological factor:*, i.e., stoppage of alcohol, stoppage of drugs causing portal cirrhosis.

◆ *Diet:* Low salt. Total daily intake of 2000 calories with protein intake of 120 g. If patient can tolerate it. Fats and carbohydrates in normal amount. Vitamin B complex.

◆ *Symptomatic treatment:*
  • For anemia vitamin B12 and folic acid is given
  • For restlessness sedatives, such as lorazepam should be given
  • For ascites low sodium diet and diuretics should be given.

Q.20. Write management of Amoebic liver abscess.
(Mar 2011, 4 Marks)

Ans.

Management of Amoebic Liver Abscess

Injection dehydroemetine 60 mg IM daily for 6 days.

Tablet Tinidazole 600 mg TDS for 7 days.

Tablet Chloroquine 500 mg TDS for 11 days.

If Amoebic liver abscess is large:

◆ The abscess should be aspirated and all fluid pus, etc., will be removed.

◆ Open drainage of pus may be undertaken if there is large amount of pus secondarily infected or if there are signs of pus, but aspiration is negative.

◆ Depending on the patient's response aspiration of abscess may be carried out.

Q.21. Describe the etiology, diagnostic criterias and management of viral hepatitis. *(Apr 2008, 15 Marks)*

Ans. Viral hepatitis is a clinical entity where systemic infection causes inflammation and hepatic cell necrosis.

Etiology

Hepatitis A,B,C,D,E, cytomegalovirus, herpes simplex virus, Epstein-barr virus and yellow fever virus.

Diagnostic Criterias

Diagnosis is based on investigations. Following are the investigation which confirm the diagnosis of viral hepatitis

Investigations

◆ **Hepatitis A:**
  • Nonspecific lab tests
    − Raised serum bilirubin within few days and remain high up to 12 weeks.
    − Serum AST and ALT levels remain high for 1 to 3 weeks.
    − Alkaline phosphatase level is mildly elevated, though it remains persistently high, it suggest hepatitis associated cholestasis.
  • Specific test
    − Hepatitis A specific IgM antibody can be detected at the onset of symptoms and at first rise in serum ALT. It peaks within first month and remain positive for 3 to 6 months.
    − IgG and hepatitis A virus become positive at onset of illness and is detectable for many years
    − Nucleic acid based test like PCR.

◆ **Hepatitis B:**
In a patient with history of severe anorexia, nausea, vomiting, fever for few days, elevated serum bilirubin and value of SGPT over 500 indicates HBV. The etiological agent is identified by serological markers.

Serological diagnosis of hepatitis B:

Stage of infection	HBsAg	Anti-HBc		Anti-HBs
		IgM	IgG	
Incubation	Positive	Positive	Negative	Negative
Acute hepatitis B				
Early	Positive	Positive	Negative	Negative
Late or established	Positive	Positive	Positive	Negative
Convalescence				
3–6 months	Negative	Positive or negative	Positive	Positive or negative
6–9 months	Negative	Negative	Positive	Positive
Post-infection				
More than 1 year	Negative	Negative	Positive	Positive
Chronic infection	Positive	--------	Positive	Negative
Immunization without exposure to infection	Negative	Negative	Negative	Positive

Markers	Interpretation
HBsAg	Indicates presence of virus in body
HBeAg	Indicates active replication of virus
HBe antibody	Indicates seroconversion and non-replicative stage
IgM anti-HBc	Indicate recent infection or acute flare of chronic infection. Low levels in chronic infection
HBs antibody	Indicates immunity against the infection either manual or following the vaccine
HBV DNA quantitative	Indicates viral load

♦ **Hepatitis C**
  • Antibodies to HCV (anti-HCV)
    – Detection of antibodies to recombinant HCV poly-peptides. Enzyme immunoassay measures antibodies against two antigens NS4 and NS3.
    – These assays can detect antibodies within 6 to 8 weeks of exposure.
    – Average time for seroconversion is 2 to 3 weeks
  • Recombinant immunoassay
  • Hepatitis C virus RNA testing qualitative test
  • Hepatitis C virus RNA testing quantitative test
  • HCV genotyping is helpful in predicting response to therapy.
♦ **Hepatitis D**
  • During Hepatitis D viral infection both IgM and IgG antibodies can be detected in serum in acute phase.
  • HDV infection can also be detected using reverse transcriptase Polymerase chain reaction (RT-PCR)
♦ **Hepatitis E:**
  • Identification of IgM antibodies to HEV from acute plasma serum samples. Antibodies detected are against ORF-2 and ORF-3
  • Peak titers for IgM are observed during first 4 weeks while onset of infection. A rising titer of IgG antibody is also diagnostic of infection.
    For management of viral hepatitis refer to Ans. 6 of same chapter.

Q.22. Write in brief the signs, symptoms and treatment of ascites.   *(Apr 2008, 5 Marks)*

Ans. Ascites is the accumulation of free fluid in the peritoneal cavity.

Symptoms

♦ Patient has sudden abdominal pain and fever may also be present.
♦ Edema over ankles and feet.
♦ Skin over abdomen is stretched.

Sign

♦ Bulging of abdomen and in flanks is present.
♦ Umbilicus is transversely stretched or everted.
♦ Presence of fluid thrill and shifting dullness.
♦ Increase in inferior vena cava pressure.

♦ Diaphragm may be pushed upwards and there can be respiratory distress.
♦ Pleural effusion on right side can be present.
♦ Urinary output is reduced.

Treatment

♦ In every case of ascites oral diuretics, i.e., furosemide 40 to 80 mg + spironolactone 25 to 100 mg is administered.
♦ Sodium intake is restricted and diet which is low in sodium is given.
♦ In case of massive ascites which produce cardiorespiratory enlargement, abdominal paracentesis is done and fluid is drained slowly. Fluid should not be drained quickly because it causes vasovagal attack.

Q.23. Write short note on fulminant hepatic failure.
    (Dec 2010, 5 Marks)

Ans. Fulminant hepatic failure is seen in a healthy person which develop acute hepatitis and goes into hepatic encephalopathy within the 8 weeks of illness.

Etiology

♦ Acute viral hepatitis
♦ Drugs—all hepatotoxic drugs
♦ Pregnancy with hepatitis
♦ Wilson's disease
♦ Due to Reye's syndrome.

Clinical Features

♦ *Cerebral features:* Poor alertness, slurred speech, drowsiness, confusion, disorientation, convulsion and coma.
♦ Jaundice is present.
♦ Fetor hepaticus
♦ Flapping tremors are present.
♦ Signs of portal hypertension are present, i.e., ascites, edema.
♦ Cerebral edema is present.

Investigations

♦ Bilirubin levels are high
♦ Serum transaminase levels are high
♦ Prothrombin time is prolonged
♦ Urine may contain urobilinogen and bilirubin
♦ Serum ammonia levels are high
♦ USG of liver shows reduced liver size.

Treatment

♦ Phenobarbitone or 5 mg IV diazepam is given to patient.
♦ Care of pulse, blood pressure, bowel and bladder is taken.
♦ 5 to 10% of glucose drip IV is given.
♦ IV vitamin K is given 10 mg for 3 days.
♦ IV vitamin C is given 500 mg daily for prevention of bleeding.
♦ IV ranitidine is given 50 mg twice daily.
♦ Encephalopathy is treated by with drawl of protein intake; Sterilization of gut by neomycin 1 g orally for 6 hours; increased fecal output of nitrogen by changing bacterial

flora with lactulose 30 to 60 mL orally after 2–3 hours till loose stool is produced.

♦ Infections should be treated with amoxicillin or ceftizoxime.

Q.24. Enumerate the causes of cirrhosis liver.

(Aug 2012, 5 Marks)

Ans.

Causes of Cirrhosis of Liver

♦ Viral hepatitis B and C
♦ Alcohol
♦ Cryptogenic
♦ *Metabolic:*
  • Hemochromatosis
  • Wilson's disease
  • $\alpha1$—antitrypsin deficiency
  • Cystic fibrosis
  • Glycogen storage disease
  • Galactosemia
♦ *Biliary obstruction:*
  • Primary biliary cirrhosis
  • Sclerosing cholangitis
  • Secondary biliary cirrhosis
♦ *Venous outflow obstruction:*
  • Budd-Chiari syndrome
  • Veno-occlusive disease
  • Congestive heart failure
♦ *Drugs:*
  • Methotrexate
  • Methyldopa
  • Oxyphenisatin
  • Amiodarone
♦ *Indian childhood cirrhosis.*

Q.25. Write short note on high-risk groups and prophylaxis of hepatitis B. *(Feb 2014, 3 Marks)*

Ans.

High-risk Groups of Hepatitis B

The hepatitis B virus can infect infants, children, teens and adults. Although everyone can be at some risk for a hepatitis B infection, there are people who are at greater risk because of their ethnic background, occupation, or lifestyle choices.

The following list is a guide for screening high-risk groups, but it certainly does not represent all potential risk factors.

♦ Healthcare providers and emergency responders
♦ Sexually active heterosexuals (more than 1 partner in the past six months)
♦ Men who have sex with men (Homosexuals)
♦ Individuals diagnosed with a sexually transmitted disease (STD)
♦ Illicit drug users (injecting, inhaling, snorting, pill popping)
♦ Sex contacts or close household members of an infected person
♦ Children adopted from countries where hepatitis B is common (Asia, Africa, South America, Pacific Islands, Eastern Europe, and the Middle East)

♦ All pregnant women
♦ Recipients of a blood transfusion before 1992
♦ Kidney dialysis patients and those in early renal failure
♦ Inmates of a correctional facility
♦ Staff and clients of institutions for the developmentally disabled
♦ Any individual who may have other risk factors not included on this list.

Prophylaxis of Hepatitis B

♦ Recombinant hepatitis B vaccine having HBsAg capable of producing active immunization.
♦ Usually three injections of vaccine should be given IM during current, first and sixth month. These vaccinations provide 90% of prophylaxis from hepatitis B virus.
♦ If patient is immunocompromised larger doses of vaccination should be given.
♦ Passive immunization is provided by IM injection of hyperimmune serum globulins which is given within 24 hours or almost within a week of exposure to infected blood.
♦ Active along with passive immunization is provided to the paramedicos who has undergone needle stick injury, to newborn babies of hepatitis B positive mothers and to regular sexual partner of hepatitis B positive patient. Dosage is 500 IU for adults and 200 IU for babies.

Precautions to be taken for Prevention from Hepatitis B

♦ Avoid infected blood transfusion, body organs, sperms and other tissues. Blood should be screened before transfusion.
♦ Strict sterilization process should be ensured in clinics.
♦ Presterilized needles and syringe should be used.
♦ Avoid injections unless they are absolutely necessary.
♦ Carrier should be told not to share razors or tooth brushes, use barrier methods of contraceptions, avoid blood donation.

Q.26. Write short note on causes and investigations of ascites. *(Feb 2014, 3 Marks)*

Ans.

Causes of Ascites

♦ Disease of peritoneum
  • Infections:
    – Tuberculous peritonitis.
    – Spontaneous bacterial peritonitis.
    – *Fungal:* Candida, histoplasma.
    – *Parasitic:* Schistosoma, enterobius.
    – *Viral:* Acute severe hepatitis.
  • *Neoplasms:*
    – Primary mesothelioma.
    – Secondary carcinomatosis, e.g., adenocarcinoma, sarcoma, teratoma, leukemia, Hodgkin's disease, lymphocytic lymphoma, myeloid metaplasia.
    – Pseudomyxoma peritonei
  • Familial paroxysmal peritonitis
  • *Miscellaneous:*
    – Vasculitis — SLE and other collagen vascular diseases, allergic vasculitis (Henoch-Schönlein purpura).

- Eosinophilic gastroenteritis.
- Whipple's disease.
- Granulomatous peritonitis — Sarcoidosis, Crohn's disease, starch peritonitis.
- Peritoneal loose bodies.
- Peritoneal encapsulation.
♦ Portal hypertension
♦ Congestive heart failure
♦ *Hypoalbuminemia:*
  • Nephrosis
  • Malnutrition
  • Protein-losing enteropathy
♦ Beriberi
♦ Myxedema
♦ *Ovarian disease:*
  • Meigs'syndrorne
  • Struma ovari
  • Ovarian overstimulation syndrome
♦ Pancreatic ascites due to retroperitoneal leakage of pancreatic enzymes from a ruptured cyst or pancreatic duct.
♦ Bile ascites
♦ Chylous ascites
♦ Epidemic dropsy

Investigations

♦ *Blood examination*: Anemia can be present. Presence of neutrophilic leukocytosis indicates infection.
♦ *Urine examination*: Massive albuminuria greater than 3.5 g per day is present in nephritic syndrome.
♦ *Stool for occult blood*: It may indicate gastrointestinal malignancy as cause for ascites.
♦ *Ultrasonography*: It detect ascites
♦ *Diagnostic paracentesis*: 50–100 mL of ascetic fluid is aspirated and biochemical analysis is done. Bacteriological examination should also be done. It should detect whether the ascetic fluid is exudate or transudate.
♦ *Serum-ascites albumin gradient*: Albumin present in serum and ascetic fluid is determined for calculating the gradient. Gradient >1.1 g/dL indicates transudative ascites and <1.1 g/dL indicate exudative ascites. Fluid protein <50% of serum protein indicates transudate while >50% is indicative of exudates.

Q.27. Describe clinical features of portal hypertension. How will you investigate and manage a case of cirrhosis of liver. *(Feb 2014, 8 Marks)*

Ans.

Clinical Features of Portal Hypertension

♦ Splenomegaly: Spleen gets enlarged to the size of 5–6 cm.
♦ Hypersplenism: It is common leading to anemia, thrombocytopenia and leukemia. Pancytopenia can also occur.
♦ Collateral vessels form at gastroesophageal junction which may rupture leading to hematemesis or malena.
♦ Ascites is present.
♦ Caput-medusae is seen around umbilicus and at times large umbilical collateral give rise to venous hum.

♦ Fetor hepaticus results from shunting of portal blood. In fetor hepaticus foul smell from breadth is present due to mercaptans.

Investigation of Case of Cirrhosis of Liver

I. **Assessment of severity of cirrhosis of liver:**
  A. *Liver biochemistry:*
    - It may be normal in compensated cirrhosis.
    - SGOT/SGPT reflect the activity of the disease, which is low when cirrhosis is established, but increased in evolution of cirrhosis due to autoimmune hepatitis.
    - Alkaline phosphatase and transaminases may be slightly raised in decompensated cirrhosis.
    - Serum albumin reflects liver cell function, its low level indicates cirrhosis.
    - Plasma bilirubin is normal in most of the cases but it gets increased in decompensated cirrhosis.
    - Low albumin, i.e., <2.5 g/L and rising bilirubin are signs of progressive liver damage and these constitute bad prognostic signs.
  B. *Hematology:*
    - Anemia, leukopenia and thrombocytopenia or pancytopenia may be seen in cirrhosis.
    - Increased prothrombin time is a bad prognostic sign.
  C. *Ascitic fluid examination:* Ascites is transudate in nature.

II. **Assessment of type or cause of cirrhosis of liver:**
  A. *Blood biochemistry*
    - Viral markers, i.e., HbSAg are of value in identification.
    - Serum autoantibodies, antinuclear, anti-smooth muscle and anti-mitochondrial antibodies level increase in cryptogenic cirrhosis and biliary cirrhosis.
    - Rise in alkaline phosphatase indicates biliary cirrhosis.
    - *Serum immunoglobins:* The IgG is increased in autoimmune hepatitis, IgA increases in alcoholic cirrhosis and IgM in primary biliary cirrhosis.
  B. *Imaging*
    - *Ultrasound examination:* USG reveals changes in size, shape and echotexture of the liver. Fatty change and fibrosis produce diffuse increases echogenicity. Presence of ascites, varices portal vein diameter and enlarge in size of spleen can be determined on ultrasound.
    - Barium meal swallow is done for esophageal varices.
    - Endoscopy can be done for detection and for treatment of varices
  C. *Liver biopsy:*
    It is also necessary to confirm the diagnosis of cirrhosis.

Management of Case of Cirrhosis of Liver

No treatment can reverse cirrhosis or even ensure that no further progression occurs, but medical therapy can improve general health and treat the symptom of disease effectively.

The Main Objectives

♦ Detect treatable causes
♦ Prevent and correct malnutrition

- Manage chronic cholestasis
- Treat the complication.
  - *Treatable causes:* The treatable causes are alcohol abuse, drug ingestion, *hemochromatosis and Wilson's disease, relief of biliary obstruction will prevent secondary biliary cirrhosis.
  - *Nutrition:* In absence of ascites, a high energy 3000 kcal/day, protein rich (80–100 g/day) diet should be advised. Salt restriction is strictly required if ascites are present. Fat intake is not restricted unless cholestasis is a feature. Complete absence of alcohol. Vitamin and other supplements are not required when good diet is taken.
  - *Drug treatment:* Any drug should be avoided because as most of the drugs are metabolized in the liver which are liable to develop toxic reaction because they will unable to get metabolize.
  - *Liver transplantation:* It is considered in all patients with chronic liver disease who develop liver failure.

Q.28. Describe hepatitis-B under following headings.

(Nov 2014, 2+2+2+2 Marks)

  a. Etiology
  b. Clinical features
  c. Diagnosis
  d. Prophylaxis

Ans. *For etiology and clinical features refer to Ans. 7 of same chapter. For prophylaxis refer to Ans. 25 of same chapter.*

Diagnosis
Serology

- HBV consists of number of antigens. The three important antigens are hepatitis B surface antigen (HBsAg), core antigen (HBeAg) and hepatitis e antigen (HBeAg).
- Appearance of hepatitis B surface antigen (HBsAg) in serum is the first evidence of infection. It normally persists for 3–4 weeks, but can persist up to 6 months. After disappearance of HBsAg, antibody against HBsAg (anti-HBs) appears and persists for years and confers immunity. Presence of anti-HBs antibody means either previous infection or vaccination.
- HBeAg is not seen in the blood. However, antibody to it (anti-HBc) appears early during the illness. Presence of IgM anti-HBc indicates acute infection and IgG anti-HBc suggests chronic infection (when HBsAg positive) or recovery (when anti-HBs positive).
- Presence of HBeAg indicates active viral replication and high degree of infectivity. Anti-HBe appears as HBeAg disappears and its presence suggests low level of viral replication and decreased infectivity. Above mentioned serological tests are done to identify the cause of hepatitis.

Viral Blood

HBV–DNA is measured by polymerase chain reaction in blood. Viral loads are in excess of 105 copies/mL in presence of active viral replication.

Other Investigations

- During early phase of hepatitis, there is an increase in more than 400 units/L increase in plasma Alanine aminotransferase and aspartate aminotransferase.
- High levels of alkaline phosphatase are suggestive of cholestasis.
- Prothrombin time is increased which indicates severe liver damage.

Q.29. Write short answer on universal precautions for a dentist working on a hepatitis B positive patient.

(Sep 2018, 3 Marks)

Ans.

Universal Precautions for a Dentist Working on a Hepatitis B Positive Patient

- Wear safety spectacles to protect eyes.
- Water proof gown to protect front and arms.
- Full boots to protect the feet
- Wear double pair of gloves
- Keep minimum surgical assistants
- Sharp instruments should be passed from scrub nurse to surgeon in a kidney tray to avoid injury.
- Put used needles in puncture resistant container and never try to replace them back in protective sheath.
- Minimize aerosol production during surgery by not using ultrasonic instrumentation, air syringe or high speed hand pieces.
- When the procedure is complete all instruments should be scrubbed and sterilized. Disposable items should be preferred as they can dispose after procedure.
- All the working surfaces should be wiped with 2% activated glutaraldehyde (cidex).

Q.30. Write long answer on etiology, sign and symptoms of acute and chronic hepatitis.   *(Sep 2018, 5 Marks)*

Ans.

Acute Hepatitis

It is an acute parenchymal disease of liver which evolve within hours, days to few weeks is known as acute hepatitis.

Etiology

Etiology of acute hepatitis can be infective or non-infective.

Infective

- Viral: Hepatitis A,B,C,D,E, cytomegalovirus, herpes simplex virus, yellow fever virus and Epstein barr virus.
- Post-viral: It is Reye's syndrome which occur in children
- Non-viral: *Toxoplasma*, *Coxiella* and Leptospira

Non-Infective

- Drugs: The drugs are halothane, paracetamol, isoniazid, rifampicin, chlorpromazine and methyldopa.
- Poisons: aflatoxin and carbon tetrachloride
- Metabolic: Pregnancy and Wilson's disease
- Vascular: Shock, oral contraceptives, Budd–Chiari syndrome

Q 27. *Hemochromatosis = A hereditary disorder in which iron salts are deposited in the tissues, leading to liver damage, diabetes mellitus, and bronze discoloration of the skin.

Sign and Symptoms

Symptoms

It is divided into following phases:

1. **Prodromal phase**
   - Development of jaundice is preceded by a prodromal phase during which nonspecific systemic symptoms, such as anorexia, nausea, vomiting, headache, fatigue, malaise, myalgia and arthralgia can occur.
   - Presence of low grade fever

2. **Icteric phase**
   - Prodromal symptoms diminish due to onset of clinical jaundice. Patient can complain about dark urine and yellow discoloration of eyes and skin. Clay colored stool and pruritus is suggestive of cholestasis.
   - Many of the patients can never enter this phase.

3. **Recovery phase**
   - It is followed by an improvement in general symptoms and diminution of jaundice.
   - Complete clinical and biochemistry recovery occur under 3 to 4 months in majority of patients with hepatitis B.

Signs

- Presence of the yellow sclera
- Because of pruritus scratch marks are seen on skin
- Tender hepatomegaly with splenomegaly is seen in 50% of cases and lymphadenopathy in 20% of cases.

Chronic Hepatitis

It is defined as any hepatitis which lasts for 6 months or more.

Etiology

- **Infective:** Due to Hepatitis B, C and D
- **Toxic causes**
  - Drugs, such as isoniazid and alpha methyldopa
  - Alcoholic steatohepatitis and non-alcoholic steato-hepatitis
- **Metabolic causes:** Hemochromatosis, Wilson's disease, α1-anti-trypsin deficiency.
- **Unknown cause:** Autoimmune hepatitis.

Sign and Symptoms

Causes of chronic hepatitis	Symptoms	Signs
Hepatitis B	• Ill health • Fatigue • Weakness • Right upper quadrant pain • Redness of palms • Poor appetite • Low grade fever	• Tender hepatomegaly • Splenomegaly • Jaundice may be mild or absent • Spider telangiectasia • Ascites

Contd…

Contd…

Causes of chronic hepatitis	Symptoms	Signs
Hepatitis C	• Malaise • Fatigue • Ill health • Poor appetite • Faulty food intolerance • Upper abdominal pain over liver	• Slight hepatomegaly

Chronic autoimmune hepatitis	Two groups are present i.e.
	1. *Menopausal group:* Either they remain asymptomatic or can have mild fatigue.
	2. *Teenage group:*
	  - Fatigue
	  - Anorexia
	  - Fever
	  - Arthralgia
	  - Epistaxis
	  - Amenorrhea
		• Presence of mild-to-moderate jaundice with other signs of chronic liver disease mainly hepatosplenomegaly.
		• Spider telangiectasia
		• Cushingoid face with acne, hirsutism, pink striae and bruises can be seen.
		• Polyarthritis, glomerulonephritis, pleurisy, hemolytic anemia, thyroiditis and Sicca syndrome

Q.31. Write short answer on chronic hepatitis.

(Apr 2019, 3 Marks)

Or

Write long answer on clinical features and management of chronic hepatitis. *(Oct 2019, 6 Marks)*

Ans. It is defined as any hepatitis which lasts for 6 months or more.

Etiology

For details refer to Ans. 30 of same chapter.

Clinical Features

For details refer to heading sign and symptoms of Ans. 30 of same chapter.

Investigations

In Chronic Hepatitis B

- SGOT and SGPT show moderate increase in serum bilirubin and transaminase.
- In advanced disease hypoalbuminemia is present.
- Mild hyperglobulinemia is also seen.
- Viral markers of hepatitis B, i.e., HbsAg, HBV DNA and HbcAg are seen in serum unless mutant virus is seen.
- Liver biopsy confirms the diagnosis. On H & E examination HbsAg is seen as ground glass appearance inside the cytoplasm of hepatocytes and this is confirmed by histochemical staining.
- In immunohistochemistry staining HbcAg is seen.

In Chronic Hepatitis C

♦ Serum bilirubin is normal or can be slightly raised.
♦ SGOT and SGPT are abnormal and provide the clue to diagnosis.
♦ Plasma albumins and globulins are normal.
♦ ELISA test: Show HCV antibody in serum.
♦ Polymerase chain reaction test: It shows HCV-RNA antibody.

In Chronic Autoimmune Hepatitis

♦ Raised serum bilirubin, globulin and transaminases.
♦ Antibodies, i.e., antinuclear, antismooth muscle and antimitochondrial are seen in high titer.
♦ Liver biopsy shows changes of chronic active hepatitis.

Management

In Chronic Hepatitis B

♦ Patients having active viral replication and HBV DNA more than 105 copies/mL or more than 20,000 IVI positive in serum with elevated aminotransferase levels can be treated by nucleoside or nucleotide analogue or by pegylated interferon – α 2a (180 μg per week for 48 hours) or recombinant human interferon α (5 millions daily or 10 million units three times a week IM for 4 to 6 weeks.
♦ Nucleoside analogue, such as entecavir 0.5 mg orally is more effective. It can be given 1 mg in patients who are resistant to lamivudine.
♦ Lamivudine 100 mg orally daily suppresses HBV DNA in serum and improve liver histology in 60% of patients and normalize enzyme levels in 40% of cases after one year of administration.
♦ Due to mutation in polymerase gene 15 to 30% of cases relapse on lamivudine treatment due to mutation in polymerase gene. In these cases Tenofovir or Adefovir 10 mg daily for 1 year should be given.

In Chronic Hepatitis C

Here main aim of the treatment is to eliminate HCV RNA to stop the progression of active liver disease to prevent development of cirrhosis and hepatocellular carcinoma.

Recent treatment is combination of peginterferon, i.e., α2a 180 μg/week or α2b 1.5 μg/kg/week SC along with Ribavirin 1000 to 1200 mg/day for genotype 1 and 1800 mg/day for genotype 2 and 3. This is given in divided doses for a year for genotype 1 and 6 months for the other genotypes. The drug should not be taken in pregnancy.

In Chronic Autoimmune (Lupoid) Hepatitis

♦ Prednisolone should be given 30 mg/day orally for 14 days which is followed by maintenance dose of 10 to 15 mg/day along with azathioprine 1 to 2 mg/kg/day for 2 years.
♦ Various other drugs, such as cyclosporine, tacrolimus and mycophenolate are tried in the resistant cases.
♦ In drug treatment failures and in patients with fulminant hepatitis liver transplantation can be done.

Q.32. Write short note on clinical features and management of portal hypertension.   *(Jan 2019, 7 Marks)*

Ans. Portal hypertension is defined as the pathologic increase in portal pressure above the upper limit of 5 mm Hg.

For clinical features of portal hypertension refer to Ans. 27 of same chapter.

Management of Portal Hypertension

♦ Identify the underlying cause and start treating it.
♦ Treatment of variceal bleeding:
  1. **Local measures:**
     a. *Sclerotherapy:* Sclerosing agents, such as sodium tetradecyl sulfate and 3% phenol in water are injected via upper GI endoscopy, around varices. It obliterates the blood vessels and stop bleeding. If bleeding recur it can be repeated. If active bleeding persists, before giving sclerotherapy, first bleeding should be controlled by balloon tamponade.
     b. *Banding:* Here variceal bleeding is stopped where varices are sucked into an endoscope accessory, which allow them to occlude with tight rubber band. Occluded vari subsequently sloughs with variceal obliteration. In acute bleeding it is less easy to apply.
     c. *Balloon tamponade:* Sengstaken–Blakemore tube is used here which posses two balloons and exert pressure in lower esophagus as well as fundus of stomach. Tube is passed via the mouth and its presence on the stomach is checked by auscultating over upper abdomen while injecting air in stomach. Provide gentle traction to maintain pressure on varices. Only gastric balloon is inflated which control the bleeding. If esophageal balloon is also inflated, it is important to deflate it for 10 minute in every 3 hours to prevent esophageal mucosal damage.
     d. *Shunt surgery:* Portacaval shunts show promising results. But here chances of hepatic encephalopathy are high and death occurs from liver failure. So, it is only used when other measures fail and done in patients with good liver functions.
  2. **Drugs:**
     a. *Vasopressin:* IV infusion is given, 0.4 units/min till bleeding stops or for 24 hours and then 0.2 units/min for further 24 hours. Since, it can cause angina, myocardial infarction and arrhythmias nitroglycerine transdermally or IV is given. ECG monitoring should go on.
     b. *Somatostatin or Octreotide:* It is the drug of choice. It should be given 50 μg IV followed by infusion of 50 μg hourly.
     c. *Terlipressin:* It is given 2 mg IV every 6 hourly till bleeding stops and then 1 mg IV for further 24 hours.
  3. **Prophylaxis:** In cases with variceal bleeding, recurrent bleeding is common which is stopped by sclerotherapy, banding, drugs, such as beta blockers or nitrates.

Propranolol 80 to 160 mg/day decreases portal venous pressure.

4. Transjugular intrahepatic portal shunt is used in patients who wait for liver transplant.

5. Liver transplant.

♦ Treatment of enlarged spleen: Splenectomy and shunt surgery is done.

♦ Treatment of ascites:

1. Salt restricted diet with diuretics, such as spironolactone and furosemide

2. Massive ascites require therapeutic tapping.

4. DISEASES OF CARDIOVASCULAR SYSTEM

Q.1. Write short note on **acute rheumatic fever.**

(Apr 2007, 5 Marks)

Or

Describe in brief about rheumatic fever.

(Dec 2015, 4 Marks)

Or

Write short answer on rheumatic fever.

(May 2018, 3 Marks)

Ans. It is an acute inflammatory disease which occurs due to infection by group A hemolytic streptococci which involves heart, joint, skin and nervous system which develops as autoimmune reaction to infecting organism.

Etiology

♦ *Predisposing causes:*
Age should be 5 to 15 years.
Sex has equal incidence

♦ *Genetic factors*: Family incidence known.

♦ *Social and economic factors*: Dampness, overcrowding and under nutrition increases incidence.

♦ Idiosyncrasy is presumably a factor since 3% of people are involved in streptococcal epidemics develop rheumatic fever.

Clinical Manifestations

♦ *Prodromal phase*: Tonsillitis or sore throat 1 to 4 weeks prior to onset of acute rheumatic fever. Besides this anorexia, pallor, fatigability and nervous irritability is present.

♦ *Latent phase*: When antibodies to preceding streptococcal infection are produced.

♦ Phase of onset of rheumatic fever/mode of onset.
Arthritis and fever 2–3 weeks after infection.

♦ Cardiac symptoms 3–6 weeks after infection is first to draw attention.

♦ *Abdominal symptoms*: Abdominal pain and tenderness, nausea, vomiting, fever and leukocytosis.

♦ Pyrexia of unknown origin

♦ Typhoid or influenzal mode of onset with fever

♦ Nodules of skin lesion.

Treatment of Acute Rheumatic Fever

♦ Bed rest is important to reduce joint pain and cardiac workload. Duration of bed rest is guided by markers of inflammation like temperature, WBC count and ESR.

♦ Benzathine penicillin 1.2 μ IM 4 hourly. If patient is allergic to penicillin, erythromycin 40–50 mg/kg for ten days is given.

♦ Aspirin usually relieves symptom of arthritis rapidly. A starting dose of 60 mg/kg body weight per day is given divided into 6 doses. The dose may be increased to 120 mg/kg body weight. This dose may produce severe symptoms like vomiting, tachypnea and acidosis. Aspirin is given till ESR comes to normal.

♦ Corticosteroids like prednisolone produces rapid symptomatic relief than aspirin and is indicated in cases with severe arthritis or carditis. Prednisolone is given in doses of 1.2 mg/kg body weight till ESR comes to normal.

Q.2. Outline the management of **acute rheumatic fever.**

(Mar 2009, 5 Marks)

Or

Discuss the management of acute rheumatic fever.

(Aug 2010, 12 Marks)

Ans.

Management

I. *Treatment of acute attack:*

• Bed rest is important to reduce joint pain and cardiac workload. Duration of bed rest is guided by markers of inflammation, such as temperature, WBC count and ESR.

• Benzathine penicillin 1.2 μ IM 4 hourly. If patient is allergic to penicillin, erythromycin 40–50 mg/kg for ten days is given.

• Aspirin usually relieves symptom of arthritis rapidly. A starting dose of 60 mg/kg body weight per day is given divided into 6 doses. The dose may be increased to 120 mg/kg body weight. This dose may produce severe symptoms, such as vomiting, tachypnea and acidosis. Aspirin is given till ESR comes to normal.

• Corticosteroids, such as prednisolone produces rapid symptomatic relief than aspirin and is indicated in cases with severe arthritis or carditis. Prednisolone is given in doses of 1.2 mg/kg body weight till ESR comes to normal.

II. *Secondary prevention:* To prevent further attack of rheumatic fever, long-term prophylaxis is needed.

• Benzathine penicillin 1.2 μ IM is injected at the interval of 21 days. Further attack is unusual after the age of 21 years and treatment can be stopped.

• To prevent chances of endocarditis prophylactic antibiotic therapy should be given.

Q.3. Describe briefly diagnosis of rheumatic fever.
(Sep 2007, 2.5 Marks)

Or

Write short notes on Jones criteria for rheumatic fever. *(Mar 2008, 3 Marks)*

Or

Write short note on Duke Jones criteria in acute rheumatic fever.
(Sep 2009, 4 Marks)

Ans. Diagnosis of rheumatic fever is made by 'Jones criteria' which is as follows:

Major Criteria

♦ **Carditis:**
  • It is pancarditis involving endocardium, myocardium and pericardium.
  • It manifests as breathlessness, palpitation and chest pain.
  • Tachycardia, cardiomegaly and new or change murmurs
  • Aortic regurgitation in 50% cases.
  • Pericarditis produces frictional rub and pericardial tenderness.
  • Cardiac failure due to myocardial infarction.
♦ **Sydenham's chorea:**
  • Late neurological manifestations that occurs at least three months after the episode of acute rheumatic fever when all signs disappear.
  • More common in female.
  • It is characterized by involuntary dancing movements of hands, feet or face.
♦ **Polyarthritis:**
  • Early feature of illness is nonspecific.
  • It is characterized by acute painful symmetric and migratory inflammation of large joints.
  • Classical presentation is acute migratory polyarthritis. Pain and swelling in involved joints subside or disappear as newer joints get affected.
♦ **Erythema marginatum:** Red macules which fade in center, but remain red at the edges and occur mainly on trunk and proximal extremities on face.
♦ **Subcutaneous nodules:** They are small, dense, firm, painless and are best felt over tendons and bones.
  • Nodules appear more than 3 weeks after onset of other manifestations.

Clinical

♦ Fever
♦ Arthralgia
♦ Previous history of rheumatic fever or rheumatic heart disease.

Laboratory

♦ Acute phase reactants (leukocytosis, raised ESR, C- reactive protein)
♦ Prolonged PR interval in ECG.

Essential Criteria

Evidence for recent streptococcal infection as evidenced by:
♦ Increase in ASO titer
  • >333 Todd units (in children).
  • >250 Todd units (in adults).
♦ Positive throat culture for streptococcal infection
♦ Recent history of scarlet fever.

Confirmation of Diagnosis

Result is based on presence of two or more major criterias or one major and two minor criteria, in the presence of essential criteria, is required to diagnose acute rheumatic fever.

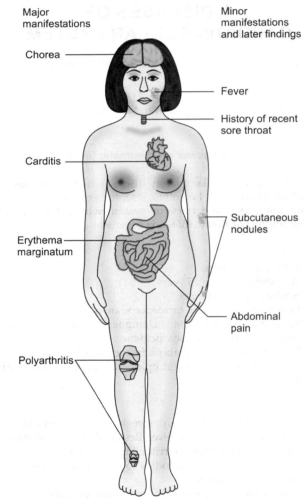

Fig. 6: Jones criteria.

Q.4. How will you diagnose and manage a case of rheumatic fever? Outline complications of rheumatic fever.
(Sep 2009, 5 Marks)

Ans. *For diagnosis refer to Ans. 3 of same chapter.*

For management refer to Ans. 2 of same chapter.

Complications

- Myocardial infarction
- Mitral stenosis
- Tricuspid regurgitation
- Aortic regurgitation
- Aortic stenosis is rare
- Mitral regurgitation.

Q.5. Enumerate the causes of Jones criteria of acute rheumatic fever. *(Mar 2001, 5 Marks)*

Ans. The causes of Jones criteria are:

- Previous streptococcal infection
- Recent scarlet fever
- Positive throat culture from streptococcal A
- Increased-antistreptolysin O titer.

Q.6. Describe clinical features, diagnosis, investigations and management of rheumatic mitral stenosis. *(Dec 2012, 8 Marks)*

Ans. Mitral stenosis is a valvular heart disease.

Rheumatic mitral stenosis occurs in elderly people and is most common in females.

Clinical Manifestations

Symptoms

- Patient complains of breathlessness and fatigue on exertion.
- Progression of stenosis lead to dyspnea on rest and even have orthopnea and paroxysmal nocturnal dyspnea.
- Acute pulmonary edema can also occur.
- Hemoptysis can be present due to rupture of pulmonary congestion and pulmonary embolism and cough due to pulmonary congestion.
- Chest pain is present due to pulmonary venous hypertension.

Signs

- Atrial fibrillation is present.
- *Auscultation:* Presence of loud first heart sound, opening snap and mid diastolic low pitched rumbling murmur best heared at the apex.
- *Signs of raised pulmonary capillary pressure:* Pleural effusion, crepitation, pulmonary edema.
- *Signs of pulmonary hypertension:* RV heave, loud P2
- *Others:* Basal crackles, ascites and pleural effusion

Investigations

- *ECG:*
  - Right ventricular hypertrophy
  - Left atrial hypertrophy
- *X-ray chest:*
  - Prominent left atrial appendage may be seen in left border of heart between pulmonary artery and left ventricle. It indicates left atrial enlargement.
  - Double shadow of enlarged left atrium on right side of spine.
  - Signs of pulmonary venous congestion
- *Echocardiogram:*
  - Show thick immobile mitral cusp
  - Decreased diastolic filling of left ventricle

- Decreased valve orifice area
- Left atrial thrombus, if it is present.
- *Cardiac catheterization:* is used to assess valvular lesions and to detect coronary artery disease.
- *Doppler:*
  - Pressure gradient across mitral valve
  - Pulmonary artery pressure
  - Left ventricular function

Diagnosis

It is based on physical signs and investigations.

Management

- **Pharmacological:**
  - Salt restriction should be done in diet or very low salt diet is given.
  - Digitalis therapy is given. In the patient with congestive heart failure Tab. digoxin 0.25 mg BD is given.
  - Diuretics can be given for controlling heart failure
  - Anticoagulants, such as heparin can be given to prevent embolism
  - Prophylactic oral penicillin V 250 mg BD is given to prevent rheumatic fever. If patient is allergic of penicillin erythromycin 250 mg daily orally is given.
- **Surgical:**

  When patient remains symptomatic despite of medical treatment or when mitral stenosis is severe, surgical intervention is needed:
  - *Mitral valvotomy:*
    - Percutaneous balloon valvotomy is indicated when mitral valve is noncalcified and without regurgitation. The procedure involves the passing of catheter across the valve and inflation of the balloon to dilate the orifice.
    - Open valvotomy is carried out in patients where balloon valvotomy is not possible or in cases with restenosis. In this procedure, the fusion of the valve is loosened and calcium deposit and thrombi are removed.
  - *Mitral valve replacement:* The mitral valve is replaced when there is critical mitral stenosis and/or there is associated mitral regurgitation. Replacement is also done when the mitral valve is severely distorted and calcified.

Q.7. Describe briefly clinical features and management of aortic regurgitation. *(Sep 2006, 5 Marks)*

Ans. Aortic regurgitation is produced due to acute rheumatic carditis which is associated with other valve involvement and infective endocarditis.

Clinical Features

Symptoms

- *In mild-to-moderate aortic regurgitation:*
  - Often asymptomatic
  - On palpitation—pounding of heart is a common symptom
  - Symptoms of left heart failure appear but late

♦ *In severe aortic regurgitation:*
- Symptoms of heart failure, i.e., dyspnea, orthopnea are present at onset.
- Angina pectoris is frequent complaint.
- Arrhythmias are uncommon.

Signs

♦ Collapsing or good volume pulse (wide pulse pressure)
♦ Bounding peripheral pulses
♦ Dancing carotids (Corrigan's sign)
♦ Capillary pulsation in nail beds (Quincke's sign)
♦ Pistol shots sound and Duroziez's sign/murmur
♦ Head nodding with carotid pulse — de Musset's sign
♦ Cyanosis (peripheral, central or both) may be present
♦ Pitting ankle edema may be present.
♦ Tender hepatomegaly if right heart failure present.

Management

♦ Treatment of underlying causes, such as endocarditis and syphilis.
♦ *Surgical:* Replacement of aortic valve should be performed before heart failure can develop. Serial evaluation of end systolic dimensions should be made and surgery considered when this exceeds 5 mm.
♦ *Medical:*
- Prophylaxis against bacterial endocarditis before and after surgery
- Therapy of heart failure if develops.

Q.8. Briefly describe subacute bacterial endocarditis.
(Apr 2010, 5 Marks) (Nov 2008, 15 Marks)

Or

Describe clinical features, investigations and management of subacute bacterial endocarditis.
(June 2010, 20 Marks)
(Sep 2008, 5 Marks) (Sep 2004, 20 Marks)

Or

Write short note on clinical features and treatment of bacterial endocarditis. *(Sep 2006, 10 Marks)*

or

Write short answer on subacute bacterial endocarditis. *(Sep. 2018, 3 Marks)*

Ans. Subacute bacterial endocarditis is defined as infection and inflammation of inner lining of heart including heart valves. It also includes infection at the site congenital heart anomaly.

Clinical Manifestations

♦ *General:* Presence of nausea, fever, anorexia, weight loss, night sweat and weakness.
♦ *Cardiovascular system:* Tachycardia, cardiac murmur, conduction defect and cardiac failure.
♦ *Blood vessels:* Loss of peripheral pulse.
♦ *Central nervous system:* Headache, hemiplegia or monoplegia and toxic encephalopathy.

♦ *Lungs:* Pleuritic pain and hemoptysis
♦ *Nails:* Osler's nodes, clubbing of finger and splinter hemorrhage.
♦ *Skin:* Purpuric spot and petechial hemorrhage.
♦ *Eyes:* Roth's spot and subconjunctival hemorrhage.
♦ *Kidney:* Hematuria and glomerulonephritis
♦ *Spleen:* Splenomegaly is present
♦ *Blood:* Anemia is present

Pathogenesis

Flowchart 5: Pathogenesis of bacterial endocarditis.

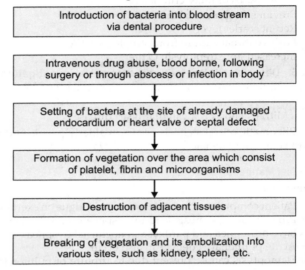

Investigations

♦ *Blood culture:* In absence of recent or concurrent antibiotic therapy, the first 3 random blood cultures are positive in most patients, and blood culture is positive by third day in 90%.
♦ *Urine:* Microscopic hematuria is the most common finding. Slight albuminuria and hyaline and granular casts also found.
♦ *Hematology:* Normocytic normochromic anemia, usually mild. May be raised ESR and raised C-reactive protein.
♦ *Chest radiograph:* May be diagnostic in right-sided endocarditis, with multiple shadows visible due to an embolic pneumonia.
♦ *ECG:* Myocardial infarction seen on ECG may be due coronary embolism, and a conduction defect may be due to development of an aortic root abscess.
♦ *Echocardiography:* Higher sensitivity in identifying vegetation with transesophageal echocardiography as compared to transthoracic echocardiography.
- *Vegetations:* An echodense structure attached to the valve or its supporting structures, or lying in the track of a turbulent jet, which is irregular in shape.
- Leaflet perforation is best seen as regurgitant jet on color flow mapping.
- Annular and periprosthetic echolucent spaces (abscesses) and fistula formation.
♦ *Chest X-ray:* Shows evidence of cardiomegaly and heart failure.

Management

Management is divided into three parts:
1. Treatment during disease process
2. Prophylaxis
3. Indication for cardiac surgery.

Treatment During Disease Process

♦ It is mainly antimicrobial treatment. Along with source of infection symptoms are removed as soon as possible.
♦ Antibiotics should preferably be bactericidal.
♦ Antibiotics should be administered parenterally to achieve high serum concentration since the vegetation is avascular.
♦ Therapy is generally of prolonged duration.
♦ Selection of antibiotics should be based on culture report and minimum inhibitory concentration (MIC) values.
♦ Empirical therapy may be initiated in acute severe cases after drawing blood samples for culture. The antibiotics are later changed based on sensitivity reports, if necessary.
♦ Treatment of infective endocarditis should be prompt and adequate. The list of antibiotics commonly used, their dosage and indications are given below in table.

Antimicrobial Therapy for Infective Endocarditis

Microorganism	Antibiotic regimen
S. viridans and Group D streptococci	Penicillin G (1.2 g IV at 4–6 hour interval for 4 weeks), then oral amoxicillin is given (6 g) daily for 2 to 6 weeks. Or Penicillin G (1.2 g IV for two weeks) + Gentamicin 1 mg/kg at 8 hours interval for 2 weeks, then oral amoxicillin (6 g) daily for 2–6 weeks. *If patient is allergic to penicillin:* Cetazolin 2.0 g IV at 6–8 hours interval for 4 weeks, Or Vancomycin 15 mg/kg IV at 12 hour interval for 4 weeks.
Enterococci or penicillin resistant S. viridans	Penicillin G (1.5 to 2 g IV for 4–6 weeks or ampicillin 2.0 g IV at 6 hours interval tor 4–6 weeks + Gentamicin 1 mg/kg at 8 hour interval IV or IM for 5–6 weeks. *If allergic to penicillin,* Vancomycin 15 mg/kg IV at 12 hours interval for 4 weeks.
Pneumococci or Group A streptococci	Penicillin G (0.6 to1.2 g IV in divided doses at 4–6 hours interval for 4 weeks). *If allergic to penicillin* Cefazolin 2.0 g IV at 6 to 8 hours interval for 4 weeks.
S. aureus	Nafcillin 2.0 g IV at 4 hours interval for 4–6 weeks Or Flucloxacillin 2.0 g IV 6 hourly for 2 weeks, then 2.0 g orally 6 hourly for 4 weeks. *If allergic to penicillin* Cefazolin 2.0 g IV at 6 to 8 hours interval for 4 weeks. Or Vancomycin 15 mg/kg IV at 12 hour interval for 4 weeks.

Contd...

Contd...

Microorganism	Antibiotic regimen
HACEK organism (rare)	Ceftriaxone 2 g/day IV as a single dose for 4 weeks or ampicillin + gentamicin may be used.
Coxiella burnetii (Rickettsia)	Tetracycline 0.5 to 1 g IV or orally Or Rifampicin (600 mg 12 hourly orally) + doxycycline (100 mg 12 hourly orally).

Prophylaxis Against Infective Endocarditis

Patients with valvular and congenital heart disease who are at high or moderate risk of endocarditis should receive prophylactic antibiotics before undergoing any procedure which may cause bacteremia.

Antibiotic regimen for prophylaxis of endocarditis in adults at moderate or high-risk is as follows:
♦ Oral cavity, respiratory tract, or esophageal procedures (in patients at high-risk, administer a half dose after the initial dose).
  • *Standard regimen:* Amoxicillin 2.0 g oral 1 hour before procedure.
  • *Inability to take oral medication of standard regimen:* Ampicillin 2.0 g IV or IM within 30 min of procedure.
  • *If patient is allergic to Penicillin:*
    Clarithromycin 500 mg or azithromycin 500 mg orally l hour before procedure.
    Or
    Cephalexin or cefadroxil 2 g orally 1 hour before procedure.
    Or
    Clindamycin 600 mg oral l hour before procedure.
  • If patient is allergic to penicillin and is unable to take oral medication.
    Clindamycin 600 mg IV 30 min before procedure.
    Or
    Cefazolin 1.0 g IV or IM 30 min before procedure.
♦ *Genitourinary and gastrointestinal tract procedures:*
  • *In high-risk patients:* Ampicillin 2 g IM or IV + Gentamicin 1.5 mg/kg IV or IM within 30 min of starting the procedure followed by ampicillin
  • *In high-risk patients allergic to penicillin:* Vancomycin 1 g IV over 1 to 2 hour + gentamicin 1.5 mg/kg IV or IM combination is given within 30 min of starting the procedure.
  • *In moderate risk patients:* Amoxicillin 2.0 g oral 1 hour before procedure
    Or Ampicillin or amoxicillin 2.0 g IV or IM within 30 min of procedure.
  • *In moderate risk patients allergic to penicillin:* Vancomycin 1 g IV over 1 to 2 hours completed within 30 min of starting procedure.

Indication for Cardiac Surgery

♦ Heart failure due to valve damage
♦ Failure of antibiotic therapy, i.e., in fungal endocarditis
♦ Large vegetation on left sided heart valves with evidence or high-risk of systemic emboli.
♦ Abscess formation

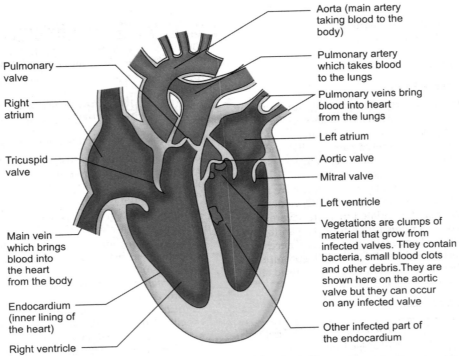

Fig. 7: Subacute bacterial endocarditis.

Q.9. Outline the management of subacute bacterial endocarditis. *(Mar 1999, 5 Marks)*

Ans. Management is divided into three parts:

1. Treatment during disease process
2. Prophylaxis
3. Indication for cardiac surgery.

For details Refer to Ans. 8 of same Chapter.

Q.10. Write short note on clinical signs of SABE.
(Mar 2000, 5 Marks)

Ans.

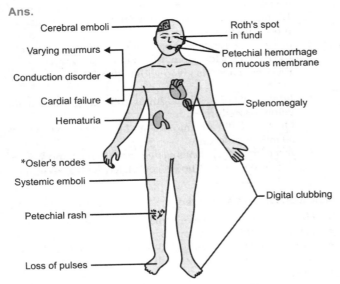

Fig. 8: Subacute bacterial endocarditis.

Q 10. *Osler's nodes = Painful red, raised lesions found on hand and feet.

♦ Cardiovascular system: Tachycardia, cardiac murmur, conduction defect and cardiac failure.
♦ Blood vessels: Loss of peripheral pulse
♦ Central nervous system: Headache, hemiplegia or monoplegia and toxic encephalopathy
♦ Lungs: Pleuritic pain and hemoptysis
♦ Nails: *Osler's nodes, clubbing of finger and splinter hemorrhage.
♦ Skin: Purpuric spot and petechial hemorrhage.
♦ Eyes: Roth's spot and subconjunctival hemorrhage.
♦ Kidney: Hematuria and glomerulonephritis
♦ Spleen: Splenomegaly is present
♦ Blood: Anemia is present

Q.11. Enumerate clinical and diagnostic features of mitral stenosis. *(Feb 1999, 5 Marks)*

Ans.

Clinical Features

♦ Patient complains of breathlessness and fatigue on exertion.
♦ Progression of stenosis lead to dyspnea on rest and even have orthopnea and paroxysmal nocturnal dyspnea.
♦ Acute pulmonary edema can also occur.
♦ Hemoptysis can be present due to rupture of pulmonary congestion and pulmonary embolism and cough due to pulmonary congestion.
♦ Chest pain is present due to pulmonary venous hypertension.

Signs

♦ Atrial fibrillation is present.
♦ *Auscultation:* Presence of loud first heart sound, opening snap and mid diastolic low pitched rumbling murmur best heared at the apex.

♦ *Signs of raised pulmonary capillary pressure:* Pleural effusion, crepitation, pulmonary edema.
♦ *Signs of pulmonary hypertension:* RV heave, Loud P2
♦ *Others:* Basal crackels, ascites and pleural effusion

Diagnostic Features
Investigations

♦ *ECG:*
  • Right ventricular hypertrophy
  • Left atrial hypertrophy
♦ *X-ray chest:*
  • Prominent left atrial appendage may be seen in left border of heart between pulmonary artery and left ventricle. It indicates left atrial enlargement.
  • Double shadow of enlarged left atrium on right side of spine.
  • Signs of pulmonary venous congestion.
♦ *Echocardiogram:*
  • Show thick immobile mitral cusp
  • Decreased diastolic filling of left ventricle
  • Decreased valve orifice area
  • Left atrial thrombus, if it is present.
♦ *Cardiac catheterization:* is used to assess valvular lesions and to detect coronary artery disease.
♦ Doppler:
  • Pressure gradient across mitral valve
  • Pulmonary artery pressure
  • Left ventricular function

Q.12. Write short note on coarctation of aorta.
(Mar 2000, 5 Marks)

Ans. Coarctation of aorta is defined as the narrowing of aorta at or distal to the subclavian artery.

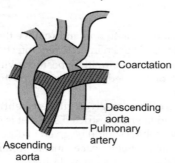

Fig. 9: Coarctation of aorta.

Clinical Features

♦ In uncomplicated cases the only symptoms are *intermittent claudication, pain, weakness and dyspnea on running.
♦ Headache and nose bleed
♦ Hypertension in upper limb
♦ Physical examination shows weak or impalpable femorals in comparison to strong radial acting pulsation.
♦ Heart size remains normal with left ventricular forcible apex.
♦ On auscultation:
  • S1 is accentuated

• S2 normal splitting delayed A2
• S3 with left ventricular filling
• S4 with hypertension.

Investigation

♦ **ECG:** It shows left axis deviation representing left ventricular failure.
♦ **X-ray:** Normal sized heart with prominent ascending aorta. Barium swallow shows characteristic E sign.
♦ **Aortography:** Show usually short narrow segment.

Treatment

♦ Medical management consists of control of congestive cardiac failure in infancy.
♦ Definitive management is operative.
♦ Operation can be done at any age, but lowest risk is between 1–10 years.
♦ Resection of narrow segment is done in operation.

Q.13. Write short note on tetralogy of Fallot.
(Mar 2008, 5 Marks) (Apr 2008, 5 Marks)

Ans. It is the commonest cyanotic congenital heart disease in children above the age of 2 years. It is characterized by four constituents:
1. Ventricular septal defect.
2. Pulmonary stenosis
3. Overriding or dextroposed aorta
4. Right ventricular hypertrophy.

Clinical Features

♦ The chief complaint is development of *anoxic spells. The anoxic spells are dangerous for children and can occur many times.
♦ It occurs prominently after walking up or following exertion.
♦ Children start crying, become dyspneic, blue than before and may loose consciousness. Convulsions may occur.
♦ Frequency varies from once in a few days to numerous attacks everyday.
♦ Each spell is life-threatening.

Physical Signs

♦ Cyanosis
♦ Clubbing of finger and toes
♦ Growth is stunted
♦ Ejection systolic murmur is present at pulmonary area.
♦ ECG may show right ventricular hypertrophy
♦ Second sound may show delayed splitting
♦ In X-ray chest boot shaped heart is seen
♦ Echocardiography shows that aorta is not juxtaposed with intraventricular septum.

Complications

♦ Syncope
♦ Cerebral abscess
♦ Stroke due to cerebral thrombosis
♦ Subacute infective endocarditis
♦ Sudden death

Q 12. *Intermittent claudication = Cramping or pain in the leg muscles brought on by the predictable amount of walking and is relieved by the rest.
Q 13. *Anoxic spells = Paroxysmal attacks of dyspnea.

Treatment

It is divided into two stages:
1. Management of anoxic spells
2. Definitive treatment.

Management of Anoxic Spells

- Knee chest position
- Humidified oxygen/moist oxygen
- *Morphine:* 0.1 to 0.2 mg/kg subcutaneous inj.
- Correction of acidosis if pH <7.1 by giving sodium bicarbonate IV
- Propranolol 0.1 g/kg IV during spells and then 0.5 to 1 mg/kg 4 to 6 hourly orally.
- *Vasopressor:* Methoxamine IM or IV
- Correct anemia
- Consider operation.

Definitive Treatment

It is operative. Operative treatment is of two varieties, i.e., papillative and definitive.

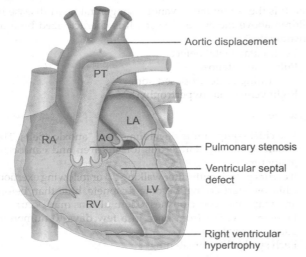

Fig. 10: Tetralogy of Fallot *(For color version, see Plate 1).*

Q.14. Outline the management of congestive cardiac failure. *(Mar 1997, 7.5 Marks)*

Ans. The management of cardiac failure aims to restore balance between metabolic demands of the body and person heart's ability to meet these demands.

- Rest: Complete bed rest is the key stone of management. When the patient is dyspneic, bed rest is given with the head end of bed raised to 45°. The legs should be kept below the pelvis to prevent the fluid present in legs to return to vascular system and precipitate pulmonary edema.
- Diet: Basic aim is to restrict sodium in the diet. Quantity of salt intake per day should not exceed 0.5 g. Salt substitutes may be used to make diet more palatable.
- Diuretics: In cardiac failure, there is always sodium and water retention. Hence, diuretics are given to increase sodium extraction. Furosemide 40 to 80 mg orally produces effect in 4 to 6 hours and on IV administration of furosemide 40 to 100 mg produces its effect in 20 minutes. Spironolactone which is potassium sparing diuretic is given

25 mg orally 4 times a day which removes the symptoms like hypokalemia due to action of furosemide. Triamterene or amiloride hydrochloride is given along with spironolactone.
- Digitalis: It increases the force of myocardial contraction and decreases work of heart. The commonly used drug is digoxin which is administered orally 0.25 mg BD. For rapid digitalization digoxin 0.5–0.75 mg is given slow IV over a period of 5 to 10 minutes under electrocardiographic control.
- Sympathomimetic amines: Dopamine at low doses of 3 to 5 µg/kg/min increases contractility of heart.
- Vasodilators: Sodium nitroprusside in the dose of 5 to 10 µg/min have balance dilator effect. Besides this hydralazine, nitrates and ACE inhibitors are used.
- Inodilator levosimendan: This is a calcium channel sensitizer. It has positive inotropic and vasodilator effect. It is given IV with loading dose of 6–12 µg/kg/min over 10 min followed by infusion 0.05 to 2 µg/kg/min infusion.
- Oxygen: It is given via Woulfe's bottle at rate of 5 to 8 lts/min.
- Miscellaneous drugs: Tranquilizers, such as diazepam 2 to 5 mg TDS are given to reduce anxiety.
- Cardiac re-synchronization therapy or biventricular pacing: It is used in patients with symptomatic refractory cardiac failure with conduction abnormality or left bundle branch block. This therapy involves pacing the right atrium, right ventricle and left ventricle to improve synchrony of the cardiac chambers.
- Left ventricular assist device: Devices, such as intra-aortic balloon pump, impella device, heart-mate, thoratic are considered when medical management fails. They are usually used as a bridge to cardiac transplant.

Q.15. Describe the management of acute left ventricular failure. *(Sep 1998, 5 Marks)*

Ans.

Management

First aim of treatment is to find and remove the precipitating cause, i.e., arrhythmia or an intercurrent infection.

- Patient should be kept in sitting position, with legs hanging along side of the bed, i.e., upright posture should be maintained.
- *Diet:* Salt free diet is given till left ventricular failure improves and later on restricted salt diet is given.
- *Sedatives:* Morphine should be given in doses of 5 to 10 mg along with an anti-emetic, i.e., metaclopramide 10 mg IV and repeat the drug as soon as desired.
- *Oxygen:* About 60% of oxygen is given by facemask under positive pressure. It should be given as 6 to 8 L/min through Wolfe's bottle.
- *Loop diuretics:* Furosemide 40 to 100 mg IV should be given.
- IV sodium nitroprusside 20 to 30 µg/min or IV nitroglycerin should be given in patients whose systolic blood pressure is more than 100 mm Hg.
- *Digitalis:* If digoxin is not used previously, the three fourth of full dose, i.e., 0.5 to 1 mg is given as IV dose.
- Bronchodilators: At times aminophylline or theophylline in dose of 250 to 500 mg IV decreases brochoconstriction.
- In cases of severe left ventricular failure inotropes can be given.
- If all the above measures failed then rotating tourniquet should be applied to extremities.

♦ *Intra-aortic balloon counterpulsation:* It is used in acute left ventricular failure during cardiac procedures or cardiac repairs.

Q.16. Write a short note on systemic hypertension.
(Mar 2008, 5.5 Marks) (Feb 2006, 5 Marks)
Or
Write about clinical features, etiology, complications and management of systemic hypertension.
(Sep 2005, 20 Marks)
Or
Describe briefly on secondary hypertension.
(Apr 2015, 4 Marks)
Or
Describe the etiology, clinical features and management of hypertension. *(Feb 2013, 15 Marks)*
Or
Write diagnosis and management of hypertension
(Jan 2017, 12 Marks)

Ans. Systemic hypertension is defined as systolic pressure equal to or above 140 mm Hg and diastolic pressure equal to or above 90 mm Hg measured on two or more different occasions.

Etiology

♦ *Renal disorders:*
  • Renovascular stenosis
  • Parenchymal renal disease, particularly glomerulone-phritis
  • Polycystic kidney disease
♦ *Endocrinal disorders:*
  • Pheochromocytoma
  • Cushing's syndrome
  • Primary hyperaldosteronism
  • Acromegaly
  • Hypothyroidism and hyperthyroidism
♦ *Drugs:*
  • Oral contraceptives
  • Corticosteroids
  • Sympathomimetic drugs
  • Cyclosporine
  • NSAIDs
♦ *Miscellaneous:*
  • Toxemia of pregnancy
  • Coarctation of aorta
  • Raised intracranial pressure
  • Obstructive sleep apnea.

Clinical Features

♦ Majority of patients remain asymptomatic and are diagnosed on routine clinical examination.
♦ Common symptoms are occipital headache, dizziness, palpitation and fatigue.
♦ Some of the patients may also present with symptoms which are related to target organ damage like epistaxis, hematuria, blurred vision, angina and breathlessness.
♦ Various symptoms pertaining to underlying cause can be present, such as weight gain (Cushing's syndrome), weight loss (thyrotoxicosis), episodic headache, palpitation, and sweating (pheochromocytoma)

♦ History taking should include age, sex, occupation, lifestyle of patient along with history of smoking, diabetes mellitus, hyperlipidemia, alcohol and drug intake and presence of hypertension in all family members.
♦ *Physical examination:* Presence of truncal obesity (Cushing's disease), palpable kidneys (polycystic kidneys), radiofemoral delay (coarctation of aorta), recurrent back pain, undiagnosed fever and recurrent urinary infections suggest (chronic pyelonephritis) abdominal bruit (renovascular), may help in identifying the secondary cause of hypertension.
♦ The signs of complications of hypertension, such as heaving apex, 4th heart sound, loud aortic second heart sound, pulmonary crackles, and retinal changes may also be present.

Complications

♦ *Central nervous system complications:*
  • Transient cerebral ischemic attacks
  • Cerebrovascular accidents (strokes)
  • Subarachnoid hemorrhage.
  • Hypertensive encephalopathy is characterized by very high blood pressure, it is characterized by transient disturbances in speech and vision, paresthesias, convulsion, disorientation, loss of consciousness and papilledema. The neurological symptoms are reversible as blood pressure comes under control.
♦ *Ophthalmic complications:*
  • *Hypertensive retinopathy:* In this, there is thickening of the walls of the retinal arterioles, diffuse or segmental narrowing of blood columns, varying width of the light reflex from vessel walls, arteriovenous nipping retinal hemorrhages, soft and hard exudates and papilledema. Severe retinopathy can cause visual field defects and blindness.
♦ *Cardiovascular complications:*
  • Coronary artery disease (angina, myocardial infarction)
  • Left ventricular failure
  • Aortic aneurysm
  • Aortic dissection
♦ *Renal complications:*
  • Proteinuria
  • Progressive renal failure
♦ *Malignant hypertension:* It is a clinical syndrome of markedly high blood pressure with retinal hemorrhages and exudates. It also includes confusion, headache, vomiting, visual disturbances and renal function deterioration.

Diagnosis

Diagnosis is based on the investigations and clinical features
Investigations
♦ Basic investigations which are done in all patients:
  • Urine examination for protein, blood and glucose
  • Serum creatinine and blood urea nitrogen for assessing the renal functions
  • Serum electrolytes, i.e., serum sodium and serum potassium
  • Hematocrit
  • Fasting and post-prandial blood glucose for hyperglycemia

- Serum potassium for hypokalemic alkalosis or diuretic therapy
- Plasma urea assessment
- Complete serum lipid profile
- ECG for left ventricular hypertrophy or ischemia
- Chest X-ray for assessing the cardiomegaly or heart failure.
- Special investigations to screen for special group of patients
  - X-ray chest and echocardiography
  - Intravenous pyelogram and renal ultrasound, if renal disease is suspected (polycystic disease)
  - Renal arteriography for renal artery stenosis, if it is suspected
  - 24-hour urine catecholamine for pheochromocytoma, if it is suspected
  - Plasma renin activity and aldosterone for Conn's syndrome, if it is suspected
  - Urinary cortisol and dexamethasone suppression test for Cushing's syndrome, if it is suspected
  - Angiography/MRI for coarctation of aorta, if it is suspected.

Management

Refer to Ans. 18 of same chapter.

Q.17. Enumerate the complications and outline the management of systemic hypertension.

(Mar 2000, 5 Marks)

Ans. *Refer to Ans. 16 of same chapter.*

Q.18. Describe briefly management of hypertension.

(Feb/Mar 2004, 5 Marks)

Ans.

Management

Nonpharmacological Treatment

- **Salt restriction:** Modest sodium restriction 2.4 g sodium or 6 g NaCl is effective in controlling hypertension.
- **Weight reduction:** In overweight persons, reduction of 1 kg may reduce 1.6 to 1.3 mm Hg of blood pressure
- **Stop smoking:** Smoking raises BP. It is an independent and most important reversible coronary risk factor.
- **Diet:**
  Lacto-vegetarian diet and high intake of poly unsaturated fish oils have high potassium levels and lower blood pressure by:
  - Increased sodium extraction
  - Decreased sympathetic activity
  - Decreased renin-angiotensin secretion and direct dilatation of removal of renal arteries
  - Adequate calcium and magnesium intake should be maintained in diet
- Limit of alcohol intake is done
- Various forms of relaxation, such as yoga, biofeedback and psychotherapy lower the blood pressure
- Regular exercise, relaxation exercise.

Pharmacological Therapy

- **Diuretics:** Commonly used diuretics are hydrochlorothiazide 100 mg per day, chlorthalidone 50–100 mg/day. The reduced potassium levels in body results in hypokalemia, potassium supplements have to be given in people on long-term diuretic therapy. Potassium sparing diuretics, i.e., spironolactone 25 mg TDS is given.
- **Beta-blockers:** Propranolol was used extensively as effective antihypertensive drug. The dose administered as 40–160 mg/day.
- **Calcium channel blockers:** Nifedipine 16 to 20 mg BD is administered. Side effects are headache, dizziness, flushing. Drug is contraindicated in acute myocardial infarction, cardiogenic shock, pregnancy and is used with caution in diabetics and edema.
  Felodipine sulfate 5 to 10 mg/day is effective in mild to moderate hypertension.
  Amlodipine 5 to 10 g is effective and is safe in hypertensives.
- **ACE inhibitors:**
  - Enalapril maleate 5 mg OD is given.
  - Captopril in combination with diuretics or a beta-blocker. 25 g TDS of captopril is administered. It is considered safe in asthmatics and diabetics.
  - Ramipril 2.5 mg daily is used to reduce hypertension.
- **Alpha-1 adrenergic blockers:** Prazosin is commonly used drug. Dose is 0.5 mg TDS.
- **Vasodilators:** Diazoxide and sodium nitroprusside are given as IV dosage.

Q.19. Outline the management of acute myocardial infarction.

(Mar 2010, 5 Marks)

Ans. The management of myocardial infarction is divided into two parts:
1. Early management.
2. Late management.

Early Management

- Aspirin 150–300 mg to be chewed earliest.
- Sublingual glyceryl trinitrate 0.4–1 mg, to be repeated, if necessary
- Oxygen through nasal cannula at a rate of 2–4 L/min.
- Procure IV line and take blood samples for glucose, lipids and complete hemogram.
- Record 12-lead ECG.
- Pain may be relieved by IV morphine (5 mg) plus metoclopramide as an antiemetic (10 mg).
- IV beta-blockers (metoprolol 5 mg every 2–5 minutes for 3 doses) for ongoing chest pain, hypertension and tachycardia provided there is no contraindication.
- Thrombolysis should be done.
- If PTCA is planned, give GP IIb/IIIa inhibitor
- After admission immediately shift the patient to ICU or ICCU

In Hospital Treatment

Hospitalization and Strict Bed Rest

- Hospitalize the patient and advice strict bed rest. As early as the patient is hospitalized, the better it is.
- Patient should be strictly admitted in ICCU.

Analgesia

- IV morphine sulfate 10 mg and an anti emetic, i.e., cyclizine 50 mg is given through IV cannula.
- The drug is repeated depending on the response till complete analgesia is received and patient feels better.

Anti-platelet Drugs

Low dose aspirin, i.e., 75 to 150 mg and clopidogrel 300 mg stat and then 75 mg orally daily is given.

Oxygen Therapy

Inhalation of oxygen increases arterial partial pressure of oxygen, so there is increase in the concentration of oxygen gradient which is responsible for diffusion of oxygen in ischemic myocardium from adjacent better perfused areas. This is given by facemask or nasal prongs for a day or two after infarction.

Thrombolysis

♦ Coronary thrombolysis helps to restore patency of coronary artery preserves left ventricular function and improves survival.
♦ The choice of drug for thrombolysis is less important than the speed of treatment.
♦ Streptokinase, 1.5 million units in 100 mL of saline given in an intravenous infusion over 1 hour, is a widely accepted method. It is a cheap, but being antigenic, sometimes, may cause serious allergic manifestations. Hence, it can be used once and therapy is changed if the patient requires second thrombolysis within few years.

Alteplase (Tissue Plasminagen Activator (tPA)

♦ It is a potent fibrinolytic drug but is expensive.
♦ It is less antigenic and does not cause hypotension.
♦ The current tPA regimen given over 90 minutes (bolus dose of 15 mg followed by 50 mg over 30 minutes and then 35 mg over next 60 minutes) is widely accepted. The other drugs include reteplase given in double dose regime, i.e., 10 million units over 2–3 minute followed by another dose of 10 million units after 30 minutes. Tenecteplase given as bolus dose of 53 mg/kg over 10 seconds. Both reteplase and tenectaplase are known as bolus fibrinolytics.

Angioplasty

Immediate angioplasty of infarct related artery is safe and is effective alternative to thrombolysis. It is done in the patients in whom the hazards of thrombolysis is high.

Anti-coagulants

♦ Sub-cutaneous heparin, i.e., 7,500 units twice a day for 7–10 days or till discharge of patient from the hospital can be employed. In patients who do not receive thrombolytic therapy to prevent venous thrombosis.
♦ Patients who receive thrombolytic therapy (tPA) should receive immediate and full doses of heparin (10,000 U bolus plus, 1000 U hourly).

Beta-Adrenergic Blockers

Acute beta-adrenoreceptors blockade intravenous atenolol (5–10 mg given over 5 minutes) or metoprolol (5–15 mg given over 5 minutes) relieves pain, reduces arrhythmias, salvages myocardium and improves short-term mortality in patients who present within 12 hours of onset of pain.

Nitrates and Other Agents

Sublingual glyceryl trinitrate 0.4 mg is useful in threatened infarction.

Sedatives

Diazepam 5 mg for three to four times a day is effective. It is given for few days.

Diet

♦ For first 4 to 5 days low calorie diet which is divided into multiple meals is given.
♦ If heart failure is present restrict the salt.
♦ From second week, food should be increased in amount.

Lipid Lowering Agent

Atorvastatin is given to reduce the LDL levels.

Late Management

♦ *Risk stratification and further investigations:* Prognosis of patient survived after myocardial infarction depends on degree of myocardial damage, any residual ischemia and presence of ventricular arrhythmias.
♦ *Life style modification:*
  • Stop smoking
  • Diet control
  • Regular exercise.
♦ *Secondary prevention*
  • Antiplatelet agents, i.e., aspirin
  • Lipid lowering agents
  • Beta-blockers and ACEI in congestive cardiac failure and hypertension.
  • Control of blood sugar in diabetes.
♦ *Rehabilitation and after care:*
  • Physical activities should be restricted for 4 to 6 weeks since infarct takes 4–6 weeks to become replaced with fibrous tissue.
  • Gradual mobilization and return to work over 6 weeks.
  • When there are complications, the regimen has to be modified accordingly.
  • Exercise within the limits set by angina and tiredness will do no harm but much good. Same limits apply to sexual activity.
  • Control of obesity, regular exercises, cessation of smoking, adoption of a less frenetic way of life and control of plasma lipids by diets and drugs.
  • Complications should be managed. Pain relief, reassurance, rest and correction of hypokalemia play a major role in prevention of arrhythmias.

Routine Drug Therapy

♦ Low dose aspirin, i.e., 75 to 150 mg daily and is continued indefinitely.
♦ Beta-adrenergic blocker should be given for 4 to 6 weeks if there is no contraindication.
♦ ACE inhibitor, i.e., captopril 25 mg TID or ramipril 2.5 to 5 mg BD
♦ Lipid lowering agent atorvastatin is given to lower the LDL levels.

Q.20. Enumerate the complications and outline the management of acute myocardial infarction.

(Mar 2000, 5 Marks)

Ans.

Enumeration of Complications of Myocardial Infarction

♦ Immediate
  • Arrhythmias and conduction disturbances
    – Sinus bradycardia
    – Ventricular ectopics
    – Ventricular tachycardia
    – Ventricular fibrillation
    – Idioventricular rhythm
    – Atrial fibrillation
    – Heart block
  • Post – myocardial angina can occur in 50% patients occur.
  • Acute circulatory failure.
  • Pericarditis
  • Mechanical complications include:
    – Papillary muscle dysfunction or rupture
    – Rupture of interventricular septum
    – Rupture of ventricle
  • Mural thrombosis and embolism
  • Sudden death
♦ *Late complications:*
  • Post-myocardial infarction syndrome (Dressler's syndrome)
  • Ventricular aneurysm.

Management

Refer to Ans. 19 of same chapter.

Q.21. Describe the clinical features, diagnosis and treatment of acute myocardial infarction.

(Mar 2001, 15 Marks)

Or

Describe the clinical features of acute myocardial infarction. (Feb 2013, 5 Marks)

Ans. Acute myocardial infarction is defined as irreversible damage to myocardium of heart as a result of occlusive thrombus due to rupture of atherosclerotic plaque in coronary artery.

Clinical Features

♦ **Symptoms:**
  • *Pain:* Chest pain is more common and is severe in comparison to angina. Pain is severe with pallor and peculiar facial expression. Pain is described as tightness, heaviness and constriction.
  • *Anxiety:* It is common and occurs when there is fear of impending death.
  • Nausea and vomiting.
  • Breathlessness due to fall in cardiac output.
  • Collapse or syncope due to arrhythmia and profound hypertension.
♦ **Signs:**
  • Signs of sympathetic activation
    – Pallor
    – Sweating
    – Tachycardia.
  • Signs of vagal stimulation
    – Vomiting
    – Bradycardia.

• Signs of impaired myocardial function
    – Hypotension and oliguria
    – Narrow pulse pressure
    – Raised jugular venous pressure
    – Third heart sound
    – Quite first heart sound
    – Lung crepitations.
• *Signs of tissue damage:* Fever and arrhythmia
• *Signs of complications:*
    – Due to mitral regurgitation
    – Due to pericarditis.
    – Ventricular ectopic beats
    – Ventricular tachycardia
    – Heart blocks.

Diagnosis

Diagnosis of acute myocardial infarction is based on history, characteristics symptoms and signs and investigations.

Investigations

♦ *Electrocardiography:*
  • ECG is the specific method for confirming the diagnosis.
  • Typical changes are seen in leads which faces the infracted area. These changes are:
    – Elevation of ST-segment
    – Pathologic Q-waves appear.
    – T waves may become tall and peaked in very early myocardial infarction. T waves are transient and last for a few hours only.
    – In contrast to transmural lesions, partial thickness or subendothelial infarction causes ST/T wave changes without Q-waves or prominent ST elevation.
    – Changes in the ECG are seen which evolve in pre-dictable fashion over next few days to weeks.
♦ *Blood test:*
  • *Plasma biochemical markers:*
    Myocardial infarction leads to detectable rise in the plasma concentration of various enzymes and proteins that are normally concentrated within the cardiac cells. Plasma enzymes (cardiac injury enzymes) are as follows:
    – Creatine kinase (CK).
    – Aspartate aminotransferase (AST).
    – Lactate dehydrogenase (LDH).
    – Myoglobin
    – Troponins (troponin I and troponin T)
  • Creatine kinase starts to rise at 4–6 hours and it peaks by about 12 hours and falls to normal in 48–72 hours. Myocardial isoenzyme of creatine kinase is more specific. It is useful for diagnosis of early myocardial infarction.
  • Aspartate aminotransferase (AST) starts to rise at about 12 hours and reaches a peak on the first or second day and returns on third and fourth day.
  • Lactate dehydrogenase (LDH) starts to rise after 12 hours, reaches a peak after 2–3 days and may remain elevated for a week. Rise in the value of LDH I (an isoenzyme of LDH) is a more sensitive indicator of myocardial infarction than total LDH. It is useful in diagnosis for patients who present several days after myocardial infarction.

- Cardiac troponins are cardiac troponin-T (cTn-T) and cardiac troponin-I (cTn-I). Sensitivity of troponins is similar to that of isoenzymes of creatine kinase. Moreover, cTn-T remains elevated for 100 to 200 hours after acute myocardial infarction and therefore, it may have particular utility in the evaluation of patients who present sufficiently long episode after the pain in chest.
  - Leukocytosis with a peak on first day.
  - ESR is raised which may remain raised for some days.
  - C-reactive protein is elevated.
- *Chest X-ray:* It can detect acute pulmonary edema or congestion. It is also helpful to detect pericardial effusion, cardiomegaly, etc.
- *Radionuclide scanning:* It shows site of necrosis and the extent of impairment of ventricular function.
- *Echocardiography:* This is done for regional wall motion abnormality and ejection fraction.

Treatment

Refer to Ans. 19 of same chapter.

Q.22. Write short note on angina pectoris.

(Mar 2000, 5 Marks)

Or

Describe clinical features, diagnosis and management of angina pectoris. *(Mar 2011, 4.5 Marks)*

Ans. Angina pectoris is a symptom complex caused by transient myocardial ischemia and constitutes a clinical syndrome rather than a disease.

Types

- Stable
- Unstable
- Nocturnal
- Prinzmetal's
- Postinfarction angina

Etiology

Acute myocardial ischemia occurs when myocardial oxygen demand exceeds supply in following:

- Coronary atherosclerotic narrowing (most cases).
- Non-atherosclerotic coronary artery disease—Coronary spasm, coronary thromboembolism, congenital anomalies, coronary vasculitis.
- Valvalar heart disease—Aortic stenosis and/or aortic regurgitation, mitral stenosis with pulmonary hypertension, mitral valve prolapse.
- Pulmonary hypertension.
- Systemic hypertension.
- Hypertrophic or dilated cardiomyopathy.
- Anemia—from tachycardia and reduction in O_2 availability.

Precipitating Causes

- Physical exertion
- Heavy metal
- Exposure to cold
- Emotion and excitement
- Hyperinsulinism in diabetic patients

- *Other causes:* Straining at stools, bathing, sexual intercourse, micturition.

Clinical Features

Symptoms

- *Anginal pain:*
  - *Site:* Most often over middle or lower sternum or over left precordium, at times in epigastrium. Sometimes discomfort is located only in left shoulder or left upper arm, occasionally in lower jaw and rarely in interscapular area.
  - *Radiation of pain:* May spread to right or left arm or both neck or jaw. Occasionally, pain starts in the wrist, upper arms or face and then spreads to the chest.
  - *Character:* Vice-like constriction or choking. Sometimes only pressure or burning pain, rarely mere weakness of one or both arms. An important characteristic is its constancy, the pain being steady while it lasts.
  - *Duration:* Most commonly 1 to 4 minutes. It may force patient to stop walking.
  - *Provocation:* By effort especially, such as walking against the wind or up a climb, hurrying after meals or unaccustomed exercise at times due to excitement anger, and fear. In advanced cases, pain is provoked by lying down (angina decubitus) or stooping.
  - Relief with sublingual nitroglycerine.
- *Dyspnea:* If it occurs before the pain suggests severe ventricular disease.
- *Other symptoms:*
  - Choking sensation in throat or feeling of impending doom.
  - Belching or passage of flatus or polyuria after an attack.
  - Dizziness, faintness or rarely syncope
  - If pain is severe sweating and nausea.

Signs

- At time, no signs are present.
- *Signs of LV dysfunction:* Atrial or third heart sound.
- Dysfunction of papillary muscle: It can lead to transient mitral regurgitation in case of ischemia.
- *Signs associated with risk factors:*
  - Hypertension.
  - Hyperlipidemia—Arcus senilis, xanthelasma, or cholesterol deposits along tendons and in skin of palms and buttocks.
  - Obesity
  - Diabetes and its accompaniments.
- *During the attack*—pallor and sweating with rise of BP often tachycardia. Pressure on carotid sinus may produce slowing of pulse and cessation of pain.

Diagnosis

Investigations

- *Resting ECG:* ECG changes of myocardial ischemia are reflected in ST-T waves. Occasionally, there is flattening of T waves in some lead in patient with angina.
- *Exercise ECG or stress test:* With continuous ECG monitoring and intermittent BP recording is performed with a treadmill

or bicycle ergometer. Standardized protocols are used (e.g. Bruce protocol), enabling performance to be assessed in same patient at different times and workload at onset of symptoms or ECG changes to be determined. An exercise ECG is abnormal, if there is horizontal or down-sloping ST segment depression of 0.1 mm or more in any lead.

♦ *Myocardial perfusion scintigraphy:* The isotope cardiovascular stress (usually thallium-201 or technetium—99m) is injected at peak exercise and images taken with a camera immediately or shortly after exercise and compared with rest images taken a few hours later following a second injection of tracer. Areas of myocardial ischemia are identified by reduced isotopic uptake in the same anatomical distribution stress images but not resting images (reversible defect).

♦ *Coronary angiography:* It is done before angioplasty or coronary bypass surgery.

Management

It is divided into three phases:
1. General measures.
2. Pharmacological treatment.
3. Invasive treatment.

General Measures

♦ Do not smoke
♦ Aim at ideal body weight
♦ Take regular exercise
♦ Avoid severe exertion, vigorous exercise and exercise in cold weather
♦ Take sublingual nitrate before taking exertion that may induce angina.

Pharmacological Treatment

Following agents are used with successful outcome.
♦ *Antiplatelet agents:*
   • Aspirin is used usually in dose of 75–150 mg daily.
   • Clopidogrel is used along with or without aspirin at dose of 75 mg daily.
♦ *Anti-anginal agents:*
   • Sublingual glyceroltrinitrat effectively abort anginal attack by causing coronary vasodilatation and reducing preload and cardiac output.
   • Beta-blockers improve cardiac efficiency and reduce oxygen consumption. Cardioselective agents, such as atenolol 25 to 50 mg, metoprolol 200 mg daily can be used.
   • Calcium-channel antagonists, i.e., amlodipine, lacidipine. They are the vasodilators and lowers myocardial oxygen demand by reducing blood pressure and myocardial contractility.
   • Potassium-channel opener, i.e., nicorandil has atrial and venous dilatation property which does not exhibit tolerance.

Invasive Treatment

♦ *Percutaneous coronary *intervention or percutaneous transluminal coronary *angioplasty is done.
♦ Coronary artery bypass grafting is done.

Q 22. *Percutaneous = Effected through skin
   *Intervention = One or more actions taken in order to modify an effect.
   *Angioplasty = Any endovascular procedure that reopens narrow blood vessels and restores forward blood flow.

Q.23. Describe briefly complete heart block.

(Feb 2014, 4 Marks)

Ans. Complete heart block is also known as third degree heart block or complete AV block.

Etiology

♦ *Congenital:*
   • Usually associated with ventricular septal defect, rarely isolated.
♦ *Acquired:*
   • Rheumatic heart disease
   • Acute infections—rheumatic fever, diphtheria
   • Drugs—digitalis, quinidine
   • Calcific aortic stenosis.
   • Trauma (penetrating).
   • Surgical procedures: After correction of ventricular septal defect, or following insertion of prosthetic valves or removal of hypertrophied septum in hypertrophic cardiomyopathy.
   • Cardiomyopathy (particularly infiltrative).
   • Syphilitic heart disease.
   • *Infiltrative masses:* Sarcoidosis, tubercles, abscesses from endocarditis, gummas, tumors, amyloidosis, hemochromatosis.
   • *Collagen diseases:* Rheumatoid arthritis, dermatomyositis.
   • *Fistulae:* Sinus of Valsalva aneurysm rupturing into right atrium.
   • *Unknown cause:* Idiopathic fibrosis.

Clinical Features

Symptoms

♦ *Due to low cardiac output:* Lassitude, fatigue, light headedness, and especially during exercise syncope. Symptoms of vertebrobasilar insufficiency and congestive heart failure may be precipitated.

♦ *Due to increased stroke volume:* Uncomfortable awareness of heart beat, or slow palpitation, if block is intermittent.

♦ *Due to transient circulatory arrest:* Stokes-Adams attacks — Symptoms depend on duration of standstill of circulation: About 5 seconds—giddiness and faintness, about 10 seconds—convulsions. Convulsions and incontinence may suggest epilepsy, but in transient asystole pallor is often striking, patient flushes during recovery, and consciousness is regained very rapidly; though some permanent impairment of cerebral function may occur after long or repeated episodes.

Signs

♦ *Slow and regular heart rate:* At 30 to 50 beats per minute, which does not usually increase significant with physical activity or exercise.

♦ *Raised Jugular venous pressure:* 'a' waves may be seen in the neck unrelated to ventricular beats.

♦ *Cannon waves:* Giant 'a' waves which are transmitted in the neck when the atrium contracts against a closed tricuspid valve.

- *Variation in intensity of first heart sound:* First heart sound is loudest when the interval between the preceding atrial beat and the ventricular beat is short, it is faintest when the interval is long. From time-to-time, there is a sharp accentuation of the first sound at the apex (cannon sound).
- *Tide pulse pressure:* Due to increased systolic pressure and low diastolic pressure. This gives rise to water hammer pulse and capillary pulsation.
- *Cardiac enlargement:* Due to increased stroke volume, hyperdynamic cardiac impulse.
- *Systolic ejection murmur:* Loudest in 2nd and 3rd left interspaces adjacent to the sternal edge, and due to increased velocity of blood flow associated with increased stroke volume.
- *Atrial sounds:* They may be heard in constant relation to first and second heart sounds.
- *Apical diastolic flow murmur:* It is occasional.
- *ECG:* There is no relation between atrial and ventricular complexes. The duration of QRS is normal.

Management

In Acute Complete AV Block

Acute onset of complete AV block occurs in acute myocardial infarction, i.e., in inferior myocardial infarction and anterior myocardial infarction.

Complete AV Block with Inferior Myocardial Infarction

- Complete AV block occurs usually in acute inferior wall infarction but are transient and less troublesome. No treatment is needed in such patients who are well and hemodynamically stable. If in such cases, clinical deterioration occurs, then atropine 0.6 mg IV can be given as a bolus and repeated, if necessary. If this treatment fails, then a temporary pacemaker may be inserted. In most of the patients, heart block disappears under 7–10 days.

Complete AV Block with Anterior Myocardial Infarction

- This occurs less commonly, is dangerous and carry poor prognosis. Asystole commonly occurs in such cases and lead to mortality. If patients develop asystole, atropine 0.6 mg IV given as bolus and repeated, if needed. Temporary pacemaker is inserted immediately. Isoprenaline infusion, i.e., 1 to 5 mg in 500 mL of 5% dextrose should be started at minimum rate to produce a satisfactory heart rhythm till temporary pacemaker is inserted.
- If block is due to drug toxicity, strictly stop the offending drug.

Chronic Complete AV block

A permanent pacemaker is indicated in patients having asymptomatic Mobitz type II complete heart block because it can improve their prognosis.

Q.24. Describe clinical features, investigation and treatment of left ventricular failure.

(Mar 2003, 15 Marks)

Or

Write short note on left ventricular failure.

(Jan 2012, 5 Marks)

Ans. Left ventricular failure is defined as failure to maintain an effective ventricular output for a given pulomonary venous or left atrial pressure or can do so only at the expense of an elevated left atrial filling pressure.

Causes

- *Left ventricular outflow obstruction:*
  - Systemic hypertension
  - Aortic valvular stenosis
  - Idiopathic hypertrophic subaortic stenosis
  - Coarctation of aorta
- *Left ventricular inflow obstruction:*
  - Mitral stenosis
  - Left atrial myxoma
  - Endomyocardial fibrosis with stiff left ventricle
- *Left ventricular volume overload:*
  - Mitral valve prolapsed
  - Mitral regurgitation
  - Aortic regurgitation (rheumatic and non-rheumatic)
  - Ventricular septal defect
  - Patent ductus arteriosus
  - High output states
  - Papillary muscle dysfunction
- *Reduced left ventricular contractility:*
  - Cardiomyopathy predominantly involving left ventricle
  - Anterior wall myocardial infarction
  - Left ventricle endocarditis

Clinical Features

- Progressive dyspnea is the earliest sign of left heart failure.
- Presence of orthopnea due to increase in venous return during recumbent position.
- Attacks of breathlessness which occur at night and awaken the patient, i.e., paroxysmal nocturnal dyspnea.
- In severe heart failure, there is a periodic respiration in which periods of hyperpnea alternate with apnea, i.e., Cheyne-Stokes respiration.
- Presence of dry cough which is disturbing.
- Presence of oliguria and nocturia.
- Presence of tachypnea because of stiff congested lungs and there is also presence of tachycardia because of hypoxia created due to pulmonary congestion.
- Presence of fatigue and weakness.
- Cerebral symptoms are present, i.e., altered mental state, difficulty in concentration, memory impairment, headache, insomnia and anxiety.

Physical Findings

- Extremities can be cold or pale.
- There is presence of tachycardia and rapid pulse rate.
- Presence of profuse sweating
- Presence of tachypnea, i.e., increased respiratory rate
- There is low pulse volume or pulsus alternans can be present.
- Presence of central cyanosis.
- Third heart sound can be heard.
- There is presence of basal pulmonary rales or crackles.
- Presence of an expiratory wheezing.
- Presence of oliguria.
- Hydrothorax or pleural effusion is present.
- Presence of anxiety and depression.

- Urine can be of high specific gravity and shows proteinuria.
- Presence of massive cardiomegaly.

Investigations

- *Electrocardiogram:*
  - Presence of left ventricular hypertrophy and left atrial hypertrophy in patients having aortic valvular diseases as well as mitral regurgitation.
  - Presence of ST-T changes in patients having disease of myocardium.
- *Chest X-ray:*
  - Presence of enlargement of cardiac shadow.
  - Presence of pulmonary venous congestion which extends from hilum to periphery.
  - There is presence of Kerley's lines because of interstitial edema.
- *Echocardiogram:*
  - Increase in the left ventricular dimensions
  - Left ventricular end diastolic pressure or volume of both can be high
  - Increase in the cardiac output and stroke volume
  - There is reduction in ejection fractions
- *Other test:* Monitor blood urea and other electrolytes.

Treatment

First aim of treatment is to find and remove the precipitating cause, i.e., arrhythmia or an intercurrent infection.

- Patient should be kept in sitting position, with legs hanging alongside of the bed, i.e., upright posture should be maintained.
- *Diet:* Salt-free diet is given till left ventricular failure improves and later on restricted salt diet is given.
- *Sedatives:* Morphine should be given in doses of 5 to 10 mg along with an anti-emetic, i.e., metoclopramide 10 mg IV and repeat the drug as soon as desired.
- *Oxygen:* About 60% of oxygen is given by facemask under positive pressure. It should be given as 6 to 8 lts/min through Wolfe's bottle.
- *Loop diuretics:* Furosemide 40–100 mg IV should be given.
- IV sodium nitroprusside 20–30 μg/min or IV nitroglycerine should be given in patients whose systolic blood pressure is more than 100 mm of Hg.
- *Digitalis:* If digoxin is not used previously, the three fourth of full dose, i.e., 0.5 to 1 mg is given as IV dose.
- *Bronchodilators:* At times, aminophylline or theophylline in dose of 250 to 500 mg IV decreases bronchoconstriction.
- In cases of severe left ventricular failure, inotropes can be given.
- If all the above measures failed, then rotating tourniquet should be applied to extrimities.
- *Intra-aortic balloon counterepulsation:* It is used in acute left ventricular failure during cardiac procedures or cardiac repairs.

Q.25. Discuss etiology, clinical features, diagnosis and management of acute myocardial infarction.

(Feb/Mar 2004, 20 Marks)

Or

Write etiology, clinical features, diagnosis and management of myocardial infarction.

(Aug 2018, 12 Marks)

Ans. Acute myocardial infarction is defined as irreversible damage to myocardium of heart as a result of occlusive thrombus due to rupture of atherosclerotic plaque in coronary artery.

Etiology

- The most important cause of myocardial infarction is coronary atherosclerosis.
- Obesity and hypertension
- Cigarette smoking
- Diabetes mellitus
- Sedentary life cycle (A life cycle involving little exercise, even of at least strenuous type)
- Dyslipidemia, i.e., increased levels of LDL.
- Hereditary susceptibility

For clinical features and diagnosis refer to Ans. 21 of same chapter.

For management refer to Ans. 19 of same chapter.

Q.26. Describe clinical diagnosis of subacute bacterial endocarditis. How will you confirm diagnosis?

(Sep 2005, 10 Marks)

Or

Write short note on diagnosis of infective endocarditis. *(Mar 2007, 5 Marks)*

Ans. For clinical diagnosis of subacute bacterial endocarditis, there is a criteria given by Duke, i.e., Duke's criteria.

Duke's Criteria for Clinical Diagnosis of SABE

Major Criteria

- *Blood culture:* Positive blood culture with typical infective endocarditis microorganisms (Viridans streptococci, *S. bovis*, HAECK group or community acquired *S. aureus* or enterococci)
- *Endocardial involvement:* New regurgitation murmur, positive ECG for SABE.

Minor Criteria

- Predisposing cardiac or IV drug abuse.
- Fever
- *Vascular phenomenon:* Emboli, mycotic aneurysms, petechiae
- Immunologic phenomenon: Glomerulonephritis and rheumatoid factor.
- *Echocardiogram:* Consistent with infective endocarditis, but not meeting major criteria.
- *Microbiology:* Positive blood cultures, but not meeting major criteria, serological evidence of active infection with possible microorganisms.

Confirmation of Diagnosis

The confirmation is of three types, i.e:

- *Definite:*
  - Pathology or bacteriology of vegetations.

    Or
  - Both major criteria

    Or

- One major and three minor criteria

  Or

- Five minor criteria

♦ *Possible:*

Neither definite nor rejected

♦ *Rejected:*

- Firm alternative diagnosis

  Or

- Resolution on less than four days of antibiotics.

Q.27. Write short note on malignant hypertension.

(Apr 2007, 5 Marks) (Feb 2002, 5 Marks)

Ans. Malignant hypertension is a complication of hypertension characterized by very elevated blood pressure and organ damage in eyes, brain, lung and kidneys.

It differs from other complication of hypertension in that it is accomplished by *papilledema.

Systolic and diastolic blood pressure are usually greater than 240 and 140 mm Hg.

Malignant hypertension is an hypertensive emergency.

Etiology

♦ Drugs, i.e., cocaine, beta-blockers and oral contraceptives
♦ Alcohol
♦ Atherosclerosis
♦ Chronic diabetes mellitus
♦ Renal failure.

Clinical Features

♦ Chest pain is present
♦ Dyspnea
♦ Neurological defect
♦ Angina and myocardial infarction
♦ Pulmonary edema
♦ Headache
♦ Cerebral hemorrhage or infarction
♦ Visual disturbance
♦ *Hypertensive encephalopathy
♦ Gastrointestinal symptoms, i.e., nausea and vomiting.
♦ Oliguria.

Diagnosis

♦ Complete blood count
♦ Coagulation profile
♦ Electrolyte profile
♦ Urine output and electrolytes
♦ TSH
♦ Renal function test
♦ Chest radiograph
♦ Head CT scan
♦ ECG to see ischemia and infarction.

Treatment

Since malignant hypertension is a medical emergency, it requires immediate treatment.

♦ Most effective agent for blood pressure reduction in an emergency is controlled IV infusion of sodium nitroprusside, i.e., 0.3 to 1.0 µg/kg/min.
♦ Alternatively diazoxide 300 mg IV or enalaprilat 1.25 mg IV is given rapidly and anti-hypertensive effect is noted under 1 to 3 min. The same dose is repeated when pressure begins to elevate.
♦ Chewing a nifedipine 10 mg capsule is often sufficient to give a graded reduction in blood pressure.
♦ Bed rest should be given to the patient.
♦ Sedation by IV diazepam is given.
♦ A potent diuretic, i.e., IV furosemide 40 mg stat can also be given.

Q.28. Describe the etiology, clinical features, complications and management of acute myocardial infarction.

(Sep 2008, 15 Marks)

Ans. Acute myocardial infarction is defined as irreversible damage to myocardium of heart as a result of occlusive thrombus due to rupture of atherosclerotic plaque in coronary artery.

Etiology

♦ The most important cause of myocardial infarction is atherosclerosis.
♦ Obesity and hypertension
♦ Cigarette smoking
♦ Diabetes mellitus
♦ Sedentary life cycle.
♦ Dyslipidemia.

For clinical features, refer to Ans. 21 of same chapter.

For complications, refer to Ans. 20 of same chapter.

For management, refer to Ans. 19 of same chapter.

Q.29. Write short note on prehypertension and its management.

(Sep 2008, 2.5 Marks)

Ans. Prehypertension is considered to be blood pressure readings with a systolic pressure from 120–139 mm Hg or a diastolic pressure from 80–89 mm Hg. Readings greater than or equal to 140/90 mm Hg are considered hypertension.

Symptoms

Prehypertension is often asymptomatic (without symptoms) at the time of diagnosis. Only extremely elevated blood pressure (malignant hypertension) can, in rare cases, cause headaches, visual changes, fatigue, or dizziness, but these are nonspecific symptoms which can occur with many other conditions. Thus, blood pressures above normal can go undiagnosed for a long period of time.

Management

Depending on one's blood pressure and risk factors for heart disease, one may only need to make a few lifestyle adjustments. Here are some strategies to help manage prehypertension:

♦ Lose weight, if one is overweight. Being overweight increases the risk of high blood pressure. However, losing

---

Q 27. *Papilledema = Edema and inflammation of the optic nerve at its point of entrance into retina.
     *Hypertensive encephalopathy = Headache, vomiting, seizure and change in mental status.

weight can lower high blood pressure. Studies show that modest weight loss can prevent hypertension by 20% in overweight people with prehypertension.

♦ *Exercise regularly:* Exercise helps to lose weight. Exercise also helps in lowering blood pressure.

♦ *Eat plenty of fruits, vegetables, whole grains, fish, and low-fat dairy:* Studies show high blood pressure can be lowered and prevented with the DASH diet. This diet is low in sodium and high in potassium, magnesium, calcium, protein, and fiber.

♦ *Cut back on dietary salt/sodium:* A diet high in sodium (salt) can increase blood pressure. A low-sodium diet can lower high blood pressure or prevent it. Aim for less than 2,300 milligrams of sodium daily (about 1 teaspoon of table salt).

♦ Eat foods low in saturated and trans fat and cholesterol. Diets high in saturated fat (meats and high-fat dairy), trans fat (some margarine, snack foods, and pastries) and cholesterol (organ meats, high-fat dairy, and egg yolks) may lead to obesity, heart disease, and cancer.

♦ *Eat a plant-based or vegetarian diet:* Add high-protein soy foods to your diet. Increase servings of fruits and vegetables by adding one serving at a time. You can add a serving of fruit at lunchtime. Then add a serving of vegetables at dinner.

♦ *Drink only in moderation:* Drinking excess alcohol can increase blood pressure. Limit drinking to not more than two drinks a day for men, and one drink a day for women.

Q.30. Write management of unstable angina pectoris.
(Mar 2011, 4 Marks)

Or

Write management of unstable angina.
(Mar 2013, 4 Marks)

Ans.

♦ To control acute disease and stabilize the thrombotic process:

♦ Hospitalization—to facilitate rapid adjustments in therapy which are usually required.

♦ Oxygen administration and sedation.

♦ Therapy with beta blockers and calcium antagonists.

♦ Sublingual nitrates for immediate relief.

♦ IV nitrates—IV Nitroglycerin 3–10 µg/min if patient does not settle on above therapy. IV nitrates produce hypotension and regular BP measurements are required and dose is increased.

♦ Aspirin 325 mg. OD and Clopidogrel 75 mg/day or Prasugrel 10 mg/day.

♦ Anticoagulation with heparin. Dose 60 U/kg IV bolus followed by 12 U/kg/hr infusion. Low molecular heparin superior to unfractionated heparin in dose of 1 mg/kg 12 hourly subcutaneous.

♦ Glycoprotein IIb/IIIa receptor inhibitors—which block the receptors that lead to platelet aggregation
- Eptifibatide 180 µg/kg IV bolus followed by 2 µg/kg/min. infusion.
- Tirofiban 0.4 pg/kg/min over 30 mins, followed by 0.1 µg/min. infusion.
- Abciximab 0.25 mg/kg IV bolus followed by 0.125 µg/kg/min. infusion.

♦ Long-term management of underlying coronary artery disease—with revascularization procedures.

Q.31. Describe types, etiology, sign, symptoms, investigations and outline treatment of infective endocarditis.
(Jan 2012, 12 Marks)

Or

Write short note on infective endocarditis.
(Dec 2010, 5 Marks)

Or

Describe risk factors clinical features, diagnosis and treatment of infective endocarditis.
(Apr 2015, 8 Marks)

Or

Discuss etiology, clinical feature and treatment of infective endocarditis.
(May 2018, 5 Marks)

Or

Discuss etiology, clinical features and treatment of infective endocarditis.
(Apr 2019, 5 Marks)

Ans. Infective endocarditis is an illness caused by microbial infection of the cardiac endothelial surface.

Types

♦ *Acute bacterial endocarditis:* Caused by virulent organisms and run its course over days to weeks.

♦ *Subacute bacterial endocarditis:* Caused by organisms of low virulence and run its course over weeks to months.

♦ *Non-bacterial thrombotic endocarditis:* Sterile vegetations occur in this type.

♦ *Surgical endocarditis:* May follow any type of surgery and is caused by *Staphylococcus epidermidis.*

Etiology

Generally, the microorganisms attack an already damaged heart. The microorganisms responsible are *Streptococcus viridans, S. faecalis* and *Staphylococcus aureus.* Below given are all the heart defects which lead to infective endocarditis.

Relatively High Risk

♦ Prosthetic heart valves.
♦ Aortic valve disease
♦ Mitral regurgitation + stenosis
♦ Congenital heart disease
♦ Previous infective endocarditis.

Intermediate Risk

♦ Mitral valve prolapse
♦ Mitral stenosis
♦ Tricuspid valve disease
♦ Pulmonary valve disease
♦ Asymmetrical septal hypertrophy
♦ Calcific aortic sclerosis
♦ Non-valvular intracardiac prosthetic implants

Very Low Risk

♦ Atrial septal defect
♦ Atherosclerotic plaques

♦ Postmyocardial infarction thrombi, atrial thrombi and ventricular aneurysms
♦ Syphilitic aortitis
♦ Cardiac pacemakers
♦ Surgically corrected cardiac lesions (without prosthetic implants)

Signs

♦ **Signs of infection:**
  • *Fever:* Variable, low grade.
  • *Anemia:* Yellow muddy discoloration of skin.
  • *Clubbing:* of fingers and toes occurs early.
  • *Splenomegaly:* after about 6 weeks of illness. Sudden enlargement with tenderness and rub if infarction of spleen. Rarely gross splenomegaly.
  • *Arthralgia:* Sudden transient pain in joints without any effusion.
♦ **Cardiac signs:**
  Murmur:
  • *Organic heart murmur:* due to valvular defect or congenital cardiovascular lesions.
  • *Development of new murmurs:* due to perforation of ventricular septum, rupture of sinus of Valsalva, acute mitral regurgitation or acute aortic regurgitation.
  • *Absence of murmur:*
    – Endocarditis involving mural thrombus complicating healed myocardial infarction.
    – Early acute endocarditis involving previously normal valve.
    – Tricuspid endocarditis when it exists, may be murmur free.
  • Cardiac failure—may occur due to toxic myocarditis.
♦ **Systemic embolism:**
  • *Arterial:*
    – Cerebral producing hemiplegia or mycotic aneurysms which may subsequently rupture.
    – Renal causing colic and hematuria.
    – Retinal with disturbing vision.
    – Of mesenteric arteries causing acute abdominal pain; splenic infarction with sudden local pain and perhaps friction.
    – Peripheral vessel resulting in gangrene of an extremity. Early prosthetic valve endocarditis.
  • *Pulmonary:* Recurrent pneumonitis (infective emboli cause abscesses) and arterial rupture.
♦ **Immunological:**
  • *Thenar and hypothenar eminences:*
    – *Osler's nodes:* Tender, pea-sized nodules on pads of fingers and toes. Often pale in the center
    – May occur in crops. Fade after few days usually without breaking down or leaving any residue.
    – Either due to minute emboli in superficial terminal vessels or due to vasculitis.
    – *Laneway lesions:* Large nontender macules on palms and soles.

• *Skin and mucous membranes:*
  – Petechial hemorrhages in palpebral conjunctivae, buccal and pharyngeal mucous membrane.
  – *Subungual:* Splinter hemorrhages
  – *Finger and toe tips:* Osler's nodes
  – *Retina-Roth spots:* Lesions with a white center and red edge. Boat-shaped hemorrhage
  – *Renal:* Glomerulonephritis leading to kidney failure.

Symptoms

♦ Patient with a known cardiac ailment may start complaining of vague ill health, fatigue, weakness and a low-grade fever.
♦ There is presence of pain and marked aches all over the body.

Investigations

♦ *Blood cultures:* In absence of recent or concurrent antibiotic therapy, the first 3 random blood cultures (2–4 hours apart) are positive in most patients, and blood culture is positive by third day in 90%.
♦ *Urine:* Microscopic hematuria most common finding. Slight albuminuria and hyaline and granular casts also found.
♦ *Hematology:* Normocytic. normochromic anemia, usually mild. May be raised ESR and raised C-reactive protein.
♦ *Chest radiograph:* May be diagnostic in right-sided endocarditis, with multiple shadows visible due to an embolic pneumonia.
♦ *ECG:* Myocardial infarction seen on ECG may be due to coronary embolism, and a conduction defect may be due to development of an aortic root abscess.
♦ *Echocardiography:* Higher sensitivity in identifying vegetation with Transesophageal echocardiography as compared to transthoracic echocardiography. (a) *Vegetations:* An echodense structure attached to the valve or its supporting structures, or lying in the track of a turbulent jet, which is irregular in shape. (b) Leaflet perforation is best seen as regurgitant jet on color flow mapping. (c) Annular and periprosthetic echolucent spaces (abscesses) and fistula formation.
♦ *Chest X-ray:* Shows evidence of cardiomegaly and heart failure.

Treatment

For treatment refer to Ans. 8 of same chapter.

Q.32. Describe etiology, diagnostic criteria, complications and management of rheumatic fever.

(Feb 2013, 12 Marks)

Ans. *For etiology refer to Ans. 1 of same chapter.*
For diagnostic criteria refer to Ans. 3 of same chapter.
For management refer to Ans. 2 of same chapter

Complications

Inflammation caused by rheumatic fever may last for a few weeks to several months. In some cases, the inflammation may cause long-term complications.

Rheumatic heart disease is permanent damage to the heart caused by the inflammation of rheumatic fever. Problems are most common with the valve between the two left chambers of the heart (mitral valve), but the other valves may be affected.

The damage may result in one of the following conditions:

♦ *Valve stenosis:* This condition is a narrowing of the valve, which results in decreased blood flow.
♦ *Valve regurgitation:* This condition is a leak in the valve, which allows blood to flow in the wrong direction.

♦ *Damage to heart muscle:* The inflammation associated with rheumatic fever can weaken the heart muscle, resulting in poor pumping function.

Damage to the mitral valve, other heart valves or other heart tissues can cause problems with the heart later in life.

Resulting conditions may include:

♦ Atrial fibrillation, an irregular and chaotic beating of the upper chambers of the heart (atria).
♦ Heart failure, an inability of the heart to pump enough blood to the body.

Q.33. Write the difference between cardiac and non-cardiac chest pains. *(Nov 2011, 4 Marks)*
Ans.

Features	Cardiac Chest Pain	Non-cardiac Chest Pain
Nature of pain	Pain is dull, constricting, choking and/or crushing	Pain may vary from burning to sharp, stabbing and prickling
Location	Pain is usually central (towards the center of the chest) and fanning outwards (diffuse)	Pain is usually localized—located at only one spot which can be clearly pinpointed by the patient
Radiation of pain	Pain radiates to the jaw, neck, shoulder, arms (either one or even both) or back	There may not often be any radiation of the pain
Precipitating factors	Exertion or emotion, large meal or even extremes of temperature, particularly cold, can trigger or exacerbate the pain	Spontaneous although it may be exacerbated by exertion, Changes in posture, deep or rapid breathing or pressure may also exacerbate the pain
Pain-relieving factors Signs and symptoms	Pain is relieved by rest and responds quickly to nitrates. • Severe shortness of breath—patient may report a feeling of suffocation • Dizziness • Fainting spells ('blackouts')	Not relieved significantly by rest, at all • Gastrointestinal: Bloating, belching, nausea vomiting and/or regurgitation • Respiratory: Shallow breathing, persistent cough, abnormal breathing sounds, difficulty breathing when lying flat, expectorating mucus or coughing up blood. (Refer to Lung Chest Pain) • Musculoskeletal: Limited range of motion, cannot tolerate pressure on the affected area • Psychological: Weepy, depressed, excited, agitated, fearful

Q.34. **Give definition, etiology, sign and symptoms, investigation and treatment of congestive cardiac failure.** *(Feb 2013, 12 Marks)*

Or

Write clinical features, investigations and treatment of congestive cardiac failure. *(Jan 2016, 12 Marks)*

Or

Write short note on congestive cardiac failure.
(Mar 2006, 10 Marks) (May/June 2009, 5 Marks)

Or

Write sign and symptoms of congestive cardiac failure. *(Jan 2012, 5 Marks)*

Or

Describe in brief congestive cardiac failure.
(Mar 2016, 4 Marks)

Ans. It is defined as a pathophysiologic state when heart is not able to maintain its cardiac output to meet the demands of metabolizing tissues or can do so only at the expense of elevating filling pressures.

In congestive cardiac failure, patient has features of both right- and left-sided heart failure.

Etiology

Left-sided Failure

♦ *Myocardial damage:*
  • Myocardial infarction
  • Myocarditis
  • Cardiomyopathy
  • Cardiac depressant drugs
♦ *Increased load:*
  • Hypertension
  • Mitral and aortic valve disease
  • Cardiac arrhythmias
  • Over transfusion

Right-sided Failure

- *Pulmonary hypertension:*
  - Secondary to left heart failure
  - Chronic lung disease
  - Pulmonary embolism
  - Left-to-right shunts.
- Primary pulmonary hypertension.
- Right ventricular infarction.
- Pulmonary and tricuspid valve disease
- Isolated right ventricular cardiomyopathy.

Signs and Symptoms/Clinical Features

Left-sided Failure

- Common respiratory signs are tachypnea (increased rate of breathing) and increased work of breathing (nonspecific signs of respiratory distress). Rales or crackles, heard initially in the lung bases, and when severe, throughout the lung fields suggest the development of pulmonary edema (fluid in the alveoli). Cyanosis which suggests severe hypoxemia, is a late sign of extremely severe pulmonary edema.
- Additional signs indicating left ventricular failure include a laterally displaced apex beat (which occurs, if the heart is enlarged) and a gallop rhythm (additional heart sounds) may be heard as a marker of increased blood flow, or increased intracardiac pressure. Heart murmurs may indicate the presence of valvular heart disease, either as a cause (e.g. aortic stenosis) or as a result (e.g. mitral regurgitation) of the heart failure.
- Backward failure of the left ventricle causes congestion of the pulmonary vasculature, and so the symptoms are predominantly respiratory in nature.
- Patient will have dyspnea (shortness of breath) on exertion and in severe cases, dyspnea at rest.
- Increasing breathlessness on lying flat, called orthopnea, occurs. It is often measured in the number of pillows required to lie comfortably, and in severe cases, the patient may resort to sleeping while sitting up.
- Another symptom of heart failure is paroxysmal nocturnal dyspnea a sudden night time attack of severe breathlessness, usually several hours after going to sleep.
- Easy fatigability and exercise intolerance are also common complaints related to respiratory compromise.
- Cardiac asthma or wheezing may occur.
- Compromise of left ventricular forward function may result in symptoms of poor systemic circulation, such as dizziness, confusion and cool extremities at rest.

Right-sided Failure

- Physical examination may reveal pitting peripheral edema, ascites, and hepatomegaly.
- Jugular venous pressure is frequently assessed as a marker of fluid status, which can be accentuated by eliciting hepatojugular reflux.
- Backward failure of the right ventricle leads to congestion of systemic capillaries. This generates excess fluid accumulation in the body. This causes swelling under the skin (termed peripheral edema or anasarca) and usually affects the dependent parts of the body first (causing foot and ankle swelling in people who are standing up, and sacral edema in people who are predominantly lying down).
- Nocturia (frequent night time urination) may occur when fluid from the legs is returned to the bloodstream while lying down at night.
- In progressively severe cases, ascites (fluid accumulation in the abdominal cavity causing swelling) and hepatomegaly (enlargement of the liver) may develop.
- Significant liver congestion may result in impaired liver function, and jaundice and even coagulopathy (problems of decreased blood clotting) may occur.

Investigation

- *Electrocardiogram (ECG)*: This will reveal arrhythmias, ventricular hypertrophy and myocardial ischemia.
- *Chest X-ray*: This will show enlargement of heart, peripheral lung congestion, presence of Kerley's lines, pulmonary edema, hydrothorax, pulmonary hypertension, double atrial shadow in mitral valve disease and calcification of valves.
- *Echocardiogram*: In this, ultrasound is used to image the heart muscle, valve structures, and blood flow patterns. The echocardiogram is very helpful in diagnosing heart muscle weakness. In addition, the test can suggest possible causes for the heart muscle weakness (for example, prior heart attack, and severe valve abnormalities). Virtually all patients in whom the diagnosis of congestive heart failure is suspected should ideally undergo echocardiography early in their assessment.
- Nuclear medicine studies assess the overall pumping capability of the heart and examine the possibility of inadequate blood flow to the heart muscle.
- *BNP or B-type natriuretic peptide level:* This level can vary with age and gender but is typically elevated from heart failure and can aid in the diagnosis, and can be useful in following the response to treatment of congestive heart failure.
- *Blood urea and electrolytes:* It is done for hypokalemia, hyponatremia and renal failure,

Treatment

- *Rest:* Complete bed rest is the key stone of management. When the patient is dyspneic, bed rest is given with the head end of bed raised to 45°. The legs should be kept below the pelvis to prevent the fluid present in legs to return to vascular system and precipitate pulmonary edema.
- *Diet:* Basic aim is to restrict sodium in the diet. Quantity of salt intake per day should not exceed 0.5 g. Salt substitutes may be used to make diet more palatable.
- *Diuretics:* In cardiac failure, there is always sodium and water retention. Hence, diuretics are given to increase sodium extraction. Furosemide 40–80 mg orally produces effect in 4–6 hours and on IV administration of furosemide 40–100 mg produces its effect in 20 minutes. Spironolactone which is potassium sparing diuretic is given 25 mg orally 4 times a day which removes the symptoms, such as hypokalemia due to action of furosemide. Triamterene or amiloride hydrochloride is given along with spironolactone.

◆ *Digitalis:* It increases the force of myocardial contraction and decreases work of heart. The commonly used drug is digoxin which is administered orally 0.25 mg BD. For rapid digitalization digoxin 0.5–0.75 mg is given slow IV over a period of 5–10 minutes under electrocardiographic control.

◆ *Sympathomimetic amines:* Dopamine at low doses of 3–5 µg/kg/min increases contractility of heart.

◆ *Vasodilators:* Sodium nitroprusside in the dose of 5–10 µg/min have balance dilator effect. Besides this hydralazine, nitrates and ACE inhibitors are used.

◆ *Inodilator levosimendan:* This is a calcium channel sensitizer. It has positive inotropic and vasodilator effect. It is given IV with loading dose of 6–12 µg/kg/min over 10 min followed by infusion 0.05 to 2 µg/kg/min infusion.

◆ *Oxygen:* It is given via Woulfe's bottle at rate of 5–8 L/min.

◆ *Miscellaneous drugs:* Tranquilizers, such as diazepam 2 to 5 mg TDS are given to reduce anxiety.

◆ *Cardiac re-synchronization therapy or biventricular pacing:* It is used in patients with symptomatic refractory cardiac failure with conduction abnormality or Left Bundle Branch Block. This therapy involves pacing the right atrium, right ventricle and left ventricle to improve synchrony of the cardiac chambers.

◆ Left ventricular assist device: Devices, such as intra-aortic balloon pump, Impella device, heart-mate, thoracic are considered when medical management fails. They are usually used as a bridge to cardiac transplant.

Q.35. Write on management of cardiac arrest.

(Feb 2013, 6 Marks)

Ans. Cardiac arrest is defined as sudden failure of heart resulting in inadequate cerebral circulation.

Management

◆ **Basic life support or basic cardiac life support**

Maintain the airway, breathing and circulation simultaneously as rapidly as possible as follows:

• *Airway:* Airway must be patent. If any of the foreign body is suspected, the patient must be rolled on one side and 4–5 forceful blows must be delivered rapidly between the shoulder blades with the heel of the hand. Now keep the patient in supine position and abdominal thrusts in an upward direction are given to the patient just below the xiphisternum. After the foreign body is excluded, patient should be kept in supine position as he may require external cardiac massage and artificial respiration. The patient's head should be lifted with one hand under the neck and the other hand pressing the forehead so that the head is tilted backwards to keep the upper airway patent.

• Breathing: Once the patency of airway is maintained, and if breathing is inadequate, artificial ventilation must be given. With the above position, the patient's nostrils must be sealed with thumb and index finger and mouth-to-mouth respiration must be given to the patient.

This is done by taking a deep inspiration and exhaling in the patient's mouth and then the patient is allowed to exhale passively. Continue this procedure at the rate of 16–18/min. In hospitals, an Ambu bag is used.

• *Circulation:* With the patient in supine position, neck extended and legs elevated a sudden sharp thrust is given on the chest wall. This may restore the effective beating of the heart especially, if the cardiac arrest is due to cardiac standstill. In absence of response, external cardiac massage is given.

◆ **Advanced Cardiac Life Support (ACLS)**

As the basic life support is maintained an ECG must be taken to determine whether the cause of cardiac arrest is ventricular asystole or ventricular fibrillation.

• If it is ventricular asystole, while electric methods of treatment like external cardiac pacemaker are made available, the following drugs are given;

– *Epinephrine (Adrenaline):* 1 mL of 1:1000 epinephrine is given intravenous followed by a bolus of dextrose.

– *Calcium:* 10 mL calcium gluconate 10% is injected IV or sometimes intracardiac. It is rarely used.

– *Sodium bicarbonate:* 10 mL of 7.5% sodium bicarbonate is infused slowly intravenously to correct metabolic acidosis. This is also rarely used.

– *Vasopressors:* Nor-epinephrine 1:1000 is initially given in the dose of 2 mL and later repeated, if hypotension persists.

• If it is ventricular fibrillation the following drugs are used in addition:

– *Lignocaine:* 50–100 mg is injected intravenously as a bolus and may be repeated after 15–20 min.

– *Propranolol:* 5–10 mg may be given intravenously as an antiarrhythmic agent.

– *Bretylium tosylate:* It is given as 5 to 10 mg/kg IV

◆ **Specific measures**

• *For ventricular asystole:* If cardiac arrest persists in spite of the above measures, external cardiac pacing is done. If this is negative or required for a long period, internal cardiac pacemaker is inserted.

• *For ventricular fibrillation:* If the above drugs do not immediately revert the cardiac rhythm, or if ventricular fibrillation is recurrent in spite of the above measures a direct current (DC) shock is given to the heart with 200 joules. It should be repeated, if required after a few minutes with 300 V Joules and then up to 400 Joules.

◆ **Management after successful resuscitation in an unconscious patient**

• Endotracheal intubation with controlled ventilation should be continued with the help of a ventilator to keep the partial pressure of oxygen at 100 mm Hg and partial pressure of carbon dioxide at 30–40 mm Hg.

• Blood pressure must be maintained at 10 mm Hg systolic, if required with the help of vasopressors like dopamine.

• Acid-base and fluid electrolyte balance should be maintained.

- Mannitol 350 to 500 mL IV or dexamethasone 4 mg 6 to 8 hourly IV should be given in presence of cerebral edema.
- Phenytoin sodium, diazepam or phenobarbitone should be given if there are convulsions.
- Aspiration pneumonia should be prevented by appropriate antibiotics.

Q.36. **Write in brief sign, symptoms and treatment of rheumatic fever.** *(Apr 2008, 5 Marks)*

Or

Write signs and symptoms of acute rheumatic fever.
(Dec 2010, 5 Marks)

Ans. It is an acute, recurrent, inflammatory disease mainly of children typically occurring 1 to 5 weeks after Group A streptococcal infection.

Symptoms

- Pyrexia of unknown origin.
- Arthralgia, i.e., pain in joints. Pain in joints is fleeting and migratory.

Signs

Carditis

- It is pancarditis involving endocardium, myocardium and pericardium.
- It manifests as breathlessness, palpitation and chest pain. tachycardia, cardiomegaly and new or change murmurs.
- Aortic regurgitation in 50% cases.
- Pericarditis produces frictional rub and pericardial tenderness.
- Cardiac failure due to myocardial infarction.

Sydenham's Chorea

- Late neurological manifestations that occurs at least three months after the episode of acute rheumatic fever when all signs disappear.
- More common in female.
- It is characterized by involuntary dancing movements of hands, feet or face.

Arthritis

- Early feature of illness and is nonspecific.
- It is characterized by acute painful symmetric and migratory inflammation of large joints.

Erythema Marginatum

Red macules which fade in center but remain red at the edges and occur mainly on trunk and proximal extremities on face.

Subcutaneous Nodules

- They are small, dense and firm and painless and are best felt over tendons and bones.
- Nodules appear more than 3 weeks after onset of other manifestations.

Respiratory

Epistaxis is an atypical manifestation.

Gastrointestinal

Mild gastroenteritis is present. Repeated vomiting spells are present.

Treatment

Refer to Ans. 1 of same chapter.

Q.37. **Write in brief sign, symptoms and treatment of hypertension.** *(May/June 2009, 5 Marks)*

Ans. Hypertension refers to increase in the blood pressure.

Symptoms

- *General:* Presence of headache, dizziness, palpitation and easy fatigability
- *Symptoms referable to systemic vascular involvement:*
  - Epistaxis
  - Hematuria
  - Blurring of vision or sudden blindness
  - Dyspnea on exertion
  - Anginal chest pain
  - Palpitations
  - Transient ischemic episodes leading to weakness or paralysis
  - Hypertensive encephalopathy
  - Tinnitus
  - Syncope
- *Symptoms related to underlying disease:*
  - Edema and puffy face due to acute nephritis
  - Weight gain, hirsutism, truncal obesity due to Cushing's syndrome
  - Weight loss, tremors, palpitation and sweating due to hyperthyroidism or pheochromocytoma
  - Joint pain, bronchospasm and peripheral vascular disease symptoms due to polyarteritis nodosa.

Signs

- Moon's face, buffalo hump and truncal obesity in Cushing's syndrome.
- Presence of puffy face, rough skin, obesity in myxedema
- Tremors, tachycardia, exophthalmos, thyroid dermopathy and goiter in hyperthyroidism
- Prognathism, clubbed hand, coarse features in acromegaly
- Palpable kidney lump in polycystic kidney
- Bruit over abdominal aorta.
- Undiagnosed fever and recurrent urinary infections in chronic pyelonephritis.

Treatment

Refer to Ans. 18 of same chapter.

Q.38. **Describe the definition, etiology, clinical features, diagnostic criteria and management of acute rheumatic fever.** *(Dec 2009, 15 Marks)*

Or

Discuss, etiology, clinical features, diagnostic criteria and management of acute rheumatic fever.
(Dec 2009, 15 Marks)

Or

Write short note on clinical features and management of acute rheumatic fever. *(Jan 2019, 7 Marks)*

Or

Describe in detail about acute rheumatic fever.

(Oct 2019, 6 Marks)

Ans. *For definition refer to Ans. 36. For etiology refer to Ans. 1 of same chapter. For clinical features refer to Ans. 2 of same chapter. For diagnostic criteria and management refer to Ans. 3 of same chapter.*

Q.39. Write short note on congenital heart disease.

(Jun 2010, 5 Marks)

Ans. Congenital heart diseases are the abnormalities of heart and great vessels due to defective development in the prenatal period.

Classification

- ♦ **Acyanotic:**
  - *Acyanotic with left to right shunt:*
    - Atrial septal defect (ASD)
    - Ventricular septal defect (VSD)
    - Patent ductus arteriosus
    - Aorto-pulmonary window
    - Common complete atrio-ventricular canal.
  - *Acyanotic without shunt:*
    - Pulmonary stenosis
    - Endocardial cushion effects
    - Aortic stenosis
    - Coarctation of aorta.
- ♦ **Cyanotic:**
  - Complete transposition of great vessels
  - Persistent truncus arteriosus
  - Tetralogy of Fallot
  - Ebstein's anomaly with right-to-left shunt
  - Common atrium.

Etiology

- ♦ *Patent ductus arteriosus:* Maternal cause, Patau's syndrome
- ♦ *Atrial septal defect:* Rubella virus, Noonan's syndrome, Holt-Oram syndrome, Down syndrome, Patau's syndrome,
- ♦ *Ventricular septal defect:* Alcohol, Holt-Oram syndrome, Down's syndrome, Edward's syndrome.
- ♦ *Tricuspid atresia:* Alcohol
- ♦ *Fallot's Tetralogy:* Down's syndrome, lesions associated with 22q11 deletions.

Features of Various Congenital Heart Diseases

- ♦ Central cyanosis and digital clubbing is present in transposition of great vessels and tetralogy of Fallot.
- ♦ Growth retardation as well as intellectual impairment is present in all congenital heart diseases.
- ♦ Syncope is present in severe right or left ventricular outflow tract obstruction.
- ♦ Short stature is commonly seen in patients with congenital heart disease.

Q.40. Describe JNC VII criteria for hypertension. Write in brief investigations and outline treatment.

(Aug 2011, 15 Marks)

Ans. JNC VII criterias is the 7th report of the Joint National Committee on Prevention Detection, Evaluation and Treatment of High Blood Pressure.

JNC VII Criteria for Hypertension

Category	Systolic Pressure (mm Hg)	Diastolic Pressure (mm Hg)
Normal	<120	<80
Pre-hypertension	120–139	80–89
Hypertension Stage1	140–159	90–99
Stage 2	>160	>100

Hypertension should be based on average of two or more readings taken at each of two or more visits after initial reading.

Investigations

- ♦ **Routine tests:**
  - *Urinalysis:* Detection of proteinuria and microscopic hematuria may indicate some degree of renal arteriolar necrosis and nephrosclerosis, or underlying intrinsic renal disease, such as polycystic kidneys, chronic pyelonephritis or glomerulonephritis.
  - *Serum biochemistry:* High sodium and low potassium may suggest primary hyperaldosteronism.
  - *Urea and creatinine:* High levels suggest a degree of renal impairment due to hypertension, or that underlying renal disease is the cause for hypertension.
  - *Lipid and glucose concentrations:* To judge cardiovascular risk status for each patient.
  - *ECG:* Detection of left ventricular hypertrophy and strain pattern is an important adverse prognostic indicator.
- ♦ **Special tests:**
  - Intravenous pyelogram and renal ultrasound, if renal disease is present.
  - Renal arteriography for renal artery stenosis
  - Plasma rennin activity and aldosterone for Conn syndrome
  - Angiography / MRI for coarctation of aorta.

Treatment

For treatment refer to Ans. 18 of same chapter.

Q.41. Describe etiology, clinical features and management of coronary artery disease. *(Jan 2012, 15 Marks)*

Ans. Coronary artery diseases are also known as ischemic heart disease.

Coronary Artery Diseases

- ♦ Angina pectoris
- ♦ Acute myocardial infarction
- ♦ Sudden cardiac death.

Etiology of Coronary Artery Diseases

- ♦ Atherosclerotic coronary artery disease
- ♦ *Other coronary artery diseases:*
  - Coronary artery spasm
  - Coronary arteritis
  - Embolism
  - Coronary AV malformation
- ♦ *Valvular diseases:*
  - Aortic stenosis and regurgitation
  - Mitral valve prolapse

♦ *Other cardiac diseases:*
- Hypertrophic cardiomyopathy
- Collagen disease
- Syphilis

♦ *Increased demands:*
- Thyrotoxicosis
- Anemia
- Beriberi

Clinical Features

♦ *Angina pectoris: Refer to Ans. 22 of same chapter.*
♦ *Acute myocardial infarction: Refer to Ans. 21 of same chapter*
♦ *Sudden cardiac arrest:* In this, a person with good health fall ill and die suddenly within minutes and few hours.
- Absence of pulses
- On auscultation, cardiac impulse is not present.
- Extremities are cold
- Cessation of respiration of patient
- Blood pressure is not measurable.

Management

♦ *Angina pectoris: Refer to Ans. 22 of same chapter.*
♦ *Acute myocardial infarction: Refer to Ans. 19 of same chapter.*
♦ *Sudden cardiac arrest: Refer to Ans. 47 of same chapter.*

Q.42. Write classification of rheumatic heart diseases and discuss the sign and symptoms of mitral stenosis.

(Aug 2012, 15 Marks)

Ans.

Classification of Rheumatic Heart Diseases

Based on the severity of rheumatic heart disease.

Priority 1 (Severe)	Severe valvular disease Or Moderate/severe valvular lesion with symptoms Or Mechanical prosthetic valves, tissue prosthetic valves and valve repairs including balloon valvuloplasty
Priority 2 (Moderate)	Any moderate valve lesion in the absence of symptoms and with normal left ventricular function Or Mild mitral regurgitation PLUS mild aortic stenosis Or Mild or moderate mitral or aortic stenosis Or Any pulmonary or tricuspid valve lesion coexisitng with a left-sided valve lesion
Priority 3 (Mild)	Acute rheumatic fever with no evidence of rheumatic heart disease Or Trivial to mild valvular disease
Priority 4 (Inactive)	Patient with the history of acute rheumatic fever (no rheumatic heart disease) for whom secondary prophylaxis has been ceased

Sign and Symptoms of Mitral Stenosis

Symptoms

♦ Patient complains of breathlessness and fatigue on exertion.
♦ Progression of stenosis lead to dyspnea on rest and even have orthopnea and paroxysmal nocturnal dyspnea.
♦ Acute pulmonary edema can also occur.
♦ Hemoptysis can be present due to rupture of pulmonary congestion and pulmonary embolism and cough due to pulmonary congestion.
♦ Chest pain is present due to pulmonary venous hypertension.

Signs

♦ Atrial fibrillation is present.
♦ *Auscultation:* Presence of loud first heart sound, opening snap and mid diastolic low-pitched rumbling murmur best heard at the apex.
♦ *Signs of raised pulmonary capillary pressure:* Pleural effusion, Crepitation, pulmonary edema.
♦ *Signs of pulmonary hypertension:* RV heave, Loud P_2
♦ *Others:* Basal crackles, ascites and pleural effusion

Q.43. Write management of atrial fibrillation.

(Dec 2012, 4 Marks)

Ans. It is the most common sustained tachyarrhythmia seen in patients.

Management

♦ Ventricular rate is reduced by giving digoxin. Digoxin 0.5 mg IV slowly is given. After this, patient is kept on oral digitalis therapy, i.e., 0.25 mg twice daily.
♦ Antiarrhythmic drugs, such as propranolol is given IV at a rate of 1 mg every 5 min followed by maintenance of oral dose of 20–40 mg three times a day.
♦ Underlying causes, such as thyrotoxicosis and acute chest infections should be treated to maintain normal sinus rhythm.
♦ Anticoagulant therapy should be given in patients with chronic atrial fibrillation.
♦ Defibrillation should be done. A DC shock of 100 joules restore normal sinus rhythm.

Q.44. Write short note on PTCA. *(Nov 2014, 3 Marks)*

Ans. Percutaneous transluminal coronary angioplasty (PTCA) is a minimally invasive procedure to open up blocked coronary arteries, allowing blood to circulate unobstructed to the heart muscle.

♦ In PTCA, balloon dilatation of coronary stenosis is done.

Method

Procedure of doing PTCA is commenced by passing a guide wire under fluoroscopic control, this wire positions the balloon dilatation center at level of stenosis, now balloon dilatation of the stenotic segment is carried out for maintaining the circulation all through.

Indications

♦ This method provides complete or partial revascularization in cases of stable angina pectoris, unstable angina pectoris or myocardial infarction.

♦ It is indicated in patients with recurrent angina after coronary artery bypass grafting (CABG).

Complications

♦ Blood vessel occlusion can occur by thrombosis.
♦ Recurrent angina pectoris
♦ Restenosis can occur.

Q.45. Describe risk factors, clinical features, diagnosis and treatment of myocardial infarction.
(Dec 2015, 8 Marks)

Or

Describe clinical features, diagnosis, primary care, treatment and complications of acute myocardial infarction. *(Apr 2017, 12 Marks)*

Ans. *For clinical features and diagnosis refer to Ans. 21 of same chapter.*

For treatment of myocardial infarction, refer to Ans. 19 of same chapter.

For complications, refer to Ans. 20 of same chapter.

Risk Factors

♦ Family history of heart disease
♦ Patient history of heart disease
♦ Diabetes or elevated blood glucose even in non-diabetics
♦ Hypertension
♦ Advanced age
♦ High lipoprotein lipids
♦ Stress, smoking, sedentary lifestyle, compulsive personality
♦ Poor diet, i.e., high sodium, high fat, high intake of alcohol; low intake of B complex vitamin, calcium, magnesium and potassium; low intake of fruit and vegetables
♦ Obesity.

Primary Care

♦ Aspirin 150–300 mg to be chewed earliest.
♦ Sublingual glyceryl trinitrate 0.4–1 mg, to be repeated, if necessary
♦ Oxygen through nasal cannula at a rate of 2–4 L/min.
♦ Procure IV line and take blood samples for glucose, lipids and complete hemogram.
♦ Record 12-lead ECG.
♦ Pain may be relieved by IV morphine (5 mg) plus metoclopramide as an antimetic (10 mg).
♦ IV beta-blockers (metoprolol 5 mg every 2–5 minutes for 3 doses) for ongoing chest pain, hypertension and tachycardia provided, there is no contraindication.
♦ Thrombolysis should be done.
♦ If PTCA is planned, give GP IIb/IIIa inhibitor
♦ After admission, immediately shift the patient to ICU or ICCU

Q.46. Write clinical features, risk factors, diagnosis and management of ischemic heart disease.
(July 2016, 12 Marks)

Ans. Ischemic heart disease occurs whenever there is an imbalance between myocardial oxygen demand and its supply.

Clinical Features

♦ Presence of asymptomatic ischemia.
♦ Angina—stable or unstable
♦ Ischemic cardiomyopathy
♦ Acute myocardial infarction
♦ Cardiac arrest
♦ Arrhythmias or conduction defects
♦ Sudden cardiac death
♦ Asymptomatic coronary artery disease detected on routine medical check-up.

Risk Factors

♦ *Age:* As age advances chances of occurrence of coronary artery diseases increases. It is due to cumulative effects of multiple risk factors overtime.
♦ *Diet:* Diet rich in fat, sugar, cholesterol leads to formation of atheroma and this leads to coronary artery diseases.
♦ *Genetic:* Positive family history of sudden death, myocardial infarction, angina are points to genetic predisposition.
♦ *Personality:* In persons having traits of aggressiveness, ambition and competitiveness chances of occurrence of coronary artery diseases increases.
♦ *Smoking:* Persons who smoke are susceptible for coronary artery diseases because of nicotine and carbon monoxide.
♦ *Diabetes mellitus:* Due to diabetes atheroma may develop in early age and patient is suffering from asymptomatic coronary artery disease.
♦ *Obesity:* It is associated with increased levels of serum cholesterol, blood pressure, serum triglycerides and serum insulin which lead to coronary artery disease.
♦ *Physical activity:* Persons who does not undergo regular physical activities, such as brisk walking or exercise have chances for coronary artery diseases.

Diagnosis

In Angina Pectoris

♦ *Resting ECG:* ECG changes of myocardial ischemia are reflected in S-T waves. Occasionally, there is flattening of T-waves in some lead in patient with angina.
♦ *Exercise ECG or stress test:* With continuous ECG monitoring and intermittent BP recording is performed with a treadmill or bicycle ergometer. Standardized protocols are used (e.g. Bruce protocol), enabling performance to be assessed in same patient at different times and work load at onset of symptoms or ECG changes to be determined. An exercise ECG is abnormal, if there is horizontal or down-sloping ST segment depression of 0.1 mm or more in any lead.
♦ *Myocardial perfusion scintigraphy:* The isotope cardiovascular stress (usually thallium-201 or technetium—99m) is injected at peak exercise and images taken with a camera immediately or shortly after exercise and compared with rest images taken a few hours later following a second injection of tracer. Areas of myocardial ischemia are identified by reduced isotopic uptake in the same anatomical distribution stress images but not resting images (reversible defect).

- *Coronary angiography:* It is done before angioplasty or coronary bypass surgery.

In Acute Myocardial Infarction

Diagnosis of acute myocardial infarction is based on history, characteristics symptoms and signs and investigations.

Investigations

- *Electrocardiography:*
  - ECG is the specific method for confirming the diagnosis.
  - Typical changes are seen in leads which faces the infracted area. These changes are:
    - Elevation of ST segment
    - Pathologic Q—waves appear.
    - T waves may become tall and peaked in very early myocardial infarction. T waves are transient and last for a few hours only.
    - In contrast to transmural lesions, partial thickness or subendothelial infarction causes ST/T wave changes without Q waves or prominent ST elevation.
    - Changes in the ECG are seen which evolve in pre-dictable fashion over next few days to weeks.
- *Blood test:*
  - *Plasma biochemical markers:*
    Myocardial infarction leads to detectable rise in the plasma concentration of various enzymes and proteins that are normally concentrated within the cardiac cells. Plasma enzymes (cardiac injury enzymes) are as follows:
    a. Creatine kinase (CK).
    b. Aspartate aminotransferase (AST).
    c. Lactate dehydrogenase (LDH).
    d. Myoglobin
    e. Troponins (troponin I and troponin T)
    - Creatine kinase starts to rise at 4–6 hours and it peaks by about 12 hours and falls to normal in 48–72 hours. Myocardial isoenzyme of creatine kinase is more specific. It is useful for diagnosis of early myocardial infarction.
    - Aspartate aminotransferase (AST) starts to rise at about 12 hours and reaches a peak on the first or second day and returns on third and fourth day.
    - Lactate dehydrogenase (LDH) starts to rise after 12 hours, reaches a peak after 2–3 days and may remain elevated for a week. Rise in the value of LDH I (an isoenzyme of LDH) is a more sensitive indicator of myocardial infarction than total LDH. It is useful in diagnosis for patients who present several days after myocardial infarction.
    - Cardiac troponins are cardiac troponin-T (cTn-T) and cardiac troponin-I (cTn-I). Sensitivity of tro-ponins is similar to that of isoenzymes of creatine kinase. Moreover, cTn-T remains elevated for 100–200 hours after acute myocardial infarction and therefore, it may have particular utility in the evaluation of patients who present sufficiently long episode after the pain in chest.

- Leukocytosis with a peak on first day.
- ESR is raised, which may remain raised for some days.
- C-reactive protein is elevated.
- *Chest X-ray:* It can detect acute pulmonary edema or congestion. It is also helpful to detect pericardial effusion, cardiomegaly, etc.
- *Radionuclide scanning:* It shows site of necrosis and the extent of impairment of ventricular function.
- *Echocardiography:* This is done for regional wall motion abnormality and ejection fraction.

Management

- *For angina pectoris, refer to Ans. 22 of same chapter.*
- *For myocardial infarction, refer to Ans. 19 of same chapter.*

Q.47. Write short answer on jugular venous pulse.

(Apr 2018, 3 Marks)

Ans. Jugular venous pulse is an important physical sign of cardiovascular disease.

This pulse is examined for pressure and wave forms.

Procedure of measuring jugular venous pulse

This is examined y reclining the patient against pillows at 450 angle, neck muscles should be relaxed, upper level of pulsation of an internal jugular vein is seen, though vein may itself be not visible.

In a normal person, jugular venous pulsation in above said position remains either behind the clavicle or below it and rarely extends beyond 2 to 3 cm above sternal angle.

Waveforms of jugular venous pulse

Waveform of jugular venous pulse in patient of sinus rhythm is:

- 'a' wave occur due to atrial systole. This is absent in atrial fibrillation but becomes large in tricuspid stenosis, right ventricle hypertrophy and pulmonary hypertension.
- 'c' wave corresponds to tricuspid closure

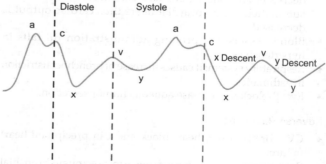

a = atrial contraction c = onset of ventricular contraction

a = Rise in ventricular pressure before opening of tricuspid value

c to x = x descent; v to y = y descent

Fig. 11: Waveforms of jugular venous pressure.

- 'v' wave result from building of pressure in right atrium during ventricular systole when tricuspid valve is closed. This wave becomes prominent in tricuspid regurgitation or congestive heart failure.
- All the above mention three waves, i.e., a, c and v waves are known as positive waves.
- There are two more waves present beside these which are known as negative waves or descents, i.e., x and y descents.
- 'x' descent correspond with atrial relaxation and downward displacement of tricuspid valve at the time of ventricular systole. It is prominent in constrictive pericarditis.
- Following the summit of 'v' wave, negative 'y' descent is produced by opening of tricuspid valve and rapid flow of blood in right ventricle.
- Prominent 'y' descent occurs in constructive pericarditis and congestive heart failure along with 'v' wave, so it is collectively known as prominent 'v' wave and 'y' descent.
- Slow 'y' descent occurs in tricuspid stenosis where 'a' wave is prominent.
- Giant 'a' wave is a large sharp systolic wave seen in venous pulse during forcible contraction of right ventricle against closed tricuspid valve. It is seen in complete heart block, atrioventricular dissociation and junctional rhythm.

Q.48. Write short answer on beta blockers.

(Apr 2018, 3 Marks)

Ans. These drugs inhibit responses mediated by the adrenergic β blockers.

Classification

- Cardioselective (β1): Metoprolol, atenolol, acebutolol.
- β2 selective: Butoxamine.
- Nonselective (β1+ β2): Propranolol, nadolol, sotalol, timolol.

Actions

- Heart: These drugs decreases force of contraction, decreases AV conduction, decreases heart rate, decreases automaticity of myocardial fibers thus cardiac output is decreased.
- Blood vessels: On prolong administration BP falls in hypertensives.
- Respiratory system: It causes increase of bronchoconstriction in asthmatics.
- Eye: β-blockers decrease aqueous humor secretion.

Adverse Reactions

- CVS: Bradycardia, heart block and can precipitate heart failure.
- Respiratory system: these drugs can precipitate bronchial asthma.

- CNS: Disturbed sleep, fatigue, hallucination and mental depression.
- Muscular weakness and tiredness
- Abrupt withdrawal can cause angina or frank myocardial infarction.

Contraindications

- They are contraindicated in asthmatics and COPD.
- They are contraindicated in patients of Prinzmetal angina.
- They are contraindicated in peripheral vascular disease.
- They are contraindicated in patients with low cardiac reserve.
- They are contraindicated in diabetic who are taking oral anti-diabetic drugs as they delay recovery from hypoglycemia.

Uses or Indications of β Blockers

- Hypertension: β blockers are used to treat all the grades of hypertension. They are also indicated in angina, myocardial infarction and cardiac arrhythmias.
- In prophylaxis of angina and myocardial infarction: β blockers decreases oxygen demand of myocardium and decreases the heart rate. These drugs reduces the frequency of angina attacks. They are indicated in acute phase of myocardial infarction so that they limit the size of infarct.
- In cardiac arrhythmias: They are indicated in atrial arrhythmias, i.e., atrial fibrillation, atrial flutter and paroxysmal supraventricular tachycardia.
- Congestive cardiac failure: Chronic usage of β blockers reduced rate of mortality during chronic heart failure.
- Pheochromocytoma: These drugs control cardiac manifestations produced by pheochromocytoma.
- Glaucoma: They decrease intraocular pressure by decreasing secretion of aqueous humor. Timolol is the choice of drug.
- In prophylaxis of migraine: They decreases the frequency of migraine headache.
- Hyperthyroidism: Sign and symptoms of hyperthyroidism decreases due to blockade of β receptors.
- Essential tremors: Propranolol provides relief in tremors.
- Anxiety: It acts as anti-anxiety drug.
- Alcohol withdrawal: Propranolol provides benefit in alcohol withdrawal.
- Dissecting aortic aneurysm: β blockers reduce cardiac contractility as well as development of pressure during systole.

Q.49. Write short answer on calcium channel blocker.

(May 2018, 3 Marks)

Ans. Following are the calcium channel blockers:

Drug	Action	Side effects	Uses
Nifedipine 10–50 mg orally or sublingually	• It is a potent calcium antagonist • It decreases oxygen consumption and reduces cardiac work by leading to peripheral vasodilatation and reducing the peripheral resistance	• Headache • Lethargy • Flushing • Tachycardia • Hypotension	**Cardiovascular uses:** • In angina pectoris • In hypertension • In peripheral vascular disease • In achalasia cardia • In Raynaud's phenomenon • In migraine • In nocturnal leg cramps • In high altitude pulmonary edema • In left ventricular hyperplasia, arrhythmias, valvular diseases, cerebrovascular diseases, post-myocardial infarction
VERAPAMIL, AMLODIPINE NICARDIPINE, ISRADIPINE, FELODIPINE, NIMODIPINE	• It leads to coronary dilatation and decreases myocardial oxygen consumption • It interferes with inward displacement of calcium and delays conduction within AV node	• Constipation • Hypotension • Vertigo • Nervousness	**Non-cardiovascular uses** • In esophageal motility disorders • In supraventricular arrhythmias • In extrinsic bronchial asthma • In biliary or renal colic • In epilepsy • In Alzheimer disease • In bone pain in transplant recipients • In subarachnoid hemorrhage, nocturnal enuresis
DILTIAZEM 30–60 mg TDS	• This drug increases the coronary blood flow, decreases myocardial contractility, reduces peripheral resistance and blood pressure, thus increasing cardiac output due to decreased afterload • It increases exercise tolerance	• Headache • Flushing • Edema and hypotension • Depression of AV nodal conduction • Bradycardia	
PERHEXILINE MALEATE 100–200 mg TDS	• Actual action is not known but it: - Reduces exercise-induced tachycardia. - Causes vasodilatation of systemic and coronary vessels, decreases left ventricular work and oxygen consumption	• Dizziness, headache • Hepatotoxicity • Impotence • Polyneuropathy, myopathy	
OXYFEDRINE 24–48 mg/day	It improves the myocardial microcirculation	• Weakness, headache, giddiness • Insomnia, nausea, constipation	

Q.50. Write short answer on anti-hypertensive drugs.

(Feb 2019, 3 Marks)

Or

Enumerate anti-hypertensive drugs.

(Oct 2019, 3 Marks)

Ans.

Enumeration of anti-hypertensive Drugs.

♦ **ACE inhibitors:** Captopril, enalapril, lisinopril, perindopril, ramipril, lisinopril, benazepril and fosinopril
♦ **Angiotensin antagonist:** Losartan, candesartan, irbesartan, valsartan, telmisartan
♦ **Calcium channel blockers:** Verapamil, diltiazem, nifedipine, felodipine, amlodipine

♦ **Diuretics:**
 • *Thiazides:* Hydrochlorothiazide, chlorthalidone, indapamide
 • *High ceiling:* Furosemide, bumetanide, torsemide
 • *K+ sparing:* Spironolactone, Amiloride, triamterene
♦ **Beta adrenergic blockers:** Propranolol, atenolol, timolol, nadolol
♦ **Beta + Alpha adrenergic blockers:** Labetalol, carvedilol
♦ **Alpha adrenergic Blockers:** Prazosin, terazosin, doxazosin, phentolamine, phenoxybenzamine
♦ **Central sympatholytics:** Clonidine and methyldopa
♦ **Vasodilators:**
 • *Arteriolar:* Hydralazine, Minoxidil and diazoxide
 • *Arteriolar + Venous:* Sodium nitroprusside.

Actions of Anti-Hypertensive Drugs

Name of anti-hypertensive drug	Action

ACE inhibitors	These drugs prevent conversion of angiotensin I into angiotensin II by inhibiting angiotensin converting enzyme thus preventing action of angiotensin II, i.e.
	• They cause dilatation of arterioles causes decrease in peripheral vascular resistance and decreases blood pressure.
	• These drugs causes decrease in aldosterone synthesis which leads to decrease in retention of sodium ion and water which causes fall in BP
	• ACE inhibitors decrease the activity of sympathetic nervous system.
	  - ACE inhibitors metabolize bradykinin which is a potent vasodilator. ACE inhibitors increase bradykinin levels causing vasodilatation and decreases blood pressure.
	  - ACE inhibitors cause stimulation of synthesis of prostaglandins which are vasodilating. This take place through bradykinin. This causes decrease in blood pressure.

Angiotensin antagonist	Losartan blocks AT1 receptors. It blocks all actions of angiotensin II like vasoconstriction and aldosterone synthesis and decreases blood pressure. It does not inhibit ACE and so bradykinin level is not increased so it decreases hypertension.

Calcium channel blockers	• **Smooth muscle relaxants**: Movement of calcium inside cardiac muscle cells released more calcium from sarcoplasmic reticulum causing excitation contraction coupling. Calcium channel blockers block all type of calcium channels and decrease availability of calcium ions thus causing relaxation of smooth muscle cell or cardiac cell. Effect is more on arterioles and less on veins.
	• **Negative, chronotropic, inotropic and dromotropic action:**
	  - Calcium channel blockers inhibit calcium movement inside cell in depolarization phase thus inhibiting contraction of cardiac muscle. Cardiac work and oxygen consumption is decreased.
	  - Calcium channel blockers inhibit refractory period of AV node, decrease SA nodal discharge suppresses ectopic foci produce Antiarrhythmic action.

Diuretics	• Diuretics cause loss of sodium and water in urine due to which there is decrease in cardiac output and hence fall in BP • Due to direct loss of sodium, arterioles respond less to noradrenaline and hence less vasoconstriction and fall in BP.

Contd…

Contd…

Name of anti-hypertensive drug	Action
Beta adrenergic blockers	On chronic therapy, these drugs reduces peripheral vascular resistance due to reduced cardiac output there is fall in both systolic and diastolic blood pressure.
Alpha adrenergic blockers	• Non-selective α blockers block α1 and α2 receptors in blood vessels which causes vasodilatation and fall in blood pressure. • Selective α blockers block selectively α1 vascular receptors due to its competitive mechanism. This causes vasodilatation and fall in blood pressure.
Central sympatholytics	• **Clonidine:** Clonidine has high affinity and high intrinsic activity at α2 receptors. Clonidine leads to stimulation of α2A receptors which causes decrease sympathetic outflow and there is fall in blood pressure and bradycardia. • **Methyldopa:** The active metabolite of methyldopa, i.e., α methyl-NA stimulates central α2 receptors to decrease the efferent sympathetic activity and decreases blood pressure.
Arteriolar vasodilator	Arteriolar vasodilators → Activate potassium channels and open them → This causes efflux of potassium ions → Hyperpolarization of vascular smooth muscle → Vasodilatation occur → Decrease in blood pressure
Arteriolar and venous dilator	Sodium nitroprusside → Causes generation of nitric oxide → Smooth muscle cell relaxation → Vasodilatation → As arteriolar dilator sodium nitroprusside → Causes blood pooling occur in veins → Decrease in venous return → Decrease in cardiac output → Decrease in blood pressure; As venodilator sodium nitroprusside → Causes decrease in peripheral vascular resistance → Decrease in afterload → Decrease in blood pressure

Indications

- Anti-hypertensive drugs, such as ACE inhibitors decreases preload and afterload in CHF.
- Anti-hypertensive drug, such as calcium channel blockers are useful in treatment of angina pectoris.
- The calcium channel blockers are also useful in treatment of arrhythmias, Raynaud's disease and in prevention of neurological damage.
- Anti-hypertensive drugs, such as hydralazine acts as vasodilators and causes fall in BP.
- Anti-hypertensive drugs mainly ACE inhibitors improve renal functions in diabetes.

Q.51. Write short answer on CPR. *(Sep 2018, 3 Marks)*

Or

Describe CPR. *(Oct 2019, 3 Marks)*

Ans. CPR means cardiopulmonary resuscitation.

- The conventional CPR ventilator technique needs that lungs should be inflated 10 to 12 times/min when there is presence of single or two rescuers.
- Main crucial factor which decides the success of cardiopulmonary resuscitation is the sufficient supply of oxygen. Since at about the 4 minutes of cardiac arrest there occurs the cerebral death.
- Look for the person's chest to rise and fall, listen to the sounds of breadth and feel the breadth of person on the cheek. If patient is responding, then his/her heart should be beating and there is no need for cardiac massage. If patient is unresponsive feel for carotid pulse, if carotid pulse is absent, cardiac massage should be started as soon as possible.
- For starting the cardiac massage, kneel at person's right side and interlock the fingers of both hands to provide external cardiac compression. Keeping the elbows straight, depress lower sternum briskly with the heel of hand 15 times for 10 seconds. Sternum should be depressed 3 to 5 cm by keeping pressure firm, controlled and applied vertically along with abrupt relaxation. Chest should be pushed down 80 to 100 times/min.
- CPR for an adult consists of 15 chest compressions and two breadths, procedure should be repeated many times in ratio of 15:2 and watch for person's chest to fall. Feel for the air being exhaled.
- If there is presence of another person, instruct him/her to set up an IV infusion and infuse 100 mL of 8.4% sodium bicarbonate at the rate of 10 mL/min.
- CPR should be continued till there is resuscitation of thee spontaneous pulse and blood pressure. Now, admit the patient to hospital.

Q.52. Write short note on clinical features and management of hypertensive emergency. *(Jan 2019, 7 Marks)*

Ans. Hypertensive emergencies constitute a group of clinical syndromes in which severe (diastolic blood pressure >120) and rarely moderate hypertension is associated with established/ongoing target organ damage.

According to JNC VI report, a hypertensive emergency was defined as severely elevated blood pressure (>220/120 mm Hg) with sign and symptoms of acute target organ damage, requiring parenteral drug treatment, close observation in the ICU and immediate reduction in blood pressure within an hour.

Clinical Features of Hypertensive Emergencies

- End organ damage:
  - Cerebrovascular: Hypertensive encephalopathy, ischemic stroke, hemorrhagic stroke.
  - Cardiovascular: Acute left ventricular failure, acute aortic dissection, unstable angina.
  - Renal-kidney failure.
- Catecholamine excess syndrome: Pheochromocytoma, clonidine withdrawal, monoamine oxidase inhibitor.
- Postoperative bleeding from suture sites.
- Eclampsia.
- Severe epistaxis.
- Grade III and IV fundal changes.

Management

- Hospitalization
- Immediate reduction of blood pressure: Parenteral and oral drugs are used.
- Vasodilators 0.25 to 10 µg/kg/min as IV infusion.
- Nicardipine hydrochloride 5 to 15 mg/IV.
- Fenoldopam mesylate 0.1–0.3 µg/kg/min IV infusion
- Nitroglycerin 5–100 ug/min IV infusion
- Enalaprilat 1.25–5 mg q6h IV
- Hydralazine hydrochloride 10–20 mg IV

Adrenergic Inhibitors

- Labetalol 20–80 mg IV bolus every 10 min 0.5 to 2 mg/min IV infusion
- Esmolol 25–50 µg/kg/min IV bolus, then 50 to 100 µg/kg/min by infusion., may repeat bolus or increase infusion to 30 pg/min
- Phentolamine 5–15 mg IV bolus
- Epistaxis: Nose packed with absorbent cotton soaked in adrenaline solution, cauterization after active bleeding has stopped or pressure fails to control bleeding. Nasal cavity pack if source of bleeding not accessible to cauterization.
- LV failure: *For details refer to Ans. 15 of same chapter.*
- Cerebral hemorrhage: Rapid reduction of pressure to prevent further bleeding.
- Dissecting aneurysm: Rapid reduction of blood pressure. Propranolol may be useful.

Surgical Treatment

1. In renovascular hypertension: Following are the indications—(a) Age 30 years or less. (b) Severe hypertension (c) BP difficult to control medically. (d) Progressive kidney failure in a hypertensive patient is due to either bilateral renal stenosis or stenosis of the artery to a single kidney. *Procedures:* (a) Bypass grafting of renal artery. (b) Percutaneous transluminal angioplasty—(i) Fibromuscular dysplasia. (ii) Single discrete atherornatous plaque in renal arterial midportion. (iii) Intrarenal arterial stenosis inaccessible to surgery. (iv) Transplant artery stenosis.
2. Surgery for coarctation of aorta.
3. Surgical removal of pheochromocytoma.

5. DISEASES OF RESPIRATORY SYSTEM

Q.1. Describe clinical features, investigations and management of lung abscess. *(Mar 2003, 15 Marks)*

Or

Write in brief sign, symptoms and treatment of lung abscess. *(May/June 2009, 5 Marks)*

Ans. It is localized pyogenic infection of the lung characterized by the *suppuration, destruction of lung parenchyma with cavitation and formation of abscess.

Clinical Features

Symptoms

- In most of the patients disease commence with high-grade fever, chills and rigors, pleuritic chest pain and cough.
- After some days, as the abscess cavity ruptures into a patent bronchus, the patient suddenly starts expectorating large quantities of sputum.
- Sputum is very large in volume, purulent, foul smelling, greenish yellow in color or it is often blood tinged. Expectoration of cough varies with posture, i.e., more in lying down position than compared to sitting position.
- In few of the cases, the lung abscess is more insidious in onset with low-grade fever, malaise, weight loss, anorexia and a deep-seated chest discomfort.
- As the disease become chronic patient starts to loose his/her weight.

Clinical Signs

- During general examination, there is presence of anemia, fever, clubbing of fingers, halitosis and oronasal sepsis.
- In most of the patients, there may be signs of consolidation, i.e., coarse crepitations/crackles or rales, dullness on percussion, increased vocal fremitus, vocal resonance, bronchial breathing and pleural rub appear.
- In case of ruptured pyogenic abscess producing amphoric or cavernous bronchial breathing heard over the area involved, signs of pleural effusion, i.e., dull percussion note with absent breath sounds will be present.
- Signs of septicemia, i.e., fever, perspiration, tachypnea and tachycardia are present.

Investigations

- *Blood examination:* There can be presence of normocytic normochromic anemia. Leukocytosis is present in infective abscess. Raised ESR is also present.
- *Examination of sputum:* It consists of isolation of infective microorganisms by Gram's stain and acid-fast bacilli by Ziehl-Neelsen stain, Aerobic and anaerobic cultures and sensitivity, malignant cells are detected by the special stains.
- *Urine examination:* This is carried out for proteinuria, pus cells and cases. Albuminuria is indicative of amyloidosis which is a complication of chronic lung abscess.
- *Chest X-ray:* It shows radiolucency in the the area of consolidation. Wall or border of cavity completely surrounds the radiolucent area and air-fluid level is seen. Associated involvement of pleura is noted by obliteration of CP angle.
- *Fiberoptic bronchoscopy:* It is done to rule out bronchogenic cause of lung abscess. It also exclude malignancy, obtain specimen for studies and for removing the secretions.
- CT scan of thorax may detect lung abscess with certainty.

Management

General Measures

- Bed rest
- Oxygen is given
- High protein diet is taken
- Exercise is avoided.

Specific Antimicrobial Treatment

- Intensive antimicrobial therapy is employed depending on the sputum culture and drug sensitivity of the organism
- Most of the patients with lung abscess respond to oral ampicillin 500 mg QDS or cotrimoxazole 960 mg BD is given. Along with this oral metronidazole 400 mg 8 hourly is given along with other antibiotics. Duration of antibiotic therapy is variable. Some of the patients require antibiotic therapy for 4 to 6 weeks. Injectables should be given in the emergency situations. Clindamycin 600 mg IV 8 hourly is given.

Postural Drainage

- *Percussion therapy* or "clapping" over the site of the abscess with the patient in the postural drainage position is often effective in dislodging and expelling secretions from the cavity.
- *Bronchoscopy:* Suction is applied to the orifices of the bronchi leading to segments presumed to be involved in the process in hope of initiating or promoting drainage. In addition any foreign material is removed and a careful search made for a tumor.
- *Oxygen inhalations:* When sputum is foul because it checks the anaerobic organisms
- *Head elevation:* Patient bed should be inclined to 45° from horizontal plane in cases of altered mentation, on mechanical ventilatory support.

Surgical Resection

If at the end of 3 weeks, there is no clinical and radiological improvement, then segmental resection of lung, lobectomy or pneumonectomy is done.

Q.2. Describe etiology, clinical features and management of lung abscess. *(Aug 2012, 15 Marks)*

Ans. Lung abscess is the localized pyogenic infection of the lung characterized by the suppuration, destruction of lung parenchyma with cavitation and formation of abscess.

Etiology

- Infection: Staphylococci, streptococci, *Pneumococcus* and *fusiform bacilli*.
- Aspiration of infected material from the oral cavity and throat.
- As a complication of pneumonia when the organism is virulent and patient's immunity is low.

Q 1.   *Suppuration = Formation of pus.

- Bronchial obstruction as in bronchogenic carcinoma.
- Embolic infection with the cavity formation.
- Necrosis and abscess formation of growth in the lung.
- Metastatic lung abscess.
- Rupture of amoebic liver abscess into lung.

Complications

- An abscess may extend to the surrounding structures producing mediastinitis and pericarditis.
- Involvement of pleura causes *pleurisy, *empyema and *pyopneumothorax.
- Pleural effusion, pneumothorax, bronchopleural fistula
- Metastatic cerebral abscess
- Severe hemoptysis may occur.
- Extrapulmonary complications include pain, abscess, *cachexia and amyloidosis.
- Aspergilloma
- A chronic form of lung abscess may leave behind bronchiectasis and chronic cavity with fibrosis.

For management and clinical features, refer to Ans. 1 of same chapter.

Q.3. Write short note on bronchial asthma.
(Dec 2008, 5.5 Marks)
Or
Describe in brief on bronchial asthma.
(Dec 2015, 4 Marks)
Or
Outline the management of allergic bronchial asthma. *(Sep 2010, 5 Marks)*
Or
Describe clinical features, diagnosis and management of bronchial asthma. *(Mar 2011, 4.5 Marks)*
Or
Describe clinical features of bronchial asthma.
(Feb 2013, 5 Marks)
Or
Discuss clinical features, complications investigations and treatment of bronchial asthma.
(Apr 2018, 5 Marks)
Or
Write short answer on bronchial asthma.
(May 2018, 3 Marks)
Or
Write etiology, clinical features, diagnosis and management of bronchial asthma. *(Ang 2018, 12 Marks)*
Or
Write short answer on management of bronchial asthma. *(Feb 2019, 3 Marks)*

Ans. Bronchial asthma consists of an increased responsiveness of bronchial tree, which is characterized by frequent attacks of dyspnea due to generalized bronchial constriction.

Etiology

- Genetic and environmental factors also cause bronchial asthma.
- Early onset asthma starts in childhood, there should be family history of atopy, i.e., external antigen and other allergic disorders, i.e., urticaria, allergic rhinitis and eczema. In this, skin tests are positive for allergies and there are high levels of IgE antibody in serum. There is positive response to provocative tests which involve in inhalation of specific antigen.
- Late onset asthma occurs in adulthood. In this, there is no effect of atopy along with no family history of allergens. Skin tests are normal and there are no increased levels of IgE antibody in serum.

Various Trigger Factors for Bronchial Asthma

- Night or early morning
- Exercise (especially running)
- Cold air, fog
- Viral respiratory tract infection
- Allergens (e.g. house dust, mite, cat fur)
- Nonspecific irritants (e.g. cigarette smoke, perfumes, paints)
- Drugs (e.g. B-blockers, aspirin, NSAIDs)
- Emotion or stress
- Occupational exposure

Clinical Features

- Symptoms of bronchial asthma can be episodic or persistent.
- Asthma is characterized by paroxysms of dyspnea, cough and wheezing commonly in children and young adults.
- Attacks can be mild or severe or may last for hours, days or rarely weeks. Between episodes, the patients become asymptomatic.
- In older patients, asthma is chronic and persistent. Symptoms get worst in the early morning.
- On examination, there is tachypnea, tachycardia as well as involvement of accessory respiratory muscles.
- Breath sound become harsh, vesicular with prolonged expiration. Prominent wheeze should be audible in both phases of respiration.
- Acute severe asthma is a life-threatening attack of asthma which is previously called as status asthmaticus. In this, patient may additionally have tachycardia, pulsus paradoxus, cyanosis and active accessory respiratory muscles. The air entry is drastically reduced with silent chest on auscultation. The patient may become confused or drowsy.

Investigations/Diagnosis

- Chest radiograph may be normal, or show signs of segmental or lobar collapse.
- Full blood count reveals eosinophilia.
- *Sputum:* On examination eosinophils, Charcot-Leyden crystals and at times Curschmann's spirals may appear

---

Q 2. *Pleurisy = Inflammation of pleural cavity
*Empyema = A collection of inflamed, infected fluid between the pleura.
*Pyopneumothorax = The presence of pus and gas in pleural cavity.
*Cachexia = A state of ill-health, malnutrition and wasting

purulent (due to eosinophilic leukocytes) in absence of infection).

♦ *Skin tests:* A patch test is done with aqueous solution of substance to be tested. Positive test indicates wheal and flare. Tests are performed with groups of substances or allergens which produce asthma.

♦ *Lung function test:* Spirometry shows reduction in FEV1, FEV1/FVC ratio and peak expiratory flow rate (PEFR). Reversibility, which is one of characteristic feature of asthma, is shown by 200 mL increase in FEV, 15 minutes after inhaled short acting β2 agonist or 2–4 weeks trial of oral corticosteroids.

♦ *Provocation (challenge) tests:* Exercise challenge tests useful in young adults and can be used to confirm diagnosis of asthma, since fall in FEV, or PEFR occurs after 5–7 minutes of vigorous exercise in most patients with asthma.

♦ *IgE and IgE specific test:* Elevation of total serum IgE supports diagnosis of atopy, and measurement of fractions of IgE specific to one allergen, radioallergosorbent test (RAST) can be useful in some patients in whom a specific allergy is suspected.

Complications of Bronchial Asthma

Following are the complications of bronchial asthma:

♦ **Respiratory**
  • From mucus plugs
    – Atelectasis lobar or lobular
    – Bronchiectasis
  • From cough
    – Subcutaneous emphysema
    – Mediastinal emphysema
    – Spontaneous pneumothorax
    – Cystic degeneration of lungs
    – Spontaneous rib fracture
  • From infection
    – Recurrent bronchitis and pneumonia
  • From uneven ventilation and pulmonary perfusion
    – Respiratory failure and cor pulmonale

♦ **Cardiac**
  • Dysrhythmias from hypoxia and stress of asthma, compounded by bronchodilator therapy with β agonist and theophylline
  • Myocardial infarction rarely in severe asthma

♦ **Hypokalemia:** Due to high dose corticosteroids, high dose β agonists, respiratory alkalosis of hypocapnia

♦ **Other complications**
  • Nausea and vomiting from theophylline
  • Acute myopathy due to high dose IV steroids

Management

♦ Identify the allergens and wherever possible, exposure to such agents must be avoided.

♦ *Drug therapy:* The drugs used in asthma can be grouped as: (a) quick relievers, which inhibit smooth muscle contraction and cause bronchodilatation and (b) long-term control medications, which prevent or reverse inflammation.

Management of Acute Severe Asthma

♦ *Treatment of severe acute asthma at home:*
  • Administer oxygen (40–60%) through mask, if available.
  • Bronchodilator: IV Aminophylline, i.e., 250–375 mg in 20 mL of saline slowly after checking blood pressure Or IV, Salbutamol 250 μg in 20 mL of saline over 10 min Or IV Terbutaline 250 μg in 20 mL of saline over 10 min.
  • *Alternatively:*
    – Salbutamol (5 mg) or terbutaline (10 mg) by nebulizer.
    – Give hydrocortisone sodium succinate 200 mg IV stat.
    – Arrange for emergency admission to a hospital in ambulance equipped with oxygen therapy.
    – Give prednisolone 60 mg orally

♦ *In hospital treatment:*
  • High concentration of oxygen, i.e., 40–60% at high flow rate should be given. It is recommended in all cases even in the presence of CO_2 retention. Oxygen supply should be started immediately through mask, and concentration adjusted according to blood gas measurement. PaO_2 of greater than 8.5 to 9.0 kPa should be maintained, if possible.
  • High doses of salbutamol, i.e., 2.5–5 mg or terbutaline 5–10 mg by nebulizer should be given initially and repeated after 30 minutes, necessary. If no improvement occurs with nebulized therapy, then 250 μg of salbutamol or terbutaline may be given by IV infusion over 10 minutes.
  • In all severe cases of acute asthma systemic corticosteroids, i.e., hydrocortisone 200 mg IV stat and then 4 to 6 hourly or oral prednisolone 40–60 mg/day to tide over the crisis.
  • Systemic bronchodilators, such as aminophylline 250 mg IV over a period of 30 minutes may be given immediately followed by either 8 hours doses or continuous infusion not exceeding total dose of 1.5 g/day.
  • Ipratropium bromide can be used in acute severe asthma in doses of 0.5 mg added to a nebulized beta-agonist.
  • Reassess the patient by PEFR and arterial blood gas analysis. If recovery is good, then continue oxygen therapy and oral prednisolone, i.e., 40 mg/day in decreasing doses is given. Nebulized β-adrenoreceptor agonist may be continued every 4–6 hours and then replaced by metered dose inhalation. IV hydrocortisone 200 mg 6 hourly may be continued for 24–48 hours in severe cases followed by oral steroids. If response is not good, then shift the patient in respiratory intensive care for assisted ventilation.
  • *Assisted ventilation:* Mechanical ventilation can be life saving in few patients who are critically ill.

Management of Chronic Asthma

For management of chronic bronchial asthma, a stepwise approach is chosen according to the severity of disease. Once the disease is controlled, a step-down therapy should be attempted.

♦ *Step 1: Use of inhaled bronchodilators:* Here inhaled short-acting β₂ adrenoreceptor agonists bronchodilators, such as salbutamol or terbutaline 100 to 200 µg are used as needed for minor symptoms.

♦ *Step 2: Use of bronchodilators with regular use of inhaled anti-inflammatory agents:* If the symptoms are not controlled by inhaled adrenergic drugs, then a low dose of inhaled steroid is added, i.e., beclomethasone dipropionate or budesonide up to 800 µg twice a day.

♦ *Step 3: Use of bronchodilators with high doses of steroids:* Dose of inhaled steroid is increased till 800–2000 µg a day.

♦ *Step 4: Use of high-dose corticosteroids and bronchodilators with therapeutic drug:* In addition to drugs used in Step 3, An inhaled long-acting adrenergic agent, such as salmeterol or formoterol can be added or sustained released theophylline can be used orally or inhaled ipratropium bromide or sodium cromoglycate are tried.

♦ *Step 5: Addition of oral steroids:* Regular oral steroid, i.e., prednisolone 20–30 mg/day in single dosage is added to Step 4 regimen to control symptoms.

Patient Education and Monitoring of Therapy

♦ Educate the patients about the nature of disease as well as its treatment. Patients are trained to recognize the severity of their disease and monitor the response to therapy with the use of peak flow meter.

♦ Demonstrate the proper use of inhalation devices, such as metered-dose inhalers (pressurized aerosol system), rotahaler (dry powder system) and nebulizers.

♦ Encourage the usage of inhaler therapy because it is effective in lower dosage together with a rapid onset of action and has less side effects.

Q.4. Write short note on status asthmaticus.

(Oct 2007, 5 Marks)

Or

Describe briefly the management of status asthmaticus. *(Dec 2012, 4 Marks)*

Ans. Status asthmaticus is a continuous state of breathlessness without any period of relief. A prolong attack of continuous asthma with fluctuations also comes under status asthmaticus.

Clinical Features

♦ Presence of repeated dry cough which causes aggravation of dyspnea and respiratory distress.

♦ Patient sweats heavily and there is also presence of tachycardia.

♦ Presence of an increased pulse rate till 120/min.

♦ Respiratory rate is 30/min

♦ Presence of pulsus paradoxus

♦ As breathlessness is present, patient is unable to speak.

♦ Peak expiratory flow is falls to less than 50%.

♦ When patient develops carbon dioxide retention, hypoxemia and acidosis, there can be occurrence of life-threatening situation.

♦ CNS effects, such as confusion, drowsiness, semiconsciousness and cyanosis develops.

♦ In critically-ill patients, chest becomes silent due to decrease in the air entry.

Management

Treatment of Severe Acute Asthma at Home

♦ Administer oxygen (40–60%) through mask, if available.

♦ Bronchodilator: IV Aminophylline, i.e., 250–375 mg in 20 mL of saline slowly after checking blood pressure Or IV, Salbutamol 250 µg in 20 mL of saline over 10 min Or IV. Terbutaline 250 µg in 20 mL of saline over 10 min.

♦ Alternatively
  • Salbutamol (5 mg) or terbutaline (10 mg) by nebulizer.
  • Give hydrocortisone sodium succinate 200 mg IV stat.
  • Arrange for emergency admission to a hospital in ambulance equipped with oxygen therapy.
  • Give prednisolone 60 mg orally

In Hospital Treatment

♦ High conc. of oxygen, i.e., 40–60% at high flow rate should be given. It is recommended in all cases even in the presence of CO_2 retention. Oxygen supply should be started immediately through mask, and concentration adjusted according to blood gas measurement. PaO_2 of greater than 8.5 to 9.0 kPa should be maintained if possible.

♦ High doses of salbutamol, i.e., 2.5–5 mg or terbutaline 5–10 mg by nebulizer should be given initially and repeated after 30 minutes, necessary. If no improvement occurs with nebulized therapy then 250 µg of salbutamol or terbutaline may be given by IV infusion over 10 minutes.

♦ In all severe cases of acute asthma systemic corticosteroids, i.e., hydrocortisone 200 mg IV stat and then 4 to 6 hourly or oral prednisolone 40–60 mg/day to tide over the crisis.

♦ Systemic bronchodilators, such as aminophylline 250 mg IV over a period of 30 minutes may be given immediately followed by either 8 hours doses or continuous infusion not exceeding total dose of 1.5 g/day.

♦ Ipratropium bromide can be used in acute severe asthma in doses of 0.5 mg added to a nebulized beta-agonist.

♦ Reassess the patient by PEFR and arterial blood gas analysis. If recovery is good, continue oxygen therapy and oral prednisolone, i.e., 40 mg/day in decreasing doses is given. Nebulized β-adrenoreceptor agonist may be continued every 4–6 hours and then replaced by metered dose inhalation. IV hydrocortisone 200 mg 6 hourly may be continued for 24–48 hours in severe cases followed by oral steroids. If response is not good, then shift the patient in respiratory intensive care for assisted ventilation.

♦ *Assisted ventilation:* Mechanical ventilation can be life saving in few patients, who are critically ill.

Patient Education and Monitoring of Therapy

♦ Educate the patients about the nature of disease as well as its treatment. Patients are trained to recognize the severity of their disease and monitor the response to therapy with the use of peak flowmeter.

♦ Demonstrate the proper use of inhalation devices, such as metered-dose inhalers (pressurized aerosol system), rotahaler (dry powder system) and nebulizers.

♦ Encourage the usage of inhaler therapy because it is effective in lower dosage together with a rapid onset of action and has less side effects.

Q.5. Mention the complications of lobar pneumonia.

(Sep 2006, 5 Marks)

Ans.

Complications of Pneumonia

In lung:

- Pleural effusion
- Pneumothorax
- Empyema
- Lung abscess
- Respiratory failure.

In Cardiac Involvement:

- Pericarditis
- Endocarditis

- Myocarditis
- Cardiac failure.

GIT complications: They are uncommon and may be in form of:

- Acute dilatation of stomach
- Paralytic ileus
- Peritonitis.

Other Complications

- Pneumococcal meningitis
- Arthritis
- Parotitis
- *Otitis media
- Nephritis
- Venous thrombosis.

(Apr 2010, 15 Marks)

Q.6. Write note on management of pneumonia.

Ans. Types of pneumonias and its management.

Primary pneumonias	Management
Pneumococcal pneumonia	• Initially oral amoxicillin should be given 500 mg 8 hourly or erythromycin 500 mg 6 hourly. • If patient is very ill or gram-negative or staphylococcal infection is present IV ampicillin 0.5 to 1 g 6 hourly + flucloxacillin 250–500 mg IV 6 hourly + gentamicin 60–80 mg every 8 hourly IV is given. • Antibiotic therapy should be given for 7 to 10 days. • Choice of antibiotic depends on the causative microorganisms. • Oxygen therapy is given in seriously-ill patients. Oxygen should be delivered at very high rate. • Analgesics, such as mefenamic acid 250–500 mg or pethidine 50–100 mg or morphine 10 to 15 mg IM or IV injections should be given. • Physiotherapy is given to patient by encouraging him to cough and to take deep breadth as pleuritic pain disappears
Staphylococcal pneumonia	• IV flucloxacillin 0.5–1 g 6 hourly or erythromycin 0.5–1 g every 6 hourly is given in cases with mild infection. • If infection is severe than IV sodium fusidate in dosage of 500 mg 6 hourly is given thrice a day in addition to cloxacillin and erythromycin. Treatment should be given for 2 weeks.
Klebsiella pneumoniae	• IV gentamicin 2–5 mg/kg is given in divided doses for every 8 hours. • IV Ceftazidime or cefotaxime 1 g 8 hourly is given or ciprofloxacin 200 mg after every 12 hours IV infusion for 30 to 60 min is choice of treatment.
Legionella pneumoniae	• Erythromycin 1 g 8 hourly IV for 13 weeks followed by 500 mg qds for 2 weeks. • Doxycycline 100 mg twice a day orally for 3 weeks. • Rifampicin 600 mg twice a day orally for 3 weeks. • In *Legionella endocarditis*, the treatment with antibiotics has to be continued for 3–12 months.
Primary atypical pneumonia	• Oral tetracycline 500 mg 6 hourly or erythromycin 500 mg 6 hourly is effective. • If severe case is present, above drugs should be given parenterally.
Viral pneumonia	• Disease is self-limiting. • Antipyretics can be given
Secondary pneumonia	**Management**
Acute broncho is pneumonia	• Oral amoxicillin 250–500 mg after every 8 hours Or cotrimoxazole 960 mg twice a day is usually effective. • In cases with severe infection, cefotaxime or ceftriaxone 1 g IV twice a day may be used. • If cyanosis is present, then oxygen therapy is given. • Physiotherapy is advised to older and debilitated patients who get recovered from acute episode.
Aspiration pneumonia	• Oral Amoxycillin 500 mg 8 hourly or Ampicillin 500 mg 6 hourly Or cotrimoxazole 960 mg twice a day is usually effective. • For anaerobes, oral metronidazole 400 mg 8 hourly is given. • Above treatment should be given for 2 weeks. • Analgesics should be given, if pain is present. • Physiotherapy and postural drainage is required in cases of lung abscess.
Nosocomial pneumonia	• In mild cases, amoxicillin with clavulanic acid 500 mg TDS is given. • In severe cases IV cefuroxime 750 mg every 8 hourly + Clarithromycin 250 mg every 8 hourly is given.
Pneumonia in immunocompromised host	• Before culture and sensitivity report is received, a third generation cephalosporine, i.e., cefotaxime 1.0 g IV twice a day or a quinolone, i.e., ciprofloxacin 200 mg IV + amoxycillin 500 mg IV after every 8 hours can be started. • At times, gentamicin 80 mg after every 8 hours may be added to the above regimen. • Metronidazole can be added is anaerobic infection is present. • After treatment, if no response is gained under a week bronchoscopy is done and lavage is sent for culture and sensitivity

---

Q 5.   *Otitis media = An infection of the air filled space behind the ear drum caused by bacteria and viruses.

Q.7. Discuss briefly the management of community acquired pneumonia. *(Feb/Mar 2004, 5 Marks)*

Ans. Community acquired pneumonia is also known as primary pneumonia.

Community acquired pneumonia is defined as an infection that begins outside the hospital or is diagnosed within 48 hours after admission to hospital in a patient who has not resided in a long-term facility for 14 days or more before the onset of symptoms.

Investigations

Blood Tests

♦ WBC count is marginally raised or is normal in patients with pneumonia caused by atypical microorganisms.

♦ Absolute neutrophil count is more than 15×10^9/L and this is indicative of bacterial etiology.

♦ A very high or low WBC count can be seen in severe pneumonia.

♦ C-reactive protein is typically elevated.

Radiological Examination

♦ A confident diagnosis should always need a chest X-ray.

♦ In pneumococcal pneumonia, a homogeneous opacity is seen localized to the affected lobe or segment which appears within 12 to 18 hours from onset of illness.

Microbiological Investigations

♦ Most of the cases of community acquired pneumonia are successfully managed, if they are not severe. So the need of microbiological investigation is based on clinical circumstances.

♦ In severe cases of community acquire pneumonia a full range of microbial tests should be carried out.

♦ If patient does not respond to the initial therapy, microbiological tests provide proper modification of therapy.

Assessment of Gas Exchange

♦ Pulse oximetry is the non-invasive method which measures the arterial oxygen saturation and monitors the response to oxygen therapy.

♦ An arterial blood gas is sampled in patients with low arterial oxygen saturation or having features of severe pneumonia to assess whether patient has evidence of ventilator failure or acidosis.

Management of Community Acquired Pneumonias

Community acquired pneumonias	
Type of pneumonia	**Management**
Pneumococcal pneumonia	• Initially oral amoxicillin should be given 500 mg 8 hourly or erythromycin 500 mg 6 hourly. • In severe hospitalized cases of community acquired pneumonia, IV ampicillin or amoxicillin should be given 500 mg 8 hourly. IV cefotaxime or ceftriaxone may be given in penicillin-resistant strains. Vancomycin is given in infections resistant to penicillin or cephalosporin • Antibiotic therapy should be given for 7–10 days. • Choice of antibiotic depends on the causative microorganisms. • Oxygen therapy is given in seriously ill patients. Oxygen should be delivered at very high rate. • Analgesics, such as mefenamic acid 250 to 500 mg or pethidine 50–100 mg or morphine 10–15 mg IM or IV injections should be given. • Physiotherapy is given to patient by encouraging him to cough and to take deep breath as pleuritic pain disappears.
Staphylococcal pneumonia	• IV flucloxacillin 0.5–1 g 6 hourly or erythromycin 0.5–1 g every 6 hourly is given in cases with mild infection. • If infection is severe than IV sodium fusidate in dosage of 500 mg 6 hourly is given thrice a day in addition to cloxacillin and erythromycin. Treatment should be given for 2 weeks.
Klebsiella pneumoniae	• IV gentamicin 2–5 mg/kg is given in divided doses for every 8 hours. • IV Ceftazidime or cefotaxime 1 g 8 hourly is given or ciprofloxacin 200 mg after every 12 hours IV infusion for 30–60 min is choice of treatment.
Legionella pneumoniae	• Erythromycin 1 g 8 hourly IV for 13 weeks followed by 500 mg qds for 2 weeks. • Doxycycline 100 mg twice a day orally for 3 weeks. • Rifampicin 600 mg twice a day orally for 3 weeks. • In *Legionella endocarditis*, the treatment with antibiotics has to be continued for 3–12 months.
Primary atypical pneumonia	• Oral tetracycline 500 mg 6 hourly or erythromycin 500 mg 6 hourly is effective. • If severe case is present, then above drugs, should be given parenterally.
Viral pneumonia	• Disease is self limiting. • Antipyretics can be given.

Q.8. Write short note on pulmonary embolism.

(May/June 2009, 5 Marks)

Or

Enumerate etiology, clinical features, investigations, complications and management of pulmonary embolism. *(Aug 2011, 15 Marks)*

Ans. Pulmonary embolism is the most common and fatal form of venous thromboembolism in which there is occlusion of pulmonary arterial tree by thromboemboli.

Etiology

Thrombotic

- Deep vein thrombosis
- Congestive heart failure
- Right-sided endocarditis
- Atrial fibrillation.

Non-thrombotic

- Fat embolism
- *Amniotic fluid embolism:* Spontaneous delivery and cesarean section
- *Tumor embolism:* Choriocarcinoma
- *Parasitic embolism:* Schistosomiasis
- *Air embolism:* Pulmonary barotraumas generally in the sea divers.

Clinical Features

In Acute Massive Embolism, i.e., Acute Cor Pulmonale

- Symptoms are of presence of acute dyspnea, tachypnea, tachycardia, hemoptysis and chest pain.
- Signs are increase in the jugular venous pressure, presence of central cyanosis, Loud P2 and narrow splitting of P2, an ejection systolic murmur in P2 area, right ventricular hypertrophy, signs of shock,

In Small- or Medium-sized Pulmonary Vessels Embolization

- Symptoms are hemoptysis, pleuritic pain and wheeze which is the triad of pulmonary infarct.
- Signs are of pleural effusion, i.e., reduced or absent chest wall movement and expansion of chest on the side involved, activity of extrarespiratory muscles is absent, position of trachea and mediastinum is shifted to opposite side, percussion note is stony dull on the side of involvement, vocal fremitus is reduced or absent on the side involved, breath sounds are absent or diminished over the area involved.

In Multiple Microembolization, i.e., Chronic Cor Pulmonale

- Symptoms are of presence of dyspnea, weakness, fatigue and syncope.
- Signs are increase in the jugular venous pressure, presence of cyanosis, edema, hepatomegaly, presence of loud P2 with the ejection systolic murmur in P2 area, presence of narrow splitting of P2, presence of parasternal heave and right ventricular atrophy.

Diagnosis

It is in the patients who had suspicion for underlying cause for emboli formation, development of pulmonary sign and symptoms as well as cardiovascular involvement, presence of thrombophlebitis in deep leg veins, prolonged bed rest, immobilization, cardiac irregularity in form of atrial fibrillation should be considered while keeping in mind clinical picture of precordial pain, breathlessness and tachycardia in patient who had recently gone for major surgery. Examination of veins is mandatory in the patients who are at high risk for development of deep vein thrombosis. These features along with investigatory features form the diagnosis. Following are the investigations:

Investigations

- *Blood examination:* If pulmonary infarct is present, there can be leukocytosis or raised ESR.
- *Chest X-ray:* In massive pulmonary embolism, there is presence of diffuse infiltrates in the lung with increased bronchovascular markings. If medium size vessels are involved, there will be triangular pleuropulmonary opacity in peripheral lung fields, there can also be pleural effusion present.
- *Arterial blood gas analysis:* Presence of hypoxemia and hypocapnia.
- *D-dimer:* It is a fibrin degradation product release in circulation in pulmonary embolism. Presence of high levels of D-dimer is suggestive of an embolism while presence of low D-dimer exclude pulmonary embolism.
- *Echocardiography:* It shows the right ventricular dilatation and presence of clot in it.
- *Spiral CT scan:* CT of chest along with the IV contrast diagnose the pulmonary embolism. It effectively diagnose the large and central pulmonary embolism. Newer scanners can also detect peripherally present emboli.
- *Pulmonary angiography:* It demonstrates the site of obstruction of all sized blood vessels.

Complications

- The foremost complication for pulmonary embolism is pulmonary hypertension.
- Right-sided heart failure
- Peripheral segmental infarctions.

Management

- In patient of massive embolism
  - If patient is in state of shock or collapse:
    - Vasopressors, such as dopamine or dobutamine are to be given.
    - Administer oxygen to the patient.
    - Correct acidosis
    - If there is failure of an initial resuscitation or there is hypotension or right ventricular dysfunction, primary therapy should be administered, i.e., dissociation of clot by thrombolysis or embolectomy.
  - If acute event is survived by the patient,
    - Streptokinase 2.5–5 lac unit IV > in dextrose or saline is given for 30 min followed by 1 lac IV for 24 hours.
    - Recombinant tissue plasminogen activator tPA, i.e., Alteplase 100 mg for 2 hours is a good alternative to thrombolytic therapy.

- Anticoagulation therapy is an initial and immediate treatment of choice.
    - Loading dose of 80–150 units/kg is given which is followed by 15 to 18 units/kg/hr as continuous infusion.
    - Warfarin should be added to heparin and is continued for 5 days.
    - After 5 days taper the heparin and administer warfarin for 6 weeks to 6 months.
    - Monitor anticoagulant therapy by PTT or INR ratio or bleeding time which should be 2–3 times than the control.
- In small embolisms
    - Analgesics, i.e., NSAIDs should be given to relieve the pain.
    - Anticoagulant is given to prevent further embolization.
    - Various preventive measures should be undertaken, such as calf muscle exercise, elastic stockings, prolong immobilization at bed, respiration exercises should be done.

Q.9. Write short note on tropical eosinophilia.

(Mar 1998, 5 Marks)

Ans. *Tropical eosinophilia:* A disease of tropical countries (India, Pakistan, Bangladesh, Sri Lanka, etc.) is characterized by chronic cough, attack of breathlessness, lassitude and weight loss with rise in eosinophilic count in blood.

Etiology

The most important cause of tropical eosinophilia is allergic reaction to filarial worm, e.g., *Wuchereria bancrofti*.

Pathology

Patients having tropical eosinophilia lack IgG blocking antibodies against the circulating microfilaria. Microfilaria is removed from peripheral circulation and is trapped in various tissue sites by IgG dependent cell-mediated effector mechanism. Antigens are released as parasites get destroyed which initiates Type I hypersensitivity reaction. Peripheral eosinophilia occurs due to a reaction which further progress to granuloma and fibrosis.

Clinical Features

- Chronic cough of several weeks or months duration is the prominent complaint.
- Cough may be dry or mucoid to mucopurulent
- There is constricting sensation in the chest.
- Patient suffers from general *debility, weight loss, low grade fever and malaise.
- Presence of lymphadenopathy and splenomegaly
- Nocturnal bronchospasm

Diagnosis

- Positive history for prolong presence of patient in endemic area.
- Lacking of microfilaria in blood, in both night as well as day samples.

Q 9.   *Debility = Weakness or lack of strength.

- Presence of high titers of filarial antibodies.
- IgE levels are 1000 units/mL.
- Peripheral eosinophilia with 3000 cells/mL.

Treatment

The drug of choice is diethyl carbamazine given in dose of 5 mg/kg body weight for 2 weeks

- In adult dosage, three tab of 50 mg four times a day for 5 days.
- In addition patient will require bronchodilators to relieve the bronchospasm.
- Corticosteroids and antihistaminics are employed.
- Recovery after therapy is good.
- Repeat course of drug may have to be given after six weeks.

Q.10. Write short note on acute respiratory failure.

(Apr 2010, 5 Marks)

Ans. Respiratory failure is defined as failure of respiratory system to maintain normal partial pressure of oxygen and carbon dioxide in the blood.

Types of Acute Respiratory Failure

- *Type I acute respiratory failure:* In this, there is acute alteration in blood gases concentration with hypoxemia and normo- or hypocapnia because of tachypnea or hyperventilation.
- *Type II acute respiratory failure:* It is also known as asphyxia. In this, there is hypercapnia and acute respiratory acidosis.

Causes

- *Type I acute respiratory failure:*
    - Acute asthma
    - Pulmonary embolism
    - Pulmonary edema
    - Acute respiratory distress syndrome
    - Pneumothorax
    - Pneumonia
- *Type II acute respiratory failure:*
    - An inhaled foreign body
    - Status asthmaticus
    - Paralysis of respiratory muscles
    - Fractured ribs
    - Brainstem ischemia
    - Overdose of narcotic drugs

Management

- Removal of underlying cause is mandatory.
- Hospitalize the patient and treat in the respiratory intensive care unit.
- Supervise coughing in a conscious patient and change the patient's position from side to side which helps in clearing airway.
- By using a rolled gauze piece clear the thick secretions in oral cavity by holding in an artery forcep.
- Secretions at back of throat or in trachea are removed by frequent secretion.

♦ High concentration of oxygen is given to the patients via ventimasks to improve hypoxemia and ventilation. For small children, oxygen tents are used. Oxygen therapy should be continued till patient achieve normal level of blood gases.

♦ In Type II, acute respiratory failure immediate reversal of precipitating factor should be done. In cases where reversal cannot occur temporary ventilator support is required.

♦ If patient get worse even after taking above-mentioned treatment, tracheostomy and endotracheal intubation is done and now the patient should be supported with intermittent positive pressure ventilation.

♦ Mucolytic agents, such as bromhexine liquefy secretion. Acetylcysteine, i.e., 1–2 mL of 20% solution is instilled via tracheostomy tube.

♦ Patients suffering from acute respiratory distress syndrome can be on positive end expiratory pressure.

♦ Intravenous fluids and electrolyte therapy is given.

♦ Underlying infection should be treated by proper antibiotics.

♦ H2 blockers are given via IV drip

♦ Patient should be slowly weaned from respirator as voluntary effort is gained from ventilation as etiology is corrected.

Q.11. Write short note on tuberculous pleural effusion.
(Mar 1997, 5 Marks)

Ans. *Pleural effusion:* Abnormal accumulation of fluid in pleural spaces.

♦ When amount of fluid is more than 300 mL.

♦ Tubercular pleural effusion occurs due to tuberculosis.

♦ In tubercular pleural effusion, the pleural fluid is exudative fluid mixed with the blood.

Clinical Features

♦ Acute form comes in the form of acute pleurisy with constitutional symptoms, such as fever, toxemia, loss of appetite and ill health.

♦ Acutely developing effusion will produce breathlessness and dry cough.

♦ Chronic forms of pleurisy present with the picture of chronic ill health, low grade fever and loss of appetite.

Physical Signs

On Inspection

♦ Presence of bilaterally symmetrical chest.

♦ Restrictions of movements of chest on the side of effusion.

On Palpation

♦ Shifting of trachea and mediastinum to opposite side on pushing.

♦ Diminishing of expansion of chest on involved side.

♦ Absence of vocal fremitus on involved side.

On Percussion

Stony dull percussion note on the involved side.

On Auscultation

♦ Absence of breath sounds or diminishing of breath sounds over area of pleural effusion.

♦ Amphoric bronchial breathing can be heard at apex of pleural effusion at interscapular region over the involved side.

♦ Absence of vocal resonance.

Investigations

♦ **Examination of pleural fluid**
  • Pleural fluid is serous or straw-colored and forms cobwebs on standing.
  • Fluid is exudates in nature.
  • On microscopic examination, prominent cell type in fluid is lymphocyte.

♦ Tuberculin test is positive.

♦ Pleural biopsy show granulomatous lesion.

♦ Culture for acid-fast bacilli is positive.

♦ Polymerase chain reaction (PCR) test for tuberculosis is positive.

♦ X-ray chest shows uniform dense opacity with upward concavity in lower and lateral part of hemithorax pushing the lung medially. Sharp angle between diaphragm and rib cage get altered.

♦ ESR is high in tubercular effusion.

♦ Ultrasound localizes and detects the effusion.

♦ **Biochemical tests:**
  • Lactate dehydrogenase get increased in tubercular effusion.
  • Adenosine deaminase activity gets increased in tuberculous pleural effusion, i.e., it is more than 40 IU/L.
  • Interferon Gamma levels are more than 140 pg/mL.

Treatment

In tuberculous pleural effusion, antitubercular therapy is started, i.e., all four drugs isonex, rifampicin, pyrazinamide and ethambutol are given for first three months and then on three drugs, i.e., isonex, rifampicin, ethambutol for six months.

♦ Aspiration of pleural fluid is done for diagnosis, for relieving dyspnea and if fever and toxemia is not subsiding after 4 weeks of antitubercular therapy.

♦ Chest physiotherapy is done to encourage expansion of lower chest.

Q.12. How will you diagnose and manage a case of pneumococcal pneumonia? *(Mar 1997, 15 Marks)*

Ans. It is defined as the inflammation of the lung parenchyma. Pneumococcal pneumonia is caused by the *Pneumococcus.*

Diagnosis of Pneumococcal Pneumonia

♦ **Physical signs:**
  • At the time of early stage of illness, there are decreased respiratory movements.
  • Impairment of percussion node
  • Breadth sounds are diminished.

- Pleural rub is present on the affected side.
- Three days after the disease, signs of consolidations are seen, i.e., high-pitched bronchial breathing and increased vocal resonance.
- At the time of resolution, numerous coarse crackles/crepitations are heard this indicate liquefaction of alveolar exudates.
- **Blood test:** It reveals marked neutrophil leukocytosis.
- **Blood culture:** It shows the presence of *Streptococcus pneumonia.*
- **Examination of sputum:** Gram staining of sputum may demonstrate pneumococci.
- **Chest radiograph:** In pneumococcal pneumonia, a homogeneous opacity is seen localized to the affected lobe or segment which appears within 12–18 hours from onset of illness.
- **Serological test:** It can detect pneumococcal antigen in the serum.
- In some of the cases, fiberoptic, bronchoscopic aspiration or transthoracic needle aspiration is required.

Management

- Initially oral amoxicillin should be given 500 mg 8 hourly or erythromycin 500 mg 6 hourly.
- If patient is very ill or gram-negative or staphylococcal infection is present IV ampicillin 0.5–1 g 6 hourly + flucloxacillin 250–500 mg IV 6 hourly + gentamicin 60–80 mg every 8 hourly IV is given.
- Antibiotic therapy should be given for 7–10 days.
- Choice of antibiotics depends on the causative microorganisms.
- Oxygen therapy is given in seriously-ill patients. Oxygen should be delivered at very high rate.
- Analgesics, such as mefenamic acid 250–500 mg or pethidine 50–100 mg or morphine 10–15 mg IM or IV injections should be given.
- Physiotherapy is given to patient by encouraging him to cough and to take deep breath as pleuritic pain disappears.

Q.13. Write short note on eosinophilia.

(Mar 2006, 10 Marks) (Mar 2008, 2.5 Marks)
(April 2008, 5 Marks)

Ans. Rise in eosinophils in blood to abnormal levels, i.e., greater than 0.4×10^9/L is known as eosinophilia

Causes/Etiology of Eosinophilia

- *Parasitic infection:* Ascariasis, Hookworm disease, *Wuchereria bancrofti*, schistosomiasis.
- *Allergic conditions:* Drug allergy, hay fever, asthma, aspergillosis
- *Skin disorders:* Psoriasis, eczema, dermatitis herpetiformis
- *Tumors:* Lymphoma and myeloproliferative disorders
- *Collagen vascular disorders:* Rheumatoid arthritis, systemic lupus erythematosus
- Hypereosinophilic syndrome
- *Miscellaneous:* Addison's disease, sarcoidosis.

Types of Pulmonary Eosinophilia

- **Cryptogenic eosinophilic pneumonia:**
  - It is seen commonly in middle age females.
  - Symptoms present are of fever, malaise, nausea, breathlessness and dry cough.
  - Chest X-ray show abnormal shadows in upper zones simulating pulmonary tubercular infiltrates.
  - Peripheral blood and sputum on examination show eosinophilia.
  - Both ESR and serum IgE levels are elevated.
  - Prednisolone is given which should be withdrawn in tapered doses after patient get normal.
- **Drug-induced bronchopulmonary eosinophilia:**
  - As the name suggests, it occur due to drugs.
  - It starts with cough and long with other symptoms, such as fever with chills and dyspnea.
  - On X-ray pulmonary infiltrates are seen.
  - Withdrawal of an offending drug and use of steroids.
- **Asthmatic bronchopulmonary eosinophilia:**
  - It is characterized by asthma.
  - Main cause is allergy to *A. fumigatus* or *Candida*
  - Presence of transient fleeting shadows on X-ray.
  - Peripheral blood and sputum on examination show eosinophilia.
- **Idiopathic eosinophilic syndromes:**
  - *Loeffler's syndrome:*
    - This is a benign acute eosinophilic pneumonia.
    - Various parasitic infestations are associated with it.
    - It is characterized by migratory pulmonary infiltrates.
    - There is also presence of cough, fever and dyspnea.
  - *Hypereosinophilic syndrome:*
    - There is presence of peripheral blood eosinophilia for 6 months or long.
    - In this disease, there is lack of presence of parasitic, allergic or other known cause of eosinophilia.
    - It leads to the multisystem organ dysfunction.
    - There is tissue infiltration by mature eosinophils as well as blood and bone marrow eosinophilia.
    - In this syndrome, organs affected are heart, lung, liver, spleen, skin and nervous system.
    - Treatment should be done by steroids.
  - *Churg-Strauss syndrome:*
    - It is a multisystem vasculitic disorder which affects skin, lungs, kidney and nervous system.
    - Patient suffers from fever, malaise, anorexia, weight loss, severe asthmatic attack.
    - Presence of pulmonary infiltrates on X-ray.
    - Peripheral blood on examination shows eosinophilia.
    - Treatment is done by steroids and immunosuppressive agents.

Clinical Features

- Cases of pulmonary eosinophilia generally have mild symptoms in the form of a cough with mucoid expectoration, breathlessness and mild fever, dyspnea or orthopnea, wheezing

♦ General weakness and exhaustion

♦ Pain in chest which is mild and diffuse.

Diagnosis

♦ Blood count shows raised eosinophilic count and IgE level.

♦ Skin test is positive.

♦ There is presence of high amount of eosinophils in the sputum.

♦ X-ray chest shows diffuse miliary mottling often stimulating tuberculosis.

Treatment

By long-term steroids, such as oral prednisolone 60 mg/day.

Q.14. Write note on prevention of bronchial asthma.

(Sep 1997, 5 Marks)

Ans. A disease of airways produced by hyper-responsiveness of tracheobronchial tree to a wide variety of stimuli resulting in reversible narrowing of air passage.

Preventive Measures

♦ *Pollen*
  • Try to avoid exposure to flowering vegetation.
  • Keep bed room windows clean.

♦ *House dust*
  Vacuum cleaning of mattress daily.
  Shake out blankets and bed sheets daily.
  Dust is removed from the bedroom thoroughly.

♦ *Animal dander*
  Avoid contact with animals especially dogs, cats, etc.
  Feathers in pillow and quilts should be substituted from foam pillows and terylene quilts.

♦ *Drugs:* Avoid all preparation of relevant drugs.

♦ *Insect web:* Do not allow the insect web to collect.

Less Common

♦ *Foods/Food items:* Identify and eliminate them from dishes, such as fish, meat, milk, etc.

♦ Chemicals, such as isocyanides and resins, etc: Avoid exposure to contact

♦ *Occupational pollutants:* Avoid pollutants and change the occupation.

  If care should be taken for these factors, asthma will be prevented, i.e., cold air, tobacco smoke, respiratory tract infection, drugs (beta-blockers, NSAIDs, aspirin, etc.), strenuous exercise (exercise induced asthma).

Q.15. Outline the clinical features of empyema.

(Sep 2005, 10 Marks)

Ans. Empyema means the presence of pus in the pleural cavity.

Clinical Features of Acute Empyema

Symptoms

♦ *Those of primary disease:* Imperfect recovery in pneumonic cases, or sudden increase in fever with rigors.

♦ *Those due to mechanical effect:* Pleuritic chest pain in early stage, dyspnea, cough and sputum.

♦ *Those due to toxemia:* Malaise, anorexia, sweats and loss of weight.

Signs

♦ Same as pleural effusion, i.e.
  • *On inspection:*
    – Presence of bilaterally symmetrical chest.
    – Restrictions of movements of chest on the side of effusion.
  • *On palpation:*
    – Shifting of trachea and mediastinum to opposite side on pushing.
    – Diminishing of expansion of chest on involved side.
    – Absence of vocal fremitus on involved side.
  • *On percussion:*
    – Stony dull percussion note on the involved side.
  • *On auscultation:*
    – Absence of breath sounds or diminishing of breath sounds over area of pleural effusion.
    – Amphoric bronchial breathing can be heard at apex of pleural effusion at interscapular region over the involved side.
    – Absence of vocal resonance.

♦ Sometimes edema of chest wall is present.

♦ Finger clubbing can develop within 2 to 3 weeks of onset.

Clinical Features of Chronic Empyema

♦ Recurrent symptoms of chest pain and fever.

♦ Loss of weight and anemia.

♦ Clubbing of fingers.

♦ Chest wall deformity from fibrosis.

♦ Chronic sinus tracts into the skin or lungs may develop.

♦ When bronchopleural fistula is present, air can be heard (or felt) blowing through a patent sinus during coughing.

Q.16. Write short note on chronic bronchitis.

(Feb 2002, 5 Marks)

Ans. Chronic bronchitis may be defined as a "condition where there is persistent productive cough for at least three consecutive months in at least two consecutive years".

Etiology

♦ Cigarette smoking

♦ Air pollution and clinical factors

♦ Infections, i.e., upper respiratory tract infection in smokers

♦ Occupation

♦ Familial and genetic factors

♦ Alpha-1 antitrypsin deficiency.

Clinical Features

Symptoms

♦ It affects male more commonly than the females

♦ Chronic bronchitis is present with recurrent attacks of cough

♦ Cough may occur in paroxysms or is more in elderly hours of morning.

♦ Cough is dry when start but later sputum is bringing out which is mucoid to mucopurulent sometimes, it is blood tinged.

♦ Patient complains sense of tightness in chest, breathlessness and asthma-like picture.
♦ Fever and toxemia appear when infection supervenes

Signs

♦ There is increase in respiratory rate.
♦ Inspiratory and expiratory ronchi and presence of crepitation at the base of lungs.

Investigation

♦ *X-ray:* In early stage, it is normal and later it shows widening of intercostal spaces, ribs placed more horizontally, diaphragm displaced downwards and some patient shows patches of pneumonia.
♦ Sputum for culture and sensitivity test is usually sterile.
♦ *Lung function tests:*
   • Decrease in FEV1
   • Subnormal FEV1/VC
   • Decrease in PEF
   • Normal lung volumes except with emphysema
   • Normal diffusing capacity.
♦ *Blood gas analysis:* In severe cases, there is increase in hypercapnia and decrease in hypoxemia.

Management

♦ Bronchial irritants should be avoided, i.e.
   • Smoking should be strictly stopped.
   • Passive smoking is stopped.
   • Gas smoke is avoided by housemakers.
   • Aerosols, such as hair spray, insecticide spray and aerosols should be avoided.
   • Polluted atmosphere should be strictly avoided.
♦ *Treatment of an infection:*
   • Ampicillin 250–500 mg every 6 hourly is given for 5 to 7 days.
   • Cotrimazole 960 mg can be given as BD dose.
   • Antibiotics should be given till purulent mucous become mucoid.
   • If necessary modify antibiotics as per culture and sensitivity test.
♦ *Bronchodilators:*
   • In mild-to-moderate chronic bronchitis oral theophylline 150 mg BD or inhaled salbutamol 200 µg 6 hourly can be given.
   • In severe bronchitis, ipratropium bromide 40–80 µg 6 hourly is added.
♦ *Mucolytic agents:* Bromhexine and carbocisteine are to be given.
♦ *Corticosteroids:* Prednisolone 30 mg/day for 2 weeks is given. If improvement occur by oral steroids, they are replaced by inhalational steroids.
♦ *Domiciliary oxygen therapy:* Long-term oxygen therapy in low concentration, i.e., 2 L/min by nasal cannula is given to reverse or to delay development of pulmonary hypertension.

Q.17. Describe clinical features and evaluate management of postprimary tuberculosis. *(Mar 1998, 15 Marks)*

Ans. Postprimary tuberculosis is also known as secondary tuberculosis.

Most of the morbidity and mortality from TB is caused by this form disease.

It occurs due to reactivation of dormant primary tuberculosis; as a progressive primary lesion; hematogenous spread to lungs.

At times tuberculosis remains symptom-free and is diagnosed on routine radiography.

Clinical Features

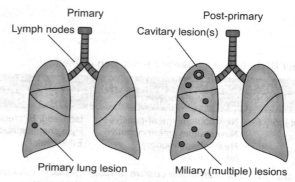

Fig. 12: Post-primary tuberculosis.

Symptoms

♦ Evening rise of temperature
♦ Night sweats
♦ Malaise and cachexia
♦ Irritability and difficulty in concentration.
♦ Cough and expectoration for more than three weeks.
♦ Pleuritic chest pain
♦ Breathlessness is the feature of advanced disease.
♦ Indigestion and dyspnea
♦ Amenorrhea often in young women
♦ Hoarseness of voice.
♦ Sputum can be mucoid, purulent or blood stained.
♦ Hemoptysis is a classical feature
♦ Presence of localized wheeze from local ulcer or narrowing of major bronchus.
♦ Presence of recurrent cold.

Physical Signs

♦ Fever and weight loss
♦ Tachycardia and tachypnea
♦ Rapid pulse rate
♦ Physical signs of collapse, consolidation, cavitation, fibrosis, bronchiectasis, pleural effusion or pneumothorax.
♦ In some cases only localized *rhonchi or rales are present.
♦ Clubbing of fingers is present in chronic disease.
♦ Most common physical sign of chest is fine crepitation in the upper part of one or both the lungs. This is heard on taking a deep breath after coughing.

Q 17. *Rhonchi or rales = A wheezing, snoring or squeaking sound heared during auscultation of chest of a person with partial airway obstruction.

- Later on, there can be presence of dullness to percussion or bronchial breathing in upper part of one or both the lungs.
- In chronic cases, there is evidence of volume loss and mediastinal shift.
- Hilar, mediastinal and cervical groups lymph nodes are enlarged with splenomegaly.

Management

Refer to Ans. 18 of same chapter.

Q.18. Write short note on chemotherapy of pulmonary tuberculosis. *(Sep 1997, 5 Marks)*

Ans.

Chemotherapy

Drugs for Primary Chemotherapy (First line antitubercular drugs)

Drug	Daily dose (Adult)	Thrice weekly dose
Rifampicin	>50 kg 600 mg <50 kg 450 mg	(10 mg/kg) (10 mg/kg)
Isoniazid	200–300 mg (in military TB 10 mg/kg)	(5 mg/kg) (10 mg/kg)
Pyrazinamide	>50 kg 2 g (25 mg/kg max 2 g) <50 kg 1.5 g	(35 mg/kg, max 3 g)
Ethambutol	25 mg/kg in initial phase	(30 mg/kg) 15 mg/kg in continuation phase

Under DOTs following treatment regimen is used

	Indication	Intensive phase		Continuation phase	
		Drugs	Duration	Drugs	Duration
Category I	New sputum smear-positive New sputum smear-negative New extrapulmonary tuberculosis	Isoniazid, Rifampicin, Pyrazinamide and Ethambutol	Thrice weekly for 2 months	Isoniazid and Rifampicin	Thrice weekly for 4 months
Category II	Sputum smear-positive relapse Sputum smear-positive failure Sputum smear-positive treatment after default	Isoniazid, Rifampicin, Pyrazinamide, Ethambutol and streptomycin	Thrice weekly for 2 months followed by		
		Isoniazid, Rifampicin, Pyrazinamide and Ethambutol	For 1 month	Isoniazid, Rifampicin and Pyrazinamide	5 months

Second-line Antituberculous Drugs

Drug	Dose
Streptomycin	20–40 mg/kg/day OD IM
Kanamycin	15–30 mg/kg/day OD IM
Amikacin	15–22.5 mg/kg/day OD IM
Capreomycin	15–30 mg/kg/day OD IM
Ofloxacin	15–20 mg/kg/day BD orally
Levofloxacin	7.5–10 mg/kg/day OD orally
Moxifloxacin	7.5–10 mg/kg/day orally
Ethionamide	15–20 mg/kg/day BD orally
Prothionamide	15–20 mg/kg/day BD orally
Cycloserine*	10–20 mg/kg/day OD or BD orally
PAS*	150 mg/kg/day BD or TDS orally

*Cycloserine and PAS are bacteriostatic others are bactericidal.

Treatment Regimen under RNTCP for MDR-TB (Multi-drug-resistant TB) and XDR-TB (Extensively drug resistant TB)

- *For MDR-TB:*
  - *Six drugs in intensive phase for 6–9 months:* Kanamycin, Levofloxacin, Ethionamide, Cycloserine, Pyrazinamide and Ethambutol.
  - *Four drugs in continuation phase for 18 months:* Levofloxacin, Ethionamide, Cycloserine and Ethambutol.
  - Reserve drug is p-aminosalicylic acid.
- *For XDR-TB:*
  - *Seven drugs in intensive phase for 6–12 months:* Capreomycin, p-aminosalicylic acid, Moxifloxacin, high-dose Isoniazid, Clofazimine, Linezolid, Amoxicillin and Clavulinic acid.
  - *Six drugs in continuation phase for 18 months:* p-aminosalicylic acid, Moxifloxacin, high dose isoniazid, Clofazimine, Linezolid, Amoxicillin and Clavulinic acid.
  - Reserve drugs: Clarithromycin, Thiacetazone

Q.19. Write short note on side effects of antitubercular drugs. *(Sep 2008, 5 Marks)*

Ans.

First line antitubercular drugs	
Name of drug	Side effects
Rifampicin	Nausea, vomiting, diarrhea, skin rashes and liver damage, influenza, such as reaction, leukopenia, eosinophilia, ataxia and dizziness
Isoniazid	Peripheral neuropathy, psychosis hepatic injury, optic neuritis convulsions and dryness of mouth
Pyrazinamide	Polyarthralgia, nausea, vomiting, malaise, toxic hepatitis, hyperuricemia, gout
Ethambutol	Blurring of vision, optic neuritis, nausea, vomiting, liver damage and peripheral neuropathy

Second line antitubercular drugs	
Name of drug	Side effects
Streptomycin	Nephrotoxicity, ototoxicity, ataxia, anaphylaxis, injection abscess, circumoral paresthesia, eosinophilia, drug fever
Kanamycin Amikacin	Ototoxicity, deafness, vertigo, nephrotoxic tinnitus, vertigo, renal damage, cutaneous reactions, hypocalcemia, hypomagnesaemia and hepatitis
Capreomycin	Psychosis, seizures, peripheral neuropathy, headache, somnolence and allergy
Ofloxacin Levofloxacin Moxifloxacin	Anorexia, nausea, vomiting, dizziness, headache, mood changes and impaired growth
Ethionamide Protionamide	Skin rash, purpura, anorexia, nausea, vomiting, headache, anaphylactic shock, postural hypotension, metallic taste, hypersalivation, hallucination, menstrual disorders.

Second line antitubercular drugs	
Name of drug	Side effects
Cycloserine	Weakness, tremor, ataxia, convulsion, slurred speech, brisk jerk, ankle clonus, insomnia and psychosis.
PAS (p-amino salicyclic acid	• Gastrointestinal symptoms: Anorexia, nausea, vomiting, diarrhea • Intolerance: Fever, skin rash and lymphadenopathy • Hemopoietic: leukopenia, eosinophilia, ataxia • Hepatic damage • Acute renal failure • Myxedema and Loeffler's syndrome

Q.20. Write short note on nosocomial pneumonia.
(Nov 2014, 3 Marks) (Mar 2007, 5 Marks)

Ans. Nosocomial pneumonia is defined as hospital acquired pneumonia.

♦ It is the secondary pneumonia.
♦ Pneumonias developing in hospital in a patient who has been admitted for more than 48 hours should be considered to be nosocomial rather than community acquired.
♦ Because of change of oropharyngeal flora in hospitalized patients, it is caused by anaerobic gram-negative organism like *E. coli*, *Klebsiella pneumoniae*, *Pseudomonas*, more frequent. *Staphylococcus aureus*, pneumococci and *H. influenza* are less frequent causative organisms.

Factors Predisposing for Nosocomial Pneumonia

♦ *Reduced host defenses against bacteria:*
  • Reduced immune defenses (e.g. corticosteroid treatment, diabetes, malignancy)
  • Reduced cough reflex (e.g. postoperative)
  • Disordered mucociliary clearance (e.g. anesthetic agents)
  • Bulbar or vocal cord palsy
♦ *Aspiration of nasopharyngeal or gastric secretions:*
  • Immobility or reduced conscious level
  • Vomiting, dysphagia, achalasia or severe reflux
  • Nasogastric intubation
♦ *Bacteria introduced into lower respiratory tract:*
  • Endotracheal intubation/tracheostomy
  • Infected ventilators/nebulizers/bronchoscopes
  • Dental or sinus infection
♦ *Bacteremia:*
  • Abdominal sepsis
  • Intravenous cannula infection
  • Infected emboli

Treatment

♦ In mild cases, amoxicillin with clavulanic acid 500 mg TDS is given.
♦ In severe cases IV cefuroxime 750 mg every 8 hourly + Clarithromycin 250 mg every 8 hourly is given.
♦ Most of the patients require ventilatory support and also need supplemental oxygen therapy.

Q.21. Write short note on aspiration pneumonia.
(Apr 2007, 10 Marks)

Ans. Aspiration pneumonia is also known as suppurative pneumonia.

Aspiration pneumonia is the consolidation of lung in which there is continued destruction of parenchyma by inflammatory cells which causes formation of microabscess.

Etiology

Aspiration pneumonia is caused by *Staphylococcus aureus*, Sterptococcal pneumonia, *Streptococcus pyogenes*, *Haemophilus influenza* as well as various other anaerobic bacterias.

Clinical Features

Symptoms

- Aspiration pneumonia occurs mostly on the right side as compared to left side.
- Patient complaints of high fever, cough and dyspnea.
- During coughing copious foul-smelling sputum is present, which is blood stained too.
- There is presence of tachycardia and restlessness.
- Weight loss is too rapid.
- There is also presence of perspiration.

Signs

- Signs of lung consolidation are seen.
- If there is formation of lung abscess, cavitation can be felt.
- There is presence of pleural rub.
- Digital clubbing is also well appreciated.

Investigations

- TLC and DLC should be carried out for checking neutrophilic leukocytosis.
- ESR is high.
- *Chest X-ray:* It shows a homogeneous opacity. If there is presence of fluid in the opacity, this indicates of an abscess.
- *Culture of sputum* is carried out to identify microorganisms.

Treatment

- In aerobic infection ampicillin 500 mg QID or amoxicillin 500 mg TID or cotrimoxazole 960 mg BD orally provides relief.
- In anaerobic infection, metronidazole 400 mg TID orally is added.
- Antibiotics should be prescribed based on the culture and sensitivity testing.
- Treatment should be continued for 10 to 15 days.
- NSAIDs should be given for pain relief.
- In subjects with lung abscess physiotherapy and postural drainage is done.

Complications

- Amyloidosis
- Empyema
- Bronchiectasis
- Septicemia
- Pulmonary fibrosis.

Q.22. Mention complications of pulmonary tuberculosis.
(Apr 2007, 5 Marks)

Ans. The complications of pulmonary tuberculosis are as follows:

I. Early complications
- Pneumonia
- Empyema
- Hemoptysis
- Laryngitis
- Pneumothorax.

II. Late complications
- Bronchiectasis
- Mycetomas in cavity
- Colonization of fibrotic lung with nontuberculous Mycobacterium
- Nonrespiratory disease, i.e., genitourinary, bone.

Q.23. Write short note on smoking-related disorder.
(Mar 2008, 2.5 Marks)

Ans. The incidence of smoking-related diseases is greater in younger than in older smokers, particularly for coronary artery disease and smokers.

- Cardiovascular disease
- Cigarette smokers are more likely than nonsmokers to develop large vessel atherosclerosis as well as small vessel disease.
- Cigarette smoking also increases likelihood of myocardial infarction and sudden cardiac death.

Cancer

Tobacco smoking causes cancer of lung, oral cavity, nose, oro and hypopharynx, nasal cavity and paranasal sinuses, larynx, esophagus, stomach, pancreas, liver, kidney, ureter, urinary bladder and uterine cervix and also causes myeloid leukemia.

Respiratory Disease

Cigarette smoking is responsible for 90% of COPD within 1–2 years of beginning of smoke regularly.

Many smokers will develop inflammatory changes in small airway due to there is reduced expiratory airflow.

Other Conditions

Smoking delays healing of peptic ulcer, increases risk of osteoporosis, senile cataract, macular degeneration, premature menopause, wrinkling in skin, gallstone, male impotence and cholecystitis in women.

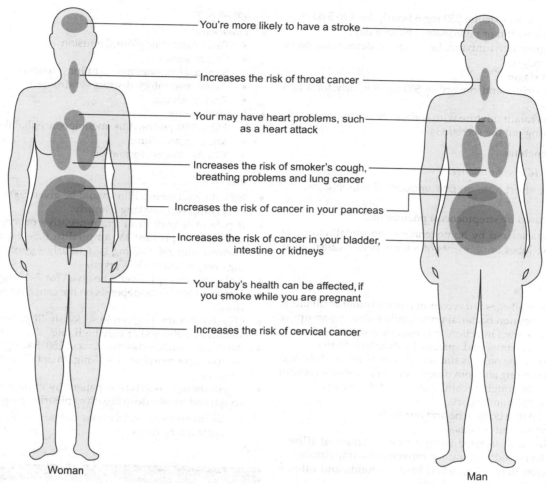

You're more likely to have a stroke

Increases the risk of throat cancer

Your may have heart problems, such as a heart attack

Increases the risk of smoker's cough, breathing problems and lung cancer

Increases the risk of cancer in your pancreas

Increases the risk of cancer in your bladder, intestine or kidneys

Your baby's health can be affected, if you smoke while you are pregnant

Increases the risk of cervical cancer

Woman

Man

Fig. 13: Smoking-related disorders.

Q.24. Write short note on bronchitis.

(Apr 2008, 5 Marks) (Mar 2008, 5.5 Marks)

Ans. Bronchitis is the infection of the bronchi.

Types

1. Acute bronchitis.
2. Chronic bronchitis.

Acute Bronchitis

It is an acute infection of the bronchi and may be caused by the infection with organisms, such as *Streptococcus*, pneumococci, *Haemophilus influenzae* or primarily viral in origin.

Causes

- *Infection:* Bacterial or viral, or descending infection from nasal sinus or throat.
- *Complicating other diseases,* such as measles and whooping cough.
- *Physical and chemical irritants:* Inhaled dust, steam, gases, such as sulfur dioxide and ether.

Symptoms

- *Toxemia:* Malaise, fever, ill health, tachycardia
- *Irritative:* Cough with expectoration, at first scanty viscid sputum is present and later on it become more copious and mucopurulent; substernal pain or raw sensation under sternum.
- *Obstructive:* Chocked up feeling, paroxysms of dyspnea following spells of coughing relieved with expectoration.

Physical Signs

Fever, tachycardia, flushing of face, respiratory rate is slightly increased. Crepitations are heard at the base when secretions collect in the lungs.

Treatment

- **In dry stage:**
  - Bed rest
  - Nutritious diet
  - Tincture benzoin inhalation
  - Application of vicks vaporub on chest

- Capsule amoxicillin 250 mg 8 hourly for 4 to 5 days.
- Tablet aspirin or paracetamol twice a day.
- Cough sedative mixture like linctus codeine to suppress dry cough.

♦ **In moist stage:**
- Amoxicillin and cloxacillin 500 mg 8 hourly for 4 to 5 days.
- Expectorant mixture with sodium or potassium iodide to bring out the secretions.

Chronic Bronchitis

Refer to Ans. 16 of same chapter.

Q.25. Write short note on pneumococcal pneumonia.
(Sep 2009, 4.5 Marks)

Ans. It is caused by streptococcal pneumonia.

It is characterized by homogeneous consolidation of one lobe or more lobes or segments of a lung, hence, called lobar pneumonia

Clinical Features

♦ It occurs at all ages but is common in early and adult life. It is most common bacterial pneumonia following an upper respiratory tract infection. It is usually a sporadic disease, common in winter and spreads by droplet infection.
♦ In children, the onset is sudden often with fever, chills and rigors, vomiting and convulsions. In adults, the onset is with fever, chills, cough, breathlessness and chest pain.
♦ Shaking chills and rigors
♦ Loss of apatite body ache and headache
♦ Hemoptysis and weakness
♦ The physical signs during an early stage of illness show decreased respiratory movements, impairment of percussion note, diminished breath sounds and often a pleural rub on the affected side.
  - Later on, usually after 3 days, signs of consolidation appear.
  - During resolution, numerous coarse crackles crepitations are heard, indicating the liquefaction of alveolar exudate.

Investigations

♦ *Blood test:* It reveals marked neutrophil leukocytosis.
♦ Blood culture: It shows the presence of *Streptococcus pneumonia.*
♦ *Examination of sputum:* Gram staining of sputum may demonstrate pneumococci.
♦ *Chest radiograph:* In pneumococcal pneumonia, a homogeneous opacity is seen localized to the affected lobe or segment which appears within 12–18 hours from onset of illness.
♦ *Serological test:* It can detect pneumococcal antigen in the serum.
♦ In some of the cases, fiberoptic, bronchoscopic aspiration or transthoracic needle aspiration is required.

Complications

♦ *Pulmonary:*
- Parapneumonic pleural effusion
- Emphysema
- Suppurative pneumonia or lung abscess
- Acute respiratory distress syndrome
- Pneumothorax

♦ *Extrapulmonary*
- Hepatitis, pericarditis, meningoencephalitis
- Multiorgan failure
- Ectopic abscess formation

Management

♦ Initially, oral amoxicillin should be given 500 mg 8 hourly or erythromycin 500 mg 6 hourly.
♦ If patient is very ill or gram-negative or staphylococcal infection is present IV ampicillin 0.5–1 g 6 hourly + flucloxacillin 250–500 mg IV 6 hourly + gentamicin 60–80 mg every 8 hourly IV is given.
♦ Antibiotic therapy should be given for 7–10 days.
♦ Choice of antibiotic depends on the causative microorganisms.
♦ Oxygen therapy is given in seriously-ill patients. Oxygen should be delivered at very high rate.
♦ Analgesics, such as mefenamic acid 250–500 mg or pethidine 50–100 mg or morphine 10–15 mg IM or IV injections should be given.
♦ Physiotherapy is given to patient by encouraging him to cough and to take deep breath as pleuritic pain disappears.

Q.26. Differentiate between pleural friction rub and crackles or rales.
(Sep 2008, 2.5 Marks)

Ans.

Pleural friction rub	Crackles or rales
A pleural friction rub is caused by the inflammation of the visceral and parietal pleurae	Crackles are the sounds you will hear in a lung field that has fluid in the small airways or if atelectasis is present
This is a low-pitched creaking, grating or rubbing sound	This is small bubbling or clicking heard with a stethoscope, it is much like the static sound heard on the radio
Sound is heard more often with inhalation than expiration	Sound is heard with breathing in or out and is not always a continuous sound
Sound occur when inflamed pleural surfaces rub together during respiration	The sounds produced are created when air is forced through respiratory passages that are narrowed by fluid, mucus, or pus

Q.27. Write short note on primary tuberculosis and its investigations.
(Sep 2009, 4 Marks)

Ans. Primary tuberculosis is the first lesion which develops in a previously unexposed non-sensitized individual irrespective of the age.

Pathology

♦ Reinfection of a sensitized person or reactivation of a primary dormant lesion is called secondary or post-primary tuberculosis.

♦ The initial lesion after ingestion of tubercle bacilli which mainly occurs in the lungs constitutes primary tuberculosis.

♦ It commonly involves children and is in the form of subpleural lesion either in the lower part of upper lobe or upper part of lower lobe.

♦ The initial entry of the bacilli initiates nonspecific inflammatory response which hardly produces any symptoms. Bacilli are transported to regional lymph nodes and parenchymal lesion in the lungs (Ghon Focus) along with enlarged lymph nodes which may calcify over a period of time and this constitutes primary complex (Ghon's complex).

♦ A case of primary tuberculosis draws attention when a child may present with a nonspecific pneumonia or bronchial obstruction because of enlarged hilar gland or low-grade fever with pleural effusion.

♦ Primary complex heals leaving a calcified lesion.

♦ Bacilli may remain for years and may become reactivated when body's immunity falls as in malnutrition, debilitating disease and following severe form of measles, whooping cough.

Clinical Features

As tuberculosis remains symptom-free and is diagnosed on routine radiography.

Symptoms

♦ Evening rise of temperature
♦ Night sweats
♦ Malaise and cachexia
♦ Irritability and difficulty in concentration.
♦ Cough and expectoration for more than three weeks.
♦ Pleuritic chest pain
♦ Breathlessness is the feature of advanced disease.
♦ Indigestion and dyspnea
♦ Amenorrhea often in young women
♦ Hoarseness of voice.
♦ Sputum can be mucoid, purulent or blood stained.
♦ Hemoptysis is a classical feature
♦ Presence of localized wheeze from local ulcer or narrowing of major bronchus.
♦ Presence of recurrent cold.

Physical Signs

♦ Fever and weight loss
♦ Tachycardia and tachypnea
♦ Rapid pulse rate
♦ Physical signs of collapse, consolidation, cavitation, fibrosis, bronchiectasis, pleural effusion or pneumothorax.

♦ In some cases, only localized *rhonchi or rales are present.
♦ Clubbing of fingers is present in chronic disease.
♦ Most common physical sign of chest is fine crepitation in the upper part of one or both the lungs. This is heard on taking a deep breath after coughing.
♦ Later on, there can be presence of dullness to percussion or bronchial breathing in upper part of one or both the lungs.
♦ In chronic cases, there is evidence of volume loss and mediastinal shift.
♦ Hilar, mediastinal and cervical groups lymph nodes are enlarged with splenomegaly.

Investigations

♦ **Sputum examination (for acid fast bacilli):** By direct smear examination (Ziehl-Neelsen stain). At least, three smears must be examined before finally reaching a conclusion. When direct smear is negative, sputum examination be done by concentration method using 24 hours collection of sputum. Further confirmation is done by sputum culture by animal inoculation which takes 4–8 weeks. If adequate amount of sputum is not available, bronchoscopic aspiration of secretions be made and submitted for smear and culture examination.

♦ **Serology:** In this ELISA, technique is used which helpful in diagnosis of tuberculosis in children. PCR technique is more specific and sensitive serological test than ELISA, but PCR is less used due to its high cost.

♦ **Chest X-ray:** Presence of multiple nodular infiltrations or ill-defined opacities in one of upper lobes is characteristic for pulmonary tuberculosis. An area of translucency in radiopacities is indicative of cavitation. Presence of cavity is indicative of an active lesion. In some of the patients multiple thick-walled cavities can be seen. At the time of fibrosis, trachea and mediastinum shift to same side. Fibrosis can also cause calcification

♦ **Pathological tests:**
  • *Blood examination:* Peripheral blood examination shows monocytosis, i.e., 8 to 12%
  • ESR is elevated.
  • *Tuberculin test:* It is a test to recognize prior tubercular infection, and is done by injecting one unit of purified protein derivative (PPD) on the forearm and readings taken after 48 hours. Induration of more than 15 mm indicates a positive test. The younger is the patient, greater is significance of positive test. A negative test does not always exclude tubercular infection since it may be negative in patients of blood malignancies, malnourishment and those on immunosuppressive therapy. Tuberculin test is nonspecific and only indicates prior infection. Its sensitivity wanes with age.

Q.28. Write difference between bronchial and cardiac asthma. *(Sep 2008, 2.5 Marks) (Sep 2011, 4 Marks)*

Ans.

	Features	Cardiac asthma	Bronchial asthma
1.	Past history	Of hypertension, aortic disease	Of previous attacks of asthma or other allergic conditions
2.	Age	Onset is after 40 years	Any age
3.	Precipitating factor	Precipitated by exertion, acute myocardial infarction or hypertension	Trigger factors may be infection, nonspecific irritants, external allergens, exercise or emotional factors
4.	*Symptoms:*		
	a. Cough	Cough and dyspnea almost simultaneous. Pink frothy sputum which increases in intensity towards end of attack	Starts with dyspnea Expectoration of thick sticky sputum
	b. Wheezing	Rare	Usual
	c. Sweating asthma	Prominent	Rare unless acute severe
5.	*Signs:*		
	a. Inspection		
	- Accessory muscles of respiration	Not active	Active
	- Shape of chest	Normal	Emphysematous
	- Respirations expiration	Rapid and shallow	Rapid with prolong
	b. Auscultation		
	- Chest	Expiration not unduely prolonged	Expiration markedly prolonged
		Rales more than ronchi in early stages at lung bases, gradually ascending up with progress of the attack	Ronchi are more than rales Signs diffuse all over the lungs
	- Heart	A2 may be loud	Normal A2
	c. Pulse	Pulsus alternans	Feeble and rapid
	d. BP	Usually elevated	Normal or low
	e. Extremities	Cold	Warm

Q.29. Write short note on respiratory failure.

(Apr 2008, 5 Marks)

Ans. Respiratory failure is defined as failure of respiratory system to maintain normal partial pressure of oxygen and carbon dioxide in the blood.

Types

- **Type I (Hypoxemic) respiratory failure:**
  - *Acute:* In this, there is acute alteration in blood gases concentration with hypoxemia and normo- or hypocapnia because of tachypnea or hyperventilation.
  - *Chronic:* Chronic alteration in blood gases occur due to slow diffusion of carbon dioxide via lungs. So there is occurrence of hypoxemia and normocapnia. Here pH and bicarbonate levels remain normal.
- **Type II (Hypercapnic) respiratory failure:**
  - *Acute:* It is also known as asphyxia. In this, there is hypercapnia and acute respiratory acidosis.
  - *Chronic:* In this, there is hypoxemia, hypercapnia but low or normal pH.
  - *Acute on chronic Type II respiratory failure:* Here there is sudden rise of carbon dioxide and there is occurrence of acidemia with acute insult from the precipitating factors. This is known as acute on chronic Type II respiratory failure.

Signs and Symptoms (Clinical Features)

Due to Hypoxemia

- *Signs:*
  - Tachycardia
  - Central cyanosis
  - Poor peripheral circulation
  - Depress level of consciousness
  - Cardiac arrhythmias.
- *Symptoms:*
  - Sweating
  - Restlessness
  - Mental confusion.

Due to Hypercapnia

- *Signs:*
  - *Effect on CNS functions:* Asterixis, mitosis, hyporeflexia, confusion and coma
  - Bounding pulse
  - Muscle twitching
  - Elevated blood pressure
  - Cardiac dysrhythmias.
- *Symptoms:*
  - Breathlessness
  - Headache
  - Warm extremities.

Management

Acute Respiratory Failure

- Removal of underlying cause is mandatory.
- Hospitalize the patient and treat in the respiratory intensive care unit.
- Supervise coughing in a conscious patient and change the patient's position from side to side which helps in clearing airway.
- By using a rolled gauze piece clear the thick secretions in oral cavity by holding in an artery forceps.
- Secretions at back of throat or in trachea are removed by frequent secretion.
- High concentration of oxygen is given to the patients via ventimasks to improve hypoxemia and ventilation. For small children, oxygen tents are used. Oxygen therapy should be continued till patient achieve normal level of blood gases.
- In Type II acute respiratory failure, immediate reversal of precipitating factor should be done. In cases where reversal cannot occurs temporary ventilator support is required.
- If patient get worse even after taking above-mentioned treatment, tracheostomy and endotracheal intubation is done and now the patient should be supported with intermittent positive pressure ventilation.
- Mucolytic agents, such as bromhexine liquefy secretion. Acetylcysteine, i.e., 1–2 mL of 20% solution is instilled via tracheostomy tube.
- Patients suffering from acute respiratory distress syndrome can be on positive end expiratory pressure.
- Intravenous fluids and electrolyte therapy is given.
- Underlying infection should be treated by proper antibiotics.
- H_2 blockers are given via IV drip
- Patient should be slowly weaned from respirator as voluntary effort is gained from ventilation as etiology is corrected.

Chronic Respiratory Failure

- Nebulized solution of salbutamol, i.e., 2.5–5 mg 4 hourly or terbutaline 5–10 mg can also be given.
- Bronchodilator such aminophylline is given in dose of 0.25 g IV diluted in 10 mL of 10–25% dextrose and is injected slowly.
- Short course of antibiotics should be given.
- Secretions should be removed by asking the patient to cough or by intermittent endotracheal catheter suction.
- If patient develops pulmonary edema or cor pulmonale.
- Oxygen therapy and assisted ventilation should be given to acute on chronic Type II respiratory failure patients till patient have acceptable levels of PaO_2 and $PaCO_2$.
- If condition of patient worsen mechanical ventilation by fixed volume, ventilators is given to deliver fix volume of oxygen.
- Ventilatory assistance is slowly withdrawn as patient returns to voluntary effort.

Q.30. Write short note on emphysema. *(Apr 2008, 5 Marks)*

Ans. It is defined as distention of the air spaces distal to the terminal bronchiole with destruction of alveolar septa.

Predisposing Factors/Etiology

- Smoking
- Environmental pollution
- Genetic predisposition due to alpha-I antitrypsin deficiency
- Bacterial
- Occupational exposure.

Types of Emphysema

- *Centriacinar:* Presence of destruction and enlargement of central or proximal part of respiratory unit. Predominant involvement of upper lobe and apices. Commonly seen in male smokers.
- *Panacinar:* Presence of uniform destruction and enlargement of acinus. It is predominant in lower basal zones. It is associated with alpha-1 antitrypsin deficiency.
- *Paraseptal:* It involves only distal acinus. Found near pleura often causes spontaneous pneumothorax
- *Irregular:* There is irregular type of acinus with scarring involvement.

Clinical Features

There are two types of patients suffering from emphysema. Type A refers to pink puffers who have minimal cough and expectoration while dyspnea is prominent and Type B refers to blue bloaters. In this, patients have marked blood gas abnormalities though the pulmonary diffusing capacity is within the normal limits.

Symptom	Type A (Pink Puffers)	Type B (Blue Bloaters)
Cough	Minimal	Predominant
Expectoration	Minimal	Copious
Dyspnea	Predominant	Mild
Cyanosis	Absent	Present
Cor pulmonale	Infrequent	Common
Edema	Not common	Edema in dependent parts
Jugular venous pressure	Not raised	Raised
Diffusing capacity of lungs	Decreased	In normal limits

Treatment

Chronic source of infection in upper respiratory airway be removed.

- Patient should be taken away from cold climate
- Smoking in any form must be stopped
- Breathing exercise be advised
- Respiratory infection be prevented and prompt antibiotic treatment, e.g., ampicillin, amoxicillin.
- Bronchodilators are used, i.e., theophylline and salbutamol.
- In severe respiratory insufficiency, corticosteroids are useful prednisolone
- Oxygen inhalation, intermittently is useful in case of emphysema.

Q.31. Enumerate antitubercular drugs—its dosage and complications.   *(Nov 2008, 10 Marks).*

Ans.

First-line antitubercular drugs		
Name of drug	**Dosage**	**Complications**
Rifampicin	>50 kg 600 mg <50 kg 450 mg	Nausea, vomiting, diarrhea, skin rashes and liver damage, influenza like reaction, leukopenia, eosinophilia, ataxia and dizziness
Isoniazid	200–300 mg (In miliary TB 10 mg/kg)	Peripheral neuropathy, psychosis hepatic injury, optic neuritis convulsions and dryness of mouth
Pyrazinamide	>50 kg 2 g <50 kg 1.5 g	Polyarthralgia, nausea, vomiting, malaise, toxic hepatitis, hyperuricemia, gout.
Ethambutol	25 mg/kg in initial phase	Blurring of vision, optic neuritis, nausea, vomiting, liver damage and peripheral neuropathy

Second line antitubercular drugs		
Name of drug	**Dosage**	**Complications**
Streptomycin	20–40 mg/kg/day OD IM	Nephrotoxicity, ototoxicity, ataxia, anaphylaxis, injection abscess, circumoral paresthesia, eosinophilia, drug fever
Kanamycin	15–30 mg/kg/day OD IM	Ototoxicity, deafness, vertigo, nephrotoxic tinnitus, vertigo, renal damage, cutaneous reactions, hypocalcemia, hypomagnesemia and hepatitis
Amikacin	15–22.5 mg/kg/clay OD IM	
Capreomycin	15–30 mg/kg/day OD I IM	Psychosis, seizures, peripheral neuropathy, headache, somnolence and allergy
Ofloxacin	15–20 mg/kg/day BD orally	Anorexia, nausea, vomiting, dizziness, headache, mood changes and impaired growth
Levofloxacin	7.5–10 mg/kg/day OD orally	
Moxifloxacin	7.5–10 mg/kg/day orally	
Ethionamide	15–20 mg/kg/day BD orally	Skin rash, purpura, anorexia, nausea, vomiting, headache, anaphylactic shock, postural hypotension, metallic taste, hypersalivation, hallucination, menstrual disorders
Prothionamide	15–20 mg/kg/day BD orally	
Cycloserine	10–20 mg/kg/day OD or BD orally	Weakness, tremor, ataxia, convulsion, slurred speech, brisk jerk, ankle clonus, insomnia and psychosis
PAS (p-aminosalicylic acid)	150 mg/kg/day BD or TDS orally	• Gastrointestinal symptoms: Anorexia, nausea, vomiting, diarrhea • Intolerance: Fever, skin rash and lymphadenopathy • Hemopoietic: leukopenia, eosinophilia, ataxia • Hepatic damage • Acute renal failure • Myxedema and Loeffler's syndrome

Q.32. Discuss etiology, clinical features, diagnosis and outline the management of acute pulmonary embolism.   *(Dec 2009, 15 Marks)*

Ans.

Etiology

♦ *Thrombotic:*
  • Deep vein thrombosis
  • Congestive heart failure
  • Right-sided endocarditis
  • Atrial fibrillation.
♦ *Non-thrombotic:*
  • Fat embolism
  • *Amniotic fluid embolism:* spontaneous delivery and cesarean section
  • *Tumor embolism:* Choriocarcinoma
  • *Parasitic embolism:* Schistosomiasis
  • *Air embolism:* Pulmonary barotraumas generally in the sea divers

Clinical Features

In Acute Massive Embolism, i.e., Acute Cor Pulmonale

♦ Symptoms are of presence of acute dyspnea, tachypnea, tachycardia, hemoptysis and chest pain.
♦ Signs are increased in the jugular venous pressure, presence of central cyanosis, Loud P2 and narrow splitting of P2, an ejection systolic murmur in P2 area, right ventricular hypertrophy, signs of shock,

In Small or Medium-sized Pulmonary Vessels Embolization

♦ Symptoms are hemoptysis, pleuritic pain and wheeze which is the triad of pulmonary infarct.
♦ Signs are of pleural effusion, i.e., reduced or absent chest wall movement and expansion of chest on the side involved, activity of extrarespiratory muscles is absent, position of trachea and mediastinum is shifted to opposite side, percussion note is stony dull on the side of involvement, vocal fremitus is reduced or absent on the side involved, breath sounds are absent or diminished over the area involved.

Diagnosis

It is in the patients who had suspicion for underlying cause for emboli formation, development of pulmonary sign and symptoms as well as cardiovascular involvement, presence of thrombophlebitis in deep leg veins, prolonged bed rest, immobilization, cardiac irregularity in form of atrial fibrillation should be considered while keeping in mind clinical picture of precordial pain, breathlessness and tachycardia in patient who had recently gone for major surgery. Examination of veins is mandatory in the patients who are at high risk for development of deep vein thrombosis. These features along with investigatory features form the diagnosis. Following are the investigations:

Investigations

♦ *Blood examination:* If pulmonary infarct is present there can be leukocytosis or raised ESR.
♦ *Chest X-ray:* In massive pulmonary embolism, there is presence of diffuse infiltrates in the lung with increased bronchovascular markings. If medium size vessels are involved, there will be triangular pleuropulmonary opacity in peripheral lung fields, there can also be pleural effusion present.
♦ *Arterial blood gas analysis:* Presence of hypoxemia and hypocapnia.
♦ *D-dimer:* It is a fibrin degradation product release in circulation in pulmonary embolism. Presence of high levels of D-dimer is suggestive of an embolism while presence of low D-dimer exclude pulmonary embolism.
♦ *Echocardiography:* It shows the right ventricular dilatation and presence of clot in it.
♦ *Spiral CT scan:* CT of chest along with the IV contrast diagnose the pulmonary embolism. It effectively diagnose the large and central pulmonary embolism. Newer scanners can also detect peripherally present emboli.
♦ *Pulmonary angiography:* It demonstrates the site of obstruction of all sized blood vessels.

Management

♦ In patient of massive embolism
  • *If patient is in state of shock or collapse:*
    – Vasopressors, such as dopamine or dobutamine are to be given.
    – Administer oxygen to the patient.
    – Correct acidosis
    – If there is failure of an initial resuscitation, or there is hypotension or right ventricular dysfunction, primary therapy should be administered, i.e., dissociation of clot by thrombolysis or embolectomy.
  • *If acute event is survived by the patient:*
    – Streptokinase 2.5–5 lac unit IV> in dextrose or saline is given for 30 min followed by 1 lac IV for 24 hours.
    – Recombinant tissue plasminogen activator tPA, i.e., Alteplase 100 mg for 2 hours is a good alternative to thrombolytic therapy.
  • *Anticoagulation therapy is an initial and immediate treatment of choice:*
    – Loading dose of 80–150 units/kg is given which is followed by 15–18 units/kg/hr as continuous infusion.

– Warfarin should be added to heparin and is continued for 5 days.
– After 5 days, taper the heparin and administer warfarin for 6 weeks to 6 months.
– Monitor anticoagulant therapy by PTT or INR ratio or bleeding time which should be 2 to 3 times than the control.
♦ In small embolisms
  • Analgesics, i.e., NSAIDs should be given to relieve the pain.
  • Anticoagulant is given to prevent further embolization.
  • Various preventive measures should be undertaken, such as calf muscle exercise, elastic stockings, prolong immobilization at bed, respiration exercises should be done.

Q.33. Write on RNTCP classification of tuberculosis.

(Dec 2009, 10 Marks)

Ans. RNTCP or the Revised National Tuberculosis Control Program is the state-run tuberculosis control initiative of the Government of India. It incorporates the principles of directly observed treatment-short course (DOTS), the global TB control strategy of the World Health Organization. The program provides, free of cost, quality antitubercular drugs across the country through the numerous Primary Health Centres and the growing number of private-sector DOTS-providers.

Objectives

♦ Detecting at least 70% of sputum positive tuberculosis patients in the community.
♦ Curing at least 85% of the newly detected sputum positive cases.

RNTCP classifies tuberculosis patients into following treatment categories.

TB Category	Patient type	Initial phase	Continuation phase	Total duration
I	New sputum positive Or New smear negative Or New case with severe form of extrapulmonary tuberculosis	$2H_3R_3Z_3E_3$	$4H_3R_3$	6 months
II	Smear positive failure Or Smear positive relapse Or Sputum positive treatment after default	$2H_3R_3Z_3E_3S_3$ + $1H_3R_3Z_3E_3$	$5H_3R_3E_3$	8 months
III	Smear negative pulmonary T.B. with limited parenchymal involvement Or Less severe form of extrapulmonary T.B.	$2H_3R_3Z_3$	$4H_3R_3$	6 months

Explanation of Standard Code

- Each antitubercular drug has standard abbreviation, i.e.
  - Isoniazid (H)
  - Rifampicin (R)
  - Pyrazinamide (Z)
  - Ethambutol (E)
  - Streptomycin (S)
  - H: Isoniazid (300 mg), R: Rifampicin (450 mg), Z: Pyrazinamide (1500 mg), E: Ethambutol (1200 mg), S: Streptomycin (750 mg).
- Patients who weigh 60 kg or more receive additional Rifampicin 150 mg.
- Patients who are more than 50 years old receive Streptomycin 500 mg. Patients who weigh less than 30 kg receive drugs as per pediatric weight band boxes according to body weight.
- Numerical before a phase is the duration of that phase in months.
- Numerical in subscript is the number of doses of that drug per week. If there is no subscript numerical, then the drug is given daily.

Treatment Regimen under RNTCP for MDR-TB (Multidrug-resistant TB) and XDR-TB (Extensively drug resistant TB)

- For MDR-TB:
  - Six drugs in intensive phase for 6–9 months: Kanamycin, Levofloxacin, Ethionamide, Cycloserine, Pyrazinamide and Ethambutol.
  - Four drugs in continuation phase for 18 months: Levofloxacin, Ethionamide, Cycloserine and Ethambutol.
  - Reserve drug is p-aminosalicylic acid.
- For XDR-TB:
  - Seven drugs in intensive phase for 6–12 months: Capreomycin, p-aminosalicylic acid, Moxifloxacin, high dose Isoniazid, Clofazimine, Linezolid, Amoxicillin and Clavulanic acid.
  - Six drugs in continuation phase for 18 months: p-aminosalicylic acid, Moxifloxacin, high dose Isoniazid, Clofazimine, Linezolid, Amoxicillin and Clavulanic acid.
  - Reserve drugs: Clarithromycin, Thiacetazone.

Second-line antituberculous drugs

Drug	Dose
Streptomycin	20–40 mg/kg/day OD im
Kanamycin	15–30 mg/kg/day OD im
Amikacin	15–22.5 mg/kg/day OD im
Capreomycin	15–30 mg/kg/day OD im
Ofloxacin	15–20 mg/kg/day BD orally
Levofloxacin	7.5–10 mg/kg/day OD orally
Moxifloxacin	7.5–10 mg/kg/day orally
Ethionamide	15–20 mg/kg/day b orally
Prothionamide	15–20 mg/kg/day BD orally
Cycloserine*	10–20 mg/kg/day OD or BD orallt
PAS*	150 mg/kg/day BD or TDS orally

*Cycloserine and PAS are bacteriostatic others are bactericidal.

Q.34. Write in brief clinical features and treatment of pneumonia. *(Jun 2010, 5 Marks)*

Or

Write sign and symptoms of pneumonia. *(Jan 2012, 5 Marks)*

Ans. Pneumonia is an accumulation of secretions and inflammatory cells in alveolar spaces of lungs caused by infection.

Clinical Features

Symptoms

- Malaise, fever, rigors, and night sweats, vomiting in the elderly confusion and disorientation.
- Dyspnea, cough, and sputum which is often blood-stained or rusty and difficult to expectorate.
- Pain aggravated by cough, deep breath or movement, usually localized to site of inflammation.

Signs

- *In early stage:*
  - Pulse rate and heart rate increases
  - Alae nasi are in action
  - Presence of herpes on the lip
  - Movements of chest are restricted.
  - Percussion over the affected area is diminished.
  - Breath sound are harsh with prolong expiration and few crypts.
- *Signs of pulmonary consolidation:*
  - Limitation of movement on affected side.
  - Increased vocal fremitus
  - Impaired percussion
  - Breathing sounds are bronchial, few crypts may be audible.
  - Vocal resonance is increased.
  - Pleural rub may be heard.
- *During the period of resolution:*
  - Bronchial breathing disappear
  - Normal breath sound appear
  - Coarse crepitations during both phases of respiration.

Treatment

For treatment refer to Ans. 6 of same chapter.

Q.35. Write short note on malignancy of lung. *(Mar 2013, 3 Marks)*

Ans. Malignancy of lung is known as lung cancer.

Predisposing Factors

- Cigarette smoking
- *Occupational exposure:* This is due to radioactive gases, asbestos, arsenic, nickel, chromates, metallic iron
- *Atmospheric pollution:* In urban areas
- *Lung diseases:* Chances of lung cancer increases in patients with cryptogenic fibrosing alveolitis.

Clinical Features

Symptoms

♦ *Nonspecific:* Weakness, tiredness, anorexia, loos of weight
♦ *Respiratory:* Presence of influenza-like illness or pneumonia distal to obstruction caused by tumor, Increased cough, mild hemoptysis, dyspnea, chest pain which is worst at night, wheeze.

Signs

♦ Clubbing of fingers
♦ Supraclavicular lymphadenopathy
♦ Mid- inspiratory crackles over a lobe, reduction of breadth sounds over a lobe and signs of lobar collapse.
♦ Wheezing sound is present
♦ Pleural effusion is present.

Diagnosis

It is based on physical examination and investigations.

Investigations

♦ Chest X-ray shows peripheral round mass. It is well defined or irregular with pseudopodia or Sun-ray projection radiating from its surface.
♦ *Sputum cytology:* On examination reveals presence of cancer cells.
♦ *Bronchoscopy:* Fiberoptic bronchoscopy is done.
♦ Thoracic CT including upper abdomen is done to see extensions of malignancy.

Management

♦ Surgery can be done.
♦ *Radiotherapy:* When resection is not carried out of tumor, radiotherapy is employed. Continuous hyperfractional accelerated radiotherapy (CHART) three times daily for 2 weeks increases chances of survival.
♦ *Chemotherapy:* Useful in patients with widespread disease and no local symptoms. Commonly used combinations are mitomycin-ifosfamide-cisplatin, Mitomycin-cisplatin-vincristine, cisplatin-gemcitabine and cisplatin-vinorelbine. Three cycles are given.

Q.36.   Write short note on first-line antitubercular drugs.

(Feb 2014, 3 Marks)

Ans. The first-line antitubercular drugs are Isoniazid, Rifampin, Pyrazinamide, Ethambutol and Strepto-mycin.

These drugs have high antitubercular efficacy as well as low toxicity and are used routinely.

Isoniazid

♦ Isoniazid is a first line antitubercular drug.
  • It acts on extracellular as well as intracellular TB and is equally effective in alkaline and acidic medium.
  • The most possible action of isoniazid is inhibition of synthesis of mycolic acids which are unique fatty acid

component of mycobacterial cell wall. The lipid content of *Mycobacterium* exposed to isoniazid is reduced.
  • Isoniazid is completely absorbed orally and penetrates all body tissues, tubercular cavities and placenta.
  • It is extensively metabolized in liver by acetylation.
  • The metabolites are excreted in urine.

Rifampin

♦ Rifampin is bactericidal to *M. tuberculosis.*
♦ Bactericidal action covers all subpopulations of TB bacilli, but acts best on slowly or intermittently dividing ones, as well as on many atypical mycobacteria.
♦ It has good sterilizing and resistance preventing actions.
♦ Rifampin inhibits DNA dependent RNA synthesis.
♦ It is well-absorbed orally, widely distributed in the body: penetrates cavities, caseous masses, placenta and meninges.
♦ It is metabolized in liver to an active deacetylated metabolite which is excreted mainly in bile, some in urine also.

Pyrazinamide

♦ It is weakly tuberculocidal but more active in acidic medium.
♦ It is more lethal to intracellularly located bacilli and to those at sites showing an inflammatory response (pH is acidic at both these locations).
♦ It is highly effective during the first 2 months of therapy when inflammatory changes are present.
♦ By killing the residual intracellular bacilli, it has good 'sterilizing' activity.
♦ It inhibits mycolic acid synthesis, but by interacting with a different fatty acid synthase encoding gene.
♦ Pyrazinamide is absorbed orally, widely distributed, has good penetration in CSF, extensively metabolized in liver and excreted in urine.

Ethambutol

♦ Ethambutol is selectively tuberculostatic and clinically as active as S. Fast multiplying bacilli are more susceptible as are many atypical mycobacteria.
♦ Ethambutol inhibits arabinosyl transferases involved in arabinogalactan synthesis and to interfere with mycolic acid incorporation in mycobacterial cell wall.
♦ Patient acceptability of ethambutol is very good and side effects are few.

Streptomycin

♦ It was the first clinically useful antitubercular drug.
♦ It is tuberculocidal, but less effective than rifampin; acts only on extracellular bacilli. Thus, host defense mechanisms are needed to eradicate the disease.
♦ It penetrates tubercular cavities, but does not cross to the CSF, and has poor action in acidic medium.
♦ Resistance developed rapidly when streptomycin was used alone in tuberculosis–most patients had a relapse.

Q.37. Describe various extrapulmonary tuberculosis and how will you treat a case of tubercular meningitis?
(Nov 2014, 8 Marks)

Ans.

Extrapulmonary Tuberculosis

In extrapulmonary tuberculosis which involves all the major organs in body from heart to gastrointestinal tract.

Following are the various types of extrapulmonary tuberculosis:

Tuberculous Pericarditis

♦ Involvement of pericardium is very common by *M. tuberculum bacteria.*
♦ It occurs in form of pericarditis, pericardial effusion and later on there is constrictive pericarditis.
♦ Its earliest sign is pericardial rub and fever.
♦ As disease exacerbate, there is formation of effusion and when it is massive cardiac tamponade may occur.

Gastrointestinal Tract

♦ There is occurrence of primary lesion due to swallowing of tubercle bacilli which lodges in the ileocecal region and produce primary hypertrophic ileocecal tuberculosis.
♦ Common manifestations are tuberculous peritonitis, tabes mesenterica, tuberculous enteritis, diarrhea and fistula.

Skeletal Tuberculosis

♦ Tuberculosis of spine, paravertebral cold abscess, sinus tract formation and involvement of weight-bearing joints, such as knees and hips.
♦ When tubercular granuloma extend to the mandible or maxilla via extraction socket by means of hematological spread, this can lead to tuberculous osteomyelitis.
♦ Early diagnosis by joint aspiration and biopsy is done to prevent disability and to avoid surgery.

Genitourinary Tuberculosis

♦ It presents as painless hematuria and sterile pyuria.
♦ In this renal parenchyma, calyces, ureter and bladder are affected in descending order.
♦ Testicular and epididymal involvement may be present which causes sterility.
♦ In females Involvement of fallopian tubes causes female infertility.

Meningeal Tuberculosis

Tuberculoma in brain and tubercular meningitis are very common complications and may leave behind number of sequelae.

Adrenal Tuberculosis

♦ It produces the picture of Addison's disease.
♦ It is seen in long standing cases of abdominal tuberculosis.

Lupus Vulgaris

When tubercle bacilli invade the skin this is known as lupus vulgaris.

Oral Tuberculosis

♦ When tubercle bacilli directly inoculated in oral tissues of a person who had not acquired the immunity to the tuberculosis.
♦ In oral cavity, there is involvement of tongue, gingiva, extraction socket and buccal mucosa.
♦ In oral cavity at above mention sites, there is presence of typical tubercular ulcer.
♦ Tuberculous gingivitis appears as diffuse, hyperemic or nodular papillary proliferation.

Treatment of a Case of Tubercular Meningitis

♦ *Antitubercular drugs:* Rifampicin 600 mg/day + Isoniazide (600 to 900 mg/day) + Pyrazinamide (1.5 g) should be given. Treatment with this regimen is given for 2 months. This is followed by rifampicin 600 mg/day + Isoniazide (600 to 900 mg/day) for 12 to 18 months.
♦ *Steroids:* Prednisolone 40–60 mg/day to reduce toxicity, pia-arachnoid adhesions and feeling of well-being.

Q.38. Write etiology, clinical features, investigations and treatment of pneumonia. *(Feb 2015, 12 Marks)*

Or

Discuss etiology, clinical features and treatment of infectious pneumonia. *(Apr 2019, 5 Marks)*

Or

Write short answer on etiology of pneumonia.
(Oct 2019, 3 Marks)

Ans. *For clinical features of pneumonia refer to Ans. 34 of same chapter.*

For treatment of pneumonia refer to Ans. 6 of same chapter.

Etiology

♦ *Bacterial:* Pneumococcus, Staphylococcus, Streptococcus, H. influenza, E. coli, Klebsiella, Pseudomonas, etc.
♦ *Atypical:* Viral, Rickettsial, mycoplasmal
♦ *Protozoal:* E. histolytica
♦ *Fungal:* Actinomycosis, aspergillosis, histoplasmosis, nocardiosis
♦ *Allergic:* Loeffler's syndrome
♦ Radiation
♦ *Collagenosis:* Systemic lupus erythematosus, rheumatoid arthritis, polyarteritis nodosa
♦ *Chemical:* Aspiration of vomitus, gases and smokes, kerosene, paraffin and petroleum.

Investigations

♦ X-ray chest is done for assessing the opacity in lung.
♦ Examination of sputum is done by Gram's and Ziehl–Neelsen stains.

♦ Sensitivity as well as sputum culture should be carried out for anaerobic and aerobic organisms.

♦ If sputum is absent, then bronchoscopic aspiration is done for both culture and sensitivity.

♦ Blood examination is done for assessing leukocytosis.

♦ Sputum, urine and serum testing should be done for identifying the pneumococcal antigen.

♦ If empyema is present, then pleural fluid aspiration is done.

♦ Blood gas analysis should be done.

Q.39. Write etiology, diagnosis and management of pulmonary tuberculosis. *(July 2016, 12 Marks)*

Or

Describe etiology, sign, symptoms and management of pulmonary TB. *(Feb 2019, 5 Marks)*

Or

Write long answer on etiology and management of pulmonary tuberculosis. *(Oct 2019, 6 Marks)*

Ans. Involvement of lungs by tuberculosis is known as pulmonary tuberculosis.

Etiology

♦ *Mycobacterium tuberculosis* leads to the pulmonary tuberculosis.

♦ In immunocompromised patients or in children tuberculosis can be caused by atypical *Mycobacterium*.

Diagnosis

It is based on clinical signs and symptoms as well as investigations.

Symptoms

♦ Evening rise of temperature

♦ Night sweats

♦ Malaise and cachexia

♦ Irritability and difficulty in concentration.

♦ Cough and expectoration for more than three weeks.

♦ Pleuritic chest pain

♦ Breathlessness is the feature of advanced disease.

♦ Indigestion and dyspnea

♦ Amenorrhea often in young women

♦ Hoarseness of voice.

♦ Sputum can be mucoid, purulent or blood stained.

♦ Hemoptysis is a classical feature

♦ Presence of localized wheeze from local ulcer or narrowing of major bronchus.

♦ Presence of recurrent cold.

Physical Signs

♦ Fever and weight loss

♦ Tachycardia and tachypnea

♦ Rapid pulse rate

♦ Physical signs of collapse, consolidation, cavitation, fibrosis, bronchiectasis, pleural effusion or pneumothorax.

♦ In some cases only localized *rhonchi or rales are present.

♦ Clubbing of fingers is present in chronic disease.

♦ Most common physical sign of chest is fine crepitation in the upper part of one or both the lungs. This is heard on taking a deep breath after coughing.

♦ Later on, there can be presence of dullness to percussion or bronchial breathing in upper part of one or both the lungs.

♦ In chronic cases, there is evidence of volume loss and mediastinal shift.

♦ Hilar, mediastinal and cervical groups lymph nodes are enlarged with splenomegaly.

Investigations

♦ *Serology:* In this ELISA, technique is used which helpful in diagnosis of tuberculosis in children. PCR technique is more specific and sensitive serological test than ELISA, but PCR is less used due to its high cost.

♦ *Chest X-ray:* Presence of multiple nodular infiltrations or ill-defined opacities in one of upper lobes is characteristic for pulmonary tuberculosis. An area of translucency in radiopacities is indicative of cavitation. Presence of cavity is indicative of an active lesion. In some of the patients multiple thick-walled cavities can be seen. At the time of fibrosis, trachea and mediastinum shift to same side. Fibrosis can also cause calcification.

♦ *Pathological tests:*
  • *Blood examination:* Peripheral blood examination shows monocytosis, i.e., 8 to 12%
  • ESR is elevated.
  • *Tuberculin test:* It is a test to recognize prior tubercular infection, and is done by injecting one unit of purified protein derivative (PPD) on the forearm and readings taken after 48 hours. Induration of more than 15 mm indicates a positive test. The younger is the patient, greater is significance of positive test. A negative test does not always exclude tubercular infection since it may be negative in patients of blood malignancies, malnourishment and those on immunosuppressive therapy. Tuberculin test is nonspecific and only indicates prior infection. Its sensitivity wanes with age.

Management

♦ *Chemotherapy: For details, refer to Ans. 18 of same chapter.*

♦ *Corticosteroids:* They are to be given in the severe cases to enable them to survive till antitubercular drugs become effective. Oral prednisolone is given in doses of 20 mg orally for 6 to 8 weeks. Steroids produce euphoria and increase appetite in the patients.

♦ *Surgery:* Surgical resection of infected lobe is feasible.

♦ *Symptomatic treatment:*
  • *Cough:* If it is irritative, linctus codeine is given. Smoking should be stopped.
  • *Laryngitis:* Rest is given to the voice. If pain is present anesthetic powders, spray and lozenges are given.

Q.40. Describe etiology, clinical features, diagnosis, complications and treatment of chronic obstructive pulmonary disease. *(Mar 2016, 8 Marks)*

Or

Write etiology, clinical features, diagnosis, and management of chronic obstructive pulmonary disease (COPD). *(Jan 2018, 12 Marks)*

Ans. Chronic obstructive pulmonary disease is characterized by irreversible obstruction to the airflow throughout lungs. It consists of two important disorders of lungs, i.e., chronic bronchitis and emphysema. These both diseases coexist in a single patient.

Etiology

- *Localized:*
  - Congenital
  - Compensatory due to lung collapse, scarring or resection
  - Partial bronchial obstruction due to neoplasm or foreign body
  - MacLeod's syndrome
- *Generalized:*
  - Idiopathic
  - Senile
  - Familial, i.e., due to alpha-l-anti-trypsin deficiency
  - Associated with chronic bronchitis, asthma or pneumoconiosis.

Clinical Features

In most of the patients, chronic bronchitis is associated with emphysema so two types clinical syndromes of chronic obstructive pulmonary disease are present i.e.

1. Predominant chronic bronchitis with emphysema, i.e., Blue bloater type
2. Predominant emphysema with some degree of chronic bronchitis, i.e., pink-puffers type

Features	Pink-puffer, i.e., prominent emphysema	Blue bloater, i.e., prominent chronic bronchitis
Onset	Dyspnea and cough	Cough without dyspnea
Build	Thin	Obese
Sputum	Scanty	Profuse, mucopurulent
Dyspnea	intense with purse lip breathing	Relatively mild dyspnea
Cough	After dyspnea starts	Before dyspnea starts
Cardiac failure (Cor pulmonale)	Rarely develop edema or overt heart failure	Often edematous and easily lapse into CHF
Weight loss	Marked weight loss	No marked weight loss except terminally
Bronchial infections	Less frequent	More frequent
Episodes of respiratory failure	Often terminal	Repeated

Contd...

Contd...

Features	Pink-puffer, i.e., prominent emphysema	Blue bloater, i.e., prominent chronic bronchitis
Pulmonary hypertension	None or mild	Moderate to severe
Course	Unrelenting downhill	Ambulatory
Chest X-ray	Signs of emphysema seen	Bronchovascular markings are prominent
Hypoxemia	Mild	Moderate to severe
Hypercapnia	Absent or mild	Present
Cyanosis	Absent or present terminally	Present and common
Secondary polycythemia	Uncommon	Common
Diffusing capacity	Decreased	Normal or increased

Diagnosis

- History of chronic progressive symptoms, i.e., cough or wheeze or breathlessness.
- *General condition:* Patient can be emaciated, cyanosed and edematous. Jugular venous pressure may show giant a-waves.
- *Chest findings:*
  - Chest wall process is barrel-shaped.
  - Movement of chest is decreased.
  - Centrally placed mediastinum
  - Percussion is hyper-resonant.
  - Breath is diminished vesicular with prolong expiration.
  - Rhonchi are heared.
  - Vocal resonance sounds are diminished.
- *Heart:*
  - Apex beat may not be visible or palpable.
  - Right ventricular heave can be present.
  - Heart sounds can be diminished. Second sound can be loud. Gallop rhythm can be heared.
  - Functional tricuspid regurgitation murmur can be present.
  - Hyperkinetic state with warm limb and water hammer pulse is present.
- *Miscellaneous:*
  - Hepatomegaly can be present.
  - Optic disc can show papilledema
- *Investigations:*
  - There is presence of post-bronchodilator FEV1/FVC less than 0.7 which confirms the presence of persistent airflow limitation and thus is diagnostic of chronic obstructive pulmonary disease.
  - Arterial blood gas show retention of carbon dioxide in emphysema.

- Serum alpha-1-anti-trypsin levels to diagnose alpha-1 anti-trypsin deficiency.
- *X-ray chest:* Presence of hypertranslucency of lung fields, wide intercoastal spaces, diaphragm is low and flat, heart is tubular shaped, presence of large hilar shadows, diminished peripheral vascular pattern, rounded areas of hypertranslucency with thin hairline shadow forming margins.

Complications

In Emphysema

- Pneumothorax due to rupture of bullae in pleural space.
- Cor pulmonale, i.e., right-sided heart failure or right ventricular hypertrophy secondary to lung disease.
- Type II respiratory failure.

In Chronic Bronchitis

- Type I and type II respiratory failure
- Cor pulmonale
- Pulmonary arterial hypertension
- Secondary infections
- Secondary polycythemia

Treatment

- Bronchial irritants should be avoided, i.e.
  - Smoking should be strictly stopped.
  - Passive smoking is stopped.
  - Gas smoke is avoided by housemakers.
  - Aerosols, such as hair spray, insecticide spray and aerosols should be avoided.
  - Polluted atmosphere should be strictly avoided.

- *Treatment of an infection:*
  - Ampicillin 250 to 500 mg every 6 hourly is given for 5–7 days.
  - Cotrimazole 960 mg can be given as BD dose.
  - Antibiotics should be given till purulent mucous become mucoid.
  - If necessary modify antibiotics as per culture and sensitivity test.
- *Bronchodilators:*
  - In mild-to-moderate chronic bronchitis oral theophylline 150 mg BD or inhaled salbutamol 200 µg 6 hourly can be given.
  - In severe bronchitis, ipratropium bromide 40 to 80 µg 6 hourly is added.
- *Mucolytic agents:* Bromhexine and carbocisteine are to be given.
- *Corticosteroids:* Prednisolone 30 mg/day for 2 weeks is given. If improvement occur by oral steroids they are replaced by inhalational steroids.
- *Domiciliary oxygen therapy:* Long-term oxygen therapy in low concentration, i.e., 2 L/min by nasal cannula is given to reverse or to delay development of pulmonary hypertension.
- If cor pulmonale is present diuretics, such as furosemide, digitalis and potassium salts might be given.
- Chest physiotherapy should be done, and proper exercises should be taught to the patient.
- Patients with COPD should receive influenza and pneumococcal vaccines.
- Non-invasive ventilation is useful in those with pronounced daytime hypercapnia.
- Lung volume reduction surgery can be done. In this parts of lungs are resected to reduce hyperinflation.

Q.41. Write short answer on antitubercular drugs.

Ans.

(Sep 2018, 3 Marks)

Name of the drug	Mechanism of action	Adverse effects	Uses

Rifampicin 400 to 600 mg/day orally	It inhibits DNA dependent RNA polymerase and so it stops the expression of bacterial genes. It is bactericidal	- Liver damage
		- Influenza like reaction
		- Intolerance
		- Orange red color to urine and feces.
			- Tuberculosis
			- Other uses
			  - Herpes zoster
			  - Leprosy
			  - Influenza
			  - Brucella
			  - Mycetoma
			  - Legionella
			  - Chlamydia

Rifabutin 150 mg/day	It inhibits the DNA dependent RNA polymerases	- GI disturbances - Fever and rash	- HIV-associated tuberculosis - In Multidrug resistance tuberculosis - In HIV-associated tuberculosis
Isonicotinic acid Hydrazide (INH) 300 mg daily for 1 to 2 years orally	- It inhibits phospholipid synthesis of bacterial cell membrane - It leads to intracellular or extracellular chelation of the calcium ions which are essential for the bacterial metabolism - It is a bactericidal drug	- Peripheral neuritis - Optic neuritis - Intolerance: Fever, malaise jaundice, skin rashes - Blood dyscrasias	Tuberculosis

Contd…

Contd...

Name of the drug	Mechanism of action	Adverse effects	Uses
Ethambutol 25 mg/kg for 12 weeks 15 mg/kg for one and a half year at night	It is bacteriostatic and acct against rapidly growing organisms	• Anaphylactic reaction • Optic nerve damage • Nausea and vomiting • Confusion and headache	First line therapy in tuberculosis
Pyrazinamide 500 to 750 mg BD	It is bactericidal	• Toxic hepatitis on day 7th • Hyperuricemia. Gout and polyarthralgia • Skin rashes and photosensitivity	In tuberculosis

Streptomycin It is used 0.75 g per day IM for 3 months in tuberculosis	• It combines with the ribosomes and interferes with mRNA ribosome combination, inducing it to manufacture peptide chains with wrong amino – acids with which destroy the bacterial cell and bind to 50S ribosomal unit.
	• It inhibits enzyme involved in Krebs cycle and xanthine oxidase. It is bactericidal drug
		• Anaphylaxis
		• Ototoxicity, tinnitus, vertigo
		• Injection abscess
		• Nephrotoxicity
		• Eosinophilia
		• Drug fever
		• Drug resistance
		• Circumoral paresthesia
			• In tuberculosis
			• Other uses
			  - Plaque
			  - Tularemia
			  - Brucellosis
			  - Urinary tract infection
			  - Respiratory tract infection
			  - Chancroid
			  - *H. influenza* meningitis

Cycloserine 1 to 2 g daily.	It inhibits the synthesis of bacterial cell wall	• Insomnia and psychosis • Weakness, tremors, convulsion, ataxia, slurred speech and ankle clonus	It is the reserve second line agent
Para-aminosalicylic acid	It interferes with the utilization of para amino benzoic acid by mycobacterium	• GI disturbances, such as anorexia, nausea, vomiting and diarrhea • Intolerance: fever, skin rash and lymphadenopathy • Hemopoietic: Leukopenia, eosinophilia, ataxia • Damage to liver • Acute renal failure • Myxedema	It is used as a reserve drug as it has low level of antituberculous activity

Q.42. **Write short answer on pleural effusion.**

(Apr 2019, 3 Marks)

Ans. Pleural effusion is the collection of fluid which is more than the normal in pleural cavity irrespective of the nature of fluid (transudate or exudates).

Etiology

♦ Pleural effusion with no involvement of pleura: It occurs because of passive transudation. Main causes are:
  • Constrictive pericarditis
  • Liver cirrhosis
  • Congestive cardiac failure
  • Nephrotic syndrome
  • Hypoproteinemia because of malnutrition or malabsorption.
♦ Pleural effusion because of involvement of pleura which leads to exudation or chylous effusion: Main cause are:
  • Tuberculosis
  • Pneumonia
  • Lymphomas
  • Rheumatoid arthritis
  • Pulmonary infarction
  • Subphrenic abscess
  • Systemic lupus erythematosus
  • Pancreatitis
  • Rupture of amoebic liver abscess
  • Miscellaneous, i.e., uremia, Meig's syndrome

Clinical Features

♦ Almost all the cases which are affected have pyrexia.
♦ Dyspnea is the earliest symptom to appear.
♦ On inspection
  • Bilaterally symmetrical chest is present.
  • Over the side of effusion movements of chest are restricted.
♦ Palpation
  • By push trachea and mediastinum are shifted to the opposite side.

- Expansion of chest gets diminished over the side which is involved.
- Vocal fremitus either get diminished or is absent over the involved side.

- Percussion: Percussion note is stony dull over the involved side. Rising dullness is seen on the axilla over the same side.
- Auscultation:
  - Over the area of pleural effusion breadth sounds are absent or markedly diminished.
  - This is occasional but amphoric bronchial breathing can be heard at the apex of pleural effusion in inter – scapular region over the involved side.
  - Vocal resonance is diminished or absent.
  - Pleural rub may be heard above effusion in some of the cases.

Investigations

- **X-ray chest:** This is diagnostic. It shows the presence of uniform dense opacity along with upper concavity in lower and the lateral part of hemithorax which pushes the lung medially. Obliteration of sharp angle is seen between diaphragm and the rib cage. Subpulmonic effusion provides the appearance of an elevated hemidiaphragm. At times effusion can be seen in interlobar fissures where it produces round opacity which resemble as lung tumor on the chest X-ray.
- **Blood examination:** It shows:
  - Normocytic normochromic anemia.
  - High ESR in tubercular effusion.
- **Ultrasonography:** It helps in detecting and localizing effusion. Aspiration can be done under the guidance of ultrasound.
- **Pleural aspiration or paracentesis:** Here 50 mL of fluid is aspirated by an aspiration needle. This fluid is sent for biochemical, bacteriological and cytological examination. Appearance of fluid should be noted. It is straw colored, hemorrhagic, purulent or chylous.
- **Pleural biopsy:** It is indicated in tubercular and malignant effusion for confirming the nature of lesion. It is done during diagnostic aspiration of pleural fluid.
- **Other investigations:**
  - Tuberculin test and examination of sputum
  - Bronchoscpoy
  - Thoracoscopy
  - Scalene lymph node biopsy
  - Serological test for anti-nuclear and rheumatoid factor
  - Ultrasound of liver

Treatment

1. **Aspiration of pleural effusion:** Dyspnea should be relieved. Not more than one liter of fluid should be removed on first occasion. Iatrogenic pneumothorax can be produced during aspiration, so X-ray chest must be performed after the aspiration.

   Indications for aspiration of pleural fluid are:
   - For diagnostic purpose
   - For relieving dyspnea if cardiorespiratory embarrassment is present.

- If there is no response to the treatment.
- If both fever and toxemia is not subsiding after 4 weeks of antitubercular therapy.

2. **Treatment of underlying cause:**
   - Antitubercular therapy should be started for treating the tuberculosis.
   - For malignant pleural effusion, repeated aspiration should be done and when it becomes unavoidable then pleurodesis can be tried by injecting mustine hydrochloride or tetracycline inside pleural space to produce adhesion in between the two layers of pleura which obliterates potential pleural space.
   - If amoebic liver abscess get ruptured in pleural space, it is treated by metronidazole, chloroquine and aspirating the pleural fluid.

Q.43. **Write short answer on treatment of ARDS.**

(Oct 2019, 3 Marks)

Ans. ARDS is acute respiratory distress syndrome.

Treatment of ARDS

- **Removal of underlying cause:** If possible, e.g., broad spectrum antibiotics for sepsis, drainage of infected fluid collections, removal of necrotic tissue.
- **Support of the injured lung:** By restoration and maintenance of adequate tissue oxygen delivery. Most patients require ventilatory support. The purpose of respiratory support is to achieve adequate arterial oxygenation without exacerbating the underlying lung injury. The usual aims are low respiratory rate (<10–14/minute), low tidal volume (6–8 mL/kg), relatively high positive end expiratory pressure (5–20 cm H_2O).
- **Additional measures:**
  - *Prone positioning:* It is most effective in early exudative phase of lung injury when it allows recruitment of alveoli, improving ventilation/perfusion matching. There are also cardiovascular benefits.
  - *Inverse ratio ventilation:* In this method, inspiratory time is increased so that it is longer than expiratory time. With decreased time to exhale, dynamic hyperinflation leads to increased end expiratory pressure.
  - *High-frequency ventilation (HFV):* It entails ventilating at extremely high respiratory rates (5–20 cycles per second) and low VTs (1–2 mL/kg).
  - *Use of partial liquid ventilation (PLV)* with perfluorocarbon (inert, high density liquid that easily solubilizes oxygen and carbon) has shown improvement in pulmonary function of ARDS patients with no survival benefit.
  - *Lung-replacement therapy with extracorporeal membrane oxygenation (ECMO)* which provides clear survival benefit in neonatal respiratory distress syndrome, may also have utility in selected adult patients with ARDS.
  - *Nitric oxide and nebulized prostacyclin:* Low concentrations (1–20 ppm) nitric oxide acts as a local vasodilator in the vicinity of ventilated alveoli reducing shunt. The same effect is achieved with nebulized prostacyclin.
  - *Corticosteroids:* These may be beneficial in ARDS caused by inflammation (e.g., acute pancreatitis) rather than sepsis. They may also hasten recovery and improve

outcome in those with severe pulmonary fibrosis or persistent ARDS.

- *Reduction of lung water:* Excessive extravascular lung water may result from over-enthusiastic fluid replacement, or from severe pulmonary leak, reflecting the severity of inflammatory insult. Hence management includes attempts to keep the patient dry; this is reasonable in well-resuscitated patients with adequate circulation, but is inappropriate in septic patients with evidence of poor tissue perfusion, in whom inadequate fluid replacement increases risk of multiorgan dysfunction.

6. DISEASES OF RENAL SYSTEM

Q.1. Write short note on acute glomerulonephritis.

(Mar 2010, 5 Marks)

Or

Write in brief sign, symptom and treatment of acute glomerulonephritis. *(June 2010, 5 Marks)*

Or

Discuss etiology, clinical features, investigations and treatment of acute glomerulonephritis.

(Aug 2011, 15 Marks)

Or

Give definition, etiology, sign, symptoms, investigations and treatment of nephritic syndrome.

(Nov 2011, 8 Marks)

Or

Write etiology, clinical features, investigations and treatment of nephritic syndrome.

(Feb 2015, 12 Marks)

Or

Write nephritic syndrome under the following headings: *(Feb 2014, 2 Marks; Each)*

a. Causes
b. Clinical features
c. Investigations
d. Treatment

Ans. Acute glomerulonephritis involves mainly the glomeruli and to lesser extent the renal tubules by an acute transient inflammatory process which manifests clinically by acute reduction in glomerular filtration rate, rapid renal failure, proteinuria and salt and water retention.

Acute glomerulonephritis is also known as acute nephritic syndrome or nephritic syndrome.

Nephritic syndrome is characterized by oliguria, hematuria, proteinuria, edema, hypertension and acute renal failure.

Etiology

- *Infectious disease:*
  - Post-streptococcal glomerulonephritis
  - Non-streptococcal post-infectious glomerulonephritis

  - *Bacterial:* Infective endocarditis, sepsis, Pneumococcal pneumonia, typhoid fever, secondary syphilis, meningococcemia
  - *Viral:* Hepatitis B, infectious mononucleosis, mumps, measles, varicella, vaccinia, echovirus and coxsackievirus
  - *Parasitic:* Malaria, toxoplasmosis
- *Multisystem disease:*
  - Systemic lupus erythematosus
  - Vasculitis
  - Henoch-Schönlein purpura
  - Goodpasture's syndrome
- *Primary glomerular disease:*
  - Mesangiocapillary glomerulonephritis
  - Mesangial proliferative glomerulonephritis
- *Miscellaneous:*
  - Gullain-Barré syndrome
  - Irradiation of Wilm's tumor
  - Diphtheria-Pertussis-Tetanus (DPT) vaccine
  - Serum sickness.
  - IgA nephropathy

Clinical Features

Symptoms

- Patient complains to puffiness over the face and edema over the feet in early hours of morning.
- In some cases, headache, vomiting and abdominal pain is present.

Signs

- Generalized anasarca is present. It is more over face.
- Oligouria is present.
- Proteinuria is present. It is less than 1 g/day.
- Hypertension is present since there is retention of salt and water.
- Hematuria is present.
- Presence of circulatory congestion.
- Occurrence of circulatory congestion due to capillaritis, increased cardiac output and short circulation time.

Investigations

- *Urine examination:*
  - Volume of urine is reduced.
  - Urine is dark in color or smoky when it is fresh and after hemolysis it becomes tea colored.
  - Proteinuria is variable which is rarely more than 2.5 g/day.
  - Red cells and red cell casts are present in urine microscopy. There is also presence of white cells, white cell casts and granular casts.
- *Blood examination:*
  - There is presence of polymorphonuclear leukocytosis
  - ESR is raised.
  - Blood urea and serum creatinine are raised.
  - C3 levels are reduced.
- *ASO titer:* It is elevated in poststreptococcal nephritis.

- Antinuclear antibody is present in significant titer in lupus nephritis.
- X-ray chest shows cardiomegaly and pulmonary edema, but it is not always present.
- Renal biopsy is indicative of glomerulonephritis

Complications

- Hypertensive encephalopathy
- Acute left heart failure
- Non-cardiogenic pulmonary edema
- Uremia

Management

- *Bed rest:* Patient should be hospitalized and rest is given till illness is resolved. In mild cases, bed rest is given for 3 weeks and in severe cases for 3 months.
- *Fluid restriction:* Avoid fluid overload. For first 24 hours only 500 mL of water or glucose or barley water should be given. If volume of urine in 24 hours is less than 400 mL teart for acute renal failure and if it is more than 400 mL limit intake of fluid to 500 mL + a volume equal to that passed in preceding 24 hours. Fruit juices rich with potassium are given with caution.
- *Diet:* Restrict dietary protein and restrict sodium and potassium intake. Monitor potassium and sodium.
- *Hypertension:* Moderate-to-severe hypertension is controlled by hydralazine, beta-blockers, such as atenolol or calcium channel blockers or ACE inhibitors. Salt restriction should be done.
- *Antibiotics:* Injection benzathine penicillin 500,000 units IM 6 hourly for 7 days.
- *Diuretics:* It is not indicated unless there is acute LVF or pulmonary edema is present. Frusemide 40 mg IV daily for few days, followed by oral substitution till diuretic phase is induced.
- In patients with progressive renal failure or if fluid overload is present, dialysis may have to be employed.

Q.2. Write short note on glomerulonephritis.

(Jan 2012, 5 Marks)

Ans. Involvement of glomeruli in the kidney either by the process of inflammation or immunologically mediated injury or part of generalized systemic diseases constitute glomerulonephritis.

Classification of Glomerulonephritis

- **Clinical:**
  Acute nephritic syndrome
  Subacute nephritis
  Chronic nephritis
  Chronic renal failure
- **Morphologically based on histological examination:**
  Minimal change disease
  Membranous glomerulonephritis
  Focal segmental glomerulonephritis
  Membranoproliferative glomerulonephritis
- **Etiologic:**
  Primary glomerulonephritis
  Secondary due to systemic disease

Hereditary disorders producing glomerulonephritis.
Also refer to Ans. 1 of same chapter.

Q.3. Enumerate the common causes of nephrotic syndrome. *(Aug 2012, 5 Marks) (Apr 2010, 5 Marks)*

Ans. It is a clinical complex with number of renal and extrarenal features

- Hypoproteinemia
- Hypoalbuminemia
- Generalized edema or anasarca
- Hypercholesterolemia
- Hypercoagulability.
- Primary glomerular diseases
  - Minimal change nephropathy.
  - Mesangioproliferative glomerulonephritis.
  - Membranous nephropathy.
  - Focal and segmental glomerulosclerosis.
  - Crescentic glomerulonephritis
- *Idiopathic*
- *Secondary to other diseases:*
  - *Infections:* Malaria, hepatitis B, herpes zoster, streptococcal and staphylococcal infections, syphilis, leprosy, schistosomiasis.
  - *Drugs:* NSAIDs, Heavy metals, such as gold, anticonvulsants, penicillamine, ACE inhibitors, heroin, rifampicin, tolbutamide and probenecid.
  - *Malignancy:* Hodgkin's disease and other lymphomas.
  - *Systemic diseases:* Diabetes mellitus, amyloidosis, systemic lupus erythematosus, Henoch-Schonlein purpura, cryoglobulinemia, polyarteritis nodosa.
  - *Familial disorders:* Congenital (neonatal) nephrotic syndrome, Alport's syndrome, Fabry's disease
  - *Miscellaneous conditions:* Reflux nephropathy, renal vein thrombosis, toxemia of pregnancy, allergic reactions to insect bites, pollens and vaccines, renal artery stenosis.

Q.4. Outline the management of nephrotic syndrome.

(Sep 2009, 5 Marks)

Ans. Management of nephrotic syndrome involves:

- Scientific treatment of underlying morphology or causative disease
- General measures to control nephritic complications
- Treatment to reduce proteinuria
  Nonspecific measures that may reduce proteinuria include ACE and NSAIDs.
  ACE-I and ARBs (angiotensin-receptor blockers) reduce proteinuria and slows the rate of progression of rate of renal failure by lowering intraglomerular pressure and preventing development of hemodynamically mediated focal segmental *glomerulosclerosis.
- Edema: Advice patient to take low sodium diet, i.e., 1 to 2 g/day. In mild edema thiazide induce gentle diuresis. In moderate edema frusemide in doses of 80 to 120 mg/day or torsemide 20 to 40 mg/day is given. In patients with severe edema frusemide 20 to 40 mg/day is combined with spironolactone 100 to 200 mg/day for complete resorption of sodium throughout the nephron.
- Hypercholesterolemia: It is treated by the lipid lowering agent especially statins. Atorvastatin 20 mg od or BD

Q 4.   *Glomerulosclerosis = Fibrosis of renal glomeruli associated with protein loss in the urine.

- Anticoagulation is needed for patient with deep vein thrombosis, arterial thrombosis and pulmonary embolism.
- Antiplatelet agents and warfarin could be advocated.
- Diet: Restricted protein diet is advised since high protein diet accelerates progression of nephritic syndrome.
- Vitamin D supplementation is advisable.
- Antibiotics: Aggressive antibiotic therapy is given in nephrotic syndrome as chances of sepsis are always present. Mainly cephalexin are given.
- Corticosteroids: Produce rapid and complete remission with clearing of proteinuria in 90% cases.

  Dose—Prednisolone 1 mg/kg/day, maximum 80 mg/day. Remission usually occurs between days 7 and 14, though some patients need up to 16 weeks therapy to achieve complete remission.

  Prednisolone dose is reduced to 0.5 mg/kg/day and then tapered slowly. An attempt to stop treatment should be made after 8 weeks. In patients who relapse, course of prednisolone should be repeated.
- Immunosuppressive drugs: In steroid-resistant patients, or in those in whom remission can only be maintained by heavy doses of steroids, cyclophosphamide 1.5–2 mg/kg/day for 8–12 weeks with concomitant prednisolone 7.5–15 mg/day.
- Levamisole: In corticosteroid-dependent children 2.5 mg/kg to maximum 150 mg on alternate days is useful in maintenance of remission.

Q.5. **Describe the clinical features and diagnostic features of nephrotic syndrome.** *(Feb 2002, 5 Marks)*

Ans.

Clinical Features

- *Age and sex:* Nephrotic syndrome is two to three times more common in childhood with peak incidence at 2–3 years. In this age group, there is a male : female ratio of 2.5 : 1, in adults, sex incidence is equal.
- *Edema:* It is peripheral involving the limbs, particularly lower limbs. In children, edema may be more obvious in the face and abdomen. Usually, massive generalized anasarca, the patient almost weighing double his true weight. Intense edema of the scrotum or vulva may occur. There may be bilateral hydrothorax. Edema may persist for many weeks or months. Spontaneous subsidence with diuresis (nephrotic crisis) may occur, to be followed again by increase of edema.
- *Gastrointestinal symptoms:* Anorexia causes severe malnutrition, Diarrhea and vomiting due to edema of intestinal wall.
- *General symptoms:* Prolonged protein loss causes anorexia, lethargy, tiredness, frequent infections and muscle wasting. Dyspnea may occur, if there is fluid in the pleural cavity.
- *Blood pressure:* There may be periods of hypertension; ultimately with development of chronic nephritis permanent hypertension may develop.

Diagnostic Features

Diagnosis is not difficult when there is massive generalized edema with albuminuria, hypoproteinemia and hypercholesterolemia.

Diagnosis is based on clinical signs and investigations.

Clinical signs

- Physical examination reveals generalized edematous person. Edema may persist for many weeks or months.
- Tachycardia is present while blood pressure is normal.
- Pitting edema is present over legs and feet, abdominal walls and lower eyelids.
- Eyelids become puffy
- At places where edema is severe ascites and pleural effusion are seen.
- Kidneys are not palpable.

Investigations

- *Urine examiation:*
  - Oliguria while edema is forming, dieresis or normal amount of urine during period of subsidence of edema.
  - Proteinuria: It is massive, usually more than 5 g/day though variable from time to time; urine becomes almost solid on boiling. Daily loss of protein may be 20–50 g.
  - 24 hour urine shows excretion of albumin or protein more than 3.5 g/day.
  - Red blood cells are absent or few are seen
  - Casts: Fatty casts, tubular cells, oval fat bodies, doubly refractile bodies are seen.
- *Blood examination:*
  - *Anemia:* It is slight normochromic.
  - *Hypoalbuminemia:* Serum albumin usually less than 3 g/100 mL. Total serum globulin concentration frequently lowered with often elevation of α_2 and β-globulins.
  - Serum lipids show increase in LDL levels and cholesterol.
  - ESR is raised due to hyperfibrinogenemia.
  - *Serum complement level:* Serum complement C3 and C4 levels get reduced.
  - Other biochemical tests, i.e., blood urea, serum creatinine, creatinine clearance and electrolytes are normal.
- *Ultrasound of abdomen:* It can show normal small or large kidneys which depends on the underlying cause. Amyloid and diabetic kidneys are large while kidney in glomerulonephritis is small.
- *Renal biopsy:* It is normal on light microscopy but electron microscopy shows typical abnormalities (effacement of epithelial cell foot processes).

Q.6. **Describe briefly investigation and management of nephrotic syndrome.** *(Mar 2001, 5 Marks)*

Ans.

Investigation of Nephrotic Syndrome

- *Urine examiation:*
  - Oliguria while edema is forming, dieresis or normal amount of urine during period of subsidence of edema.
  - *Proteinuria:* It is massive, usually more than 5 g/day though variable from time to time; urine becomes almost solid on boiling. Daily loss of protein may be 20–50 g.
  - 24-hour urine shows excretion of albumin or protein more than 3.5 g/day.
  - Red blood cells are absent or few are seen

- Casts: Fatty casts, tubular cells, oval fat bodies, doubly refractile bodies are seen
♦ *Blood examination:*
  - *Anemia:* It is slight normochromic.
  - *Hypoalbuminemia:* Serum albumin usually less than 3 g/100 mL. Total serum globulin concentration frequently lowered with often elevation of α_2 and β-globulins.
  - Serum lipids show increase in LDL levels and cholesterol.
  - ESR is raised due to hyperfibrinogenemia.
  - *Serum complement level:* Serum complement C3 and C4 levels get reduced.
  - Other biochemical tests, i.e., blood urea, serum creatinine, creatinine clearance and electrolytes are normal.
♦ *Ultrasound of abdomen:* It can show normal small or large kidneys which depends on the underlying cause. Amyloid and diabetic kidneys are large while kidney in glomerulonephritis is small.
♦ *Renal biopsy:* is normal on light microscopy but electron microscopy shows typical abnormalities (effacement of epithelial cell foot processes).

For management refer to Ans. 4 of same chapter.

Q.7. Enumerate the complications and outline the management of nephrotic syndrome.

(Mar 2000, 5 Marks)

Ans.

Complications of Nephrotic Syndrome

♦ *Protein malnutrition:* Due to protein loss
♦ Ascites, pleural and pericardial effusion
♦ Accelerated atherosclerosis and coronary artery disease
♦ Pulmonary thromboembolism, stroke, deep vein thrombosis due to hypercoagulability
♦ Vitamin D deficiency is responsible for hypocalcemia
♦ Microcytic hyperchromic anemia
♦ Hypothyroidism due to depressed thyroxin level due to loss of thyroxin, binding globulin.
♦ Chronic renal failure eventually leading to end stage renal diseases and require hemodialysis and renal transplantation

For management refer to Ans. 4 of same chapter.

Q.8. Write short note on nephrotic syndrome.

(Mar 2016, 3 Marks) (Mar 2007, 2 Marks)

Or

Write note on nephrotic syndrome.

(Dec 2009, 10 Marks)

Ans. Nephrotic syndrome is defined as the presence of heavy proteinuria and hypoalbuminemia in association with varying degrees of edema, lipiduria and hyperlipidemia.

Causes

♦ *Primary glomerular diseases:*
  - Minimal change nephropathy.
  - Mesangioproliferative glomerulonephritis.
  - Membranous nephropathy.
  - Focal and segmental glomerulosclerosis.
  - Crescentic glomerulonephritis

♦ Idiopathic
♦ Secondary to other diseases:
  - *Infections:* Malaria, hepatitis B, herpes zoster, streptococcal and staphylococcal infections syphilis, leprosy, schistosomiasis.
  - *Drugs:* NSAIDs, heavy metals, such as gold, anti – convulsants, penicillamine, ACE-inhibitors, heroin, rifampicin, tolbutamide and probenecid.
  - *Malignancy:* Hodgkin's disease and other lymphomas.
  - *Systemic diseases:* Diabetes mellitus, amyloidosis, systemic lupus erythematosus, Henoch-Schonlein purpura, cryoglobulinemia, polyarteritis nodosa.
  - *Familial disorders:* Congenital (neonatal) nephrotic syndrome, Alport's syndrome, Fabry's disease
  - *Miscellaneous conditions:* Reflux nephropathy, renal vein thrombosis, toxemia of pregnancy, allergic reactions to insect bites, pollens and vaccines, renal artery stenosis.

Clinical Features

♦ *Age and sex:* Nephrotic syndrome is two to three times more common in childhood with peak incidence at 2–3 years. In this age group, there is a male: female ratio of 2.5 : 1, in adults, sex incidence is equal.
♦ *Edema:* It is peripheral involving the limbs, particularly lower limbs. In children, edema may be more obvious in the face and abdomen. Usually, massive generalized anasarca, the patient almost weighing double his true weight. Intense edema of the scrotum or vulva may occur. There may be bilateral hydrothorax. Edema may persist for many weeks or months. Spontaneous subsidence with diuresis (nephrotic crisis) may occur, to be followed again by increase of edema.
♦ *Gastrointestinal symptoms:* Anorexia causes severe malnutrition, Diarrhea and vomiting due to edema of intestinal wall.
♦ *General symptoms:* Prolonged protein loss causes anorexia, lethargy, tiredness, frequent infections and muscle wasting. Dyspnea may occur, if there is fluid in the pleural cavity.
♦ *Blood pressure:* There may be periods of hypertension; ultimately with development of chronic nephritis permanent hypertension may develop.

Investigations

♦ *Urine examination:*
  - Oliguria while edema is forming, dieresis or normal amount of urine during period of subsidence of edema.
  - *Proteinuria:* It is massive, usually more than 5 g/day though variable from time to time; urine becomes almost solid on boiling. Daily loss of protein may be 20–50 g.
  - 24 hour urine shows excretion of albumin or protein more than 3.5 g/day.
  - Red blood cells are absent or few are seen
  - Casts: Fatty casts, tubular cells, oval fat bodies, doubly refractile bodies are seen
♦ *Blood examination:*
  - *Anemia:* It is slight normochromic.
  - *Hypoalbuminemia:* Serum albumin usually less than 3 g/100 mL. Total serum globulin concentration frequently lowered with often elevation of α_2 and β-globulins.

- Serum lipids show increase in LDL levels and cholesterol.
- ESR is raised due to hyperfibrinogenemia.
- *Serum complement level:* Serum complement C3 and C4 levels get reduced.
- *Other biochemical tests,* i.e., blood urea, serum creatinine, creatinine clearance and electrolytes are normal.
- *Ultrasound of abdomen:* It can show normal small or large kidneys which depends on the underlying cause. Amyloid and diabetic kidneys are large while kidney in glomerulonephritis is small.
- *Renal biopsy:* It is normal on light microscopy but electron microscopy shows typical abnormalities (effacement of epithelial cell foot processes).

Treatment

- *Edema:* Advice patient to take low sodium diet, i.e., 1–2 g/day. In mild edema thiazide induce gentle dieresis. In moderate edema, frusemide in doses of 80–120 mg/day or torsemide 20–40 mg/day is given. In patients with severe edema frusemide 20–40 mg/day is combined with spironolactone 100–200 mg/day for complete resorption of sodium throughout the nephron.
- *Corticosteroids:* Produce rapid and complete remission with clearing of proteinuria in 90% cases. Dosage is Prednisolone 1 mg/kg/day, maximum 80 mg/day. Remission usually occurs between days 7 and 14, though some patients need up to 16 weeks therapy to achieve complete remission.
- Prednisolone dose is reduced to 0.5 mg/kg/day and then tapered slowly. An attempt to stop treatment should be made after 8 weeks. In patients who relapse, course of prednisolone should be repeated.
- *Immunosuppressive drugs:* In steroid-resistant patients, or in those in whom remission can only be maintained by heavy doses of steroids, cyclophosphamide 1.5–2 mg/kg/day for 8–12 weeks with concomitant prednisolone 7.5–15 mg/day.
- *Levamisole:* In corticosteroid dependent children 2.5 mg/kg to maximum 150 mg on alternate days is useful in maintenance of remission.
- *Antibiotics:* Aggressive antibiotic therapy is given in nephrotic syndrome as chances of sepsis are always present. Mainly cephalexins are given.

Q.9. Write short note on urine examination of renal failure.
(Oct 2003, 10 Marks)

Ans. Reduction in glomerular filtration rate and rise in nitrogenous and nonnitrogenous substance in blood as a result of degenerated renal function is known as renal failure.

For Acute Renal Failure

- Volume of urine is less (Oliguria) or absent, i.e., anuria.
- Albumin content in urine depends on the underlying causes.
- Urine osmolality is more than 600 mOsm/L; urinary sodium excretion is less than 20 mmol/L; urine/plasma urea ratio is more than 10:1
- Dipstick for blood, protein or both is suggestive of renal inflammatory process.

- *Urine microscopy:* Presence of red cell cast is suggestive of glomerulonephritis.

For Chronic Renal Failure

- Volume of urine passed daily is in the form of polyuria.
- Appearance and color is normal.
- There is no odor present
- Specific gravity of urine is low and fixed.
- Albuminuria is present
- Microscopically, there are hyaline and broad cell cast in urine
- Serum creatinine increases

Q.10. How will you diagnose and investigate a case of nephrotic syndrome? *(Sep 2005, 10 Marks)*

Ans. Diagnosis is based on clinical signs and investigations:

Clinical Signs

- Physical examination reveals generalized edematous person. Edema may persist for many weeks or months.
- Tachycardia is present while blood pressure is normal.
- Pitting edema is present over legs and feet, abdominal walls and lower eyelids.
- Eyelids become puffy
- At places where edema is severe ascites and pleural effusion are seen.
- Kidneys are not palpable.

Investigations

- *Urine examination:*
  - Oliguria while edema is forming, dieresis or normal amount of urine during period of subsidence of edema.
  - *Proteinuria:* It is massive, usually more than 5 g/day though variable from time to time; urine becomes almost solid on boiling. Daily loss of protein may be 20–50 g.
  - 24 hour urine shows excretion of albumin or protein more than 3.5 g/day.
  - Red blood cells are absent or few are seen
  - Casts: Fatty casts, tubular cells, oval fat bodies, doubly refractile bodies are seen
- *Blood examination:*
  - *Anemia:* It is slight normochromic.
  - *Hypoalbuminemia:* Serum albumin usually less than 3 g/100 mL. Total serum globulin concentration frequently lowered with often elevation of α_2 and β-globulins.
  - Serum lipids show increase in LDL levels and cholesterol.
  - ESR is raised due to hyperfibrinogenemia.
  - *Serum complement level:* Serum complement C3 and C4 levels get reduced.
  - Other biochemical tests, i.e., blood urea, serum creatinine, creatinine clearance and electrolytes are normal.
- *Ultrasound of abdomen:* It can show normal small or large kidneys which depends on the underlying cause. Amyloid and diabetic kidneys are large while kidney in glomerulonephritis is small.

♦ *Renal biopsy:* It is normal on light microscopy but electron microscopy shows typical abnormalities (effacement of epithelial cell foot processes).

Q.11. Outline the management of urinary tract infection.
(Apr 2010, 5 Marks)

Ans. Infection of kidneys, ureter or bladder by microorganism that either ascends from the urethra or spread to kidney from bloodstream.

Management

♦ Rest should be given to the patient.
♦ Mild-to-moderate cases should be treated by giving antibiotics, i.e., nitrofurantoin, ciprofloxacin, gentamicin, cotrimoxazole, norfloxacin.
♦ In severe cases, parenteral antibiotics, i.e., inj. carbenicillin is given.
♦ Fluid intake should be high, alkalization of urine with potassium citrate solution to alleviate symptoms
♦ To reduce pain, antispasmodic drug is given.

Q.12. Outline the management of acute gout.
(Feb 1999, 5 Marks)

Ans. Gout is an abnormality of metabolism which results in the deposition of monosodium urate crystals in joints and other tissues.

Management

Management of Acute Attack

♦ *NSAIDs:* Any of the NSAID should be given except aspirin as it causes uric acid retention. Selective COX-2 inhibitors, e.g., Etoricoxib 120 mg OD or Valdecoxib 20–40 mg BD can be given. Colchicine 0.5 mg postoperatively every 2 hours, up to 4–6 mg/day is now reserved for patients without renal, hepatic or marrow disease, in whom the more effective NSAIDs contraindicated or poorly tolerated.
♦ *Corticosteroids:* Methyl prednisolone acetate 5–25 mg per joint as Intra-articular injection is given. Systemic oral prednisolone 20 mg/day tapered off over 4–10 days or IM triamcinolone 60 mg/day repeated in 1–4 days, are highly effective relatively safe alternatives.
♦ Restrict allopurinol or uricosuric drugs till the acute attack has settled for 2–3 weeks as they can prolong the acute attack or trigger their episodes. Patients should be advised to avoid diuretics and/or salicylates.

Long-term Management

♦ *Diet:* It should given low in purine and fats.
♦ Weight reduction in obese patient, avoid alcohol.
♦ *Anti-hyperuricemic therapy:*
  • *Hypouricemic drug:* Allopurinol 300 mg daily with a NSAID or colchicines 0.5 mg BD.
  • Febuxostat 40 mg OD to reduce and maintain serum uric acid levels below 6 mg/dL. If serum uric acid levels are more than 6 mg/dL after 2 to 4 weeks treatment with the drug 80 mg/day, dose is increased to 120 mg/day.

• Probenecid 0.5 to 1 g BD or Sulfinpyrazone 100 mg TDS as an alternative to allopurinol with colchicines if renal function is not impaired.
• Benzbromarone 100 mg daily in patients with moderate renal impairment where other uricosuric agents are ineffective.
• If patient do not tolerate or fail the full dose of other treatments IV pegloticase is given 8 mg for every 2 weeks. It dramatically reduces the serum uric acid.

Q.13. Write the investigation and management of proteinuria.
(Mar 2000, 5 Marks)

Ans. Proteinuria is defined as presence of protein usually albumin in the urine, this finding may be transient and entirely benign or a sign of severe renal disease.

Investigations of Proteinuria

♦ *Heat coagulation method:* This is done by heating upper portion of urine in a test tube. White coagulum present at top of the urine is suggestive of proteinuria.
♦ *Dipstick test:* This is a bedside test, which patient can perform by himself if his/her color vision is normal. Color change in strip is compared to the color on bottle which quantify loss of proteins.
♦ *Electrophoresis of proteins:* It detects the globulins in urine.
♦ *Immunoelectrophoresis:* It is carried out to identify fragments of immunoglobulins when there is a monoclonal peak on routine urine paper electrophoresis.
♦ *24 hours urine for proteinuria:* It is done to separate the cases of nephrotic syndrome, i.e., massive proteinuria more than 3.5 g/day from other etiology of proteinuria in which there is mild proteinuria, i.e., 1 to 2 g/day.
♦ *Radioimmunoassay:* This test is done for detection of microalbuminuria.

Management of Proteinuria

Proteinuria is not a specific disease. So its treatment depends on identifying and managing its underlying cause.

♦ Angiotensin-converting enzyme (ACE) inhibitors and angiotensin receptor blockers (ARBs) reduce intraglomerular pressure by inhibiting angiotensin II mediated efferent arteriolar vasoconstriction. These groups of drugs have a proteinuria-reducing effect independent of their antihypertensive effect.
♦ When treatment with an ACE inhibitor or ARB does not adequately control proteinuria in a patient with chronic kidney disease (e.g. diabetic nephropathy), a further reduction in proteinuria can be achieved by adding a mineralocorticoid receptor antagonist (MRA), such as eplerenone or spironolactone.
♦ Immunosuppressants, such as cyclophosphamide and azathioprine should be reserved for patients with progressive renal insufficiency or with vasculitic lesions on renal biopsy.
♦ Patients with moderate-to-severe proteinuria are usually fluid overloaded and require diuretic therapy along with dietary salt restriction.

♦ There are recommendations for no restrictions or only mild restriction in protein intake, i.e., 0.8–1 g/kg daily.

Q.14. Write short note on renal failure. *(Mar 2007, 2 Marks)*

Ans. The deterioration of renal function resulting in decline in GFR and rise in urea and non-nitrogenous substances in blood is called renal failure.

Types

1. Acute renal failure.
2. Chronic renal failure.

Acute Renal Failure

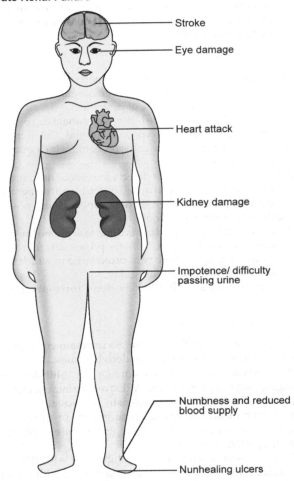

Fig. 14: Renal failure.

♦ There is acute fall in GFR over days or weeks.
♦ Invariable reversible
♦ Causes of acute renal failure may be pre renal, renal or postrenal.
♦ Oligouria and anuria are characteristics.
♦ Symptoms and signs of uremia are of recent onset.
♦ Parameters of acute reduction of GFR, i.e., edema, hypertension, salt and water retention are presenting features.
♦ Broad casts or renal failure casts are absent.

♦ Specific gravity of urine is high
♦ Dialysis is rewarding required for short period.

Chronic Renal Failure

♦ GFR falls gradually over a period of months or years.
♦ Invariably irreversible
♦ Causes are mostly renal but may be extrarenal.
♦ Polyuria and nocturia are commonly seen.
♦ Symptoms and signs of uremia are of more than three months of duration.
♦ Proof of chronicity is present, such as long duration of symptoms and signs of uremia, small sized kidney, anemia, hypertension, renal osteodystrophy.
♦ Broad casts or renal failure casts present.
♦ Specific gravity of urine is low and fixed.
♦ Repeated chronic maintenance and dialysis is required.
♦ Renal transplantation is final answer.

Q.15. Write briefly clinical features and management of nephrotic syndrome. *(Apr 2007, 5 Marks)*

or

Write short note on clinical features and management of nephrotic syndrome. *(Jan 2019, 7 Marks)*

Or

Describe sign, symptom and management of nephrotic syndrome. *(Feb 2019, 5 Marks)*

Ans. *For clinical features refer to Ans. 5 and for management refer to Ans. 4 of same chapter.*

Q.16. Write short note on UTI. *(Sep 2007, 2 Marks)*

Ans.

UTI- Urinary Tract Infection

The urinary tract infection is divided into two general anatomic categories:

1. Lower tract infection (Urethritis and cystitis).
2. Upper tract infections (Acute pyelonephritis, prostatitis, intra renal and perinephric abscess).

Etiology

Gram-negative organisms are mainly responsible, i.e., *E. coli, Proteus, Klebsiella, Enterobacter,* etc.

♦ UTI is more common in females as compared to males.
♦ Pain is the most common sign. It can be mild, constant or intense and colicky.
♦ There is also abrupt onset of frequency of micturition and dysuria.
♦ Patient suffers from fever with rigors and chills, malaise, loss of appetite and vomiting.
♦ There is presence of scalding pain in urethra during micturition.
♦ After urinary bladder get empty, there is desire to pass more urine.
♦ Hematuria can occur.
♦ In chronic infection, there are periods of acute exacerbation in addition to malaise, low-grade fever and ill health.
♦ In acute cases, tachycardia and tenderness develops on deep palpation on renal region.

Investigations

♦ *Urine examination:* A mid stream specimen is taken for examination. A heavily infected urine may look hazy to naked eye. It may have a fishy smell in *E. coli* infection and ammoniacal in Proteus infection. Reaction of urine usually is acidic. Albumin is present in traces. Microscopic examination will show clumps of pus cells. Urine should be cultured for type of organisms. Colony count done and sensitivity of the organism to various drugs.

♦ Plain X-ray abdomen is done for renal/bladder/ureteric calculi

♦ Intravenous pyelography for any congenital anomalies, calculi.

♦ Ultrasonography for renal size, calculi and any other abnormality.

Management

♦ Rest should be given to the patient.

♦ Mild-to-moderate cases should be treated by giving antibiotics, i.e., nitrofurantoin, ciprofloxacin, gentamicin, cotrimoxazole, norfloxacin.

♦ In severe cases, parenteral antibiotics, i.e., inj. carbenicillin is given.

♦ Fluid intake should be high. Alkalization of urine with potassium citrate solution to alleviate symptoms.

♦ To reduce pain, antispasmodic drug is given.

Q.17. Differentiate acute and chronic nephritis.

(Mar 2008, 2.5 Marks)

Ans.

Features	Acute nephritis	Chronic nephritis
1. Onset	Acute	Insidious
2. History	History of sore throat or skin infection in previous weeks	History of acute or subacute nephritis
3. Clinical features	Puffiness of face, minimal edema, pallor, hypertension, cardiomegaly	Pallor, hypertension, cardiomegaly and no ascites
4. Urine	Smoky and dark colored and specific gravity is raised	Polyuria, specific gravity is low and fixed, albumin is traced
5. Blood chemistry level are normal	Serum protein and cholesterol levels are increased	Blood urea and creatinine
6. Ultrasonography	Kidney is normal	Kidney is small

Q.18. Define nephrotic syndrome its etiology, clinical features, pathological blood and urine findings and management. *(Nov 2011, 8 Marks)*

Or

Describe the etiology, clinical features and management of nephrotic syndrome. *(Dec 2010, 15 Marks)*

Ans. This syndrome refers to massive proteinuria more than 3.5 g/day mainly of albumin, reduced albumin concentration, edema, hyperlipidemia, lipiduria and hypercoagulability.

♦ For etiology refer to Ans. 3 of same chapter.
♦ For clinical features refer to Ans. 5 of same chapter.
♦ For blood and urine findings refer to Ans. 6 of same chapter.
♦ For management refer to Ans. 4 of same chapter.

Q.19. Describe causes, clinical features and management of chronic renal failure. *(Sep 2009, 4.5 Marks)*

Ans. Persistent impairment of tubular and glomerular function of gradual onset so that kidneys are unable to maintain their normal physiological functions constitutes chronic renal failure.

Causes

♦ *Congenital or heredofamilial disorders:* Polycystic disease of kidney, Alport syndrome

♦ *Vascular diseases of kidney:* Vasculitis, polyarteritis nodosa, systemic lupus erythematosus.

♦ *Glomerular diseases:* Proliferative glomerulonephritis, Crescentic glomerulonephritis, membranous glomerulonephritis, glomerulosclerosis, diabetic nephropathy.

♦ *Tubulointerstitial diseases:* Chronic pyelonephritis, tuberculosis of kidney, analgesic nephropathy

♦ *Obstructive renal diseases:* Pelvic tumor, benign enlargement of prostrate, retro-peritoneal fibrosis

Clinical Features

♦ Cases of chronic renal failure may remain asymptomatic for a long time and it is often either an intercurrent infection or exacerbation of the disease process or some complications which draw attention to the patients illness. Symptoms are varied and involve all the major systems of body.

♦ Patient has got marked weakness, lethargy and restlessness. There is anorexia, nausea and vomiting.

♦ Sleep rhythm is disturbed. Nausea, retching is most marked in the early hours of morning.

♦ Patient develops revulsion towards food. Dehydration is invariably present.

♦ Neurological features include headache, lassitude, neuropathy, muscular weakness. In those with severe degree of hypertension, convulsions, muscular twitchings, irritability and in late stages of renal failure, loss of consciousness even leading to coma.

♦ Hypertension is invariably present in chronic renal failure. Patient may develop hypertensive heart failure, myocarditis or pericarditis.

♦ Patient has acidotic breathing.

♦ Repeated chest infections are common. Uremic lung develops soon.

♦ Skin has a yellowish-brown pigmentation and patient complains of intractable itching.

♦ Because of disturbances in calcium metabolism (osteomalacia, osteoporosis, renal osteodystrophy) and development of secondary hyperparathyroidism, patient has aches and pains in the bones.

♦ Cases of chronic renal failure suffer from anemia which is normocytic normochromic. Bleeding tendency is often present and patient may bleed from various sources.

♦ Menstrual irregularities in women (amenorrhea, infertility) are common while men may complain of impotence.

- Physical examination reveals generally an ill, looking person, anaemic, pale. Skin is shallow with a peculiar earthy color.
- Tongue is brown, dry and furred.
- Breath has a peculiar ammoniuremic smell (uraemic fetor).
- Hiccough is present.

Management

- The aim is to delay the progression of renal failure and main thought is to correct water and electrolyte disturbances, prevent endogenous breakdown of protein and retention all its end products as well as controlling blood pressure levels and improving the quality of life.
- *Diet:* Adequate caloric intake by encouraging patient to consume high caloric, carbohydrate foods, such as sweetened rice, sugar, sweetened biscuits, corn-flour, bread, etc. Restriction of dietary proteins (15–18 g per day) essential to reduce the rate of production of nitrogenous waste products. High carbohydrate diet gives energy and so it is essential that patient takes adequate amount of calories.
- *Fluids and electrolytes:* Patients in chronic renal failure have to maintain balance in their salt and water intake. Fluid intake should be sufficient so that patient passes at least 2–2.5 liters of urine per day. Overhydration as well as dehydration must be prevented. Salt intake has to be restricted in presence of edema, hypertension and congestive cardiac failure. Intake of potassium has to be restricted.
- *Anemia:* Anemia in chronic renal failure requires fresh blood transfusions. It is better to use packed cells.
- *Renal bone disease:* There is hypocalcemia along with features of hyperparathyroidism. Calcium orally is given to act as phosphate binder from the gut. Large doses of vitamin D or D3 are taken to help in the absorption of calcium from the gut.
- *Hypertension:* Control of hypertension is essential, since it shall worsen the renal failure as well as produce various complications. Angiotensin converting enzyme (ACE) inhibitors are the one which, are preferred for treating renal hypertension.

Q.20. Write about diet in renal failure. *(Nov 2008, 10 Marks)*

Ans.

Diet in Renal Failure

- Adequate caloric intake by encouraging patient to consume high caloric, carbohydrate foods, such as sweetened rice, sugar, sweetened biscuits, corn-flour, bread, etc.
- Restriction of dietary proteins (15–18 g per day) essential to reduce the rate of production of nitrogenous waste products.
- High carbohydrate diet gives energy and so it is essential that patient takes adequate amount of calories.
- Patients in chronic renal failure have to maintain balance in their salt and water intake.
- Fluid intake should be sufficient so that patient passes at least 2–2.5 liters of urine per day. Overhydration as well as dehydration must be prevented. Salt intake has

to be restricted in presence of edema, hypertension and congestive cardiac failure.
- Intake of potassium has to be restricted if levels of serum potassium are high.
- Diet consists of whole meal bread, marmalade or honey, small quantity of fish, fruits and vegetables.
- Milk about 200 mL per day is permitted.
- Patient can take good quantities of sugar, jam, honey, tea and lemonade.

Q.21. Write about causes of anasarca and define and discuss nephrotic syndrome. *(Nov 2008, 15 Marks)*

Ans. Anasarca is a form of generalized edema. There is massive collection of fluid in the subcutaneous interstitial spaces and the various sacs of the body.

The various causes of anasarca are:

Causes of Anasarca

- Heart disease—right heart failure.
- Kidney disease—nephritis. nephrosis
- Severe anemia—tropical diseases (epidemic dropsy)
- Nutritional causes—wet beri-beri, hypoproteinemia
- Endocrine disorder—myxedema
- In congenital—general edema.
  For nephrotic syndrome, refer to Ans. 8 of same chapter.

Q.22. Write in brief on sign, symptoms and treatment of nephrotic syndrome. *(May/Jun 2009, 5 Marks)*

Ans. Nephrotic syndrome is a clinical complex with number of renal and extra-renal features.

Symptoms

- Gradual onset of generalized edema with puffiness of eyelids.
- Patient complains of loss of appetite, malaise and generalized weakness.
- Swelling over abdomen is present
- Breathlessness is present
- Diarrhea is also present.
- Amount of passing of urination is decreased in 24 hours.

Signs

- Physical examination reveals generalized edematous person.
- Tachycardia is present while blood pressure is normal.
- Pitting edema is present over legs and feet, abdominal walls and lower eyelids.
- Eye lids become puffy
- At places where edema is severe ascites and pleural effusion are seen.
- Kidneys are not palpable.

Treatment

Refer to Ans. 8 of same chapter.

Q.23. Write sign and symptoms of uremia. *(Dec 2010, 5 Marks)*

Ans. Following are the signs and symptoms of uremia:

Symptoms

♦ Malaise, weakness, lethargy and fever.
♦ Nausea, vomiting, anorexia, diarrhea
♦ Polyuria and breathlessness when patient gets exerted.
♦ Headache, confusion and disorientation
♦ Irregular menstrual cycle and loss of libido.

Signs

♦ Presence of fluid and electrolyte disturbances.
♦ *Neurological:* Cramps, lethargy, myopathy, seizures and coma
♦ *Cardiovascular:* hypertension, pulmonary edema, pericarditis
♦ *Gastrointestinal tract:* Gastritis and enteritis
♦ *Hematological:* Anemia and bleeding diathesis
♦ *Endocrinal:* Secondary hyperparathyroidism, amenorrhea, osteodystrophy.

Q.24. Write short note on acute nephritis.

(Nov 2011, 3 Marks)

Ans. If the kidneys suddenly become inflamed, a condition is developed called acute nephritis. Acute nephritis can lead to kidney failure.

Types

There are several types of acute nephritis.

Interstitial Nephritis

In interstitial nephritis, the spaces between the renal tubules that form urine become inflamed. The kidneys swell from the inflammation.

Pyelonephritis

Pyelonephritis is an infection in the bladder that travels up the ureters and spread into the kidneys.

Glomerulonephritis

This type of acute nephritis produces inflammation in the glomeruli. Inflamed glomeruli may not filter the blood properly.

Symptoms

♦ Pain in the pelvis
♦ Pain or a burning sensation while urinating
♦ Frequent need to urinate
♦ Cloudy urine
♦ Blood or pus may be present in urine
♦ Pain in the kidney area and/or abdomen
♦ Swelling in the body, commonly in the face, legs, and feet
♦ Vomiting
♦ Fever.

Diagnosis

Various diagnostic tests may be needed to confirm a case of acute nephritis. These tests include the following:

♦ A biopsy of the kidneys. A biopsy is a small tissue sample taken from an organ and examined in a laboratory setting.

♦ Urine and blood testing. These tests may detect and locate bacteria and signs of infection. Abnormal blood cells may be present to show signs of infection.
♦ A CT scan may be used to take pictures of your pelvis and abdomen.

Treatment

♦ **Medications:**
  • Antibiotics and pain relievers may be, used if pyelonephritis is present.
  • If high blood pressure is present, calcium channel blockers should be taken.
  • Corticosteroids or other immune suppressing medications should also be given.
♦ **Home Care:**
  • *Drink more and more water:* Water helps your kidneys flush out any waste products that may be hampering the recovery.
  • Eat less sodium to prevent fluid retention.

Q.25. Write short note on clinical features and treatment of post-streptococcal glomerulonephritis.

(Mar 2013, 3 Marks)

Ans. It follows an acute streptococcal infection of throat or skin by Group-A beta hemolytic streptococci.

Clinical Features

♦ It is commonly seen in children.
♦ In morning, there is presence of puffiness over the face and edema over the feet.
♦ Presence of headache, vomiting and abdominal pain
♦ Oligouria is present.
♦ Proteinuria is less, i.e., 1 g/day
♦ Hypertension is present.
♦ Circulatory congestion can occur.

Treatment

♦ *Bed rest:* Patient should be hospitalized and rest is given till illness is resolved. In mild cases, bed rest is given for 3 weeks and in severe cases for 3 months.
♦ *Fluid restriction:* Avoid fluid overload. For first 24 hours only 500 mL of water or glucose or barley water should be given. If volume of urine in 24 hours is less than 400 mL teart for acute renal failure and if it is more than 400 mL limit intake of fluid to 500 mL + a volume equal to that passed in preceding 24 hours. Fruit juices rich with potassium are given with caution.
♦ *Diet:* Restrict dietary protein and restrict sodium and potassium intake. Monitor potassium and sodium.
♦ *Hypertension:* Moderate-to-severe hypertension is controlled by hydralazine, beta-blockers, such as atenolol or calcium-channel blockers or ACE inhibitors. Salt restriction should be done.
♦ *Antibiotics:* Injection benzathine penicillin 500,000 units IM 6 hourly for 7 days.

- *Diuretics:* It is not indicated unless there is acute LVF or pulmonary edema is present. Frusemide 40 mg IV daily for few days, followed by oral substitution till diuretic phase is induced.
- In patients with progressive renal failure or if fluid overload is present, dialysis may have to be employed.

Q.26. Write about acute renal failure under following headings.   *(Apr 2015, 2 + 2 Marks)*
    a. Causes
    b. Management

Ans.

Causes

- *Pre-renal causes:* The causes for renal hypoperfusion are septicemia, hypovolemia, hemorrhage, shock, burn, crushing injury, hemolysis inside the vessels, rhabdomyolysis.
- *Intrarenal causes:* The causes for intrinsic renal disease are renovascular obstruction, glomerulonephritis, vasculitis, tubulointerstitial nephritis, acute tubular necrosis.
- *Obstructive causes:* Obstruction of the urinary tract at any place.

Management

Management of acute renal failure is divided into three phase, i.e.

- **Oligouric phase:**
    - Water and electrolyte balance should be maintained. One liter of fluid should be started and CVP is also maintained. Fluids which are to be replaced should be calculated by loss to urine output of yesterday.
    - Proteins should be given, i.e., 20–40 g of proteins per day are given.
    - In cases of infections, antibiotics are to be given based on culture and sensitivity test.
    - Sodium bicarbonate should be given.
    - Dialysis should be done when in oliguria is present, hyperkalemia, metabolic acidosis etc.
- **Diuretic phase:**
    - Fluid and electrolytes should be replaced.
    - IV glucose or glucose saline is given.
    - 70–80 g of protein per day is given.
    - Patient is told to have plenty of fruit juices.
- **Recovery phase:** After 7–20 days recovery occurs.

Q.27. Write in detail about nephrotic syndrome under the headings:
    a. Definition
    b. Etiology
    c. Clinical features
    d. Diagnosis
    e. Treatment

Ans.
a. **Definition:** Nephrotic syndrome is defined as the presence of heavy proteinuria and hypoalbuminemia in association with varying degrees of edema, lipiduria and hyperlipidemia.

b. For etiology *refer to Ans. 3 of same chapter.*
c. For clinical features *refer to Ans. 5 of same chapter.*
d. For diagnosis *refer to Ans. 10 of same chapter.*
e. For treatment *refer to Ans. 8 of same chapter.*

Q.28. Write long answer on etiopathology and treatment of nephrotic syndrome.   *(Oct 2019, 6 Marks)*

Ans.

Etiopathology of Nephrotic Syndrome

- Lesion in the nephrotic syndrome occur in glomeruli which causes damage to its permeability leading to the filtration of large amount of albumin or high molecular proteins which is the main hallmark of disease.
- Sustained proteinuria is followed by hypoalbuminaemia which occur because of excessive urinary losses, increased renal catabolism and due to the inadequate hepatic synthesis of albumin.
- Hypoalbuminemia leads to decrease in the plasma oncotic pressure which produces disturbances in Starling's forces across capillaries producing the shift of fluids from intravascular compartment to interstitial space which causes edema.
- Fluid collection extracellularly causes reduction in effective blood volume which leads to stimulation of renin angiotensin aldosterone system and ADH which potentiates edema because of retention of the sodium and water.
- Decreased plasma oncotic pressure because of hypoalbuminemia causes stimulation of lipoprotein synthesis in liver producing hyperlipidemia which is the frequent accompaniment of nephrotic syndrome.
- Low density lipoproteins and cholesterol get elevated which is followed by triglycerides. Oval fat bodies or the fatty casts are seen in the urine known as lipiduria.

For treatment of nephrotic syndrome *refer to Ans. 8 of same chapter.*

---

7. DISEASES OF BLOOD

Q.1. Write short note on anemia.   *(Feb 2006, 5 Marks)*

Or

Write clinical features, type and management of anemia.   *(July 2016, 12 Marks)*

Ans. Anemia is a state in which the hemoglobin concentration falls below the accepted normal range depending on age and sex.

Classification of Anemia/Types of Anemia

Etiological Classification of Anemia

- *Blood loss:*
    - Post-hemorrhagic
    - Chronic blood loss due to piles, hematemesis, menorrhagia
    - Hookworm disease

- **Deficiency of hemopoietic factors**
  - Iron deficiency
  - Folate and vitamin B12 deficiency
  - Protein deficiency, i.e., diarrhea, malabsorption
- **Bone marrow aplasia**
  - Aplastic anemia
  - Pure red cell aplasia
- **Anemia due to systemic infections or systemic disorders:**
  - Anemia due to chronic infection
  - Anemia due to chronic renal disease
  - Anemia due to chronic liver disease
  - Disseminated malignancy
  - Endocrinal diseases
- **Anemia due to bone marrow infiltration**
  - Leukemias
  - Lymphomas
  - Myelofibrosis/myelosclerosis
  - Multiple myeloma
  - Congenital sideroblastic anemia
- Anemia due to increased red cell destruction (hemolytic anemias)
  - Intracorpuscular defect (hereditary or acquired)
  - Extracorpuscular defect (acquired)

Morphological Classification of Anemia

Based on the red cell size, hemoglobin content and red cell indices, anemias are classified into 3 types:

1. *Microcytic, hypochromic:* MCV, MCH, MCHC are all reduced, e.g., in iron-deficiency anemia and in certain noniron deficient anemias (sideroblastic anemia, thalassemia, anemia of chronic disorders).
2. *Normocytic, normochromic:* MCV MCH, MCHC are all normal, e.g., after acute blood loss, haemolytic anemias, bone marrow failure, anemia of chronic disorders.
3. *Macrocytic:* MCV is raised, e.g., in megaloblastic anemia due to deficiency of vitamin B12 or folic acid.

Physiological Classification

This is based on the reticulocyte production index:
- Anemia with reticulocyte production count less than 2.5
  - *Normocytic-normochromic:* Iron deficiency anemia, aplastic anemia, anemia of inflammatory, renal and endocrine disease.
  - Microcytic or macrocytic
  Microcytic: Sideroblastic, thalassemia
  Macrocytic: Vitamin B12 or folate deficiency
- *Anemia with reticulocyte production count more than 2.5*
  Hemolytic/hemorrhagic: Anemia due to blood loss, Hemoglobinopathies, autoimmune hemolytic, etc.

Clinical Features

Symptoms

- *General:* Lassitude and fatigue
- *Gastrointestinal tract:* Nausea, weight loss, anorexia, flatulence and constipation

- *Cardiovascular symptoms:* Palpitations, exertional dyspnea, angina, throbbing in head and ear.
- *Central nervous system symptoms:* Tinnitus, headache, dizziness, insomnia, numbness, tingling sensation in hand and feet.
- *Genitourinary tract:* Amenorrhea or menorrhagia, loss of libido.

Signs

- Presence of polarity on skin, mucous membrane and conjunctiva.
- Tachycardia
- Presence of collapsing pulse
- Midsystolic flow murmur across aortic and the pulmonary valves.
- In severe anemia, there is presence of cardiomegaly and congestive heart failure.
- Edema can be present.

Investigations

Every case of anemia should have the following investigations to detect degree and cause of anemia:
- Hemoglobin count decreases.
- RBC count, packed cell volume, mean corpuscular volume and mean corpuscular hemoglobin concentration (MCHC). Total leukocyte count and differential leukocyte count.
- Peripheral blood film for type of anemia and shape of RBCs and presence of any abnormal cells.
- Clotting time and bleeding time in hemolytic anemia.
- Blood platelets.

Bone marrow examination is done when cause of anemia requires further investigation especially to detect type of erythropoiesis.

Other Investigations

- *Stools for parasites:* Test for presence of blood and stools is done in patients suspected to chronic blood loss.
- Urine for albumin, bile salt, pigments and urobilinogen
- *Gastric analysis:* Histamine fast achlorhydria in pernicious anemia and megaloblastic anemia.
- Studies for detecting steatorrhea and malabsorption studies.
- Schilling test for vitamin B12 absorption in megaloblastic and dimorphic anemias.
- FIGLU test is done to assess folic acid deficiency. About 15 g of histidine hydrochloride is given by mouth and the urine in which it is excreted it is collected over next eight hours. Normal excretion is 1–17 mg

Management

- Correction of dietary deficiency, i.e., faulty dietary habits, chronic alcoholism and malnourishment.
- Treatment of underlying cause, i.e., ankylostomiasis, piles, menorrhagia, infection, chronic kidney failure, leukemia, liver disease, collagen disease or endocrine deficiency, surgical correction of intestinal abnormalities, e.g., blind loop.

♦ Removal of toxic chemical agent or drug, i.e., in some cases of hemolytic anemia or aplastic anemia.
♦ *Blood transfusion:* Its chief value is its immediate effect.
♦ Administration of substances specifically lacking, i.e.
  • Hematinic should be started only after adequate blood examination, since response to a hematinic may obscure the blood picture.
  • The specific hematinic should be given alone.
  • The hematinic should be given in adequate doses for a sufficient period of time.

Q.2. Write note on iron-deficiency anemia.
(Apr 2010, 5 Marks) (Mar 2011, 3 Marks)
Or
Write short note on clinical features and investigations of iron deficiency anemia. *(Mar 2007, 5 Marks)*
Or
Write iron-deficiency anemia under following headings: *(Dec 2012, 2 Marks each)*
a. Etiology
b. Clinical Features
c. Investigations
d. Treatment
Or
Write etiology, clinical features and treatment of iron deficiency anemia. *(Jun 2014, 12 Marks)*
Or
Define and classify anemia write about the management of iron deficiency anemia.
(Sep 2018, 5 Marks)
Or
Write short answer on iron deficiency anemia.
(Feb 2019, 3 Marks)
Or
Write signs and symptoms of iron deficiency anemia.
(Dec 2010, 5 Marks)

Ans. *For definition and classification of anemia refer to Ans. 1 of same chapter.*

Iron deficiency anemia is commonest cause of anemia and is a microcytic hypochromic anemia.

Causes/Etiology

♦ *Due to increased blood loss:*
  • *Gastrointestinal:* Peptic ulcer, piles, hookworm manifestation, Carcinoma of stomach, acute erosive gastritis, ulcerative colitis
  • *Lung:* Due to hemoptysis
  • *Renal:* Hemoglobinuria and hematuria
  • *Uterine:* Menorrhagia, postmenopausal uterine bleeding.
  • *Nose:* Epistaxis
♦ *Due to increased body demands:*
  • In adolescence
  • During prematurity
  • In pregnancy and lactation.
♦ Due to inadequate dietary intake:
  • In low socioeconomic status

  • In elder patients with loss of teeth
  • Anorexia of pregnancy.
♦ Decreased absorption:
  • In achlorhydria
  • In patients with malabsorption
  • In cases with gastrectomy.

Clinical Features

Symptoms

♦ Tiredness
♦ Weakness
♦ Lethargy
♦ Loss of appetite
♦ Headache and bodyache
♦ Inability to concentrate, giddiness
♦ Breathlessness
♦ Epigastric discomfort.

Signs

♦ Pallor
♦ Palpitation
♦ Angular stomatitis
♦ Atrophic gastritis
♦ Flattening or spoon-shaped nails, i.e., platynychia and koilonychia
♦ Tongue is pale and smooth
♦ Glossitis
♦ Hepatosplenomegaly
♦ Pulmmer-Vinson syndrome, i.e., dysphagia and cricoid webs.

Investigations

♦ *Blood picture and red cell indices:*
  • *Hemoglobin:* Fall on hemoglobin concentration.
  • *Red cells:* RBCs in blood film are hypochromatic and microcytic and there is anisocytosis, poikilocytosis and elliptocytosis.
  • *Reticulocyte count:* Normal or reduced.
  • *Absolute values:* MCV, MCH and MCHC are decreased.
  • *Leukocytes:* Usually normal
  • *Platelets:* Usually normal but raised if bleeding is cause of anemia.
  • *ESR:* Value of ESR is low.
♦ *Bone marrow findings:*
  • *Marrow cellularity:* Marrow cellularity is increased due to erythroid hyperplasia.
  • Erythropoiesis: Normoblastic erythropoiesis.
  • Marrow iron is deficient.
♦ *Biochemical findings:*
  • Serum iron level is low.
  • Total iron-binding capacity is high.
  • Serum ferritin is very low.

Management

♦ Proper physical and mental rest.
♦ Good nourishing diet with supplementation of foods rich in iron.
♦ *Oral iron therapy:* Ferrous sulfate 200 mg TID is given in between the meals. If after taking the drug, there is any

abdominal pain, nausea, vomiting or constipation, the salt is changed to ferrous gluconate or ferrous fumarate. Oral iron therapy should be given for 6 months.

♦ *Parenteral iron therapy:* Iron sorbitol ciric acid complex 1.5 mg/kg body weight is given as IM or Iron dextran in 5% glucose is given as IV

♦ *Blood transfusion:* Packed red cells are transfused.

Q.3. Write short note on hemolytic anemia.

(Sep 2006, 5 Marks) (Sep 2009, 4 Marks)

Or

Write causes of hemolytic anemia.

(Feb 2013, 6 Marks)

Or

Define and classify anemia. Discuss clinical features, investigation and treatment of hemolytic anemia.

(Apr 2018, 5 Marks)

Ans. *For definition and classification of anemia refer to Ans. 1 of same chapter.*

Hemolytic anemia is a reduction in number of circulating red cells from there premature destruction.

Etiological Classification or Causes

♦ **Acquired or Extracorpuscular**
  • *Immunohemolytic anemia:*
    – Autoimmunohemolytic anemia
      » Warm antibody autoimmune hemolytic anemia
      » Cold antibody autoimmune hemolytic anemia
    – Drug-induced immunohemolytic anemia
    – Iso immune hemolytic anemia
  • *Mechanical trauma:* Micro-angiopathic hemolytic anemia
  • *Direct toxic effect:* Malaria, bacteria, infection and other agents
  • *Acquired red cell membrane abnormalities:* Paroxysmal nocturnal hemoglobinuria.
  • Splenomegaly.

♦ **Hereditary or Intracorpuscular**
  • *Abnormalities of red cell membrane:*
    – Hereditary spherocytosis
    – Hereditary elliptocytosis
    – Hereditary stomatocytosis.
  • *Disorders of red cell interior:*
    – *Red cell enzyme defect:*
      » *Defects in HMP shunt:* G6PD deficiency
      » *Defects in glycolytic pathway:* Pyruvate kinase deficiency.
    – *Disorders of hemoglobin:*
      » Structurally abnormal hemoglobin, sickle syndrome and other hemoglobinopathies.
      » *Reduced globin chain synthesis:* Thalassemias.

Clinical features

♦ There is presence of high fever, toxemia, marked *prostration, shock and hemoglobinuria

♦ Acute renal failure may develop

♦ Chronic form includes jaundice varying from mild to severe form, mongoloid faces, splenomegaly, chronic leg ulcers and pigment stones in gallbladder.

Investigations Or Diagnosis for Hemolytic Anemia

Test of Increased Red Cell Breakdown

♦ Blood film shows normocytic normochromic or dimorphic anemia.

♦ Unconjugated serum bilirubin is raised

♦ Urine urobilinogen is raised but bilirubinuria is absent

♦ Serum hepatoglobin is reduced

♦ Plasma LDH is increased

♦ There is evidence of intravascular hemolysis, i.e., hemoglobinemia, hemoglobinuria, methemoglobinemia, hemosiderinuria.

Test of Increased Red Cell Production

♦ Reticulocyte count get increased

♦ Blood film shows macrocytosis, polychromasia and presence of normoblasts

♦ Bone marrow examination shows erythroid hyperplasia with raised iron store.

♦ X-ray of bones show expansion of marrow space in bones, such as skull.

Test of Damage to Red Cells

♦ Blood film show microspherocytes and fragmented RBCs.

♦ Osmotic fragility is increased.

♦ Electrophoresis test is done for abnormal hemoglobin

♦ Estimation of Hemoglobin A2 should be done

♦ Estimation of Hemoglobin F should be done

♦ Test for sickling is done

♦ Screening test for G6PD deficiency is done

Test for Shortened Red Cell Survivor

♦ Chromium labeled method show short red cell life span.

Treatment of Hemolytic Anemia

♦ Patients with compensated hemolytic process need no treatment.

♦ Mainly management is general and specific.

♦ Folic acid 5 mg is given routinely and lifelong in patients with inherited hemolytic disorders

♦ Patients having hereditary spherocytosis may undergo splenectomy if they have moderate to severe disease or have experienced episodes of hemolytic crisis or gall stones.

Q.4. Enumerate causes of agranulocytosis.

(Sep 2008, 2.5 Marks)

Ans. It is defined as an acute disease marked by a deficit or absolute lack of granulocytic WBCs, i.e., neutrophils, basophils and eosinophils.

Causes

♦ Endocrinal causes like hyperpituitarism, hypoadrenalism.

Q 3.   *Prostration = Absolute exhaustion

♦ Agranulocytosis due to drugs: This is a very important cause and is related to dosage of drugs as well as sensitivity reaction. The main drugs are:
  • Anti-cancer drugs
  • Anti-inflammatory drugs
  • Phenothiazines and tranquilizers
  • Sulfonamides and cotrimoxazole
  • Anti-thyroid drugs
  • Anti-diabetic drugs
  • Anti-histaminics
  • Anti-epileptic drugs
  • Anti-microbial agents
♦ Diuretics:
  • Deficiency of vitamin B12 and folate
  • It is caused due to obliteration of bone marrow due to myelofibrosis, lymphoma and sarcoma.
    It is caused due to bone marrow damage due to X-ray radiation.
♦ Due to viral infections, i.e., hepatitis, HIV, influenza, EBV
♦ Due to bacterial infections, i.e., enteric fever, tuberculosis and gram-negative bacterial septicemia
♦ Due to protozoal diseases, i.e., malaria and kala-azar.
♦ Due to autoimmune diseases, i.e., SLE, chronic autoimmune neutropenia
♦ Congenital, i.e., in Kostmann's syndrome

Q.5. Describe clinical manifestations and management of agranulocytosis. *(Mar 2003, 10 Marks)*

Ans. It is defined as an acute disease marked by a deficit or absolute lack of granulocytic WBCs, i.e., neutrophils, basophils and eosinophils.

Clinical Manifestations

♦ Females are more commonly affected than males
♦ Early manifestations of agranulocytosis are may be in form of sore throat or pain.
♦ There may be fever going up to 130°F, sometimes coming with rigor chills, body ache and pain and extreme degree of prostration.
♦ In large number of cases ulceromembranous lesions appear on throat, tonsils, gum, tongue and genitalia
♦ These are often covered with grayish black exudates and may become gangrenous.
♦ Lymph gland generally cervical groups and in some, there are generalized lymphadenopathy
♦ Liver and spleen may become enlarged.
♦ As disease progresses severe toxemia develops and patient may go into shock.

Management

♦ Firstly, the cause is removable which is identifiable.
♦ Secondly, the infection is controlled and patient is put on isolation ward and barrier nursing is done.
♦ Anti-bacterial drugs, such as penicillin 5 mega units IM or IV 4 hourly or ciprofloxacin 500 mg IV 4 hourly is started immediately.

♦ In addition metrogyl 500 mg every 6 hourly to take care of infection
♦ Anabolic steroids are also given.
♦ In cases where toxemia is severe corticosteroids are employed, i.e., injection dexamethasone 4 mg IV 6 hourly.
♦ Granulocytes transfusion is given to tide over crisis. This is given daily for 5–7 days.

Q.6. Describe briefly diagnosis of agranulocytosis.
(Apr 2010, 5 Marks)

Ans. The diagnosis of agranulocytosis is based on clinical history and physical examination.

♦ Person with history of sore throat, fever with rigor and chills, body ache and extreme degree of prostration (absolute exhaustion).
♦ In large number of cases ulceromembranous lesions are present on throat, tonsil, gums, tongue and genitalia. The lesions are covered with grayish black exudates and become gangrenous.
♦ Confirmation of diagnosis is made by laboratory investigations.
♦ Peripheral blood film shows complete absence of neutrophils.
♦ Bone marrow is hypocellular and there is depletion of myeloid elements.

Q.7. Discuss in short neutropenia. *(Mar 1997, 5 Marks)*

Ans. The presence of abnormally small number of neutrophils in the blood usually less than 1500 to 2000 per micro liter.

Causes

♦ Starvation and *debility.
♦ Overwhelming infections and toxemia in older people.
♦ *Infections:* Typhoid, measles, malaria, kala-azar, hepatitis, influenza, HIV and miliary TB.
♦ Hypersplenism, liver cirrhosis.
♦ *Bone marrow failure:* In aplastic anemia, leukemia and myelofibroma
♦ *Drugs:* Sulfonamides, antibiotic, analgesics, anti-thyroids, anti-convulsants, etc.
♦ Anaphylactic shock.

Clinical Manifestations

♦ Females are more commonly affected as compared to males
♦ Early manifestations of agranulocytosis are may be in form of sore throat or pain.
♦ There may be fever going up to 130°F, sometimes coming with rigor chills, body ache and pain and extreme degree of prostration.
♦ In large number of cases ulceromembranous lesions appear on throat, tonsils, gum, tongue and genitalia
♦ These are often covered with grayish black exudates and may become gangrenous.
♦ Lymph gland generally cervical groups and in some, there are generalized lymphadenopathy
♦ Liver and spleen may become enlarged.

Q 7. *Debility = Weakness

♦ As disease progresses severe toxemia develops and patient may go into shock.

Investigations

♦ Peripheral blood film show complete absence of neutrophils.
♦ Bone marrow is normocellular and show decrease mature neutrophils.

Management

♦ Firstly, the cause is removable which is identifiable.
♦ Secondly, the infection is controlled and patient is put on isolation ward and barrier nursing is done.
♦ Anti-bacterial drugs, such as penicillin 5 mega units IM or IV 4 hourly or ciprofloxacin 500 mg IV 4 hourly is started immediately.
♦ In addition metrogyl 500 mg every 6 hourly to take care of infection
♦ Anabolic steroids are also given.
♦ In cases where toxemia is severe corticosteroids are employed, i.e., injection dexamethasone 4 mg IV 6 hourly.
♦ Granulocytes transfusion is given to tide over crisis. This is given daily for 5 to 7 days.

Q.8. Write note on hemophilia. *(June 2010, 5 Marks)*
(Sep 2007, 5 Marks) (Feb 2006, 5 Marks)

Ans. Hemophilia is an inherited disorder which affects males and is transmitted by females.

♦ It is a X-linked recessive disorder caused by deficiency of factor VIII. This type of hemophilia is called classic hemophilia.
♦ The another disorder is hemophilia B or Christmas disease which involves males inherited to X-linked recessive trait. It is caused due to deficiency of factor IX.

Clinical Features

♦ *At birth:* Newborn with hemophilia is usually healthy, though bleeding from cord and cephalohematoma may occur.
♦ *In infant:* Hemophilia is asymptomatic till 6 to 12 months, when bruising becomes more obvious. Bleeding from the mouth is common.
♦ *During childhood:* In severely affected individuals, spontaneous bleeding may occur in joint and muscles, including psoas muscle.
♦ *In adults:* Frequency of spontaneous bleeding decreases, but joints may already have been damaged. Intracranial hemorrhage is a life-threatening complication. Spontaneous bleeds are common in mildly affected individuals, but after injury bleeding occurs till appropriate therapy has begun.

Investigations

♦ APTT is prolonged in hemophilia A and B, but PT is normal.
♦ Specific factor assay demonstrate reduced factor VIII c in hemophilia A and factor IX in hemophilia B. If the clinical history is strongly suggestive of hemophilia, normal APTT does not exclude the diagnosis.

Treatment

♦ It is done by fresh blood transfusion when bleeding is in the large mass.
♦ Factor VIII concentrate is employed in case of hemophilia A and factor IX concentrate is employed in case of hemophilia B.
♦ A hemophilic will require treatment before any dental procedure. Such patient is managed by IV infusion or cryoprecipitate or factor VIII combined with aminocaproic acid 4 to 6 g QDS.
♦ For any major surgery or periodontal surgeries or extraction of tooth hemophilic patient should be hospitalized. Infusion of factor VIII concentrate is given before surgery and is continued for 48 to 72 hours. Antibiotic should also be given to the patient.

Complications of Hemophilia

♦ Hepatitis in patients who received multiple transfusion of FFP or cryoprecipitate.
♦ AIDS in a patient not screened for HIV and treated with FFP or cryoprecipitate.
♦ Anemia from excessive bleeding.
♦ Contractures in muscles following intramuscular hematomas.
♦ Spontaneous intracranial hemorrhage in severe hemophilia.

Q.9. Write short note on bleeding disorders in dental practice. *(Sep 2008, 7 Marks)*

Or

Write short note on bleeding disorder.

(Aug 2012, 5 Marks)

Ans. *Bleeding disorders:* Bleeding disorders or hemorrhagic diatheses are a group of disorders characterized by defective hemostasis with abnormal bleeding.

Bleeding Disorders

Idiopathic Thrombocytopenic Purpura

Etiology

♦ Impaired platelet production
♦ Accelerated platelet destruction
♦ Splenic sequestration
♦ Dilution loss

Oral Manifestations

♦ Excessive bleeding after tooth extraction.
♦ Extensive spontaneous gingival bleeding may be seen.
♦ Petechiae do not blench on pressure

Management

♦ Corticosteroids that is prednisolone 60 mg/dL.
♦ Splenectomy, if there is no response to prednisolone to prednisolone in 3–4 days.
♦ Local hemostatics.

Hemophilia

Etiology

- It is a hereditary disorder.
- It occurs due to the deficiency to reduce activity of factor VIII in hemophilia A or factor IX in hemophilia B.

Oral Manifestations

- Prolonged bleeding after tooth extraction hematoma of floor of mouth and larynx with subsequent respiratory embarrassment.
- Physiological process of tooth eruption may be associated with severe and prolonged hemorrhage.

Management

- It is done by fresh blood transfusion when bleeding is in the large mass.
- Factor VIII concentrate is employed in case of hemophilia A and factor IX concentrate is employed in case of hemophilia B.
- A hemophilic will require treatment before any dental procedure. Such patient is managed by IV infusion or cryoprecipitate or factor VIII combined with aminocaproic acid 4 to 6 g QDS.
- For any major surgery or periodontal surgeries or extraction of tooth hemophilic patient should be hospitalized. Infusion of factor VIII concentrate is given before surgery and is continued for 48 to 72 hours. Antibiotic should also be given to the patient

von Willebrand's Disease

Etiology

Hereditary coagulation disorder occurring due to qualitative or quantitative defects in von Willebrand factor.

Oral Manifestations

- Gingival bleeding and postextraction bleeding
- Disease may be discovered after dental extraction.

Management

- Mild episodes of bleeding can be treated with desmopressin which increases vWF level which leads to secondary increase in Factor VIII.
- For more serious bleeds during dental procedure hemostasis is achieved by Factor VIII concentrate which contain considerable quantities of vWF in addition to factor VIII.

Hereditary Hemorrhagic Telangectasia

It is transmitted as autosomal dominant trait and is characterized by bleeding from mucous membrane.

Management

- In patient having repeated attacks of epistaxis septal dermoplasty should be done. In septal dermoplasty, involved mucosa get removed and skin grafting is done.
- If spontaneous hemorrhages are present or nasal bleeding is present during dental procedure, it is controlled by giving pressure packs.

- Sclerosing agents, i.e., sodium tetradecyl sulfate if injected intra lesionally stop bleeding.
- Electrocautery is done. It helps in arresting bleeding.

Disseminated Intravascular Coagulation

It is a condition that results when the clotting system is activated in all or a major part of vascular system. Despite widespread fibrin production the major clinical problem is bleeding not thrombosis. Disseminated intravascular coagulation (DIC) is associated with a number of disorders, such as infection, obstetric complications, cancer and snakebite.

Management

- Correction of hemodynamic instability by fluid therapy, transfusion of packed cells or whole blood.
- *Factor replacement:* This is the specific therapy, in this fresh-frozen plasma, cryoprecipitate, platelet concentrate transfusions are essential. Fresh-frozen plasma is given at the dose of 15 mL/kg. Platelet is transfused at the dosage of 0.1 unit/kg.

Q.10. Write short note on leukemia.   *(Sep 2008, 7 Marks)*

Ans. Leukemia is defined as clone of malignant cells derived from myeloid or lymphoid stem cells.

Etiology

- Genetic factors, such as familial, identical twins, congenital disorders.
- Environmental factors, i.e., atomic radiation and pollution
- Ionizing radiations
- Retroviruses
- Chemical agents, i.e., alkylating agents, cytotoxic drugs.

Types of Leukemias

Acute Leukemia

- Acute lymphoblastic leukemia
- Acute myeloid leukemia

Chronic Leukemia

- Chronic lymphatic leukemia chronic myeloid leukemia.

Clinical Features

- Anemia
- Fatigue and lethargy
- Fever
- Bone and joint pain
- Combination of pallor, petechiae or purpura is present.
- Mucus membrane is bleeding
- Hepatomegaly, splenomegaly and renomegaly is present.
- There is tenderness over other bones.

Investigations

- Bone marrow picture shows hypercellular reaction is present with premature and primitive cells.
- There is presence of biochemical changes with presence of Philadelphia chromosome.

- Peripheral blood film show normocytic normochromic picture with an abundance of neutrophil, myelocyte, metamyelocyte.
- White cell counts are elevated

Treatment

- Chemotherapy, bone marrow transplantation or both should be done.
- New regimes are derived regularly and are tailored to specific illness
- Treatment is given in several phases, with a period of induction chemotherapy to induce remission followed by maintenance and consolidation phases.
- This multiphase treatment is designed for further deplete malignant cells from bone marrow to achieve complete cure.

Q.11. Describe the etiology, clinical features and management of acute leukemia. *(Feb 2013, 15 Marks)*

Ans. Acute leukemia is defined as an uncontrolled growth of immature hemopoietic cells at the exposure normal marrow tissue.

Etiology

- *Radiation:* Association between radiation-induced genetic damage to the hemopoietic progenitors and development of myelodysplasia and acute leukemia is seen after nuclear disease.
- *Chemical and drugs:* Chronic benzene exposure and use of cytotoxic and immunosuppressive agents.
- Oncogens and cytogenic abnormalities
- Genetic factors, i.e., genetic disorders, such as Down's syndrome, Klinefelter's syndrome, etc.
- *Viruses:* Infection by human lymphotrophic virus (HTLV-1).

Clinical Features

- Symptoms due to anemia, i.e., tiredness, weakness and marked pallor.
- *Hemorrhagic manifestation:* Petechiae, bleeding from gums and nose, persistent bleeding after tooth extraction.
- *Infection:* It causes infective lesions of mouth and throat, i.e., ulceration of mouth and pharynx, herpes simplex infection of face and infection of respiratory tract, such as bronchitis and pneumonia.
- Symptoms of cellular hyperviscosity
- There are tissue deposits of leukemic cells causing gum hypertrophy which is common in myelomonocytic and monocytic variety of AML.
- Lymphadenopathy and splenomegaly are common in acute lymphoid leukemia.
- Signs of organ infiltration are present, i.e.
  - *CNS:* Meningeal involvement occurs in children with acute lymphocytic leukemia.
  - *Skin:* Bluish nodules or dusky red patches are present.
  - *Kidneys:* Presence of kidney failure.
  - *Other sites:* Testes, ovary, liver, gut and serous membranes, such as pleura and peritoneum.

- Bone pain are present, i.e., tenderness of sternum, osteolytic bone lesions and pathologic fractures may occur.
- Constitutional symptoms, i.e., fever, malaise and prostration.
- Roth's spot, i.e., presence of white central retinal hemorrhages in acute myeloid leukemia.

Management

Chemotherapy

- **Induction phase:** Initial high dose chemotherapy in order to reduce leukemic cells below the levels of morphogenic detection.
  Treatment regimen for acute lymphoblastic leukemia:
  - Vincristine 1.4 mg/m² IV weekly for 4 weeks.
  - Prednisolone 60 mg/day for 4 weeks.
  - L- Asparaginase 50–200 ku/kg IV for 4 weeks.
  - Daunorubicin 30 mg/m² IV daily for two weeks.
  Treatment regimen for acute myeloid leukemia:
  - Daunorubicin IV alternate days 3 doses.
  - Cytosine arabinoside IV BD for 10 days
  - Thioguanine oral BD for 10 days.
  - In this, blood transfusion and platelet transfusion are required.
- **CNS prophylaxis:** Intrathecal methotrexate is given in acute lymphoblastic leukemia
- **Consolidation:** Another dose of chemotherapy to reduce leukemic burden
  In acute lymphoblastic leukemia
  - IV daunorubicin
  - IV cytosine arabinoside
  - IV Etoposide
  - Methotrexate, 6-thioguanine
  - Dexamethasone
  In acute myloid leukemia:
  - High dose IV Cytosine arabinoside is given
- **Maintenance:** Low dose chemotherapy for 18 months to 2 years
  In acute lymphoblastic leukemia:
  - Oral Prednisolone
  - IV Vincristine
  - Oral 6 – mercaptopurine
  - Oral Methotrexate
  In acute myeloid leukemia:
  Post-remission therapy is given, i.e., myeloablative therapy followed by bone marrow transplantation in relapse or those with high-risk chromosomal changes.
- **Bone marrow transplantation**
  In acute lymphoblastic leukemia: Allogenic bone marrow transplantation is an option in acute lymphocytic leukemia patients entering first remission who have an HLA – identical sibling, provided the sibling is fit and is less than 55 years.
  In acute myeloid leukemia: In adult patient-high dose chemotherapy with autologus transplantation of hemopoietic stem cells derived from peripheral blood or bone marrow can be done.

♦ **Supportive care:**
- Hemoglobin level should not allow falling below 8 g/dL by transfusing 4 units of packed RBCs. This is done to avoid anemia.
- If bleeding is present, then there is transfusion of pooled or single donor platelets.
- Good nursing, prophylactic gastrointestinal tract decontamination, antibiotics and attention to fluid balance are given to prevent infections.
- If disseminated intravascular coagulation is present, then fibrinogen replacement, platelet transfusion twice daily and anticoagulants are given.
- *Pneumocystis jiroveci* pneumonia is a risk during the treatment of acute lymphocytic leukemia maintenance therapy.
- Hyperuricemia is prevented by adequate hydration and pretreatment with allopurinol which should be continued till peripheral blood is cleared of blast cells.

Q.12. Write short note on chronic myeloid leukemia.

(Feb/Mar 2005, 5 Marks) (Apr 2010, 4 Marks)

Ans. Chronic myeloid leukemia is a clonal disorder of pluripotent stem cell.

The most important characteristic feature of chronic myeloid leukemia is demonstration of Philadelphia chromosome in leukemic blast cells.

Clinical Features

Common Features

♦ *Nonspecific:* Loss of weight, fatigue, malaise, excessive perspiration.
♦ *Splenomegaly:* Size of spleen is enlarged
♦ Bleeding, excessive menstrual or other bleeding.
♦ Anemia
♦ *Bone pain:* It is due to extension of hemopoiesis through long bones.

Rare Features

♦ Splenic infarction
♦ Leukostasis
♦ Gout
♦ Retinal hemorrhage
♦ Fever.

Etiology

Chronic myeloid leukemia results from translocation of genetic material between chromosome 9 and 22.

The translocation result in production of abnormal tyrosine kinase that makes affected cell immortal.

Investigations

♦ *Peripheral blood:* WBC count is 10–500 × 10^9/L, with excess of neutrophils, myelocytes and blasts. Basophilia and eosinophilia are prominent and thrombocytosis is common.

♦ Bone marrow is hypercellular with marrow fibrosis and gaucher like cells. High myeloid to erythroid ratio, i.e., 15 to 20 : 1.
♦ Neutrophil alkaline phosphatase is low.
♦ Serum vitamin B12 is increased.
♦ Serum uric acid is increased.

Treatment

Chronic Phase

♦ Tyrosine kinase inhibitor therapy with Imatinib 400 mg OD as first line.
♦ *Other second generation:* Tyrosine kinase inhibitor advocated in first line therapy.
♦ Ponatinib used in case of resistant to first and second generation tyrosine kinase inhibitor.
♦ Zinatinib is now used in cases of very high counts.
♦ Allogenic stem cell transplant with HLA-atched-related or unrelated donor, in case of tyrosine kinase inhibitor intolerance
♦ Omacetaxine can also be given.
♦ Alpha-interferon therapy can be given to maintain remission in chronic phase of disease in patient less than 70 years of age. It is given either intramuscularly or subcutaneously in dose of 3 to 9 mega units daily, then dose is reduced and majority of patients tolerate the dose of 3 mega units/3 times a week without any side effect.

Advanced Phase Disease

♦ *Treatment of lymphoid blast crisis is done:* Treatment similar to acute lymphoblastic leukemia is done.
♦ *Myeloid crisis:* Prognosis is poor and few of drugs used in treatment of AML offer more than temporary relief.

Q.13. Write short note on oral manifestation of leukemia.

(Mar 1998, 5 Marks)

Ans.

Oral Manifestations of Acute Leukemia

♦ Bleeding from gingiva is present. Gingiva becomes boggy, edematous and red in color.
♦ Presence of paresthesia of lower lip.
♦ Crustation over lips is seen.
♦ Mobility of permanent teeth is present.
♦ Oral mucosa appears pale with ulceration along with petechiae and ecchymosis.

Oral Manifestations of Chronic Leukemia

♦ Gingival hypertrophy is present. Ulceration of gingiva with necrosis is present.
♦ Tongue is dark and is swollen.
♦ Presence of mobility of teeth is seen.
♦ Necrosis of PDL is seen
♦ Alveolar bone destruction is also present.

Q.14. Write short note on splenomegaly.

(Dec 2010, 5 Marks) (Jan 2016, 6 Marks)

Or

Write short answer on splenomegaly.

(Apr 2018, 3 Marks)

Or

Enumerate the causes of splenomegaly.

(Dec 2010, 5 Marks) (Aug 2012, 5 Marks)

Or

Enumerate five causes of splenomegaly.

(Dec 2009, 5 Marks)

Or

Write short answer on causes of splenomegaly.

(Feb 2019, 3 Marks)

Ans. Splenomegaly is defined as the enlargement of the spleen. Spleen can be mildly, moderately and massively enlarged.

Classification of Splenomegaly as Per its Size

♦ Mild splenomegaly: In it spleen is mildly enlarged and weighs up to 500 g.
♦ Moderate splenomegaly: In it the spleen is moderately enlarged weighs up to 500 to 1000 g.
♦ Massive splenomegaly: In it the spleen is massively enlarged and weighs up to greater than 1000 g.

Causes of Splenomegaly

Infections

♦ *Bacterial:* Septicemia, typhoid, infective endocarditis, TB, syphilis.
♦ *Viral:* Hepatitis, infectious mononucleosis.
♦ *Protozoan:* Malaria and kala-azar.
♦ *Parasitic:* Hydatid.

Circulatory

♦ Congestive cardiac failure
♦ Portal hypertension
♦ Hepatic or portal vein thrombosis
♦ Splenic vein obstruction.

Hematological

♦ *Hemolytic disorders:* Hereditary spherocytosis, elliptocytosis, pyruvic kinase deficiency, etc.
♦ *Hematological malignancies:* Acute leukemia, chronic myeloid leukemia and lymphomas
♦ *Myeloproliferative disorders:* Polycythemia vera
♦ Inflammatory and collagen disorders: Acute rheumatic fever, lupus erythematosus
♦ *Granulomatous disorders:* Sarcoidosis and berylliosis
♦ *Metabolic storage diseases,* i.e., Gaucher's disease
♦ *Splenomegaly of unknown etiology:* Tropical splenomegaly, non-tropical splenomegaly.

Q.15. Enumerate the causes of generalized lymphadeno-pathy.

(Dec 2010, 5 Marks)

Or

Enumerate the causes of lymphadenopathy.

(Jan 2012, 5 Marks)

Ans.

♦ **Infectious Diseases:**
  • *Viral infections:*
    – Infectious hepatitis
    – Infectious mononucleosis
    – AIDS
    – Rubella
    – Varicella
    – Herpes zoster.
  • *Bacterial infections:*
    – Streptococci
    – Staphylococci
    – *Salmonella*
    – *Brucella*
    – *Listeria monocytogenes.*
  • *Fungal infections:*
    – Coccidioidomycosis
    – Histoplasmosis
    – Chlamydial Infections
    – Lymphogranuloma venereum
    – Trachoma.
  • *Mycobacterial infections:*
    – Tuberculosis
    – Leprosy
    – Parasitic infestations
    – Microfilariasis
    – Toxoplasmosis.
  • *Spirochetal diseases*
    – Syphilis
    – Yaws
    – Leptospirosis.
♦ **Immunologic Diseases:**
  • Rheumatoid arthritis
  • Systemic lupus erythematosus
  • Dermatomyositis
  • Serum sickness
  • Drug reactions: Phenytoin, hydralazine
  • Primary biliary cirrhosis
  • Chronic active hepatitis.
♦ **Malignant Disorders:**
  • Haematologic disorders:
    – Hodgkin's lymphoma
    – Myeloid leukemia—blastic crisis
    – Chronic lymphatic leukemia
  • Metastatic tumors:
    – Melanoma
    – Kaposi's sarcoma
    – Tumors
    – Lung
    – Breast
    – Prostate
    – Kidney
    – Head and neck
    – Gastrointestinal tract.

♦ **Endocrine disease:**
  • Hyperthyroidism.
♦ **Lipid Storage disease:**
  • Gaucher's disease
  • Niemann-Pick disease.
♦ **Miscellaneous disorders:**
  • Sarcoidosis
  • Amyloidosis
  • Sinus histiocytosis.

Q.16. Describe the clinical and diagnostic features of chronic myeloid leukemia. *(Feb 2002, 5 Marks)*

Ans. *For clinical features, refer to Ans. 12 of same chapter.*

Diagnostic Features

Diagnosis is based on the clinical findings and investigations.

Investigations

♦ Normocytic-normochromic anemia
♦ Mean WBC count is 220×10^9/L (range 9.5 to 600×10^9/L) or (2–6 lakhs/μL.)
♦ Mean platelet count is 445×10^9/L (range 162–2000 × 10^9/L)
♦ Leukocyte alkaline phosphatase: Absent in granulocytes in CML
♦ Plasma uric acid and alkaline phosphatase are increased
♦ Serum B12 level is increased due to increase in transcobalamin III which is present in neutrophil granules.
♦ Bone marrow shows increased cellularity especially myeloid and megakaryocytic. Marrow and blood show basophilia, eosinophilia and monocytosis.
♦ Disease acceleration is denoted by
  • Blasts 10–19% in blood or bone marrow
  • Basophils >20% in blood or bone marrow
  • Platelets <100,000/μL unrelated to therapy or = 10,00,000/μL. unresponsive to therapy
  • Increasing splenic size
  • Increasing WBC count unresponsive to therapy
  • Cytogenetic clonal evolution
  • Progressive anemia.
♦ Blastic crisis is established by:
  • Blasts >20% in bone marrow or peripheral blood smear
  • Extramedullary blast formation.
  • Large foci or clusters of blasts in bone marrow.
♦ All patients have evidence of translocation by cytogenetics, fluorescent in situ hybridization, or by molecular methods.

Q.17. Write short note on approach to investigate a case of lymphadenopathy. *(Sep 2004, 5 Marks)*

Or

How will you investigate a case of lymphadeno-pathy? *(Feb/Mar 2004, 5 Marks)*

Or

Write short answer on lymphadenopathy. *(May 2018, 3 Marks)*

Ans.

History

♦ **Age:** Tuberculous lymphadenitis in childhood, secondary carcinoma in old age.
♦ **Occupation:** Tularemia in hunters and butchers; sporotrichosis in farmers and gardeners.
♦ **Duration:**
  • Acute swelling of a few days duration mostly pyogenic.
  • Subacute lymphadenitis of 3–4 weeks duration may be due to streptococcal infection, tuberculosis, secondary syphilis, infectious mononucleosis or tularemia.
  • Chronic lymphadenopathies include tuberculosis, lymphomas, leukemia, primary lymphatic tumors and secondary carcinoma. History of previous radiation treatment or operative removal.

Physical Examination

Local

♦ *Number of glands:* Single gland may appear to be affected for some time in tuberculosis, Hodgkin's and secondary carcinoma. Multiple in tuberculosis, Hodgkin's disease, leukemia.
♦ *Site:*
  • Neck usual site for tuberculous lymphadenitis, lymphosarcoma, and most other lymphadenopathies.
  • Inguinal gland enlargements may be due to syphilis, lymphogranuloma inguinale or chancroid.
  • The infraclavicular glands are seldom so enlarged as to be palpable except in secondary cancer or Hodgkin's disease.
  • Supratrochlear (epitrochlear) lymphadenopathy in non-Hodgkin's lymphoma, chronic lymphocytic leukemia, infectious mononucleosis, secondary syphilis, sarcoidosis, IV drug abuse.
  • Hilar and superior mediastinal lymphadenopathy in tuberculosis, histoplasmosis, sarcoidosis, pneumoconiosis, malignancy and cryptococcosis.
♦ *Character:* Discrete in Hodgkin's disease and leukemia, primary tumors of lymphatic tissue and so called "lymphadenoid" form of tuberculous lymphadenitis. Moveable, discrete and painless in sarcoidosis. Matted together in tuberculosis and lymphogranuloma.
♦ *Cold abscess:* In tuberculosis, lymphogranuloma, tularemia and sporotrichosis. Tuberculous glands may break through to give a typically indolent ulcer with undermined edges.
♦ *Primary cause:* In the area drained by the enlarged glands;, e.g., scalp if occipital or posterior auricular glands, fauces and pharynx in upper anterior cervical group, etc. Healed scar at portal of entry, scar of operative removal, or of radiation treatment.

Systemic

♦ *Skin:*
  • Cutaneous tumors mostly on the face, usually in chronic lymphatic leukemia. Sometimes generalized erythroderma, polymorphic rashes and purpura.

- Rash of secondary syphilis.
- Painless papules without surrounding erythema may be found on face, arms and legs in sarcoidosis.
- Eruption of lupus erythematosus.

♦ *Lungs:* Pulmonary or mediastinal tuberculosis, lesions of sarcoidosis or metastatic or primary deposits in carcinoma.

♦ *Abdomen:* Abdominal glands may be palpable in tuberculosis. Enlargement of spleen and liver in leukemia and Hodgkin's disease.

♦ *Genitalia:* Scar of primary sore of syphilis, or "chancre" in lymphogranuloma.

♦ *Icterus:* Jaundice with lymphadenopathy may be met with in viral hepatitis (cervical glands), lymphoma, acute lymphocytic leukemia, disseminated TB.

♦ *Temperature:* Raised in Hodgkin's disease, infectious mononucleosis and tularemia.

Investigations

♦ *Blood picture:* For diagnosis of leukemia and infectious mononucleosis. Positive ANA and reduced complement C4 levels in SLE.

♦ *Special tests:* Serologic tests for syphilis. Paul-Bunnell or monospot test for infectious mononucleosis, Agglutination reaction and animal inoculation in tularemia. Autoantibodies in SLE.

♦ Liver biopsy useful in sarcoidosis and infectious mononucleosis. Serological tests for HIV infection.

♦ Radiography of lungs and gastrointestinal tract. Skeletal changes in Boeck's sarcoid and sporotrichosis (multiple small areas of decalcification).

♦ *Biopsy:* Needle aspiration biopsy is useful for initial evaluation of superficial lymphadenopathy. It is however not helpful in diagnosis of lymphomas and other hematologic malignancies. Lymph-node biopsy tissue should be processed for culture of appropriate organisms, frozen in liquid nitrogen for lymphocyte typing or special studies for malignant cell types, and for routine histological studies.

♦ CT scan of abdomen in lymphoma.

♦ Lymphangiography of value in diagnosing site, extent, and, in certain cases, even the nature of primary lymph node enlargement.

Q.18. How will you investigate a case of anemia?

(Feb/Mar 2004, 5 Marks)

Ans. Every case of anemia should have the following investigations to detect degree and cause of anemia:

♦ Hemoglobin count decreases.

♦ RBC count, packed cell volume, mean corpuscular volume and mean corpuscular hemoglobin concentration (MCHC). Total leukocyte count and differential leukocyte count.

♦ Peripheral blood film for type of anemia and shape of RBCs and presence of any abnormal cells.

♦ Clotting time and bleeding time in hemolytic anemia.

♦ Blood platelets.

Bone marrow examination is done, when cause of anemia requires further investigation, especially to detect type of erythropoiesis.

Other Investigations

♦ *Stools for parasites:* Test for presence of blood and stools is done in patients suspected to chronic blood loss.

♦ Urine for albumin, bile salt, pigments and urobilinogen

♦ *Gastric analysis:* Histamine fast achlorhydria in pernicious anemia and megaloblastic anemia.

♦ Studies for detecting steatorrhea and malabsorption studies.

♦ Schilling test for vitamin B12 absorption in megaloblastic and dimorphic anemias.

♦ FIGLU test is done to assess folic acid deficiency. 15 gram of histidine hydrochloride is given by mouth and the urine in which it is excreted it is collected over next eight hours. Normal excretion is 1–17 mg.

Q.19. Enumerate the causes of iron deficiency anemia. How will you treat iron deficiency anemia?

(Sep 2005, 10 Marks)

Ans. *For enumeration of causes of iron deficiency anemia refer to Ans. 3 of same chapter.*

Treatment of Iron Deficiency Anemia

♦ *Oral iron therapy:* Ferrous sulfate 200 mg TID is given in between the meals. If after taking the drug, there is any abdominal pain, nausea, vomiting or constipation, the salt is changed to ferrous gluconate or ferrous fumarate. Oral iron therapy should be given for 6 months. Iron absorption is enhanced by combining iron salts with hydrochloric acid, ascorbic acid, succinic acid, fructose, cysteine, isonine and cobalt. Administration of iron after food minimizes gastric upset.

♦ *Parenteral iron therapy:* Iron sorbitol ciric acid complex 1.5 mg/kg body weight is given as IM or Iron dextran in 5% glucose is given as IV A small test dose should be given IV before giving total dose. Total dose of iron should not exceed 2.5 g.

♦ *Blood transfusion:* Packed red cells are transfused.

Q.20. Discuss causes of bleeding. *(Feb/Mar 2004, 5 Marks)*

Ans.

♦ Bleeding can be the result of inability to form a temporary clot or the inability to form a definitive clot.

♦ Inability to form a temporary clot results from inadequate platelet count, i.e., thrombocytopenia or abnormal platelet function, i.e., thrombocytopathy.

♦ Inability to form a definitive clot results from abnormalities in clotting factor.

♦ Disseminated intravascular coagulation and hemophilia results in bleeding.

♦ Idiopathic thrombocytopenic purpura

♦ Aplastic anemia

♦ Leukemia.

Q.21. Write short note on massive splenomegaly.

(Sep 2005, 5 Marks)

Ans. A clinically palpable spleen is called splenomegaly and it may be mild, moderate and massive.

When weight of spleen is over 1000 g, it is massive.

Causes

- Chronic myeloid leukemia
- Chronic malaria
- Kala-azar
- Myelofibrosis
- Hairy cell leukemia
- Banti's disease (tropical splenomegaly)
- Myeloid metaplasia
- Gaucher's disease
- Hepatic vein obstruction.

Q.22. Write short note on differential diagnosis of massive splenomegaly. *(Sep 2006, 5 Marks) (Mar 2010, 5 Marks)*

Ans. When there is enlargement of spleen with its weight greater than 1000 g, it is known as splenomegaly.

Differential Diagnosis

- **Cirrhosis of liver:**
  - *Symptoms and signs of hepatocellular failure:* Spider nevi, liver palms, alopecia, gynecomastia and testicular atrophy in males, icterus, *Fetor hepaticus.* Palpable enlarged liver.
  - *Evidence of portal hypertension:* Ascites, prominent veins on abdomen, hematemesis, piles.
  - *Diagnosis by liver biopsy* demonstration of esophageal varices by barium swallow, laparoscopy and scanning.
- **Infections, subacute and chronic:**
  - *Chronic malaria:*
    - History of fever with rigors with classical features of the attack like cold stage, hot stage, sweating stage.
    - Spleen very large and firm.
    - Liver may be enlarged.
    - Severe anemia.
    - Malarial parasites in peripheral blood or sternal marrow.
    - Leukopenia.
    - Therapeutic test with adequate dose of anti-malarial drug during fever.
  - Kala-azar:
    - Residence in endemic area.
    - *Splenomegaly:* which may be massive.
    - *Recurrent fever:* Double rise of temperature in 24 hours may be seen.
    - Liver enlarged but not grossly like spleen.
    - Anemia.
    - Loss of hair and pigmentation of skin.
    - Generalized lymphadenopathy especially in children. Nodes are soft, nontender.
    - Other features are cough, hemorrhagic features
    - LD bodies—on stained material from bone marrow or splenic aspirate.
  - *Subacute infective endocarditis:*
    - Unexplained fever.
    - Presence of cardiac murmur.
    - Presence of petechiae, anemia, peripheral emboli, clubbing of fingers.
    - Red cells in urine.
    - Positive blood culture.

- *Brucellosis:*
  - History of ingestion of raw milk, or occupation hazard in veterinary surgeons, laboratory personnel or slaughter house workers.
  - Patient not toxic in spite of high fever.
  - Spleen of moderate size, rarely massive.
  - Liver may be enlarged, particularly, if spleen is very large.
  - Back pain common.
  - Culture of organism from blood or bone marrow. Complement fixation and anti-human globulin tests in chronic infection.
- *Tuberculous splenomegaly*: In rare cases, tuberculous enlargement of spleen occurs with little involvement of other organs. Blood picture shows anemia, leukopenia or thrombocytopenia either single or in combination. Weakness, lassitude, loss of weight and often pyrexia. Bleeding may occur. X-ray of spleen may demonstrate areas of calcification.

Q.23. Write short note on hemophilia A. *(Sep 2006, 5 Marks)*

Ans. It is the most common congenital disorder of coagulation caused by reduction of factor VIII.

- It is a sex-linked disorder with factor VIII gene located on X-chromosome.
- Women are the carrier and males are affected.

Clinical Features

- *At birth:* Newborn with hemophilia is usually healthy, though bleeding from cord and cephalohematoma may occur.
- *In infant:* Hemophilia is asymptomatic till 6 to 12 months, when bruising becomes more obvious. Bleeding from the mouth is common.
- *During childhood:* In severely affected individuals, spontaneous bleeding may occur in joint and muscles, including psoas muscle.
- *In adults:* Frequency of spontaneous bleeding decreases, but joints may already have been damaged. Intracranial hemorrhage is a life-threatening complication. Spontaneous bleeds are common in mildly affected individuals, but after injury bleeding occurs till appropriate therapy has begun.

Investigations

- APTT is prolonged in hemophilia A, but PT is normal.
- Specific factor assay demonstrate reduced factor VIII in hemophilia A.

Management

- It is done by fresh blood transfusion when bleeding is in the large mass.
- Factor VIII concentrate is employed in case of hemophilia A
- A hemophilic will require treatment before any dental procedure. Such patient is managed by IV infusion or cryoprecipitate or factor VIII combined with aminocaproic acid 4 to 6 g QDS.
- For any major surgery or periodontal surgeries or extraction of tooth, hemophilic patient should be hospitalized.

Infusion of factor VIII concentrate is given before surgery and is continued for 48 to 72 hours. Antibiotic should also be given to the patient.

♦ Desmopressin 0.3 µg/kg IV is combined with an anti-fibrolytic agent which increases Factor VIII levels in hemophilia A and may ne used to avoid treatment with blood products.

Complications of Hemophilia A

♦ Hepatitis in patients who received multiple transfusion of FFP or cryoprecipitate.
♦ AIDS in a patient not screened for HIV and treated with FFP or cryoprecipitate.
♦ Anemia from excessive bleeding.
♦ Contractures in muscles following intramuscular hematomas.
♦ Spontaneous intracranial hemorrhage in severe hemophilia.

Q.24. Write short note on purpura.   *(Apr 2007, 5 Marks)*

Ans. Any rash in which blood cells leak into the skin or mucus membrane, usually at multiple sites. Purpuric rashes are often associated with disorders of coagulation or thrombosis.

Pin point purpuric lesions are called as petechiae, large hemorrhage into the skin are called as ecchymoses.

Types of Purpura

♦ *Allergic purpura:* Any of a group of purpuras caused by a variety of agents, including bacteria, drugs and food.
♦ *Anaphylactic purpura or Henöch-Schönlein purpura:* A form of small vessel vasculitis that affects children more commonly than adults, it is marked by abdominal pain, polyarticular joint disease and purpuric lesions of the lower extremities.
♦ *Idiopathic thrombocytopenic purpura or hemorrhagic purpura:* It is hemorrhagic autoimmune disease in which there is destruction of circulating platelets, caused by auto-antibodies that bind with antigen on the platelet membrane.

Symptoms

♦ Bleeding from nose, the gums or the gastrointestinal tract.
♦ Physical findings include petechiae, especially on the lower extremities and ecchymoses.

Laboratory Findings

Platelet count is usually less than 100, 000 per cumm.

Treatment

♦ If patient are asymptomatic and platelet count is about 40,000 per cumm, treatment is unnecessary.
♦ For symptomatic patients, treatment regimen include high dose corticosteroid, IV immunoglobulin, splenectomy.

Q.25. Write short note on thrombocytopenia.

(Mar 2008, 5.5 Marks)

Or

Write short answer on thrombocytopenia.

(Apr 2018, 3 Marks) (May 2018, 3 Marks)

Ans. Thrombocytopenia means decreased platelet count, i.e., less than 1,50,000 per cumm.

Etiology

♦ *Impaired platelet production:*
   • *Due to impaired platelet production:*
      – *Bone marrow failure:*
         » Aplastic anemia
         » Leukemia
         » Megaloblastic anemia
         » Myelofibrosis
         » Marrow infiltration.
      – Selective suppression of platelet production
         » Drugs, such as sulfa drugs, rifampicin, thiazides, etc.
♦ Increased consumption or destruction of platelets.
   • Disseminated intravascular coagulation
   • Thrombotic thrombocytopenic purpura
   • Idiopathic thrombocytopenic purpura
   • Gram-negative septicemia
   • Viral infection.
♦ Increased splenic sequestration.
   • Hypersplenism
      – Lymphoma
      – Liver diseases.

Clinical Features

♦ As the count of platelets is above 1 lakh per cumm of blood, patient remain asymptomatic and bleeding time is also normal.
♦ As count of platelets is in between 50,000 and 1 lakh per cu mm of blood, bleeding is increased. At this stage, bleeding occur with severe trauma.
♦ As count of platelets reaches below 50,000, bruising is present along with purpura. At this stage, bleeding occur along with minor trauma.
♦ Platelet count less than 20,000 per cu mm of blood causes spontaneous bleeding.

Q.26. Describe drug treatment of AML.   *(Oct 2007, 5 Marks)*

Ans.

Drug Treatment

♦ *Induction of remission*
   Daunorubicin IV alternate days 3 doses
   Cytosine arabinoside IV BD for 10 days
   Thioguanine oral BD for 10 days
♦ *Consolidation phase:* Repeat cycle of drugs used for inducing remission, consolidation phase ranges up to 2 years.
♦ *Cranial prophylaxis:* Not required since cranial involvement only in few cases.
♦ *Maintenance phase:* Generally maintenance therapy is not required since intensive treatment in remission and consolidation phase sufficient to give relief. If relapse occurs use of ablative therapy supported by allogenic or autologous bone marrow transplantation.

Q.27. Write short note on thalassemia.   *(Nov 2011, 3 Marks)*

Ans.

♦ Thalassemias are genetic disorders of hemoglobin synthesis in which there is reduced production of one or more chains of hemoglobin.

♦ This results in a relative excess production of either α chains or β chains, which without their partner chains are unstable and precipitate in RBCs or their precursors.

♦ The inclusion bodies produced by this process increase the rigidity of RBCs and result in their destruction, either in the marrow or the circulation or both. Hence the anemia of thalassemia results from ineffective erythropoiesis due to intramedullary RBC destruction, and a shortened RBC survival caused by hemolysis.

♦ Thalassemias are classified according to the particular globin chain that is ineffectively produced.

♦ In alpha thalassemia, there is reduced rate of chain synthesis.

♦ Beta thalassemias are associated with synthesis of beta chains.

♦ Beta thalassemias is divided into two forms, i.e., thalassmias minor and thalassemia major.

Clinical Features

♦ Onset: Affected children fail to thrive from about third month and become progressively more anemic.

♦ Increasing pallor is present

♦ Splenomegaly: Hemosiderosis with extramedullary hematopoiesis

♦ Facies: Frontal bossing due to thickening of cranial bones and prominent cheek bones due to overgrowth of zygomatic bones.

♦ Mild hemolytic jaundice

♦ Increased susceptibility to infections

♦ Hepatomegaly: Due to extramedullary hemopoiesis in first 3–4 years. Later on further enlargement due to hemosiderin deposits in Kupffer cells.

♦ Cardiac involvement: Myocardial hemosiderin may result in arrhythmias and cardiac failure.

♦ Endocrines:
  • Stunted growth from growth hormone deficiency
  • Delayed puberty due to hypothyroidism
  • Hypoparathyroidism can cause osteoporosis and fractures
  • Diabetes mellitus due to iron deposits in Islet of Langerhans

Investigations

♦ *Hematological:*
  • Anemia: It is moderate-to-severe with 10 to 12 g/dL. RBCs are microcytic hypochromic. Target cells are present and basophilic stippling is common. Also presence of tear drop, elliptical, fragments in red cells and at times red cell with Howell-Jolly body.
  • Reticulocytosis is present.
  • Leukocytosis with few metamyelocytes and myelocytes

♦ *Biochemical:*
  • Reduced serum haptoglobins
  • Bilirubin (unconjugated) increased and urine urobilinogen increased
  • Iron status
    – Serum iron and ferritin markedly increased.
    – Total iron binding capacity (TIBC) is reduced.

♦ *Bone marrow:*
  • Erythroid hyperplasia with reversed M : E ratio
  • Normoblastic erythropoiesis
  • Ineffective erythropoiesis — Some normoblasts die in the marrow without maturing into red cells
  • Myelopoiesis and megakaryopoiesis
  • Increased bone marrow iron

♦ *Other special tests:*
  • HbF levels are high.
  • *Hb electrophoresis:* Bands of both HbA and HbF in β-thalassemia.
  • *Global chain synthesis:* α-β globin chain synthesis ratio altered (normal 1 : 1) due to lack of synthesis of β chains.
  • DNA analysis-useful for predicting disease severity and diagnosis.
  • Liver spectrometry for detecting hemosiderosis of liver.

Management

♦ Blood transfusions should be done to keep level of hemoglobin between 9–11 g%, if infant's Hb. 6–7 g% and failure to thrive. Transfusions are given every 2 to 4 weeks.

♦ Chelating agent, such as desferrioxamine as SC infusion using a syringe driver pump/infuser.

♦ *Splenectomy:* Hypersplenism due to splenomegaly causes neutropenia and increased need for blood transfusion. Splenectomy reduces severity of neutropenia and subsequent infections. Splenectomy should be done as late as possible.

♦ *Bone marrow transplantation:* Indication for bone marrow transplantation in cases where matched siblings are available in a family, if not available, to look for a matched related donor. This is curative for the patient.

♦ Folic acid supplements should be given to the patient.

Q.28. Describe various bleeding disorders and their management in detail. *(Apr 2008, 15 Marks)*

Or

Write notes on bleeding disorders.
(Aug 2011, 10 Marks)

Ans.

Etiology of Bleeding Disorders

♦ **Vascular Defects**
  Bleeding disorders caused by vascular defects may be caused by structural malformation of vessels. Hereditary disorders of connective tissue and acquired connective tissue disorders. Vascular defects rarely cause serious bleeding. Bleeding into skin or mucous membrane starts immediately alter trauma but ceases within 24 to 48 hours. The vascular defects are hereditary hemorrhagic telangiectasia, Henoch-Schönlein purpura.

♦ **Platelet Disorder:**
  It can be of two types:
  • Reduction in number—Thrombocytopenic purpura. If the total number of circulating platelets falls below 50,000 per mm³ of blood the patient can have bleeding. In some cases, the total platelet count is reduced by unknown mechanism, this is called primary or

idiopathic thrombocytopenic purpura (ITP). Chemicals, radiation and various systemic disease (e.g. leukemia) may have direct effect on the bone marrow and may result in secondary thrombocytopenia.

- *Defect in quality:* Nonthrombocytopenic purpura, e.g., von Willebrand's disease, Bernard-Soulier disease, Glanzmann's thrombasthenia von Willebrand's disease (pseudohemophilia) is the most common inherited bleeding disorder. Unlike hemophilia, it can occur in females. This is a disease of both coagulation factors and platelets. It is caused by an inherited defect involving platelet adhesion. Platelet adhesion is affected because of a deficiency of von Willebrand's factor.

- Various drugs, such as carbamazepine, aspirin, methyldopa, phenytoin can also lead to platelet disorders.

- **Coagulation Defects**
  - *Hemophilia A:* It is the most common coagulation defect. It is inherited as X-linked recessive trait. The hemostatic abnormality in hemophilla A is caused by a deficiency/defect of factor VIII. Until recently, factor VIII was thought to be produced by endothelial cells and not by the liver as most of coagulation factors. The defective gene is located on the X-chromosome.
  - *Hemophilia B (Christmas disease):* Factor IX is deficient or defective. It is inherited as X-linked recessive trait. Like Hemophilia A, the disease primarily affects males and the clinical manifestations of the two are identical.
  - *Disseminated intravascular coagulation (DIC):* It is a condition that results when the clotting system is activated in all or a major part of vascular system. Despite widespread fibrin production the major clinical problem is bleeding not thrombosis. DIC is associated with a number of disorders, such as infection, obstetric complications, cancer and snakebite.

Management of Bleeding Disorders

Hereditary Hemorrhagic Telangiectasia

It is transmitted as autosomal dominant trait and is characterized by bleeding from mucous membrane.

Management

- In patient having repeated attacks of epistaxis septal dermoplasty should be done. In septal dermoplasty, involved mucosa get removed and skin grafting is done.
- If spontaneous hemorrhages are present or nasal bleeding is present, then it is controlled by giving pressure packs.
- Sclerosing agents, i.e., sodium tetradecyl sulfate, if injected intralesionally stop bleeding.
- Electrocautery is done. It helps in arresting bleeding.

Idiopathic Thrombocytopenic Purpura (ITP)

Steroid Treatment Protocol

- *Initial steroid treatment protocol for ITP:* Initial steroid treatment protocol l mg/kg/day prednisone, PO for 2–6 weeks.
- *Subsequent steroid treatment protocol for ITP:* Prednisone dose is individualized for every patient. Usually, the dose

of prednisone is tapered to less than 10 mg per day for 3 months and then withdrawn. Splenectomy is done, if discontinuation of prednisone causes a relapse.

- *Follow* the 'rule of twos' for major dental treatment and provide extra steroids prior to surgery, if the patient is currently on steroids or has used steroids for 2 weeks longer within the past 2 years.

Minor Surgery

- Hemostasis after minor surgery is usually adequate, if platelet levels are above 50,000 cells/mm³.
- Platelets can be replaced or supplemented by platelet transfusions; though sequestration of platelets occurs rapidly. Platelet transfusion is indicated for established thrombocytopenic bleeding.
- When given prophylactically platelets should be given half before surgery to control capillary bleeding and half at the end of the operation to facilitate the placement of adequate sutures.
- Platelets should be used within 6–24 hours after collection and suitable preparations include platelet rich plasma (PRP), which contains about 90% of the platelets from a unit of fresh blood and platelet-rich concentrate (PRC), which contains about 50% of the platelets from a unit of fresh whole blood.
- PRC is thus the best source of platelets. Platelet infusions carry the risk of isoimmunization, infection with blood-borne viruses and, rarely, graft-versus-host disease.
- Where there is immune destruction of platelets (e.g. in ITP), platelet infusions are less effective.
- The need for platelet transfusions can be reduced by local hemostatic measures and the use of Desmopressin or tranexamic acid or topical administration of platelet concentrates.
- Absorbable hemostatic agents, such as oxidized regenerated cellulose (Surgical), synthetic collagen (Instat) or microcrystalline collagen (Avitene) may be put in the socket to assist clotting in postextraction socket.
- Drugs that affect platelet function, such as gentamicin, antihistamines and aspirin should be avoided.

Major Surgery

For major surgery platelet levels over 75,000 cells/mm³ are desirable.

Hemophilia

It is a hereditary disorder of blood coagulation characterized by excessive hemorrhage due to increased coagulation time. It is of two types, i.e., hemophilia A and hemophilia B.

Management

- Local anesthesia is contraindicated. So intrapulpal anesthesia, intraligamentary anesthesia should be used. Sedation with diazepam or NO_2-O_2 sedation can be given.
- Endodontic procedures should be carried out and care is taken not to do instrumentation beyond apex. If hemorrhage is present, it should be controlled by 1:1000 aqueous epinephrine on paper point.

- Restorative treatments can be carried out by proper application of rubber dam for avoiding trauma to gingiva and other soft tissues. In case if rubber dam is not present an epinephrine impregnated hemostatic cord is kept in gingival sulcus before preparation of crown or inlay margin.
- Complete dentures and removable partial dentures can be given to hemophilic patients and are well tolerated by them. Patient has to take care for proper maintenance of hygiene of prosthesis.
- Conservative periodontal treatment should be done rather than attempting for periodontal surgeries.
- In case, if oral surgical procedures are to be done local hemostatic agents should be used, pressure surgical packs should be employed, sutures, topical thrombin is used. After removal of tooth, socket is packed with mechanical splint. Postoperative use of antifibrinolytic agent is used to support clot maintenance.
- In cases of Hemophilia A Human freeze-dried factor VIII concentrate or new recombinant factor VIII is used.
- In hemophilia B human dried factor IX concentrate is supplied as power which is to be mixed with distill water and administer IV.

von Willebrand Disease

- It is the most common inherited bleeding disorder. It is inherited as autosomal dominant but a severe form of disease may be inherited as a sex-linked recessive trait.
- It is caused due to the deficiency or defect in Von Willebrand factor.
- Types of Von-Willebrand diseases are: Type I, Type II A and II B, Type III

Management

- Surgical procedures can be performed in patients with mild von Willebrand disease by using DDAVP and EACA. Patients with severe Von Willebrand disease requires cryoprecipitate and Factor VIII concentrate.
- Bleeding should be controlled by using local measures, such as pressure packs, gelfoam with thrombin, tranexamic acid, etc.
- Aspirin and NSAIDs are avoided and acetaminophen can be given to patients.
- In majority of patients with von Willebrand disease hemostatic defect is controlled with desmopressin via nasal spray.
- Type I von Willebrand disease is treated with desmopressin while Type II A and B and Type III require clotting factor replacement.

Disseminated Intravascular Coagulation

Management

- Correction of hemodynamic instability by fluid therapy, transfusion of packed cells or whole blood.
- *Factor replacement:* This is the specific therapy, in this fresh frozen plasma, cryoprecipitate, platelet concentrate transfusions are essential. Fresh-frozen plasma is given at

the dose of 15 mL/kg. Platelet is transfused at the dosage of 0.1 unit/kg.

Q.29. Discuss causes, diagnosis and management of iron deficiency anemia. *(May/June 2009, 15 Marks)*

Ans. *For causes and management refer to Ans. 2 of same chapter.*

Diagnosis

It is based on the clinical signs and symptoms and investigations.

Clinical Signs and Symptoms

Symptoms

- Tiredness
- Weakness
- Lethargy
- Loss of appetite
- headache and bodyache
- Inability to concentrate
- Giddiness
- Breathlessness
- Epigastric discomfort.

Signs

- Pallor
- Palpitation
- Angular stomatitis
- Atrophic gastritis
- Flattening or spoon-shaped nails, i.e., platonychia and koilonychia
- Tongue is pale and smooth
- Glossitis
- Hepatosplenomegaly
- Plummer-Vinson syndrome, i.e., dysphagia and cricoid webs.

Investigations

- Blood picture and red cell indices
  - *Hemoglobin:* Fall on hemoglobin concentration.
  - *Red cells:* The RBCs in blood film are hypochromatic and microcytic and there is anisocytosis, poikilocytosis and elliptocytosis
  - *Reticulocyte count:* Normal or reduced.
  - *Absolute values:* MCV, MCH and MCHC are decreased.
  - *Leukocytes:* Usually normal
  - *Platelets:* Usually normal but raised if bleeding is cause of anemia
  - *ESR:* value of ESR is low
- *Bone marrow findings:*
  - *Marrow cellularity:* The marrow cellularity is increased due to erythroid hyperplasia.
  - *Erythropoiesis:* Normoblastic erythropoiesis.
  - Marrow iron is deficient.
- *Biochemical findings:*
  - Serum iron level is low.
  - Total iron binding capacity is high.
  - Serum ferritin is very low.

Q.30. Write notes on oral manifestations of hematological disorder.
(Aug 2011, 10 Marks)

Ans. Following are the oral manifestations of hematological disorders:

Hematological disorder	Oral manifestation
Leukemias	• Enlargement, bleeding and necrosis of gingiva • Necrosis and ulceration of oral mucosa • Ecchymosis • Profuse bleeding on trauma or following extraction of tooth
Agranulocytosis	• Gangrenous ulceration of gingiva, buccal mucosa, soft palate and lip. • Wound healing is delayed
Polycythemia	• Hematoma formation and ulceration of mucosa, gingiva and tongue. • Petechiae and ecchymosis • Spontaneous gingival bleeding • Purplish-red discoloration of tongue, cheek and lips
Iron deficiency anemia	• Mucosal atrophy • Pallor • Bald tongue • Atrophic glossitis • Angular cheilitis • Glossodynia
Pernicious anemia	• Erythematous oral mucosa with burning sensation. • Beefy red tongue with depapillation or Hunter's glossitis • Focal areas of atypical mucosal erythema • Xerostomia is present
Folic acid deficiency anemia	• Depapillation of tongue with glossitis • Glossodynia • Aphthous-like ulceration
Aplastic anemia	• Presence of purpura • Spontaneous gingival bleeding • Gingival hyperplasia • Ulceration • Halitosis • Severe mucosal pallor
Thalassemia	• Protrusion of upper teeth. • Maxillary teeth have spacing in between. • Prominent premaxilla and cheek bones • Mongoloid faces
Sickle cell anemia	• Mucosal pallor • Pain in mandible • Lip paresthesia • Delayed eruption of teeth
Hemophilia	• Petechiae • Prolonged bleeding after tooth extraction • Excessive bleeding on physiologic eruption and exfoliation of tooth
Erythroblastosis Fetalis	• Black, brown and bluish pigmentations of teeth • Protrusion of upper teeth • Enamel hypoplasia

Q.31. Classify anemia and discuss nutritional anemias.
(Aug 2012, 12 Marks)

Or

Write short answer on causes and treatment of macrocytic anemia. *(Oct 2019, 3 Marks)*

Ans.

Classification of Anemia

Etiological Classification of Anemia (By Lea and Febiger, 1981)

♦ **Loss of blood:**
  • Acute posthemorrhagic anemia
  • Chronic posthemorrhagic anemia.

♦ **Excessive destruction of red blood corpuscles:**
  • *Extracorpuscular causes:*
    – Antibodies
    – Infections like malaria
    – Splenic sequestration and destruction
    – Associated diseases like lymphomas
    – Drugs, chemical and physical agents
    – Trauma to RBC.
  • *Intracorpuscular hemolytic diseases:*
    – Hereditary
      » Disorders of glycolysis
      » Faulty synthesis or maintenance of reduced glutathione
      » Qualitative or quantitative abnormalities in the synthesis of globulin
      » Abnormalities in RBC membrane
      » Erythropoietic porphyria.
  • Acquired
    – Paroxysmal nocturnal hemoglobinuria
    – Lead poisoning

♦ **Impaired blood production resulting from deficiency of substances essential for erythropoiesis:**
  • Iron deficiency
  • Deficiency of various B vitamins: Vitamin B12 and folic acid (pernicious anemia and megaloblastic anemia); pyridoxine responsive anemia
  • Protein deficiency
  • Possibly ascorbic acid deficiency.

♦ **Inadequate production of mature erythrocytes:**
  • Deficiency of erythroblast
    – *Atrophy of bone marrow:* Aplastic anemia
      » Chemical or physical agents
      » Hereditary
      » Idiopathic.
    – Isolated erythroblastopenia
      » Thymoma
      » Chemical agents
      » Antibodies.
  Infiltration of bone marrow:
    – Leukemia, lymphomas
    – Multiple myeloma

- Carcinoma, Sarcoma
  - Myelofibrosis.
- *Endocrine abnormalities:*
  - Myxedema
  - Addison's disease
  - Pituitary insufficiency
  - Sometimes hyperthyroidism.
- Chronic renal failure.
- *Chronic inflammatory disease:*
  - Infectious
  - Noninfectious including granulomatous and collagen disease.
- Cirrhosis of liver.

Morphological Classification of Anemia

Based on the red cell size, hemoglobin content and red cell indices, anemias are classified into 3 types:

1. *Microcytic, hypochromic:* MCV, MCH, MCHC are all reduced, e.g., in iron deficiency anemia and in certain non-iron deficient anemias (sideroblastic anemia, thalassemia, anemia of chronic disorders).
2. *Normocytic, normochromic:* MCV MCH, MCHC are all normal, e.g., after acute blood loss, hemolytic anemias, bone marrow failure, anemia of chronic disorders.
3. *Macrocytic:* MCV is raised, e.g., in megaloblastic anemia due to deficiency of vitamin B12 or folic acid.

Nutritional Anemias

Following are the nutritional anemias:

- ♦ Iron deficiency anemia
- ♦ Macrocytic anemia.

For iron deficiency anemia in detail refer to Ans. 2 of same chapter.

Macrocytic Anemia

Macrocytosis is the rise in mean cell volume or red cells above the normal range. It is due to vitamin B12 deficiency or folic acid deficiency.

Etiology/causes

- ♦ **Vitamin B12 deficiency**
  - *Inadequate intake:*
    - In strict vegetarians
    - In poor diet.
  - *Due to malabsorption:*
    - *Gastric:*
      - » Pernicious anemia
      - » Congenital intrinsic factor deficiency
      - » Gastrectomy.
    - *Small intestinal disease:*
      - » Topical and Non-topical sprue
      - » Crohn's disease
      - » Fish tapeworm.
    - Increased requirement
      - » In pregnancy.
- ♦ **Folic acid deficiency**
  - Inadequate intake
    - Infancy
    - Old age
    - Poverty

- Alcoholism
  - Kwashiorkor.
- Malabsorption
  - Celiac Disease
  - Topical sprue
  - Congenital folate malabsorption.
- Increased utilization or loss
  - Physiological
    - » Prematurity
    - » Pregnancy and lactation.
  - Pathological
    - » Blood disorders
    - » Malignancy
    - » Dialysis.
  - Anti-folate Drugs
    - » Methotrexate
    - » Pyrimethamine
    - » Trimethoprim
    - » Anti-convulsant drugs.

Clinical features

- ♦ **Due to anemia:** Shortness of breath, anemia and pallor.
- ♦ **Gastrointestinal:** Diarrhea, loss of weight and appetite
- ♦ **Neurological:** Vitamin B12 neuropathy and neural tube defects due to deficiency of folic acid.
- ♦ **Gonadal dysfunction:** It is due to deficiency of both Vitamin B12 and folic acid
- ♦ **Epithelial cell changes:** Glossitis and other epithelial surfaces show cellular abnormalities.

Investigations

- ♦ **Vitamin B12 Deficiency:**
  - Hemoglobin levels are decreased below normal range.
  - Mean corpuscular volume is raised.
  - Peripheral blood film examination reveals macrocytosis, poikilocytosis and hypersegmentation of the neutrophils
  - Bone marrow examination reveals hypercellular marrow with megaloblastosis, giant metamyelocytes and platelets
  - Serum iron and serum ferritin levels are raised.
  - Schilling's test is positive.
- ♦ **Folic acid deficiency:**
  - Serum folate levels are low
  - Red cell folate levels are low
  - Figlu test is positive.

Treatment

- ♦ **Vitamin B12 Deficiency:**
  - Hydroxycobalamine 1000 μg IM is given, i.e., 6 injections in 2 to 3 weeks.
  - Since rapid regeneration of blood deplete marrow iron stores, so ferrous sulfate 200 mg daily is given after starting the therapy.
  - Maintenance dose of 500–1000 μg IM is given for every 3 months.

♦ **Folic acid deficiency:**
- Initially Folic acid 5 mg daily orally for 4 months is given.
- Maintenance dose is 5 mg folic acid once a week.

Q.32. Write Hodgkin's lymphoma under following headings:
(Mar 2013, 2 Marks each)
- a. **Clinical Features**
- b. **Investigations**
- c. **Staging**
- d. **Treatment**

Ans. Hodgkin's disease is a clinically and histologically distinct chronic lymphoproliferative disorder of unknown etiology.

Clinical Features

Local Signs

- ♦ *Lymphadenopathy:* Superficial lymph nodes in neck are first to enlarge at first one side and then other. On palpation, lymph nodes are painless, leathery and discrete. In advanced cases there is a pyramidal swelling with base at clavicle and apex at angle of the jaw.
- ♦ *Splenomegaly:* Moderate enlargement is present.
- ♦ *Hepatomegaly:* Moderate and nontender

Systemic Symptoms

- ♦ Presence of cachexia and loss of weight
- ♦ Fever is present. It can be of mild grade or undulant for several days or can be continuous.
- ♦ Night sweats are present
- ♦ Anemia can be present
- ♦ Generalized or refractory pruritus

Features Due to Metastatic Growth

- ♦ *In skin:* pruritus, erythema, herpes zoster
- ♦ *In bones:* localized pain and tenderness
- ♦ *Nervous system:* Paresthesia and pain
- ♦ *Respiratory tract:* Paralysis of larynx, Collapse of lung, pleural effusion
- ♦ *Gastrointestinal:* Jaundice and ascites
- ♦ *Genitourinary:* Hematuria, retention of urine and pain in back.

Due to Immunologic Changes

- ♦ Lowering of resistance to infection
- ♦ Homolytic anemia

Investigations

- ♦ *Blood test:*
  - Nonspecific anemia of chronic disease is common
  - Lymphopenia is present.
  - ESR is elevated
- ♦ *Lymph node biopsy:*
  - Show presence of reed-sternberg cells.
- ♦ *Imaging:*
  - Chest X-ray to look for mediastinal lymph nodes and pleural effusion.

- CT is valuable in detecting intrathoracic and abdominal lymphadenopathy. It can also detect presence or absence of bone marrow involvement after chemotherapy.
- *Bone marrow:* Aspiration biopsy is indicated in stage II disease and higher staging.

Staging

Ann Arbor Staging Classification of Hodgkin's Disease

Stage I (A or B)	I, I$_E$	Involvement of a single lymph node region Involvement of a single extralymphatic organ or site
Stage II (A or B)	II, II$_E$	Involvement of two or more lymph node regions on the same side of the diagphragm (or) with localized contiguous involvement of an extranodal organ of site
Stage III (A or B)	III, III$_E$, III$_S$, III$_{ES}$	Involvement of lymph node regions on both sides of the diaphragm (or) with localized contiguous involvement of an extranodal organ or site (or) with involvement of spleen (or) both features of III$_E$ and III$_S$
Stage IV (A or B)	IV	Multiple or disseminated involvement of one or More extralymphatic organs of tissues with or without lymphatic involvement

A: asymptomatic; B: presence of constitutional symptoms;
E: extranodal involvement; S: splenomegaly

Treatment

Stage I and II

- ♦ Mainly radiotherapy is given, i.e., external high cobalt radiotherapy.
- ♦ Above the diaphragm, Y field therapy is given.
- ♦ Below the diaphragm, mantle or inverted Y field therapy is given
- ♦ Chemotherapy should also be given.
- ♦ Involved field radiation therapy is given to all sites of bulky disease post-ABVD

Stage III and IV

- ♦ Mainly chemotherapy is given
- ♦ Drugs used are MOPP combination, i.e.
  - Mustine—6 mg/m^2 IV daily on days 1 and 8
  - Oncovine—1.4 mg/m^2 IV daily on days 1 and 8
  - Procarbazine—100 mg/m^2 orally on days 1–14
  - Prednisolone—40 mg/m^2 orally on days 1–14
- ♦ Give 6 courses with 2 weeks rest between the end of one course and beginning of next.
- ♦ ABVD combination is popular these days, i.e.
  - *Adriamycin:* 25 mg/m^2 IV on days 1 and 15
  - *Bleomycin:* 10 mg/m^2 IV on days 1 and 15
  - *Vinblastine:* 6 g/m^2 IV on days 1 and 15
  - *Dacarbazine:* 150 mg/m^2 IV on days 1 to 5
  - Alternating MOPP with ABVD gives excellent response.

Q.33. Describe mechanism of coagulation. Write hemophilia under following headings:

a. Definition
b. Clinical features
c. Treatment *(Nov 2014, 3 + 1 + 2 +3 Marks)*

Ans. Coagulation is the spontaneous arrest of the bleeding.

Following are the factors which are involved in the mechanism of coagulation of blood:

Factor I—Fibrinogen
Factor II—Prothrombin
Factor III—Thromboplastin (Tissue factor)
Factor IV—Calcium ions

Factor V—Labile factor
Factor VI—Presence not approved
Factor VII—Stable factor
Factor VIII—Anti-hemophilic factor
Factor IX—Christmas factor
Factor X—Stuart-Prower factor
Factor XI—Plasma thromboplastin antecedent
Factor XII—Hegman factor
Factor XIII—Fibrin-stabilizing factor
Factor XIV—Prekallikrein
Factor XV—Kallikrein
Factor XVI—Platelet factor

Coagulation Occurs in Three Stages

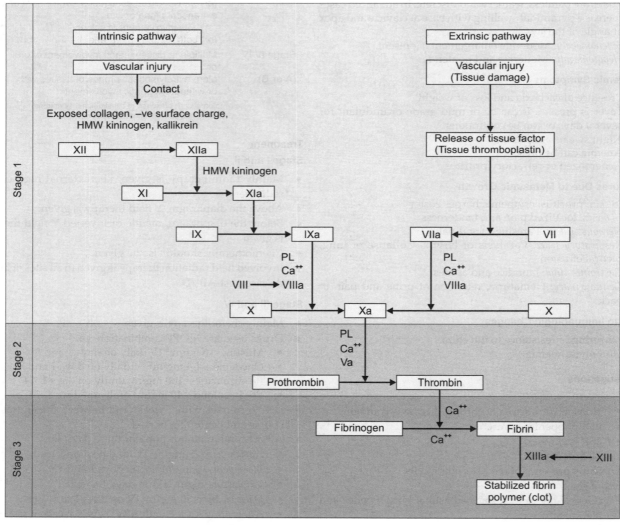

Fig. 15: Coagulation of mechanism.

Mechanism of coagulation

Blood coagulation occurs in three major stages:
- Stage 1: Activation of Stuart-Prower factor (formation of prothrombin activator)
- Stage 2: Formation of thrombin from prothrombin
- Stage 3: Formation of fibrin from fibrinogen

Activation of Stuart-Prower Factor (Factor X)

Activation of Stuart-Prower factor or factor X is the key to blood coagulation. Factor Xa is called prothrombin activator as it activates prothrombin to form thrombin. Therefore, this process is also called prothrombin activation.

This is achieved by two pathways: the intrinsic pathway and the extrinsic pathway.

Intrinsic Pathway

Intrinsic mechanism of prothrombin activation occurs in four steps:

Step 1 (activation of factor XII)

Activation of intrinsic pathway starts with contact of Hageman factor with a negatively charged surface or exposed collagen of the injured vessel wall.

1. High molecular weight kininogen and kallikerin act as cofactors to facilitate the activation of factor XII
2. Exposed collagen stimulates platelet adhesion and aggregation before initiating blood coagulation.

Step 2 (activation of factor XI)

Activated factor XII (XIIa) converts factor XI to its active form (XIa). This step is accelerated in the presence of high molecular weight kininogen.

Step 3 (activation of factor IX)

Factor XIa then converts factor IX to IXa, which is accentuated by factor VIIa. Calcium accelerates this process.

Step 4 (activation of factor X)

Final step in activation of prothrombin activator is activation of factor X. Factor IXa causes activation of factor X to Xa, the activated Stuart-Prower factor. The membrane phospolipid, calcium and activated factor VIII act as cofactors for the activation of Stuart-Prower factor is crucial in Stage 1. Formation of factor VIIIa is the key to the process of activation of factor X

Extrinsic Pathway

Extrinsic pathway of blood coagulation occurs in three steps:

Step 1 (release of tissue thromboplastin)

Key to the clotting mechanism is the release of tissue thromboplastin from the injured tissue. As tissue thromboplastin is the tissue factor which is viewed as extrinsic to circulating blood, this system of blood coagulation is called extrinsic system of clotting.

Step 2 (activation of VII)

Tissue thromboplastin converts factor VII to its active form (VIIa). This is the key step in extrinsic mechanism. Factor VIIa

directly activates not only factor X, but also factor IX. Thus it also influences intrinsic mechanism of activation of factor X.

Step 3 (activation of X)

Factor VIIa converts X to Xa. This process is accelerated in the presence of calcium, platelet phospholipid and tissue thromboplastin.

Formation of Thrombin from Prothrombin

This is the second stage of blood coagulation in which activated Stuart-Prower factor (Xa) converts prothrombin to thrombin, in the presence of platelet phospolipid, calcium and activated factor V (Va). Factor Va acts as cofactor for acceleration of this process. Therefore, it is also called proaccelerin or accelerator globulin.

Formation of Fibrin from Fibrinogen

This is the final stage of blood coagulation in which thrombin acts as an enzyme to convert fibrinogen to fibrin. In this process, first, the fibrin monomers are formed and afterward, they are polymerized to fibrin thread (blood clot). This occurs in three steps:

1. Proteolysis of soluble fibrinogen
2. Polymerization of fibrin monomers
3. Stabilization of fibrin polymer

Proteolysis of Soluble Fibrinogen

Fibrinogen has three domains: two peripheral (D) domains and one central (E) domain.

1. Thrombin binds with central domain and proteolytically releases two fibrinopeptides A and B from amino-terminals of $A\alpha$ and $B\beta$ chains of each fibrinogen molecules.
2. Release of fibrinopeptides leads to the formation of fibrin monomer.

Mechanism of Fibrin Stabilization

Flowchart 6: Mechanism of fibrin stabilization.

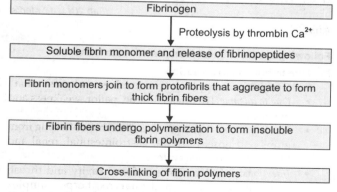

Polymerization of Fibrin Monomers

Fibrin monomers join to form protofibrils.

1. About 15 to 20 protofibrils aggregate to form thick fibers of fibrin.

2. Protofibrils also branch out to form into a meshwork of interconnected thick fibrin fibers. This is called polymerization of fibrin monomers.
3. Thrombin initiates the process of polymerization and simultaneously activates factor XIII.
4. Factor XIIIa completes the process of polymerization.

Stabilization of Fibrin Polymer

Fibrin stabilizing factor (XIIIa) stabilizes the fibrin polymers by cross-linking them.
1. Factor XIII is converted to XIIIa by thrombin.
2. Calcium acts as a cofactor for this conversion.
3. Covalent cross-linking of fibrin polymers provides adequate strength to the fibrin thread and to the fibrin meshwork.
4. The stabilized fibrin meshwork is the blood clot.
5. Red cells and platelets are trapped inside the fibrin meshwork to give the volume to the clot.

Definition of Hemophilia

Hemophilia is an inherited disorder which affects males and is transmitted by females. It is an X-linked recessive disorder caused by deficiency of factor VIII.

Clinical Features

For clinical features, refer to Ans. 8 of same chapter.

Treatment

For treatment refer to Ans. 8 of same chapter.

Q.34. Write short note on agranulocytosis.
(Nov 2014, 3 Marks)

Ans. It is defined as an acute disease marked by a deficit or absolute lack of granulocytic WBCs, i.e., neutrophils, basophils and eosinophils.
- *For etiology or causes refer to Ans. 4 of same chapter.*
- *For Clinical manifestations and management refer to Ans. 5 of same chapter.*
- *For diagnosis refer to Ans. 6 of same chapter.*

Q.35. Write clinical features of acute leukemia.
(Feb 2015, 12 Marks)

Ans.

Following are the clinical features of acute leukemia:

I. Due to bone marrow failure
- *Constitutional symptoms:* Fever, malaise and prostration
- *Due to anemia:* Tiredness, fatigue, pallor, weakness and dyspnea.
- *Bleeding manifestations:* Bruises, Petechiae, bleeding from gums and nose, purpura, gastrointestinal, renal and bleeding in nervous system.
- *Infections:* Infective lesions of oral cavity and throat, ulcers in oral cavity and pharynx, herpes simplex infection, Infections of respiratory tract, such as bronchitis and pneumonia, infections of skin, such as cellulitis and boils.

II. Due to organ infiltration
- *CNS:* Hemorrhage, meningeal infiltration and multiple cranial nerve palsies.
- *Skin:* Bluish nodules or dusky red patches.
- *Kidneys:* Renal failure
- *Heart:* Cardiomyopathy and pericarditis
- *Fundus:* Roth spots and papilledema
- *Testes:* Swelling present in acute lymphoid leukemia
- Bony tenderness is present especially in sternum
- Presence of hepatosplenomegaly and lymphadenopathy.

III. Due to leukemic cells
- Tissue deposits of leukemic cells leads to gum hypertrophy.
- Symptoms of cellular hyperviscosity are headache, confusion, fits, focal neurological signs and coma.
- In promyelocytic variant of acute myeloid leukemia the release of cytoplasmic granular contents activates coagulation and fibrinolytic systems which leads to acute hemostatic failure.

Q.36. Write short note on folic acid. *(Apr 2015, 2 Marks)*
Ans. Folic acid is a combination of glutamic acid, para-aminobenzoic acid and pteridine nucleus.

Sources

Sources of folic acid are yeast, fresh green vegetables, cereals, liver, kidney, meat.

Daily Requirement

50 to 100 µg.

Deficiency of Folic Acid

Deficiency of folic acid leads to megaloblastic anemia, glossitis, diarrhea, weight loss and weakness.

Indications
- In megaloblastic anemia caused due to folate deficiency, folic acid is given in dose of 1–5 mg/day and is continued till 3–4 months.
- In pregnancy due to increase demand, it is given 0.5 mg/day from first trimester.
- Folic acid antagonizes methotrexate toxicity.

Q.37. Write down common coagulation disorders. Write down the clinical features, investigations and management of idiopathic thrombocytopenic purpura. *(June 2015, 12 Marks)*
Ans. Coagulation disorders deal with disruption of the body's ability to control blood clotting.

Common coagulation disorders are:
- Hemophilia, or hemophilia A (Factor VIII deficiency), an inherited coagulation disorder. This genetic disorder is carried by females but most often affects males.

- Christmas disease, also known as hemophilia B or Factor IX deficiency, is less common than hemophilia A with similar in symptoms.
- Disseminated intravascular coagulation disorder, also known as consumption coagulopathy, occurs as a result of other diseases and conditions. This disease accelerates clotting, which can actually cause hemorrhage.
- Thrombocytopenia is the most common cause of coagulation disorder. It is characterized by a lack of circulating platelets in the blood. This disease also includes idiopathic thrombocytopenia.
- Von Willebrand's disease is a hereditary disorder with prolonged bleeding time due to a clotting factor deficiency and impaired platelet function. It is the most common hereditary coagulation disorder.
- Hypoprothrombinemia is a congenital deficiency of clotting factors that can lead to hemorrhage.
- Other coagulation disorders include factor XI deficiency, also known as hemophilia C, and factor VII deficiency. Hemophilia C afflicts one in 100,000 people and is the second most common bleeding disorder among women. Factor VII is also called serum prothrombin conversion accelerator (SPCA) deficiency. One in 500,000 people may be afflicted with this disorder that is often diagnosed in newborns because of bleeding into the brain as a result of traumatic delivery.

Idiopathic Thrombocytopenic Purpura

It is considered to be the autoimmune disease of platelets.

Clinical Features

Acute idiopathic thrombocytopenic purpura

- It is seen commonly in children who are recovering from the viral disease.
- Onset of the disorder is sudden and symptoms are seen 2 to 3 weeks after the viral infection with appearance of purpura or at times epistaxis.

Chronic idiopathic thrombocytopenic purpura

- This is seen during 2nd to 4th decades of life.
- It has female predilection.
- Patient has purpura or epistaxis.
- There is presence of ecchymoses and menorrhagia
- Internal bleeding can also be present.
- Splenomegaly can be present.

Investigations

- Bleeding time becomes prolonged.
- Platelet count get decreased
- Bone marrow examination reveals increase in the number of megakaryocytes indicating peripheral destruction of platelets.

Management

In children

- Mild idiopathic thrombocytopenic purpura requires no treatment.

- In moderate-to-severe idiopathic thrombocytopenic purpura prednisolone 2 mg/kg daily oral administration is advised.
- Platelet transfusion can be given.
- After giving steroidal therapy, if bleeding persist immunoglobulins should be given.

In adults

- In adults, prednisolone should be given 1 mg/kg as standard regimen and is continued for 2 to 4 weeks, after this drug should be slowly withdrawn.
- If bleeding is high platelet infusion should be done.
- IV immunoglobulin should be given, i.e., 1 g/kg. This is to be given in the patients who are not responding to prednisolone therapy.
- If patient has more than two remissions of the disease splenectomy should be done.

Q.38. Describe the etiology, classification, clinical features, approach to diagnosis and treatment of anemias.

(Dec 2015, 10 Marks)

Ans. *For classification of anemias, refer to Ans. 31 of same chapter.*

Etiology

For etiology of iron deficiency anemia, refer to Ans. 2 of same chapter.
For etiology of macrocytic anemia, refer to Ans. 31 of same chapter.
For etiology of folic acid deficiency anemia, refer to Ans. 31 of same chapter.
For etiology of hemolytic anemia refer to etiological classification in Ans. 3 of same chapter.

Clinical Features

For clinical features of iron deficiency anemia, refer to Ans. 2 of same chapter.
For clinical features of macrocytic anemia, refer to Ans. 31 of same chapter.
For clinical features of folic acid deficiency anemia, refer to Ans. 31 of same chapter.
For clinical features of hemolytic anemia, refer to Ans. 3 of same chapter.

Approach to Diagnosis

For diagnosis of iron deficiency anemia, refer to Ans. 29 of same chapter.
For diagnosis of macrocytic anemia, refer to Ans. 31 of same chapter.
For diagnosis of folic acid deficiency anemia, refer to Ans. 31 of same chapter.
For diagnosis of hemolytic anemia, refer to Ans. 3 of same chapter.

Treatment

For treatment of iron deficiency anemia refer to Ans. 2 of same chapter.
For treatment of macrocytic anemia refer to Ans. 31 of same chapter.
For treatment of folic acid deficiency anemia refer to Ans. 31 of same chapter.
For treatment of hemolytic anemia refer to Ans. 3 of same chapter.

Q.39. Describe iron deficiency anemia under following headings: *(Mar 2016, 2+2+2 Marks)*
   a. Iron metabolism
   b. Investigations
   c. Treatment

Ans.

Iron Metabolism

Average diet consists of 10–15 mg of iron out of which 5–10% is normally absorbed. Iron required for hemoglobin synthesis is derived from two primary sources, i.e., ingestion of food containing iron and recycling of iron from senescent red cells. Iron is absorbed from duodenum and upper jejunum in ferrous form (Fe^{2+}) and plays role in absorption. Iron absorbs better from heme diet. Iron from heme is released in mucosa of small intestine after absorption for its utilization. Iron is consumed from the diet and recycling of iron released is done by catabolism of hemoglobin derived from destroyed senescent red cells. Transfer of iron to bone marrow is by iron-binding globulin, i.e., transferrin. Iron is stored in reticuloendothelial cells, hepatocytes and skeletal muscle cells as two iron protein complexes, i.e., ferritin which is water soluble and hemosiderin which is water insoluble. Iron is also present in myoglobin and cytochrome enzymes.

Total of 0.5–2 mg of iron is absorbed daily by normal human male or non-menstruating female. Out of which 0.5–1 mg of iron is lost in sweat, urine, stool and in mensis. 2 mg of iron is utilized in pregnancy. 0.5 mg is utilized in growth and lactation women.

For investigations and treatment in detail for iron deficiency anemia, refer to Ans. 2 of same chapter.

Q.40. Write short note on clinical features and diagnosis of acute myeloid leukemia. *(Apr 2017, 6 Marks)*

Ans.

Clinical Features of Acute Myeloid Leukemia

♦ It occurs in adults and it age ranges from 15–40 years.
♦ It comprises of 20% of childhood leukemia.
♦ Symptoms due to anemia, i.e., tiredness, weakness and marked pallor.
♦ *Hemorrhagic manifestations:* Petechiae, bleeding from gums and nose, persistent bleeding after tooth extraction.
♦ Infection: It causes infective lesions of mouth and throat, i.e., ulceration of mouth and pharynx, herpes simplex infection of face and infection of respiratory tract, such as bronchitis and pneumonia.
♦ Symptoms of cellular hyperviscosity
♦ There are tissue deposits of leukemic cells causing gum hypertrophy which is common in myelomonocytic and monocytic variety of AML.
♦ Lymphadenopathy and splenomegaly are present
♦ Signs of organ infiltration are present, i.e.
   • *Skin:* Bluish nodules or dusky red patches are present.
   • *Kidneys:* Presence of kidney failure.

• *Other sites:* Testes, ovary, liver, gut and serous membranes, such as pleura and peritoneum.
♦ Bone pain are present, i.e., tenderness of sternum, osteolytic bone lesions and pathologic fractures may occur.
♦ Constitutional symptoms, i.e., fever, malaise and prostration.
♦ Roth's spot, i.e., presence of white central retinal hemorrhages in acute myeloid leukemia

Diagnosis of Acute Myeloid Leukemia

♦ Peripheral blood picture shows increase in number of typical or atypical myeloblasts. Auer rods may be found in cytoplasm.
♦ Bone marrow aspirate shows more than 30% blast cells. Marrow is entirely replaced by myeloblasts and promyelocytes.
♦ There is presence of low to high WBC count.
♦ Thrombocytopenia is moderate.
♦ *Cytochemical stains:* Myeloperoxidase and Sudan black are positive.

Q.41. Write short answer on megaloblastic anemia.
(Apr 2018, 3 Marks) (May 2018, 3 Marks)

Or

Write short note on clinical features and management of megaloblastic anemia. *(Jan 2019, 7 Marks)*

Ans. Megaloblastic anemias are characterized by macrocytic blood picture (MCV >100 fl) and megaloblastic bone marrow.

Causes of megaloblastic anemia

I. Due to Vitamin B12 deficiency

♦ Inadequate intake: In strict vegetarians, poor quality diet, in elderly
♦ Impaired absorption
   • Gastric
      – Pernicious anemia
      – Congenital intrinsic factor deficiency
      – Gastrectomy
   • Small intestinal disease
      – Bacterial overgrowth
      – Crohn's disease and resection of terminal ileum
      – Tropical sprue and non-tropical sprue
      – Selective ileal malabsorption of B12 .
      – Fish tapeworm disease
      – Coeliac disease (folic deficiency more common)
      – Miscellaneous — HIV infection, severe pancreatic disease, drugs
♦ Increased requirement: In pregnancy and disseminated cancer

II. Due to folic acid deficiency

♦ Inadequate intake: In malnutrition, old age, poverty, alcoholism, Goat's milk, Kwashiorkor
♦ Impaired absorption: Celiac disease, dermatitis herpetiformis, tropical sprue, congenital folate malabsorption and oral contraceptives

◆ Increased requirement: Infancy, pregnancy and hyperplastic marrow due to hemolytic anemia

◆ Impaired utilization: Folic acid antagonists, methotrexate, pyrimethamine, trimethoprim, anticonvulsant drugs

◆ Increased loss (combined folic acid and vitamin B12 deficiency): Tropical sprue, non-tropical sprue and hemodialysis.

Clinical Features

◆ Due to anemia: Shortness of breath, dyspnea, pallor and in older subjects angina or cardiac failure.

◆ Gastrointestinal: Diarrhea, loss of appetite and weight. Sore tongue due to glossitis and angular cheilosis. Mild jaundice may give the patient a lemon yellow tint.

◆ Neurological
  • Vitamin B12 neuropathy: Due to symmetrical damage to peripheral nerves and posterior and lateral columns of spinal cord, the legs being more affected than arms. Psychiatric abnormalities and visual disturbances may occur (from folate deficiency).
  • Neural tube defects: Folic acid supplements during pregnancy have been shown to reduce incidence of spina bifida, encephalocele and anencephaly in the fetus.

◆ CVS disease: Raised serum homocysteine concentrations have been associated with arterial obstruction and venous thrombosis.

◆ Gonadal dysfunction: Deficiency of either B12 or folic acid may cause sterility, which is reversible with appropriate vitamin supplements.

◆ Knuckle pigmentation

Laboratory Diagnosis

◆ **Blood Film**
  • Macrocytosis: Hemoglobin content in red cells is proportionately increased hence normal MCHC.
  • Peripheral smear: It shows
    – Oval macrocytes
    – Anisopoikilocytosis.
    – Few tear drop cells and normocytes.
    – Few nucleated RBCs.
    – Macrocytes without central pallor.
    – Evidence of dyserythropoiesis: basophilic stippling, Cabot ring and Howell-Jolly bodies.
  • Hemoglobin is decreased.
  • Hypersegmented neutrophils may be the first evidence of megaloblastic anemia.
  • Iron ferritin level increases.

◆ **Bone marrow**
  • Hypercellularity with marked erythroid hyperplasia.
  • Megaloblasts are larger than normoblasts and have sieve like nuclear chromatin. Evidence of dyserythropoiesis.
  • Myelopoiesis — Giant metamyelocytes and giant band forms with abnormal nuclear shapes.
  • Megakaryocytes with hyperlobulation and immature nucleus.

• Dimorphic anemia — Macrocytes and hypochromic microcytes in cases of combined B12/Folate and iron deficiency.

◆ **Biochemical estimations**
  • Serum folate levels: Decrease determined by isotope dilution method, microbiologic assay.
  • Serum vitamin B12 levels — Decrease determined by isotope dilution technique or microbiological assay.
  • Increased levels of methylmalonic acid in serum and urine in B12 deficiency.
  • FIGLU excretion in urine in excess in folic acid deficiency.
  • Deoxyuridine suppression test for deficiency of both vitamin B12 and folate.
  • Schillings test of vitamin B12 absorption. Radioactive vitamin B12 is used to assess intrinsic factor and Vitamin B12 to distinguish megaloblastic anemia due to intrinsic factor deficiency (pernicious anemia) from other causes of B12 deficiency.
  • Serum homocysteine levels - increased in folate and B12 deficiency.

Diagnosis of Megaloblastic Anemia

◆ Oval macrocytes in peripheral smear.
◆ Hypersegmented neutrophils.
◆ Megaloblastic erythropoiesis in bone marrow.
◆ Response to B12/Folate therapy.

Treatment

◆ **Vitamin B12 deficiency:**
  • Initially: Hydroxycobalamin 1000 µg IM, 6 injections in 2–3 weeks.
  • Maintenance dose is 500–1000 µg IM every three months for life.
  • For patients sensitive to B12 injections or those who refuse injections, oral B12 (cyanocobalamin) in large daily doses (100 µg or more).
  • Since rapid regeneration of blood deplete marrow iron stores, so ferrous sulfate 200 mg daily is given after starting the therapy.

◆ **Folate deficiency:**
  • Initially folic acid 5 mg daily orally for at least 4 months. Folic acid in such big doses should not be given until B12 deficiency has been excluded, since folic acid may precipitate B12 neuropathy in a severely deficient B12 patient.
  • Maintenance: Need depends on whether the underlying cause can be reversed, e.g., gluten-free diet in celiac disease.

Q.42. Describe the coagulation pathway. Discuss the clinical features, pathogenesis and treatment of hemophilia. *(May 2018, 5 Marks)*

Ans. *For coagulation pathway refer to Ans. 33 of same chapter.*

Pathogenesis of Hemophilia

◆ Hemophilia is caused by quantitative reduction of factor VIII in 90% of cases, while 10% cases have normal or increased level of factor VIII with reduced activity.

- Factor VIII is synthesized in hepatic parenchymal cells and regulates the activation of factor X in intrinsic coagulation pathway.
- Factor VIII circulates in blood complexed to another larger protein, von Willebrand's factor (vWF), which comprises 99% of the factor VIII— vWF complex.
- Normal hemostasis requires 25% factor VIII activity. Though occasional patients with 25% factor VIII level may develop bleeding, most symptomatic haemophilic patients have factor VIII levels below 5%.

For clinical features and treatment of hemophilia refer to Ans. 8 of same chapter.

Q.43. Write short answer on sickle cell anemia.

(Apr 2019, 3 Marks)

Ans. Sickle cell anemia is characterized by presence of HbS – sickle hemoglobin which give sickle shape to RBC in the state of reduced oxygen tension.

Sickle cell anemia is from about third month of life, sine HbS is more than 70% in red cells.

Inheritance

- It is transmitted as incomplete autosomal dominant disease.
- There are always 1:4 chances with each pregnancy that offspring will have sickle cell anemia when both the parents have heterozygous state.

Pathogenesis

Clinical problems in sickle cell anemia relate to veno-occlusion caused by polymerization of deoxygenated hemoglobin S. This results in the pathognomonic change in the shape of erythrocytes to the sickle shape that stiffen the RBC membrane, increase viscosity and cause dehydration due to potassium leakage and calcium influx. The most common clinical feature is the painful vaso-occlusive crisis resulting from blockage of small vessels. However, large vessels disease also occurs, resulting in thrombotic cerebrovascular accidents, acute sickle chest syndrome, and placental infarction.

Clinical Features

Sickle cell anemia usually manifest in two ways i.e.

Chronic Anemia

- Symptoms appear after 6 months of life when most of the hemoglobin F is replaced by hemoglobin S in red cells.
- Hemolytic anemia is present.
- Secondary folate deficiency is common and exacerbate anemia which leads to growth retardation and delayed puberty.
- Symptoms of chronic severe hemolytic anemia, i.e., fatigue, lassitude, breathlessness, cardiomegaly and increased susceptibility to infection are present.
- Due to hyperplasia in bone marrow inside the skull there is frontal bossing, malar prominence during the first year of life.

- Other physical signs are mild jaundice, splenomegaly and poor healing ulcers over the legs.

Vaso-Occlusive Crisis

- It is a painful crisis which occurs due to blockage of small or large vessels known as infarction crisis.
- It is common in bone and spleen.
- In infants finger and toes are affected which produce large swelling, pain and tenderness.
- At any age mesenteric infarction with acute abdominal colic, renal infarction with painless hematuria may occur.
- Presence of aseptic necrosis of head of femur is common in adults and is a distressing complication.
- Cerebral infarction and pulmonary infarction are commonly seen.
- Attacks of pain and infarction can occur spontaneously or are due to infection, dehydration and chilling.
- Onset of the pain is rapid and can be severe during first 24 hours and then subside in next few days.

Investigations

- Hemoglobin level: It is low usually 6 to 8 g%.
- Unconjugated bilirubin: It is high.
- Blood film: It show sickle cells, target cells, polychromasia, Howell – Jolly bodies. Reticulocytosis is also present over the age of 7 years.
- Sickling test: It is positive with reducing substance, i.e., sodium metabisulfite.
- Family study to differentiate whether patient is homozygous or heterozygous for sickle cell disease.
- Hemoglobin electrophoresis: It confirms the diagnosis. HbS is present in 80 to 95% of patients with no HbA.

Management

There is no cure for the disease as genetic makeup of patient cannot be changed.

Management should be aimed at:

- Symptoms should be relieved and life style is improved by folic acid supplements.
- Removal of infection is by antibiotics. Prophylaxis in young children by phenoxy benzyl 250 mg once a day.
- Lifelong prophylaxis against malaria by antimalaria drugs.
- Infections and dehydration should be treated. Avoid chilling.
- Aspirin, paracetamol, mefenamic acid are used for pain.
- Blood transfusion is given in emergency cases, i.e., before surgery or when hemoglobin falls below 5 g/dL.
- Allogenic transplantation has given hope in treating patients of sickle cell anemia. But it is very costly and its exact role has to be defined.

Q.44. Discuss in detail about multiple myeloma.

(Oct 2019, 5 Marks)

Ans. Multiple myeloma is a malignant disease of plasma cells in the bone marrow. It is characterized by excess production of a monoclonal immunoglobulin molecule, which can be detected in the serum, urine or both, and is associated with bone pain, anemia and kidney failure, hypercalcemia.

Its incidence increases with the age and most of the patients are over the age of 60 years.

Pathogenesis

For unknown reasons, one clone of plasma cells overgrows and produces one particular immunoglobulin molecule.

1. Proliferation of plasmoblasts plasma cells.
2. IL—6: It plays an important role in proliferation of plasma cells and also lytic lesions of bones. It is also responsible for anemia due to inhibition of erythropoiesis.
3. Kaposi sarcoma associated herpes virus (KSHV) in dendritic cells secret IL-6.
4. Pre-existing MGUS (monoclonal gammopathy of uncertain significance) predisposes to development of malignant myeloma.
5. Chronic exposure to low dose irradiation, e.g., in workers of nuclear power plants, uranium mines.

In 80% of patients, there is a paraprotein in the serum, usually of the IgG or IgA class. The abnormal cells may also produce free light chains, small enough to cross the glomerulus, and pass into the urine as Bence–Jones protein, often causing tubular damage.

In 20% of patients, free light chains are only produced (Bence–Jones-only myeloma) and there is no paraprotein in the serum (free light chain disease). Non-secretory myelomas are now known to consist of excess free light chain disease and are usually seen in elderly patients.

Clinical Features and Complications

- Bone disease:
  - Bone pain is the most common presenting symptom.
  - Pathological fractures
  - Generalized osteoporosis may lead to compression fractures of vertebrae causing back pain and occasionally cord compression.
- Anemia is a common presenting feature.
- Kidney failure. It is most commonly caused by Bence–Jones protein, which damages the tubules as it passes through the kidneys. Other factors that can cause or contribute to renal failure include hypercalcemia, infection, and dehydration.
- Infections: Due to impaired humoral and cell-mediated immunity leading to increased susceptibility to bacterial and virus infection. Chest infections are common.
- Neurologic: Spinal cord/root compression.
- Due to M-proteins
  - Cryglobulinemia
  - Hyperviscosity affects CNS, retina, CVS
  - Bleeding tendency: Due to adhesion and aggregation of platelets
  - Coagulation cascade affection from formation of complexes with factors V, VII, VIII, I, II.
- Amyloidosis: About 10% of patients develop primary (AL) amyloidosis. The kidney is usually affected; deposition of amyloid in the glomeruli leads to generalized proteinuria and nephrotic syndrome. Peripheral neuropathy (particularly carpal tunnel syndrome) and congestive heart failure may occur.

- Metabolic disturbances If there is acute rheumatic fever — hypernatremia, hyperphosphatemia.
- Constitutional symptoms: Weight loss, fever, malaise
- Asymptomatic patients: Diagnosis following finding of raised ESR or abnormal protein electrophoresis on routine screening or investigation for an unrelated problem.

Investigations

1. Blood:
   - Reduced hemoglobin, TLC and PLT usually normal.
   - Rouleaux formation due to increased globulins.
   - Serum B12 microglobulin is useful prognostic marker and is usually raised
   - Hypercalcemia.
   - Kidney function tests: Raised serum urea, cretinine, uric acid and potassium.
2. Bone marrow:
   - Increased number of myeloma cells >10% diagnostic. Myeloma cell is large in size with round to oval eccentric nucleus and pale blue cytoplasm. But may be normal as bone marrow investigation is usually patchy. Bone marrow biopsy is difficult due to extremely soft and spongy nature of the bones.
   - Some cases show "flame cells" with peripheral cytoplasm sowing flare, "grape cells" showing rounded immunoglobulin inclusions and "Russel bodies" in the cytoplasm.
3. Skeletal survey with X-rays of long bones, skull, vertebrae.
4. Serum and urine protein electrophoresis: M-band seen on serum protein electrophoresis. Bence Jones proteins (free light chains) in urine found in 2/3rd of patients.
5. Serum immunofix and free light chain ratio.
6. 24-hour urine for immunofixation.
7. Bence–Jones protein in urine.

Diagnostic Criteria for Multiple Myeloma
Major Criteria

1. Plasmacytoma on tissue biopsy
2. Bone marrow plasmacytosis with >30% plasma cells
3. Monoclonal globulin spike on serum electrophoresis: IgG >35%, IgA >20 g/L. Light chain excretion on urine electrophoresis 1 g/24 hrs in absence of amyloidosis.

Minor Criteria

1. Bone marrow plasmolysis with 10–30% plasma cells.
2. Monoclonal spike present, but less than levels defined
3. Lytic bone lesions
4. Normal IgM <500 mg/L, IgA <1 g/L or IgG <6 g/L

Diagnosis of myeloma needs minimum of one major and one minor criteria which must include 1+2.

Differential Diagnosis

- Cirrhosis, tuberculosis, angioimmunoblastic lymphadenopathy with dysproteinemia.
- Monoclonal gammopathy of uncertain significance.
- Waldenstrom's macroglobulinemia

Management

♦ **Immunomodulation:** It is done with drugs, such as Pomalidomide, lenalidomide. Thalidomide is now used usually in combination with Bortezomib, and Dexamethasone.

♦ **Proteosome inhibitors:** Bortezomib (first generation), Corplazomib (second generation). Lenalidomide 25 mg/day in patients with newly diagnosed multiple myeloma is highly effective.

Recommended combinations

• Bortezomib + Lenalidomide + Dexamethasone or Bortezomib + Thalidomide + Dexamethasone

• Other drugs used in combination

Melphalan, Liposonasonabid, Doxorubicin + Cyclophosphamide

♦ Autologous transplant: For second line therapy in refractory case. Can be used as alternative to above agents with similar results.

♦ Bisphosphonates: They are used monthly as part of all treatment regimes in myeloma patients.

♦ Autologous bone marrow transplantation carries a low risk and is suitable for patients up to 65 years of age. Duration of remission and survival appear to be prolonged compared with conventional chemotherapy.

♦ Stem cell transplantation: Peripheral blood cell accelerate myelopoiesis.

With new drugs available, transplant can now be used as salvage therapy, as survival rates are equivalent.

8. DISEASES OF ENDOCRINE SYSTEM

Q.1. Write short note on acromegaly. *(Dec 2012, 3 Marks)*

Ans. If the excess of growth hormone occur after the fusion of epiphysis, then enlargement of acral parts, i.e., hands, finger, feet and toes occur leading to increase in their width rather than length.

Etiology

♦ In 95% of cases, it is pituitary adenoma.

♦ Excessive secretion of growth hormone releasing hormone from carcinoid tumors and adrenal tumors.

♦ Excessive growth hormone-secreting pancreatic islet cell tumors.

♦ As a part of multiple endocrine neoplasia type I.

Clinical Features

♦ *General:* Fatigue, weight gain, heat intolerance, increased sweating

♦ *Skin changes:* Thickening of skin. Skin is coarse and greasy, perspiration, hypertrichosis

♦ *Soft tissues:* Thickening of lips and nose, macroglossia, increase in heel pad, hypertrophy of muscular system in initial stages, mammary hyperplasia.

♦ *Skeletal changes:* Arthropathy of joints; Enlargement of hands, feet, supraorbital ridges, facial bones; prognathism is present; spacing apart of teeth; thick clavicles; Changes in spine, i.e., osteoporosis, kyphosis, lordosis and scoliosis; carpal tunnel syndrome; prominent ridges and furrows on skull; Large frontal and maxillary sinus.

♦ *Cardiovascular:* Hypertension, cardiac failure or acromegalic cardiomyopathy, coronary artery disease, Arrhythmias

♦ *Respiratory:* Deep voice due to enlargement of larynx, Lungs enlarge proportionately with thorax

♦ *Ophthalmologic:* Visual field defects are present, such as bitemporal hemianopia or scotomas

♦ *Metabolic:* Impaired glucose tolerance is present.

♦ *Malignancy:* Prevalence of malignant disease, i.e., probability of colonic cancer increased.

Investigations

♦ *Imaging:*

• *Radiography:*

– X-ray skull shows enlarged sella turcica, enlarged frontal sinus, increase thickness of skull, macrognathia and wide space teeth.

– There is arrow head tufting of finger tips

– *Heel pad sign:* Heel pad >23 mm thick.

• *CT scan:* A large adenoma is easily seen on CT scan taken after IV contrast.

– *MRI:* Sagittal view is useful in identifying the relationship between suprasellar and infrasellar structures.

♦ *Biochemical diagnosis:*

• Growth hormone levels are increased.

• *Glucose tolerance test:* It is the accepted diagnostic method measuring glucose and growth hormone. In healthy individuals growth hormone is undetectable during the test.

• *Insulin-like growth factor-I (IGF–I) levels:* Growth hormone stimulates production of IGF–I predominantly in liver. IGF-I levels assess disease activity in acromegalics, reflecting overall growth hormone secretion.

Management

♦ **Surgical:** Surgery is the treatment of choice. Surgical removal of tumor is done by transsphenoidal route followed by radiotherapy.

♦ **Radiotherapy:** It is advised when initial attempts at surgery do not reduce growth hormone levels to 5 MU/L. Implantation of radioactive isotope. Yttrium-90 causes major reduction in growth hormone levels.

♦ **Medical therapy:**

• Bromocriptine 20–30 mg/day orally in divided doses is given.

• Octreotide decreases the growth hormone levels. Its dose is 100 μg TDS and can be increased up to 1500 μg/day. *Sandostatin:* LAR is a sustained release formulation of octreotide. It is given as 30 mg IM for 6 weeks which decreases growth hormone levels and also decreases pituitary tumor size.

- Growth hormone receptor antagonist, i.e., Pegvisomant is given S C as 40 mg/day followed by self-administration of 10 mg/day. Liver function needs monitoring.

Q.2. Outline the management of thyrotoxicosis.
(Apr 2010, 5 Marks)

Or

Write short answer on drugs used in thyrotoxicosis.
(Oct 2019, 3 Marks)

Ans. The management of thyrotoxicosis is divided into four parts as follows:

1. **General:**
   - Allow the patient to take mental and physical rest.
   - Maintain nutrition of patient by giving nutritious diet.
   - If patient is anxious alprazolam 0.25 to 0.5 mg BD is given.
2. **Drug therapy:**
   - Anti-thyroid drugs, such as carbimazole, i.e., 40 to 60 mg/day, methimazole, i.e., 100 to 150 mg 8 hourly and propylthiouracil, i.e., 300 to 450 mg/day can be given depending on the severity of the disease. Drugs should be gradually decreased for 4 to 8 weeks based on FT4 levels. When FT4 levels are normal, the carbimazole 5 to 15 mg/day or propylthiouracil 50 mg/day is given. Drugs can be given for 1 to 2 years by regular checking of FT4 and TSH levels.
   - For symptomatic relief, beta-blockers, such as propranolol 80–160 mg daily is given. It is given for 2 to 3 weeks along with anti-thyroid treatment. It relieves symptoms, such as anxiety, tremors and tachycardia.
   - Dexamethasone 8 mg/day may be used to inhibit conversion of T4 to T3 in severe form of thyrotoxicosis.
   - Lithium carbonate 300–450 mg TDS inhibit thyroid hormone secretion temporarily in patients who are allergic to iodides and thioamides.
   - Potassium perchlorate 500 mg BD inhibits iodine uptake by thyroid gland. It is combined with thioamides.
3. **Surgery:** Subtotal thyroidectomy is done in severely affected cases. Before surgery patient should be made euthyroid by beta blockers and anti-thyroid drugs. Two weeks before the surgery drugs should be stopped and lugol iodine is given to reduce the vascularity.
4. **Radioiodine treatment:** Radioactive iodine, i.e., 131I leads to the destruction of thyroid cells and is given with anti-thyroid drugs to prevent thyroid storm.
   - Anti-thyroid drugs must be stopped for minimum of 3 to 5 days before ^{131}I to allow uptake of isotope 555 MBq to ablate thyroid.
   - High doses are needed for large goiter in severely thyrotoxic patients.

Q.3. Write short note on Grave's disease.
(Mar 2001, 5 Marks)

Ans. Grave's disease is an autoimmune disease caused by production of autoantibodies that stimulate thyroid-stimulating hormone receptor on thyroid cell membrane resulting in excessive synthesis and secretion of thyroid hormone.

Risk Factors

- *Genetic susceptibility:* Role of hereditary factors is evidenced by increased incidence of other autoimmune disorders in members of patient's families.
- Emotional stress
- *Gender:* Females more prone than men (7 to 10:1) ratio.
- *Pregnancy:* iodine-containing drugs
- *Iodine and drugs:* Amiodarone and iodine-containing contrast media may precipitate Graves' disease.
- Irradiation, e.g., radioactive iodine for multinodular goiter.

Clinical Features

Symptoms

- Weight loss with increased appetite
- Heat intolerance and sweating
- Fatigue and weakness
- Hyperactivity, irritability, dysphoria, insomnia
- Dyspnea
- Oligomenorrhea, loss of libido
- Diarrhea/Defecation hyperclefecation
- Polyuria

Signs

- Tremor, hyperreflexia
- Tachycardia, atrial fibrillation in elderly
- Warm moist skin
- Lid retraction, lid lag (causing a stare)
- **Thyroid ophthalmopathy is a specific feature for Grave's disease for which signs and symptoms are as follows:**

Symptoms	Signs
Xerophthalmia	*Lid signs:* Lid lag and lid retraction resulting in staring look
Puffy eyelids	*Soft tissue signs:* Eyelid edema, Conjunctival erythema and chemosis
Proptosis	*Proptosis:* It is combined with lid retraction
Eyelid retraction	Exposure keratitis
Diplopia especially at extreme gaze	External ophthalmoplegia
Loss of vision	Absence of wrinkling on looking upwards
Field loss	*Mösbius sign:* Failure of convergence
Dyschromatopsia	
Ocular pressure on pain	
Lacrimation	

Investigations

- T3 and T4 both are elevated.
- Low TSH or become undetcetable

♦ ^{131}I uptake is increased, i.e., greater than 35% at 5 hours
♦ Serum cholesterol is low
♦ ECG shows tachycardia, arrhythmias, ST-T changes
♦ Ultrasonography of thyroid shows diffuse goiter.

Management

Treatment for Discomfort

♦ Artificial tears should be given for the day, i.e., methylcellulose is given.
♦ Simple eye ointment should be given for the night
♦ Patient should use dark glasses with side frames.
♦ No smoking

Medical Therapy

♦ Reduction of morning lid edema by sleeping on bed with its head slightly raised.
♦ Prednisolone 60 mg daily is given.
♦ Anti-thyroid drugs, such as carbimazole, i.e., 40–60 mg/day, methimazole, i.e., 100–150 mg 8 hourly and propylthiouracil, i.e., 300–450 mg/day can be given depending on the severity of the disease. Drugs should be gradually decreased for 4 to 8 weeks based on FT4 levels. When FT4 levels are normal carbimazole 5–15 mg/day or propylthiouracil 50 mg/day is given. Drugs can be given for 1–2 years by regular checking of FT4 and TSH levels.
♦ For symptomatic relief beta blockers, such as propanolol 80–160 mg daily is given. It is given for 2–3 weeks along with anti -thyroid treatment. It relieves symptoms, such as anxiety, tremors and tachycardia.
♦ Radioactive iodine, i.e., ^{131}I leads to the destruction of thyroid cells and is given with anti-thyroid drugs.

Surgery

♦ Subtotal thyroidectomy is done in severely affected cases. Before surgery patient should be made euthyroid by beta-blockers and anti-thyroid drugs. Two weeks before the surgery drugs should be stopped and lugol iodine is given to reduce the vascularity.

Q.4. Write short note on hyperthyroidism.
(Oct 2007, 10 Marks) (June 2010, 5 Marks)
(Sep 2009, 4 Marks)

Ans. Hyperthyroidism is defined as increased secretion of thyroid hormone with increase in level of T3 and T4.

Etiology

♦ *Common causes:*
  • Grave's disease
  • Toxic nodular goiter
    – Multinodular
    – Solitary nodule
♦ *Less common:*
  • Thyroiditis
  • Drug-induced
  • Factitious
  • Iodine excess
♦ *Rare:*
  • Pituitary or ectopic TSH
  • Thyroid carcinoma

Clinical Features

♦ Goiter is present, i.e., either diffuse or nodular.
♦ *Gastrointestinal features:* Vomiting, diarrhea and weight loss
♦ *Cardiovascular features:* Arrhythmia, i.e., atrial fibrillation, dyspnea, wide pulse pressure
♦ *Dermatological manifestations:* Clubbing, loss of hair, palms become red, increased sweating
♦ *Reproductive features:* Amenorrhea, infertility, abortion, impotence
♦ *Ophthalmological features:* Exophthalmos, Diplopia, lid retraction, staring look, excessive watering from eyes
♦ *Neuromuscular features:* Tremors in hand, psychosis, irritability, restlessness, nervousness, high tendon reflexes
♦ *Miscellaneous:* Fatigue, polydipsia, heat tolerance

Investigations

♦ Serum TSH level is decreased and is the initial diagnostic test. Normal TSH levels exclude clinical hyperthyroidism.
♦ Serum total and unbound (free) T3 and T4 are increased in hyperthyroidism.
♦ In some cases, only T3 levels are raised whereas T4 is normal (T3 toxicosis).
♦ TSH-R antibodies levels are increased in about 75% cases. ESR may be increased in subacute thyroiditis.
♦ Uptake of radioactive iodine by thyroid is increased in Graves' disease and toxic nodular goiter, whereas it is low in subacute thyroiditis.
♦ Ultrasonography of thyroid gland reveals diffuse enlargement of thyroid gland which helps in differentiating Graves' disease from nodular goiter.

Management

Drug Therapy

♦ Anti-thyroid drugs, such as carbimazole, i.e., 40–60 mg/day, methimazole, i.e., 100–150 mg 8 hourly and propylthiouracil, i.e., 300–450 mg/day can be given depending on the severity of the disease. Drugs should be gradually decreased for 4–8 weeks based on FT4 levels. When FT4 levels are normal carbimazole 5–15 mg/day or propylthiouracil 50 mg/day is given. Drugs can be given for 1–2 years by regular checking of FT4 and TSH levels.
♦ For symptomatic relief beta-blockers, such as propranolol 80–160 mg daily is given. It is given for 2–3 weeks along with anti–thyroid treatment. It relieves symptoms, such as anxiety, tremors and tachycardia.
♦ Dexamethasone 8 mg/day may be used to inhibit conversion of T4–T3 in severe form of thyrotoxicosis.
♦ Lithium carbonate 300–450 mg TDS inhibit thyroid hormone secretion temporarily in patients who are allergic to iodides and thioamides.
♦ Potassium perchlorate 500 mg BD inhibits iodine uptake by thyroid gland. It is combined with thioamides.

Surgery

Subtotal thyroidectomy is done in severely affected cases. Before surgery patient should be made euthyroid by beta- blockers and anti-thyroid drugs. Two weeks before the surgery drugs should be stopped and lugol iodine is given to reduce the vascularity.

Radioactive Iodine

- Radioactive iodine, i.e., ^{131}I leads to the destruction of thyroid cells and is given with anti-thyroid drugs to prevent thyroid storm.
- Anti-thyroid drugs must be stopped for minimum of 3–5 days before ^{131}I to allow uptake of isotope 555 MBq to ablate thyroid.
- High doses are needed for large goiters in severely thyrotoxic patients.

Q.5. Describe clinical manifestations and management of myxedema. *(Mar 2003, 10 Marks)*

Or

Write short note on treatment of myxedema. *(Feb 2013, 5 Marks)*

Ans. Myxedema is a clinical condition resulting from decreased circulating levels of T3 and T4. It is characterized by deposition of mucinous material causing swelling of skin and subcutaneous tissue.

Clinical Features

- *General:* There is tiredness, *somnolence, weight gain, cold intolerance and goiter.
- *Skin and subcutaneous tissue:* Coarse dry skin, puffiness of face with malar flush, baggy eyelids with swollen edematous appearance of supraclavicular regions, neck and lacks of hand and feet.
- *Cardiovascular and respiratory features:* Bradycardia, angina, cardiac failure, pericardial effusion and pleural effusion.
- *Neuromuscular features:* Aches and pains, cerebellar syndrome with slurred speech and ataxia, muscle cramps and stiffness.
- *Gastrointestinal features:* Constipation and ascites
- *Developmental:* Growth and mental retardation
- *Reproductive system:* Infertility, menorrhagia, hyperprolactinemia and galactorrhea.

Investigation

- Serum T3 and T4 are decreased.
- Serum TSH level is high
- Creatinine level increases
- Serum cholesterol level is increased
- BMR is low
- Iodine uptake by thyroid is poor
- ECG can show bradycardia, low amplitude of QRS and ST-T changes.
- Blood picture shows macrocytic anemia.
- X-ray chest can be normal or shows cardiomegaly.
- Photomotogram reveals delayed ankle jerk.

Management

- In patient of myxedema adequate ventilation is maintained along with electrolyte balance and slow warming.
- Principle of therapy is replacement of deficient thyroid hormones.
- Treatment of myxedema is the life-long replacement of thyroid hormones by L-thyroxine.

Q 5. *Somnolence = Excessive sleepiness.

- Initial starting dosage is 50–100 µg daily as a single dose empty stomach in the morning for first 3 to 4 weeks. After some time, dosage can be increased to 150 µg/day. Adjustment of final dosage should be done after assessing TSH levels.
- Maximum dosage of L–thyroxine is 300 µg/day.
- In geriatric patients or the patients suffering with ischemic heart disease, low dose of L–thyroxine 25 µg/day can be started and is increases after assessing the levels of TSH.
- Since plasma half-life of L–thyroxine is 7 days so increase and decrease in dose should be done at an interval of 2 weeks.

Q.6. Write short note on hypothyroidism. *(May/June 2009, 5 Marks) (Feb 2006, 5 Marks)*

Or

Write in brief on hypothyroidism. *(Mar 2016, 4 Marks)*

Or

Write signs and symptoms of hypothyroidism. *(Jan 2012, 5 Marks)*

Or

Write all clinical features of hypothyroidism. *(Jun 2014, 5 Marks)*

Or

Write clinical features, diagnosis, and management of hypothyroidism. *(Jun 2018, 12 Marks)*

Or

Discuss clinical features, complications, investigations and treatment of hypothyroidism. *(May 2018, 5 Marks)*

Or

Describe sign, symptoms and management of hypothyroidism. *(Feb 2019, 5 Marks)*

Or

Write short answer on hypothyroidism. *(Apr 2019, 3 Marks)*

Ans. Hypothyroidism is defined as the clinical condition caused by the low level of circulating thyroid hormones.

Types

- *Primary:* When the cause lies in thyroid
- *Secondary:* When hypothyroidism occurs due to disease of anterior pituitary.

Clinical Features

Symptoms

- Feeling of tiredness
- Weight gain
- Cold intolerance
- Hoarseness of voice and lethargy
- Somnolence
- Goiter
- Hyperlipidemia.

Signs

♦ *Skin and subcutaneous tissues:* Dry skin, puffiness of face with malar flush, baggy eyelids, alopecia, vitiligo
♦ *Cardiovascular:* Bradycardia, angina, heart failure
♦ *Respiratory:* Pericardial effusion, pleural effusion
♦ *Psychiatric:* Depression and psychosis
♦ *Neuromuscular:* Ache and pain, cerebellar ataxia, myalgia, delayed relaxation of reflexes, carpal tunnel syndrome
♦ *Gastrointestinal:* Constipation, ascites, ileus
♦ *Hematological:* Iron deficiency anemia, macrocytic anemia, pernicious anemia, normochromic normocytic anemia
♦ *Reproductive:* Infertility, impotence, menorrhagia
♦ *Development:* Growth retardation, mental retardation and delayed puberty.

Investigations

♦ Serum T3 and T4 levels are low.
♦ Serum TSH level is high in primary hypothyroidism and low in secondary hypothyroidism.
♦ Serum cholesterol levels are high.
♦ ECG shows bradycardia, low amplitude of QRS and ST-T changes.
♦ Blood picture shows macrocytic anemia.
♦ X-ray chest can be normal or show cardiomegaly

Treatment

♦ Treatment of hypothyroidism is life long.
♦ Thyroid hormones are replaced by L-thyroxine
♦ Initial starting dosage is 50–100 µg daily empty stomach as single dose in morning for first 3 to 4 weeks. Later dose is increased to 150 µg daily.
♦ Final dose adjustment is done by TSH levels. TSH levels are maintained in normal range by increasing the dosage.
♦ Maximum dose of L-thyroxine is 300 µg.

Complications of hypothyroidism

Untreated hypothyroidism can lead to a number of health problems:

♦ **Goiter:** Constant stimulation of thyroid to release more hormones may cause the gland to become larger — a condition known as a goiter. Hashimoto's thyroiditis is one of the most common causes of a goiter. Although generally not uncomfortable, a large goiter can affect appearance and may interfere with swallowing or breathing.
♦ **Heart problems:** Hypothyroidism may also be associated with an increased risk of heart disease, primarily because high levels of low-density lipoprotein (LDL) cholesterol — the "bad" cholesterol — can occur in people with an underactive thyroid. Even subclinical hypothyroidism, a mild or early form of hypothyroidism in which symptoms have not yet developed, can cause an increase in total cholesterol levels and impair the pumping ability of heart. Hypothyroidism can also lead to an enlarged heart and heart failure.
♦ **Mental health issues:** Depression may occur early in hypothyroidism and may become more severe over time. Hypothyroidism can also cause slowed mental functioning.

♦ **Peripheral neuropathy:** Long-term uncontrolled hypothyroidism can cause damage to peripheral nerves— the nerves that carry information from brain and spinal cord to the rest of body. Signs and symptoms of peripheral neuropathy may include pain, numbness and tingling in the area affected by the nerve damage. It may also cause muscle weakness or loss of muscle control.
♦ **Myxedema:** This rare, life-threatening condition is the result of long-term, undiagnosed hypothyroidism. Its signs and symptoms include intense cold intolerance and drowsiness followed by profound lethargy and unconsciousness. A myxedema coma may be triggered by sedatives, infection or other stress on your body. If in an individual shows signs or symptoms of myxedema, he/she need immediate emergency medical treatment.
♦ **Infertility:** Low levels of thyroid hormone can interfere with ovulation, which impairs fertility. In addition, some of the causes of hypothyroidism, such as autoimmune disorder— can also impair fertility.
♦ **Birth defects:** Babies born to women with untreated thyroid disease may have a higher risk of birth defects than babies born to healthy mothers. These children are also more prone to serious intellectual and developmental problems. Infants with untreated hypothyroidism present at birth are at risk of serious problems with both physical and mental development. But if this condition is diagnosed within the first few months of life, the chances of normal development are excellent.

Q.7. Discuss thyroid function tests. *(Oct 2003, 15 Marks)*

Ans. A laboratory thyroid profile includes measurement of:

♦ Serum T4
♦ Resin T3 uptake
♦ T4 binding ratio
♦ Free T4 index
♦ Thyroid-stimulating hormone.

Serum T4

Measured total serum T4 reflects hormone which both binds to thyroid-binding globulin and free hormone. The normal range of serum T4 is 5–11.5 µg/DL. Hence, changes in either free hormone level or concentration in thyroid-binding globulin will alter total serum T4 but not affect free hormone level. Therefore, increased secretion of thyroid-binding globulin increases total serum T4 whereas decrease in TBG lowers total serum T4.

Resin T3 Uptake

It reflects the thyroid-binding globulin concentration and is reported as percentage, i.e., 25 to 35%. A present amount of radioactive T3 is added to patient's sample of serum. Radioactive T3 binds to all liable binding sites on thyroid-binding globulin and left over is bound to resin and is measured.

T4 Binding Ratio

The resin T3 uptake is converted to T4 binding ratio by dividing the measured resin T3 uptake by reference serum mean resin T3 uptake which is 30%. The resin T3 uptake and to T4 binding ratio are low and high in hypothyroidism and hyperthyroidism, respectively.

Free T4 Index

It represents a calculated free T4 hormone concentration. It is calculated by multiplying total serum T4 by T4 binding ratio. The free T4 index is low and high in hypothyroidism and hyperthyroidism.

Thyroid-Stimulating Hormone (TSH)

It is secreted from anterior pituitary and has negative feedback relationship with circulating T4 and T3. It is the single best test for diagnosing primary hypothyroidism and hyperthyroidism. In former condition, serum TSH is increased and in later condition it is decreased.

Q.8. Write briefly on Addison's disease.

(Apr 2010, 5 Marks)

Ans. Addison's disease or primary hypoadrenalism results from destruction of adrenal cortex by variety of pathological processes.

Etiology

- It is caused due to autoimmune adrenalitis.
- Infections, i.e., TB, cytomegalovirus and fungal infection associated with AIDS.
- By tumors
- Inherited disorders, i.e., adrenoleukodystrophies and familial isolated glucocorticoid deficiency.

Clinical Features

- *Pigmentation of skin and mucus membrane:* There is bluish black discoloration of lips, gums and posterior aspect of palate.
- *Gastrointestinal symptoms:* Anorexia, nausea and vomiting. Constipation with intermittent diarrhea, achlorhydria and abdominal pain
- *Cardiovascular system:* Postural hypotension, faintness may result. Dyspnea is also present.
- *Muscular system:* Muscular weakness and wasting with creatinuria. Sometimes cramp in muscles is present.
- *Mental and nervous:* Muscle weakness and lassitude (exhaustion) are first symptoms to appear. Loss of memory and drowsiness.
- *Genital system:* Impotence and *amenorrhea are present.
- *Renal system:* Renal function is impaired and the excretion of urine is diminished.

Investigation

- Serum sodium and chloride level are decreased
- Blood sugar level is decreased
- Blood urea increases
- Urine secretion of chloride is increased.
- Urinary secretion decreases
- BMR is decreased
- Abdominal X-ray shows calcification of adrenal gland.

Treatment

- *Cortisone substitution:* Hydrocortisone 20 mg TDS for 72 hours. For maintenance, dose is 20 mg in morning and 10 mg in evening.

Q 8.   *Amenorrhea = Absence of monthly periods in females.

- *Aldosterone substitution:* Fludrocortisone 50 μg BD is started.
- *Salt:* Patients with diarrhea or profuse sweating should be given an additional 3–6 g of sodium chloride daily.

Q.9. Write short note on thyrotoxicosis (Clinical features).

(Sep 2004, 3.5 Marks) (Mar 2009, 5 Marks)

Or

Write short note on thyrotoxicosis.

(Sep 2006, 10 Marks)

Or

Write short answer on thyrotoxicosis.

(Apr 2018, 3 Marks)

Ans. For *clinical features of thyrotoxicosis, refer to Ans. 4 of same chapter.*

Q.10. Describe the clinical findings of hyperthyroidism.

(Sep 2005, 10 Marks)

Or

Describe the clinical findings, diagnosis and management of hyperthyroidism.

(Sep 2004, 20 Marks)

Ans. For *clinical finding and management refer to Ans. 4 of same chapter.*

Diagnosis

The case with signs like exophthalmos, tremors, tachycardia and thyroid enlargement and symptoms, i.e., sweating, intolerance to heat, restlessness, increased appetite, diarrhea and weight loss can be diagnosed as hyperthyroidism. In anxiety state, the hands are cold and moist while in hyperthyroidism, they are warm and moist.

Thyroid function test: There is raised T3 and T4 levels.

Diagnosis is solely based or investigations. *For details of investigations refer to Ans. 4 of same chapter.*

Q.11. Write short note on parathyroid hormone.

(Feb 2002, 5 Marks)

Ans. Parathyroid hormone is secreted by chief cells of parathyroid gland.

Action

- Primary function of parathyroid hormone is to maintain the blood calcium level within the range of 9 to 11 mg%.
- Parathyroid hormone maintains blood calcium level by acting on bone, kidney and GIT; by increasing the resorption of calcium from bones, by decreasing excretion of calcium through kidneys, by increasing absorption of calcium through GIT.
- The increased activity of parathyroid glands lead to excessive secretion of parathormone which leads to the disorder known as hyperparathyroidism and decreased synthesis of parathormone is called hypoparathyroidism.

Q.12. Write short note on investigations in a case of Cushing's syndrome. *(Mar 2007, 5 Marks)*

Ans. Cushing's syndrome is caused by the excessive production of cortisol.

Investigations

♦ Urinary excretion of 11 oxysteroids and 17 ketosteroids is increased. Dexamethasone suppression test showing failure of significant plasma cortisol suppression favors adrenal tumor as the cause.

♦ Glucose tolerance test, such as diabetes.

♦ X-ray chest for evidence of thymic carcinoma.

♦ X-ray skull for pituitary edema is not helpful since a pituitary basophilic adenoma does not expand and so sella turcica and glenoid processes are normal.

♦ X-ray dorsal spine may show collapse of vertebrae producing fish spine appearance.

♦ IV *pyelography for adrenocortical tumor. *Perirenal insufflation, *tomography, USG and CT scan and MRI to detect adrenal hyperplasia.

Q.13. Write in brief clinical features and management of thyroid nodules. *(Apr 2007, 5 Marks)*

Ans. The term "thyroid nodule" refers to any abnormal growth that forms a lump in the thyroid gland.

Clinical Features

♦ Voice hoarseness

♦ Rapid increase in size, there are compressive symptoms, such as dyspnea or dysphagia

♦ Lymphadenopathy

♦ Sudden, unexplained weight loss

♦ Nervousness

♦ Rapid or irregular heartbeat.

Management

♦ Surgery should be performed in the following instances:
  • Reaccumulation of the nodule despite 3 to 4 repeated FNACs
  • Size in excess of 4 cm
  • Complex cyst on thyroid ultrasound (showing solid and cystic components)
  • Compressive symptoms
  • Signs of malignancy (vocal cord dysfunction, lymphadenopathy)

♦ Oral thyroxine therapy to suppress pituitary secretion of thyroid-stimulating hormone, thereby removing an important growth factor for thyroid follicle cells.

9. NUTRITION AND METABOLIC DEFECTS

Q.1. Write short note on vitamin A deficiency.
(Feb 2006, 5 Marks) (Mar 2009, 5 Marks)
Or
Describe the clinical features of vitamin A deficiency.
(Feb 2013, 5 Marks)

Ans. Deficiency of vitamin A causes interference with growth, reduced resistance to infections and interference with nutrition of cornea, conjunctiva, trachea, hair follicle and renal pelvis.

♦ Vitamin A deficiency interferes with ability of eyes to adapt to darkness and impairs visual affinity.

♦ Children with vitamin A deficiency will experience impaired growth and development.

Causes

♦ Poor intake

♦ Malabsorption

♦ Disease of liver and intestine.

Clinical Features

♦ Earliest sign of deficiency of vitamin is difficulty in reading or sewing at night or finding anything in darkness.

♦ Conjunctiva becomes dry and small grayish white raised spots appear. Bitot's spots form grayish white triangular plaques on conjunctival surface lateral to cornea.

♦ Microcytic anemia.

♦ Cornea subsequently becomes dry and lusterless, and if there is lack of treatment changes are irreversible.

♦ *Keratomalacia involving the cornea leading to the ulceration and blindness may result.

♦ Children with vitamin A deficiency not only have retarded growth but also increased tendency to chest infection.

♦ Skin become dry and rough

♦ Imperfect enamel formation of teeth.

♦ *Hemeralopia:* Patient is unable to see bright light.

♦ Asteatosis, i.e., persistent dry scaling of the skin is the earliest manifestation.

♦ Phrynoderma, i.e., toad skin. Brown to dark brown, dry, rough, hyperkeratotic follicular papules with central keratotic horny spurs. Bilateral and symmetrical distribution in anterolateral aspects of thighs, posterolateral aspects of arms.

Treatment

♦ Prevention of vitamin A deficiency by giving good nutrition, intake of fresh leafy green vegetables and addition of vitamin A to food stuffs.

♦ Single dose of oral retinol palmitate 60 mg or 200,000 IU should be given. In cases of diarrhea, 50 mg IV may be given. Second dose is repeated next day and the third and last dose is given at the time of follow-up visit.

♦ Various other associated conditions, such as diarrhea, dehydration, electrolytic imbalance, protein energy malnutrition should be treated by appropriate measures.

♦ For local treatment of eyes patient should be sent to ophthalmologist.

♦ If primary or secondary infections are present, antibiotics should be given to the patient.

Q 12. *Pyelography = X-ray photography of kidneys, renal pelvis, ureters and urinary bladder after injection with radiopaque contrast dye.
*Perirenal insufflation = The obsolete technique of instilling air into the perirenal space in order to visualize the adrenal gland better on radiographic studies.
*Tomography = A raddiographic technique that selects a level in the body and blurs out structures above and below that plane, leaving a clear image of selected anatomy. It is accomplished by moving the X-ray tube in the opposite direction from a imaging device around a stationary fulcrum defining the plane of interest.

Q 1. *Keratomalacia = Softening of cornea in early childhood due to deficiency of vitamin A.

Q.2. Write short notes on beriberi. *(Sep 1999, 5 Marks)*

Ans. Beriberi is caused due to the deficiency of vitamin B1, i.e., thiamine.

Deficiency of vitamin B1 affects growth, nutrition and carbohydrate metabolism.

Etiology

Deficiency of vitamin B1 occurs due to:

♦ Chronic alcohol intake
♦ Severe malnutrition
♦ Chronic debilitating diseases

Pathogenesis

Thiamine forms an essential part of two coenzymes which are important in oxidative decarboxylation of alpha-ketoacidosis. Deficiency of vitamin leads to accumulation of alpha- ketoacidosis whose toxic effects results in production of beriberi.

Types of Beriberi

♦ *Wet Beriberi or cardiovascular beriberi:* Beriberi is wet when there is cardiac involvement.
♦ *Dry beriberi or neuritic type:* Beriberi is dry when there is CNS involvement.

Clinical Features

♦ *Beri-beri*
  • *Wet beriberi:* Palpitation, dyspnea, Cardiomegaly, warm extremities, anasarca (severe generalized edema), signs of congestive heart failure in late stage.
  • *Dry beriberi:* Cramps, tingling and numbness in the limbs, nystagmus (cyclic movements of eyes), wrist and foot drop, ataxia, loss of equilibrium, paresthesia and confusion.
♦ *Wernick's encephalopathy:* There is involvement of brain which is characterized by ataxia, ophthalmoplegia, confusion and disorientation.
♦ *Korsakoff psychosis:* It occurs due to involvement of mammillary bodies and confabulates with amnesia.
♦ Presence of angular stomatitis.

Diagnosis

♦ Blood thiamine is low
♦ Raised pyruvate and lactate levels.
♦ Low urinary excretion of thiamine and its metabolites
♦ Measuring of whole blood or erythrocyte transketolase activity before and after addition of thiamine. In this there is low transketolase activity which increases by 15% after addition of thiamine confirm the diagnosis.
♦ There is clinical improvement after single dose of thiamine, i.e., 50 mg IM with increase in diastolic blood pressure and decrease in heart rate is another diagnostic criteria.

Treatment

♦ Vitamin B1 (50–100 mg daily) IM or IV is given.

♦ As acute crisis is over, patient has given small dose of 5 mg daily along with nourishing diet.
♦ Diet consists of high B complex and protein content like eggs, milk, nuts and green vegetables.
♦ Wet beriberi with cardiac involvement require digoxin and diuretics, if congestive heart failure is present.

Q.3. Describe briefly vitamin D deficiency.
(Mar 2010, 5 Marks)

Ans. Vitamin D deficiency leads to rickets in growing child and osteomalacia in adults.

Vitamin D is essential in calcium and phosphorus metabolism. It is required for normal development of bones and teeth.

Deficiency of vitamin D causes imperfect skeletal formation, bone disease, rickets and caries.

Vitamin D Deficiency Rickets

It occurs generally in growing children.

Clinical Features

♦ In first six months of life tetany and convulsions are common. These above manifestations are due to hypocalcaemia.
♦ Wrist and ankles are swollen
♦ Changes in bone are found in epiphyseal plates, metaphysis and shaft.
♦ Localized area of thinning are sometime present in skull so that a finger can produce indentation. This condition is called craniotabes.
♦ Pigeon breast is present.
♦ Developmental abnormalities of dentin and delayed eruption.
♦ Higher caries index.
♦ Hypoplasia of enamel is present.
♦ Pulp chamber is large.
♦ Malocclusion of teeth is present.

Investigations

♦ *Radiological:* Radiograph of wrist show widening of distal ends of shaft of both radius and ulna. Zone of epiphyseal cartilage get thickened. As these changes get completely developed, they cause saucer shaped deformity.
♦ *Biochemical changes:*
  • Low plasma calcium and phosphate levels
  • High serum alkaline phosphatase levels
  • Plasma 25 dehydroxy cholecalciferol is low or absent.

Vitamin D Deficiency Osteomalacia

It is also known as adult rickets. Only flat bones and diaphysis of long bones are affected.

Clinical Features

♦ Pelvic deformities are seen in females.
♦ Remodeling of bone occur in absence of adequate calcium resulting in softening and distortion of skeleton.
♦ Bone pain and muscle weakness is present.
♦ Severe periodontitis is present.

Management of Rickets and Osteomalacia

♦ Dietary enrichment of vitamin D in form of milk.

♦ If tetany is present give IV calcium gluconate. Daily dose is 1000–2000 IU of vitamin D combined with 500–1000 mg of calcium.

♦ Curative treatment includes 2000–4000 IU of calcium daily for 6–12 weeks followed by daily maintenance dose of 2000–4000 IU for long period.

♦ Patients with osteomalacia require large dose of vitamin D and calcium, i.e., 40,000–1,00,000 IU of vitamin D and 15–20 g of calcium lactate per day.

Q.4. **Write short note on protein calorie malnutrition.**
(Jan 2012, 5 Marks)

Ans. Protein calorie malnutrition leads to marasmus.

Marasmus

It is seen in infants and young children.

In marasmus, there is total deficiency of calories including protein deficiency.

Causes

♦ Poor intake of breastfeeds and or inadequate supply of milk and other nutrients.

♦ Lack of digestion

♦ Impaired absorption of protein.

♦ Protein is absorbed but cannot be metabolized satisfactorily.

♦ Protein is metabolized but not properly utilized.

Clinical Features

It occurs below the age of 1 year

♦ There is progressive loss of subcutaneous fat.

♦ Child is irritable and cries excessively.

♦ Typical appearance of monkey face.

♦ Sunken and lusterless eyes.

♦ Delay in sitting, standing and walking.

♦ Abdomen may be *distended or sunken and it does not has fat in wall

♦ Lack of playful movements and persistent crying.

♦ Gross degree of muscle wasting is present

♦ Limbs are thin, look like sticks and buttocks do not contain fat.

♦ Head is large for body and ribs are visible.

Management

♦ Correction of fluid, electrolytes, acidosis, hypoglycemia, hypothermia.

♦ Look for the infections and treat them from proper antibiotic therapy.

♦ Diet is given to the child which is rich in proteins, energy and essential nutrients. Diet therapy should be continued till the child attains normal weight as well as nutritional status.

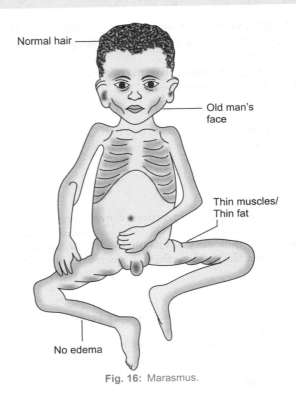

Fig. 16: Marasmus.

Labels: Normal hair · Old man's face · Thin muscles/Thin fat · No edema

Q.5. **Write causes and management of malnutrition in India.** *(Oct 2003, 5 Marks)*

Ans.

Causes of Malnutrition

♦ *Due to defective intake of food:*
  • Loss of appetite due to depression, anxiety, anorexia nervosa, etc.
  • Due to persistent vomiting
  • Alcohol intake
  • Unbalanced therapeutic diet
  • Administration of prolong IV fluids, parenteral fluids in hospitalized patients

♦ *Maldigestion and disordered absorption:*
  • In hypochlorhydria or achlorhydria
  • In steatorrhea
  • Intestinal hurry due to surgical resection
  • Due to prolong use of antibiotics

♦ *Defective utilization:*
  • In cirrhosis of liver
  • In malignancy
  • In infections
  • In renal failure
  • Due to inborn error of metabolism, i.e., Hartnup's disease
  • Due to drugs, such as anti-epileptics

Q 4. *Distended = To stretch out.

◆ *Loss of nutrients from body:*
- Proteinuria in nephrotic syndrome leads to hypoproteinemia.
- In diabetes mellitus, glycosuria causes loss of energy and undernutrition
- Due to excessive menstrual blood loss
- Hypokalemia due to severe persistent diarrhea.

◆ *Due to increased demands:*
- In pregnancy, lactation, adolescence, illness and heavy manual work.
- In fever and thyrotoxicosis
- In burn, surgery and trauma, there is increase in catabolism of proteins and vitamin C.
- Malignant cachexia causes loss of weight due to increased demand.

Treatment of Malnutrition

In Adults

◆ For mild starvation, adequate supplementation of nutrients is necessary
◆ In moderately starved people, extra-feeding is needed
◆ In severely starved persons, food is given in small amount at frequent intervals. Food should be staple meal, i.e., cereal with some sugar, milk and oils, salt is restricted. Potassium, magnesium and vitamins are adequately given. This is continued till patient feel active.

In Children

◆ **Diet**
- **Diet for mild-to-moderate cases:** Diet should be easily digestable. It should be rich in proteins, minerals and vitamins with extra calories. Milk should be given. Egg is a good flip with milk and water as a source of first class protein. Plant protein mixtures, such as corn, soya, diet milk can be given. Additional fats should be included. If there is lactose intolerance dal, rice and butter can be given.
- **Diet for acute cases:** Protein intake should be 3 to 4 g/kg/day and energy intake of 150 kcal/kg/day. If child is unable to take diet from mouth go for nasogastric intubation. Care must be taken to take suffieicnt amount of plant, animal proteins and fats to maintain the weight.

◆ **Vitamins and mineral supplementations**
- Vitamin A, D, B complex and C are given at therapeutic dosages.
- In vitamin A deficiency 30 mg of vitamin A should be given for 3 days.
- 0.5–1 g of potassium chloride dissolve in feeds or water should be given daily in divided dosages.

◆ **Maintenance of body temperature**
For maintenance of body temperature at night blankets or room heaters are useful.

◆ **Skin care**
- In cases of dermatoses skin should be kept clean and protected.

◆ **In hospital treatment**
- Correction of dehydration, electrolyte disturbances, hypoglycemia, acidosis and hypothermia.
- Parenteral therapy with half of saline and 2.5% glucose before diet therapy.
- In anemia, packed erythrocyte infusion is given.

Q.6. Write short note on osteoporosis.

(Oct 2007, 5 Marks)

Ans. Osteoporosis is a group of skeletal disorders characterized by reduction in bone mass per unit bone volume, which results in increased risk of fracture, even in absence of noticeable injury.

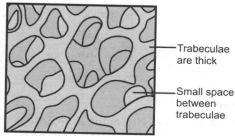

Fig. 17: Normal cancellous bone.

- Trabeculae are thick
- Small space between trabeculae

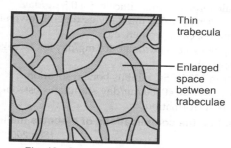

Fig. 18: Osteoporotic cancellous bone.

- Thin trabecula
- Enlarged space between trabeculae

Causes

◆ *Dietary calcium deficiency: E*specially in case of women both premenopausal and postmenopausal. Apart from increased requirements, degree of calcium absorption from intestine decreases with age.
◆ Excessive alcohol or caffeine.
◆ Genetic influences.

Other disorders affecting mineral homeostasis:

◆ *Endocrine:* Cushing syndrome, hyperthyroidism, type I diabetes mellitus, hypogonadism and acromegaly
◆ *Drugs:* Glucocorticoids, thyroxin and diuretics.

Clinical Features

◆ Bone loss progresses for many years without causing symptoms.
◆ Shortened heights, bone pain, low back pain, difficulty in getting up from chair are complaints in women at menopause with osteoporosis.
◆ Signs of osteoporosis include deformities of skeleton, such as kyphosis (Dowager's hump) and loss of height especially in vertebral compression fracture.

Diagnosis

♦ *History of fracture:* Fractures associated with osteoporosis are vertebral fractures, hip fractures and Colle's fracture of distal radius.

♦ *Radiograph:* It shows prominence of vertical trabeculae, generalized loss of contrast between bone and soft tissue.

♦ *Bone density measurement:* Dual energy X-ray absorptiometry is the gold standard. It is performed in spine, both hips and both wrists. Bone densities are then plotted against normal database to provide standard deviation from normal, i.e., T score. For post-menopausal women, T score values are:

1 to 0	is normal
0 to –1	is normal
–1 to –2.5	is osteopenia
<2.5	is osteoporosis

Management

♦ Active physical activity helps to maintain strength, flexibility and coordination of body improves.

♦ Calcium 1.5–2 g/day, if calcium malabsorption is there, cholecalciferol 0.25 mg, alfacalcidol 0.5 μg/day.

♦ *Estrogen therapy:* 0.635 mg daily estrogen is given in small thin women, early women, etc.

♦ Biphosphates, i.e., etidronate 400 mg/day for 2 weeks inhibit bone resorption.

♦ Calcitonin 100 IU SC inhibits bone resorption.

♦ Sodium fluoride 40–60 mg/day stimulates osteoblasts and causes bone formation.

Q.7. Mention the complications of diabetes mellitus.

(Sep 2006, 5 Marks)

Or

Write short note on complications of diabetes mellitus. *(Mar 2016, 3 Marks) (Apr 2010, 5 Marks)*

(Mar 2011, 4 Marks)

Or

Enumerate the complications of diabetes mellitus.

(Feb/Mar 2005, 5 Marks)

Or

Write notes on ten complications of diabetes mellitus. (Only names) *(Dec 2009, 10 Marks)*

Ans. Diabetes mellitus is collection of disorders that have hyperglycemia as hallmark.

Complications

Acute or Immediate Complications

♦ Diabetic ketoacidosis or coma

♦ Hypoglycemia or hypoglycemic coma

♦ Non-ketotic hyperosmolar diabetic coma

♦ Lactic acidosis

First two complications occur in Type I diabetes mellitus and other two occur in Type II diabetes mellitus.

Diabetic Ketoacidosis

♦ It is an exclusive complication of type I diabetes. It can develop in patients with severe insulin deficiency combined with glucagon excess. Failure to take insulin and exposure to stress are precipitating causes.

♦ As the ketogenesis continues the excess ketone bodies produced cannot be degraded by the muscles and other tissues resulting in ketosis, which manifests as anorexia, nausea, vomiting, deep and fast breathing, mental confusion and coma. However, most of the patients recover.

Hypoglycemia

♦ It is defined as fall in blood glucose concentration below 3.1 mmol/L.

♦ It is seen in type I diabetes patients due to excessive administration of insulin, missing a meal or due to stress.

♦ As the hypoglycemia continues, it can lead to comma, cardiac arrhythmias and is fatal.

♦ This can lead to worsening of control of diabetes and rebound hyperglycemia.

Nonketotic Hyperosmolar Diabetic Coma

♦ It is common in type II diabetes mellitus.

♦ The clinical hallmark is hyperglycemia, hyperosmolality and dehydration without ketoacidosis.

♦ Precipitating features are infection, myocardial infarction, drugs, such as thiazides, steroids, diphenylhydantoin.

♦ Loss of glucose in urine is so intense that the patient is unable to drink sufficient water to maintain urinary fluid loss.

♦ Because of high viscosity of blood, thrombotic and bleeding complications are frequent. Mortality rate is high in this complication.

Lactic Acidosis

♦ It is seen in type II diabetes mellitus.

♦ It is caused due to excess lactate production and/or inadequate utilization.

♦ This can be precipitated by metformin or other systemic disorders, such as liver or renal failure, pancreatitis or leukemia.

♦ Cardiovascular collapse leads to mortality.

Chronic or Late Onset Complications

These complications are due to changes in small blood vessels, i.e., microangiopathy or in large blood vessels, i.e., macroangiopathy.

Microvascular are retinopathy, neuropathy, nephropathy and miscellaneous.

Macrovascular are atherosclerosis, hypertension, peripheral vascular disease and diabetic foot ulcer.

The chronic complications occur more frequently in Type II diabetes mellitus rather than Type I diabetes mellitus.

Diabetic Retinopathy

♦ This is the very important cause of blindness in diabetic patients.

- Dilatation of retinal capillaries is earliest sign. Besides these there is also presence of microaneurysms, retinal hemorrhage, neovascularization, hard and soft exudates, vitreous hemorrhage and fibrosis.
- Frequency, onset and severity of retinopathy vary in diabetic patients.
- Background retinopathy is most common and proliferative retinopathy is less common.

Diabetic Neuropathy

- It can involve any part of nervous system except the brain.
- Neuropathy is an early and common complication which leads to morbidity and disability.
- Poor glycemic control and long duration of diabetes is associated with high incidence of neuropathy.
- Sign and symptoms are of peripheral nervous system.
- Main pathological changes in peripheral nerves are axonal degeneration of myelinated and non-myelinated fibers, Segmental demyelination, Schwann cell injury.

Diabetic Nephropathy

- This is the most common cause of mortality and morbidity in diabetic patients.
- About 40 to 50% of type II diabetes patient develop it and 25% patients with type I diabetes develop end stage renal disease and die of it.
- It is divided into three stages, in first stage patient is asymptomatic but has high GFR, in next stage there is renal hypertrophy which leads to microalbuminuria. In advance stage, patient develop macroproteinuria and passes onto nephrotic syndrome.
- About 25% of patients with diabetic nephropathy can go directly at end stage renal disease with hypertension and undergo chronic renal failure.

Miscellaneous

It consists of various infections, gastroparesis, arthropathy.

Atherosclerosis

- In diabetic patient development of atheroma is faster as compared to normal individual.
- Hyperlipidemia, decreased HDL levels, increased platelet adhesiveness, obesity and associated hypertension are contributory factors for atherosclerosis.
- Atherosclerosis leads to coronary artery disease, silent myocardial infarction, cerebral stroke and gangrene of toes and feet.

Diabetic foot ulcer

- This is the frequent site of complication in diabetes.
- Pathogenic components of diabetic foot are neuropathy, peripheral vascular disease causing ischemia and secondary infection causing ulceration.

Q.8. Write short note on treatment of diabetes mellitus.

(Apr 2017, 6 Marks)

Ans.

Management

I. Diet Management

- Restoration of normal blood glucose and optimum levels.
- Maintenance of blood glucose levels as near to physiologic levels to prevent onset or progression of complications.
- Maintenance of normal growth rate in children and adolescents as well as attainment and maintenance of reasonable body weight in adolescents and children.
- Provision of adequate nutrition for pregnant women and fetus during lactation.
- Consistency in timing of meals and snacks to prevent inordinate swings in blood glucose level.
- Motivation to have small frequent meals.
- Determination of meal plan appropriate for individual and based on dietary history to have good compliance.
- Management of weight reduction for obese individuals with NIDDM.
- Improvement in the overall health of patients with diabetes through optimal nutrition.

Total Calories

Requirements are determined by the patients activity:

- Overweight NIDDM should be encouraged to establish their weight within a desirable range. A reduction of approximately 500 kcal/day can result in loss of 1–2 kg/month.
- *Carbohydrates:* Carbohydrates should be taken in form of starch and complex sugars. 100–300 g of carbohydrates should be spreaded over 3 meals, i.e., 60 g each and 3 snacks, i.e., 30 g each with half liter of milk. Unrefined carbohydrates should be substituted by refined carbohydrates to the extent possible.
- *Proteins:* Recommended dietary allowance of 0.85 g/kg body weight for adult is an appropriate guide.
- *Fat:* Fat intake should be 50–150 g daily divided between the meals. Replacement of saturated with polyunsaturated fat is desirable to reduce cardiovascular risk. Cholesterol intake should be <300 mg/day.
- *Fiber:* Increased consumption of dietary fiber especially soluble fiber are associated with lower levels of blood glucose and serum lipids. The water insoluble fibers, such as cellulose, lignin and most hemicelluloses found in whole grain breads, cereals and wheat bran affect gastrointestinal transit time and fecal bulk with little impact on plasma glucose. However highly viscous water soluble fibers, such as pectins, gums and storage polysaccharide found in fruits, legumes, lentils roots, tubers, oat and oat bran, when eaten in purified form, reduce serum levels of glucose and insulin. Ideal recommended amount of fiber in patient's diet is 35–40 g/day.
- *Alternative sweeteners:* Both nutritive and non-nutritive sweeteners are acceptable in diabetes management.
- *Sodium:* It should be restricted to 1000 mg/1000 kcal, not to exceed 3000 mg/day to minimize symptoms of hypertension.

♦ *Alcohol:* It should be taken in moderation and may need to be restricted entirely by person with diabetes and insulin—induced hypoglycemia, neuropathy, poor control of glucose and lipids, or obesity.

♦ *Vitamins, minerals and antioxidants:* intake should be encouraged.

Forbidden foods: Sugar, jam, jellies, honey, jaggery, tinned fruits and juices, sweets, chocolate, ice creams, pastries, glucose drinks, foods made with sugar, pudding, sauces.

Foods allowed in moderation: Bread of all kinds and *chapattis* made from wheat or millets, plain biscuits, all fresh fruits, baked beans, breakfast cereals.

Free foods: All meat, fish, eggs (not fried), clear soup or meat extracts; tea or coffee; vegetables, such as cabbage, cauliflower, spinach, pumpkin, brinjal, lady's finger, turnip, French beans, cucumber, lettuce, tomato, spring onions, radish, asparagus. Spices, salt, pepper and mustard; butter and margarine. Sugar substitutes for sweetening.

II. Oral Hypoglycemics

These drugs are used in patients of Type II diabetes mellitus (NIDDM) who do not respond to dietary management and who would otherwise require treatment with insulin in later situation, so they are also used as adjuvant drugs to insulin in overweight diabetes patients.

♦ Insulin secretagogues, i.e., drugs increasing secretion of insulin
- Sulfonylureas

Name of drug	Intial daily dose (mg)	Dose/ day	Comment
First generation			
Acetohexamide	250 mg	1–2	Has diuretic and uricosuric activity
Chlorpropamide	100 mg	1–2	Can potentiate ADH
Tolazamide	100 mg	1–2	Disulfiram-like action with alcohol in 1/3rd of patients, Has diuretic activity
Second generation			
Glibenclamide	2.5–20 mg	1–2	Hypoglycemia can be severe
Gliclazide	40–320 mg	1–2	Metabolism/excretion by liver/kidney
Glipizide	5 mg	1–2	Mild diuretic activity
Glyburide	2.5 mg	1–2	Highest risk of hypoglycernia
Glimepiride	1 mg	1	Excreted in urine and bile

- *Meglitinides:*
  - Repaglinide, i.e., 0.5–4 mg three times a day
  - Nateglinide, i.e., 60–120 mg three times a day 15 to 30 min before each meal

- Voglibose, i.e., 0.2–0.3 mg, 15–30 min before each meal.

♦ Insulin sensitizers, i.e., drugs sensitizing action of insulin and overcome insulin resistance
- Biguanides, i.e., metformin should be given 1.5–2.5 g/day in three divided doses after meals.
- Thiazolidinediones, i.e., rosiglitazone should be given 2–8 mg or pioglitazone 15–45 mg in a single or two divided doses. They can be combined with sulfonylureas or metformin

♦ Alpha glucosidase inhibitors, i.e., Acarbose 25 to 100 mg TDS or Voglibose 0.2–5 mg TDS taken orally in three main meals. It can be given in combination with metformin 500 mg for increased efficiency.

♦ *DPP-4 inhibitor:* Vildagliptin 50–100 mg daily in two dived doses with meals ot saxagliptin 2.5 to 5 mg OD.

♦ *Pramlintide:* Initial dose is 15 µg before each meals in Type I diabetes mellitus and 60 µg in Type II diabetes mellitus.

III. Insulin

Following are the indications for insulin therapy:
♦ In type I diabetes mellitus
♦ In gestational diabetes
♦ Hyperglycemia despite maximum doses of oral agents
♦ Decompensation due to intercurrent events, such as infection, acute injury or stress
♦ Development of severe hyperglycemia with ketosis
♦ Perioperative in patients undergoing surgery
♦ Kidney or hepatic disease

Various Insulin Preparations

Insulin preparation	Onset (Hours)	Peak (Hours)	Duration (Hours)
Rapid acting			
Regular	½–1	2–4	6–8
Lispro (analogue)	¼–½	1–2	3–5
Intermediate acting			
NPH (isophane)	1–4	8–10	12–20
Lente (insulin zinc suspension)	2–4	8–12	12–20
Long acting			
Ultralente (Extended insulin zinc suspension)	3–5	10–16	18–24

Treatment Strategies with Insulin

♦ *Single dose regimen:* Daily injection of intermediate-acting insulin given before breakfast. The starting dose 0.3–0.4 U/kg/day; increased gradually to obtain glucose values in acceptable range. Regular insulin can be added to decrease the glucose level that follows breakfast.

♦ *Twice daily regimen:* Combination of regular and intermediate acting insulin BD, i.e., before breakfast and before dinner ("Split mix" regimen).

♦ *Multiple daily injections:* For achievement of more tight control of blood glucose which requires administration of at least 3 injections per day. These can be given with use of mixture of intermediate- and short-acting insulins (pre-mixed insulin) in the morning before breakfast, with regular insulin before supper- and intermediate-acting at bedtime; or again a combination of regular and intermediate-acting before dinner. Divide the total daily into 2 equal doses following 1:1 transfer from basal insulin. Give half before breakfast and other half before dinner. The largest meal will require larger proportion of insulin. Reduce total dose by 20%, if patient experiences recurrent hypoglycemia.

♦ *Insulin concentrations:* The insulins are available in many concentrations. In India, the commonly used is 40 U/mL

♦ *Insulin purity:* The impurities which may be contained are proinsulin, insulin intermediates and contaminating proteins from islet tissue or exocrine pancreas, such as glucagon, somatostatin and pancreatic polypeptides. Standard insulins currently have only 10–20 PPM of proinsulin and purified monocomponent insulins less than 1 PPM.

Best sites for the insulin injection are subcutaneous fat on abdomen, buttock, anterior thigh and dorsal area of arm.

IV Exercise

♦ Exercise must be adjusted to patient's preference and existing medical condition.

♦ Aerobic exercise is preferred, i.e., swimming, cycling, walking, running. etc

♦ Addition of moderate resistance should be considered.

♦ Duration should be 20–45 minutes per session.

♦ Frequency is 3–4 sessions per week is required to observe beneficial metabolic effects. 4–5 sessions per week for weight reduction.

♦ ADA recommends 150 min/week of moderate aerobic physical activity with no gaps longer than 2 days.

♦ Program of exercise should be:
  • Stretching for 5–10 min
  • Warm up for 5–10 min
  • Exercise for 20–45 min
  • Warm down for 10 min at 30% of full exercise intensity.

Q.9. Write short note on insulin. *(Feb 2006, 5 Marks)*

Ans. Insulin is required for proper control of diabetes and to keep blood sugar within limits.

Following are the indications for insulin therapy:

♦ In type I diabetes mellitus
♦ In gestational diabetes
♦ Hyperglycemia despite maximum doses of oral agents
♦ Decompensation due to intercurrent events, such as infection, acute injury or stress
♦ Development of severe hyperglycemia with ketosis
♦ Perioperative in patients undergoing surgery
♦ Kidney or hepatic disease

Various Insulin Preparations

Insulin preparation	Onset (Hours)	Peak (Hours)	Duration (Hours)
Rapid acting			
Regular	½–1	2–4	6–8
Lispro (Analogue)	¼–½	1–2	3–5
Intermediate acting			
NPH (Isophane)	1–4	8–10	12–20
Lente (Insulin zinc suspension)	2–4	8–12	12–20
Long acting			
Ultralente (Extended insulin zinc suspension)	3–5	10–16	18–24

Treatment Strategies with Insulin

♦ *Single dose regimen:* Daily injection of intermediate acting insulin given before breakfast. The starting dose 0.3–0.4 U/kg/day; increased gradually to obtain glucose values in acceptable range. Regular insulin can be added to decrease the glucose level that follows breakfast.

♦ *Twice daily regimen:* Combination of regular and intermediate acting insulin BD, i.e., before breakfast and before dinner ("Split mix" regimen).

♦ *Multiple daily injections:* For achievement of more tight control of blood glucose which requires administration of at least 3 injections per day. These can be given with use of mixture of intermediate- and short acting insulins (pre-mixed insulin) in the morning before breakfast, with regular insulin before supper- and intermediate- acting at bedtime; or again a combination of regular and intermediate acting before dinner. Divide the total daily into 2 equal doses following 1:1 transfer from basal insulin. Give half before breakfast and other half before dinner. The largest meal will require larger proportion of insulin. Reduce total dose by 20%, if patient experiences recurrent hypoglycemia.

♦ *Insulin concentrations:* The insulins are available in many concentrations. In India, the commonly used is 40 U/mL

♦ *Insulin purity:* The impurities which may be contained are proinsulin, insulin intermediates and contaminating proteins from islet tissue or exocrine pancreas, such as glucagon, somatostatin and pancreatic polypeptides. Standard insulins currently have only 10–20 PPM of proinsulin and purified monocomponent insulins less than 1 PPM.

Site of Insulin Injection

Best sites for the insulin injection are subcutaneous fat on abdomen, buttock, anterior thigh and dorsal area of arm.

Insulin Delivery System

♦ Insulin pens are used in both Type I and Type II diabetes mellitus.

♦ Continuous insulin infusion systems are used in Type II diabetes mellitus.

Complications

Following are the complications of insulin therapy:

♦ *Hypoglycemia:* It is the most frequent and most serious reaction. Hypoglycemia can occur in any diabetic following inadvertent injection of large doses, by missing a meal or by performing various exercises

♦ *Local reaction:* Swelling, erythema and stinging sometimes occurs especially in beginning. *Lipodystrophy occurs at injection site after long usage.

♦ *Insulin allergy:* This is infrequent and is due to contaminating proteins. Urticaria, angiedema and anaphylaxis are manifestations.

♦ *Edema:* Some patients develop short-lived dependent edema when insulin therapy is started.

♦ *Weight gain:* Patients on long-term insulin therapy gain weight.

Q.10. Outline management of diabetic comma.

(Feb 1999, 5 Marks)

Ans. Diabetic ketoacidosis or diabetic comma is the exaggeration or deranged energy metabolism due to deficiency of insulin which results in accumulation of acid metabolites and ketone bodies.

Management

Following is the management of diabetic comma

♦ **Admission of patient**
- Diagnosis is confirmed by examination of blood glucose and ketone measurements.
- Initial assessment of dehydration, hyperosmolality, serum potassium, acidosis and kidney function is done.
- Fluid loss is measured by subtracting admission weight by last known stable weight.
- Patient should be evaluated for sepsis.

♦ **Management during hour 1**
- If patient is hypovolemic and hypotensive fluid administration is done, i.e., normal saline is administered and if necessary colloids should be given. Rate of administration is necessary to restore circulatory function. As blood pressure become normal and urine output becomes adequate rate of administration of normal saline is 1000 mL/h.
- Continuous IV infusion of regular insulin 5–10 units/h is given.
- IV, infusion of potassium is done at 10–40 mmol/hour during initiation of insulin therapy.
- Sodium bicarbonate IV is given in cases with acidosis. Dose is 50–100 mmol/L sodium bicarbonate in 0.45% saline for 30–60 minutes. Additional potassium should also be given with bicarbonate therapy.

♦ **Management during hour 2**
- Normal saline should be continued at 500 mL/hour. Plasma osmolality should be greater than 285 mmol/L during first 12 hours. If serum sodium is greater than 150 mmol/L switch to 0.45% saline.
- Blood glucose should be checked and insulin is adjusted to 5 mmol/L/h. Blood glucose should not fall below 11.1–14.0 mmol/L. Anion gap is decreasing and blood pH is increasing.

- Serum potassium should be maintained at 4–5 mmol/liter by addition of potassium to IV fluids.

♦ **Management during hours 3 to 4**
- Management should be continued as given in second hour.
- Cognitive and neurological symptoms should be observed for 12 hours.

♦ **Management during hours 5 to 8**
- Normal saline should be continued at 250 mL/hour. As blood glucose reaches 11.1–14 mmol/L, change IV fluid to 500 mL/h normal saline with 5% glucose.
- Insulin should be continued at maintenance dose until ketoacidosis is cleared.
- Potassium should be continued at 10–40 mmol/hour, since ketoacidosis is cleared.
- Phosphate replacement is done at 6 hours, if serum phosphate is <2 mg/dL

♦ **Management during hours 8 to 24**
- IV repletion is continued with 0.45% saline with or without 2.5% or 5% glucose as needed.
- As diabetic comma is subsided, patient should be switched to subcutaneous insulin and stop IV and IM insulin.

Q.11. Differentiate between diabetic comma and hypoglycemic comma.

(Feb 2006, 3 Marks) (Sep 2008, 2.5 Marks)

Ans.

Feature	Diabetic comma	Hypoglycemic comma
Onset	Slow and insidious	Rapid and quick
History	Too little or no insulin	Regular dose of insulin and no food
Precipitating factor	Due to untreated or hidden infection	In severe unaccustomed exercise
Cause	Due to inadequate insulin	Due to excess of insulin
Symptoms	Frequent vomiting with abdominal pain	No vomit/occasional vomit
Signs	• Tongue and skin are dry • Weak or feeble pulse • Breathing is rapid and shallow • Presence of air hunger • Smell of acetone is present • Tendon reflexes are diminished • Plantars are normal	• Tongue and skin are moist • Bounding pulse • Normal breathing • Absence of air hunger • Smell of acetone is absent • Tendon reflexes are brisk • Plantars are extensor
Urine	Glucose and ketone bodies are present	Glucose and ketone bodies are absent
Blood	Low blood glucose, bicarbonate and pH levels are normal	High blood glucose, low bicarbonate and pH
Treatment	Response to treatment is slow	Response to treatment is quick and is very rapid to IV glucose

---

Q 9.   *Lipodystrophy = Abnormal distribution of fat in the body.

Q.12. Write short note on hypoglycemia.

(Sep 2010, 5 Marks)

Ans. Hypoglycemia is defined as fall in blood glucose concentration below 2.5 mmol/L.

It can be present as asymptomatic, mild, severe or may be present as coma.

Etiology

♦ Postprandial
♦ Alcohol ingestion
♦ Starvation, prolonged exercise, infection
♦ Non-islet cell tumors, e.g., hepatoma, adrenal carcinoma, mesothelioma, etc.
♦ Iatrogenic, i.e., drug induced due to oral hypoglycemic, salicylism, due to propranolol.

Clinical features

♦ *Cardiovascular system:* Palpitation, tachycardia, anxiety, cardiac arrhythmias
♦ *Central nervous system:* Tremors, confusion, headache, tiredness, difficulty in concentration, in coordination, slurred speech, drowsiness, convulsion and coma.
♦ *Gastrointestinal tract:* Nausea and vomiting
♦ *Skin:* Sweating and hypothermia

Diagnosis

♦ *In hypoglycemia state:*
  • Suggestive history
  • Dramatic response to IV glucose during attack
  • Low plasma level glucose during attack
  • C-peptide concentration >200 pmL/L
♦ *Of cause:*
  • Clinical: Exclude hypopituitarism, Addison's disease, liver cirrhosis or failure, sarcoma, alcohol ingestion after fasting, self administration of insulin or sulfonylurea.
  • *Investigations for insulinomas:*
    – Overnight fasting plasma glucose and insulin measurements will demonstrate spontaneous hypoglycemia and raised plasma insulin
    – Low plasma C-peptide with high plasma insulin.
    – High fasting plasma proinsulin.

Management

♦ *In acute attack:*
  • Administration of rapidly absorbable carbohydrate
  • In mild reaction, orange juice (100 mL) or corn syrup or candy taken orally sufficient.
  • In unconscious or uncooperative patients 50 mL of 50% glucose IV if vein not available glucagon 1 mg SC or IM will cause sufficient increase in blood sugar to allow the patient to become rational and cooperative.
  • When recovery is slow, e.g., after overdose of insulin or sulfonylurea therapy, constant infusion of 10–20% dextrose is given to maintain the blood sugar.
♦ *Conservative treatment and prevention of acute attacks*
  • *Diet:* Carbohydrate not more than 150 g in slowly absorbable form like cereals, bread, fruits and vegetables. Liberal protein because glucose derived from it is liberated slowly; fat to make up calories. In hepatogenic type bedtime meal to prevent early morning hypoglycemia.
  • Restriction of physical exercise.
♦ *Surgical measures:*
  • Removal of islet cell tumors, or partial resection of pancreas
    – In fulminating cases where convulsions are not controlled by glucose.
    – In severe, chronic cases not controlled by diet.
    – Patients with marked, neuropsychiatric symptoms.
♦ *Drugs*
  • *Glucagon:* The efficacy depends on size of hepatic glycogen stores. The drug has little effect on blood glucose in patients who have been fasting or are hypoglycemic for long periods. IM injection of 1mL of glucagon is given, if hypoglycemia is insulin induced.
  • *Diazoxide and Octreotide* may be used to control symptoms while the patient is awaiting surgery or when the patient is not a candidate for surgery.

Q.13. Write short note on vitamin B12 deficiency.

(Feb 2002, 5 Marks)

Ans. It is also known as Wonder vitamin and cyanocobalamin.

Causes of Vitamin B12 Deficiency

♦ Due to inadequate dietary intake
♦ Due to malabsorption
  • Intrinsic factor deficiency in pernicious anemia, gastrectomy, congenital lack of intrinsic factor
  • Intestinal causes, i.e., tropical sprue, Ileal resection, Crohn's disease
  • Removal of vitamin B12 from intestines, i.e., in tapeworm infestation and due to bacterial proliferation in intestinal blind loop syndrome
  • Drugs, such as neomycin, PAS and colchicine.

Clinical Features

♦ *Blood:* Megaloblastic anemia
♦ *General features:* Pallor, anorexia, diarrhea
♦ *Oral manifestations:* Glossitis, glossodynia, angular stomatitis, xerostomia
♦ *Nervous system manifestations:*
  • *Subjective sensory disturbances:* Paresthesia, Tingling and numbness in toes, tips of fingers, rarely simultaneously in both upper and lower extremities. Sometimes burning or stabbing pains or even lightning pains like tabes.
  • *Objective sensory loss:* Sense of vibration, posture and passive movement affected first in lower, later in upper limbs. Glove and stocking type of superficial sensory loss. Tenderness of calf muscles.
  • *Motor symptoms:* Pyramidal weakness and ataxia develop at variable interval after onset of sensory disturbances.
  • *Reflexes:* Ankle jerks lost, knee jerks may be absent. Both exaggerated, if lateral column lesion predominates. Plantars extensor.

- *Sphincter disturbances:* First difficult or precipitate micturition, later retention of urine or incontinence. Impotence is early.
- *Mental changes:* Mild dementia, impaired memory. Confusional psychosis or irritability or depression.
- Bilateral primary optic atrophy in 5%.

Diagnosis

- Presence of low hemoglobin
- Macrocytosis,
- High MCHC
- Megaloblastic bone marrow
- Gastric achlorhydria
- Serum vitamin B12 less than 100 pg/mL
- Elevated homocysteine

Treatment

- Vitamin B12 deficiency especially in those with megaloblastic anemia is treated by giving hydroxocobalamin 1000 microgram IM twice a week for first week. This is followed by 1000 µg weekly for 6 weeks.
- Replacement therapy is given throughout the life in dosage of hydroxocobalamin 1000 µg IM for every three months.
- For patients sensitive to injections, Oral B$_{12}$ in large daily doses is given, i.e., 100 µg or more.

Q.14. Write short note on scurvy.

(Dec 2012, 3 Marks) (Feb/Mar 2004, 5 Marks)

Ans. Deficiency of vitamin C leads to scurvy.

Due to vitamin C deficiency, there is defective collagen formation.

Etiology

- In artificially fed infants
- It is precipitated by febrile disease, infections and diarrhea

Clinical Features

- Onset of the disease is usually gradual, there is fretfulness and increasing pallor, or tenderness of legs which causes child to cry whenever touched, anorexia and loss of weight. First symptom is inability of the child to use his legs.
- *Symptoms due to hemorrhages:*
  - *Under periosteum of long bones:* "Pithed frog posture" with thighs flexed and abducted and knees flexed, sometimes diffuse swelling above or below the knee; in severe cases, infiltration of muscles with blood causing edematous limbs, i.e woody leg; hemorrhage between diaphysis and epiphysis causes separation of epiphysis from shaft.
  - Perifollicular hemorrhage.
  - In orbit, there is proptosis with swelling of eyelids
  - *Hematuria:* May be an early symptom and is only microscopic.
  - Scorbutic beading of the ribs
- Presence of anemia
- Keratosis of hair follicles with 'corkscrew' hair
- Failure of wound healing

Oral Manifestations

- It chiefly affects the gingival and periodontal region.
- The interdental and marginal gingiva becomes bright red, swollen, smooth, shiny producing appearance known as scurvy bud. In fully developed scurvy, gingiva becomes boggy, ulcerated and bleeds easily
- There is a typical fetid breath of a patient with fusospirochetal stomatitis.
- Color of the gingiva changes to violaceous red.
- In severe cases, hemorrhage and swelling of periodontal ligament membrane occur followed by loss of bone and loosening of teeth which are exfoliated.

Diagnosis

- Low ascorbic acid level in platelets and plasma
- Anemia is mild-to-moderate but may be severe.
- X-ray shows characteristic features, such as
  - Pencilled cortex
  - White lines of Frankel
  - Zone of Trummerfeld
  - Halo sign of Wimberger
  - Subperiosteal hematoma
  - Joint effusion
  - Scorbutic rosary

Management

- About 3 to 4 ounces of fresh orange juice or tomato juice daily.
- Ascorbic acid 100 mg or more orally or parenterally twice or thrice daily for 10 to 15 days.

Q.15. Write short note on balanced diet.

(Feb/Mar 2004, 5 Marks) (Apr 2008, 5 Marks)
(June 2010, 5 Marks) (Aug 2012, 5 Marks)

Or

Write notes on balanced diet.   *(Aug 2011, 10 Marks)*

Or

Write about balanced diet.   *(Mar 2006, 10 Marks)*

Or

Write short answer on balanced diet.

(Sep 2018, 5 Marks)

Ans. A diet adequate in energy providing substances, i.e., carbohydrates and fats, tissue building compounds, i.e., proteins, inorganic chemical, i.e., water and mineral salts, agents that regulate or catalyze metabolic process, i.e., vitamins and substances for certain physiological processes, such as bulk for promoting peristaltic movement of digestive tract known as balanced diet.

- For proper growth, maintenance and development of our body an ideal combination of essential nutrient, vitamins and minerals should be aimed.
- An average Indian diet is poor in quality as well as quantity in meeting the daily needs.
- A balanced diet should contain 30 kcal/kg optimum body weight.

- Balanced diet should contain 60–70% carbohydrates of total calories, 12–18% protein of total calories, 20–25% fats of total calories.
- Diet should contain as much as of fresh fruits, vegetables which provide nutrients.
- Fiber is an important part of the food.
- Milk is an ideal food and contains or proximate the principles of balanced diet.
- A balanced diet not only looks after the well-being of person but may have role to play in prevention of certain diseases.
- So while planning a balanced diet, care should be taken that all essential ingredient in diet are adequately incorporated with fresh fruits, vegetables and fiber diet.
- Food should be palatable, properly cooked and well balanced providing a balance between food intake and energy output.

Q.16. Write note on pellagra. *(Dec 2009, 10 Marks)*

Ans. It is the clinical condition produced due to the deficiency of nicotinic acid or niacin.

Etiology

- Inadequate intake or absorption of niacin.
- Restricted or limited diet in which single serial grain, i.e., corn is consumed without consumption of wheat, eggs, beef and another niacin rich food.
- In chronic alcoholism.

Clinical Features

- Pellagra is triad of dermatitis, diarrhea and dementia.
- Dermatitis is bilaterally symmetrical and occur in parts exposed to sunlight. In acute cases skin lesions may produce vesiculation, cracking, exudation, crusting with ulceration and desquamation. In chronic cases, dermatitis occurs.
- Gastrointestinal manifestations: Presence of anorexia, nausea, dysphagia. Glossitis precede the skin lesions. Diarrhea is also present.
- Mental features consists of apathy, insomnia, fatigue followed by encephalopathy characterized by confusion, disorientation, loss of memory and hallucination.
- Other features: Loss of appetite, irritability and burning sensation in different areas of body.

Oral Manifestations

- Oral mucosa is fiery red and is painful.
- Glossitis is present. Tongue is red, swollen and beefy. In early stage, only the tip and margins of tongue are swollen and red but in advance cases, tongue looses the papillae and reddening is intense.
- Presence of angular stomatitis
- Superimposed acute necrotizing ulcerative gingivitis is present involving gingiva, tongue and mucosa.

Diagnosis

- NAD and NADP levels are low in RBCs in patients with pellagra.
- Plasma tryptophan is low.

Treatment

Initially by injection nicotinamide 50–100 mg IM daily for a week. Maintenance dose of 50 mg orally per day.

Q.17. Write in brief clinical features and management of diabetic ketoacidosis. *(Apr 2007, 5 Marks)*

Ans. Diabetic ketoacidosis or diabetic comma is the exaggeration or deranged energy metabolism due to deficiency of insulin which results in accumulation of acid metabolites and ketone bodies.

Clinical Features

Symptoms

- Polyuria
- Thirst
- Weight loss
- Weakness
- Nausea
- Vomiting
- Leg cramps
- Blurred vision
- Abdominal pain.

Signs

- Dehydration
- Hypotension
- Tachycardia
- Confusion
- Drowsiness
- Comma.

For management, refer to Ans. 10 of same chapter.

Q.18. Write short note on metabolic syndrome X / dysmetabolic syndrome. *(Apr 2007, 5 Marks)*

Ans. Metabolic syndrome is a combination of medical disorders that increase one's risk for cardiovascular disease and diabetes. It affects a large number of people in a clustered fashion.

It is known under various other names, such as (metabolic) syndrome X, insulin resistance syndrome, Reaven's syndrome or CHAOS.

Clinical Features

Symptoms

- Fasting hyperglycemia
- High blood pressure
- Central obesity (also known as visceral, male pattern or apple-shaped adiposity), overweight with fat deposits mainly around the waist.
- Weakness, fatigue and restlessness.

Signs

- Fatty liver (especially in concurrent obesity),
- Non-alcoholic fatty liver disease
- Polycystic ovarian syndrome
- Hemochromatosis (iron overload);
- Acanthosis nigricans (a skin condition featuring dark patches).

Treatment

The main treatment is lifestyle, i.e., caloric restriction and physical activity. However, drug treatment may occasionally be necessary. Generally, the individual diseases that comprise the metabolic syndrome are treated separately, e.g., diuretics and ACE inhibitors for hypertension. Cholesterol drugs may be used to lower LDL cholesterol and triglyceride levels, if they are elevated.

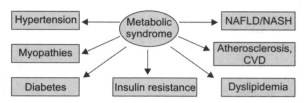

Fig. 19: Metabolic syndrome.

Q.19. Write short note on diabetic ketoacidosis.

(May/June 2009, 5 Marks) (Sep 2007, 5 Marks)
(Dec 2010, 5 Marks)

Or

Write clinical features, etiology diagnoses and management of diabetic ketoacidosis.

(Aug 2018, 12 Marks)

Ans. Diabetic ketoacidosis a state of acidemia induced by excess production of ketoacids. Dehydration and hyperglycemia are the rule and lactic acidosis may also be present.

Pathophysiology

Diabetic ketoacidosis is caused by severe insulin deficiency and is accentuated by excessive glucagon secretion. This leads to major clinical and laboratory abnormalities seen in diabetic ketoacidosis, which includes excess mobilization of free acids from adipose tissue, increased glucose production from the liver, impaired glucose uptake and utilization by muscle. The two major effects of uncontrolled diabetes are:

- Increased glucose production which causes hyperglycemia, osmotic diuresis, electrolyte depletion and dehydration
- Increased ketogenesis, resulting in metabolic acidosis

Precipitating Causes/Etiology

- Acute infection viral or bacterial single most common cause.
- Omission of insulin or inadequate dosage.
- Vomiting.
- Diarrhea.
- Prolonged neglect of diabetes.
- Indiscretions in diet.
- Surgical operations.
- Trauma.
- Myocardial infarction.
- Pregnancy.
- Thyrotoxicosis.
- Resistance to insulin.
- Unnoticed interruption of insulin delivery in diabetics treated with continuous subcutaneous insulin infusion.

Clinical Features

Refer to Ans. 17 of same chapter.

Diagnosis

The cardinal features are:

- Acidosis, i.e., arterial pH ≤ 7.3
- Plasma anion gap ≥ 16 mmol/L
- Serum ketone is positive
- Serum bicarbonate ≥ 15 mmol/L
- Hyperglycemia, i.e., Plasma glucose ≥ 11.1 mmol/L

Management

Refer to Ans. 28 of same chapter.

Q.20. Write short note on vitamin D.

(Feb 2014, 3 Marks) (Mar 2008, 7 Marks)

Ans. Vitamin D are a group of sterol and commonly found in animals mainly there are two types of active form:

D2 - Ergosterol/Ergocalciferol

D3 - 7- dehydrocholesterol.

Source

Fish liver oil, egg yolk, butter milk, the cheapest source is sun light which forms vitamin D3 from its precursor present in the skin.

Physiological Functions

- Vitamin D increases the absorption of Ca and P.
- It increases the calcification of bones in children and adult. So, it is essential for the development of bones and normal growth of body.
- It increases the excretion of phosphate by kidney and helps in lowering of serum phosphate concentration.
- It increase the citrate levels of blood, bone, kidney and heart tissues.
- It decreases the pH in the lower intestinal tract which helps in increasing the absorption of calcium and phosphate.

Daily Requirements

Infants and children:	400 IU
Adult:	200 IU
Pregnant and lactating women:	400 IU

Deficiency of Vitamin D

- *Rickets:* Due to defect in bone growth and calcification of long bones in children.
- *Osteomalacia:* Due to defective calcification of steroid tissue in adult.

Causes of Deficiency of Vitamin D

- Dietary insufficiency or insufficient exposure to sunlight.
- Gastrointestinal disorder.
- Chronic obstructive jaundice.
- Prolonged treatment with anticonvulsant drugs.

Toxicity or Excess of Vitamin D

There is presence of anorexia, lassitude, vomiting, diarrhea, profuse sweating, polydipsia, polyuria and headache. Hypercalcemia causes calcium deposition in tissues and kidneys which leads to renal failure.

Q.21. Write short note on vitamin C.

(Mar 2008, 5.5 Marks) (Mar 2011, 4 Marks)

Ans. Vitamin C was named ascorbic acid owing to its anti-ascorbic properties.

♦ Ascorbic acid is a white crystalline water-soluble substance with sour taste.
♦ It is easily destroyed by cooking.

Absorption and Storage

♦ Ascorbic acid is easily absorbed from the small intestine, peritoneum and subcutaneous tissues.
♦ It is not stored in any particular organ and is spread throughout the body.

Sources

Amla, citrus fruits, tomatoes, guava, green peppers.

Physiological Functions

♦ It is involved in oxidation reaction of cell.
♦ It is required for the metabolism of amino acid, e.g., tyrosine and tryptophan.
♦ It is also involved in conversion of folic acid into its active coenzyme.
♦ It is required for iron absorption and also for the formation of collagen fibers and mucopolysaccharides of connective tissue.

Daily Requirements

♦ Infants: 35 mg
♦ Children: 40 mg
♦ Adults: 45 mg
♦ Pregnant and lactating women 80 mg.

Deficiency Manifestations

♦ Severe ascorbic acid deficiency produces—**Scurvy.**
♦ *For scurvy in detail refer to Ans. 14 of same chapter.*

Q.22. Write short note on Thiamin (Vitamin B1).

(Sep 2009, 4.5 Marks)

Ans.

Thiamine (Vitamin B1)

Synonyms: Anti-beriberi factor, anti-neuritic vitamin, aneurin.

Properties

♦ Thiamine is readily soluble in water
♦ It is stable in acid medium.
♦ It is destroyed when autoclave at 120°C for 30 minutes.

Source

♦ *Rich sources*: Polishing rice, wheat jaw and yeast
♦ *Good source*: Cereals, pulses, nuts, oil seeds
♦ *Fair sources*: Meat, fish, egg, milk, vegetable and fruit.

Daily Requirement

♦ *Infants:* 0.3 to 0.5 mg
♦ *Children:* 0.7 to 1.2 mg
♦ *Adults:* 1 to 1.5 mg
♦ *Pregnant woman:* 1.3 to 1.5 mg.

Physiological Role

♦ Thiamine is essential for growth.
♦ It is essential for maintaining the nerves in normal condition.

Deficiency Manifestations

♦ *Beri-beri:* It is a nutritional disorder.
  • Wet-beriberi
    – Edema is the most prominent feature
    – Anorexia and dyspepsia are present.
  • Dry beriberi
    – Essential feature is polyneuropathy
    – Muscles become wasted and weak and difficulty in walking.
  • Infantile Beriberi.
♦ *Wernick's encephalopathy:* There is involvement of brain which is characterized by ataxia, ophthalmoplegia, confusion and disorientation.
♦ Korsakoff psychosis: It occurs due to involvement of mammillary bodies and confabulates with amnesia.
Presence of angular stomatitis.

Q.23. Write short note on diabetic diet. *(Nov 2011, 3 Marks)*

Ans. The golden rule for a diabetic on diet therapy should be to eat little and more often.

♦ A heavy meal is not desirable since it gives rise to rise in blood lipids.
♦ One must time the meals, food must have variety and monotony in diet be avoided.
♦ Foods should be adjusted in such a way that they form part of the family ratios.

Requirements are Determined by the Patient's Activity

♦ Overweight NIDDM should be encouraged to establish their weight within a desirable range. A reduction of approximately 500 kcal/day can result in loss of 1–2 kg/month.
♦ *Carbohydrates:* Carbohydrates should be taken in form of starch and complex sugars. 100–300 g of carbohydrates should be spreaded over 3 meals, i.e., 60 g each and 3 snacks, i.e., 30 g each with half liter of milk. Unrefined carbohydrates should be substituted by refined carbohydrates to the extent possible.
♦ *Proteins:* Recommended dietary allowance of 0.85 g/kg body weight for adult is an appropriate guide.
♦ *Fat:* Fat intake should be 50 to 150 g daily divided between the meals. Replacement of saturated with polyunsaturated fat is desirable to reduce cardiovascular risk. Cholesterol intake should be <300 mg/day.
♦ *Fiber:* Increased consumption of dietary fiber especially soluble fiber are associated with lower levels of blood glucose and serum lipids. The water insoluble fibers, such as cellulose, lignin and most hemicelluloses found in whole grain breads, cereals and wheat bran affect gastrointestinal

transit time and fecal bulk with little impact on plasma glucose. However, highly viscous water soluble fibers, such as pectins, gums and storage polysaccharide found in fruits, legumes, lentils roots, tubers, oat and oat bran, when eaten in purified form, reduce serum levels of glucose and insulin. Ideal recommended amount of fiber in patient's diet is 35–40 g/day.

♦ *Alternative sweeteners:* Both nutritive and non-nutritive sweeteners are acceptable in diabetes management.

♦ *Sodium:* It should be restricted to 1000 mg/1000 kcal, not to exceed 3000 mg/day to minimize symptoms of hypertension.

♦ Alcohol: It should be taken in moderation and may need to be restricted entirely by person with diabetes and insulin—induced hypoglycemia, neuropathy, poor control of glucose and lipids, or obesity.

♦ Vitamins, minerals and antioxidants — intake should be encouraged.

Forbidden foods: Sugar, jam, jellies, honey, jaggery, tinned fruits and juices, sweets, chocolate, ice creams, pastries, glucose drinks, foods made with sugar, pudding, sauces.

Foods allowed in moderation: Bread of all kinds and *chapattis* made from wheat or millets, plain biscuits, all fresh fruits, baked beans, breakfast cereals.

Free foods: All meat, fish, eggs (not fried), clear soup or meat extracts; tea or coffee; vegetables, such as cabbage, cauliflower, spinach, pumpkin, brinjal, lady's finger, turnip, French beans, cucumber, lettuce, tomato, spring onions, radish, asparagus. Spices, salt, pepper and mustard; butter and margarine. Sugar substitutes for sweetening.

Q.24. Give definition, etiology, sign, symptoms, complication and management of diabetes mellitus.
(Feb 2013, 12 Marks)

Ans. Diabetes mellitus is a group of metabolic diseases characterized by hyperglycemia resulting from defects in insulin secretion, insulin action or both.

Etiology

♦ *Heredity:* It is inherited as mendelian type of recessive trait and is predominant in children born to parents who are diabetic. Every person who has a history of diabetes in his or her family is a carrier of disease. The risk percentage in first degree relatives is generally up to 20% while in second degree relatives it is about 5% and the overall percentage of diabetes among the children of diabetics goes up to 10%. Identical twins of a diabetic have almost 40% chances of developing the disease.

♦ *Obesity:* Obese people are more prone to suffer from diabetes probably because obesity imposes strain on the islets of Langerhans and there is a relative deficiency of insulin. Obese also show a relative resistance to insulin due to reduction in the number of insulin receptors on target cells. Obesity results due to uninhibited indulgence in food and lack of physical activity and imposes a constant stress on the pancreas. Thus these people are more prone to get diabetes.

♦ *Race:* All races are involved and suffer from diabetes though a number of factors operate in one ethnic group or the other. Jewish race has been known to be more commonly affected than others. Some communities are known to have less incidence of diabetes as compared to others, but here the role of diet, physical exercise and environmental factors come into play. A certain community in Japan (Ainus) was known to have practically no or little diabetes probably due to undernourishment and poverty, but with the rapid industrialization and boom in the economy of the community, the incidence of diabetes among them has gone up.

♦ *Social and environmental factors:* Diabetes has been considered a disease of civilization and its prevalence is closely related to the economic affluence. Diabetes occurs more in richer and affluent classes of society though the poorer class of people are equally liable to suffer from early onset diabetes. Diabetes in richer class of people is closely related to their eating habits, lack of physical effort and obesity.

♦ *Exercise:* Lack of physical effort and exercise promotes obesity and indirectly predisposes to diabetes. Physical effort and leading an active life goes a long way in keeping one self-trim and helps in the proper utilization of body glucose and maintains a homeostatic balance.

♦ *Diet:* Excessive intake of carbohydrates and refined sugars produces strain on the pancreas and this combined with sedentary occupation goes a long way in predisposing to diabetes.

♦ *Parity:* Women with repeated pregnancies are more liable to develop diabetes since too many pregnancies are a strain on the carbohydrate metabolism and often there is hormonal imbalance.

Sign and Symptoms/Clinical Features

In Type I Diabetes Mellitus

Symptoms

♦ Polydipsia, polyuria and polyphagia
♦ Weight loss
♦ Weakness and lassitude.

Sign

♦ Severe emaciation with wasting of muscles
♦ Ribs are prominent.
♦ In such patients if diabetic ketoacidosis is severe patient develop mental apathy, confusion and undergo coma.

In Type II Diabetes Mellitus

Symptoms

Patient remains asymptomatic in the beginning. Disease is detected during routine checkup.

Sign

In this multiple systems are affected, so considering this various signs are:

♦ *Eyes:* Errors of refraction leads to frequent change in spectacles, premature formation of cataract, retinopathy, recurrent sty.

♦ *Skin:* Abscess, carbuncle, boils, nonhealing wounds.

♦ *Gastrointestinal tract:* Chronic diarrhea, malabsorption and dilatation of stomach.

♦ *Cardiovascular system:* Hypertension, ischemic heart disease, diabetic foot, cold extremities.

♦ *Respiratory system:* Pneumonia, tuberculosis and lung abscess.

♦ *Nervous system:* Autonomic neuropathy and peripheral neuritis.

♦ Urinary tract: Nephrotic syndrome, urinary tract infection.

♦ Genital tract: Pruritus vulvae, menstrual irregularity and infertility.

For complications refer to Ans. 7 and for management refer to Ans. 8 of same chapter.

Q.25. Write briefly on sign, symptoms and treatment of protein malnutrition. *(May/June 2009, 5 Marks)*

Ans. Protein malnutrition is caused due to deficiency of proteins in body.

Symptoms

♦ Patient has high urge for food and water.

♦ Patient becomes weak, exhausted and fatigued.

♦ Presence of loss of libido

♦ Patient feels cold

♦ Amenorrhea is present.

♦ Patient looks old and mature and face is expressionless.

♦ Diarrhea may occur.

♦ Patient in inactive and is depressed.

♦ There is loss of libido

Signs

♦ Muscle wasting is present.

♦ Extremities of patient are cold.

♦ Skin is dry, lusterless and become fissured.

♦ Subcutaneous fat is absent and bony prominences are prominent.

♦ Circumference of arm is subnormal.

♦ In females edema is present which is not due to hypoalbuminemia.

♦ Body temperature is subnormal

♦ Tendon jerks become diminished.

♦ Pulse of patient is slow and blood pressure becomes low.

♦ Abdominal distention is commonly present.

Treatment

In Adults

♦ For mild starvation adequate supplementation of nutrients is necessary

♦ In moderately starved people extra-feeding is needed

♦ In severely starved persons food is given in small amount at frequent intervals. Food should be staple meal, i.e., cereal with some sugar, milk and oils, salt is restricted. Potassium, magnesium and vitamins are adequately given. This is continued till patient feel active.

In Children

♦ **Diet**
  • *Diet for mild-to-moderate cases:* Diet should be easily digestible. It should be rich in proteins, minerals and vitamins with extra calories. Milk should be given.

Egg is a good flip with milk and water as a source of first class protein. Plant protein mixtures, such as corn, soya, diet milk can be given. Additional fats should be included. If there is lactose intolerance dal, rice and butter can be given.

  • *Diet for acute cases:* Protein intake should be 3 to 4 g/kg/day and energy intake of 150 kcal/kg/day. If child is unable to take diet from mouth go for nasogastric intubation. Care must be taken to take sufficient amount of plant, animal proteins and fats to maintain the weight.

♦ **Vitamins and mineral supplementations:**
  • Vitamin A, D, B complex and C are given at therapeutic dosages.
  • In vitamin A deficiency 30 mg of vitamin A should be given for 3 days.
  • 0.5 to 1 g of potassium chloride dissolve in feeds or water should be given daily in divided dosages.

♦ **Maintenance of body temperature**
  For maintenance of body temperature at night blankets or room heaters are useful.

♦ **Skin care**
  In cases of dermatoses skin should be kept clean and protected.

♦ **In hospital treatment:**
  • Correction of dehydration, electrolyte disturbances, hypoglycemia, acidosis and hypothermia.
  • Parenteral therapy with half of saline and 2.5% glucose before diet therapy.
  • In anemia packed erythrocyte infusion is given.

Q.26. Discuss the clinical features, diagnosis and management of diabetes mellitus.
(Jan 2018, 12 Marks)(Jun 2010, 15 Marks)

Ans. *For clinical features refer to sign and symptoms of Ans. 24 of same chapter. For management refer to Ans. 8 of same chapter.*

Diagnosis

Diagnosis is based on symptoms, signs and laboratory tests. In presence of signs and symptoms, confirmation is done by finding random blood glucose higher than 200 mg/dL.

Investigations

♦ **Blood sugar estimation:** Both fasting and post-prandial (2 hours after a meal) levels of blood sugar be estimated. Mean value of blood sugar in healthy adults is 70 to 80 mg%. When fasting blood sugar level exceeds 110 mg% diagnosis is clear. Post-prandial blood sugar level is further screening test, if value exceeds 120 mg% it is strongly suggestive of diabetes mellitus. Random blood sugar estimation is not of much help as screening test. Value exceeding 160 mg% in presence of glycosuria is suggestive but values about 200 mg% is diagnostic.

♦ **Oral glucose tolerance test:** In this, first sample is taken after an overnight fast of 8 hours following which patient is given glucose 1 g/kg body weight. Blood is then collected at 30, 60, 120 and 180 minutes. In diminished glucose tolerance, level of blood glucose is raised at 180 minutes.

♦ **Glycosylated hemoglobin:** It measures the long-term glycemic control. Slow non-enzymatic attachment of glucose to hemoglobin result in formation of glycosylated hemoglobin.

♦ **Microalbumin:** Patients with microalbuminuria are on greater risk in developing kidney failure as well as cardiovascular damage.

♦ **Urine protein/creatinine ratio:** It provides information of proteinuria in patients with diabetic nephropathy. More is the ratio greater is the damage.

♦ **Insulin levels:** Elevated blood glucose levels with low insulin levels indicate insufficient insulin levels for adequate control of blood glucose. High insulin levels with low blood glucose indicate change in dosage of drug.

♦ **Insulin antibody test:** In this, there is quantitative determination of antibodies against insulin in serum.

♦ **GAD – 65 antibody:** These antibodies are common in newly diagnosed diabetic patient and often appear years before clinical onset in the disease. Presence of this antibody is the strong predictive marker for onset of type I diabetes mellitus.

Criterias given by WHO in 1999

♦ Presence of classic symptoms of diabetes and causal plasma glucose greater than or equal to 200 mg/dL. Causal is any time of day without regard to time since last meal. Classic symptoms of diabetes include polyuria, polydipsia and unexplained weight loss.

Or

♦ Fasting plasma glucose greater than or equal to 126 mg/dL. Fasting is defined as no caloric intake for 8 hours.

Or

♦ Two hours plasma glucose greater than or equal to 200 mg/dL during an oral glucose tolerance test. Test is performed as described by World Health Organization by using glucose load containing equivalent of 75 g anhydrous glucose dissolved in water.

In absence of unequivocal hyperglycemia with acute metabolic decompensation above criterias are confirmed by repeated testing on other days.

Q.27. Write sign and symptoms of diabetes mellitus.

(Aug 2012, 5 Marks)

Or

Describe clinical features of diabetes mellitus.

(Feb 2013, 5 Marks)

Or

Write short answer on sign and symptoms of diabetes mellitus. *(Sep 2018, 3 Marks)*

Ans. *Refer to Ans. 24 of same chapter.*

Q.28. Write management of diabetic ketoacidosis.

(Mar 2013, 4 Marks)

Ans. Following is the management of diabetic ketoacidosis

♦ Admission of patient
  • Diagnosis is confirmed by examination of blood glucose and ketone measurements.

• Initial assessment of dehydration, hyperosmolality, serum potassium, acidosis and kidney function is done.

• Fluid loss is measured by subtracting admission weight by last known stable weight.

• Patient should be evaluated for sepsis.

♦ Management during hour 1
  • If patient is hypovolemic and hypotensive fluid administration is done, i.e., normal saline is administered and if necessary colloids should be given. Rate of administration is necessary to restore circulatory function. As blood pressure become normal and urine output becomes adequate rate of administration of normal saline is 1000 mL/h.

  • Continuous IV infusion of regular insulin 5–10 units/h is given.

  • IV infusion of potassium is done at 10–40 mmol/h during initiation of insulin therapy.

  • Sodium bicarbonate IV is given in cases with acidosis. Dose is 50–100 mmol/L sodium bicarbonate in 0.45% saline for 30–60 minutes. Additional potassium should also be given with bicarbonate therapy.

♦ Management during hour 2
  • Normal saline should be continued at 500 mL/h. Plasma osmolality should be greater than 285 mosmol/L during first 12 hours. If serum sodium is greater than 150 mmol/L switch to 0.45% saline.

  • Blood glucose should be checked and insulin is adjusted to 5 mmol/L/h. Blood glucose should not fall below 11.1–14.0 mmol/L. Anion gap is decreasing and blood pH is increasing.

  • Serum potassium should be maintained at 4–5 mmol/L by addition of potassium to IV fluids.

♦ Management during hours 3 to 4
  • Management should be continued as given in second hour.

  • Cognitive and neurological symptoms should be observed for 12 hours.

♦ Management during hours 5 to 8
  • Normal saline should be continued at 250 mL/h. As blood glucose reaches 11.1–14 mmol/L, change IV fluid to 500 mL/h normal saline with 5% glucose.

  • Insulin should be continued at maintenance dose until ketoacidosis is cleared.

  • Potassium should be continued at 10–40 mmol/h since ketoacidosis is cleared.

  • Phosphate replacement is done at 6 hours if serum phosphate is <2 mg/dL.

♦ Management during hours 8 to 24
  • IV repletion is continued with 0.45% saline with or without 2.5% or 5% glucose as needed.

  • As ketoacidosis is subsided patient should be switched to sub-cutaneous insulin and stop IV and IM insulin.

Q.29. Write classification, clinical features, investigations and treatment of diabetes mellitus.

(Jun 2014, 12 Marks)

Ans. Diabetes mellitus is a clinical syndrome of hyperglycemia with glycosuria due to lack of insulin or insulin resistance is termed as diabetes mellitus.

Classification

Primary Diabetes

♦ Type I insulin dependent diabetes mellitus (IDDM). It is sub-divided:
  • Immune mediated (islet cell antibodies).
  • Non-immune (no antibody).
♦ Type II non-insulin dependent diabetes mellitus (NIDDM) It is sub-divided:
  • Obese (insulin resistance with relative insulin deficiency).
  • Non-obese (insulin secretory detect with insulin resistance).

Secondary Diabetes

♦ Pancreatic diabetes due to pancreatitis.
♦ Hormonal or endocrinal abnormalities, i.e., acromegaly, Cushing's syndrome, pheochromocytoma, etc.
♦ Drugs induced (Iatrogenic) due to steroids and thiazides.
♦ Insulin receptors antibodies.
♦ Genetic syndromes, i.e., Lipodystrophies, muscular dystrophies, Klinefelter's syndrome, Turner's syndrome, Down's syndrome, DIDMOAD (Diabetes insipidus, diabetes mellitus, optic atrophy and deafness) syndrome.

Clinical Features

For clinical features refer to Ans. 24 of same chapter.

Investigations

♦ *Blood sugar estimation:* Both fasting and post-prandial (2 hours after a meal) levels of blood sugar be estimated. Mean value of blood sugar in healthy adults is 70 to 80 mg%. When fasting blood sugar level exceeds 110 mg% diagnosis is clear. Post-prandial blood sugar level is further screening test, if value exceeds 120 mg% it is strongly suggestive of diabetes mellitus. Random blood sugar estimation is not of much help as screening test. Value exceeding 160 mg% in presence of glycosuria is suggestive but values about 200 mg% is diagnostic.
♦ *Oral glucose tolerance test:* In this, first sample is taken after an overnight fast of 8 hours following which patient is given glucose 1 g/kg body weight. Blood is then collected at 30, 60, 120 and 180 minutes. In diminished glucose tolerance, level of blood glucose is raised at 180 minutes.
♦ *Glycosylated hemoglobin:* It measures the long-term glycemic control. Slow non-enzymatic attachment of glucose to hemoglobin result in formation of glycosylated hemoglobin.
♦ *Microalbumin:* Patients with microalbuminria are on greater risk in developing kidney failure as well as cardiovascular damage.
♦ *Urine protein/Creatinine ratio:* It provides information of proteinuria in patients with diabetic nephropathy. More is the ratio greater is the damage.
♦ *Insulin levels:* Elevated blood glucose levels with low insulin levels indicate insufficient insulin levels for adequate control of blood glucose. High insulin levels with low blood glucose indicate change in dosage of drug.

♦ *Insulin antibody test:* In this, there is quantitative determination of antibodies against insulin in serum.
♦ *GAD-65 antibody:* These antibodies are common in newly diagnosed diabetic patient and often appear years before clinical onset in the disease. Presence of this antibody is the strong predictive marker for onset of type I diabetes mellitus.

Treatment

For treatment refer to Ans. 8 of same chapter.

Q.30. Write short note on obesity. *(Feb 2013, 5 Marks)*

Ans. Obesity is the condition in which there is excessive accumulation of body fat.

Obesity is the common disorder of the nutrition of affluent societies.

Etiology

♦ *Genetic and Environmental factors:* Genetic and environmental factors play important role in causing the obesity. Familial predisposition is also seen. Overeating and other factors also cause obesity. If both the parents of a child are overweight then chances of child being obese are 80%.
♦ *Socioeconomic status:* Obesity is the disorder of affluent societies. Some occupations also predisposes to obesity, such as cooks. In some of the societies obesity is considered as the sign of heritage.
♦ *Energy intake:* Minute excess of calories causes accumulation of fat. If there is lag of physical activity, this also causes obesity.
♦ *Drugs:* Various drugs, such as steroids, oral contraceptives, etc., causes increase in appetite, this leads to weight gain.
♦ *Endocrine:* During pregnancy there is increase in the body fat which is under hormonal influence. Obesity can also occur in hypothyroidism due to decrease calorie demands.

Clinical Features

♦ Type II diabetes mellitus, gallbladder stones, gout and various other metabolic disorders are associated with obesity.
♦ Varicose vein, hernia and osteoarthritis are the mechanical disorders associated with obesity.
♦ Various respiratory infections are also associated with the obesity along with the sleep disorders.
♦ Hypertension, atherosclerosis and ischemic heart diseases are the cardiovascular diseases which are associated with the obesity.

Management

♦ *Diet:* Calories uptake should depend on the age, sex, occupation and urgency of the weight reduction. An obese person should spare from fats, butter, ghee, cream dry fruits (nuts) vegetables (potatoes and peas). Person should follow strict diet regime and maintain discipline in choice of foods to which he/she takes and the amount of calories consumed per day. Food should be taken in intervals, chewed slowly.
♦ *Exercise:* Habit of regular physical exercise should be cultivated by an obese person. An obese person should do

morning and evening walks, jogging, stretch exercise and taking part in outdoor games.

♦ *Drug therapy:* In this, recent era serotonergic drugs are used. DL-fenfluramine which was the first generation drug was used to reduce weight. These days it is replaced by second generation drugs dL-fenfluramine, fluoxetine which is a slow releasing serotonin antagonist, sibutramine which is a slow serotonin and noradrenaline reuptake inhibitor. These drugs increase the satiety and potentiate serotonin in hypothalamus.

♦ *Surgical treatment:* This method is employed in the persons having severe obesity. The surgical methods employed are:
  • *Wiring of jaws:* This is carried out to prevent eating and only taking liquids. This method is good but as wires are removed patient regains the weight.
  • *Gastric plication:* In this, stomach is reduced by creating a small pouch due to stapling of stomach to abdominal wall. Good results can be attained.
  • *Bariatric surgery:* It is done in persons with extreme obesity.

Q.31. Write short note on gestational diabetes.

(Nov 2014, 3 Marks) (Dec 2015, 3 Marks)

Ans. Gestational diabetes is defined as development of hyperglycemia, first time in pregnancy.

♦ It occurs in women who are genetically predisposed to type 1 and type 2 diabetes.
♦ The condition is asymptomatic.
♦ Repeated hyperglycemia in every pregnancy lead the women to undergo suffering from permanent diabetes.
♦ Gestational diabetes can occur in any women, so at the time of pregnancy during each trimester random blood sugar screening is done by oral glucose tolerance test. In this test blood glucose is more than 126 mg%.

Obstetric Complications Associated with Gestational Diabetes Mellitus

♦ Maternal risk
  • Maternal hypertension
  • Eclampsia
  • Nephropathy, retinopathy and vascular complications can worsen.
♦ Fetal risk
  • Stillbirth
  • Neonatal hypoglycemia
  • Neonatal hypocalcemia
  • Macrosome
  • Hyaline membrane disease
  • Growth retardation
  • Congenital anomalies

Diagnostic Criteria

Condition	Glucose load	FBS	PDG (Oral glucose tolerance test)
IGT	75 g	NA	140 mg/dL
DM	75 g	140 mg/dL	200 mg/dL

A two-step strategy has been proposed for establishment of diagnosis of gestational diabetes. First step is to give 50 mg oral glucose and measure serum glucose at 60 min; if glucose is found less than 140 mg then test is normal and if found greater than 140 mg, then it warrants second step of administration of 100 g glucose and measure the serum glucose in fasting state and at 1, 2 and 3 hrs. Normal plasma glucose concentration is given below:

♦ Fasting <105 mg/L.
♦ At 1 hr <190 mg/L.
♦ At 2 hr <165 mg/L
♦ At 3 hr <145 mg/L.

Deviations from the normal indicate gestational diabetes mellitus.

Management

♦ High dietary protein intake. Salt restriction if edema is present.
♦ Exercise should be done regularly
♦ Insulin therapy is essential.
♦ Oral hypoglycemic should be avoided except metformin which is effective in women with PCOD to aid conception.

Q.32. Describe briefly on Type II diabetes.

(Apr 2015, 4 Marks)

Ans. Type II diabetes is also known as non-insulin dependent diabetes mellitus.

Etiology

♦ *Genetic:* It is inherited as mendelian type of recessive trait and is predominant in children born to parents who are diabetic. Every person who has a history of diabetes in his or her family is a carrier of disease. The risk percentage in first degree relatives is generally up to 20%t while in second degree relatives it is about 5%. Type II diabetes is caused due to abnormal insulin secretion and insulin resistance.
♦ *Due to pancreatic beta cell failure:* In Type II diabetes, there is reduction of pancreatic beta cell mass with reduction in insulin levels. As beta cells decreases alpha cells secrete glucagon and this causes hyperglycemia.
♦ *Environmental factors:* Physical inactivity and obesity are the factor leading to type II diabetes in genetically susceptible individuals.
♦ *Age:* Type II diabetes occur after age of 30 years.

Clinical Features

Symptoms

Patient remains asymptomatic in the beginning. Disease is detected during routine checkup.

Sign

In this multiple systems are affected, so considering this various signs are:

♦ *Eyes:* Errors of refraction leads to frequent change in spectacles, premature formation of cataract, retinopathy, recurrent sty.

- *Skin:* Abscess, carbuncle, boils, nonhealing wounds.
- *Gastrointestinal tract:* Chronic diarrhea, malabsorption and dilatation of stomach.
- *Cardiovascular system:* Hypertension, ischemic heart disease, diabetic foot, cold extremities.
- *Respiratory system:* Pneumonia, tuberculosis and lung abscess
- *Nervous system:* Autonomic neuropathy and peripheral neuritis
- *Urinary tract:* Nephrotic syndrome, urinary tract infection.
- *Genital tract:* Pruritus vulvae, menstrual irregularity and infertility.

Management

- Low energy and weight reducing diet is given to the patient of obese type II diabetes mellitus.
- Non-obese type II diabetes should have to maintain their weight, so they have to take weight maintenance diet.

These drugs are used in patients of Type II diabetes mellitus (NIDDM) who do not respond to dietary management and who would otherwise require treatment with insulin in later situation, so they are also used as adjuvant drugs to insulin in overweight diabetes patients.

- Insulin secretagogues, i.e., drugs increasing secretion of insulin
  - Sulfonylureas

Name of drug	Intial daily dose (mg)	Dose/ day	Comment
First generation			
Acetohexamide	250 mg	1 – 2	Has diuretic and uricosuric activity
Chlorpropamide	100 mg	1 – 2	Can potentiate ADH
Tolazamide	100 mg	1 – 2	Disulfiram-like action with alcohol in 1/3rd of patients, has diuretic activity
Second generation			
Glibenclamide	2.5 to 20 mg	1 – 2	Hypoglycemia can be severe
Gliclazide	40 to 320 mg	1 – 2	Metabolism/excretion by liver/kidney
Glipizide	5 mg	1 – 2	Mild diuretic activity
Glyburide	2.5 mg	1 – 2	Highest risk of hypoglycemia
Glimepiride	1 mg	1	Excreted in urine and bile

- Meglitinides
  - Repaglinide, i.e., 0.5 to 4 mg three times a day
  - Netaglinide, i.e., 60 to 120 mg three times a day 15 to 30 min before each meal
  - Voglibose, i.e., 0.2 to 0.3 mg, 15 to 30 min before each meal.

- Insulin sensitizers, i.e., drugs sensitizing action of insulin and overcome insulin resistance
  - Biguanides, i.e., metformin should be given 1.5 to 2.5 g/day in three divided doses after meals.
  - Thiazolidinediones, i.e., Rosiglitazone should be given 2 to 8 mg or pioglitazone 15 to 45 mg in a single or two divided doses. They can be combined with sulfonylureas or metformin.
- *Alpha glucosidase inhibitors,* i.e., Acarbose 25 to 100 mg TDS or Voglibose 0.2 to 5 mg TDS taken orally in three main meals. It can be given in combination with metformin 500 mg for increased efficiency.
- *DPP-4 inhibitor:* Vildagliptin 50 to 100 mg daily in two dived doses with meals ot saxagliptin 2.5 to 5 mg OD.
- *Pramlintide:* Initial dose is 15 µg before each meals in Type I diabetes mellitus and 60 µg in Type II diabetes mellitus.

Q.33. Write short note on tetany.

(Apr 2015, 3 Marks)(Mar 2016, 3 Marks)

Ans. Tetany is a clinical condition with low levels of ionized calcium causing increased neuromuscular excitability.

Etiology

Low levels of calcium, potassium, magnesium causes tetany.

- *Hypocalcemia:* This is due to following factors, i.e., malabsorption of calcium, osteomalacia, hypoparathyroidism, acute pancreatitis, anti-convulsant drugs.
- *Hypokalemia:* This is caused due to repeated vomiting, excessive intake of alkali, due to acute anion load, primary hyperaldosteronism, due to acute anion load.
- Acute hypocalcemia is caused by sepsis, burns, alkalosis, parathyroid surgery, malignancy, hypomagnesemia, etc.

Clinical Features

- In children, there is presence of triad of symptoms, i.e., carpopedal spasm, stridor and convulsion.
- In carpopedal spasm, the hands adopt a posture in which flexion occurs at metacarpophalangeal joint and extension at interphalangeal joint and opposition of thumb occur.
- Stridor occurs due to closure of glottis.
- In case of adults tingling sensation occur in peripheral part of limbs and around the mouth.
- *Trousseau's sign:* Increasing the blood pressure by the inflation of sphygmomanometer cuff at above the systolic level leads to carpopedal spasm in 2 to 5 minutes.

Chvostek's sign: Tapping at the facial nerve especially at angle of mandible leads to twitching of facial muscles.

Management

In management etiological factor leading to tetany is eliminated and hypocalcemia and alkalosis should be treated.

Treatment of Hypocalcemia

About 10% calcium gluconate 20 mL IM is given. For longlasting effect 10 mL of drug is given additionally.

Treatment of Alkalosis

♦ If vomiting is present IV isotonic saline should be given.
♦ If alkali is the etiological factor, alkalis should be withdrawn, after withdrawal if effect is not proper ammonium chloride 2 g orally is given after every 4 hours.
♦ If hyperventilation is the etiological factor, patient is asked to inhale 5% carbon dioxide in oxygen.

Q.34. What are the non-communicable diseases. Write down the diagnostic criteria of diabetes mellitus, complication and management of type-2 diabetes mellitus. *(June 2015, 12 Marks)*

Ans. Non-communicable disease is a medical condition or disease that is noninfectious or non-transmissible. Non-communicable disease can refer to chronic diseases which last for long periods of time and progress slowly.

The most non-communicable diseases are obesity, diabetes, cancer, cardiovascular, chronic respiratory and neurological diseases.

For diagnostic criteria of diabetes mellitus refer to Ans. 26 of same chapter.

For complications of diabetes mellitus refer to Ans. 7 of same chapter.

For management of diabetes mellitus refer to Ans. 32 of same chapter.

Q.35. Write diagnosis, clinical features and complications of diabetes mellitus. *(Jan 2016, 12 Marks)*

Ans. *Diagnosis is based on investigations, for investigations in detail refer to Ans. 29 of same chapter and for criteria of diagnosis refer to Ans. 26 of same chapter*

For clinical features of diabetes mellitus refer to Ans. 24 of same chapter.

For complications of diabetes mellitus refer to Ans. 7 of same chapter.

Q.36. Write short answer on protein energy malnutrition. *(Feb 2019, 3 Marks)*

Ans. Protein energy malnutrition occurs both in adults and children.

Protein Energy Malnutrition in Adults

Protein energy malnutrition in adults is known as undernutrition and starvation.

Starvation is defined as undernutrition of severe magnitude, warranting inpatient treatment inside the hospital.

Undernutrition is the state of negative energy balance.

Etiology

♦ **Due to defective intake of food:**
  • Loss of appetite in anxiety, expression, anorexia nervosa etc.
  • In alcoholics
  • In cases with persistent vomiting
  • Unbalanced therapeutic diet
  • In prolonged intravenous or parenteral fluids therapy
♦ **Due to maldigestion and disordered absorption:**
  • In hypochlorhydria or achlorhydria.

• Steatorrhea causes malabsorption of fats.
• Intestinal hurry due to surgical resection.
• Prolonged use of antibiotics

♦ **In defective utilization:**
  • In renal failure
  • In liver cirrhosis
  • In infections
  • In malignancy
  • Inborn errors of metabolism
  • Various drugs, such as antiepileptics antagonize folate and Vitamin D

♦ **Loss of nutrients from body:**
  • Proteinuria in nephrotic syndrome leads to hypoproteinemia
  • In diabetes mellitus, produces loss of energy and unernutrition.
  • In excessive menstrual blood loss
  • Hypokalemia because of severe persistent diarrhea.

♦ **Because of increased demands:**
  • In pregnancy, lactation, adolescence, heavy manual work needs extra energy and normal diet is not sufficient.
  • In burns, surgery and trauma where there is increase in catabolism of proteins as well as Vitamin C.
  • In both fever and thyrotoxicosis where metabolism get increased and require lot of energy.

Clinical Features

Symptoms

♦ There is high urge for both food and water.
♦ Presence of weakness, exhaustion and fatigue
♦ Patient feels cold
♦ Presence of nocturia
♦ There is presence of amenorrhea and loss of libido
♦ Patient looks mature and old.
♦ Patient has expressionless face.
♦ Diarrhea can be present
♦ Patient becomes introvert, depressive and less active.

Sign

♦ Skin becomes lusterless, fissured and dry.
♦ Extremities of patient are cold.
♦ Subcutaneous fat gets degraded and bony prominence become prominent.
♦ Wasting of muscles.
♦ Arm circumference and body temperature becomes subnormal
♦ Slow pulse and low blood pressure
♦ Diminishing of tendon jerks.
♦ Abdominal distention is present.

Investigations

♦ Body weight is markedly decreased which depends on degree of starvation. Depending on reduction in the weight and body mass index starvation is subdivided as:
  • Mild undernutrition: Weight for height comes down from 90% to 81% of standard BMI (20 to 18)

- Moderate undernutrition: Weight for height comes down from 80% to 71% of standard BMI (18 to 16)
- Severe undernutrition: Weight for height is ≤70% of standard BMI (≤16)
- Plasma free fatty acids are increased.
- Plasma glucose gets decreased, insulin secretion is decreased. Levels of glucagon and cortisol are high.
- Normal plasma albumin
- Resting BMR decreases due to reduced body mass.
- Fixed specific gravity of urine.
- Anemia, Leukopenia, thrombocytopenia can be seen. ESR is normal but it can be increased due to the presence of infections.
- ECG is indicative of sinus bradycardia and low voltage.
- Skin hypersensitivity test can give false negative results.

Treatment

Grading should be done before starting the therapy.

- Mild starvation needs proper supplementation of nutrients. Moderate starvations needs extra feeding while severe starvation require hospitalization.
- Food should be bland in the form of staple meal, i.e., a cereal with some of the sugar, milk and oils.
- Restriction of salt is mandatory. Potassium, magnesium, vitamins should be adequately provided.
- At the time of refeeding, gain of 5% weight per month indicates satisfactory response. It is to be given till patient feels active.

Protein Energy Malnutrition in Children

Protein energy malnutrition in children form spectrum of disease where at one end there is protein malnutrition, i.e., Kwashiorkor and at other end there is total deficiency of calories which includes protein deficiency, such as marasmus.

Marasmus

For marasmus in detail refer to Ans. 4 of same chapter.

Kwashiorkor

It is protein energy malnutrition where there is deficiency of proteins or amino acids.

Etiology

It occurs in children at the age of 2 years, when the child is weaned from the breast onto traditional family diet deficiency in protein. There is very less amount of milk and limited supply of cereal food in such families. If there is presence of customary diet of the child in families which are low in protein and energy to minimum requirements, child can maintain moderate health but will develop protein malnutrition in health and stress. So in these areas gastroenteritis, malaria, typhoid, measles, nutritional deficiency and kwashiorkor becomes an endemic. Now food supply become short each year because of limited resources, so hunger grips them and kwashiorkor incidence gets increase.

Signs and Symptoms

- **Growth:** It declines, child remain lean and thin. There is also presence of generalized edema because of hypoalbuminemia.
- **Mental changes:** Child becomes miserable, apathetic and has characteristic mewing cry.
- **Muscles and fat:** Presence of wasting of muscles of chest, hips, upper arm, legs.
- **Hair:** Presence of fine, straight, sparse pigmentation, change in the color from black to bond, red or gray.
- **Mucosal changes:** There is presence of angular stomatitis, smooth tongue, cheilosis and ulceration around anus.
- **Skin changes:** These are seen in the severe cases. They occur in form of thickening, pigmentation, desquamation and ulceration. In severe cases, child appears as it is burnt. In moderate cases dermatosis with fissuring occur in moderate cases.
- **Gastrointestinal tract:** There iss presence of anorexia and diarrhea. Due to fatty changes liver become enlarged and fatty.
- **Blood:** Presence of moderate degree of anemia.
- **Vitamins:** Presence of vitamin A deficiency keratomalacia, xerosis, etc. Folate deficiency is common. Deficiency of vitamin A leads to purpura and bleeding.

Treatment

In mild-to-moderate cases

Easily digestible and palatable diet rich in proteins, minerals and vitamins should be along with extra calories is very essential. Milk should be given to child in adequate amount. Plant protein mixtures, i.e., corn, soya, dried milk can also be used. Additional fast should be included.

Diet for acute cases

- In all the regimes in acute cases protein intake of 3 to 4 g/kg/day and energy intake of 150 kcal/kg/day is mandatory.
- If child is inable to take feed, nasogastric intubation can be done.
- If lactose intolerance is seen, mixture of casilan, cream, glucose, cereal is a good choice.
- Care should be taken that the child should contain sufficient amount of plant and animal proteins and fats to maintain weight gain.

Vitamin and mineral supplementation

- Vitamin A, D, B complex and C and therapeutic doses of iron should be given routinely.
- If vitamin A deficiency is suspected, it is necessary to provide 30 mg of vitamin A everyday.
- Potassium should be given every day to children orally. 0.5 to 1 g of potassium chloride dissolve in water or feeds given daily in divided doses.

Body temperature

It should be controlled by heating rooms or by electric blankets.

Care of skin

If dermatosis is present, skin should be cleaned and carefully protected.

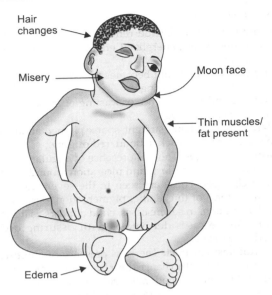

Hair changes

Misery

Moon face

Thin muscles/ fat present

Edema

Fig. 20: Kwashiorkor.

Q.37. Write short note on clinical features and management of osteomalacia. *(Jan 2019, 7 Marks)*

Ans. Osteomalacia is the disorder of mineralization of adult skeleton in which epiphyseal growth plates are already closed.

Clinical Features

♦ Here skeletal abnormalities are dominant features.
♦ Patient complaints of boy tenderness and diffuse skeletal pain.
♦ There can be mild backache to severe pain around hip.
♦ Muscle weakness is present.
♦ Waddling gait is present.
♦ Tetany can occur in few cases with carpopedal spasm.
♦ Spontaneous fractures can occur.
♦ If rib involvement is present severe pseudofractures can occur.
♦ Pseudofractures or the looser's zones are the translucent bands which are seen due to the rarefaction of the bone which commonly occur at point of stress and are symmetrical.
♦ These pseudofractures are visible in flat bones or at the end of long bones and if such fractures are present, they are suggestive of osteomalacia.
♦ If chronic renal failure is the cause of osteomalacia there may be subperiosteal bony erosion in middle phalanges and sclerosis of vertebral end plate (rugger jersey spine).

Management

Diagnosis

♦ **Biochemistry:**
  • Plasma calcium level is low or normal.
  • Serum phosphate levels are raised
  • Alkaline phosphatase levels are raised

♦ **Radiography:** Looser's zone, linear areas of defective mineralization mainly in long bones, pelvis and ribs.

Treatment

♦ Vitamin D 1000 to 5000 IU daily should be given for 6 to 12 weeks which is followed by daily dosage of 200 to 400 IU for few months.
♦ If patient is unable to take medicine orally, vitamin D should be given by IM route.
♦ If the osteomalacia is secondary because of renal pathology alfacalcidol, i.e., I- hydroxycholecalciferol 0.25 µg daily can be given.

10. DISEASES OF NERVOUS SYSTEM

Q.1. Enumerate causes of facial pain.
(Sep 2008, 2.5 Marks)

Ans.

Causes of Facial Pain

♦ Neuritis of cutaneous nerves of face and scalp.
♦ Arthralgia of temporomandibular joint
♦ Trigeminal neuralgia.
♦ Post herpetic neuralgia.
♦ Temporal arthritis.
♦ Miscellaneous causes:
  • Facial neuralgia: It is a form of inflammation of nerve of face and scalp. It generally occurs as complication of septic state or due to involvement of neurotrophic virus. The pain is confined to face and scalp.
  • Arthralgia of TMJ: It is in the form of rheumatic arthritis or ankylosing spondylitis (a chronic progressive inflammatory disorder unlike other rheumatological disorders) when there is pain and swelling of joint.
  • Trigeminal neuralgia: This is a disease seen commonly in middle and elderly individuals and is characterized by attacks of severe pain in distribution of trigeminal nerve and its branches especially in maxillary and mandibular branches.
  • Postherpetic neuralgia: Herpes zoster commonly involves the ophthalmic division of 5th nerve, characterized by vesicular eruption on the face.
  • Temporal arthritis: It is a form of collagen disorder of unknown etiology which involves mainly the arteries. It occurs in elderly age group. Patient may complain of pain on the face, jaw, mouth and tongue in distribution of branches of external carotid artery.
  • Miscellaneous causes: These include lesions of trigeminal nerve in brain stem, *syringobulbia and thrombosis of posterior inferior cerebellar artery. Tabes dorsalis is another cause of pain coming in attacks over the face.

Q 1.   *Syringobulbia = It is a medical condition in which fluid filed cavities affect brainstem. It results from congenital abnormality, trauma or tumor growth.

Q.2. Write short note on trigeminal neuralgia.

(Apr 2007, 5 Marks)
(Feb 2013, 5 Marks) (Sep 2007, 5 Marks)
(Apr 2017, 6 Marks) (Mar 2011, 4 Marks)

Or

Write short answer on trigeminal neuralgia.

(Sep 2018, 3 Marks)

Or

Write the clinical features and management of trigeminal neuralgia. *(Jan 2019, 7 Marks)*

Or

Write short answer treatment of trigeminal neuralgia.

(Oct 2019, 3 Marks)

Ans. Trigeminal neuralgia is also called as Tic Douloureux.

A disorder characterized by the *paroxysmal attacks of neuralgic pain with affection of one or more division of trigeminal nerve. The pain involves the third and second divisions equally and rarely the first.

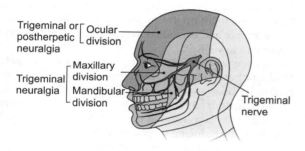

Fig. 21: Trigeminal neuralgia.

Clinical Features

♦ Pain is unilateral and is confined to one of the three divisions of nerve. Pain is sharp and onset is sudden. The pain is only of a few seconds.
♦ During the attacks there is flushing of face, i.e., redness of the face.
♦ Dilatation of pupil is present.
♦ There is excessive lacrimation
♦ After repeated attacks skin becomes shiny and hair in the area becomes gray.
♦ Sometimes secretion of nasal mucus and saliva may occur in the side of pain.

Etiology

Trigeminal neuralgia is spontaneous and following exposure to cold wind, blow on face, or chewing or eating, drinking hot or cold fluid and washing the face.

Management/Treatment

♦ Elimination of all possible sources of infection.
♦ Drugs:
  • *Analgesics:* Potent analgesics must be used with caution because of danger of habituation.
  • *Carbamazepine:* 100–200 mg BD a day and increasing the dose to 600–800 mg per day.
  • *Phenytoin sodium:* 0.1 g TDS when carbamazepine is not tolerated.
  • *Vitamin B12:* 1000 μg IM daily for two weeks.
♦ *Injection of alcohol:* It is given in affected nerve, or gasserian ganglion. If more than one division is affected inject 10 minims of 90% alcohol after local anesthesia with 2–3 drops of procaine.
♦ *Microvascular decompression:* In this, there is separation of blood vessels is done which are in contact with trigeminal nerve roots. There is also insertion of nonabsorbable sponge which provide relief of pain in most of the patients.
♦ *Radiofrequency thermocoagulation:* This procedure is carried out at the trigger spot or site of pain origin which is localized by electric stimulation of needle inserted in trigeminal ganglion and leads to permanent relief.
♦ *Surgery:* In this selective or complete preganglionic section of trigeminal root is done. This technique can lead to disadvantages, such as permanent dysesthesiae. Another better technique is percutaneous electrocoagulation of preganglionic rootlets corresponding to trigger zone, the temperature of probe being so regulated as to coagulate small thinly myelinated pain fibers but preserving most heavily myelinated touch fibers.

Q.3. Write short note on facial palsy.

(Mar 2008, 7 Marks) (Sep 2005, 5 Marks)

Ans. Facial palsy refers to the paralysis of facial muscles.

It is of two types:

1. Upper motor neuron palsy
2. Lower motor neuron palsy or Bell's palsy:

Upper Motor Neuron Palsy

♦ It affects mainly muscles of lower part of face and is never complete.
♦ It is seldomly isolated palsy.
♦ The emotional movements are preserved.
♦ There is no muscle *contracture.
♦ There is no reaction of degeneration.
♦ Electromyography and nerve conduction is normal.

Lower Motor Neuron Palsy or Bell's Palsy

Refer to Ans. 4 of same chapter.

Q 2.   *Paroxysmal attacks = Sudden recurrence or intensification of symptoms, such as a spasm or seizure.
Q 3.   *Contracture = It is a fixed tightening of muscle, tendons, ligaments or skin. It prevent normal movement of associated body part like in burn.

Q.4. Write short note on Bell's palsy.

(Dec 2013, 3 Marks) (Apr 2015, 3 Marks)
(Dec 2010, 5 Marks) (Sep 2006, 5 Marks)

Or

Write causes and clinical features of Bell's palsy.

(Jan 2012, 6 Marks)

Ans. Bell's palsy is an acute apparently isolated, lower motor neuron facial palsy.

Etiology

♦ *Cold:* It usually occurs after exposure to cold.
♦ *Trauma:* Extraction of teeth or injection of local anesthetic may damage to the nerve and subsequent paralysis.
♦ *Surgical procedure:*, such as removal of parotid gland tumor in which the facial nerve is sectioned can also cause facial paralysis.
♦ *Tumors:* Tumors of the cranial base, parapharyngeal space and infratemporal fossa after cause 7th nerve palsy.
♦ *Familial:* Familial and hereditary occurrence is also reported in case of Bell's palsy.
♦ Facial canal and middle ear neoplasm.
♦ Herpes simplex—viral infection.

Clinical Features

♦ **Symptoms:**
   • Sudden following exposure to chill or without any apparent precipitating causing, maximum paralysis in 24 hours.
   • Postauricular pain is common.
   • Spontaneous complaints of loss of sense of taste, *hyperacusis.
   • Sweating is less on the affected side.
♦ **Signs:**
   • Forehead is not wrinkled and frowning is lost.
   • Eye of the affected side is not closed and on attempting closure eyeball turns upwards and outwards.
   • On showing teeth the lips do not separate on the affected side. Whistling is not possible. Nasolabial fold is flattened out. Angle of mouth on affected side droops with dribbling of saliva.
   • Cheeks puff out with the expiration because of buccinator paralysis and food collects between the teeth and paralyzed cheek. Fluid runs out while drinking.
   • Base of tongue is lowered.
   • Deafness may result.

Investigations

Electromyography is of prognostic importance.

♦ If signs of denervation are present after 10 days, i.e., axonal degeneration is present and recovery is incomplete or delayed.
♦ If there is incomplete denervation in less than 7 days the prognosis is good.
♦ Fibrillation potential after 2 weeks is suggestive of Wallerian degeneration.

Management

♦ *Local heat:* Infrared or moist heat over the face or parotid region or both if there is tenderness of nerve trunk.
♦ *Local treatment of muscles:* The patient should massage the facial muscles with bland oil for twice a day for 5 min. The massaging movements should start from the chin and lower lip and are directed upwards. With return of function the patient should practice movements of various muscles of face before a mirror.
♦ *Prevention of facial sagging:* Application of strips of adhesive tape is done to lift up the angle of mouth. Tape is attached to the temple and extends down in a V shaped fashion to upper and lower lips.
♦ *Protection of eye:* It is done with dark glass or eye patch. Mild zinc boric solution is used to wash the eye to prevent conjunctivitis.
♦ *Corticosteroids:* If seen under a week of onset. Prednisolone 40 mg/day for 4 days and in tapering doses for over next 6 days helps by reducing secondary edema.
♦ *Antivirals:* Acyclovir, valacyclovir or famciclovir in combination with steroids, if started within 3 days of onset.
♦ *Surgery:* Decompression of facial nerve in second or third week cannot influence favorably natural course of Bell's palsy. Cases which fail to recover after 9 months in them anastomosis of facial nerve with accessory or preferably hypoglossal nerve is considered, or plastic surgery in cases of total paralysis with atrophy of muscle.

Q.5. Write short note on migraine.

(Dec 2015, 3 Marks) (Mar 2009, 5 Marks)

Or

Write short answer on migraine. *(Feb 2019, 3 Marks)*

Ans. Migraine is defined as recurrent attacks of headache varied in intensity frequency and duration and is commonly unilateral in onset and is associated with anorexia and sometimes with nausea and vomiting.

Q 4. *Hyperacusis = Highly debilitating and rare hearing disorder characterized by increased sensitivity to certain frequencies and volume ranges of sound.

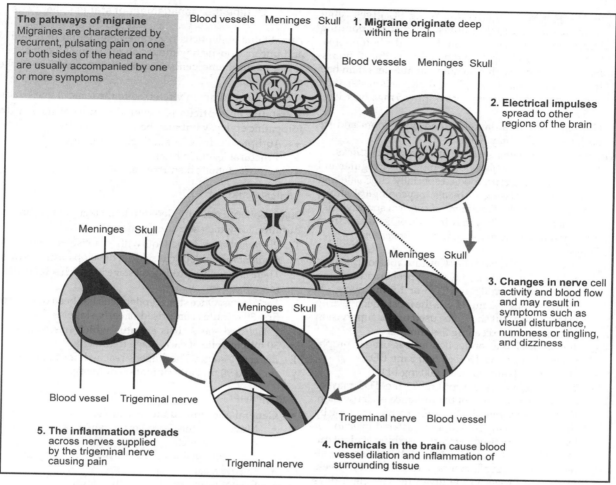

The pathways of migraine
Migraines are characterized by recurrent, pulsating pain on one or both sides of the head and are usually accompanied by one or more symptoms

Blood vessels Meninges Skull

1. Migraine originate deep within the brain

Blood vessels Meninges Skull

2. Electrical impulses spread to other regions of the brain

Meninges Skull

Meninges Skull

3. Changes in nerve cell activity and blood flow and may result in symptoms such as visual disturbance, numbness or tingling, and dizziness

Meninges Skull

Blood vessel Trigeminal nerve

Trigeminal nerve Blood vessel

5. The inflammation spreads across nerves supplied by the trigeminal nerve causing pain

Trigeminal nerve

4. Chemicals in the brain cause blood vessel dilation and inflammation of surrounding tissue

Fig. 22: Pathways of migraine.

Clinical Features

♦ The headache follows and the pain is confined on one side by occasionally it may be bilateral.
♦ Nausea and vomiting may be present and last for the few hours.
♦ Light and noise sensitivity is present.
♦ Fatigue and stress are present in the case.
♦ There is presence of polyuria.

Simplified Diagnostic Criteria for Migraine

Repeated attacks of headaches lasting for 4 to 72 hours which have features:
♦ Normal physical examination
♦ No other reasonable cause for headache
♦ *At least two of:*
  • Unilateral pain
  • Throbbing pain
  • Aggravation of pain by movement
  • Moderate or severe intensity

♦ At least one of:
  • Nausea or vomiting
  • Photophobia or phonophobia

Management

♦ *During attack*
  • *Analgesics:* NSAIDs, e.g., diclofenac can be given orally or im and is particularly useful when severe vomiting is a feature. Sublingual Piroxicam has significant analgesic effects in acute migraine without aura with excellent tolerability.
  • *Ergotamine:* Ergotamine tartrate 0.25 to 0.5 mg IM or orally 1–2 mg. tablet preferably in combination with 100 mg caffeine –2 tablets at onset followed by l tablet after 30 minutes, if necessary, or Dihydroergotamine 1 mg IM, or 1–2 mg by mouth. Whichever preparation is used, a high dose often causes nausea and vomiting. These may be prevented by giving cyclizine 50 mg. or chlorpromazine 25 mg.

- *5-HT1 agonists:* Sumatriptan 6 mg SC gives relief from headache in 60 minutes, with corresponding improvement in nausea, vomiting and photophobia. Oral dose of 100 mg provides relief within 2 hours. Headaches recur within 48 hours in little less than half the patients. Rizatriptan given orally acts faster than sumatriptan. Zolmitriptan nasal spray 5 mg gives relief in 5 minutes.
- *General:* Lying in a darkened and quiet room and ice pack to the head may help.

♦ *Reducing frequency and severity of subsequent attacks*
- *Elimination of trigger factors:* Sleeping late, irregular and hurried meals, certain foods, especially chocolate and fried food, or missing of meals, psychological stress, contraceptive pills. Treatment of cervical spondylosis.
- *Relaxation exercises:* They may include biofeedback from a temporalis electromyogram. *Yoga, Pranayama.*
- *Drugs:*
  - *Serotonin (5-HT) inhibitors:* Calcium antagonists, such as Flunarizine 10 mg/day Or Cyproheptadine 4 mg tds. Or Pizotifen 0.5 mg TDS or 1.5 mg nocte. Or Methysergide 1–2 mg TDS is the most effective drug in this group, but should be used under supervision in courses not exceeding 3–4 months.
  - *Topiramate:* It is an antiepileptic drug used in prophylaxis of migraine, Dose: 2.5 to 5 mg BD
  - Divalproex (valproic acid) 200 mg BD
  - *Tricyclic agents:* Amitryptiline 25 mg TDS may be effective irrespective of the presence of depression.
  - *Ergotamine tartrate:* For histamine cephalgia 1 mg by mouth or 0.25 mg by self-administered injection or by suppository used regularly last thing at night can be continued for many weeks without harmful effects, 2 days being left without treatment each week.
  - *Hormones:* Progesterone given for last eight days may be useful for migraine occurring in the immediate premenstrual period or at beginning of catamenia. When migraine begins or becomes worse at the time of menopause, estrin, given in small doses as continuous therapy sometimes helpful.
  - *Schedule:*
    » Propranolol 40–160 mg/day or Flunarizine 5–10 mg/day as first line of therapy.
    » In patients with episodic and chronic migraine Topiramate 50–100 mg/day.
    » In patients with episodic migraine Divalproex 250–750 mg/day.
    » For mixed migraine and tension type headache: Amitriptyline 10–25 mg/day.
    After 6–12 months of prophylaxis gradual withdrawal should be considered.

Q.6. Write short note on **status epilepticus.**

(Sep 2006, 5 Marks)

Or

Write management of status epilepticus.

(Nov 2011, 4 Marks) (Mar 2011, 4 Marks)

Or

Outline the management of status epilepticus.

(Feb 2002, 5 Marks)

Ans. Status epilepticus is an alternate period of convulsions and unconsciousness without any intervening normal period. It is a medical emergency because if not rapidly controlled it may be fatal.

It is most commonly referred to the tonic clonic seizures.

Status epilepticus is never the presenting feature of idiopathic epilepsy but may be precipitated by:
♦ Abrupt withdrawal of antiepileptic drugs.
♦ Structural lesion in brain
♦ Acute metabolic disturbance.

Clinical Features

Status epilepticus is divided into four stages depending on the duration for which seizures continue.

1. *Prodromal phase:* In patients with established epilepsy, tonic-clonic status epilepticus seldom develops without warning. There is usually a prodromal stage in which seizures become more frequent.
2. *Early status:* Once status epilepticus has been developed the first 30 minutes comprised of early stage.
3. *Established status:* It is a status which has continued for 30 min in spite of early stage treatment.
4. *Refractory status:* The stage is reached, if seizures continue for 60 to 90 min after initiation of therapy.

Management

♦ **General and immediate measures:**
- Move away the person from danger, such as fire, water, machinery, etc.
- After convulsions cease, turn into recovery position.
- Ensure clear airway
- Do not insert anything in the mouth.
- If convulsions continue for more than 5 minutes urgent medical attention is required.
- Patient should not be left alone until he is recovered.
- Establish intravenous access in large veins. Take blood for electrolytes, glucose, calcium, magnesium, full blood count, antiepileptic drug levels, alcohol and toxicology screen and cultures as appropriate. Urea and electrolytes, blood glucose, calcium and phenytoin levels are obtained urgently.
- Check glucose and immediately correct any hypoglycemia with 50% glucose up to 50 mL IV over 1 to 2 min in a large vein.
- If poor nutrition or alcohol abuse is suspected, administer thiamine 250 mg IV over 10 min.
- Check for the blood gases.

♦ **Pharmacological management**
- Lorazepam 4 mg IV over 2–3 minutes or IV Diazepam 5 mg IV. Repeat dose, if necessary. If IV access not possible give Midazolam 10 mg intranasally or IM.
- Give IV phenytoin 15–20 mg/kg or IV Fosphenytoin 20 mg/kg in infusion at rate of less than 50 mg/min (phenytoin).

- Alternatives to IV phenytoin are valproate 500–1000 mg IV bolus or levetiracetam 1 g bolus.

  Refractory status—if seizures continue (more than 20 minutes), then intubate and give one of the following:
- Midazolam drip IV. Load with 0.2 mg/kg and infuse at rate of 0.03–0.2 mg/kg/hr

  Or
- Propofol IV. Load 1–2 mg/kg repeat every 5 mins till seizures stop, followed by IV infusion 2–10 mg/hr.

  Or
- Phenobarbitone IV bolus 6–8 mg/kg at a rate not more than 60 mg/min.

  Partial (local) minor status epilepticus consists of frequent seizures involving an extremity or facial muscles with preservation of consciousness and no tendency for generalization.
- Phenytoin orally during an 8 to 12 hours period followed by maintenance dose of 300 to 400 mg/day.

Q.7.　Write short note on temporal epilepsy.

(Mar 2003, 5 Marks) (Apr 2010, 5 Marks)

Ans. Temporal epilepsy is the form of epilepsy where aura (A subjective, but recognizable sensation that precedes and signals the onset convulsion) is either auditory, visual, olfactory or gustatory.

Clinical Features

- There is feeling of unusual smell, an emotional feeling or *hallucinations.
- Motor activity stops and patient looks vacant.
- There is unilateral dystonic posturing of the limb.
- There is temporary cessation of the activity followed by lip smoking, chewing movements or the patient may walk aimlessly. When seizure and amnesia is present.

Management

- *General:*
  - Avoid physical exertion, regular habits of eating and sleeping.
  - Avoid alcohol.
- *Pharmacological:*
  - Clonazepam 1.5 mg/day reduces excitability of neurons.
  - Methsuximide 500 mg daily is effective.
  - Clobazam 10 to 20 mg has antiepileptic activity.
  - Gabapentin 300 mg TDS is used to control epilepsy.
  - Lamotrigine 50 mg daily for two weeks followed by 100 mg/day given in two divided doses for 2 weeks. After dose is increased by 100 mg every 1 to 2 weeks till response is obtained.

Q.8.　Write short note on syncope.

(Mar 2016, 3 Marks) (Feb 2014, 3 Marks)
(Nov 2008, 10 Marks) (Aug 2012, 5 Marks)
(May/June 2009, 5 Marks)

Or

Write short answer on syncope *(Sep 2018, 3 Marks)*

Ans. Syncope is a transient loss or impairment of consciousness with inability to maintain postural tone due to acute decrease in cerebral blood flow.

Causes

- Due to decreased cerebral perfusion
  - Inadequate vasoconstrictive mechanisms
    - Vasovagal
    - Postural hypotension
    - Carotid sinus syncope
    - Antihypertensive drugs, i.e., hydralazine, etc.
  - Hypovolemia
    - Hemorrhage (blood loss)
    - Addison's disease
  - Reduction of venous return
    - Cough
    - Micturition
    - Mediastinal compression
    - Straining at stool evacuation (defecation)
  - Reduced cardiac output
    - Aortic stenosis or hypertrophic subaortic stenosis
    - Myocardial infarction
    - Cardiac tamponade due to pericardial effusion
    - Pulmonary embolism
  - Arrhythmias
    - AV blocks (2nd degree and 3rd degree or complete AV block)
    - Ventricular asystole
    - Ventricular tachycardia and fibrillation
    - Supraventricular tachycardia
  - Cerebrovascular disturbance
    - Transitory ischemic attack
    - Hypertension
    - Vertebrobasilar insufficiency
- Noncirculatory causes
  - Hypoxia
  - Anemia
  - Prolonged bed rest
  - Anxiety neurosis

Types of Syncope

Vasovagal Syncope

- This is the most common syncope.
- It tends to occur at the time of emotional stress or after an injury or accident or severe pain.
- It involves cardiac slowing because of vagal stimulation and sudden reduction in systemic peripheral resistance due to withdrawal of sympathetic tone.

Postural Hypotension with Syncope

- It occurs in patients who have chronic illness or instability of vasomotor reflexes.

Q 7.　*Hallucinations = A perception of having seen, heared, touched, tasted or smelled something that wasn't actually there.

- Fall in blood pressure is present in erect posture due to loss of vasoconstrictive reflexes leading to pooling of blood in capacitance vessels of lower limbs.
- It usually occurs on sudden arising from supine position or in the standing position.

Micturition Syncope

- It is seen in elder patients during or after urination mainly after arising from sitting position.
- It occurs due to the release of intravesical pressure at the time of micturition which leads to sudden vasodilatation which become augmented by standing causing syncope.

Cardiac Syncope

- It occurs due to reduction in sudden cardiac output.
- It occurs due to abnormal decrease or increase in the heart rate.
- Supraventricular tachycardias, cerebrovascular disease, valvular heart disease can cause syncope.

Carotid Sinus Syncope

- It is due to vagal mediated cardiac slowing or due to fall in blood pressure due to depressor response.
- Carotid sinus is sensitive to stretch, so it is induced in sensitive patient by turning head to one side or by tight fitting cervical collar.
- It last for few seconds to few minutes.

Cough Syncope

- It occurs in patients with chronic bronchitis or chronic obstructive pulmonary disease.
- It happens due to the decrease venous return to heart due to rise in intra-thoracic pressure at the time of coughing.

Syncope of Cerebrovascular Disease

- It occurs due to narrowing of large arteries.
- This is the manifestation of vertebrobasilar insufficiency.
- Excessive physical activity or exercise decreases blood flow to upper part of brainstem leading ot syncope.

Clinical Features

- Tingling or numbness in the limbs, sudden darkness before eyes and patient has feeling of *blacking out.
- The patient is cold and sweating and fall suddenly to ground and become unconsciousness.
- Patient's respiration+Pulse of the patient is slow and limbs are cold and clammy.
- Pupils may retract to light.

Management

- All the medical/dental procedure or treatment is stopped.
- Remove instruments from oral cavity, such as rubber dam, gauze, cotton, etc.
- Patient is kept in Trendelenburg position, i.e., patient is kept in a head low and feet up position.
- Loose tighten clothing of patient.

- Aromatic fumes inhalation is given or sprinkle cold water on face of patient for reflex stimulation.
- If recovery is gained escort patient home.
- If recovery is not gained Injection Atropine 0.6 mg IM or IV is given.
- If still recovery is not gained look for hypoglycemia and Addison's crisis
- Start basic life support
- Summon medical help.

Q.9. **Enumerate the cause of epilepsy.** *(Feb 2006, 2 Marks)*
Ans.

Causes of Epilepsy in Different Age Groups

In Neonates (0 to 2 years)

- Perinatal hypoxia, or ischemia
- Birth injury
- Acute infections, i.e., meningitis, encephalitis metabolic disturbance, i.e., hypoglycemia, hypocalcemia, hypomagnesemia structural lesions, such as congenital vascular malformations.
- Familial or genetic disorders.

In Children (2 to 12 years)

- Idiopathic
- Acute infections, i.e., meningitis, encephalitis, toxoplasmosis, cerebral abscess
- Head injury or trauma
- Febrile convulsions

In Adolescents (12 to 18 years)

- Idiopathic
- Head trauma
- Drugs, i.e., amphetamines, antidepressants, phenothiazines, etc.
- Alcohol withdrawal
- Arteriovenous malformations
- Infections, i.e., meningitis, encephalitis, cerebral abscess, toxoplasmosis

In Person of Age 18 to 35 years

- Head injury or trauma
- Alcoholism
- Brain tumors, cysts, hydrocephalus, aneurysms, AV malformations
- Inflammatory disorders, such as sarcoidosis, multiple sclerosis, SLE.

In Older Adults and Old Persons

- Brain tumors
- Cerebrovascular accidents (thrombosis, infarction, hemorrhage)
- Alcoholism
- Uremia
- Hepatic encephalopathy

Q 8.   *Blacking out = Period of alcohol-induced amnesia during which a person actively engages in behavior like walking or talking.
     *Sighing = Deep audible breadth.

♦ Hypertensive encephalopathy
♦ Electrolyte disturbances
♦ Hypoglycemia

Q.10. Write short note on pyogenic meningitis.

(Oct 2007, 10 Marks)

Or

Describe briefly clinical features and management of pyogenic meningitis. *(Sep 2006, 5 Marks)*

Ans. Inflammation of the meninges is called as meningitis.

Pyogenic meningitis occurs due to *Streptococcus pneu-moniae, staphylococcus aureus, Haemophilus influenzae*.

Pathology: Infection once it reaches the protective wall of meninges, rapidly spread over the surface of brain, spinal cord and ependymal lining of ventricles.

♦ Brain and spinal cord are swollen and congested.
♦ Cortical veins become congested and convolutions on the surface of brain become flattened because of internal hydrocephalus which is due to inflammatory adhesions obstructing outflow of CSF from fourth ventricle, whole of CSF become turbid and purulent.

Clinical Features

Symptoms

♦ Fever coming with rigors.
♦ Headache which is very severe (bursting in character) mainly in frontal region radiating down to back.
♦ Vomiting
♦ Convulsion in children
♦ Malaise
♦ Severe photophobia
♦ *Ptosis:* Due to raised intracranial tension
♦ Stiffness in neck and back
♦ Pain in neck
♦ Impairment of consciousness, i.e., confusion, delirium and coma.

Signs

♦ Head retraction is present in infants and children.
♦ Neck rigidity, i.e., bending of neck causes pain and spasm of neck muscles or it is difficult to bend the neck.
♦ Kernig's sign is positive
♦ Brudzinski's sign is also positive if patient is conscious.
♦ Presence of papilledema
♦ Presence of cranial nerve palsies

Investigation

Blood count: Leukocytosis with rise in polymorph count.

CSF Examination

♦ CSF pressure is raised.
♦ It is turbid and purulent pus like.
♦ Formation of coagulum
♦ Protein content is markedly increased.
♦ Glucose content is decreased.
♦ CSF protein is raised
♦ Gram staining of CSF is positive

Complications

♦ Cranial nerve paralysis
♦ Deafness
♦ Mental retardation
♦ Epilepsy.

Treatment

Empirical treatment should be given before CSF culture and Gram stain report. Treatment should be directed to the most common microorganism present in particular age group.

Antibiotic Treatment

♦ Ceftriaxone or cefotaxime is given against *S. pneumonia, H. influenzae*, Group B streptococci and *N. meningitides*. In this vancomycin can be added to cover cephalosporin resistant *S. pneumonia*. Ampicillin can be added to cover *L. monocytogenes* in neonates of less than 3 months and more than 55 years of age.
♦ Ceftazidime is active against *P. aeruginosa* and is preferred over ceftriaxone or cefotaxime in hospital acquired meningitis.
♦ Choice of empirical antibiotics in pyogenic meningitis is:
  • *In neonates or infants of less than 3 months:* Ampicillin 100 to 50 mg/dL + Ceftriaxone 500 to 1000 mg/kg/day or cefotaxime 50 mg/kg
  • *In children and adults:* Ceftriaxone 500 to 1000 mg/kg/day or cefotaxime 50 mg/kg + vancomycin 60 mg/kg
  • Adults more than 55 years: Ampicillin 3 g tds or QDS + Ceftriaxone 2 g BD or cefotaxime 50 mg/kg + vancomycin 1 g 8 hourly
  • In hospital acquired meningitis, post-traumatic or post-surgical, immunocompromised patients— Ampicillin 3 g tds or qds + Ceftazidime 2 g 8 hourly + vancomycin 1 g 8 hourly.

Duration of Antibiotic Therapy

♦ One week for *H. influenzae* and *N. meningitides* infection
♦ *S. pneumonia* for two weeks
♦ *L. monocytogenes* and gram-negative bacilli infections for 3 weeks.

Adjunctive Therapy

Dexamethasone 0.4 mg/kg BD for 4 days with first dose of antibiotic.

Supportive Therapy

♦ Patients having raised intracranial pressure should be treated in ICU.
♦ IV mannitol, hyperventilation and elevation of patient's head to 30° is done to decrease raised intra-cranial pressure.

Q.11. Enumerate the etiological factors of bacterial meningitis. Describe clinical features, complications and management of a case of meningococcal meningitis. *(Sep 2009, 5 Marks)*

Ans.

Etiology of Bacterial Meningitis

Bacterial meningitis is caused by various bacteria which are as follows:

♦ **In neonates or infants**
  - Gram-negative bacilli, i.e., *E. coli* and *B. proteus*
  - Group B streptococci
  - *Listeria monocytogenes*
♦ **In adolescents or adults**
  - *Streptococcus pneumoniae*
  - *Neisseria meningitidis*
  - *Mycobacterium tuberculosis*
  - *Staphococcus aureus*
  - *Haemophilus influenzae*
♦ **In old age**
  - *Haemophilus influenzae*
  - *Neisseria meningitides*
  - *Streptococcus pneumoniae*
  - *Mycobacterium tuberculosis*
♦ **In immunocompromised**
  - *Listeria monocytogenes*
  - *Gram-negative bacilli*
  - *Staphylococcus pneumoniae*
  - *Mycobacterium tuberculosis*
  - *Cryptococcus neoformans*

Clinical Features of Meningococcal Meningitis

♦ Meningococcal rash, petechial rash on skin, mucus membrane and conjunctiva.
♦ Acute fulminant illness with adrenal insufficiency.
♦ Hypotension, shock and patient go quickly in comma. This is called as Water house–Friderichsen syndrome.
♦ It is due to necrosis in adrenal gland during course of meningococcal septicemia.
♦ Signs of meningeal irritation, i.e., Kernig's and Brudzinski's sign are positive.
♦ In children and adults it is mainly present.
♦ Neck rigidity
♦ Vomiting
♦ Fever with rigor
♦ Dilatation of pupil.

Complications of Meningococcal Meningitis

♦ Neurological defect like hemiplegia, aphasia, ocular anterior, hemianopia, blindness and deafness.
♦ Mental deterioration
♦ Cerebritis, brain abscess
♦ Focal fits
♦ Auditory impairment
♦ Sub-dural empyema
♦ Internal hydrocephalus
♦ Spinal cord compression due to arachnoiditis.

Management of Meningococcal Meningitis

♦ For adult patients penicillin G 5 to 10 million units IV 6 hourly.
♦ Cephalosporins, i.e., cefotaxime 2 g IV or ceftriaxone 2 g IV OD is also effective.
  Patients allergic to penicillin are treated with chloramphenicol 1 g IV 6 hourly
♦ Treatment is continued for 7 to 10 days.

♦ For raised intracranial tension IV mannitol is given which is accompanied by high doses of dexamethasone 4 mg IV 6 hourly.
  The supportive treatment is to maintain nutrition, fluid and electrolytic balance.

Q.12. Differentiate between tubercular meningitis and pyogenic meningitis. *(Feb 2006, 2.5 Marks)*

Ans.

Tubercular meningitis	Pyogenic meningitis
• Most common organism for causing tubercular meningitis is *M. tuberculum*	• Most common organism for causing pyogenic meningitis is *S. pneumoniae*
• It is common in childhood	• It is most common in adults
• Neck rigidity, vomiting and convulsions are lower in intensity	• Neck rigidity, vomiting and convulsions are higher in intensity. Muscular spasm is more common
• It is associated with infection in lungs, bowel and mesenteric glands	• It is associated with infection in pneumonia, chronic otitis media, sinusitis and head injury
• CSF is clear or slightly opalescent and is under pressure. Cob web forms are seen if it is allowed to stand overnight. In it mainly lymphocytes are seen in CSF	• CSF is thick, greenish fluid. It is turbid and pus like. The CSF pressure is raised. Polymorphs are the most common cells found
• In it antitubercular treatment is given	• Penicillin G or cefotaxime for at least 7 days is given
• Not specific vaccine is available or present for tubercular meningitis	• Vaccination with Hib vaccine reduces the incidence

Q.13. Describe the clinical and diagnostic features of tuberculous meningitis. *(Feb 2002, 5 Marks)*

Ans.

Clinical Features

Symptoms

♦ Headache
♦ Vomiting
♦ Low grade fever
♦ Lassitude, i.e., weariness or exhaustion
♦ Depression
♦ Confusion
♦ Behavior changes

Signs

♦ Meningism may be present
♦ Occulomotor palsies
♦ Papilledema
♦ Depression of conscious level
♦ Focal hemisphere signs.

Diagnostic Features

♦ Person with history of contact with tubercular patient presenting with low grade fever, ill health, weight loss, odd behavior, headache should make one suspect tubercular meningitis.

♦ Diagnosis shall be confirmed by the lumbar puncture.

CSF examination reveals following results:

♦ CSF is straw colored, clear but when allowed to stand, a fine clot, i.e., spider web is formed.
♦ Lymphocyte count is high
♦ Protein content is high
♦ Glucose is low
♦ In acute cases, polymorphs may predominate
♦ AFB stain can be positive. Culture or AFB is positive in 80% of cases
  CT or MRI brain may show meningeal enhancement or hydrocephalous

Q.14. Outline the management of migraine.

(Mar 2009, 5 Marks)

Ans.

♦ *During attack:*
  • *Analgesics:* NSAIDs, e.g., diclofenac can be given orally or IM and is particularly useful when severe vomiting is a feature. Sublingual Piroxicam has significant analgesic effects in acute migraine without aura with excellent tolerability.
  • *Ergotamine:* Ergotamine tartrate 0.25 to 0.5 mg IM or orally 1–2 mg. Tablet preferably in combination with 100 mg caffeine—2 tablets at onset followed by 1 tablet after 30 minutes, if necessary, or Dihydroergotamine 1 mg IM, or 1–2 mg by mouth. Whichever preparation is used, a high dose often causes nausea and vomiting. These may be prevented by giving cyclizine 50 mg. or chlorpromazine 25 mg.
  • *5-HT1 agonists:* Sumatriptan 6 mg SC gives relief from headache in 60 minutes, with corresponding improvement in nausea, vomiting and photophobia. Oral dose of 100 mg provides relief within 2 hours. Headaches recur within 48 hours in little less than half the patients. Rizatriptan given orally acts faster than sumatriptan. Zolmitriptan nasal spray 5 mg gives relief in 5 minutes.
  • *General:* Lying in a darkened and quiet room and ice pack to the head may help.
♦ Reducing frequency and severity of subsequent attacks
  • Elimination of trigger factors:, e.g., sleeping late, irregular and hurried meals, certain foods, especially chocolate and fried food, or missing of meals, psychological stress, contraceptive pills. Treatment of cervical spondylosis
  • *Relaxation exercises:* They may include biofeedback from a temporalis electromyogram. *Yoga, Pranayama.*
  • *Drugs:*
    – Serotonin (5-HT) inhibitors: Calcium antagonists, such as Flunarizine 10 mg/day Or Cyproheptadine 4 mg t.d.s. Or Pizotyfen 0.5 mg t.d.s. or 1.5 mg nocte. Or Methysergide 1–2 mg t.d.s. is the most effective drug in this group but should be used under supervision in courses not exceeding 3–4 months.
    – *Topiramate:* It is an antiepileptic drug used in prophylaxis of migraine. *Dose:* 2.5 to 5 mg BD

    – Divalproex (valproic acid) 200 mg BD
    – *Tricyclic agents:*, e.g., amitriptyline 25 mg TDS may be effective irrespective of the presence of depression.
    – *Ergotamine tartrate*—for histamine cephalalgia 1 mg by mouth or 0.25 mg by self-administered injection or by suppository used regularly last thing at night can be continued for many weeks without harmful effects, 2 days being left without treatment each week.
    – Hormones: Progesterone given for last eight days may be useful for migraine occurring in the immediate premenstrual period or at beginning of catamenia. When migraine begins or becomes worse at the time of menopause, estrin, given in small doses as continuous therapy sometimes helpful.
    – *Schedule:*
      » Propranolol 40–160 mg/day or flunarizine 5–10 mg/day as first line of therapy.
      » In patients with episodic and chronic migraine Topiramate 50–100 mg/day.
      » In patients with episodic migraine Divalproex 250–750 mg/day
      » For mixed migraine and tension type headache— amitriptyline 10–25 mg/day.
      After 6–12 months of prophylaxis gradual withdrawal should be considered.

Q.15. Describe causes, clinical features, treatment and complication of meningitis. *(Sep 2004, 20 Marks)*

Ans. Inflammation of the meninges is called as meningitis.

Causes

♦ *Infectious causes:*
  • *Bacterial:*
    – *Common: N. meningitides, S. pneumoniae, H. influenza, M tuberculosis*
    – *Neonatal:* Group *B streptococcus, E. coli, L. monocytogenes*
    – *Uncommon: S. aureus, P. Aeruginosa*
    – *Rare: Salmonella, Shigella, N. gonorrhea*
  • *Viral:*
    – *Common:* Mumps, Echovirus, Coxsackie virus A and B, Genital herpes virus 1 and 2
    – *Neonatal:* Other herpes virus, Epstein-Barr virus, Varicella zoster virus
    – *Uncommon: Cytomegalovirus, HIV, Lymphocytic choriomeningitis virus*
    – *Rare: Adenovirus Types 3 and 7, Arbovirus*
  • *Protozoa: Naegleria*
  • *Fungal: Cryptococcus neoformans, Candida*
  • *Spirochaetal:* Leptospirosis, Syphilis and Lyme disease
  • *Rickettsial:* Typhus fever
♦ Noninfectious causes
  • *Malignant:* Leukemic meningitis
  • *Other noninfectious causes:* Sarcoidosis, connective tissue disease, systemic lupus erythematosus, Sjögren's syndrome
  • *Vasculitis:* Granulomatous polyangiitis, eosinophilic granulomatous polyangiitis, CNS vasculitis

Clinical Features

Symptoms

- Fever coming with rigors
- Headache which is severe mainly in frontal region radiating down to back
- Vomiting
- Convulsion in children
- Malaise
- Severe photophobia
- Ptosis—due to raised intracranial tension
- Stiffness in neck and back
- Pain in neck
- Impairment of consciousness, i.e., confusion, delirium and coma

Signs

- Head retraction is present in infants and children.
- Neck rigidity, i.e., bending of neck causes pain and spasm of neck muscles or it is difficult to bend the neck.
- Kernig's sign is positive
- Brudzinski's sign is also positive if patient is conscious.
- Presence of papilledema
- Presence of cranial nerve palsies

Treatment

Empirical treatment should be given before CSF culture and Gram stain report. Treatment should be directed to the most common microorganism present in particular age group.

Antibiotic Treatment

- Ceftriaxone or cefotaxime is given against *S. pneumonia, H. influenzae,* Group B streptococci and N. meningitides. In this vancomycin can be added to cover cephalosporin resistant *S. pneumonia.* Ampicillin can be added to cover *L. monocytogenes* in neonates of less than 3 months and more than 55 years of age.
- Ceftazidime is active against *P. aeruginosa* and is preferred over ceftriaxone or cefotaxime in hospital acquired meningitis.
- Choice of empirical antibiotics in pyogenic meningitis is:
- *In neonates or infants of less than 3 months:* Ampicillin 100 to 50 mg/dL + Ceftriaxone 500 to 1000 mg/kg/day or cefotaxime 50 mg/kg
- *In children and adults:* Ceftriaxone 500 to 1000 mg/kg/day or cefotaxime 50 mg/kg + vancomycin 60 mg/kg
- *Adults more than 55 years:* Ampicillin 3 g TDS or QDS + Ceftriaxone 2 g BD or cefotaxime 50 mg/kg + vancomycin 1 g 8 hourly
- In hospital acquired meningitis, post-traumatic or post-surgical, immunocompromised patients: Ampicillin 3 g TDS or QDS + Ceftazidime 2 g 8 hourly + vancomycin 1 g 8 hourly.

Duration of Antibiotic Therapy

- One week for *H. influenzae* and *N. meningitides* infection
- *S. pneumoniae* for two weeks
- *L. monocytogenes* and gram-negative bacilli infections for 3 weeks

Adjunctive Therapy

Dexamethasone 0.4 mg/kg BD for 4 days with first dose of antibiotic.

Supportive Therapy

- Patients having raised intracranial pressure should be treated in ICU.
- IV mannitol, hyperventilation and elevation of patient's head to 30° is done to decrease raised intracranial pressure.

For treatment of tubercular meningitis refer to Ans. 23 of same chapter

Complications

- *Neurological deficiencies:* Hemiplegia, aphasia, hemianopia, blindness, deafness.
- Mental deterioration
- Cerebritis, brain abscess, focal fits, auditory impairments, sub-dural empyema, internal hydrocephalus.

Q.16. Discuss causes and management of unconsciousness. *(Feb/Mar 2004, 10 Marks)*

Ans.

Causes of Unconsciousness

- Decrease in the cerebral perfusion:
  - Inadequate vasoconstriction mechanism
    - Postural hypotension
    - Vasovagal shock
    - Anti-hypertensive drugs
    - Carotid sinus syncope.
  - Hypovolemia:
    - Addison's disease
    - Due to blood loss, i.e., hemorrhage.
  - Decrease in the venous return
    - Mediastinal compression
    - Micturition
    - Cough
    - Straining during defecation.
  - Decrease in cardiac output
    - Myocardial infarction
    - Pulmonary embolism
    - Aortic stenosis
    - Cardiac tamponade.
  - Arrhythmias
    - In AV blocks
    - Supraventricular tachycardia
    - Ventricular asystole
    - Ventricular tachycardia.
  - Cerebrovascular disturbances
    - Hypertension
    - Transitory ischemic attack
    - Vertebrobasilar insufficiency.
- Non-circulatory causes:
  - Anemia
  - Anxiety neurosis
  - Hypoxia.

For management refer to Ans. 8 of same chapter.

Q.17. Describe the CSF picture of pyogenic meningitis and tubercular meningitis.
Ans. *(Sep 2005, 10 Marks)*

Content	Normal value	Pyogenic meningitis	Tubercular meningitis
Glucose	40–70 mg/dL	Low <40 mg/dL	Low or normal
Lactate	10–20 mg/dL	Low	Low or normal
Protein	Up to 45 mg/dL	Elevated	Elevated
Albumin	6.6–42.2 mg/dL	Elevated	Elevated
Ammonia	25–80 µg/dL	Elevated	Elevated
CSF pressure	50–180 mm/Hg	Raised and turbid	Normal
CSF volume	150 mL	Raised	Raised
Gram staining	—	Positive	Negative
Lymphocyte	60–70%	Normal	Raised
Polymorphs	None	Present	—

Q.18. Discuss the causes of headache.

(Feb/Mar 2004, 5 Marks)

Ans. The causes of headache are:
- *Intracranial and local extracranial*
  - Trauma leads to contusional or post-traumatic headache
  - *Intracranial inflammations:* Meningitis, encephalitis, cerebral abscess.
  - *Vascular headaches:* Hypertension, cerebral or subarachnoid hemorrhage, intracranial aneurysm; vasodilator drugs like nitrites and histamine, adrenaline.
  - *Menopausal:* Alcohol hangover or withdrawal, coffee withdrawal. Giant cell arteritis (temporal arteritis), thrombosis of intracranial venous sinus.
  - *Traction headache:* Pain produced by intracranial arterial displacement and distortion of the dura, usually caused by space occupying lesions or raised intracranial pressure or low intracranial pressure (intracranial hypotension).
  - *Post-lumbar puncture headache:* Low CSF pressure headache.
  - *Cough headache:* A benign syndrome of severe headache which accompanies coughing, straining or sneezing can be due to posterior fossa tumor.
- *Cranial neuritis and neuralgias:* This is of sensory nerves of scalp, e.g., orbital neuralgia, or neuralgia of auriculotemporal, posterior auricular or great occipital nerves, herpes of Gasserian ganglion.
- General or systemic causes
  - *Anoxemia:* Anemia, carbon monoxide or carbon dioxide poisoning.
  - *Toxic:* Fevers, uremia, eclampsia, metallic poisoning, "alcoholic" hangover, post-convulsive, drugs, such as quinine, tobacco, cocaine, morphine, sulfonamides. Pelvic or gallbladder disease, constipation, intestinal stasis. Nervous exhaustion.
  - *Metabolic factors:* Hypoglycemia, alkalosis or acidosis.
  - *Hemopoietic factors:* Essential polycythemia, thrombasthenia.

- *Referred pain*
  - *Eyes:* Errors of refraction, glaucoma, iritis, etc.
  - *Ears:* Otitis, mastoiditis, vestibular nerve lesions, Eustachian tube block, tumors of middle and inner ear.
  - *Teeth:* Impacted teeth, infected tooth sockets and dental roots.
  - *Paranasal sinuses:* Infection of paranasal sinuses may cause localized pain.
  - *Neck:* Diseases of upper cervical spine may be associated with both occipital and frontal pain.
- *Psychogenic:* Common cause of headache in depression.
- *Tension (muscle contraction) headache:*
  Pain resulting from sustained contraction of skeletal muscles of the neck, frontalis, occipital muscles due to emotional tension.
- *Exertional headache:*
  Headache may come on during exertion and persist for few hours afterwards.
- *Other primary headaches:*
  - Hypnic headache syndrome is a late onset disorder and usually wakes up the patient from sleep at around the same time every night. The headache is usually treatable with flunarizine and lithium.
  - Exploding head syndrome can occur any time during day or night.

Q.19. Write short note on definition and classification of epilepsy. *(Mar 2007, 5 Marks)*

Ans. Epilepsy is defined as condition characterized by the recurrent episodes primarily of cerebral origin in which there is disturbance of movement, sensation, behavior and consciousness.

Classification

Classification of epileptic seizures modified in 1981
- *Partial or focal seizures:*
  - Simple partial seizures (awareness preserved)
    Depending on the concomitant signs, they are:
    - Motor
    - Sensory

– Visual
– Versive
– Psychomotor
  • Complex partial seizures (awareness lost)
    Depending on the area involved due to spread, they are:
    – Temporal lobe
    – Frontal lobe
  • Secondary generalized partial seizures
♦ *Primary generalized seizures:*
  • Tonic-clonic (grand mal)
  • Tonic
  • Absence (petit mal)
  • Akinetic
  • Myoclonic
  • Infantile spasms
♦ *Unclassified seizures:*
  Seizures which do not fit into above two categories;
  • Neonatal seizures
  • Infantile spasms

Q.20. Write short note on panic attack. *(Mar 2007, 5 Marks)*
Ans. Panic attacks are discrete episodes of paroxysmal severe anxiety and are characterized by severe and frightening autonomic symptoms, i.e., shortness of breath, palpitations, excessive perspiration; dizziness, faintness and chest pain. Many patients believe they are in immediate danger of death or collapse and seek urgent medical attention.

Typical Feature of Panic Attack

♦ It is of sudden onset and short duration
♦ It shows rapidly escalating physical and psychological symptoms
♦ Presence of incapacitating symptoms of breathness and/ or palpitations
♦ Fear of impending death, collapse or loss of control
♦ Rapid escape from situation where attack is occurred
♦ Sometimes panic attacks are labeled nocturnal when they occur at night only
♦ Panic attack in social phobia is restricted to feared social situations
♦ Panic attack in panic disorder occurs unexpectedly in social encounters and when person is alone.

Diagnostic Guideline for Panic Attack

A panic attack is characterized by all of the following:
♦ A discrete episode of intense fear or discomfort
♦ It starts abruptly
♦ It reaches maximum intensity within a few minutes
♦ It lasts for at least several minutes
♦ At least four symptoms are present (including at least one autonomic symptom)
♦ The attack is not caused by a physical disease, an organic mental disorder, or another condition, such as schizophrenia, mood disorder or somatoform disorder.
♦ Panic attack may accompany any anxiety disorder, but a specific diagnosis of panic disorder can be made if they occur frequently and unexpectedly.

Management
♦ *Psychological:*
  • Helping patients to understand that their symptoms are not caused by serious physical ailment.
  • Relaxation training can be helpful, but severely ill patients are more likely to benefit from cognitive behavior therapy.
  • Exposure therapy can be formed under supervision of a behavior therapist.
♦ *Drugs:*
  • High dose benzodiazepines, e.g., alprazolam are effective but can cause substantial depression and should be prescribed in severely-ill patients who have not responded to other treatment approaches.
  • Antidepressant drugs, i.e., imipramine, clomipramine and selective serotonin re-uptake inhibitors, i.e., paroxetine are as efficacious in reducing anxiety symptoms, lessening agoraphobia and minimizing overall impairment.

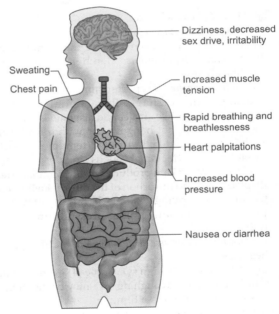

Fig. 23: Panic attack.

Q.21. Write short note on depression. *(Sep 2007, 5 Marks)*
Ans. Depression is defined as depressed mood on a daily basis for a minimum duration of two weeks.

Depression is present in a quarter to half of all mental patients.

Etiology
♦ **Genetic factors:** They play a major role in mood disorders and their effect is stronger in patients with more severe biological symptoms. In twin studies of bipolar disorder, average concordance rate is 65% in monozygotic twins and 14% in dizygotic twins.

- **Social factors:** Events associated with depression are generally 'loss events', such as loss of a job, relative or tend, money, health or status. Other factors that adversely affect the response to the events can be, a working class background, lack of confiding relationship with a spouse, unemployment, loss of a parent before 11 years of age.
- **Biological markers for depression:** They show strong associations, particularly with the somatic (endogenous) syndrome. False-positive results occur in the presence of various medical disorders. Dexamethasone suppression test is the most important biological marker.
- **Circadian rhythms and related markers:** They have also been found abnormal in depression. This is suggested by the diurnal variations in mood, early morning waking and the sometimes periodic course, for example, yearly attacks of illness.
- **Psychological factors:** Repeated trauma, stressful life events and disturbed marital and interpersonal relationships.

Clinical Features

- *General:* Hopelessness, helplessness, low mood, low self-esteem, reduced energy, suicidal thoughts, loss of interest, poor concentration, guilt, pessimism, depersonalization.
- *Somatic:* Appetite disturbance, weight change, constipation, amenorrhea, low libido, sleep disturbance
- *Anxiety:* Tension, apprehension, phobias.

Management

- Antidepressants are used in all phases of the treatment of major depression, acute management, continuation therapy and maintenance or prophylactic treatment.
- *Tricyclic drugs:* They increase recovery rate significantly, but have a wide range of side effects. These lead to non-compliance and limit usefulness in illnesses of mild to moderate severity. The dose of tricyclics should be initially low and increased gradually.
- *Selective serotonin re-uptake inhibitors:* They are effective drugs and are better tolerated at therapeutic doses than other compounds.
- If patient is not responding to antidepressant drugs ECT treatment should be given. Usually 6 to 10 ECTs are effective in resolving acute depression. As course is completed prophylactic treatment should be given to prevent relapse
- Cognitive psychotherapy should also be done.

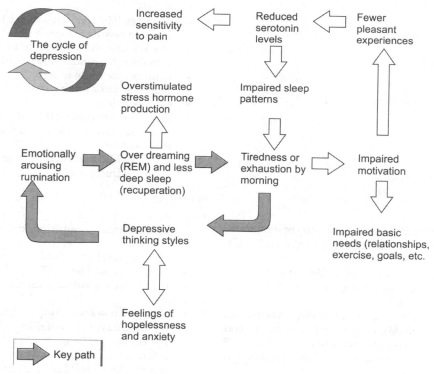

Fig. 24: Cycle of depression.

Q.22. Write short note on anxiety neurosis.

(Mar 2008, 7 Marks) (Feb 2013, 5 Marks)

Ans. Anxiety is a normal response to threat or stressful events and is usually short lived and controllable. It probably functions as an 'alarm mechanism' to prepare an individual for a physical response to perceived danger (the fight or—flight' response). Anxiety symptoms are considered clinically significant when they:

- Are abnormally severe
- Are unusually prolonged
- Occur in absence of stressful circumstances
- Impair physical, social or occupational functioning

Features of Anxiety Neurosis

Psychological

- Fear and apprehension
- Inner tension and restlessness
- Irritability
- Impaired ability to concentrate
- Increased startle response
- Increased sensitivity to physical sensations
- Disturbed sleep

Physical

- Increased muscle tension
- Tremor
- Sweating
- Palpitations
- Chest tightness and discomfort
- Shortness of breath
- Dry mouth
- Difficulty in swallowing
- Diarrhea
- Frequency of micturition
- Loss of sexual interest
- Dizziness
- Numbness and tingling
- Faintness

Management

Definitive need for treatment depends on severity of symptoms, degree of personal distress, level of occupational and social impairment.

- Benzodiazepines are effective anxiolytic drugs but can cause sedation and have potential for dependence. They should be given in short courses.
- Other drugs include certain tricyclic antidepressants, e.g., imipramine (50–300 mg/d), buspirone (15–45 mg/d) and venlafaxine (serotonin—noradrenaline reuptake inhibitor 75 mg/d) none of which have same potential for psychological or physical dependence.
- Behavior therapy in form of relaxation training, systemic desensitization and cognitive therapy. Psychotherapy and family education is must.

Q.23. Describe clinical features, diagnosis and management of tubercular meningitis. *(Mar 2011, 4.5 Marks)*

Ans.

Clinical Features

Symptoms

- Headache
- Vomiting
- Low grade fever
- Lassitude, i.e., weariness or exhaustion
- Depression
- Confusion
- Behavior changes.

Signs

- Meningism may be present:
- Oculomotor palsies
- Papilledema
- Depression of conscious level
- Focal hemisphere signs.

Diagnosis

- Person with history of contact with tubercular patient presenting with low grade fever, ill health, weight loss, odd behavior, headache should make one suspect tubercular meningitis.
- Diagnosis shall be confirmed by the lumbar puncture. CSF examination reveals following results:
  - CSF is straw colored, clear but when allowed to stand, a fine clot, i.e., spider web is formed.
  - Lymphocyte count is high
  - Protein content is high
  - Glucose is low
  - In acute cases, polymorphs may predominate
  - AFB stain can be positive. Culture or AFB is positive in 80% of cases
    - CT or MRI brain may show meningeal enhancement or hydrocephalous

Management

- General management
  - Maintenance of nutrition, hydration and electrolyte balance.
  - Case of bowel and bladder
  - Nursing should be good
  - If there are convulsions, anticonvulsants are given.
- Treatment
  - *Antitubercular drugs:* Antitubercular drugs—Rifampicin 600 mg/day + Isoniazide (600 to 900 mg/day) + Pyrazinamide (1.5 g) should be given. Treatment with this regimen is given for 2 months. This is followed by rifampicin 600 mg/day + Isoniazide (600 to 900 mg/day) for 12 to 18 months.
  - *Steroids:* Prednisolone 40–60 mg/day to reduce toxicity, pia-arachnoid adhesions and feeling of well-being.

Q.24. Write short note on examination of cerebrospinal fluid.

(Sep 2009, 4 Marks)

Ans. Normal CSF is colorless, clear.

♦ Presence of blood indicates either local trauma or subarachnoid hemorrhage especially fresh.

♦ Xanthochromia or yellowish coloration of CSF is found in cerebral hemorrhage and when pus is present in CSF in considerable amount.

♦ Turbidity when present indicates excess of polymorphonuclear cells (meningitis).

♦ A clot or cob web may form in cases of tuberculous meningitis.

♦ Of the biochemical tests, protein content is 30–40 mg/dL and sugar 80 mg/DL.

♦ Normal CSF contains a small number of cells mostly lymphocytes (0–5/cumm).

♦ Excess of cells in the CSF indicate meningeal irritation.

♦ In cases of meningitis, CSF is examined for bacteria by gram's staining.

♦ A culture examination of CSF is often carried out in suspected infective process for identifying the causal organism.

♦ CSF examination has an important role in diagnosing bacterial and viral diseases, but its role in cases of cerebral hemorrhage is now being taken over by CT scan because of hazards involved.

♦ Colloidal reactions in the form of colloidal gold reaction is of value in cases of general paralysis of insane (GPI) and differentiates it from other form of neurosyphilis.

♦ Serological reactions like Wassermann reaction are also of help in cases of neurosyphilis.

Q.25. Differentiate between syncope and epilepsy.

(Sep 2008, 2.5 Marks)

Ans.

Features	Epilepsy	Syncope
Precipitant	Unusual	Emotional, painful and stressful event
Circumstances	Any	Usually upright posture, crowded or hot environment
Onset	Usually abrupt	Usually gradual with feeling of faintness, nausea, sweating and grayishness of vision
Skin color	Pale or flushed	Pale
Breathing	Stertorous, foaming	Shallow
Incontinence	Common	Unusual
Tongue biting	Common	Unusual
Vomiting	Unusual	Common
Injury	Common	Unusual
Postictal	Drowsy, confused, headache, sleep	Rapid recovery
Duration of unconsciousness	Minutes	Seconds

Q.26. Write short note on obsessive compulsive disorder.

(Sep 2009, 4 Marks)

Ans. Obsessive-compulsive disorder (OCD) is an anxiety disorder characterized by intrusive thoughts that produce uneasiness, apprehension, fear, or worry; by repetitive behaviors aimed at reducing the associated anxiety; or by a combination of such obsessions and compulsions.

Etiology

♦ *Genetic:* Obsessive compulsive disorder is widely accepted to result from genetic vulnerability and/or chemical changes in some areas of the brain. The precise pathogenesis is not completely understood. Twin studies show concordance rates as high as 87% in monozygous twins compared with 47% in dizygous pairs.

♦ *Neurobiology:* In OCD, patients have shown abnormalities in orbitofrontal cortex, cingulate cortex and caudate nucleus. In some children and adolescents, OCD develops after β hemolytic streptococcal infection, an autoimmune reaction similar to that of rheumatic fever.

♦ *Psychological theories:* In cognitive behavioral theory, obsessions are considered anxiogenic. OCD patients cannot escape this anxiety and therefore develop compulsion in an attempt to reduce or prevent the feared consequences. Reduction of anxiety reinforces the compulsive behavior.

Symptoms and Signs

Common obsessive thoughts in obsessive-compulsive disorder (OCD) include:

♦ Fear of being contaminated by germs or dirt or contaminating others.

♦ Fear of causing harm to yourself or others.

♦ Intrusive sexually explicit or violent thoughts and images.

♦ Excessive focus on religious or moral ideas.

♦ Fear of losing or not having things you might need.

♦ *Order and symmetry:* The idea that everything must line up "just right."

♦ Superstitions; excessive attention to something considered lucky or unlucky.

Common compulsive behaviors in obsessive-compulsive disorder (OCD) include:

♦ Excessive double-checking of things, such as locks, appliances, and switches.

♦ Repeatedly checking in on loved ones to make sure they're safe.

♦ Counting, tapping, repeating certain words, or doing other senseless things to reduce anxiety.

♦ Spending a lot of time washing or cleaning.

♦ Ordering or arranging things "just so."

♦ Praying excessively or engaging in rituals triggered by religious fear.

♦ Accumulating "junk", such as old newspapers or empty food containers.

Diagnostic Criteria

♦ Obsessional thoughts, compulsive acts or both should be present on most days for at least two weeks.
♦ They are recognized by patients as their own
♦ Patients have tried to resist unsuccessfully at least one obsessive thought or compulsive act.
♦ The thoughts or act are not pleasurable.
♦ The thoughts, images, impulses and acts are unpleasantly repetitive.

Management

Behavioral Therapy

The specific technique used in BT/CBT is called exposure and ritual prevention (also known as "exposure and response prevention") or ERP; this involves gradually learning to tolerate the anxiety associated with not performing the ritual behavior. Exposure ritual/response prevention (ERP) has a strong evidence base. It is considered the most effective treatment for OCD. However, this claim has been doubted by some researchers criticizing the quality of many studies.

More recent behavioral work has focused on associative splitting.

Medication

♦ Medications as treatment include selective serotonin reuptake inhibitors (SSRIs), such as paroxetine (60 mg/day), sertraline, fluoxetine, escitalopram and fluvoxamine and the tricyclic antidepressants, in particular clomipramine (150–300 mg/day). SSRIs prevent excess serotonin from being pumped back into the original neuron that released it. Over a period of several weeks, the increased levels of serotonin downregulate the receptors, making them less responsive to 5-HT. This downregulation is concurrent with the onset of any therapeutic benefits from SSRIS, from 2–3 weeks.
♦ The atypical antipsychotics olanzapine, quetiapine, and risperidone have also been found to be useful as adjuncts to an SSRI in treatment-resistant OCD. However, these drugs are often poorly tolerated, and have significant metabolic side effects that limit their use.

Cognitive Behavior Therapy

Main approach in OCD is graded exposure and self-imposed response prevention. This require patient's to face their feared obsessions without undoing them with their compulsions. Exposure should be of sufficient duration to be effective. An effective method known as thought stopping may also be used.

Combined Therapy

Combination of cognitive behavior therapy and medication can be more effective than either alone.

Psychosurgery

For some, medication, support groups and psychological treatments fail to alleviate obsessive-compulsive symptoms. These patients may choose to undergo psychosurgery as a last resort. In this procedure, a surgical lesion is made in an area of the brain (the cingulate cortex).

Q.27. Write short note on transient ischemic attack.

(Sep 2009, 5 Marks)

Ans. These are transient attacks of loss of function of one part of the brain coming suddenly and lasting for variable period of time ranging from minutes to hours.

♦ Since arteries supplying the brain are end arteries so any pathology which produces obstruction to the flow of that vessel shall produce symptoms in the distribution of that blood vessel.
♦ Internal carotid artery is one of the commonest cerebral vessel which is involved by atherosclerosis and patient complains of transient disturbances due to localized cortical ischemia in the form of confusion contralateral hemiparesis and sensory loss. There may be aphasia (if lesion on left side) and hemianopic visual loss.
♦ Most commonly occlusion is in the common carotid artery and one may be able to appreciate diminished pulsation in the vessel in the neck. When obstruction is severe a bruit may be auscultated at the site.
♦ Obstruction of other arteries, such as anterior cerebral artery, middle cerebral artery and posterior cerebral artery produce picture almost, such as above except for little variations depending on the occlusion site.
♦ On the other hand involvement of posterior circulation (basilar artery, vertebral artery, post- inferior cerebellar artery) produces a picture of crossed hemiplegia, hemisensory loss and hemianopic visual loss. In addition patient has impairment of consciousness, small fixed pupils, pseudobulbar palsy and quadriplegia seen mainly.
♦ In basilar artery lesions while cases with posterior inferior cerebellar artery involvement are associated with severe vertigo, vomiting, dysphasia and diplopia. In addition, there is some degree of cerebellar deficiency with hypotonia and incoordination on the side of lesion, analgesia and thermoanesthesia on the face on the side of lesion and on the trunk and limbs on opposite side.
♦ Again neurological deficits shall be depending on which branch of the vessel is involved.

Q.28. Write short note on facial pain. *(Nov 2011, 3 Marks)*

Ans. Various number of conditions are involved in the pain localized to face. These may range from pain arising from diseases of teeth, gums, sinuses, temporomandibular joint to various causes.

Facial Neuritis

♦ It is a form of inflammation of the nerve of the face and scalp.
♦ It generally occurs as a complication of a septicemic estate or due to involvement by a neurotropic virus.
♦ Onset is usually acute and pain is confined to the face and scalp, occurring in paroxysms lasting for several hours and very often till the end of the day when the patient is exhausted.
♦ If the character of pain is dull aching which is intensified by exposure to cold and often occurs in the form of shooting

pains in the distribution of the nerve. Sometimes, the pain is so severe that the patient is unable to sleep.

♦ Physical examination shows presence of hyperalgesia in the distribution of nerves including face and scalp. Nerve trunk is tender on pressure.

Myofascial Pain

♦ It is a form of dull constant pain with local tenderness of the muscles of jaw.

♦ There is often pain and difficulty in opening the mouth.

♦ This pain is related to bad and improper habits of clenching and grinding of teeth. This type of habit is present amongst hysterical persons especially women who often clench and grind their teeth.

♦ There is no physical finding in such people except that these people have an emotionally labile personality and often suffer from depression.

♦ Treatment consists in giving them assurance, analgesics and tricyclic antidepressants.

Trigeminal Neuralgia

Refer to Ans. 2 of same chapter.

Post-Herpetic Neuralgia

♦ Herpes zoster commonly involves the ophthalmic division of the 5th nerve characterized by vesicular eruption on the face and pain. When herpes heals it leave behind neuralgic pain in the distribution of previous eruptions.

♦ It is a form of continuous aching or burning pain at that site on face and patient is often in great agony.

♦ Treatment is by analgesics. Sometimes codeine phosphate may have to be given.

♦ In some severe cases the course of post herpetic neuralgia may be prolonged one.

Migrainous Neuralgia

♦ It is often called 'Facioplegic migraine' where there are attacks of severe pain especially at night and the pain is confined to face and around one eye. This form of disease is common in men especially middle aged and the attack may be brought on after a bout of alcohol.

♦ The pain may last for an hour. Because of associated vomiting and paroxysmal nature of disease it is called 'migrainous neuralgia' or 'facioplegic migraine. There is headache and patient complains of some degree of congestion in the face.

♦ Treatment is by analgesics but response is poor.

Arthralgia of Temporomandibular Joint

♦ It may be in the form of rheumatoid arthritis or ankylosing spondylitis when there is pain and swelling of the joint.

♦ Movements at the joint are limited and patient complains of pain at the site as well as along the jaw confined to face.

♦ Involvement of other joints in the body shall favor the diagnosis.

♦ Treatment is by heat and anti-inflammatory drugs as well as by exercises of the joint involved with adequate periods of rest.

Temporal Arteritis

♦ It is a form of collagen disorder of unknown etiology which involves mainly the arteries.

♦ It commonly occurs in elderly age group.

♦ Patient may complain of pain on the face, jaw, mouth and tongue in the distribution of branches of external carotid artery.

♦ This pain worsens off if on eating and opening of the mouth.

♦ Since temporal arteritis is a collagen disorder there is a form of inflammation of the arteries.

Q.29. Write short note on temporal lobe epilepsy.

(Mar 2011, 3 Marks) (Dec 2012, 3 Marks)

Ans. Temporal lobe epilepsy is a form of focal epilepsy, a chronic neurological condition characterized by recurrent seizures.

Temporal lobe epilepsy (TLE) is the most common single form causing refractory epilepsy.

Temporal lobe epilepsies are a group of medical disorders in which humans and animals experience recurrent epileptic seizures arising from one or both temporal lobes of the brain.

Types

Two main types are internationally recognized:

1. *Medial temporal lobe epilepsy (MTLE):* arises in the hippocampus, parahippocampal gyrus and amygdala which are located in the inner aspect of the temporal lobe.

2. *Lateral temporal lobe epilepsy (LTLE):* arises in the neocortex on the outer surface of the temporal lobe of the brain.

Symptoms and Signs

♦ Simple partial seizures (SPS) involve small areas of the temporal lobe, such as the amygdala or the hippocampus. The term "simple" means that consciousness is not altered. In temporal lobe epilepsy SPS usually only cause sensations. These sensations may be mnestic, such as déjà vu (a feeling of familiarity), jamais vu (a feeling of unfamiliarity), a specific single or set of memories, or amnesia. The sensations may be auditory, such as a sound or tune, gustatory, such as a taste, or olfactory, such as a smell that is not physically present. Sensations can also be visual, involve feelings on the skin or in the internal organs. The latter feelings may seem to move over the body. Dysphoric or euphoric feelings, fear, anger, and other sensations can also occur during SPS. Often, it is hard for persons with SPS of TLE to describe the feeling. SPS are often called "auras" by lay persons who mistake them for a warning sign of a subsequent seizure. In fact, they are actual seizures in and of themselves. Persons experiencing only SPS may not recognize what they are or seek medical advice about them. SPS may or may not progress to the seizure types listed below.

♦ Complex partial seizures (CPS) by definition are seizures which impair consciousness to some extent. This is to say that they alter the person's ability to interact with his or her environment. They usually begin with an SPS, but then the seizure spreads to a larger portion of the temporal lobe resulting in impaired consciousness. Signs may include motionless staring, automatic movements of the hands or mouth, altered ability to respond to others, unusual speech, or unusual behaviors.

♦ Seizures which begin in the temporal lobe but then spread to the whole brain are known as secondarily generalized Tonic-Clonic Seizures (SGTCS).

Treatment

♦ In temporal lobe epilepsy, the most commonly used drugs are phenytoin, carbamazepine, primidone, valproate and phenobarbital.

♦ Newer drugs, such as gabapentin, topiramate, levetiracetam, lamotrigine, pregabalin, tiagabine, lacosamide, and zonisamide promise similar effectiveness, possibly with fewer side-effects.

♦ For patients with medial TLE whose seizures remain uncontrolled after trials of several antiepileptic drugs, resective surgery should be considered.

Q.30. Write in brief signs, symptoms and treatment of epilepsy. *(Apr 2008, 5 Marks)*

Or

Write short note on epilepsy. *(Jan 2016, 5 Marks)*

Ans. Epilepsy is defined as the group of disorders in which there are recurrent episodes of altered cerebral functions associated with paroxysmal and hypersynchronous electrical discharge of cerebral neurons.

Symptoms

♦ Aura is present which means there is warning of the attack.
♦ Loss of consciousness
♦ Patient fall over the ground
♦ Irritability
♦ Depression and abnormal feelings
♦ Giddiness and abdominal cramps
♦ When patient awakes he complains of headache

Signs

♦ Tonic contraction of muscles and epileptic cry produced by forceful expiration through the partly closed vocal cords.
♦ Tonic convulsions of two sides of the body occur with head and eyes rotated to one side.
♦ Tonic phase followed by clonic phase, i.e., after completion of tonic phase patient remain unconscious for few minutes to half an hour.
♦ Frothing of mouth and increased salivation from the mouth.
♦ During clonic phase patient may bite his tongue and pass urine and stools.

Treatment

Treatment of epilepsy is directed at the elimination of the cause of seizures, suppressing the expression of seizures and dealing with psychosocial consequences.

♦ *Immediate treatment of a seizure:*
  • Patient should always be migrated to the safer place.
  • Loose the clothes around the neck and move people away from the place so that patient can breathe fresh air easily.

• At the time of convulsion, helpers are not allowed to put the fingers inside the mouth. Tongue biting should be prevented by putting tightly rolled piece of cloth in mouth.
• As convulsion ceases, patient is turned into semiplane position and make air passage clear.
• Patient is advised to consult the doctor for medical advice.

♦ *Drug therapy:*
Choice of the drug depends on type of seizure.

• In localization related epilepsy first line prophylactics are lamotrigine, carbamazepine (slow-release), oxcarbazepine, levetiracetam.
• In primary generalized, symptomatic generalized and unclassified epilepsies, initial therapy should be lamotrigine or valproate (broad spectrum gents). Valproic acid is useful in absences and benzodiazepines in myoclonic jerks.
• Patients with refractory generalized epilepsy may benefit from adjunctive treatment with topiramate or levetiracetam, zonisamide, clonazepam, pregabalin.
• Various antiepileptic drugs along with their dosages used in epilepsy are:

Name of the drug	Dosage
In generalized tonic clonic (grand mal) or partial (focal) seizures	
Phenytoin	200 to 400 mg Adult 3 to 5 mg/kg given in BD dose
Carbamazepine	600 to 1200 mg TDS
Valproic acid	800 to 2000 mg TDS
Phenobarbital	60 to 180 mg BD
Primidone	750 to 1500 mg TDS
Lamotrigine	200 to 500 mg BD
Topiramate	200 to 400 mg BD
Oxcarbazepine	900 to 1800 mg BD
Levetiracetam	1000 to 3000 mg BD
Zonisamide	200 to 600 mg BD
Pregabaline	150 to 180 mg BD
Absence (Petit mal) seizures	
Ethosuximide	500 to 1500 mg TDS
Valproic acid	1500 to 2000 mg TDS
Clonazepam	1 to 6 mg OD or BD
Myoclonic seizures	
Valproic acid	1500 to 2000 mg TDS
Clonazepam	1 to 6 mg OD or BD

Plan of Treatment

♦ *Initial regimen:* The drug selected must be used in monotherapy. The drug should be introduced in small doses, since rapid introduction may cause side effects.

♦ *Maintenance treatment:* The aim should be to find the lowest dose which achieves complete seizure control without side effects which may be either idiosyncratic or due to intoxication, or chronic. Serum anticonvulsant levels are a useful guide to therapy—phenytoin (40–80), carbamazepine (20–50), phenobarbitone (40–170), ethosuximide (20–600). Valproate 300–600, oxcarbazepine 50–125, lamotrigine 4–60 mmol/L. If the optimum level of a single, first line drug does not control seizures, or if side-effects develop, the initial drug should be substituted with another first line anticonvulsant. If the second drug also fails to control seizures monotherapy with a third anticonvulsant, or combination therapy with two first line drugs should be tried.

If a combination of two first-line drugs is unsuccessful, one of the second-line drugs may be considered.

Drug Withdrawal

It should take place slowly over 2 to 3 months. If patient is receiving more than one drug, each drug should be withdrawn individually.

Q.31. **Write in brief signs, symptoms and treatment of facial palsy.** *(Apr 2008, 5 Marks)*

Or

Write signs and symptoms of facial palsy.
(Aug 2012, 5 Marks)

Ans. It is the paralysis of the facial nerve.

Symptoms

♦ Post-auricular pain is common and may precede paralysis by 2 days.
♦ Spontaneous complains of loss of taste sensation, hyperacusis and watering of eyes.
♦ Sweating is less over the affected side.

Signs

♦ Forehead cannot be wrinkled; frowning lost.
♦ Eye of affected cannot be closed. On attempting closure, eyeball turns upwards and outwards (Bell's phenomena).
♦ On showing the teeth, the lips do not separate on affected side. Whistling not possible. Articulation of labial components difficult. Nasolabial fold flattened out. Angle of mouth on affected side droops with dribbling of saliva.
♦ Cheek puffs out with expiration because of buccinator paralysis. Food collects between teeth and paralyzed cheek. Fluid runs out while drinking.
♦ Base of tongue is lowered.
♦ Vesicles within the external auditory meatus and ear drum in Ramsay Hunt syndrome. Pain may precede facial weakness. Deafness may result.

Treatment

♦ *Local heat:* Infrared or moist heat over the face or parotid region or both if there is tenderness of nerve trunk.
♦ *Local treatment of muscles:* The patient should massage the facial muscles with bland oil for twice a day for 5 min. The massaging movements should start from the chin and lower lip and are directed upwards. With return of function the

patient should practice movements of various muscles of face before a mirror.
♦ *Prevention of facial sagging:* Application of strips of adhesive tape is done to lift up the angle of mouth. Tape is attached to the temple and extends down in a V-shaped fashion to upper and lower lips.
♦ *Protection of eye:* It is done with dark glass or eye patch. Mild zinc boric solution is used to wash the eye to prevent conjunctivitis.
♦ *Corticosteroids:* If seen under a week of onset. Prednisolone 40 mg/day for 4 days and in tapering doses for over next 6 days helps by reducing secondary edema.
♦ *Antivirals:* Acyclovir, valacyclovir or famciclovir in combination with steroids, if started within 3 days of onset.
♦ *Surgery:* Decompression of facial nerve in second or third week cannot influence favorably natural course of Bell's palsy. Cases which fail to recover after 9 months in them anastomosis of facial nerve with accessory or preferably hypoglossal nerve is considered, or plastic surgery in cases of total paralysis with atrophy of muscle.

Q.32. **Write on causes of meningitis and discuss in detail bacterial meningitis.** *(Nov 2008, 15 Marks)*

Or

Describe the etiology, clinical features and management of bacterial meningitis.
(Dec 2010, 15 Marks)

Or

Write in brief sign, symptoms and treatment of bacterial meningitis. *(Jun 2010, 5 Marks)*

Ans.

Causes of Meningitis

♦ Neonates: *E. coli*
♦ Children:
  • *H. influenzae*
  • *S. pneumoniae*
  • *N. meningitidis.*
♦ Adults:
  • Young people: *Meningococcus*
  • Older people: *S. pneumonia.*
♦ Elderly and immunocompromised persons:
  • *Pneumococcus*
  • *Listeria*
  • Tuberculosis
  • Gram-negative organism
  • *Cryptococcus.*
♦ Viral:
  • Enterovirus
  • Herpes simplex virus
  • Mumps virus
  • Influenza virus
  • Japanese encephalitis virus
  • Arboviruses
  • Rabies virus
  • HIV.
♦ Nosocomial and post-traumatic meningitis:
  • *Klebsiella pneumoniae*
  • *E. coli*

- *Pseudomonas aeruginosa*
- *S. aureus.*
- Meningitis in special situation:
  - CSF shunts—staphylococcal
  - Spinal procedures—*Pseudomonas.*

Bacterial Meningitis

Pathophysiology

- Transmission, colonization and invasion of nasopharyngeal epithelium.
- Survival in the blood stream by evading host immune response.
- Meningeal invasion. Bacteremia may be rapidly followed by seeding of meningeal pathogens and secondary infection of the meninges.
- CSF inflammatory response.
- Cerebral edema and thrombosis.
- Bacterial meningitis causes loss of cerebrovascular anticoagulation.

Clinical Features

Symptoms

- Fever, malaise headache and vomiting.
- Pain over the neck
- Stiffness over the neck
- Confusion, delirium and coma.

Signs

- Kernig's sign is positive.
- Neck rigidity, i.e., when neck is bended there is presence of pain and there is spasm of neck muscles.
- Brudzinski's sign is also positive.
- Photophobia is present
- Cranial nerve palsies most commonly IIIrd, IVth, VIth and VIIth.
- Focal neurological deficits, such as nystagmus, aphasia, ataxia and peripheral nerve palsies.
- Partial or generalized seizures tend to be more common in *Strep. pneumoniae* and HIV meningitis.
- Purpura or petechiae in meningococcal meningitis, with or without features of septic shock.

Diagnosis

- Examination of CSF
  Typical CSF findings in acute bacterial meningitis:
  - Raised WBC count (usually 100–60,000 cells/mL (predominantly neutrophils)
  - Reduced CSF glucose (30–40% serum glucose level)
  - Raised CSF protein (0.5–5g/L)
  - Gram-staining of CSF is positive in over 90% of cases of hematologically acquired meningitis.
- Blood culture should be performed in all patients with suspected meningitis, and latex agglutination bacterial antigen test or polymerase chain reaction analysis (to detect bacterial DNA) may be performed on blood or CSF to try to obtain a diagnosis. Such tests remain positive for several days after administration of antibiotics. Laboratory markers of poor prognosis include low peripheral WBC count, thrombocytopenia, absence of CSF pleocytosis and high CSF protein levels.

Management

- For adult patients penicillin G 5 to 10 million units IV 6 hourly.
- Cephalosporins, i.e., cefotaxime 2 g IV or ceftriaxone 2 g IV OD is also effective.
  Patients allergic to penicillin are treated with chloramphenicol 1 g IV 6 hourly
- Treatment is continued for 7 to 10 days.
- For raised intracranial tension IV mannitol is given which is accompanied by high doses of dexamethasone 4 mg IV 6 hourly.
  The supportive treatment is to maintain nutrition, fluid and electrolytic balance.

Q.33. Enumerate five causes of headache.
(Dec 2009, 5 Marks)

Or

Enumerate causes of headache. *(Jan 2012, 5 Marks)*

Ans.

The Causes of Headache

- Intracranial and local extracranial
  - Trauma
  - Intracranial inflammations
  - Vascular headaches: Hypertension, cerebral or subarachnoid hemorrhage, intracranial aneurysm, vasodilator drugs, such as nitrites and histamine, adrenaline.
  - Traction headache: Pain produced by intracranial arterial displacement and distortion of the dura
  - Post-lumbar puncture headache: Low CSF pressure headache.
  - Cough headache: A benign syndrome of severe headache which accompanies coughing, straining or sneezing can be due to posterior fossa tumor.
- Cranial neuritis and neuralgias of sensory nerves of scalp, e.g., orbital neuralgia, neuralgia of auriculotemporal, posterior auricular or great occipital nerves.
- General or systemic causes:
  - Anoxemia: Anemia, carbon monoxide or carbon dioxide poisoning.
  - Toxic: Fever, uremia, metallic poisoning, "alcoholic" hangover, etc.
  - Metabolic factors: Hypoglycemia, alkalosis or acidosis
  - Hematopoietic factors: Essential polycythemia, thrombasthenia.
- Referred pain
  - Eyes: Errors of refraction, glaucoma, iritis, etc.
  - Ears: Otitis, mastoiditis, vestibular nerve lesions,
  - Teeth: Impacted teeth, infected tooth sockets and dental roots
  - Paranasal sinuses: Infection of paranasal sinuses may cause localized pain
  - Neck: Diseases of upper cervical spine may be associated with both occipital and frontal pain.

- **Psychogenic:**
  Common cause of headache in depression.
- **Tension (muscle contraction) headache:** Pain resulting from sustained contraction of skeletal muscles of the neck, frontalis, occipital muscles due to emotional tension.
- **Exertional headache:** Headache may come on during exertion and persist for few hours afterwards.

Q.34. Enumerate causes of meningitis and describe clinical features, complications and treatment of tubercular meningitis. *(Aug 2011, 15 Marks)*

Ans. *For causes of meningitis refer to Ans. 32 of same chapter.*

For clinical features and management of tubercular meningitis refer to Ans. 23 of same chapter.

Complications

- Infection spreads in parenchyma of brain causing meningoencephalitis.
- Involvement of cerebral vessel causes obliterative endarteritis
- Thrombosis of cerebral vessels lead to cerebral infarction
- Delayed complications are development of hydrocephalus optic atrophy, spinal cord compression and cranial nerve palsy.

Q.35. Write notes on facial pain. *(Aug 2011, 10 Marks)*

Ans. *For various types of facial pains refer to Ans. 34 of same chapter.*

Differential Diagnosis of Facial Pain

- **Symptomatic trigeminal neuralgia**
  - Neuralgia indistinguishable from the idiopathic variety may occur as a result of compression of trigeminal root or ganglion, e.g., meningioma, acoustic neuroma, aneurysm of basilar artery, arteriovenous malformations, basilar invagination, epidermoid cholesteatomas in the cerebellopontine angle, as a result of Paget's disease or osteomalacia.
  - *Paratrigeminal neuralgia (Raeder's syndrome):* Severe pain in and around one eye accompanied by Horner's syndrome on the affected side. It is continuous and progressive and is usually caused by a structural lesion, often malignant in the base of the skull involving the paratrigeminal region.
  - *Multiple sclerosis:* Diagnosis of multiple sclerosis should always be suspected in a young patient with trigeminal neuralgia.
  - *Syringobulbia.*
  - Painful superior orbital fissure syndrome (Tolosa-Hunt syndrome) caused by granulomatous tissue involving nerves III, IV and VI. Pain with development of ocular palsies and loss of first division trigeminal sensation.
- **Referred pain:** Paranasal sinuses, toothache, aural infection. Temporomandibular joint dysfunction (Costen's syndrome) — abnormality of bite and aggravated by chewing.
- **Vascular pain:**
  - Migraine: Episodes of severe and continuous pain, often burning in character in or behind one eye, or in cheek, forehead and temple. Often suffusion of conjunctiva and blocking of nostril on that side.

- Temporal arteritis: Pain of dull, throbbing nature with associated scalp tenderness. Thickened temporal arteries with reduced or absent pulsations.
- **Other neuralgias**
  - *Post-herpetic neuralgia:* Pain is continuous in nature. Vesicles and scars of herpetic infection.
  - *Glossopharyngeal neuralgia:* Pain in tonsillar fossa, back of throat and larynx; may radiate to ear on affected side. Swallowing is the stimulus most likely to produce pain.
- **Atypical facial pain**
  Intermittent but long-lasting pain of aching character which affects the cheek and upper jaw, often bilateral and occurs almost exclusively in young and middle-aged women. Generally believed to be a manifestation of depression or anxiety.
- **Miscellaneous**
  - *Clonic facial spasm:* Sometimes painful, usually associated with intermittent twitching of eyelid and face on one side. Platysma usually involved in twitching.
  - *Neuralgic pain:* Occasionally associated with facial hemiatrophy.
  - *Idiopathic trigeminal neuropathy:* It is commonly associated with muscle wasting of masseter.

Q.36. Write short note Grand mal epilepsy.

(Jan 2012, 5 Marks)

Ans. It is a type of a primary generalized seizure.

- It is a true seizure.
- It is also known as tonic clonic seizure.
- Grand mal epilepsy comes suddenly without warning in some patients while in others it is preceded by various phases or symptoms.
- Following are the phases:
  - Prodromal phase: In this phase patient become uneasy and irritable for some hours to days before an attack.
  - Aura: It is seen when partial seizure become generalized so the symptoms of partial seizures, such as flashing of light, hallucination of hearing words or sounds, Tingling or numbness sensation, pain in epigastrium and unnatural sensations in some part of the body. Aura is warning of an attack and is produce by an activation of epileptic discharge in brain. It remains for some seconds or minutes.
  - Tonic clonic phase: Tonic convulsions of two side of body occur with head and eyes rotated to one side. Tonic Phase occur for 10–30 seconds and there is presence of flexion of arms, tonic contraction of muscles, a cry due to spasm of respiratory muscles and extension of legs. Tonic phase is followed by clonic phase which last for 1–5 minutes. In clonic phase, there is violent jerking of face and limbs, biting of tongue and passing of urine and stools. Clonic phase is followed by unconsciousness which lasts for few minutes to half an hour.
  - Postictal phase: This phase last for few minutes to hours. There is presence of unconsciousness with flaccid limbs, corneal reflexes are lost and plantar extensor response may occur during this phase. In this patient has severe headache, confusion and automatic behavior.

Diagnosis of Grand mal Epilepsy

♦ Diagnosis of grand mal epilepsy is made by careful assessment of patient's history documented by the diagnostic studies.

♦ These include blood test to assess for the metabolic disarray, brain imaging using MRI or CT scan and EEG. Normally EEG shows series of small alpha waves about 10 per second and occasionally small beta waves, but during attack in Grand mal epilepsy series of sharp spikes is present. Between the attacks 3 Hz 5W interictal epileptiform activity there is presence of intermittent irregular slow waves in grand mal epilepsy.

♦ It also depends upon its onset and symptoms like biting of tongue, passing of urine in clothes, injury to the patient, loss of consciousness and postepileptic features.

Management

♦ **Immediate treatment of an attack of fit.**
  • Patient should be protected from the injury. He should be moved away from fire and sharp and hard object.
  • Padded mouth gag is inserted between the teeth to avoid tongue injury.
  • Clear airway should be maintained.
  • Diazepam 5 to 10 mg slow IV injection is given.

♦ **Long-term drug therapy.**
  • Phenytoin sodium 200 to 400 mg daily.
  • Carbamazepine 600 to 1800 mg daily in divided dose.
  • Sodium valproate 0.25 to 1 mg daily.
  • Phenobarbitone 60 to 180 mg daily.
  • Primidone 750 to 1500 mg daily in divided dose.

♦ **Social and psychological aspects.**
  • Patients and relatives should be told about the illness, its precipitating factors and consequences.
  • Restriction should be in children as they are more likely to be in danger. Cycling, driving and swimming is avoided.
  • Patient should be advised to take occupation in which neither he nor the community is on risk.

Q.37. Write short note on clinical features and management of syncope. *(Jan 2019, 7 Marks)*

Ans. Syncope refers to generalized weakness of muscles, loss of postural tone, inability to maintain erect posture and loss of consciousness while faintness implies only lack of strength and sense of impending loss of consciousness.

Clinical Features

Basically, clinical features depend on the type of vasovagal syncope:

Vasovagal Syncope

♦ Patient appears pale.
♦ Patient has a slow pulse, low blood pressure
♦ Presence of dilated pupils.
♦ Reduction in systemic peripheral resistance due to withdrawal of sympathetic tone.

Postural Syncope

♦ Presence of decrease in blood pressure in the erect posture.
♦ Patient feels fainting when suddenly arising from supine position and in standing position.

Cerebral Syncope

♦ Presence of recurrent attacks of syncope more the erect posture.
♦ In subclavian steal syndrome, exercise of involved arm is followed by syncope.

Situational Syncope

♦ In cough syncope, it occurs after paroxysms of cough mainly in patients with cough especially in patients with bronchitis and emphysema and is due to intrathoracic pressure which occurs with coughing and impedes venous return to heart.
♦ It occurs in men with lower urinary tract obstruction straining excessively to pass urine mainly at night. There is postural fall in blood pressure, reflex vagal activity which is stimulated by full bladder and decreased venous return due to straining.

Cardiac Syncope

♦ Presence of abnormal decrease in heart rate, i.e., AV block or increase in heart rate, i.e., supraventricular or ventricular tachycardia.
♦ Presence of cardiac standstill which is occurring from reflex vagal activity.

Management of Syncope

For details refer to Ans. 8 of same chapter.

Q.38. Discuss in detail about multiple sclerosis.
(Apr 2019, 5 Marks)

Ans. Multiple sclerosis is an inflammatory demyelinating disease of CNS (brain and spinal cord) that is disseminated in time and space (i.e. neuroanatomical location).

Pathogenesis

♦ An acute multiple sclerosis plaque develops when primed leukocytes cross the blood-brain barrier into the brain and activate macrophages. Inflammation is initiated and myelin is stripped off nearby nerve axons. Demyelinated axons lose the ability to conduct nerve impulses in normal manner, and axonal conduction is further impeded by the direct effect of soluble inflammatory mediators, such as nitric oxide. The rapid disappearance of these mediators when inflammation subsides may account for the rapid resolution of symptoms sometimes seen after an attack. It is now recognized that axons may degenerate as a secondary response to demyelination, and the axonopathy contributes to disease progression.

♦ **Autoimmune disease:** The female predominance and its weak association with specific HLA types (particularly HLA DR15 and DQ6) suggest that multiple sclerosis may be an autoimmune disease. In 20% of patients, multiple sclerosis affects one other family member.

♦ **Genetic predisposition:** Multiple sclerosis is also suggested by the racial variation in prevalence and the higher concordance risk in identical compared with non-identical twins. Hence, expression of multiple sclerosis probably depends on the interplay of an inherited risk with an environmental trigger; this may be an infective agent, such as human herpes virus 6 and *Chlamydia pneumoniae*.

Clinical Features

Symptoms

♦ *Lhermitte's symptom:* Neck flexion induces an 'electric shock' sensation running down the back, caused by a plaque in the cervical cord.

♦ *Optic neuritis:* Patients experience pain in one eye, particularly on eye movement, and dimming of vision in that eye, often described as looking through a dirty window or water.

♦ Spasticity, particularly in spinal cord lesions, may lead to stiffness, flexor spasms, cramps or spontaneous clonus.

♦ Ataxia of the limbs may be caused by a lesion of the cerebellum or its connections, or by deafferentation from a dorsal column spinal plaque.

♦ Fatigue is often prominent.

♦ Neuropathic pain may occur as part of a spinal cord syndrome or alone as in symptomatic trigeminal neuralgia.

♦ Mood disturbance: Euphoria with advanced multiple sclerosis, but depression is more common.

♦ Bladder dysfunction: It can be either detrusor hyperreflexia or detrusor sphincter dyssynergia.

♦ Symptom patterns: Symptoms caused by demyelination emerge over several days, reach a plateau and then usually resolve over days or weeks. Characteristically symptoms reappear transiently or worsen with an increase in body temperature (Uhthoff phenomenon).

Signs

Depending of the site of involvement

♦ *Spinal cord:* Spasticity, pyramidal weakness, hyperreflexia, absent abdominal reflexes, extensor plantar, spinal sensory level.

♦ *Brainstem:* Internuclear ophthalmoplegia, nystagmus, gaze palsies, facial sensory loss, rubral tremor.

♦ *Cerebellum:* Gait and limb ataxia, dysarthria, nystagmus.

♦ *Optic nerve:* Relative afferent pupillary defect, lost color vision/acquity, optic atrophy.

♦ *Cerebrum:* Dementia

Types of Multiple Sclerosis

Depending on Clinical course there are Four Subtypes of multiple sclerosis
1. Relapsing/remitting MS (RRMS)
2. Secondary progressive MS (SPMS)
3. Primary progressive MS (PPMS)
4. Progressive/relapsing MS (PRMS)
1. **Relapsing/remitting MS (RRMS):** It accounts for 85–90% of cases at onset, characterized by discrete attacks that generally evolve over days to weeks followed by substantial or complete recovery over the ensuing weeks to months. Between attacks, patients are neurologically stable.

2. **Secondary progressive MS (SPMS):** It always begins as RRMS. The clinical course changes so that the patient experience a steady deterioration in function unassociated with acute attacks. SPMS produces a greater amount of reduced neurologic disability than RRMS.

3. **Primary progressive MS (PPMS):** Patients do not experience attacks but only a steady functional decline from disease onset.

4. **Progressive/relapsing MS (PRMS):** It overlaps PPMS and SPMS and accounts for 5% of multiple sclerosis patients.

Investigations

1. **To demonstrate involvement of disseminated anatomical sites:**
   • MRI most sensitively reveals asymptomatic lesions. Serial MRI demonstrates dissemination of lesions in time more rapidly than clinical events
   • Visual evoked potentials: A unilateral delay is the most sensitive index of previous subclinical optic neuritis.
   • BAER (brainstem auditory evoked responses) to demonstrate auditory pathway subclinical lesions.

2. **To demonstrate inflammatory demyelination:**
   • CSF: Presence of oligoclonal bands in CSF but not serum indicates inflammation confined to the CSF and is seen in 95% of patients with clinically definite multiple sclerosis.
   • Evoked potentials are usually delayed and their amplitude relatively preserved.

3. **To exclude other conditions mimicking multiple sclerosis:** Often structural lesions must be excluded by MRI.

Management

No effective curative treatment.
1. **Treatment modifying the course of disease:**
   • IFNβ, Ia, Ib — has many potential sites of action, but probably acts mainly by inhibiting the effects of preinflammatory cytokines on microglial activation, thus preventing amplification of immune response. The drug is given by SC or IM injection 1–3 times weekly, and may be useful in those who suffer frequent or disabling relapses. Interferon-β is not recommended during pregnancy.
   • Glatiramer acetate — is a mixture of synthetic polypeptides and may act by specifically blocking immune responses to myelin basic protein, an autoantigen in multiple sclerosis. Dose: 20 mg SC daily.
   • Natalizumb: It is an humanized antibody directed against the α4 subunit of α4β1 integrin, a cellular adhesion molecule expressed out of the surface of lvmphocytes. It prevents lymphocytes from penetrating the BBB and entering the CNS. It is effective in reducing the attack rate and significantly improves all measures of disease severity in multiple sclerosis.

2. **Acute relapse:** Methylprednisolone 1 g/day for 3 days or prednisolone 60 mg p.o. for 1 week, then 40 mg for 1 week, followed by 20 mg for 1 week.

3. **Symptomatic treatment**

Spasticity

- Baclofen 10 mg/day, increased to maximum 80–100 mg/day in divided doses. It acts on α—aminobutyric receptors to suppress reflex arcs that have been released from higher inhibitory control.
- Tizanidine — 2 mg/day and increased slowly to maximum 20 mg/day. It acts through α2 cord receptors to moderate presynaptic release of excitatory amino acids. It is less sedating than baclofen, and associated with less muscle weakness.
- Dantrolene has a direct effect on skeletal muscles and is a second line drug.

Bladder Problems

If post—micturition bladder volume is more than 100 mL, failure to empty the bladder is the primary problem and clean, intermittent catheterization is recommended. If bladder empties but stores poorly oxybutynin 5 mg TDS.

Fatigue

Amantadine may help.

Depression

Tricyclic antidepressants should be prescribed.

---

11. TROPICAL AND INFECTIOUS DISEASES

Q.1. Enumerate the causes of enteric fever.

(Mar 1998, 5 Marks) (Apr 2010, 5 Marks)

Ans. Enteric fever is an infectious disease.

Causative Agent

- *Salmonella typhi* and *Salmonella paratyphi*
- The organisms are gram-negative nonspore forming bacilli.

Predisposing Factors

- *Organisms:* A large number of organisms are ingested by the healthy person to suffer from typhoid. Smaller inocula may produce the disease. If the organisms are very virulent or if the resistance of host is poor.
- *Stomach acidity:* Acid in the stomach destroys *Salmonella*. Hence, patients having achlorhydria or who take large amount of antacids to neutralize the acid in stomach suffer more often from the typhoid.
- *Intestinal flora:* Normal intestinal flora produces short chain fatty acids which are lethal to *Salmonella*. When these are reduced by antibiotics the patient is more prone to typhoid.

Q.2. Describe clinical signs and symptoms of enteric fever. *(Sep 1998, 5 Marks)*

Ans. Clinical signs and symptoms of enteric fever.

Invasion (1st Week)

- *Onset:* Lassitude, headache, bodyache and anorexia.
- Tongue is coated with raw tips and edges.
- Abdominal discomfort and distention occurs with nausea, vomiting and constipation which are followed by diarrhea.
- Hepatomegaly
- *Fever:* It may show step ladder rise.
- Signs of bronchitis are common. Epistaxis may occur.
- *Pulse:* Relative bradycardia and *dicrotic pulse.

Advance (2nd Week)

- **General state:** Listlessness and *apathy.
- **Abdomen:**
  - Spleen become palpable
  - Increased abdominal distention and discomfort
  - Usually there is diarrhea.
- **Temperature:** It is high with slight morning remissions.
- **Rash (Rose spots):** These are erythematous maculopapular lesions 2–4 mm in diameter which *blanch on pressure usually seen on the upper abdomen, back and chest.

Decline (3rd Week)

Mild case: Toxemia *abates and gradual fall of temperature.

Severe case: Increased toxemia, intestinal hemorrhage or perforation.

Q.3. Describe briefly complications of enteric fever and their management. *(Oct 2007, 5 Marks)*

Ans. Complications of enteric fever with their management.

Hemorrhage

Seen at the end of 2nd week and early 3rd week from gastric ulcer.

Treatment

- Absolute bed rest.
- Repeated blood transfusion
- Morphine 15 mg SC.

Shock

Treatment

- Plasma transfusion
- Oxygen
- Vasopressor drugs
- IV hydrocortisone or dexamethasone.

Perforation

It is most dangerous complication leading to peritonitis.

Treatment

- Gastric suction
- IV fluids
- Broad spectrum gram-negative agents.

Q 2.   *Dicrotic pulse = It is an abnormal carotid pulse found in conjunction with certain conditions characterized by low cardiac output. It is distinguished by two palpable pulsations, second of which is diastolic and immediately follows the second heart sound.

     *Apathy = Lack of interest, enthusiasm

     *Blanch = Become pale

     *Abates = Become less intense or widespread

Hepatitis

♦ It is represented by hepatomegaly and jaundice.
♦ Treatment is symptomatic.

Cholecystitis

Salmonella typhi has affinity for gallbladder and can produce inflammation.

Treatment

Ampicillin or ciprofloxacin is required.
Cholecystectomy is done if above treatment fails.

Toxemia

Treatment

Hydrocortisone 200 mg or Dexamethasone 8 mg parenterally followed by 45 mg prednisolone.

Meningitis

Treatment

Cefotaxime 2 g IV 4 hourly or ceftazidine 2 g 6 hourly and gentamicin.

Q.4.　Write short note on typhoid. 　　*(Feb 2006, 3 Marks)*

Or

Write short note on enteric fever.

(Dec 2010, 5 Marks) (Apr 2008, 5 Marks)

Or

Write short answer on treatment of enteric fever.

(Oct 2019, 3 Marks)

Ans. Typhoid is an acute systemic illness caused by infection due to *S. typhi.*

Epidemiology

Typhoid germs are contracted from food or drink contaminated with excreta from carriers or patients. Spread is facilitated by poor environmental hygiene.

Clinical Features

Invasion (1st Week)

♦ *Onset:* Lassitude, headache, bodyache and anorexia.
♦ Tongue is coated with raw tips and edges.
♦ Abdominal discomfort and distention occurs with nausea, vomiting and constipation which are followed by diarrhea.
♦ Hepatomegaly
♦ *Fever:* It may show step ladder rise.
♦ Signs of bronchitis are common. Epistaxis may occur.
♦ *Pulse:* Relative bradycardia and *dicrotic pulse.

Advance (2nd Week)

♦ *General state:* Listlessness and *apathy.
♦ *Abdomen:*
  • Spleen become palpable
  • Increased abdominal distention and discomfort
  • Usually there is diarrhea.
♦ *Temperature:* It is high with slight morning remissions.

♦ *Rash (Rose spots):* These are erythematous maculopapular lesions 2–4 mm in diameter which blanch on pressure usually seen on the upper abdomen, back and chest.

Decline (3rd Week)

♦ *Mild case:* Toxemia *abates and gradual fall of temperature.
♦ *Severe case:* Increased toxemia, intestinal hemorrhage or perforation.

Investigations

First Week

♦ Normochromic normocytic anemia, leukopenia and albuminuria
♦ Blood culture may be positive in 70–90% of cases.

Second Week

♦ Anemia, leukopenia may persist
♦ Widal test become positive, may show four fold rise in agglutinins against somatic 'O' antigen. It is not specific but rising titers are diagnostic.
♦ Blood culture may be positive only in 50%.

Third Week

♦ Anemia and leukopenia persist. Leukocytosis occur in severe septicemia
♦ Blood culture is positive in 30–45% of cases.
♦ Positive WIDAL test with rising titers
♦ Positive stool culture and urine test for *S. typhi.*

Complications

Following are the complications of typhoid fever:

♦ Intestinal complications:
  • Hemorrhage
  • Perforation
  • Paralytic ileus
  • Peritonitis
♦ *Extraintestinal complications:*
  • Meningitis
  • Bone and joint infection
  • Cholecystitis
  • Encephalopathy
  • Pneumonia
  • Granulomatous hepatitis
  • Nephritis
  • Myocarditis

Treatment

Specific

♦ *Ciprofloxacin:* It is given in the dose of 500 mg BD for 7 to 10 days it is avoided in children because of risk of cartilage damage and tendonitis. If absolutely required, low dose can be used for not more than 3 days.
♦ *Ceftriaxone:* It is 3rd generation cephalosporin and improves the condition rapidly. It is given in the dose of 1 g BD for 10 to 14 days.
♦ *Azithromycin:* 1 g OD for 5 days.

Supportive Treatment

- Treatment of fever—paracetamol
- Good nursing care.
- Nutritious diet should be given. 3000 calories per day should be given
- Fluid and electrolyte balance should be maintained.
- *For severe toxemia and peripheral circulatory failure:* Dexamethasone 3 mg/kg stat followed by 8 doses of 1 mg/kg 6 hourly for 48 hours each given by IV infusion over 30 min.

Treatment of Carrier

Patients who are asymptomatic, but constantly releases bacteria in stool because bacteria are persisting in gallbladder.

- Ampicillin 500 mg QID for six weeks.
- Ciprofloxacin 500 mg BD for 2 to 4 weeks.
- Cholecystectomy if above measure fails.

Q.5. Describe briefly typhoid vaccination.

(Sep 1999, 3 Marks)

Ans.

Typhoid Vaccinations

- Anti-triple typhoid vaccine containing in each mL. 1000 million typhoid organisms, 250 million each of para-typhoid 'A' and 'B' organisms. Course of 3 injections of 0.5 mL, 1 mL and 1 mL subcutaneously at intervals of not less than 7 days or not more than 28 days. Immunity lasts for about 12 months.
- *V1 capsular polysaccharide typhoid vaccine:* 25 mg in each dose. Single dose (0.5 mL) SC or IM gives protection for 3 years. However, the V1 antigen does not invariably provoke V1 antibody. Booster every 2 years.
- *TY21a—oral vaccine:* TY21a is a galactose epimerase mutant *S. typhi* given as oral enteric coated capsules. The bacilli invade mononuclear cells and undergo 4–5 cell divisions in intestinal tract. This stimulates immunity, but the bacilli do not survive within the cells, as they lack the essential enzyme UDP—galactose-4 epimerase and are therefore avirulent. The vaccine stimulates cell mediated immunity and also stimulates intestinal IgA.
- *Dose:* One capsule on days 1, 3 and 5 irrespective of age one hour before meal with milk or water. Not recommended for children under 6 years of age. Protection commences 2 weeks after last capsule and lasts for at least 3 years. Booster is given every 5 years.

Q.6. Write short answer on treatment of malaria.

(Feb 2019, 3 Marks)

Or

Write short note on treatment of malaria.

(Feb 2013, 5 Marks)

Ans. Malaria is a common topical disease caused by protozoa, *Plasmodium*.

Acute febrile illness characterized by paroxysms of fever as a result of asexual production of *Plasmodium* within the red cells.

Management

General Management

- Measurement of glucose and if possible lactate and arterial blood gases.

- Fluid balance should be maintained because both dehydration and overhydration can occur as a result of disease or treatment.
- Treatment of convulsions with diazepam.
- Attention should be given to hypoglycemia and hyponatremia.
- Blood should be taken for cross-matching and coagulation studies
- Parameters for monitoring treatment include twice daily parasite counts, regular pH and blood gas measurements and when appropriate, measurement of glucose (during iv quinine therapy), lactate, CRP and kidney function.

Specific Treatment

- **Treatment of chloroquine susceptible *P. vivax*, *P. falciparum*, *P. ovale*, *P. malariae* chloroquine:**
  This is given in the dose of 600 mg base followed by 300 mg at 6th, 24th and 48th hours. It is useful in trating all types of malaria. It is curative for *P. falciparum* malaria, but cannot prevent relapses due to exoerythrocytic cycles of *P. vivax* malaria.
- Treatment of chloroquine resistant *P. falciparum*:
  - Quinidine IV 10 mg/kg dissolved in 300 mL normal saline infused over 1 to 2 hour.
  - Quinine hydrochloride: 600 mg TDS for 3–7 days is useful.
    If required for cerebral malaria, this drug can given IV the dose is 7 mg/kg over 30 min, followed by 10 mg/kg over 4 hours and then 10 mg/kg over 8 hours or until the patient can complete a week of oral treatment.
  - *Mefloquine:* It provides rapid schizonticidal action in single dose of 15 mg/kg orally maximum dose is 1000 to 1250 mg.
  - *Halofantrine:*
    Dosage: Adult 500 mg BD for 4–6 days.
    Children: 8 mg/kg
  - *Artemether:* This drug is rapidly acting, safe and is effective against multidrug resistant infections. Artemether 3.2 mg/kg IM is given followed by 1.6 mg/kg IM every 12 to 24 hours until patient wakes up. Artesunate 2 mg/kg IV stat followed by 1 mg/kg 12 hourly.
  - *Sulfadoxine and pyrimethamine:* Combination of sulfadoxime 1500 mg and pyrimethamine 25 mg helps to cure an acute attack of chloroquine resistant malaria.
- **Treatment of chloroquine resistant *P. vivax***
  Oral mefloquine and halofantrine.
- **Treatment of persistent hypnozoites in P. vivax or P. ovale infection**
  - *Primaquine:* It is given in the dose of 7.5 mg BD for 14 days usually after doing a G6PD test
  - *Bulaquine:* It is given 25 mg OD for 5 days.

Q.7. Outline the management of F. malaria.

(Feb 1999, 4 Marks)

Ans.

- **Treatment of chloroquine susceptible *P. falciparum***
  Chloroquine: This is given in the dose of 600 mg base followed by 300 mg at 6th, 24th and 48th hours.

♦ **Treatment of chloroquine resistant** *P. falciparum*:
  • Quinidine IV 10 mg/kg dissolved in 300 mL normal saline infused over 1 to 2 hours.
  • *Quinine hydrochloride:* 600 mg TDS for 3–7 days is useful.
  • *Mefloquine:* It provides rapid schizonticidal action in single dose of 15 mg/kg orally maximum dose is 1000 to 1250 mg.
♦ **Treatment of complicated** *P. falciparum* **malaria**
  • Cerebral malaria caused by *P. falciparum* infection is a medical emergency. So depending on prevailing sensitivity of *P. falciparum* to anti-malarial drugs, i.e., quinine or chloroquine is given as an intravenous infusion over 2 to 4 hours to avoid acute circulatory failure or acute malarial encephalopathy. Quinine should be used in chloroquine-resistant cases. The starting dose of chloroquine is 5 mg/kg and of quinine is 10 mg/kg. The dose should be repeated at intervals of 8–12 hours until the patient can take the drug orally. The total dose of chloroquine is 25 mg/kg. The quinine is continued orally in the same dose for 7–10 days. Recently artemisinin (artemether) has become first line treatment of severe malaria as mentioned by WHO. Artesunate 2.4 mg/kg IV then 1.2 mg/kg/day or artemether 3.2 mg/kg, then 1.6 mg/kg IM daily is given for 3–5 days.
  • Single dose of parenteral phenobarbitone 5–20 mg/kg is given to prevent convulsion.
  • If severe anemia is present then transfusion with packed red cells is done.
  • If oliguria develops, frusemide or an infusion of mannitol is given to prevent renal failure.
  • Intravenous fluids are given, if necessary should be guided by central venous pressure because pulmonary edema may develop if the patient is over-infused.
  • Exchange blood transfusions is life saving in complicated very severe infection (over 10% of RBCs are infected).
  • Hypoglycemia and septicemia may be treated appropriately. All patients treated with quinine should be monitored for blood sugar and should receive 5–10% glucose as continuous infusion during treatment.
  • If renal failure develops dialysis should be done.
  • Care of unconscious patient or if patient undergo coma.

Q.8. Write short note on diphtheria. *(Apr 2007, 5 Marks)*

Ans. Diphtheria is an acute infectious disease caused by *Corynebacterium diphtheriae* and is characterized by the local exudates on the mucous membrane of nose, throat and larynx and systemic toxemia.

For complications refer to Ans. 9 of same chapter.

Types of Diphtheria

Pharyngeal Diphtheria

♦ It is characterized by the toxemia, *congestion and edema of palate.
♦ There is formation of a membrane in pharynx which is generally thin glistening pearly white in early stage and become thick, grayish and opaque later on.
♦ There is lymphadenopathy in neck and breath is foul smelling.

♦ In second week, there is lethargy and restlessness. Pulse becomes irregular. Respiration is rapid and shallow. Repeated vomiting takes place.

Nasal Diphtheria

♦ There is presence of unilateral and bilateral nasal discharge, at first serous and often blood stained, later thick, mucopurulent and foul smelling.
♦ Thick membrane may be visible on the mucosa of the anterior part of nasal septum.

Laryngeal Diphtheria

♦ It is common in young children
♦ It is characterized by the hoarseness, brassy cough followed by attack of inspiratory stridor and laryngeal spasm
♦ Membrane is usually limited to larynx.

Cutaneous Diphtheria

When corneum bacteria enters into the abrasion or wounds they produced punched out ulcers which is covered by the grayish membrane.

Facial Diphtheria

♦ *Mild:*
  • Reddening of one or both the tonsils.
  • Small membrane formation on one or both the tonsils.
♦ *Moderate:*
  • Membrane on both tonsils.
  • Localized tonsillar lymph node enlargement.
♦ *Severe:*
  • Rapidly spreading firmly membrane on the palate and roof of the mouth.
  • There is gross edema of facial and palatal tissue.

Conjunctival Diphtheria

♦ Due to direct involvement of the eyes by the organism or spread from the nose.
♦ It is characterized by the severe congestion in the eyes and discharge.

Clinical Features

♦ Patient complains of presence of sore throat.
♦ Low grade fever is present.
♦ Presence of headache and malaise.
♦ Hoarseness of voice, dyspnea in cases with laryngeal diphtheria.
♦ Presence of gross cervical lymphadenopathy.
♦ Formation of bluish white or grayish green pseudomembrane at the site of infection.
♦ Punched out ulcerations are present if skin is involved.
♦ Foul smelling serosanguinous discharge in cases of nasal diphtheria.
♦ Cyanosis is seen in cases with laryngeal diphtheria.

Management of Diphtheria

♦ *Bed rest:* Usually bed rest is required for 3 to 6 weeks
♦ *Antitoxin:* Anti-diphtheria serum is given subcutaneously or IM in the dose of 10,000–1,00,000 units depending on the severity of the disease.

Q 8.   *Congestion = Abnormal or excessive accumulation of body fluid.

A test dose is usually given before giving the injection to exclude hypersensitivity.

♦ *Antibiotics:* A course of ampicillin or erythromycin 500 mg 6 hourly should be given to eradicate the diphtheria bacillus.

♦ **General management:**
  • *Diet:* In mild cases, normal diet may be allowed
    – In moderate to severe cases initially fluids are given orally.
    – If there is palatal palsy semisolid diet is preferred to liquids because liquids may be regurgitate from nose.
    – If swallowing is affected, feeding should be with Ryle's tube.
  • *Care of Mouth:* The mouth should be cleaned.

♦ **Treatment of complication:**
  • *Cardiac failure:* Diuretics and digitalis may have to be given.
  • *Palatal palsy:* Head low position may be given to drain secretion of the mouth.
  • *Laryngeal obstruction:* Tracheostomy may be required.
  • Respiratory paralysis: Oxygen and ventilator may be required.

♦ **Prophylaxis:** Acute immunization should be given to all the children at age of 4th, 5th and 6th month in form of DPT.

Q.9. Mention the complications of diphtheria.

(Sep 1999, 5 Marks)

Ans.

Complications

Acute Circulatory Failure

♦ Toxic myocarditis.
♦ It is characterized by the tachycardia, feeble heart sounds, cardiac enlargement, tic-tac rhythm and arrhythmias.
♦ Sudden death may occur.
♦ Congestive heart failure.

Respiratory Complications

♦ Bronchitis
♦ Bronchopneumonia
♦ Respiratory obstruction
♦ Respiratory paralysis.

Toxic Neurological Damage

♦ Paralysis of palate
♦ Paralysis of accommodation
♦ Facial paralysis
♦ Bulbar paralysis
♦ Paralysis of muscles of respiration
♦ Peripheral neuropathy.

Renal Complications

♦ Toxic nephritis.
♦ Vascular involvement especially middle cerebral artery leading to a picture of thrombosis or monoplegia.
♦ Other complication include otitis media and arthritis.

Q.10. Enumerate the causes of hyperplasia of gums.

(Feb 1999, 4 Marks)

Ans. According to etiologic factors and pathologic changes, gingival enlargements are:

Inflammatory Enlargement

♦ Chronic
♦ Acute.

Drug-induced Enlargement

Enlargement Associated with Systemic Disease

♦ *Conditional enlargement:*
  • Pregnancy
  • Puberty
  • Vitamin C deficiency
  • Plasma cell gingivitis
  • Nonspecific conditional enlargement.
♦ *Systemic diseases causing gingival enlargement:*
  • Leukemia
  • Granulomatous disease.

Neoplastic Enlargement

♦ Benign tumors
♦ Malignant tumors

False Enlargement

♦ **According to location and distribution gingival enlargement are classified as:**
  • *Localized:* Gingival enlargement limited to one or more teeth.
  • *Generalized:* Entire mouth, gingiva is enlarged.
  • *Marginal:* Limited to marginal gingiva.
  • *Papillary:* Confined to interdental papilla.
  • *Diffuse:* Involves all parts of gingiva that is marginal, attached and interdental.
  • *Discrete:* Isolated sessile or pedunculated tumor like enlargement.
♦ **According to degree of gingival enlargement**
  • *Grade 0:* No sign of gingival enlargement.
  • *Grade I:* Enlargement confirmed to interdental papilla.
  • *Grade II:* Enlargement involves papilla and marginal gingiva.
  • *Grade III:* Enlargement covers three quarters or more of the crown.

Q.11. Enumerate causes of bleeding gums.

(Oct 2007, 5 Marks)

Or

Enumerate five causes of gum bleeding.

(Dec 2009, 5 Marks)

Ans.

Causes

♦ *Local Cause:*
  • Minor injury: Use of hard new tooth brush may cause minor local injury to gums and leads to bleeding.
  • Dental caries: It may be obvious or hidden between the teeth and get irrigating the gums.
  • Tartar
  • Pyorrhea alveolitis is the result of septic infection extending down into the sockets, loosening the teeth, causing the gum margins to recede by erosion and leading to purulent discharge. In severe cases, gums bleed on the slightest touch.

- Tuberculous gingivitis
- Stomatitis.
♦ **General conditions:**
  - Scurvy: Spongy bleeding of the gums, teeth covered by exuberant blood is the prominent feature of scurvy due to lack of vitamin C.
  - Syphilis: In second stage will produce bleeding from the gums.
  - Purpura
  - Blood dyscrasis.

Q.12. Outline the treatment of hookworm infestation.

(Mar 2010, 5 Marks)

Ans.

Treatment

♦ This consists of expulsion of the worms and treatment of anemia. If anemia is severe, it should be treated first.
♦ *Anemia:* Anemia should be treated with oral iron therapy along with vitamin B complex and folic acid. If it is severe blood transfusion should be given.

Effective Drugs

♦ Tetrachloroethylene 5 mL is given after an overnight fast and may be repeated in heavy infestations.
♦ Bephenium hydroxynaphthoate 5 g is given orally with fruit juices because it is very bitter.
♦ Mebendazole 100 mg twice daily is given for 3 days.

Q.13. Outline the management of tapeworm infestation.

(Feb 1999, 4 Marks)

Ans. Tapeworms are ribbon like segmented worms.

The common tapeworm affecting human are *Taenia saginata*, *Taenia* solium.

Humans are definitive host.

Clinical Features

♦ Mild abdominal pain
♦ Nausea
♦ Change in appetite
♦ Weakness
♦ Weight loss.

Management

♦ *Niclosamide:*
  Adults: Single dose of 2 g.
  Children: 0.5 to 1 g
  The tablets should be given on empty stomach, chewed thoroughly and washed down with a little water.
  A purgative is recommended if the dead segments are not passed out within few years.
♦ *Praziquantel:* Single dose of 5–10 mg/kg after a light breakfast.
♦ For cerebral cysticercosis praziquantel 50 mg/kg/day for 15 days or albendazole 15 mg/kg/day for 30 days.

Q.14. Write short note on chickenpox prevention.

(Oct 2003, 10 Marks)

Ans. Chickenpox is an acute infectious disease.

Etiological Agent

Chickenpox is caused by varicella virus which is closely related to the herpes simplex virus, cytomegalovirus and Epstein-Barr virus.

Prevention of Chickenpox

Varicella-zoster immunoglobin is given to the following, i.e.

Indication

♦ Following significant exposure to chickenpox in immuno-compromised and susceptible children.
♦ Susceptible adolescents and adults particularly pregnant women.
♦ Newborn infants mothers have chickenpox within 5 days before delivery.
♦ Premature infants of less then 28 weeks gestation.
♦ Premature infants whose mother do not have a history of chickenpox
♦ *Dose:* 125 units per 10 kg body weight IM within 48 hours and not later than 96 hours after exposure
♦ Maximum suggested dose is 625 units.

Vaccine

♦ Live attenuated Varicella-zoster.
♦ Safe and highly protective in both healthy and immuno-compromised children.
♦ *Dose:* In children of 2 to 12 years, who have not had chickenpox, two doses are recommended first at 12 to 15 months of age and second at 4 to 6 years of age.

Q.15. Write short note on measles. *(Feb 2006, 3 Marks)*

Ans. It is highly infective disease.

Measles are caused by RNA paramyxovirus group.

Clinical Features

♦ **Prodromal stage (4 to 5 days)**
  - Fever is present and there is abrupt rise in temperature to 400°C.
  - *Catarrh: *Coryza, conjunctivitis, photophobia and hacking cough
  - *Koplik's spots:* They appear on second day as minute pin point bluish white specks with slight reddish mottled areola around them, on buccal mucosa usually opposite to lower molars. They looks like grain of salt. They are variable in number. These spots begin to fade with appearance of rash. Red blotches may be seen on soft palate. Koplik's spots may sometime occur on lover lip in front of lower incisors, in severe cases of palate and rest of mucosa are peppered with these spots.
  - *Laryngeal involvement:* Hoarseness and laryngeal stridor is present.
  - *Gastrointestinal:* Persistent vomiting and diarrhea.
  - *Fleeting rashes:* Either urticarial or erythematous.

Q 15. *Catarrh = An excessive build up of mucouss in an airway or cavity of the body.
  *Coryza = Catarrhal inflammation of the mucous membrane in the nose, caused especially by cold or by hay fever.

♦ **Exanthematous stage:**
- On 5th day red macules appear first behind the ear, along hair line, posterior part of cheeks and spread rapidly in few hours all over the body. Macules appear in crop which by confluence form blotches with crescentric or thumb nail edge.
- In severe disease rashes are confluent, face get swollen and disfigured and along with photophobic eyes creates typical measly appearance.
- *Mucous membrane involvement:* It includes conjunctivitis, rhinitis, stomatitis, laryngitis, tracheitis and bronchitis.

♦ **Stage of Defervescence**
- Temperature falls by crisis or rapid lysis in 24 to 48 hours.
- Rashes fade from face and leaves brown staining followed by branny desquamation.
- At times normal rash of measles instead of fading become deep purple and this can persists for week or two.

Types of Measles

♦ *Toxic:* This is malignant form of disease and is manifested by high fever, delirium, circulatory, fever and may be fatal.
♦ *Pulmonary:* Respiratory infection with high temperature and rapid respiration.
♦ *Hemorrhage:* It is rare. There is hemorrhage into the mucus membrane, skin and subcutaneous tissue.

Laboratory Findings

♦ Leukopenia is frequent. If leukocytosis is present, it is indicative of superadded bacterial infection.
♦ In stained smears of sputum or nasal secretions or urine there is presence of multinucleated giant cells in which measles virus is isolated on appropriate cell cultures.
♦ Measles antigen is detected by fluorescent antibody test in stained respiratory or urinary epithelial cell.
♦ In patient having encephalitis along with measles, CSF examination is done which show rise in protein with cell count along with normal range. CSF shows lymphocytosis.

Management

♦ Bedrest is given.
♦ Frequent fluid intake.
♦ Paracetamol for the fever.
♦ Irrigation of eyes with the boric lotion.
♦ Cough linctus to suppress the dry cough.
♦ Antibiotics, such as amoxicillin if there are complications, such as otitis media or pneumonia.
♦ Vitamin A 200,000 IU orally for 2 days will prevent ocular complication and respiratory infections.

Q.16. Write short note on mumps.

(Oct 2007, 5 Marks) (Apr 2008, 5 Marks)
(Nov 2008, 10 Marks) (Sep 2009, 4 Marks)
(Dec 2009, 10 Marks) (Nov 2011, 3 Marks)

Ans. Mumps is a widely prevalent infectious disease.

Etiology

It is caused by mumps virus which belongs to group of paramyxovirus. Humans are the only natural host and infection spreads by droplet infection as well as by direct contact with respiratory secretions of the patient. Incubation period usually ranges from 12 to 22 days average being 16–18 days.

Clinical Features

♦ **Onset of disease:**
- Presence of moderate fever, sore throat, drawing or puckering feeling at angle of jaw.
- Swelling of face first draw the attention.
- Onset with rigor or convulsion.
- Onset with meningeal reaction, i.e., cerebral mumps

♦ **Early signs:**
- Presence of pain or tenderness on pressure beneath angle of lower jaw.
- Redenning of parotid duct orifice

♦ **Other features:**
- Usually one parotid gland is affected followed by the other gland after varying interval or only one gland is affected throughout. Swelling reaches to its maximum in 3 days, remain its peak for 2 days and slowly receds. Lobe of ear is in center of swelling which is tender on pressure.
- After appearance of parotitis fever rise to 400°C. Fever falls by lysis in 3 to 7 days.
- Other symptoms are diminished salivation, furred tongue and foul breadth.
- Enlargement of parotid may cause trismus and deafness.

Diagnosis

♦ *Viral isolation:* From saliva or nasopharynx in acute illness or from CSF in mumps meningitis.
♦ *Antibody titer:* Four fold rise in 1 to 2 weeks after infection.

Treatment

♦ It is mainly supportive and symptomatic.
♦ Child is put to bed rest.
♦ Mouth hygiene must be maintained meticulously.
♦ Analgesics and antipyretics are the main stay of treatment, i.e., paracetamol/nimulid syrup 1–2 teaspoonful two to three times a day
♦ Diet should be soft, bland and preferably in liquid form.
♦ In cases where complications like orchitis or neurological complications develop, prednisolone 40–60 mg per day in divided doses for about seven days is given along with antibiotics, i.e., Ampicillin/Amoxycillin/Cefazolin/Ceftizoxime.

Complications

♦ *Common complications:*
- Orchitis and epididymitis: It is unilateral. Common in young adults, may occur without parotitis. Fever return and go up to 40–50°C. Testis is swollen, tender and tense with/without epididymitis. Last for 10 days. Can result in sterility.

- Meningitis: It follows parotitis and can occur at same time or before salivary gland enlargement.
- Oophoritis: It is less common than orchitis.
- Acute pancreatitis: Occur in 2nd week. Occasionally disease can be present with pancreatitis without salivary gland involvement.

♦ *Rare complications:*
  - *Neurological:* Meningoencephalitis, cranial nerve involvement, polyneuritis, other CNS problems, i.e., cerebellar ataxia, facial palsy, transverse myelitis, hydrocephalus, flaccid paralysis and behavioral changes.
  - Arthritis: Occassionally one or more large joints, but there is no permanent damage.
  - Mastitis: Mild and transient enlargement of breasts.
  - Prostatitis in males
  - Thyroiditis
  - Nephritis
  - Fetal endocardial fibroelastosis

Q.17. Write differential diagnosis of lock jaw.

(Oct 2003, 10 Marks)

Ans. Lock jaw or tetanus is caused by the powerful neurotoxin, i.e., tetanospasmin which is released by the *C. tetani.*

This disease is characterized by the muscular rigidity and spasms.

Differential Diagnosis

♦ *Other causes of trismus:* Irritant local lesions of teeth, throat, temporomandibular joint, masseter muscle and cervical lymph nodes.

♦ *Meningitis:* Neck rigidity can occur in both tetanus and meningitis, signs of meningeal irritation, diagnostic CSF.

♦ *Rabies:* Dysphagia associated with spasms of inspiratory and pharyngeal muscles also occur in rabies. History of dog bite is present.

♦ *Tetany:* Spasm starts in periphery with carpopedal spasm.

♦ *Drug dystonia:* Dystonic relations to drug, such as phenothiazines and metoclopramide. Grimacing, spasmodic and neck retraction and torticollis, wide opening of mouth and eyes. Dystonia prolong muscular contractions that may cause twisting of body parts, repetitive body movements and increased muscular tone.

♦ *Acute peritonitis:* Board like abdominal rigidity as in tetanus, but in tetanus there is little or no tenderness.

♦ *Functional muscle spasms:* Bizarre movement of posture, absence of constant rigidity of involved muscles, history of previous personal disorders.

♦ *Catatonic schizophrenia:* It might cause confusion in absence of background information.

Q.18. Write clinical examination of tetanus patient.

(Mar 2000, 10 Marks)

Ans. Tetanus initially presents with muscle stiffness. The distribution may vary with the type of tetanus. The masseter muscles are commonly involved with an accompanying headache. Neck stiffness, difficulty swallowing, generalized muscle spasms including the abdominal and back muscles and sweating may be seen later in the disease. In severe cases, respiratory paralysis may develop, which presents with apnea, hypoxia and hypercapnia.

Physical examination of a patient with tetanus may reveal the following:

General Appearance

♦ Severe muscular spasm (location varies with the type)
  - Opisthotonos
  - Leg extension with arm flexion
  - Risus sardonicus
♦ May be in respiratory distress

Vitals

♦ Fever
♦ Tachycardia
♦ Elevated blood pressure

Musculoskeletal

♦ Spasms of the diaphragm and intercostals
♦ Stiff abdominal wall

Respiratory

♦ Tachypnea
♦ Dyspnea

Cardiovascular

♦ Normal S1 and S2
♦ Hypertension
♦ Arrhythmia

Autonomic

Intervals of bradycardia and hypotension are accompanied by that of tachycardia and hypertension.

Abdominal

Stiffening of the abdominal muscles.

The physical examination may vary according to the type of tetanus. Specific findings associated with the various types of tetanus may include:

Local Tetanus

♦ Limited area of spasm
♦ The affected area is in close proximity to a contaminated wound
♦ Contraction is usually painful and associated with swelling
♦ Generalized tetanus may follow localized tetanus

Cephalic Tetanus

♦ Ear infection or head injury may be seen
♦ Trismus
♦ Signs of CN III, IV, VI, VII and XII involvement including:
  - Tilting of the mouth
  - Inability to close the eye
  - Inability to move the tongue
  - Diplopia
♦ *Abnormal eye movements:* Dysphagia
♦ Confusion
♦ Symptoms of stroke

Generalized Tetanus

♦ Descending spasm
♦ Trismus may present initially:
  • Followed by stiffness of the neck
  • Difficulty in swallowing
  • Stiffness of abdominal muscles
♦ Other symptoms include:
  • Elevated temperature
  • Sweating
  • Elevated blood pressure
  • Episodic rapid heart rate
♦ Spasms may occur frequently and last for several minutes
♦ Spasms may continue for 3–4 weeks
♦ Complete recovery may take months

Neonatal Tetanus

♦ Unhealed, unhygienic umbilical stump
♦ Trismus (spasm of masseter muscle)
♦ Risus sardonicus (spasm of facial muscles)
♦ Clenched hands
♦ Dorsiflexion of the feet
♦ Opisthotonus (spasm of spinal muscles)

The Spatula Test

The "spatula test" is a clinical test for tetanus that involves touching the posterior pharyngeal wall with a sterile, soft-tipped instrument, and observing the effect. A positive test result is the contraction of the jaw (biting down on the "spatula"), and a negative test result would normally be a gag reflex attempting to expel the foreign object.

Q.19. How will you differentiate tetany from tetanus?

(Aug 2005, 5 Marks)

Ans.

Tetany	Tetanus
• It is the hyperexcitability of nervous system causing spasmodic, painful contraction with spasm of muscles	• It occurs in three forms, i.e., mild, moderate and severe It is a local muscle rigidity leading to trismus, change in facial expression, pain of spine of muscle
• Numbness and stiffness around the mouth with muscle cramping	• Dysphagia and trismus of jaw
• It is caused due to low calcium serum level, i.e., 4–8 mg%	• No effect on calcium serum level
• Elevated serum phosphorus levels	• No effect on serum phosphorus levels
• It is caused due to deficiency of calcium	• It is caused due to bacterial infection by *Clostridium tetani*
• Loss of hair, nail, enamel defects in teeth, severe headache diminished vision and mental retardation is present	• No such signs are present in patient
• It is treated by IV infusion or tetanus toxoid	• It is treated by giving ATS of calcium

Q.20. How will you differentiate rheumatoid arthritis from rheumatic arthritis? *(Aug 2005, 5 Marks)*

Ans.

Characteristic feature	Rheumatoid arthritis	Rheumatic arthritis
• Age of onset	20–45 years	2–15 years
• Causative factor	Autoimmunization	*S. hemolyticans*
• Onset	Insidious	Rapid
• Number of joint involved	Multiple	Multiple but not migratory
• Other symptoms	Weakness, fatigue, low fever	Fever, chills, pallor, low anemia
• Stiffness of joint	Mild to moderate	Usually not marked
• Swelling and effusion	Fusiform swelling of finger joints and effusion of bigger joints	Present
• Muscle atrophy	Marked in later stage	Absent
• Skin changes	Skin may be smooth and shiny	Red due to inflammation
• Deformities	Flexion deformity, ulnar duration of hand, later fibrous or bony ankylosis	Absent
• Distribution	Bilateral and symmetrical proximal interphalangeal are commonly involved	Multiple migratory flitting involvement of elbows, wrists, knees and ankles

Q.21. Write short note on viral exanthema.

(Sep 2008, 2.5 Marks)

Ans. Viral infections associated with skin lesions are known as viral exanthems.

Viral exanthems lead to maculopapular rashes sparing palms as well as soles.

Following are the viral exanthems:

♦ Measles
♦ Rubella
♦ Varicella-zoster infection, i.e., chickenpox and shingles
♦ Exanthem infectiosum
♦ Exanthem subitum
♦ Enteroviruses
♦ Infectious mononucleosis
♦ Adenovirus
♦ Reovirus
♦ Arbovirus.

Exanthematous Stage in Measles

♦ In exanthematous stage on 5th day the red macules appear behind the ear, along hair line and on posterior parts of cheeks and spread rapidly in a few hours all over the body. Macules appear in the crops which by confluence from bloatches with crescentric or thumbnail edge. Fully erupted rash deepens in color, petechiae may occur. In severe measles rash is confluent, the face is swollen and disfigured and together with photophobic eyes create typical measly appearance.

♦ *Mucous membrane involvement:* It consists of conjunctivitis, rhinitis, stomatitis, laryngitis, tracheitis and bronchitis.

Exanthema in Chickenpox

♦ *Evolution:* In form of crops, first at back, then chest, abdomen, face and lastly limbs.
♦ *Character:* At first macule appear then in few hours dark pink papule which soon turn into vesicle. They also get collapsed if pierced and vesicles turn into pustules in 24 hours and to scabs in 2 to 5 days.
♦ *Distribution:* It is centripetal, i.e., more on upper arm and thighs, upper part of face and in concavities and flexures.
♦ *Cropping:* Rash mature quickly and most spots dry up within 48 hours of appearance. For 2 to 3 days new spots continue to appear on any area of body vesicles, pustules and scabs are found side by side.

Exanthema in Rubella

In exanthema rash occurs more often in older children and adults on first or second day of illness, first on face and behind the ears, and then spreads downwards to trunk and limbs. The rash is variable, but commonly starts as discrete, pink, punctate, erythematous, perifollicular macules that rapidly become confluent. Alternatively, there may be blotchy pink rash or confluent blush. Rash seldom persists for more than 4 days and is not followed by staining or desquamation. Rubella without rash is common in young children. In a dark skinned patient all that may be seen is prominence of hair follicles giving a goose pimpled appearance.

Q.22. Describe briefly AIDS.   *(Sep 2008, 7 Marks)*
                    Or
Write short note on AIDS.   *(Feb 2006, 5 Marks)*
                                       (Dec 2015, 3 Marks)
                    Or
Describe etiology, sign and symptoms of AIDS.
                                       (Feb 2019, 5 Marks)

Ans. AIDS stands for acquired immunodeficiency syndrome.

A CD4 count less than 200/μL in HIV infected individual is defined as AIDS.

Etiology

Both HIV–1 and HIV–2, members of lentivirus family of retroviruses causes AIDS, but HIV–2 appears to be less virulent progress slowly and is less commonly transmitted vertically.

Transmission

♦ *Sexual:* Most HIV infection occurs in homosexual man. Multiple heterosexual contacts often prostitutes.
♦ Contacts with blood and body fluids, contaminated blood and blood products.
♦ Contaminated needles and syringes.
♦ Through organ and tissue donation
♦ *From mother to child:* In uterus at birth, breast milk.

Stages of HIV Infection by WHO (Sign and Symptoms)

Primary HIV Infection

♦ Asymptomatic
♦ *Acute retroviral syndrome:* Fever with maculopapular rash primarily on trunk with small aphthous lesions on oral and genital mucosa.

Clinical Stage 1

♦ Asymptomatic
♦ Persistent generalized Lymphadenopathy

Clinical Stage 2

♦ Unexplained moderate weight loss (<10% of presumed body weight)
♦ Infections
♦ Recurrent respiratory tract infections
♦ Herpes zoster
♦ Fungal infections of finger nails: Oral lesions
♦ Recurrent oral ulcerations
♦ Angular cheilitis: Itchy dermatosis
♦ Papular pruritic eruptions
♦ Seborrheic dermatitis

Clinical Stage 3

Conditions where a presumptive diagnosis can be made on the basis of clinical signs or simple investigations.

♦ Unexplained symptoms:
  • Chronic diarrhea for >1 month
  • Persistent fever, intermittent or constant for >1 month
♦ Severe weight loss (>10% of presumed or measured body weight)
♦ *Infections:*
  • Severe presumed bacterial infections
  • Pulmonary tuberculosis diagnosed in last 2 years
♦ *Oral lesions:*
  • Oral candidiasis
  • Oral hairy leukoplakia
  • Acute necrotizing ulcerative stomatitis, gingivitis or periodontitis
♦ Conditions where confirmatory diagnostic testing is necessary
  • Unexplained anemia (<8 g/L or neutropenia (<500 μL) or thrombocytopenia (<50,000 μL) for >1 month

Clinical Stage 4

Conditions where a presumptive diagnosis can be made on the basis of clinical signs and simple investigations

♦ HIV wasting syndrome
♦ Infections
  • *Pneumocystis pneumoniae*
  • Recurrent severe or radiological bacterial pneumonia
  • Chronic herpetic simplex infection (oral, labial, genital or anorectal of >1 month duration).
  • Esophageal candidiasis
  • Extrapulmonary tuberculosis
♦ Neoplasms: Kaposi's sarcoma
♦ Neurological disease
  • CNS toxoplasmosis
  • HIV encephalopathy

Laboratory Diagnosis

♦ **Investigations for the diagnosis of HIV infection:**
  • *HIV-ELISA:* This is the most commonly used screening test for HIV infection. If this test is positive confirmation should be done by western blot test.
  • *HIV-rapid antibody test:* They are for rapid diagnosis, i.e., within 10 to 15 minutes. It is also a screening test, as if this test comes positive confirmation is done by western blot.
  • *Western blot:* It is the confirmatory test for HIV infection.
  • *Blood cell count:* Since neutropenia, anemia and pancytopenia are associated with HIV infection, this test is done.

♦ **Investigations for monitoring progress of HIV infection:**
  • *Absolute CD4 lymphocyte count:* This is most commonly used. As its count decreases occurrence of opportunistic infection and malignancy is high, i.e., if count is less than 200 cells/μL.
  • CD4 lymphocyte percentage: In this if count is less than 14% occurrence of opportunistic infection and malignancy is high, if treatment is not given to patient.

♦ **Investigations for virological monitoring:** In this, HIV viral load tests are done, such as HIV–RNA by PCR, HIV–RNA by bDNA, HIV–RNA by NASBA. These all tests measure the actively replicating HIV virus. These cells also deflect the response of antiretroviral drugs. These test are excellent for diagnosis of acute HIV infection before its seroconversion.

Treatment

The medical management of AIDS is done by HAART, i.e., highly active antiretroviral therapy.

It causes suppression of HIV replication and prolonging life as well as improving the quality of life of the patient.

The drugs used are:
♦ Nucleoside reverse transcriptase inhibitors
  • Zidovudine: Dose: 600 mg daily in two divided doses
  • Didanosine: Dose: 400 mg OD. To be taken before meals
  • Zalcitabine: It is used in combination with zidovudine: Dose is a 0.75 mg TDS.
  • Lamivudine 150 mg orally BD
♦ Nucleotide reverse transcriptase inhibitors
  • Tenofovir: Dose: 300 mg orally OD
♦ Non-nucleoside reverse transcriptase inhibitors
  • Nevirapine: 200 mg orally daily for two weeks and then 200 mg BD
  • Efavirenz: 600 mg orally daily
♦ Protease inhibitors
  • Amprenavir—1200 mg orally BD
  • Atazanavir—400 mg orally daily
  • Indinavir—800 mg orally TDS
♦ Protease inhibitors boosted with ritonavir
  • Lopinavir R–6 capsules per day
  • Fosamprenavir—700 mg + 100 mg ritonavir twice daily
  • Ritonavir—100 mg BD orally

♦ Fusion inhibitors
  • Enfuvirtide—90 mg SC injection twice daily.

Q.23. **Write clinical examination of advanced HIV disease in patient.**   *(Mar 2000, 10 Marks)*

Ans. Clinical examination of advanced HIV disease.

External Examination

Patient is markedly cachectic with:
♦ Generalized lymphadenopathy
♦ Nodular skin lesion all over the body.
♦ White patches in the oral cavity.

Internal Examination

♦ *Skull:* Meninges are congested and inflamed.
♦ *Thorax:* There was presence of dense adhesion between the pleura and the chest wall. Mediastinal lymph nodes were enlarged and matted. Both lungs show marked destruction of parenchyma.
♦ *Abdomen:* Serosal surfaces of liver, spleen and kidney were studded with tubercle. Mesenteric lymph nodes were enlarged and matted.
♦ *Urinary bladder:* Serosal surface shows presence of tubercles.
♦ *Genital system:* It is studded with tubercles.
♦ *Adrenals:* Enlarged, congested, shows presence of multiple tubercles.

Q.24. **Write short note on chickenpox.**
        (Sep 2004, 5 Marks) (Sep 2009, 5 Marks)

Ans. It is an erythematous or vesiculopapular lesion caused by varicella-zoster virus.

It spreads through aerosol route.

Its incubation period is of 14 to 15 days.

Clinical Features

♦ **Stage of invasion or prodromata:**
  • Presence of headache, sore throat and fever for 24 hours.
  • Erythematous or urticarious prodromal rashes are seen.
♦ **Stage of eruption:**
  • *Enanthem:* Earliest lesions are on buccal and pharyngeal mucosa.
  • *Exanthem*
    – *Evolution:* In form of crops, first at back, then chest, abdomen, face and lastly limbs.
    – *Character:* At first macule appear then in few hours dark pink papule which soon turn into vesicle. They also get collapsed if pierced and vesicles turn into pustules in 24 hours and to scabs in 2 to 5 days.
    – *Distribution:* It is centripetal, i.e., more on upper arm and thighs, upper part of face and in concavities and flexures.
    – *Cropping:* Rash mature quickly and most spots dry up within 48 hours of appearance. For 2 to 3 days new spots continue to appear on any area of body vesicles, pustules and scabs are found side by side.

♦ **Other symptoms:**
- Pruritus of varying degree.
- Generalized lymphadenopathy may occur.
- Enlargement of suboccipital and posterior cervical lymph nodes.

Laboratory Diagnosis

♦ A Tzanck smear, performed by scraping the base of an acute lesion and staining with Giemsa or Papanicolaou's stain may demonstrate multinucleated giant cells having intranuclear inclusions.

♦ Other tests are fluorescent antibody against membrane antigen, immune adherence hemagglutination and ELISA.

Complications

♦ Cerebral ataxia
♦ Myocarditis
♦ Hepatitis
♦ Acute glomerulonephritis
♦ Pneumonia
♦ Arthritis
♦ Corneal lesion
♦ Bleeding diathesis.

Management

♦ No need to confine patient to bed unless symptoms are severe.

♦ For pruritus Calamine lotion with or without phenol (0.4%) and sedative antihistaminics by mouth. If there is much scabbing, gauze soaked in 1 in 5,000 solution of potassium permanganate which is changed every 4 hours may be applied to areas most affected.

♦ For secondary infection antibiotics should be given.

♦ For true varicella pneumonia oxygen is given.

♦ For encephalitis oxygen and corticosteroids are given

♦ Paracetamol is given for fever.

♦ Oral acyclovir should be initiated within 24 hours of rash results in a decrease in the duration and magnitude of the fever, and in the number and duration of skin lesions. Dose is 20 mg/kg qds with maximum of 800 mg qds.

Q.25. Write short note on oral manifestations of HIV/AIDS.
(Sep 2006, 5 Marks)

Or

Describe oral manifestations of HIV.
(Feb 2013, 5 Marks)

Or

Write long answer on oral manifestations of HIV.
(Sep 2018, 5 Marks)

Ans. Classification of Oral Manifestations By EC-Clearinghouse

Group 1: Strongly Associated With HIV Infection

♦ *Candidiasis:* Erythematous, pseudomembranous, angular cheilitis
♦ Hairy leukoplakia
♦ Kaposi's sarcoma

♦ Non-Hodgkin's lymphoma
♦ *Periodontal diseases:* Linear gingival erythema, necrotizing gingivitis, necrotizing periodontitis.

Group 2: Less Commonly Associated with HIV Infection

♦ *Bacterial infections: Mycobacterium avium-intracellulare, Mycobacterium tuberculosis*
♦ Melanotic hyperpigmentation
♦ Necrotizing ulcerative stomatitis
♦ *Salivary gland disease:* Dry mouth, unilateral or bilateral swelling of major salivary glands
♦ Thrombocytopenia purpura
♦ Oral ulcerations NOS (not otherwise specified)
♦ *Viral infections:* Herpes simplex, human papillomavirus, varicella-zoster

Group 3: Seen in HIV Infection

♦ *Bacterial infections: Actinomyces israelii, Escherichia coli, Klebsiella,* pneumonia
♦ Cat-scratch disease (*Bartonella henselae*)
♦ Epithelioid (bacillary) angiomatosis (*Bartonella henselae*)
♦ *Drug reactions:* Ulcerative, erythema multiforme, lichenoid, toxic epidermolysis
♦ Fungal infections other than candidiasis: *Cryptococcus neoformans, Geotrichum candidum, Histoplasma capsulatum, Mucoraceae* (mucormycosis/zygomycosis), *Aspergillus flavus*
♦ *Neurologic disturbances:* Facial palsy, trigeminal neuralgia
♦ Recurrent aphthous stomatitis
♦ *Viral infections: Cytomegalovirus, Molluscum contagiosum*

Description of Oral Manifestations

♦ Candidiasis is the most common oral manifestation of HIV infection. All the three types., i.e., erythematous, pseudomembranous and hyperplastic forms are seen. Erythematous candidiasis is seen when the CD4 count drops below 400 cells/mm³ and pseudomembranous develop when CD4 count drop below 200 cells/mm³.

♦ *Hairy leukoplakia:* Presence of soft painless plaque on the lateral border of tongue with corrugated surface.

♦ *Kaposi's sarcoma:* Single or multiple bluish swellings are seen with or without ulceration over gingiva and palate.

♦ *Angular cheilitis:* Linear fissures or linear ulcers are seen at the angle of mouth.

♦ *Linear gingival erythema:* It is fiery red band along the gingival margin and attached gingiva with profuse bleeding.

♦ *Necrotizing ulcerative gingivitis:* Destruction of interdental papillae is seen.

♦ *Necrotizing ulcerative periodontitis:* There is advanced necrotic destruction of periodontium, rapid bone loss, loss of periodontal ligament and sequestration.

♦ *Oral ulcerations:* Single or multiple major recurrent aphthous ulcers are seen with white pseudomembrane surrounding the erythematous halo.

♦ *Non-Hodgkin's lymphoma:* It is the malignancy of HIV infected individuals. It occurs in extranodal locations and

CNS is the common site. Intraosseous involvement is also seen.

- *Mycobacterial infection:* Mycobacterial infection in form of tuberculosis is seen. When present tongue is affected most commonly. Affected areas show common ulcerations.
- *Herpes simplex virus:* Recurrent or secondary herpes simplex infection is seen in the patients. Herpes simplex lesions increase when CD4 cell count drops below 50 cells/mm³.
- *Herpes zoster:* It is common in HIV infected individuals. Orally, involvement is severe and leads to sequestration of bone as well as loss of teeth.
- *Histoplasmosis:* It is the fungal infection caused by histoplasma capsulatum. Sign and symptoms of disease are fever, weight loss, splenomegaly and pulmonary infiltrate.
- *Molluscum contagiosum:* It is caused by pox virus. Lesions are small, waxy, dome-shaped papules which demonstrate central depressed crater.

Q.26. Write short note on HIV importance in dental practice. *(Mar 2007, 2 Marks)*

Ans. The HIV is the virus which results in the causation of the AIDS.

Prophylactic measures to be adopted by dental healthcare workers while treating AIDS patient.

- Care in handling sharp objects, such as needles, blades.
- All cuts and abrasions in an HIV patient should be covered with a waterproof dressing
- Minimal parenteral injections
- Equipments and areas which are contaminated with secretions should be wiped with sodium hypochlorite solution or 2% glutaraldehyde.
- Contaminated gloves, cottons should be incinerated.
- Equipments should be disinfected with glutaraldehyde.
- Disposable equipments (drapes, scalpels, etc.) should be used whenever possible.
- Walls and floor should be cleaned properly with soap water.
- Separate operation theater and staff to do surgeries to HIV patients is justifiable
- Avoid shaving whenever possible before surgery in HIV patients.
- All people inside the theater should wear disposable gowns, plastic aprons, goggles, overshoes and gloves.
- Surgeons, assistants and scrub nurse should wear in addition double gloves.
- Suction bottle should be half-filled with freshly prepared glutaraldehyde solution.
- Soiled body fluids should be diluted with glutaraldehyde.
- Accidental puncture area in surgeon or scrub nurse should immediately washed with soap and water thoroughly.
- Theater should be fumigated after surgery to HIV patient.

Q.27. Write short note on HIV. *(Sep 2007, 2 Marks)*

Or

Write on mode of transmission and clinical features of HIV. *(Apr 2018, 5 Marks)*

Or

Write short answer on HIV. *(Apr 2019, 5 Marks)*

Ans. HIV disease is an infectious disease caused by human immunodeficiency virus.

Late stage of HIV infection is AIDS when CD4⁺ T lymphocyte count is <200/μL.

Etiology

Both HIV–1 and HIV–2, members of lentivirus family of retroviruses causes AIDS, but HIV–2 appears to be less virulent progress slowly and is less commonly transmitted vertically.

Transmission

- *Sexual:* Most HIV infection occurs in homosexual man. Multiple heterosexual contacts often prostitutes.
- Contacts with blood and body fluids, contaminated blood and blood products.
- Contaminated needles and syringes.
- Through organ and tissue donation
- *From mother to child:* In uterus at birth, breast milk.

Pathogenesis of HIV Infection

- HIV virus infects target cells (CD4⁺ T cells, monocytes, macrophages and dendrite cells) through CD4 receptors.
- On entering T cells, the virus integrates its RNA genome into the host cell genome by first transcribing this genome into DNA (HIV provirus) with the help of enzyme reverse transcriptase.
  - Provirus is then transcribed and translated along with the host cell DNA to synthesize specific viral components, which eventually assemble to produce complete virus particles.
  - At this time patient is seronegative, i.e., antibodies against the virus are not present. But patient is highly infectious. This period is labeled "window period".
  - Although some virions are killed, HIV continues to multiply infecting increasing number of CD4 cells.
- In early stages of immune destruction, the patient is asymptomatic.
- As the immunosuppression progresses over a period of time patient becomes symptomatic.

Stages of HIV Infection by WHO

Primary HIV Infection

- Asymptomatic
- *Acute retroviral syndrome:* Fever with maculopapular rash primarily on trunk with small aphthous lesions on oral and genital mucosa.

Clinical Stage 1

- Asymptomatic
- Persistent generalized lymphadenopathy

Clinical Stage 2

- Unexplained moderate weight loss (<10% of presumed body weight)
- Infections
- Recurrent respiratory tract infections
- Herpes zoster

♦ Fungal infections of finger nails
  • Oral lesions
♦ Recurrent oral ulcerations
♦ Angular cheilitis
  • Itchy dermatosis
♦ Papular pruritic eruptions
♦ Seborrheic dermatitis

Clinical Stage 3

Conditions where a presumptive diagnosis can be made on the basis of clinical signs or simple investigations.

♦ *Unexplained symptoms*
  • Chronic diarrhea for >1 month
  • Persistent fever, intermittent or constant for >1 month
♦ Severe weight loss (>10% of presumed or measured body weight)
  • Infections
♦ Severe presumed bacterial infections
♦ Pulmonary tuberculosis diagnosed in last 2 years
  • Oral lesions
♦ Oral candidiasis
♦ Oral hairy leukoplakia
♦ Acute necrotizing ulcerative stomatitis, gingivitis or periodontitis
  • Conditions where confirmatory diagnostic testing is necessary
♦ Unexplained anemia (<8 g/L or neutropenia (<500 µL) or thrombocytopenia (<50,000 µL) for >1 month

Clinical Stage 4

Conditions where a presumptive diagnosis can be made on the basis of clinical signs and simple investigations

♦ HIV wasting syndrome
♦ Infections
  • *Pneumocystis pneumonia*
  • Recurrent severe or radiological bacterial pneumonia
  • Chronic herpetic simplex infection (oral, labial, genital or anorectal of >1 month duration).
  • Esophageal candidiasis
  • Extrapulmonary tuberculosis
♦ Neoplasms
  • Kaposi's sarcoma
♦ Neurological disease
  • CNS toxoplasmosis
  • HIV encephalopathy

Q.28. **Give definition, etiology, signs, symptoms, diagnosis, differential diagnosis and complications of enteric fever.** *(Jan 2012, 12 Marks)*

Ans. It is an acute systemic illness caused by infection due to *salmonella typhi*. Typhoid fever is characterized by fever, malaise, pain abdomen, rash, splenomegaly and leukopenia. The untreated patients may develop complications during 2nd and 3rd week due to toxemia and septicemia. In some cases it may be fatal.

For etiology refer to Ans. 1 of same chapter.

For sign and symptoms refer to Ans. 2 of same chapter.

For complications refer to Ans. 4 of same chapter.

Diagnosis

First Week

♦ Normochromic normocytic anemia, leukopenia and albuminuria
♦ Blood culture may be positive in 70–90% of cases.

Second Week

♦ Anemia, leukopenia may persist
♦ Widal test become positive, may show four fold rise in agglutinins against somatic 'O' antigen. It is not specific but rising titers are diagnostic.
♦ Blood culture may be positive only in 50%.

Third Week

♦ Anemia and leukopenia persist. Leukocytosis occur in severe septicemia
♦ Blood culture is positive in 30–45% of cases.
♦ Positive Widal test with rising titers
♦ Positive stool culture and urine test for *S. typhi*.

Differential Diagnosis

♦ **Paratyphoid fever:** Mode of onset often acute and atypical; Wider remissions of temperature; Eruption is more profuse; less toxemia; sweating and rigors more common; Intestinal complications rare.
♦ **Short fever:** A fever lasting for 8 to 10 days; no associated signs, probably of viral origin. Subside spontaneously. No complications.
♦ **Amoebic liver abscess:** Pain in right hypochondrium and lower chest, moderate fever, enlarged tender liver or compression tenderness over right lower intercostal spaces. Right hemidiaphragm may be elevated and immobile on fluoroscopy.
♦ **Viral hepatitis:** In preicteric stage there is marked nausea and vomiting, hepatic tenderness, high colored urine.
♦ **Tuberculous meningitis:** Absence of abdominal discomfort, greater frequency of vomiting, persistence of headache after first week, irritability, irregular pupils, CSF changes.
♦ **Miliary tuberculosis:** Increased respirations, irregular temperature, tachycardia, cough and cyanosis, symptoms referable to alimentary tract less pronounced. Early loss of flesh. Diagnostic CXR.
♦ **Heat fever:** Not uncommon in children and aged. Fever may be continuous or touch normal for some hours every day. Absence of other physical signs. Response to lowered temperature.
♦ **Subacute infective endocarditis:** Fever seldom continuous or high; Frequent chills with septic type of temperature; cardiac signs; anemia; embolic phenomenon; positive blood culture.
♦ *E. coli infection:* Pyelitis or septicemia—high fever, though not of continuous type. May last for 2–3 weeks. Leukocytosis, tenderness in loins, pus in urine or positive blood culture.
♦ **Malaria:** Sudden onset, wide diurnal variation, early splenic enlargement, malarial parasites in blood, response to antimalarial drugs.

Q.29. Write short note on WHO criteria for diagnosis of AIDS. *(Mar 2008, 2.5 Marks)*

Ans. WHO criteria for diagnosis of AIDS.

Primary HIV Infection

◆ Asymptomatic
◆ *Acute retroviral syndrome:* Fever with maculopapular rash primarily on trunk with small aphthous lesions on oral and genital mucosa.

Clinical Stage 1

◆ Asymptomatic
◆ Persistent generalized lymphadenopathy

Clinical Stage 2

◆ Unexplained moderate weight loss (<10% of presumed body weight)
◆ Infections
◆ Recurrent respiratory tract infections
◆ Herpes zoster
◆ Fungal infections of finger nails
  • Oral lesions
◆ Recurrent oral ulcerations
◆ Angular cheilitis
  • Itchy dermatosis
◆ Papular pruritic eruptions
◆ Seborrheic dermatitis

Clinical Stage 3

Conditions where a presumptive diagnosis can be made on the basis of clinical signs or simple investigations.

◆ Unexplained symptoms
  • Chronic diarrhea for >1 month
  • Persistent fever, intermittent or constant for >1 month
◆ Severe weight loss (>10% of presumed or measured body weight)
  • Infections
◆ Severe presumed bacterial infections
◆ Pulmonary tuberculosis diagnosed in last 2 years
  • Oral lesions
◆ Oral candidiasis
◆ Oral hairy leukoplakia
◆ Acute necrotizing ulcerative stomatitis, gingivitis or periodontitis
  • Conditions where confirmatory diagnostic testing is necessary
◆ Unexplained anemia (<8 g/L or neutropenia (<500 µL) or thrombocytopenia (<50,000 µL) for >1 month

Clinical Stage 4

Conditions where a presumptive diagnosis can be made on the basis of clinical signs and simple investigations

◆ HIV wasting syndrome
◆ *Infections*
  • *Pneumocystis pneumonia*
  • Recurrent severe or radiological bacterial pneumonia
  • Chronic herpetic simplex infection (oral, labial, genital or anorectal of >1 month duration).

• Esophageal candidiasis
• Extrapulmonary tuberculosis
◆ *Neoplasms*
  • Kaposi's sarcoma
◆ Neurological disease
  • CNS toxoplasmosis
  • HIV encephalopathy

Q.30. Write short note on risk factors for candidiasis. *(Sep 2008, 3 Marks)*

Ans. Following are the risk factors for candidiasis.

Any condition that weakens the immune system, such as:

◆ Diabetes
◆ Organ transplant
◆ Chemotherapy
◆ AIDS
◆ Daily corticosteroid use
◆ Breaks in the skin or mucous membranes
◆ Kidney dialysis
◆ Intravenous catheters
◆ Intravenous drug abuse
◆ Obesity
◆ Peptic ulcer disease
◆ Severe burns
◆ Urinary catheters

Q.31. Enumerate etiology, clinical features, investigations, complications and management of enteric fever. *(Nov 2008, 15 Marks)*

Or

Discuss clinical feature, complication and management of enteric fever. *(May/Jun 2009, 15 Marks)*

Or

Write etiology, clinical features, investigations, treatment and complications of enteric fever (Typhoid). *(Jun 2014, 12 Marks)*

Or

Describe the complications and treatment of enteric fever. *(Sep 2005, 10 Marks)*

Or

Write enteric fever under following headings: *(Dec 2012, 2 Marks Each)*

a. **Etiology**
b. **Clinical features**
c. **Complications**
d. **Treatment**

Or

Write etiology, clinical features, investigation and treatment of enteric fever. *(Jan 2016, 12 Marks)*

Or

Describe enteric fever under following headings: *(Mar 2016, 1+2+1+2 Marks)*

a. **Etiology**
b. **Clinical features**

c. Complications

d. Treatment

Or

Write etiology, clinical features, diagnosis and management of enteric fever. *(Jan 2018, 12 Marks)*

Or

Write long answer on sign, symptoms and management of enteric fever. *(Sep 2018, 5 Marks)*

Ans. *For etiology refer to Ans. 1 of same chapter.*

For clinical features (sign and symptoms) refer to Ans. 2 of same chapter.

For investigations or diagnosis refer to Ans. 28 of same chapter.

For complications refer to Ans. 4 of same chapter.

Treatment

Specific

- *Ciprofloxacin:* It is given in the dose of 500 mg BD for 7 to 10 days it is avoided in children because of risk of cartilage damage and tendonitis. If absolutely required, low dose can be used for not more than 3 days.
- *Ceftriaxone:* It is 3rd generation cephalosporin and improves the condition rapidly.
  It is given in the dose of 1 g BD for 10 to 14 days.
- *Azithromycin:* 1 g OD for 5 days.

Treatment of complications: Refer to Ans. 3 of same chapter.

Supportive Treatment

- Treatment of fever—paracetamol
- Good nursing care
- Nutritious diet should be given
- Fluid and electrolyte balance should be maintained.
- For severe toxemia and peripheral circulatory failure. corticosteroids may be used, i.e., Dexamethasone 3 mg/kg stat followed by 8 doses of 1 mg/kg 6 hourly for 48 hours each given by IV infusion over 30 min.

Treatment of Carrier

Patients who are asymptomatic, but constantly releases bacteria in stool because bacteria are persisting in gallbladder.

- Ampicillin 500 mg QID for six weeks.
- Ciprofloxacin 500 mg BD for 2 to 4 weeks.
- Cholecystectomy if above measure fails.

Q.32. Write in brief on gum hypertrophy.

(Nov 2008, 10 Marks)

Ans. Gum hypertrophy means increase in the size of gums.

Classification

According to etiologic factors and pathologic changes, gingival enlargements are:

Inflammatory Enlargement

- Chronic
- Acute.

Drug-induced Enlargement

Enlargement Associated with Systemic Disease

- Conditional enlargement
  - Pregnancy
  - Puberty
  - Vitamin C deficiency
  - Plasma cell gingivitis
  - Nonspecific conditional enlargement.
- Systemic diseases causing gingival enlargement
  - Leukemia
  - Granulomatous disease.

Neoplastic Enlargement

- Benign tumors
- Malignant tumors

False Enlargement

- **According to location and distribution gingival enlargement are classified as:**
  - *Localized:* Gingival enlargement limited to one or more teeth.
  - *Generalized:* Entire mouth, gingiva is enlarged.
  - *Marginal:* limited to marginal gingiva.
  - *Papillary:* Confined to interdental papilla.
  - *Diffuse:* Involves all parts of gingiva that is marginal, attached and interdental.
  - *Discrete:* Isolated sessile or pedunculated tumor like enlargement.
- **According to degree of gingival enlargement:**
  - *Grade 0:* No sign of gingival enlargement.
  - *Grade I:* Enlargement confirmed to interdental papilla
  - *Grade II:* Enlargement involves papilla and marginal gingiva.
  - *Grade III:* Enlargement covers three quarters or more of the crown.

Clinical Features

- Presence of slight ballooning of interdental papilla and marginal gingiva
- The enlargement progress slowly and painlessly
- It occurs as a discrete sessile or pedunculated mass resembling a tumor, it may be inter proximal or on marginal or attached gingiva
- The lesions are slow growing masses
- The lesions undergo spontaneous reduction in size, followed by exacerbation and continued enlargement
- Painful ulceration sometimes occur in fold between mass and adjacent gingiva.

Treatment

- **Scaling and curettage:** If the size of enlargement does not interfere with complete removal of deposits, the enlargement caused due to inflammation is treated by scaling and curettage.

- **Surgical removal:** Indicated for two reasons.
  - In enlargement with significant fibrotic component that does not undergo shrinkage following shrinkage and curettage.
  - If size of enlargement interferes with access to root surface deposits.

Q.33. Write in brief signs, symptoms and treatment of diphtheria. *(May/June 2009, 5 Marks)*

Ans. Diphtheria is an acute infectious disease caused by non-motile, non-sporing generally aerobic Gram-positive rods *C. diphtheriae*.

Symptoms

- Patient complains of presence of sore throat.
- Low-grade fever is present.
- Presence of headache and malaise.
- Hoarseness of voice, dyspnea in cases with laryngeal diphtheria.

Signs

- Presence of gross cervical lymphadenopathy.
- Formation of bluish white or grayish green pseudomembrane at the site of infection.
- Punched out ulcerations are present if skin is involved.
- Foul smelling serosanguinous discharge in cases of nasal diphtheria.
- Cyanosis is seen in cases with laryngeal diphtheria.

Treatment

Refer to Ans. 8 of same chapter.

Q.34. Write in brief clinical features and treatment of syphilis. *(Jun 2010, 5 Marks)*

Ans. Syphilis is a sexually transmitted disease caused by *Treponema palladium*.

Clinical Features

I. Congenital Syphilis

- It is transmitted via transplacental route from syphilitic mother to the fetus.
- But in modern era it is rare due to the screening of mothers in antenatal clinics and in early treatment of pregnant women.
- Clinical manifestations seen here are both early and late.
- Early manifestations appear under 2 years of life and resemble as mucocutaneous lesions of secondary syphilis of adults. Early lesions consist of mucocutaneous lesions, anemia, hepatosplenomegaly, lymphadenopathy, jaundice, thrombocytopenia and rarely nephrotic syndrome.
- Late manifestations occur after 2 years. Late lesions are keratitis, arthropathy, symptoms and signs of neurosyphilis which are similar to adults, gumma of palate and nasal septum leading to perforation.
- Late stigmata consists of Hutchinson's teeth and mulberry molars, idiotic facies, optic atrophy, nerve deafness and corneal opacities.

II. Acquired Syphilis

Acquired syphilis is divided into three stages, based on this clinical features are as follows:

1. **Early syphilis**
   - Primary syphilis
     - A single painless macule is seen over penis which later on become papular and then ulcerates forming punched out ulcer with well-defined margins, indurated base and fail to bleed on trauma. It is known as chancre.
     - In men, the ulcer is found on the coronal sulcus or on glans penis and in women on vulva, vaginal walls or cervix.
     - Bilateral inguinal lymphadenopathy occur. Lymph nodes are discrete, rubbery in consistency and are nontender.
     - In very short time, generalized lymphadenopathy occurs and as the lesion heals lymphadenopathy persists for a longer time.
     - Untreated ulcers resolve spontaneously in 3 to 8 weeks, usually without leaving a scar.
   - Secondary syphilis
     - In one-third of patients, primary lesions are still evident when secondary manifestations occur.
     - One to three months after appearance of primary chancre secondary stage develops.
     - Patient complains of malaise, headache and fever.
     - A maculopapular rash appears over trunk and extremities which is symmetrical, dull red in color and is nonitchy.
     - Condylomata lata are seen over round the anus, on labia, between buttocks, on lateral aspect of scrotum and other warm moist areas of body.
     - Ulcers are seen over mucous membrane of mouth, these ulcers may coalesce to form snail track ulcers.
     - Laryngeal lesions involving the vocal cords may give rise to hoarseness of voice
     - Either regional or generalized lymphadenopathy is present.
2. **Latent syphilis:** After some months, secondary stage of syphilis disappears in untreated patients followed by appearance of features of latent syphilis. Period of latency is from 2 to 4 years. Latent syphilis is of two types, i.e.,
   a. Early latent syphilis: It is diagnosed if there is presence of seroconversion of four fold rise in non-treponemal titers in past one year.
   b. Late latent syphilis: It is noninfectious and diagnosis is serological.

Treatment

Primary, Secondary and Early Latent Syphilis

- Benzathine penicillin G 2.4 million units IM usually in two sites (4 mL in each buttock) at a single visit. Additional dosages of 2.4 million units should be given 7 to 14 days later for latent syphilis of unknown duration.

♦ If patient is allergic to penicillin give ceftriaxone 125 mg IM OD for 10 days and azithromycin 1 g orally OD Or oral doxycycline 100 mg BD for 14 days.

3. **Late syphilis:** It is divided into two, i.e., tertiary syphilis and Quaternary syphilis

   a. *Tertiary syphilis:*
      - It takes years to develop.
      - Gumma is a painless round swelling which is rubbery in consistency and involves deeper tissues, such as muscle or bone and later on manifests as solitary, deep punched out mucosal ulcer.
      - Mucosal gummas affect submucous tissues of mouth, throat, palate, larynx, pharynx and nasal septum. They can ulcerate with punched out appearance and lesions have a sloughy base.
      - Bony gummas are diffuse subperiosteal reactions which often occur in long bones, particular in anterior margin of tibia.
      - Formation of lytic lesions can lead to perforation of hard palate or nasal septum which causes collapse of nasal bridge.

   b. *Quaternary syphilis:*
      - It takes 10 to 15 years to occur and produces irreversible damage to brain as well as heart.
      - Neurosyphilis consists of meningovascular and parenchymal disease. It also includes tabes dorsalis and generalized paralysis of insane.
      - Cardiovascular syphilis varies from asymptomatic aortitis to symptomatic aortic dilatation or aneurysm.

Treatment

Late Syphilis, i.e., Tertiary or Quaternary

♦ *Cardiovascular or neurosyphilis:* Procaine penicillin G 1.2 g IM daily for 4 weeks Or if patient is allergic to penicillin Oxytetracycline 500 mg 6 hourly for 4 weeks.

♦ *Benign tertiary syphilis:* Benzathine penicillin G 2.4 million units IM weekly for three weeks Or if patient is allergic to penicillin give oral doxycycline 100 mg 8 hourly for 4 weeks.

Q.35. Write short note on gonorrhea. *(Jan 2012, 5 Marks)*

Ans. It is a sexually transmitted disease caused by *Neisseria gonorrhoea.*

Clinical Features

♦ **In males:**
   - Earliest symptom present is burning or tingling sensation in urethra followed by discharge which becomes mucopurulent.
   - Dysuria is presence and increased frequency of micturition.
   - Pus is greenish yellow in color.

♦ **In females:**
   - Presence of dysuria, vaginal discharge, abnormal menstrual bleeding and rectal discomfort are the symptoms.

   - Leukorrhea is present and feature of pelvic infection are present. Pelvic infection may lead to abscess formation and toxemia.
   - Extension of infection leads to salpingitis, bartholinitis and abdominal pain.

Diagnosis

♦ History of sexual contact with pus discharge from urethra in males and from vagina in females make diagnosis more likely.

♦ It is made by demonstration of intracellular gram-negative diplococcic in smears obtained from urethral discharge and staining with Gram stain.

♦ Immunofluorescent antibody test gives quick diagnosis

♦ ELISA is done to detect gonococcal antigens.

Complications

♦ **In males:**
   - Local complications
      - Epididymitis
      - Prostatitis
      - Inguinal lymphadenitis
      - Periurethral abscess and later on periurethral fistula.
   - Systemic complications
      - Arthritis
      - Bacteremia.

♦ **In females:**
   - Local complications
      - Premature birth
      - Salpingitis
      - Pelvic infection.
   - Systemic complications
      - Perihepatitis
      - Pustular eruption.

Treatment

♦ IM injection of 2.4 g of procaine penicillin with 1 g of probenecid orally.

♦ Alternative therapy oral amoxicillin or ampicillin 3 g as single dose with 1 g of probenecid orally Or cotrimoxazole 4 g in single dose.

♦ For penicillin resistant gonorrhea ciprofloxacin is given 250 to 500 mg orally as single dosage Or Cefotaxime 0.5 to 1 g IM as single dosage.

♦ For complicated gonorrhea patient is hospitalized. Penicillin G IV 10 million units is given for 5 days; ciprofloxacin 500 mg BD for 5 days; ceftriaxone 1 g IV for 5 days is given.

Q.36. Write short note on risk factors and prophylaxis of HIV infection. *(Mar 2013, 3 Marks)*

Ans. Following are the risk factors of HIV infection

Risk Factors

♦ People who have unprotected vaginal or anal sex.

♦ People who have sex with many partners, thereby increasing the chance that they will encounter a partner who is HIV infected.

- People who share needles, for example for intravenous drug use, tattooing or body piercing
- Babies of mothers who are HIV infected.
- People who have another STD, especially STDs that cause open sores or ulcers, such as herpes, chancroid or syphilis.
- Hemophiliacs and other people who frequently receive blood products (this risk is now very much diminished, but there are still countries where blood is not adequately screened)
- Healthcare workers, where precautions are neglected or fail for example through not wearing gloves or accidental needle stick injuries.

Prophylaxis

- Practice safer sex. This includes using a condom unless you are in a relationship with one partner who does not have HIV or other sex partners.
- Never share intravenous (IV) needles, syringes, cookers, cotton, cocaine spoons, or eyedroppers with others if you use drugs.
- Do not donate blood, plasma, semen, body organs, or body tissues.
- Do not share personal items, such as toothbrushes, razors, or sex toys, that may be contaminated with blood, semen, or vaginal fluids.
- The risk of a woman spreading HIV to her baby can be greatly reduced if she: is on medicine that reduces the amount of virus in her blood to undetectable levels during pregnancy; continues treatment during pregnancy; Does not breast-feed her baby.
- Healthcare workers should take universal precautions while treating HIV positive patient.

Q.37. Discuss the signs, symptoms, diagnosis and treatment of malaria. *(Aug 2012, 12 Marks)*

Or

Write short note on malaria.

(Mar 2016, 3 Marks) (Dec 2015, 3 Marks)

Or

Write short answer on clinical features of malaria.

(Mar 2016, 3 Marks) (Oct 2019, 3 Marks)

Ans. Malaria is the acute febrile illness which is characterized by paroxysms of fever as a result of asexual reproduction of plasmodia in red cells.

Symptoms and Signs (Clinical Features)

Onset of malaria is with lassitude, anorexia, headache and fever with chills.

Three clinical stages are present:

- *Cold Stage:* It remains for half an hour. Patient feels intense cold and shivers from head to foot, teeth of patient chatter. Patient cover himself with blanket. Fever raises rapidly and is as high as 41°C.
- *Hot stage:* It follows cold stage and last for 3 to 4 hours. Patient feels intense heat and throws blanket. Patient has flushed face, headache, vomiting, dry skin.
- *Sweating Stage:* Patient has excessive perspiration, temperature is declined and patient feels relief.

Diagnosis

- *Clinical:* Periodic fever with chills, sweating, anemia and splenomegaly.
- *Blood film:* Malarial parasites are identified in thick and thin blood smears. Common microscopic characters of falciparum malaria are high concentration of parasites, predominant thin ring-shaped trophozoites
- *Malarial antigen spot test using parasite LDH:* P. falciparum antigens are taken from blood by finger prick and are exposed to monoclonal antibodies to detect antigens and read out color bands.
- Immunofluorescent microscopy and PCR (Polymerase chain reaction)
- Latex agglutination assay.

Treatment

- Treatment of chloroquine susceptible *P. vivax, P. falciparum, P. ovale, P. malariae* chloroquine:
  This is given in the dose of 600 mg base followed by 300 mg at 6th, 24th and 48th hours. It is useful in treating all types of malaria. It is curative for *P. falciparum* malaria but cannot prevent relapses due to exoerythrocytic cycles of P. vivax malaria
- **Treatment of chloroquine resistant *P. falciparum*:**
  - Quinidine IV 10 mg/kg dissolved in 300 mL normal saline infused over 1 to 2 hour.
  - *Quinine hydrochloride:* 600 mg TDS for 3–7 days is useful. If required for cerebral malaria, this drug can given IV the dose is 7 mg/kg over 30 min, followed by 10 mg/kg over 4 hours and then 10 mg/kg over 8 hour or until the patient can complete a week of oral treatment.
  - *Mefloquine:* It provides rapid schizonticidal action in single dose of 15 mg/kg orally maximum dose is 1000 to 1250 mg.
  - *Halofantrine*
    Dosage: Adult 500 mg BD for 4–6 days.
    Children: 8 mg/kg
  - *Artemether:* This drug is rapidly acting, safe and is effective against multidrug resistant infections. Artemether 3.2 mg/kg IM is given followed by 1.6 mg/kg IM every 12 to 24 hours until patient wakes up. Artesunate 2 mg/kg IV stat followed by 1 mg/kg 12 hourly.
  - Sulfadoxine and pyrimethamine: Combination of sulfadoxime 1500 mg and pyrimethamine 25 mg helps to cure an acute attack of chloroquine resistant malaria.
- **Treatment of Chloroquine resistant *P. vivex***
  Oral mefloquine and halofantrine.
- **Treatment of persistent hypnozoites in *P. vivex* or *P. ovale* infection**
  - *Primaquine:* It is given in the dose of 7.5 mg BD for 14 days usually after doing a G6PD test
  - *Bulaquine:* It is given 25 mg OD for 5 days.

Q.38. Write short note on clinical features and treatment of *P. vivex* malaria. *(Dec 2012, 3 Marks)*

Ans.

Clinical Features

Onset of malaria is with lassitude, anorexia, headache and fever with chills.

Three clinical stages are present:

♦ *Cold Stage:* It remains for half an hour. Patient feels intense cold and shivers from head to foot, teeth of patient chatter. Patient covers himself with blanket. Fever raises rapidly and is as high as 41°C.

♦ *Hot stage:* It follows cold stage and last for 3 to 4 hours. Patient feels intense heat and throws blanket. Patient has flushed face, headache, vomiting, dry skin.

♦ *Sweating Stage:* Patient has excessive perspiration, temperature is declined and patient feels relief.

Treatment

♦ *Treatment of chloroquine susceptible P. vivax:*
  • *Chloroquine:* This is given in the dose of 600 mg followed by 300 mg at 6th, 24th and 48th hours.
♦ *Treatment of Chloroquine resistant P. vivax:*
  • Oral mefloquine with dosage of three 250 mg tablets which are repeated after 6 hours.
♦ *Treatment of persistent hypnozoites in P. vivax infection:*
  • Primaquine 30 mg per day orally for 14 days is given.

Q.39. Write short note on causes and treatment of bleeding gums. *(Feb 2014, 3 Marks)*

Ans.

Causes of Bleeding Gums

Following are the causes of bleeding gums:

♦ Gingivitis and gingivostomatitis
♦ Bleeding disorders, i.e., thrombocytopenia, hemophilia, leukemia and anticoagulants.
♦ Abnormalities of vessel wall: Scurvy, Henoch Schönlein purpura, dysproteinemia
♦ Connective tissue disorders: Ehlers-Danlos syndrome, pseudoxanthoma elasticum.

Treatment of Bleeding Gums

♦ Bleeding gums can be treated by the removal of the source of bacteria.
♦ Proper maintenance of the teeth by the patient is a must.
♦ Sore and bleeding gums can be aggravated by citrus fruits and juices, rough or spicy food, alcohol, and tobacco.
♦ Take vitamin C supplements, if citrus fruits and juices cannot be taken.
♦ If dentures make gums bleed, wear them only during meals.
♦ Gum bleeding can be controlled by applying pressure with a gauze pad soaked in ice water directly to the bleeding gums.
♦ Brush teeth gently after every meal. Use a soft brush, or a special vibrating brush to clean the teeth without irritating the gums.
♦ Use gum paint regularly to control bleeding from the gums.

Q.40. Write short note on herpes zoster infection. *(Feb 2013, 5 Marks)*

Or

Write short answer on herpes zoster infection. *(Apr 2018, 3 Marks)*

Ans. It is also known as shingles.

Herpes zoster is the secondary form of infection.

After primary infection virus remains dormant in the dorsal root or cranial nerve ganglia. The disease recurs in the localized form which remains to its dermatome innervated by spinal or cranial sensory ganglion or it can affect the motor nerve causing facial nerve palsy.

Predisposing Factors

Herpes zoster is more common in people with diminished cell mediated immunity. This includes elderly people, patients with lymphoma receiving chemotherapy or steroids, and individual with HIV.

Clinical Features

♦ It consists of two stages, i.e.
  • *Pre-eruptive stage:* Pain with hyperesthesia along the course of the nerve and fever.
  • *Eruptive stage:* May be the first manifestation of disease in some cases.
♦ There are several edematous patches along the course of a nerve with intervening clear areas, these are very tender and painful.
♦ A few hours later these patches are surmounted with small vesicles in cluster. Vesicles occur in crops. The contents may become purulent. The vesicles crust over, and in absence of secondary infection, clear within a week.
♦ Chronic ulcerative lesions may be seen in HIV-infected patients.
♦ Regional glands are painful and tender.
♦ An attack lasts for 2–3 weeks.
♦ The rash is usually unilateral and leaves behind pigmentation and scarring.
♦ Thoracic and lumbar dermatomes are the sites most commonly affected.
♦ An eruption in the mandibular and maxillary distribution of trigeminal nerve is associated with oral, palatal and pharyngeal lesions. If there is involvement of ophthalmic division, there can be keratitis or uveitis with presence of vesicles over the nose.

Complications

♦ Post-herpetic neuralgia
♦ Keratitis and corneal ulceration
♦ Neurological, i.e., encephalitis, meningitis and myelitis.

Management

♦ Acyclovir 800 mg orally five times a day for a week is given. Acyclovir cream can be applied over the lesions also.
♦ Prednisolone 40–60 mg in tapering doses is given for 3 weeks.

♦ Calamine lotion or cream is given to the patient for prevention of irritation in the lesion.

♦ Anti-septic powder can also be applied for preventing the secondary infection. This should be applied after vesicles break

♦ Analgesics can be given as per need.

♦ For post-herpetic neuralgia analgesics, amitriptyline, gabapentin, pregabalin, tramadol and carbamazepine is given.

Q.41. Write short note on postexposure prophylaxis in HIV/ AIDS. *(Nov 2014, 3 Marks)*

Or

Write post exposure prophylaxis in AIDS.
(Apr 2015, 4 Marks)

Ans. Following is the postexposure prophylaxis in HIV/AIDS:

♦ HIV postexposure prophylaxis is started within an hour or two.

♦ Depending on the type and seriousness of the exposure either a basic regimen, i.e., zidovudine with lamivudine is followed or expanded drug regimen, i.e., zidovudine + lamivudine + Indinavir is given.

♦ Following is the recommended HIV postexposure prophylaxis:

Exposure type	Small volume, i.e., few drops splashed	Large Volume, i.e., major blood splash
HIV positive class I, i.e., asymptomatic HIV infection	Consider zidovudine with lamivudine	Zidovudine + lamivudine + Indinavir
HIV positive class II, i.e., symptomatic HIV infection, AIDS, acute seroconversion	Recommended zidovudine with lamivudine	Expanded zidovudine + lamivudine + indinavir
Exposure type	Less severe	More severe
Source HIV status known	No postexposure prophylaxis is warranted. Consider zidovudine with lamivudine for source with HIV risk factors	No postexposure prophylaxis is warranted
Unknown source	No postexposure prophylaxis is warranted. Considerte zidovudine with lamivudine in settings where exposure to HIV-infected person is likely	--------

Q.42. Write etiology, clinical features, investigations and complications of HIV infection. *(Feb 2015, 12 Marks)*

Ans. The presence of a reliably diagnosed disease, i.e., at least moderately indicative of an underlying defect in cell-mediated immunity occurring in a person with no known cause for immunodeficiency other than the presence of HIV.

Etiology

♦ HIV infection is caused by the infection with virus HIV-1 and HIV-2.

♦ HIV-1 is most common worldwide. It has many strains due to the mutation.

♦ HIV-2 has 40% sequence homology with HIV-1 and is very closely related to simian immunodeficiency virus.

Clinical Features

Clinical features of HIV infection as per its stage are as follows:

Stage of HIV infection	Clinical features
Acute HIV syndrome	• Fever • Headache • Pharyngitis • Malaise • Lymphadenopathy • Diffuse cutaneous erythematous rash
Chronic asymptomatic infection	• Headache • Diffuse reactive lymphadenopathy
Early symptomatic disease	• Fever • Night sweat • Chronic diarrhea

Contd…

Contd…

Stage of HIV infection	Clinical features
	• Fatigue • Minor oral infections • Headache • Anorexia • Weight loss • Nausea • Vomiting
Late symptomatic disease	Symptoms of *Pneumocystis carinii* pneumonia and other opportunistic infections
Advanced disease	Symptoms of AIDS, i.e., protozoal, fungal, viral and bacterial infections.

Investigations

♦ **Investigations for the diagnosis of HIV infection**

• HIV-ELISA: This is the most commonly used screening test for HIV infection. If this test is positive confirmation should be done by western blot test.

• *HIV-rapid antibody test:* They are for rapid diagnosis, i.e., within 10 to 15 minutes. It is also a screening test, as if this test comes positive confirmation is done by western blot.

• *Western blot:* It is the confirmatory test for HIV infection.

• *Blood cell count:* Since neutropenia, anemia and pancytopenia are associated with HIV infection, this test is done.

♦ **Investigations for monitoring progress of HIV infection**

• *Absolute CD4 lymphocyte count:* This is most commonly used. As its count decreases occurrence of opportunistic infection and malignancy is high, i.e., if count is less than 200 cells/μL.

- *CD4 lymphocyte percentage:* In this, if count is less than 14% occurrence of opportunistic infection and malignancy is high, if treatment is not given to patient.
♦ **Investigations for virological monitoring**
In this, HIV viral load tests are done, such as HIV–RNA by PCR, HIV–RNA by bDNA, HIV–RNA by NASBA. These all tests measure the actively replicating HIV virus. These cells also deflect the response of antiretroviral drugs. These test are excellent for diagnosis of acute HIV infection before its seroconversion.

Complications

System	Complications
Neuropsychiatric	Primary central nervous system lymphoma, Chronic psychiatric disorders
Head and neck	Gingivitis, dental and salivary gland disease
Cardiovascular	Cardiovascular disease, endocarditis
Pulmonary	Chronic obstructive pulmonary disease, lung cancer (including Kaposi's sarcoma and lymphoma)
Gastrointestinal	Viral hepatitis, lymphoma, Kaposi's sarcoma, HPV- related malignancies
Renal/genitourinary	Chronic kidney disease not caused by HIV-associated nephropathy
Musculoskeletal	Osteopenia, osteoporosis, osteonecrosis
Hematologic or oncologic	Lymphoma, multiple myeloma
Dermatologic	Papulosquamous disorders, molluscum contagiosum, Kaposi sarcoma

Q.43. Write herpes simplex under following headings:

(Apr 2015, 2+2+2 Marks)

　a.　**Causative organism**

　b.　**Manifestations/Clinical features**

　c.　**Treatment**

Or

Write short answer on herpes simplex.

(May 2018, 3 Marks)

Ans.

Causative Organism

Herpes simplex is caused by a DNA virus. Virus consists of two strains, i.e., Type 1 and Type 2. Type 1 virus enters through the mouth while Type 2 virus is sexually transmitted and leads to anorectal or genital infections.

Manifestations or Clinical Features

♦ Primary infection by herpes simplex
　• *Mucous membranes:*
　　– *Acute gingivostomatitis:* It is characterized by soreness of mouth, salivation, fever and malaise. Vesicles are present in the mouth.
　　– *Keratoconjunctivitis:* The condition is painful and is unilateral. Ulceration of cornea can occur which leads to chronic scarring.

　　– *Genital herpes:* In females, vesicles are present over the vulva, cervix or vagina. In males, vesicles are seen on glans penis or less commonly urethritis.
　• *Skin:*
　　– *Disseminated herpes simplex:* Seen in new born infants. Brain, liver, lungs and other vital organs are affected.
　　– *Eczema herpeticum:* In cases with atopic dermatitis, herpes simplex develops in varicelliform.
　　– *Herpetic whitlow:* It manifest as indolent inflammatory arising at site of minor skin trauma on finger in form of deep, painful multiple vesicles over the finger tip.
　　– *Anal infection:* In homosexuals, there is intense pain, tenesmus and local vesicles are present.
　• Recurrent infection
　　– *Herpes labialis:* Lesions appear on vermilion border of lip and surrounding skin. These lesions are gray or white vesicles which rupture quickly leaving small red ulcerations with slight erythematous halo on lip covered by brown crusts.
　　– *Eye infection:* Recur as superficial keratitis.
　　– *Genital infection:* They are mild and short as compared to its primary form.

Treatment

♦ About 5% acyclovir cream, is applied in every 4 hours.
♦ For severe infection oral acyclovir 200 mg 5 times a day is given. Reduce the dose to half in children.
♦ IV acyclovir 5 mg/kg for every 8 hours by slow infusion is given.
♦ Antibacterial therapy is given in mucocutaneous herpes to reduce risk of secondary infection.

Q.44. Write short note on rose spots. *(Apr 2015, 2 Marks)*

Ans. Rose spots are the clinical sign for typhoid fever.

♦ As first week of typhoid fever is over rose spots appear.
♦ Rose spots appear over the trunk. They can also be seen over back and chest.
♦ They are small macules which are 2–4 mm in diameter, red in color and on applying pressure they show blanching.
♦ Rose spots lasts for 2–3 days.

Q.45. Write in short treatment of esophageal candidiasis.

(Apr 2015, 2 Marks)

Ans. Treatment of esophageal candidiasis

♦ Oral fluconazole systemically 200 mg/day for 14–21 days is given.
♦ In cases with severe dysphagia, IV administration of Fluconazole is done.
♦ Patients who had previous infection of esophageal candidiasis, patient should be given Fluconazole 100–200 mg daily for prophylaxis.

Q.46. Write short note on infectious mononucleosis.

(Dec 2015, 3 Marks)

Ans. It is also known as glandular fever.

♦ Infectious mononucleosis is caused by Epstein-Barr virus (EBV).
♦ Incubation period for virus is 7–20 days.

Pathogenesis

EBV undergo replication in lymphoid tissues of throat and is transmitted to healthy person via saliva.

Clinical Features

- There is presence of acute onset of fever with chills, core throat, headache, malaise and tiredness.
- Lymph nodes become enlarged, discrete and slightly tender affecting cervical and submandibular lymph nodes.
- Nontender splenomegaly is present.
- Petechial rash can occur at the junction of hard and soft palate on 4th day and can persist for 3–4 days.

Investigations

- Peripheral smear shows leukocytosis with atypical lymphocytosis.
- Paul-Bunnell test can be positive in 1:32 dilution.
- Liver transaminases are raised.

Complications

- Fatigue
- Hemolytic anemia
- Hepatitis
- Meningoencephalitis
- Thrombocytopenia.

Management

- In acute phase of disease, patient should be on bed rest. Condition resolve in 4 weeks.
- Short course of steroids can be used, i.e., 10 mg prednisolone thrice daily with tapering dosages.
- Gargles with soluble aspirin are helpful for relieving sore throat.
- Antibiotics, i.e., erythromycin can be given, if secondary infection is present.
- Interferon-α administration, cytotoxic chemotherapy and radiation therapy can also be used.

Q.47. Write short note on complications of enteric fever.

(Sep 2006, 10 Marks)

Ans.

- **Intestinal complications**
  - Hemorrhage may occur at the end of the second week and is characterized by black stools, tachycardia, hypotension and diarrhea. There is no abdominal pain or rigidity or obliteration of liver dullness like in intestinal perforation. Transfusions may be needed, if there is massive blood loss.
  - Perforation may occur at the end of the second week or in the third week. It is characterized by acute pain in the lower abdomen, vomiting, abdominal distension, hypotension and tachycardia. Liver dullness may be obliterated and the abdomen becomes tender, rigid and silent (absent peristalsis).
  - Tympanitis
  - Cholecystitis
  - Splenic infarction

- Rarely, appendicitis, intussusception and pyogenic liver abscess
- **Extraintestinal complications**
  - Myocarditis, endocarditis
  - Osteomyelitis, arthritis, typhoid spine and Zenker's degeneration of rectus abdominis
  - Pulmonary infection and embolism
  - Thrombophlebitis
  - Electrolyte imbalance, shock and acute renal failure
  - *Neurological:* Meningoencephalitis, meningism, cranial nerve palsies, myelitis, ascending paralysis, Parkinsonism, athetosis, cerebellar ataxia, neuritis
  - *Typhoid state:* This is characterized by coma vigil, muttering delirium, carphologia (picking up clothes in bed) and subsultus tendinosis
  - Psychosis

Q.48. Enumerate the complications of typhoid fever.

(Feb. Mar 2005, 5 Marks)

Ans. Following are the complications of typhoid fever:

- *Intestinal complications*
  - Hemorrhage
  - Perforation
  - Paralytic ileus
  - Peritonitis
- *Extraintestinal complications:*
  - Meningitis
  - Bone and joint infection
  - Cholecystitis
  - Encephalopathy
  - Pneumonia
  - Granulomatous hepatitis
  - Nephritis
  - Myocarditis

Q.49. Write etiology, clinical features, diagnosis and management of malaria. Mention complications of falciparum malaria. *(Jan 2017, 12 Marks)*

Ans. Malaria is a common tropical disease.

Etiology

It is caused by protozoa, Plasmodium through the bite of a female anopheles mosquito.

Requirements for the causation of malaria are:

- Presence of suitable female anopheles mosquito
- Reservoir of malaria infection in the particular area.
- Suitable non-immune or partly immune hosts
- An environmental temperature with suitable humidity
  For clinical features, diagnosis and management of malaria refer to Ans. 38 of same chapter.

Complications of Falciparum Malaria

- *Central nervous system:* Cerebral malaria, i.e., convulsions and coma
- *Renal system:* Black water fever, acute renal failure
- *Blood:* Severe anemia, disseminated intravascular coagulation
- *Respiratory:* Adult respiratory distress syndrome
- *Metabolic:* Hypoglycemia, metabolic acidosis

- ◆ *Gastrointestinal tract and liver:* Diarrhea, jaundice, splenic rupture
- ◆ *Miscellaneous:* Hypotensive shock, hyperpyrexia
- ◆ *Pregnancy:* Maternal death, abortion, stillbirth and low birth weight

Q.50. Write short note on cutaneous and oral manifestations of AIDS. *(Apr 2017, 6 Marks)*

Or

Write short note on oral manifestations in AIDS patients. *(Jan 2019, 7 Marks)*

Or

Write short answer on oral manifestations of AIDS. *(Oct 2019, 3 Marks)*

Ans.

Cutaneous Manifestations of AIDS

Following are the cutaneous or dermatological manifestations of AIDS:

- ◆ *Superficial fungal infection:* Candidiasis, dermatophytosis, pityrosporum infection
- ◆ *Disseminated fungal and protozoal infection: Cryptococcus neoformans* infections, histoplasmosis, sporotrichosis, dermal leishmaniasis, coccidioidomycosis
- ◆ *Bacterial and mycobacterial infections:* Staph. aureus, *M. avium* intracellulare, *M. tuberculosis*, actinomycosis.
- ◆ Viral: HPV infection, molluscum contagiosum, herpes simplex virus, varicella and herpes zoster, cytomegalovirus, EB virus.
- ◆ *HIV-related rash:* Acute HIV exanthem, papular rash of HIV
- ◆ *Pruritic papular and follicular eruptions:* Folliculitis Eosinophilic pustular, pityrosporum, demodectic, insect bite reaction, Prurigo nodularis.
- ◆ *Papulosquamous disorders:* Seborrheic dermatitis, psoriasis, Reiter's syndrome, atopic dermatitis, lichen planus
- ◆ *Malignancies:* Kaposi's sarcoma, squamous cell and basal cell carcinoma, malignant melanoma
- ◆ *Miscellaneous dermatoses:* Acquired ichthyosis, chronic photosensitivity, granuloma annulare, vitiligo, immunobullous disorders, Sjögren's syndrome, porphyria, telangiectases, leukocytoclastic vasculitis, scabies (Norwegian), hidradenitis suppurativa, palmoplantar keratoderma.

Oral Manifestations of AIDS by EC-Clearing House

Group 1: Strongly Associated with HIV Infection

- ◆ *Candidiasis:* erythematous, pseudomembranous, angular cheilitis
- ◆ Hairy leukoplakia
- ◆ Kaposi's sarcoma
- ◆ Non-Hodgkin's lymphoma
- ◆ Periodontal diseases: Linear gingival erythema, necrotizing gingivitis, necrotizing periodontitis.

Group 2: Less Commonly Associated with HIV Infection

- ◆ *Bacterial infections: Mycobacterium avium-intracellulare, Mycobacterium tuberculosis* Melanotic hyperpigmentation

- ◆ Necrotizing ulcerative stomatitis
- ◆ *Salivary gland disease:* Dry mouth, unilateral or bilateral swelling of major salivary glands
- ◆ Thrombocytopenia purpura
- ◆ Oral ulcerations NOS (not otherwise specified)
- ◆ *Viral infections:* Herpes simplex, human papillomavirus, varicella-zoster

Group 3: Seen in HIV Infection

- ◆ *Bacterial infections: Actinomyces israelii, Escherichia coli, Klebsiella pneumoniae*
- ◆ Cat-scratch disease (*Bartonella henselae*)
- ◆ Epithelioid (bacillary) angiomatosis (*Bartonella henselae*)
- ◆ *Drug reactions:* Ulcerative, erythema multiforme, lichenoid, toxic epidermolysis
- ◆ *Fungal infections other than candidiasis: Cryptococcus neoformans, Geotrichum candidum, Histoplasma capsulatum, Mucoraceae* (mucormycosis/zygomycosis), Aspergillus flavus
- ◆ Neurologic disturbances: Facial palsy, trigeminal neuralgia
- ◆ Recurrent aphthous stomatitis
- ◆ *Viral infections:* Cytomegalovirus, molluscum contagiosum

Q.51. Write short answer on candidiasis.

(May 2018, 3 Marks)

Ans. Candidiasis is a fungal infection caused by an opportunistic fungus known as candida albicans.

Predisposing factors

- ◆ *Changes in oral flora:* Marked changes in oral flora occur due to administration of antibiotics, excessive use of antibacterial mouth rinses, xerostomia secondary to anticholinergic agent or salivary gland disease. These changes result in inhibiton of competitive bacteria leading to candidiasis.
- ◆ *Local irritant:* Chronic local irritants, i.e., dentures, orthodontic appliances, etc.
- ◆ *Drug therapy:* Various drugs, i.e., corticosteroids, cytotoxic drugs, immunosuppressive agents and radiation to head and neck.
- ◆ Acute and chronic diseases, such as leukemia, diabetes, tuberculosis etc.
- ◆ Malnutrition states, such as low serum vitamin A, pyridoxine and Vitamin A.
- ◆ *Endocrinopathy:* Such as hypothyroidism, hyperparathyroidism and Addison's disease
- ◆ Immunodeficiency states, such as AIDS, hypogammaglobulinemia.

Clinical features

- ◆ It occur in both infants and adults. In infants, oral lesion occurs between 6th and 10th day after birth.
- ◆ Common sites for infection to occur are roof of mouth, retromolar area and mucobuccal fold.
- ◆ It is more common in women as compared to man.
- ◆ Patient can complain for burning sensation.
- ◆ Lesion appears as white plaque which is pearlish white or blue white in color and are present on the oral mucosa. Lesions resemble as cottage cheese or curdled milk.

Mucosa adjacent to the lesion appears red in color and is moderately swollen.

- White patches are easily wiped out with wet gauze which leaves normal or erythematous area. This area can be painful. Deep invasion of an organism leave an ulcerative lesion on removal of patch.
- In severe infection, the involvement of pharynx and esophagus cause dysphagia.
- The fungus may travel to lower respiratory passage and may involve lungs in fulminant infection.

Investigations

- On staining with periodic acid Schiff (PAS) method, candidal hyphae are readily identified. Organisms are identified by bright magenta color. The candidal hyphae are 2μm in diameter, vary in length and may show branching.
- About 10–20% KOH is also used to identify organisms readily.
- Cultures can be obtained readily on Sabouraud's medium and on ordinary bacteriological culture media. Colonies are creamy white, smooth with a yeasty color.
- On corn-meal agar medium *C. albicans* form chlamydospores.

Diagnosis

Clinically the white lesion can be scraped off by wet gauze.

Treatment

- Treatment includes antiseptic mouth wash with antiseptic solution for 4–5 days.
- Nystatin tablets may be retained locally in the mouth 3–4 times daily or may be crushed or mixed with glycerine for local application.
- Oral administration of nystatin is needed in severe or systemic infection. Nystatin is given 250 mg TDS for two weeks followed by 1 troche per day for third week.

Q.52. Write short answer on syphilis. *(Feb 2019, 3 Marks)*

Ans. *For clinical features and treatment of syphilis refer to Ans. 34 of same chapter.*

Classification of Syphilis

- Congenital
  - Early
  - Late
- Acquired
  - Early
    - Primary syphilis
    - Secondary syphilis
  - Latent (WHO)
    - Early (Less than 1 year)
    - Late (More than 1 year)
  - Late
    - Tertiary syphilis
    - Quaternary syphilis

Mode of Transmission

- Sexual contact with the infected lesion.
- Non-sexual contact due to kissing and personal contact.
- Due to transfusion of blood and blood products
- Transplacental from mother to fetus.

Laboratory Diagnosis

- **Dark field microscopic examination:** *T. palladium* is seen in primary lesion or in mucus patches of secondary syphilis. Exudate taken from the lesions or aspirated from lymph node is examined under dark field microscope. Spirochetes are not seen in late syphilitic lesions.
- **Immunofluorescent antibody staining technique:** It demonstrates *T. palladium* in dry smear of fluid which are taken from early syphilitic lesions.
- **Serological tests:** After the four weeks of infection, they provide the positive results in secondary stage and at birth in congenital syphilis. Syphilis produces two types of antibodies, i.e., nonspecific reagenic antibodies and specific anti-treponemal antibody, these are measured by nonspecific and specific tests.
  - *Nonspecific tests for screening and diagnosis:* Here flocculation of antigen suspension occurs i.e.
    - Venereal disease laboratory test (VDRL): This is the slide test.
    - Rapid plasma regain test (RPR): In microscope, flocculation is seen. It provides rapid serological diagnosis.
  - *Specific test for confirmation of diagnosis:*
    - *T. palladium* hemagglutination assay
    - Fluorescent *T. palladium* antibody absorption
    - Immobilization test
    - Treponemal EIA test: This test, if it is positive, it is followed by other tests.

False positive results occur with non–specific tests in other infections and connective tissue disorders. Confirmation of syphilis is by specific tests.

- **Other investigations:** Done in tertiary syphilis
  - Chest skiagram for calcification of aorta in cardiovascular syphilis
  - CSF examination in neurosyphilis
- **EIA-based screening algorithm:** It starts with an automated treponemal test, i.e., EIA or CLIA and is followed by nonspecific RPR or VDRL test if results of treponemal test are positive.
- **Polymerase chain reaction (PCR):** It is used to demonstrate *T. palladium* from genital ulcer.

Q.53. Write short answer on heat stroke.

(Apr 2019, 3 Marks)

Ans. Heat stroke is also known as sunstroke or heat hyperpyrexia.

- It is characterized by sudden loss of consciousness which may be preceded by prodromal signs typical of cerebral irritation, i.e., headache, dizziness, nausea, convulsions, and visual disturbances.
- Failure of the heat regulating center gives rise to high fever and cessation of sweating.
- On examination the skin is hot and flushed and dry, pulse rapid, irregular and weak and low blood pressure.
- Temperature may reach as high as between 105°–107°F.

- If the patient is not treated the temperature continues to rise and a state of hyperpyrexia supervenes.
- Rhabdomyolysis, cardiac dysrhythmias, acute renal failure and coagulopathy ensue and contribute to the high mortality rate.

Management

- Cooling by fanning after sprinkling water. Immersion in cold water or use of ice packs or ice water enemas.
- Massage of extremities to maintain the circulation
- Sedatives are contraindicated unless convulsions are present.
- Normal saline 1000 mL IV slowly if there is presence of hydration or cramps.

Q.54. Write short note on clinical features and management of hemorrhagic fever. (Jan 2019, 7 Marks)

Ans. Hemorrhagic fever is also known as viral hemorrhagic fever.

It is an acute illness characterized by fever and in most severe cases, shock and bleeding.

Clinical Features

- Insidious onset with influenza like symptoms.
- Abdominal pain, diarrhea and vomiting may occur.
- Common physical signs are fever, pharyngitis and conjunctival injection.
- In severe cases, bleeding begins towards end of first week.
- Hypotension and shock, encephalopathy and ARDS is seen in very severe cases.

Treatment

Ribavirin reduces mortality if given in first week in Lassa fever Dose: 30 mg/kg IV loading dose, then 16 mg/kg IV 6 hourly for 4 days, then 8 mg/kg IV 8 hourly for 6 days. Total duration of treatment is 10 days.

Q.55. Write short answer on swine flu. *(Apr 2019, 3 Marks)*

Ans. Swine flu is also known as H1N1 influenza, hog flu and pig flu which is caused by swine influenza virus (SIV), that usually infects pigs and is endemic in pigs.

Swine flu results from one of the three types of influenza virus, i.e., A,B or C which are classified in the family orthomyxoviridae.

These are structurally and biologically single—stranded RNA viruses which vary antigenically. A distinctive feature of influenza viruses is that mutations occur frequently and unpredictably in the eight gene segments and especially in the hemagglutinin gene. The emergence of an inherently virulent virus during the course of a pandemic can never be ruled out.

Transmission

Infection occurs after transfer of respiratory secretions from an infected individual to an immunologically susceptible individual. If the virus is not neutralized by secretory antibodies, it invades airways and respiratory tract cells. Once it enters the host cells, it leads to cellular dysfunction and degeneration, along with viral replication and release of viral progeny.

Communicability of Virus

A patient is infectious to others from 1 day before to 7 days after onset of symptoms. If infection persists for more than 7 days, chances of communicability may persist till resolution of illness. Children are likely to spread the virus for longer period.

Clinical Features

- After an incubation period of 18–72 hours, systemic symptoms ensue.
- Abrupt onset with varying degrees of fever.
- Sore throat may be severe, may be associated with rhinitis.
- Myalgias range from mild to severe.
- Ocular symptoms may develop and include photophobia, burning sensation and/or pain on motion.
- Weakness and severe fatigue may prevent patients from normal activities.
- Cough and other respiratory symptoms may be initially minimal but progress as the infection evolves.
- Cough may be unproductive and associated with pleuritic chest pain, and dyspnea.

Complications

- **Pulmonary:** Primary viral pneumonia, secondary bacterial pneumonia and exacerbation of COPD and bronchial asthma.
- **Extrapulmonary:** Myositis, rhabdomyolysis, myoglobinuria, myocarditis and pericarditis.
- At times CNS complications may occur including encephalitis, transverse myelitis and GB syndrome and Rae syndrome.

Laboratory Findings

- Leukopenia and relative lymphopenia are typical findings, there may be thrombocytopenia.
- Specimens for viral studies viz. RTP CR and viral culture should be stored at 4°C before and during transportation within 48 hours.

Management

- **Critical measures:**
  - Avoid crowding patients together.
  - Hand hygiene.
  - Wear personal protective equipments which include high efficiency masks (ideally N95 mask or triple layer surgical mask), gowns, goggles, gloves, cap and shoe cover.
  - If suspected swine flu, isolation of infected individuals and house-hold contacts.
- **Antiviral drug therapy:** Two H1N1 influenza drugs are neuraminidase inhibitors.
  - Oseltamivir is the recommended drug for prophylaxis and treatment. It inhibits neuraminidase which is a glycoprotein on the surface of influenza virus that destroys an infected cell's receptor for viral hemagglutinin. The drug must be administered within 48 hours of symptom onset.
  - Zanamivir is a sialic acid analogue that potentiates and specifically inhibits the neuraminidases of influenza A

and B viruses. Inhaled zanamivir for the prevention and treatment for influenza virus infections. Early treatment with dose 10 mg BD for 5 days of febrile influenza in ambulatory adults and children aged 5 years and older shortens the time of illness resolution by 1–3 days and in adults reduces by 40% risk of lower respiratory tract complications.

♦ **Discharge policy:** Adult patients should be discharged 7 days after symptoms have subsided, and children 14 days after. The family of patients discharged should be educated on personal hygiene and infection control measures at home.

♦ **Vaccines:**
  • H1N1 nasal vaccine.
  • Injectable vaccine: The vaccine takes up to 3 weeks for antibodies to develop. Indication for prophylactic vaccination in high risk category i.e.
    1. Pregnant women because of higher risk of complications and can provide protection to infants.
    2. Household contacts and caretakers for infants <6 months old, because of higher risk of complications.
    3. Healthcare services workers.

12. MISCELLANEOUS

Q.1. Write short note on anaphylactic shock.

(Sep 2006, 5 Marks)

Or

Write notes on anaphylaxis.   *(Aug 2011, 10 Marks)*

Or

Discuss anaphylaxis and its management in detail.

(Jan 2017, 12 Marks)

Or

Write short answer on anaphylactic shock.

(Sep 2018, 3 Marks)

Or

Describe briefly management of drug, induced anaphylaxis.   *(Feb/Mar 2004, 5 Marks)*

Or

Outline treatment of anaphylaxis shock.

(Jan 2012, 6 Marks)

Or

Write management of anaphylaxis.

(Nov 2011, 4 Marks)

Ans. Anaphylaxis is an acute and dramatic life-threatening immunological reaction to a drug or other stimulus.

Etiology

♦ *Antibiotics:* Penicillin and streptomycin.
♦ Radio contrast media
♦ Anesthetic agent, i.e., lignocaine
♦ Blood and blood products including sera.
♦ *Hormones:* Insulin and growth hormone.

♦ *Venoms:* Bees, spiders and wasps
♦ *Others:* NSAIDs, narcotic agents, heparin and thrombolytic agents.

Clinical Features

♦ Onset may be instantaneous or within a few minutes after the IV injection and 30 minutes after exposure.
♦ *Cardiovascular:* Tachycardia, arrhythmia, hypotension and circulatory collapse.
♦ *Respiratory:* Laryngeal obstruction, angiedema, bronchospasm or pulmonary edema may occur singly or in combination.
♦ *Nervous:* Syncope and seizures.
♦ *GIT:* Diaphoresis, abdominal pain and diarrhea may occur.
♦ *Skin:* Wheel and erythematous lesions are seen which are circumscribed, round, discrete, erythematous areas with irregular borders and blanched centers.
♦ Lesions are very pruritic.
♦ If not treated death may occur.

Management

♦ *Airways:* Endotracheal intubation or perform tracheostomy, if intubation is not possible.
♦ Oxygen is given in high concentration.
♦ Injection adrenaline 0.5 to 1 mL of 1:1000 solution IM
♦ *Fluids:* 0.5 or 1 liter of fluid restores blood pressure but 6–9 liters is required for adequate restoration of blood volume.
♦ Hydrocortisone 300 mg IV.
♦ Aminophylline 250 mg IV in 20 mL dextrose to revert bronchospasm.
♦ Diphenhydramine 50 mg IV slowly.
♦ Dopamine, if hypotension persists.
♦ IV atropine and glucagon.
♦ Ventilatory support is necessary, if patient is critical.

Q.2. Write short note on drug interactions.

(Aug 2012, 5 Marks)

Ans. Drug interaction has been defined as action of an administered drug upon the effectiveness or toxicity of another drug administered earlier, simultaneously or later.

When two or more drugs are prescribed either simultaneously or in quick succession, they may exhibit either a synergistic or antagonistic action.

Types of Interaction

There are three types of interactions:

Pharmacokinetic Interactions

These results in alterations in delivery of drugs to their sites of action, i.e., impaired GI absorption, induction of hepatic enzymes and inhibition of cellular uptake.

Pharmacodynamic Interactions

In this, the responsiveness of the target system or organ is modified by other agents.

Pharmacodynamic and Other Interactions between Drugs

They are usually therapeutically useful interactions in which combined effect of two drugs is greater than that of the either drug.

For example: Amlodipine + Atenolol and Sulfonamides + Trimethoprim

The first two interactions are detrimental while last one is useful interaction employed in therapeutic medicine.

Q.3. Write short note on urticaria. *(Feb 2006, 3 Marks)*

Ans. Urticaria is a vascular reaction characterized by transient, evanescent, pruritic wheals occurring on any site of the body.

It is type I hypersensitivity reaction of skin to variety of exogenous or endogenous agents.

When the subcutaneous tissue involves, it is known as angiedema.

Etiology

♦ *Exogenous causes:*
  • Ingestants, i.e., drugs and foods
  • Inhalants, i.e., pollen, plant, dust, etc.
  • Injectants, i.e., penicillin, insulin, antisera, vaccines.
  • Contactants, i.e., bee sting and bug bites.
♦ *Endogenous causes:*
  • Infections, i.e., urinary tract infection, respiratory tract infection and candida infections.
  • Infestants, i.e., helminths, amoebiasis and giardiasis
  • Systemic disease, i.e., systemic lupus erythematosus and lymphomas.
  • Psychogenic, i.e., emotional stress.

Management

Histamine-mediated Urticaria

♦ *First line treatment:*
  • Loratadine 10 mg/day
  • Tricyclic anti-depressant doxepine 10 mg TDS or ranitidine 150 mg BD
♦ *Second line treatment*
  • Prednisolone 0.5 mg/kg 1 to 2 weeks.
♦ *Third line treatment:*
  • Cyclosporine A
  • IV immunoglobin
  • Plasmapheresis.

Immune Complex-mediated Urticaria

♦ Dapsone 75–100 mg/day
♦ Indomethacin 25–50 mg TDS
♦ Hydroxychloroquine 200–400 mg/day.

Q.4. Describe briefly side effects of corticosteroids.

(Sep 2008, 5 Marks)

Ans.

Side Effects

♦ In hyperglycemia they cause precipitation of diabetes and glucosuria.
♦ They cause muscular weakness.

♦ They cause thinning of skin, fragile skin and purple striae hirsutism.
♦ They cause Cushing's habitus in which there is moon face, narrow mouth and obesity of trunk with thinning of lungs.
♦ They increase susceptibility to infection, i.e., TB and opportunistic infection may flare up.
♦ They cause delayed healing of wound and surgical incisions.
♦ They causes peptic ulcer.
♦ They causes osteoporosis, glaucoma and growth retardation in children.
♦ At high doses, they causes psychiatric disturbance.
♦ They cause suppression of hypothalamopituitary axis.

Q.5. Write short note on differential diagnosis.

(Mar 2000, 5 Marks)

Ans. Identification of disease by comparison of illness that share features of present illness but differ in some critical ways is known as differential diagnosis.

It is given on the basis of determination of cause and pathogenic condition.

This is done by evaluating the history of disease process, sign and symptoms, laboratory test and special test, such as radiography and ECG.

For example of differential diagnosis, refer to Ans. 22 of chapter Diseases of Blood.

Q.6. Write short note on total parenteral nutrition.

(Mar 2000, 5 Marks)

Ans. The intravenous provision of dextrose, amino acids, fats, trace elements, vitamin and minerals to patients who are unable to assimilate adequate nutrition to mouth.

Patient with many illness become malnutritioned, if they are unable to eat a balanced diet for more than few weeks, however only a small percentage of these patients clearly benefit from parenteral nutrition support.

Patient who benefit most from total parenteral nutrition are those at extremes of nutritional deficiency.

Q.7. Write short note on leukorrhea. *(Mar 2007, 2 Marks)*

Ans. Leukorrhea is strictly defined as an excessive normal vaginal discharge.

♦ The excess secretion is evident from persistent vulval moistness or staining of undergarments or need to wear a vulval pad.
♦ It is non-purulent and non-offensive.
♦ It is non-irritant and never causes pruritus.
♦ The physiological basis involve in normal vaginal secretion in development of an endogenous estrogen level.
♦ *Excessive secretion is due to:*
  • Physiological excess: Normal secretion is expected to increase in condition when the estrogen level becomes high. The condition is during puberty, during menstrual cycle, pregnancy and during sexual excitement.
  • Cervical cause or cervical leukorrhea: Noninfective cervical lesion may produce excess secretion which produces out at vulva.
  • Vaginal cause or vaginal leukorrhea: Increase vaginal transudation during the uterine prolapse.

Treatment

♦ Improvement of general health
♦ Cervical factor requires surgical treatment, such as electrocautery, cryosurgery
♦ Pelvic lesion producing vaginal leukorrhea requires appropriate therapy for pathology.
♦ Pills users stop the pill temporarily
♦ Local hygiene is to be maintained meticulously.

Q.8. Write short note on acne vulgaris. *(Mar 2007, 2 Marks)*

Ans. Acne vulgaris is a disease in which the pilosebaceous follicle becomes oversensitive to normal levels of testosterone.

Etiology

♦ Androgens
♦ Follicular keratinization
♦ Hereditary
♦ *Propionibacterium acnes*
♦ Immunological factors
♦ Environmental factors

Exacerbating Factors

Acne worsens with stress and in premenstrual period.

In patients with aggressive or recalcitrant acne, underlying cause may be a virilizing syndrome in women, acromegaly, occupational exposure to acnegenic agents.

Drugs that worsen acne are steroids, hormones (androgen and progesterone), antiepileptic drugs, iodides; can follow facial massage.

Genetic and hormonal factors also play a role.

Grading

♦ **Mild disease:** Open (black heads) and closed (white heads) comedones with sparse inflammatory lesions. Some comedones are deep-seated (submarine comedones).
♦ **Moderate:** Numerous papules and pustules
♦ **Severe:** Polymorphic eruption with comedones, papules, pustules, nodules and cysts.

Management

♦ **Topical therapies are the mainstay of treatment for mild acne:**
  • Benzoyl peroxide 5% has antibacterial and keratolytic properties. It treats both inflamed and non-inflamed lesions.
  • Topical antibiotics, i.e., 1% clindamycin and 2% erythromycin are used.
  • Topical retinoids, i.e., tretinoin cream or gel (0.25 to 1%), Adelphane (0.1%) cream or gel or solution applied in night to entire face and leave it for 20–30 minutes and then wash off with mild soap
  • Sulfate calamine lotion can be used.
  • Salicylic acid can be used as adjunctive therapy.
  • Azelaic acid (20%) cream possess anti–microbial, anti – inflammatory and comedolytic properties.

♦ **Systemic therapy**
  • *Antibiotics:* Therapy is given for 3–6 months. Tetracycline 500 mg BD or doxycycline 100 mg BD for 2 weeks to 10 months. If tetracycline is not tolerated by the patient erythromycin 500 mg BD can be given
  • *Corticosteroids:* Prednisolone or dexamethasone once at night is useful in patients with severe acne unresponsive to conventional therapy.
  • *Other drugs:* Oral contraceptives, spironolactone, flutamide help in young women
  • *Adjunctive therapy:* Intralesional steroids for neurocystic lesions. Comedone extraction, chemical peels, dermabrasion, LASER and light therapy.

Q.9. Write short note on SLE. *(Mar 2007, 2 Marks)*

Or

Write short answer on systemic lupus erythematosus.
(Apr 2019, 3 Marks)

Ans. The full form of SLE is systemic lupus erythematosus.

It is an autoimmune disorder characterized by the destruction of tissue due to deposition of antibodies and immune complexes within it.

SLE produces lesion in the skin and oral mucous membrane and beside this it also involves certain body systems.

Clinical Features

♦ Skin lesions of SLE are characterized by the development of fixed erythematous rashes that have a butterfly configuration over the malar region and across the bridge of the nose.
♦ Skin rashes produce itching or burning sensation.
♦ Disease often causes hyperpigmentation of skin.
♦ Patchy or extensive loss of hair from the scalp is very common clinical findings.
♦ There is severe burning sensation in the oral mucosa and the affected area is extremely tendered to palpation.
♦ Formation of hemorrhagic macules in the oral mucosa that becomes frequently ulcerated.
♦ Fever, fatigue, malaise, vomiting, diarrhea and anorexia are present.
♦ Dysphagia and depression
♦ Splenomegaly and lymphadenopathy.

Treatment

Systemic steroid therapy is the treatment of choice.

Q.10. Write note on emergency drug tray.
(Mar 2000, 5 Marks)

Ans. Medical emergencies in dental practice are of common occurrence and a dental surgeon must well prepare to meet them since correct and early management cannot only prevent morbidity but also mortality in such patients.

For management of any medical emergency dental clinic must consist of emergency drug tray.

Emergency tray contains IV fluids, administration set, disposable syringe and needles, stethoscope, BP apparatus, sterilized pad must be available.

A fair amount of emergency drugs, such as the following must be readily available in the emergency drug tray.

- Inj. adrenaline
- Inj. atropine
- Inj. avil
- Inj. aminophylline
- Inj. methenamine
- Inj. dopamine
- Inj. lidocaine
- Inj. digoxin
- Inj. propranolol
- Inj. diazepam
- Inj. dilantin
- Inj. stemetil
- Inj. isoproterenol
- Inj. pethidine
- Inj. pentazocine
- Inj. morphine
- Inj. analgin
- Inj. diclofenac sodium
- Inj. dexamethasone
- Oxygen
- Capsule nifedipine
- Inj. serpasil
- Inj. glucose Or 5% dextrose saline.
- Inj. calcium carbonate
- Dextrose 50%
- Aromatic salts.

Q.11. Write short note on sepsis syndrome.

(Apr 2007, 5 Marks)

Ans. It is defined as the inflammatory response infection in which there is fever, tachycardia, tachypenia and evidence of inadequate blood flow to internal organs.

The syndrome is the common cause of death in severely-ill patients.

Etiology

- It is caused due to combined effect of virulent infection and the powerful host response to the infection.
- Infection of lungs, abdomen and urinary tract.
- Infections at other body sites.

Complications

- Shock
- Organ failure
- Disseminated intravascular coagulation
- Altered mental status
- Jaundice
- Metastatic abscess formation.

Treatment

Eradication of underlying cause of infection and support of failing organ systems.

- Maintaining an open airway.
- IV fluid is given.
- Adrenaline should be given to the patient.

- Draining or debriding abscess, if present.
- Heparin is given to lessen the risk of venous thrombosis.
- Antibiotics, such as cephalosporins or penicillin are given.

Q.12. Mention complications of drug reaction.

(Apr 2007, 5 Marks)

Ans. The term adverse drug reaction has been defined as any noxious which is suspected to be due to a drug occur at doses normally used require treatment or decrease in dose or indicates caution in future use of same drug.

Adverse effect of drug have been classified as:

- **Predictable reaction:** These are related to the pharmacological effect of a drug. They include:
  - *Side effects:* These are unwanted but often unavoidable pharmacodynamic effect that occurs at therapeutic doses.
    - A side effect may be based on the same action of the drug, for example, dryness of the mouth with atropine.
    - A side effect may be based on a different facet of action, for example estrogen causes nausea.
    - An effect may be therapeutic in one contact but side effect in another contact, for example, codeine used for cough, produces constipation as a side effect.
  - *Secondary effect:* These are indirect consequences of a primary action of a drug, for example, suppressing of bacterial flora by tetracyclines can result in super infection.
  - *Toxic effects:* These effects are result due to over dosage or prolong use of drugs, for example, comma by barbiturates, complete AV block by digoxin.
  - *Drug habituation and dependence:* Drugs capable of altering the moods and feeling, are liable to repetitive use to derive a feeling of euphoria to escape from the reality, social adjustment, etc.
  - *Drug withdrawal reaction:* Sudden withdrawal or stoppage of certain drugs can result in a type of adverse reaction, e.g., withdrawal of beta blockers can precipitate an effect of myocardial infarction.
    - Withdrawal of phenytoin can precipitate status epilepticus.
  - *Teratogenic effect:* This refers to the ability of drug to cause congenital abnormality in the fetus, when given during pregnancy, e.g., cleft palate following the use of corticosteroids.
  - *Drug-induced disease or iatrogenic diseases:* When certain drugs are used chronologically, they can produce disease, e.g., chronic use of aspirin can lead to production of peptic ulcer.
- **Unpredictable reactions:** These are based on the peculiarities of the patient and not on the drug action.
  - *Drug allergy:* It is an immunologically mediated reaction producing stereotype symptoms which are unrelated to the effect of drug or its doses, e.g., anaphylactic reactions resulting in urticaria, etching, angiedema, asthma.
  - *Photosensitivity:* It is a cutaneous reaction, resulting from drug-induced sensitization of the skin to UV radiation.

Drugs that causes such reactions are demeclocycline, chloroquine.

- *Idiosyncrasy:* It is generally determined as abnormal reactivity to a chemical. Certain adverse effects of some drugs are restricted to individuals with a particular genotype, e.g., barbiturates causes excitement and mental confusion in some person.

Q.13. Write short note on eczema.   *(Sep 2007, 2 Marks)*

Ans. Eczema is defined as an itchy red rash that initially weep or oozes serum and may become crusted, thickened or scaly.

Classification of Eczema

- Atopic
- Seborrheic
- Discoid
- Irritant
- Allergic
- Asteatotic
- Gravitational
- Lichen simplex
- Pompholyx.

Symptoms of Eczema

- *Acute symptoms:*
  - Redness and swelling with ill-defined margins.
  - Papules, vesicles and more rending large blister.
  - Exudation and cracking
  - Scaling.
- *Chronic symptoms:*
  - Less vascular and exudative lichenification, i.e., a dry lathery thickening with increased skin margins, secondary to rubbing and scratching
  - Fissures and stretch marks
  - Pigmentation change.

Diagnostic Criteria

Itchy skin and at least three of the following:

- History of itch in skin creases
- History of asthma/hay fever.
- Dry skin
- Visible flexural eczema.

Management

- *General:*
  - Explanation, reassurance and encouragement
  - Avoidance of contact with irritants
  - Regular use of greasy emollients
- *Medical:*
  - Topical steroids, i.e., prednisolone and hydrocortisone are used.
  - Topical immunosuppressants are used.
  - Blend emollients are used regularly both directly on skin and in bath.
  - Sedative antihistaminics, i.e., alimemazine tartrate or trimeprazine tartrate, if sleep is interrupted.

Q.14. Write short note on basic life support.

(Mar 2008, 2.5 Marks)

Ans. The aim of basic life support is to maintain the circulation, until more definitive treatment with advanced life support can be administered.

- The management of the collapsed patient requires prompt assessment and restoration of the airway, breathing and circulation (ABC) using basic life support, with the aim of maintaining the circulation until more definitive treatment with advanced life support can be administered.

Basic Life Support

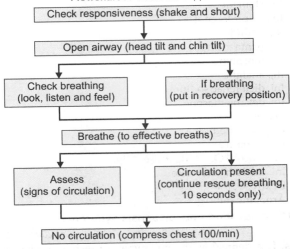

Flowchart 7: Basic life support.

Q.15. Write short note on needle stick injury.

(Mar 2008, 2.5 Marks)

Ans. Needle stick injuries are wounds caused by needles that accidentally puncture the skin.

- Needle stick injuries are a hazard for people who work with hypodermic syringes and other needle equipment.
- These injuries can occur at any time: during use, disassembling or disposal.
- Needle stick injuries transmit infectious diseases, especially blood-borne viruses.
- In recent years, concern about AIDS, hepatitis B and hepatitis C has prompted research to find out the causes of these injuries and develop measures to prevent them.
- Despite published guidelines and training program, needle stick injuries remain an ongoing problem.
- Accidental punctures by contaminated needles can inject hazardous fluids into the body through the skin. There is potential for injection of hazardous drugs, but injection of infectious fluids, especially blood, is by far the greatest concern.
- Even small amounts of infectious fluid can spread certain diseases effectively. Accidental injection of blood-borne viruses is the major hazard of needle stick injuries, especially the viruses that cause AIDS (HIV), hepatitis B and hepatitis C.

Causes

♦ *Equipment design:* Safer innovative devices using protected needle devices or needle-free systems with self-sealing ports would alleviate many of these injuries. Syringes with safety features reduce needle stick injuries.

♦ *Recapping:* Recapping can account for 25 to 30% of all needle stick injuries. Often, it is the single most common cause.

♦ *Improper disposal:* Virtually all needle stick injuries are from needles that have either been lost in the workplace or thrown into regular garbage. Janitors and garbage handlers can also experience needle stick injuries or cuts from 'sharps' when handling trash that contains needles or scalpels.

Management

♦ Stop all operative procedures.
♦ Identify and examine the wound
♦ Immediately wash but do not scrub the injury
♦ Encourage bleeding
♦ Blood specimen for both patient and health care worker is taken for specimen.

Q.16. Differentiate Type A and Type B adverse drug reaction. *(Mar 2008, 2.5 Marks)*

Ans.

Type A Adverse Drug Reaction	Type B Adverse Drug Reaction
1. These are based on pharma-cological properties of the drug	1. These are based on peculia-rities of the patient and not on drug's known action
2. It includes side effect, toxic effects and consequences of drug withdrawal	2. It includes allergy and idiosy-ncrasy
3. They are more common	3. They are less common
4. These are dose related	4. These are often non-dose related
5. Mostly these are preventable	5. Generally more serious and drug

Q.17. Describe treatment of septic shock.

(Oct 2007, 4 Marks)

Ans.

Septic Shock

This type of shock is mostly due to release of endotoxins in blood, which causes wide spread vasodilation of blood vessels resulting in fall in the cardiac output. Fall in the cardiac output is not initial feature and vasoconstriction is not observed.

Bacteria responsible for release of endotoxins are *E. coli*, *Pseudomonas proteus*, etc.

Clinical Features

♦ Restlessness, anxiety
♦ Cyanosis
♦ Cold and clammy skin

♦ Tachycardia
♦ Oliguria or anuria
♦ Acidotic breathing.

Management

♦ *Sedation with diazepam*
♦ IV fluids
♦ Blood culture and sensitivity
♦ *Antimicrobial agents:* Combination of penicillin or cephalosporins and aminoglycosides and metronidazole
♦ Injection hydrocortisone.

Q.18. Write short note on management of shock, while doing dental surgery. *(Oct 2007, 5.5 Marks)*

Ans. In such case, there following shock occurs:

Neurogenic or Vasovagal Shock

This is response to sudden fear or severe pain and the effects from slight fainting fit to death.

♦ This type of shock is also known as neurogenic or psychogenic shock.
♦ There is sudden pooling of blood in the capacitance vessels of legs and splanchnic arterial bed. This causes hypoxia of vital center.

Clinical Features

♦ History of emotional stress or pain of a sudden nature.
♦ Bradycardia or pallor.
♦ Tachypnea
♦ Fainting
♦ Reflexes are usually intact.

Management

♦ Place the patient flat or in head low position.
♦ Ensure potency of airway
♦ IV atropine may be needed for persistent or increasing bradycardia.

Hypovolemic Shock, i.e., Hemorrhagic Shock

Management

♦ Control hemorrhage.
♦ IV fluid is to restore circulating blood volume.
♦ Blood transfusion.
♦ Rising of foot end of bed.
♦ Oxygen inhalation.
♦ If acidosis develops. Sodium bicarbonate is infused till pH is normalized.
♦ Recovery is indicated by improvement in consciousness, dry and warm skin, CVP is more than 5 cm of H_2O, distended veins and increased in urinary output.

Q.19. Write short note on ACE inhibitors.

(Sep 2009, 4 Marks)

Ans. The ACE inhibitors are Captopril, Enalapril and Ramipril.

Mechanism of Action

♦ These drugs prevent conversion of angiotensin I into angiotensin II by inhibiting angiotensin-converting enzyme thus preventing action of angiotensin II, i.e., vasoconstriction and aldosterone synthesis and causes fall in BP
♦ ACE metabolizes bradykinin which is a potent vasodilator.
♦ ACE inhibitors increase bradykinin levels causing vasodilatation.

Pharmacological Actions

♦ ACE inhibitors decrease total peripheral resistance, and hence, there is decrease in systolic and diastolic blood pressure.
♦ ACE inhibitors increase blood supply to renal, cerebral and coronary arteries.
♦ ACE inhibitors causes decrease in aldosterone synthesis, and hence, there is decrease in sodium and water retention.

Adverse Effects

ACE inhibitors produce hypotension, hyperkalemia, dry persistent cough, loss of taste sensation, urticaria, angiedema, etc.

Uses

♦ *Hypertension:* ACE inhibitors are first line drugs to be used in the treatment of hypertension. They are used alone or in combination with other drugs. These drugs are more effective in renovascular hypertension.
♦ *Congestive heart failure:* ACE inhibitors decreases preload and afterload in CHF.
♦ *Diabetics:* In diabetics, renal functions are improved.
♦ *Myocardial infarction:* In myocardial infarction motility is reduced.

Q.20. Write short note on ABCD rule. *(Nov 2011, 4 Marks)*
Ans. This rule is given for diagnosis for malignant melanoma and skin cancers

♦ **A is for ASYMMETRY:** Half of a mole or birthmark does not match the other.
♦ **B is for BORDER:** The edges are irregular, ragged, notched, or blurred.
♦ **C is for COLOR:** The color is not the same all over, but may have differing shades of brown or black, sometimes with patches of red, white, or blue.
♦ **D is for DIAMETER:** The area is larger than 6 millimeters (about ¼ inch) across, or the area has been growing.

Q.21. Write short note on statins. *(Mar 2011, 4 Marks)*
Ans. They are also known as HMG-CoA reductase inhibitors.

The statins are Lovastatin, Simvastatin, Pravastatin, Atorvastatin, Rosuvastatin.

The statins are the hypolipidemic drugs.

Mechanism of Action

♦ They decrease cholesterol synthesis by inhibition of 3-hydroxy-3-methylglutaryl coenzyme A (HMG-CoA).

♦ Statins also decrease low density lipids (LDL) and triglycerides. They increases high density lipids (HDL).

Uses

♦ Used in hyperlipidemia with raised LDL and total cholesterol levels.
♦ Used in secondary hypercholesterolemia caused due to diabetes and nephritic syndrome.

Adverse Effects

♦ Headache, nausea, bowel upset and rashes
♦ Sleep disturbances
♦ Rise in serum transaminase
♦ Muscle tenderness can occur
♦ Myopathy can occur.

Q.22. Write short note on clinical uses and side effects of prednisolone. *(Mar 2011, 3 Marks)*
Ans. Prednisone is a synthetic corticosteroid drug, i.e., particularly effective as an immunosuppressant drug. It is used to treat certain inflammatory diseases (such as moderate allergic reactions) and (at higher doses) some types of cancer, but has significant adverse effects.

Clinical Uses

♦ In asthma, chronic obstructive pulmonary disease (COPD), chronic inflammatory demyelinating polyradiculoneuropathy (CIDP), rheumatic disorders, allergic disorders, ulcerative colitis and Crohn's disease, adrenocortical insufficiency, hypercalcemia due to cancer, thyroiditis, laryngitis, severe tuberculosis, urticaria (hives), lipid pneumonitis, pericarditis, multiple sclerosis, nephrotic syndrome, myasthenia gravis, and as part of a drug regimen to prevent rejection post-organ transplant.
♦ Prednisone has also been used in the treatment of migraine headaches and cluster headaches and for severe aphthous ulcer.
♦ Prednisone is used as an antitumor drug.
♦ Prednisone is important in the treatment of acute lymphoblastic leukemia, non-Hodgkin lymphomas, Hodgkin's lymphoma, multiple myeloma and other hormone-sensitive tumors, in combination with other anticancer drugs.
♦ Prednisone is also used for the treatment of the Herxheimer reaction, which is common during the treatment of syphilis, and to delay the onset of symptoms of Duchenne muscular dystrophy and also for uveitis.
♦ Prednisone also could be used in the treatment of decompensated heart failure.

Side-effects

Major

♦ Increased blood sugar for diabetics
♦ Difficulty controlling emotion
♦ Difficulty in maintaining train of thought
♦ Immunosuppression

- Weight gain
- Facial swelling
- Depression, mania, psychosis, or other psychiatric symptoms
- Unusual fatigue or weakness
- Mental confusion/indecisiveness
- Blurred vision
- Abdominal pain
- Peptic ulcer
- Infections
- Painful hips or shoulders
- Steroid-induced osteoporosis
- Stretch marks
- Osteonecrosis
- Insomnia
- Severe joint pain
- Cataracts or glaucoma
- Anxiety
- Black stool
- Stomach pain or bloating
- Severe swelling
- Mouth sores or dry mouth
- Avascular necrosis
- Hepatic steatosis.

Minor

- Nervousness
- Acne
- Skin rash
- Appetite gain
- Hyperactivity
- Increased thirst
- Frequent urination
- Diarrhea
- Reduced intestinal flora
- Leg pain/cramps
- Sensitive teeth

Q.23. Write short note on drug reactions.

(Apr 2008, 5 Marks) (June 2010, 5 Marks)
(Jan 2012, 5 Marks)

Ans. While achieving therapeutic levels drug produce unwanted side effects or toxicity. This is known as adverse drug reaction.

- Drug reactions are divided in two types, i.e., predictable reactions in the form of side effects, overdosage, toxicity and unpredictable reactions in form of idiosyncrasy and hypersensitivity reactions.
- *Following are the adverse drug reactions:*
  - Side effect: Undesirable effects which accompany therapeutic effects of drug so does not necessitate stoppage of drug, e.g., anticholinergics in treatment of peptic ulcer cause xerostomia.
  - Toxic effect: They develop when drug is used for the longer period in therapeutic doses, e.g., patient

taking isoniazid for tuberculosis develop peripheral neuropathy.

- Poisoning: It occurs when large doses of drug are consumed for prolonged periods.
- Drug intolerance: Some people are intolerant to the drug in small therapeutic doses, It is due to low threshold of the person to the drug, e.g., Chloroquine in usual doses cause nausea and vomiting while in an intolerant person it causes vomiting with single tablet.
- Idiosyncrasy: It is an abnormal reaction to any drug which occur in individuals who are genetically predisposed to it.
- Drug allergy: Allergy to any drug is independent of its dose. These reactions are based on humoral factor or cell mediated.
- Photosensitivity: Exposure of skin to ultraviolet rays of sun results in cutaneous reactions from drug induced sensitization.
- Teratogenicity: A drug is teratogenic when it harms the fetus. Such types of drugs should not be given to pregnant ladies.

Q.24. Evaluation for the case of general anesthesia.

(Nov 2008, 10 Marks)

Or

Write a short note on evaluation for the case of general anesthesia. *(Aug 2012, 5 Marks)*

Ans.

History of Patient

- Detailed history of patient is taken about any major ailment in the past and recently. Confirm the type of treatment given and if any residual effects of disease are still persisting.
- History of alcohol intake and addiction to other narcotic agents is taken.
- Some patients are allergic to certain drugs and general anesthesia. It must be thoroughly ascertained, if the person is allergic to any of these drugs.
- If a patient is chronic smoker, he/she is likely to have chronic cough and this has to be considered when giving general anesthesia.
- If there is presence of hypertension, the drugs being taken must be ascertained and recorded. Anesthetist should assess degree of hypertension and its effect on the heart as well as any interaction of the anti-hypertensive drugs with the anesthetic agents.
- If the patient is suffering from cardiac insufficiency the heart must be evaluated and certain emergency drugs must be kept at hand during operative procedure. A detailed history about all drugs the patient is on anticoagulants, digoxin, nitrates, diuretics or any other drug must be enquired and recorded.

Physical Examination

♦ A detailed general physical examination must be done preoperatively.

♦ Look for anemia and state of nutrition. Patient who is severely anemic is not fit for general anesthesia. Anemia must be corrected before. If emergency operation is to be done, blood transfusion is given.

♦ Pulse rate should be in between 60–80 beats per minute. If the pulse rate is either high or slow, cause must be found out, and if possible it should be corrected.

♦ Blood pressure must be evaluated carefully. Neither high or low blood pressure is desirable. An hypertensive must be treated before going for general anesthesia and blood pressure levels brought to normal or near normal levels. But if complications are present, such as cardiomegaly, renal or lung complications or features of left heart or congestive failure, then great caution has to be employed.

♦ Lungs are examined for evidence of chronic bronchitis with/without emphysema and other lung diseases. Look for clubbing, cyanosis and emphysema. Patient's respiratory functions must be evaluated. A chronic smoker is likely to be at disadvantage. For this breadth holding test is done. In such patients, it is desirable to institute breathing exercises for at least a week before operation and the patient is encouraged to continue with these exercises as soon as he regains consciousness. In this way, many pulmonary complications are avoided. Breathing exercises program must be carried out under the guidance of a physiotherapist with advice from the physician.

♦ Abdomen should be examined for hepatomegaly, splenomegaly, ascites and any organomegaly. Lymph glands in the body should be palpated for evidence of any disease of reticuloendothelial system.

♦ Bleeding tendencies must be looked into. History of bleed from any source after any simple injury or bruising should be considered.

♦ Oral cavity must be carefully examined, and if any loose teeth are present or if there is any great degree of sepsis these should be taken care of before operation. In patients using dentures these must be removed before administering premedication since failure to do this may choke the patient.

♦ Patient color should be carefully examined and if any signs of anemia or polycythemia are present they must be attended to.

♦ Urine should be carefully tested, and if any evidence of diabetes is present, blood sugar estimations be done. Urine be examined not only for sugar but also for albumin and ketone bodies. Diabetes must be controlled beforehand with insulin. In the presence of ketone bodies, it is usual to institute 10% glucose drip neutralizing with 25 units of soluble insulin in each bottle. This infusion is given till urine is ketone free. It is preferable in any diabetic patient who is on oral antidiabetic drugs, to switch on to soluble insulin 48 hours before operation. On the day of operation, patient is put on 5% or 10% glucose drip neutralized with soluble insulin. After operation, patient has to be continued on insulin injections till the wound has healed. This may have to be carried out for 10–14 days. Once recovery is complete and patient is ambulatory he can be switched on to oral antidiabetic drugs.

♦ If urine contains considerable amount of albumin, this indicates renal pathology and anesthetist in consultation with the physician must evaluate the risks and the type of anesthesia.

♦ Heart size must be evaluated. Position of apex beat, presence of abnormal pulsations over the precordium and cardiac murmurs must be assessed.

♦ Look for patient veins especially over the ankles and antecubital fossa. Suitable veins must be identified for intravenous purposes.

Investigations

In every patient due for general anesthesia following investigations be carried out:

♦ Hemoglobin to assess anemia.

♦ Total and differential leukocyte count.

♦ Bleeding time (BT) and clotting time (CT) for bleeding disorders.

♦ *Platelet count:* Low platelet count indicates thrombocytopenia.

♦ Complete urine examination for albumin, sugar, ketone bodies and presence of any casts and cells.

♦ Blood sugar (fasting and postprandial) to exclude diabetes.

♦ Prothrombin time for bleeding disorders.

♦ *X-ray heart (PA view) for heart size:* It shall also assess any pathology in the lungs.

♦ Electrocardiogram for any myocardial damage or insufficiency or presence of any arrhythmia.

♦ Pulmonary function tests to evaluate the lung functions.

Patient preparation before giving general anesthesia

♦ On the day of surgery, patient should be empty stomach.

♦ Little bowel enema is given to patient so that his/her bowels are empty.

♦ Breathing exercises are performed a week before.

♦ Smokers should stop smoking 2 to 3 weeks before general anesthesia for preventing pulmonary complications during and after anesthesia.

♦ Sleeping pill is given to a patient in night so that proper sleep is taken

♦ Preanesthetic medication is given which helps in induction of general anesthesia.

Q.25. Write about medical emergencies in dental practice.

Or

(Dec 2009, 10 Marks)

Write short note on medical emergencies in dental practice.

(Jun 2010, 5 Marks) (Aug 2012, 5 Marks)

Ans.

Medical Emergencies in Dental Practice

Medical emergency	Clinical features	Treatment
Syncope	• Feeling of giddiness • Weakness • Paleness and sweating	• The operator should discontinue any procedure in progress, and lower the chair back while the patients legs are slightly elevated, thus placing the patient in a semi-reclining position • This position aids venous return from the lower portions of the body while preventing venous congestion in the upper body • If the patient is conscious, then he should be instructed to take a few deep breadth • If any time a patient loses consciousness unexpectedly in the dental chair the pulse, then respiration and color should be checked • If there is any significant change in the respiratory pattern or pallor or tachycardia or bradycardia, then patients respiration should be maintained with artificial ventilation. Give supplemental oxygen • If breathing is present, take some ammonia salt solution in a cotton and hold it under the patient's nose to retrieve consciousness • Escort patient to his home
Hyperventilation	• Presence of giddiness • Presence of rapid breathing • Presence of numbness of finger and toes • Palpitations are present	• Patient is told to breathe slowly in a paper bag and rebreath the exhaled air • Above method is not for diabetics

Asthma	• Wheezing is audible
	• Extremities remain blue
	• Presence of breathlessness
		• In acute condition, i.e., pulse rate more than 110/min, respiratory rate more than 45/min, in such cases 4-metered dosage of bronchodilator is indicated
		• In life-threatening condition, following is the treatment
		  - High flow oxygen
		  - Salbutamol is given, i.e., one puff in a large volume
		  - Prednisolone 40–60 mg orally
		  - Puff is repeated in every 15 min

Angina pectoris	• Difficulty in swallowing • Pulse is bounding • Presence of moderate-to-severe crushing chest pain which radiates to left arm	• Stop dental treatment • Sublingual glyceryl trinitrate Tablet ie 0.6 mg is given • Repeat same dosage in 5 min after checking blood pressure • Repeat again after 5 min, if pain continues • If improvement is not present after 15 min, condition now is treated as acute myocardial infarction
Acute myocardial infarction	• Presence of moderate-to-severe crushing chest pain which radiates to left arm which is not relieved after taking glyceryl trinitrate	• Ambulance should be called • 100% oxygen is given • Tab Aspirin 300 mg is given in dissolved form and one glyceryl trinitrate dosage repeat another in 5 min • Opioids are given for controlling of pain
Cardiac arrest	• Presence of sudden unconsciousness • Breathing is not present • Nonpalpable to irregular pulse	• Ambulance should be called • Cardiopulmonary resuscitation initiated • Oxygen is given • Early defibrillation is done • Medical management is started with appropriate drugs
Epilepsy	• Presence of sudden unconsciousness • Presence of apnea and cyanosis • Involuntary movement of body	• Remove all the dental equipments from the mouth as well as remove all the equipment surrounding the patient • Tight clothing should be loosened • Restraining of patient should be avoided • Patient should be turned in stable lateral position after the attack is stopped • Clear airway is maintained • Aspiration is avoided

Contd…

Contd…

Medical emergency	Clinical features	Treatment
Hypoglycemia	• Patient is confused • Behavior is altered • Speech is slurred • Patient has features of sweating, hunger, tremor, drowsiness • Loss of consciousness • There is rapid fall in blood pressure if treatment is not done	• Administer glucose • In cases with loss of consciousness, glucose or glucagon is given parenterally
Hyperglycemia	• Presence of polydipsia and polyuria • Patient is dehydrated • Reduction in the conscious level and patient may undergo comma and urinary cessation	• Ambulance should be called • Hydrate the patient
Adrenal crisis	• Presence of sudden loss of consciousness • Impalpable pulse is present • There is rapid fall in blood pressure	• Patient should be kept in supine position with raised legs • Airways should be cleared and oxygen is given • Ambulance is called • IV hydrocortisone is given

Anaphylaxis	• Patient has sneezing and breathlessness
	• Presence of circulatory collapse and cardiac arrest
		• Adrenaline hydrochloride inj (1:1000) 0.3 and 0.5 mg SC/IM
		• IV fluids to correct hypotension
		• Glucocorticoids: Hydrocortisone hemisuccinate 100 mg IV
		• Antihistaminic drugs: Chlorpheniramine 10–20 mg slow IV it is given after adrenaline
		• Bronchodilators:
		  - Salbutamol or IV aminophylline is given in patients with bronchospasm
		  - Supportive therapy with oxygen or assisted ventilation

Q.26. Write short note on anaphylactic shock with diagnosis and management. *(Jan 2012, 5 Marks)*

Ans. Anaphylaxis is defined as a state of rapid developing immune response to an antigen mediated by IgE antibodies.

Diagnosis

Diagnosis is based on physical examination and investigations.

Physical Examination

♦ Presence of immediate respiration difficulty, laryngeal edema with stridor and wheeze is audible.
♦ Wheal and erythematous lesions are seen which are circumscribed, round, discrete, erythematous areas with irregular borders and blanched centers.
♦ Lesions are very pruritic.

Investigations

♦ *Skin-Prick test:* When an allergen is injected into the skin and is observed for the development of wheal and induration within 15 minutes. There is a good correlation between diameter of wheal and levels of specific IgE antibodies in serum.
♦ In vitro radioallergosorbent test (RAST) is done to detect allergen specific IgE for a variety of food, insect bites/stings, venom, latex and some drugs.
♦ Serum tryptase levels are done for detection of recent anaphylaxis.

Management

Refer to Ans. 1 of same chapter.

Q.27. Discuss the clinical presentation and management of anaphylactic shock. *(Aug 2012, 12 Marks)*

Ans.

Clinical Presentation

♦ Onset may be instantaneous or within a few minutes after the IV injection and 30 minutes after exposure.
♦ Cardiovascular: Tachycardia, arrhythmia, hypotension and circulatory collapse.
♦ Respiratory: Laryngeal obstruction, angiedema, bronchospasm or pulmonary edema may occur singly or in combination.
♦ Nervous: Syncope and seizures.
♦ GIT: Diaphoresis, abdominal pain and diarrhea may occur.
♦ Skin: Wheel and erythematous lesions are seen which are circumscribed, round, discrete, erythematous areas with irregular borders and blanched centers.
♦ Lesions are very pruritic.
♦ If not treated death may occur.

Management

Refer to Ans. 1 of same chapter.

Q.28. Write short note on aspirin. *(Feb 2013, 5 Marks)*

Ans. Chemical name of aspirin is acetyl salicylic acid.

Pharmacological Action

- It decreases the temperature by bringing temperature regulating center to normal when it becomes deranged.
- Aspirin block pain center in thalamus. It also inhibits synthesis of prostaglandins and prevent sensation of pain receptors to histamine, bradykinin and 5 hydroxytryptamine, mediators of pain and inflammation.
- Aspirin inhibits platelet aggregation by inhibiting ADP release from platelets and inhibiting the synthesis of prostaglandin, endoperoxidase and thromboxane A2.

Indications

- It acts as keratolytic, fungistatic and mild antiseptic.
- As analgesic, antipyretic and antirheumatic.
- It prevents platelet aggregation.

Side Effects

- Nausea and vomiting
- Increases prothrombin time.

- Fatty infiltration of liver and kidney.
- *Salicylism:* Headache, dizziness, vertigo, tinnitus, diminished hearing and vision.
- It causes respiratory depression.

Q.29. Write about:　　　　　　*(Apr 2015, 2+2+2+2+2 Marks)*
　　　a. **What is anaphylaxis**
　　　b. **Write etiology**
　　　c. **Causes**
　　　d. **Symptoms and Signs**
　　　e. **Treatment**

Ans.

a. Anaphylaxis is defined as state of rapid developing immune response to an antigen mediated by IgE antibodies.

b. *Etiology: For details refer to Ans. 1 of same chapter.*

c. *Causes: For details refer to Ans. 1 of same chapter.*

d. *Symptoms and signs: For details refer to Ans. 1 of same chapter.*

e. *Treatment: For details refer to Ans. 1 of same chapter.*

Q.30. Tabulate the differences, clinical features and management of anaphylactic shock and vagal shock.

(June 2015, 12 Marks)

Ans. Tabulation of differences between anaphylactic shock and vagal shock.

Sign and symptoms	Anaphylactic shock	Vagal shock
Interval (after injection)	Sometimes before, usually after a few seconds to a few minutes after the injection	Within 30 minutes after injection; the most severe reactions begin with the first 15 minutes
Consciousness	Fainting sensation, dizziness, loss of consciousness	Anxiety, which may progress to unconsciousness in severe cases
Breathing	Slow, with a few seconds of apnea in some cases	Respiratory difficulties; coughing, sneezing, wheezing, stridor
Pulse	Slow and weak, but regular	Rapid, weak and irregular
Skin	Diaphoresis, clammy skin, pallor	• Warm skin, progressing to clammy and pallor • Pruritis and urticaria • Swelling of face and tongue
Blood pressure	Hypotension	Hypotension (systolic pressure <90 mm Hg), which may progress to cardiovascular collapse
Gastrointestinal system	Nausea and vomiting	Nausea, vomiting, abdominal pains, diarrhea
Management	**Anaphylactic shock**	**Vagal shock**
	• Airways: Intubation or perform tracheostomy if intubation is not possible • Oxygen is given in high concentration • Injection adrenaline 0.5 to 1 mL of 1:1000 solution IM • Fluids: 0.5 or 1 L of fluid restores blood pressure but 6–9 L is required for adequate restoration of blood volume. • Hydrocortisone 300 mg IV • Aminophylline 250 mg IV in 20 mL dextrose to reveal broncheospasm • Diphenhydramine 50 mg IV slowly • Dopamine, if hypotension persists • IV atropine and glucagon • Ventilatory support is necessary, if patient is critical	• Place patient in a recumbent position and elevate legs above head • Ventilate the room well • Place cold, damp cloth on face • Give reassurance

Q.31. **Write down and discuss six common comorbid diseases where you should take medical consultation before dental extraction.** *(June 2015, 12 Marks)*

Ans. Comorbidity is the presence of one or more additional disorders or diseases co-occurring with a primary disease or disorder; or the effect of such additional disorders or diseases. The additional disorder may also be a behavioral or mental disorder.

Following are the six comorbid diseases for which one should take medical consultation before dental extraction:

1. Diabetes mellitus
2. Seizure
3. AIDS
4. Cardiovascular risks
5. Respiratory disorders
6. Blood dyscrasias.

Diabetes Mellitus

There are three types of diabetes: Type I is considered insulin dependent, 5–10% of cases; Type II is when the body does not produce enough insulin and, therefore diet and medication may be regulated; Gestational diabetes occurs during pregnancy and is reversed after delivery. If the patient indicates that they have diabetes, the type must be noted in the history.

Patients with uncontrolled diabetes have low resistance to infection and are prone to periodontal disease. They have poor healing response, including excessive bleeding, and may experience hypoglycemia or hyperglycemia during dental treatment. Patients who are undiagnosed diabetics may report the following symptoms: excessive thirst and hunger, increased urination, and higher birth weights in babies.

When reviewing a health history, the following questions should be asked of diabetic patients:

♦ Is your diabetes well controlled?
♦ When is the last time your blood glucose was checked?
♦ Are you currently taking oral anti-diabetic medications or insulin injections?
♦ When was the last time you ate?
♦ Did you take your medication on time today?

It is advisable to keep sources of sugar on hand for hyper or hypoglycemic episodes. Glucose gel from a pharmacy, granulated sugar packets, honey packets, or tubes of cake icing can be easily stored and used in the case of an emergency.

When questioning diabetic patients before treatment and you find out they have not eaten or taken their insulin, their appointment should be rescheduled. Make sure they understand the importance of these steps to maintain a normal blood sugar level during dental treatment. After approximately 8 hours of fasting, an average range is between 70–99 mg/dL. If they have eaten an average level should be less that 140 mg/DL. A strategy for making a dental appointment for a diabetic patient is to keep it short and in the early to mid-morning hours when sugar levels are more stable.

Seizure

Seizure disorder is caused by an electrical disturbance in the brain. Any person can experience a seizure in a stressful situation and approximately half of all seizures are considered idiopathic. Epilepsy is a condition commonly associated with a syndrome of associated seizure types.

When a known epileptic patient is scheduled for treatment, the dental team should determine, if the patient has taken his/her antiseizure medication. These patients should be scheduled for short appointments, when they are well rested. Patients often report an aura before experiencing a seizure. This aura can be a sound, feeling, or smell. Shining a bright light in the patient's eyes should be avoided, since this has been known to trigger a seizure.

Patients who are taking oral anticonvulsant medications, such as Dilantin, Zarontin, or Depacon, may experience gingival hyperplasia. Emphasis must be placed on meticulous home care to prevent serious periodontal problems and the increased need for regular dental visits.

Cardiovascular Risks

Patients who state that they have experienced chest pain, shortness of breath, pain that radiates down their neck or arm, have swollen ankles, and/or have high blood pressure are at risk for cardiovascular disease. They may or may not have been diagnosed by a physician. If this patient also indicates that they are a smoker and/or are overweight, the risk is increased. It is recommended that a medical consultation or evaluation be obtained for all patients who indicate some type of cardiovascular disease on their health histories. Additionally, medical consultations should also be obtained for patients who are reporting or exhibiting symptoms of cardiovascular disease, but have not had a definitive diagnosis. Preventing medical crises during dental treatment is the best method of protecting patients who are medically compromised.

Rheumatic heart disease is a result of rheumatic fever and can cause deformities in the heart valves. Some patients will report taking antibiotics on a regular basis, although this is not a required practice. If the patient reports a history of rheumatic fever, the dental practice must consult with the patient's physician to determine the extent of the heart involvement. This assessment will determine the need for antibiotic prophylaxis.

Congenital heart defects place the patient at high risk for bacterial endocarditis. Again, a statement from a physician is advisable to determine the type of defect and to verify the need for prophylactic antibiotics.

Coronary artery disease results from atherosclerosis. Patients may report having been diagnosed with angina pectoris, or having chest pain after some type of physical activity or stress. These patients may be taking several medications, particularly vasodilators, such as nitroglycerin; or beta-blockers, such as propranolol. The stress of a dental visit may cause an angina attack, therefore it is important to minimize patient stress, maximize patient comfort and make certain that the patient has his/her medications available, particularly nitroglycerin. In addition, it is recommended that local anesthetic without epinephrine or other vasoconstrictors be used for these patients, to avoid further constriction of the blood vessels. Patients with unstable or uncontrolled angina should wait for at least 30 days after their angina is stabilized to receive dental treatment.

Myocardial infarction is more commonly known as a heart attack. Patients who have experienced a recent myocardial infarction should not receive any dental treatment for a minimum of 6 months after the heart attack. Most fatalities from myocardial infarction occur within 3–4 months after the attack. Stressful situations, like dental treatment can cause a rupture in the area of infarct, leading to further health problems and possible death.

Hypertension is a common condition characterized by high blood pressure. Patients with uncontrolled hypertension are at risk for a stroke, kidney failure, or heart attack. Since stress will increase blood pressure, dental treatment is contraindicated in patients with severe hypertension. Patients presenting with a systolic pressure between 120–139 mm Hg should be advised to monitor their readings for improvement and see their physician for assessment. As a rule, patients with a systolic pressure greater than 160 mm Hg and/or a diastolic pressure greater than 95 mm Hg should be referred for medical consultation and treatment, dental treatment should be delayed.

It is relatively common for patients to have undiagnosed hypertension, making it very important for the dental team to monitor patient's vital signs during their dental visits. A patient who reports having frequent dizziness, nosebleeds, or headaches may have high blood pressure and may be in need of medical intervention with antihypertensive drugs and/or diuretics.

Heart failure was more commonly known as "congestive heart failure" but the American Heart Association has recently renamed and shortened the title to characterize a broader spectrum of the disease. Depending on the type of heart failure, patients will typically have swollen ankles and shortness of breath, due to poor circulation and fluids backing up in the lungs. These patients may indicate that they must sleep upright or with several pillows. In these cases, placing them in a supine position for dental treatment may cause them acute distress. Heart failure patients are usually taking one or more diuretic medications to remove fluid. Supplemental oxygen may be needed for these patients and use of nitrous oxide analgesia is contraindicated.

Respiratory Disorders

Asthma is a chronic respiratory disorder that results in a narrowing of airways. An asthma attack can be triggered in several ways including environmental allergens, medications, or exercise. Patients with asthma may be prone to an attack or episode brought on by the stress of dental treatment, or exposure to an allergen-like latex. The patient must always be instructed to bring his/her medication/inhaler to each appointment. When the health history is reviewed at the beginning of treatment, the patient should be able to produce the medication or inhaler just in case it is needed.

Chronic Obstructive Pulmonary Disease (COPD)

The two most common forms of COPD are emphysema and chronic bronchitis. Emphysema is the irreversible enlargement of the air sacs in the lungs making it hard to expel all oxygen during breathing. Chronic bronchitis is characterized as the irreversible condition of narrowed airways. Like patients with heart failure, those with either of these types of COPD may not be able to breathe easily in a supine position or after walking certain distances. Due to prolonged steroid use to treat COPD, these patients may have *Candida* infections. Before dental extraction medical consultation of such patients is necessary.

Tuberculosis (TB) is a bacterial infection that occurs primarily in the lungs, but can occur in other organ systems in the body. It is spread through airborne particles, when an infectious patient coughs, sneezes, talks, or sings. TB is most easily spread in small confined spaces where infectious people share the same airspace with others. Because TB is highly infectious and its airborne transmission is difficult to control, CDC has issued specific guidelines to help protect healthcare workers when treating patients.

In the case of TB, these guidelines state that elective, (non-emergency) dental treatment should be postponed for patients who have or are suspected of having an active, infectious TB case. If these patients can be referred for treatment in a facility that is specifically designed to treat TB patients (e.g. a hospital setting), it is acceptable for the dental practice to make this referral and not be liable for discriminatory practices.

In addition to asking patients on their health history if they have had TB, the patients should also be asked if they have experienced any of the following symptoms: night sweats, unexplained fever, weight loss, or a prolonged or bloody cough. If a patient has experienced any of these symptoms, refer them to a physician for evaluation before proceeding with anything but emergency palliative treatment.

If emergency treatment must be performed on a patient suspected of having infectious TB, the following precautions should be taken:

- Schedule the patient at the end of the day, as the last patient treated.
- All team members present in the treatment room must wear a HEPA or NIOSH N95 mask.
- High volume evacuation and dental dam isolation must be used to reduce aerosols.

AIDS

AIDS is a viral infection that impairs a patient's immune system, making the patient highly susceptible to other infectious diseases. It is transmitted through blood and other body fluids, which puts dental healthcare workers at some risk of infection from treating patients. Again, the practice of standard precautions must be followed, since many patients will not disclose their HIV positive status for fear of humiliation or rejection. Remember that information about a patient's HIV positive status is highly sensitive and must be protected. The dental team must take every precaution to protect the confidentiality of that patient's health history.

Although some dental health care workers are fearful of treating AIDS patients, it is illegal not to accept them into a dental practice or to refer them to another practice, unless the type of treatment is not performed in that practice. For example, if a general dental practice does not perform periodontal surgeries, it is legal to refer HIV positive or AIDS patients to a periodontist, since non-HIV or non-AIDS patients are referred as well. However, if only the HIV positive or AIDS patients are referred for periodontal surgery, this would be considered discriminatory.

When treating patients with full blown AIDS, who are typically immunosuppressed, the dental team should take extra precautions to protect the patient from opportunistic infections. These may include wearing sterile surgical gloves rather than non-sterile exam gloves, having the patient use a pre-treatment rinse of chlorhexidine gluconate or other mouthwash to prevent bacteremia, and using only sterile water for irrigation rather than from the air/water syringe, which may contain some bacterial contamination.

Blood Dyscrasias

Anemia is a deficiency of red blood cells, caused by vitamin or iron deficiency or bone marrow problems. An anemic patient may have problems with slow wound healing and excessive bleeding. They may report feeling weak and fatigued, and may appear very pale. If a patient exhibits these symptoms a medical evaluation should be recommended before dental extraction.

Leukemia is a type of blood cancer, where there is an overgrowth of white blood cells. These white blood cells may displace red blood cells, used to transport oxygen in the blood. These patients may exhibit oral signs, often before other symptoms of their disease. These signs typically include excessive gingival irritation in the absence of other causative agents, such as heavy plaque or calculus.

Patients with leukemia are very prone to infections, including periodontal infections. In addition, the chemotherapeutic agents used to treat the disease have many side effects, most notably xerostomia (dry mouth). Consult the treating physician before proceeding with dental treatment.

Hemorrhagic disorders are ailments in which patients experience excessive bleeding, due to a deficiency of clotting factors in their blood. Common bleeding disorders are hemophilia A and B, factor II, V, VII, X, XII, and von Willebrand's disease. A patient with one of these disorders will bruise very easily, may experience spontaneous, excessive bleeding, including unprovoked epistaxis (bleeding from the nose).

Dental treatment, such as extractions, that may cause bleeding can be risky for these patients. Close monitoring by the physician is necessary before dental extraction. Extraction should be confined to specific areas (e.g. one tooth or quadrant at a time) and transfusion with clotting factors may be necessary prior to treatment. Aspirin must never be prescribed for pain control for these patients, since, it is a natural blood thinner and increases bleeding.

Q.32. Write short answer on shock.

(Feb 2019, 3 Marks) (Apr 2018, 3 Marks)

Ans. Shock is defined as an acute clinical syndrome characterized by a significant, systemic reduction in tissue perfusion, resulting in decreased tissue oxygen delivery and insufficient removal of cellular metabolic products, resulting in tissue injury and severe dysfunction of vital organs.

It can occur either because the function of the heart itself is impaired, or because heart is inadequately filled.

Classification of Shock

Following is the classification of shock:
- Hypovolemic shock
- Cardiogenic shock
- *Distributive shock:*
  - Septic shock
  - Anaphylactic shock
  - Neurogenic shock
- Obstructive shock.

Clinical features
- Cold clammy skin, profuse sweating
- Hypotension (systolic BP <100 mm Hg)
- Tachycardia with thready pulse
- Rapid, shallow respiration
- Restlessness, drowsiness, confusion
- Oliguria, may progress to anuria
- Jugular venous pressure elevated in cardiogenic shock, reduced in hypovolemic and anaphylactic shock, variable in septic shock
- Multiorgan failure

Stages of Shock

Stage 1: Stage of compensatory shock—by neuroendocrine response to maintain the perfusion of the vital organs like brain, heart, kidney, liver.

Stage 2: Stage of decompensatory shock—where there is progressive shock causing persistent shock with severe hypotension (with mean arterial pressure <65 mm Hg); oliguria, tachycardia.

Stage 3: Stage of irreversible shock—with severe hypoxia and multiorgan dysfunction syndrome (MODS).

Causes of Shock

Hypovolemic shock
- *Due to reduction in total blood volume. It may be due to:*
  - Hemorrhage:
    - External from wounds, open fractures
    - Internal from injury to spleen, liver, mesentery or pelvis.

- Severe burns, which results in loss of plasma
- Peritonitis, intestinal obstruction
- Vomiting and diarrhea of any cause
♦ *Cardiac causes:*
  - Acute myocardial infarction, acute carditis
  - Acute pulmonary embolism wherein embolus blocks the pulmonary artery at bifurcation or one of the major branches
  - Drug induced
  - Toxemia of any causes
  - Cardiac surgical conditions, such as valvular diseases, congenital heart diseases
  - Cardiac compression causes:
    - Cardiac tamponade due to collection of blood, pus, fluid in the pericardial space which prevents the heart to expand leading to shock.
    - Trauma to heart.
♦ *Septic shock*—is due to bacterial infections which release toxins leading to shock.
♦ *Neurogenic shock*—due to sudden anxious or painful stimuli causing severe splanchnic vessel vasodilatation. Here patient either goes for cardiac arrest and dies or recovers fully spontaneously—spinal cord injury/anesthesia can cause neurogenic shock.
♦ *Anaphylactic shock*—is due to type I hypersensitivity reaction
♦ *Respiratory causes:*
  - Atelectasis (collapse) of lung
  - Thoracic injuries
  - Tension pneumothorax
  - Anesthetic complications.
♦ *Other causes:*
  - Acute adrenal insufficiency (Addison's disease)
  - Myxedema

Investigations and Monitoring of Shock

♦ Regular monitoring with blood pressure, pulse, heart rate, respiratory rate, urine output measurement (hourly) should be done. Urine output should be more than 0.5 mL/kg/h. Pulse oximetry should be used.
♦ Central venous pressure (CVP), pulmonary capillary wedge pressure (PCWP—an accurate assessment of left ventricular/ function) monitoring should be done. ICU care is needed during monitor period. But both CVP and PCWP are not accurate method of assessing tissue perfusion.
♦ Complete blood count, ESR, pH assessment, serum electrolyte estimation, chest X-ray (to rule out acute respiratory distress syndrome/pulmonary problems).
♦ Pus/urine/blood/bile/sputum cultures depending on the focus and need in sepsis.
♦ Serum lactate estimation is an important prognostic factor. Level >2 mEq/L suggest tissue ischemia.
♦ USG of a part, CT/MRI of the location of pathology of standard focus should be done; often may require repetition of these imaging to assess progress.
♦ Blood urea, serum creatinine, liver function tests, prothrombin time (PT), activated partial thromboplastin time (APTT), ECG monitoring are also should be done.

♦ All these tests including platelet count and arterial blood gas (ABG) should be repeated at regular intervals.

Treatment of Shock

♦ Treat the cause, e.g., arrest hemorrhage, drain pus.
♦ Fluid replacement: Plasma, normal saline, dextrose, Ringer's lactate, plasma expander (haemaccel). Dosage is maximum l liter can be given in 24 hours. Initially crystalloids then colloids are given. Blood transfusion is done whenever required.
♦ Ionotropic agents: Dopamine, dobutamine, adrenaline infusions—mainly in distributive shock like septic shock.
♦ Correction of acid-base balance: Acidosis is corrected by using 8.4% sodium bicarbonate intravenously.
♦ Steroid is often lifesaving. 500–1000 mg of hydrocortisone can be given. It improves the perfusion, reduces the capillary leakage and systemic inflammatory effects.
♦ Antibiotics in patients with sepsis; proper control of blood sugar and ketosis in diabetic patients.
♦ Catheterization to measure urine output (30–50 mL/h or >0.5 mL/kg/h should be maintained).
♦ Nasal oxygen to improve oxygenation or ventilator support with intensive care unit monitoring has to be done.
♦ Central venous pressure line to perfuse adequately and to monitor fluid balance. Total parenteral nutrition is given when required.
♦ Pulmonary capillary wedge pressure to monitor very critical patient.
♦ Hemodialysis may be necessary when kidneys are not functioning.
♦ Control pain—using morphine (4 mg IV).
♦ Ventilator and ICU/critical care management.
♦ Injection ranitidine IV or omeprazole IV or pantoprazole IV.
♦ Activated protein even though costly is beneficial as it prevents the release and action of inflammatory response.
♦ MAST(Military Anti-shock Trouser) provides circumferential external pressure of 40 mm Hg. lt is wrapped around lower limbs and abdomen, and inflated with required pressure. It redistributes the existing blood and fluid towards center. It should be deflated carefully and gradually.

Q.33. Write short answer on cardiogenic shock.

(Apr 2019, 3 Marks)

Ans. Cardiogenic shock is an acute circulatory failure with the raised central venous pressure.

Occurrence of cardiogenic shock is due to cardiac conditions where left side or right side of heart or pulmonary circulation is involved.

It occurs due to acute myocardial infarction, acute massive pulmonary embolism, massive pericardial effusion, valvular heart disease and sometime dissecting aneurysm of aorta.

Etiopathogenesis

♦ **Acute myocardial infarction:** It leads to circulatory failure and shock is obvious from ECG, occasionally ECG changes in ischemia due to circulatory failure from pulmonary embolism can produce confusion. Circulatory failure because of myocardial infarction is associated with acute pulmonary edema, so signs of pulmonary edema help in establishing the diagnosis and exclude pulmonary embolism which causes right heart failure.

- **Massive pericardial effusion:** It causes cardiac tamponade and acute circulatory failure is characterized by raised jugular venous pressure, pulsus paradoxus, oliguria, hepatomegaly with sign and symptoms of circulatory failure. Due to effusion heart sounds are not audible. Echocardiogram confirms the diagnosis and indicates the best site for paracentesis.
- **Progressive acute fulminant myocarditis:** It is either viral or because of acute rheumatic fever, it is also sometimes present as an acute circulatory failure. Chest X-ray shows cardiomegaly. ECG changes consist of conduction changes and ST–T changes or arrhythmia.
- **Acute valvular diseases:** They can lead to circulatory failure by leading to pulmonary edema.
- **Acute pulmonary embolism:** It is a sequel to leg vein or the pelvic vein thrombosis. ECG reveals acute right ventricular hypertrophy and the strain. Echocardiography will reveal dilated right ventricle and often small forceful contracting left ventricle.
- **Dissecting aneurysm of aorta:** It produces acute pain between two shoulder blades. There can be an early diastolic murmur because due to aortic regurgitation and pulses of both extremities of unequal volume.

Clinical Features

- Features of acute circulatory failure are apprehension, sweating, altered sensorium, hypotension, oliguria.
- Presence of raised jugular venous pressure.

- Evidence of pulmonary edema with respiratory compromise in setting of left heart failure.
- Physical signs are tachycardia, tachypnea, Cheyne–Stokes respiration.

Diagnosis

- Examination of cardiovascular system shows quite heart, feeble heart sounds, S3 gallop and murmurs depending on cause.
- Rales and crackles are audible because of pulmonary edema.

Treatment

- Patient should be shifted to ICU.
- Monitor ECG, CVP and blood gases
- For relief of pain and to allay anxiety, give morphine or pethidine.
- Oxygen inhalation is given to combat hypoxemia.
- Vasopressors: Dobutamine 2 to 10 µg/kg/min infusion in combination with dopamine from 2 to 5 µg/kg/min.
- Intra-aortic balloon counterpulsations together with a sympathomimetic amine, i.e., dobutamine may be used but left ventricular filling pressure should be kept below 20 mm Hg.
- In cardiogenic shock, fluid therapy should be given slowly under the guidance of pulmonary capillary wedge pressure and left atrial pressure. Swan–Ganz catheter is best means for continuous monitoring ventricular filling pressure. CVP is measured initially. If CVP is >6 mm Hg, 100 mL of fluid should be given. If CVP is <6 mm Hg, 250 mL of fluid should be given. Further IV fluid therapy is given slowly keeping CVP below 10 mm of Hg.

MULTIPLE CHOICE QUESTIONS

As per DCI and Examination Papers of Various Universities

1 Mark Each

1. Migraine is precipitated by:
   a. Bacteria
   b. Fungus
   c. Flash of light

2. Drug of choice in *P. falciparum* malaria is:
   a. Choloroquine
   b. Primaquine
   c. Artemether

3. Deficiency of vitamin D causes:
   a. Increased thickness of bones
   b. Osteoporosis
   c. Diarrhea

4. Lymphoma is type of:
   a. Disease of lymphatic vessels
   b. Disease of lymph nodes and spleen
   c. Causes increased neutrophils

5. Factor VIII deficiency causes:
   a. Anemia
   b. Hemophilia
   c. Clotting disorder

6. In acute nephritis urine contains:
   a. RBCs
   b. Factor VIII
   c. None of A and B

7. Vitamin B12 is:
   a. Fat soluble
   b. Water soluble
   c. None of a and b

8. Chronic hepatitis is caused by:
   a. Hepatitis B virus
   b. Hepatitis C virus
   c. Both of a and b

9. Vitamin K helps:
   a. To stop bleeding
   b. To stop clotting
   c. None of a and b

10. Mumps is caused by:
    a. Bacteria
    b. Virus
    c. Parasite

11. Which valve is least affected in rheumatic fever?
    a. Mitral valve
    b. Aortic valve
    c. Pulmonary valve
    d. Tricuspid valve

12. True about autonomic neuropathy are all, *except*:
    a. Resting tachycardia
    b. Silent MI
    c. Orthostatic hypotension
    d. Bradycardia

13. Man takes peanut and develops stridor neck swelling, tongue swelling and hoarseness of voice, most probable diagnosis is:
    a. Foreign body bronchus
    b. Parapharyngeal abscess
    c. Foreign body larynx
    d. Angioneurotic edema

14. The amino acid associated with atherosclerosis:
    a. Lysine
    b. Cystein
    c. Homocysteine
    d. Alanine

15. A 45-year-old female patient suffering from T2DM with hypertension, which of the following anti-hypertensive should not be used?
    a. Lisinopril
    b. Losartan
    c. Thiazide
    d. Trandolapril

16. In stable angina;
    a. CK-MB is elevated
    b. Troponin T and I is elevated
    c. All is elevated
    d. Nothing is elevated

17. An obese patient is presented in causality in an unconscious state. His blood sugar is 400 mg% urine tested positive for sugar and ketone bodies. Drug most useful in management is:
    a. Glibenclamide
    b. Pioglitazone
    c. Miglitol
    d. Insulin

Answers:
1. c. Flash of light
2. c. Artemether
3. b. Osteoporosis
4. b. Disease of lymph...
5. b. Hemophilia
6. a. RBCs
7. b. Water soluble
8. c. Both of a and b
9. b. To stop clotting
10. b. Virus
11. c. Pulmonary valve
12. d. Bradycardia
13. d. Angioneurotic...
14. c. Homocysteine
15. a. Lisinopril
16. d. Nothing is elevated
17. a. Glibenclamide

18. All are features of Cushing syndrome, *except*:
    a. Central obesity
    b. Glucose intolerance
    c. Episodic hypertension
    d. Easy bruising

19. The best marker to diagnose thyroid-related disorder is:
    a. T3
    b. T4
    c. TSH
    d. Thyroglobin

20. A 5-year-old girl always have to wear worn socks even is summer season, on physical examination it was noticed that she had high blood pressure and her femorals are weak as compared to radials and carotid pulse. Chest X-ray showed remarkable notching of ribs along with lower borders. This was due to:
    a. Femoral artery thrombosis
    b. Reynaud's disease
    c. Coarctation of aorta
    d. Takayasu's arteritis

21. The most important diagnostic method for enteric fever is:
    a. Widal test
    b. Blood culture
    c. X-ray abdomen
    d. Ultrasonography of abdomen

22. Peptic ulceration is strongly associated with:
    a. Family history
    b. Irregular dietary habits
    c. Hurry, worry and curry
    d. *Helicobacter pylori* infection

23. All the following can cause acute gastritis, *except*:
    a. Antihypertensives
    b. Nonsteroidal anti-inflammatory drugs
    c. Salicylates
    d. Corticosteroids

24. Palatal palsy is a complication of:
    a. Syphilis
    b. Rubella
    c. Diphtheria
    d. Mumps

25. All are clinical features of cirrhosis of liver, except:
    a. Increased libido
    b. Ascites
    c. Jaundice
    d. Palmar erythema

26. Which of the following is not characteristic of congenital syphilis?
    a. Interstitial keratitis
    b. Mulberry molars
    c. Notched incisors
    d. Ghon's complex

27. Macrocytic anemia is due to deficiency of:
    a. B1
    b. B2
    c. B6
    d. B12

28. The Best test for assessment of iron status is:
    a. Transferrin
    b. Plasma ferritin
    c. Serum iron
    d. Hemoglobin

29. Thiamin deficiency causes:
    a. Ophthalmoplegia
    b. Cardiomyopathy
    c. Peripheral neuropathy
    d. All the above

30. "CD4 count" term is used with which disease:
    a. Hepatitis B
    b. AIDS
    c. Pernicious anemia
    d. Falciparum malaria.

31. Which of the following drug is used in the treatment of hyperkalemia in acute renal failure?
    a. Amlodipine
    b. Captopril
    c. Insulin
    d. Atenolol

32. A boy presents with headache, vomiting, fever, neck stiffness the most important investigation is:
    a. Complete blood counts
    b. X-ray skull
    c. CSF Examination
    d. MRI Brain

33. In cardiology department, RMO makes a diagnosis of mitral stenosis. The most important sign on which diagnosis is based is:
    a. Ejection systolic murmur
    b. Mid diastolic murmur
    c. Pansystolic murmur
    d. Third heart sound

Answers:

18. c. Episodic...	19. c. TSH	20. c. Coarctation of aorta	21. a. Widal test
22. d. *Helicobacter...*	23. d. Corticosteroids	24. c. Diphtheria	25. a. Increased libido
26. d. Ghon's complex	27. d. B12	28. a. Transferrin	29. d. All the above
30. b. AIDS	31. c. Insulin	32. c. CSF examination	33. b. Mid diastolic...

34. A 15-year-old boy who is IDDM presents with pain in abdomen, vomiting and shortness of breath. He also gives history of fever and sore throat two days back. The most likely cause of his symptoms:
    a. Renal failure
    b. Gastritis
    c. Diabetic ketoacidosis
    d. Non-ketotic hyperosmolar coma

35. A patient of pulmonary tuberculosis is taking ATT, presents with joint pain and raised uric acid level. The most likely cause of symptoms is side effect of:
    a. INH
    b. Pyrazinamide
    c. Streptomycin
    d. Ethambutol

36. The most important investigation to confirm diagnosis of bronchial asthma is:
    a. X-ray chest
    b. Lung function test
    c. Serum IgE level
    d. CBC

37. A 18-year-old boy with hypertension, examination of CVS reveals radiofemoral delay. The most likely cause of hypertension in this patient is:
    a. Coarctation of aorta
    b. Conn's syndrome
    c. Renal artery stenosis
    d. Diabetic nephropathy

38. Gait of a patient suffering from parkinsonism is likely to be:
    a. Normal
    b. Shuffling
    c. Hemiplegic
    d. Drunken

39. In thalassemia, peripheral smear for RBC morphology shows:
    a. Normochromic normocytic
    b. Sickle cells
    c. Hypochromic microcytic
    d. Macrocytosis

40. A patient of thromboembolic stroke is taking warfarin. He comes to dental OPD for tooth extraction. The most useful investigation to see effect of warfarin is:
    a. Hematocrit
    b. Platelet count
    c. Prothrombin time
    d. Bleeding time

41. Hepatitis B spreads through:
    a. Blood transfusion
    b. Alcohol consumption
    c. Feco-oral route
    d. Droplet infection

42. Following are the causes of cirrhosis of liver, *except*:
    a. Alcoholism
    b. Wilson's disease
    c. Hepatitis E
    d. Hemochromatosis

43. Chronic diarrhea is a feature of infection by:
    a. *Bacillus cereus*
    b. Cholera
    c. Giardiasis
    d. *Campylobacter*

44. Koilonychia is a feature of:
    a. Vitamin B12 deficiency
    b. Iron deficiency
    c. Protein deficiency
    d. Folic acid deficiency

45. Schilling's test is performed to detect deficiency of:
    a. Vitamin B1
    b. Vitamin B2
    c. Vitamin B6
    d. Vitamin B12

46. Exanthematous fever characterized by vesicular eruption is:
    a. Measles
    b. Mumps
    c. Rubella
    d. Varicella

47. Cerebral malaria is caused by:
    a. *P. Falciparum*
    b. *P. vivax*
    c. *P. malariae*
    d. *P. ovale*

48. The most common mode of transmission of HIV worldwide is:
    a. Mother to fetus
    b. Injection drug use
    c. Homosexuals
    d. Heterosexuals

49. Intrinsic factor is secreted by:
    a. Parietal cells
    b. Chief cells
    c. Mucous cells
    d. Endocrine cells

Answers: 34. c. Diabetic... | 35. b. Pyrazinamide | 36. c. Serum IgE level | 37. a. Coarctation of...
38. b. Shuffling | 39. c. Hypochromic... | 40. c. Prothrombin time | 41. a. Blood transfusion
42. c. Hepatitis E | 43. a. *Bacillus cereus* | 44. b. Iron deficiency | 45. d. Vitamin B12
46. a. Measles | 47. a. *P. Falciparum* | 48. d. Heterosexuals | 49. a. Parietal cells

50. Following are vitamin K dependent clotting factors, *except*:
    a. Factor VII
    b. Factor VIII
    c. Factor IX
    d. Factor X

51. A 40-year-old male present in emergency department with central chest pain. His BP is 100/60 mm of Hg and pulse is 110 BPM, low volume. He is pale and sweating profusely. The most likely diagnosis is:
    a. Esophagitis
    b. Myocardial infarction
    c. Pleural effusion
    d. Pneumothorax

52. In rheumatic fever, the treatment of choice for symptoms is:
    a. Aspirin
    b. Paracetamol
    c. Morphine
    d. Ibuprofen

53. A 40-year-old female presents with the cold intolerance, swelling all over body, hoarseness of voice and goiter. The most likely finding on CNS examination is:
    a. Hyperreflexia
    b. Hypotonia
    c. Ataxia
    d. Delayed relaxation of ankle jerk

54. In a patient of centripetal obesity, acne and hirsutism the most likely diagnosis is:
    a. Hypogonadism
    b. Simple obesity
    c. Hypothyroidism
    d. Cushing's syndrome

55. An epileptic girl is having gingival hypertrophy in dental OPD. Antiepileptic drug which she is most likely taking is:
    a. Na valproate
    b. Phenytoin
    c. Carbamazepine
    d. Gabapentin

56. A 50-year-old man is admitted in ICCU with acute myocardial infarction. Which of the following drugs is used in reperfusion therapy?
    a. Warfarin
    b. Aspirin
    c. Streptokinase
    d. Heparin

57. A 18-year-old boy present with chronic diarrhea. Which of the following features suggests that he has irritable bowel syndrome:
    a. Anemia
    b. Abdominal pain relieved by defecation
    c. Nocturnal symptoms
    d. Blood in stool

58. In a patient with history of muscle cramps and carpopedal spasm. Which of the following serum electrolyte level is likely to be low?
    a. Calcium
    b. Sodium
    c. Chloride
    d. Potassium

59. The most common side effect of quinine is:
    a. Coma
    b. Deafness
    c. Headache
    d. Tremors

60. A young boy presents with fever, skin rash and diarrhea. Examination of oral cavity shows Koplik spots on mucosa. The most likely diagnosis is:
    a. Measles
    b. Chickenpox
    c. Smallpox
    d. Typhoid

61. One of the following is true about herpes zoster:
    a. Itching vesicles appear around lips
    b. Systemic viral infection causes vesicles around penile area
    c. Burning discomfort occurs in affected dermatome where discrete vesicles appear 3–4 days later
    d. Vesicular eruptions begin on mucosal surface first followed by centripetal distribution

62. Pernicious anemia is due to:
    a. Gastric atrophy
    b. Vitamin B1 deficiency
    c. Vitamin B12 deficiency
    d. Folic acid deficiency

63. Deficiency of coagulation factor IX is associated with:
    a. Hemophilia A
    b. Hemophilia B
    c. Henoch-schönlein purpura
    d. All the above

Answers: 50. b. Factor VIII   51. b. Myocardial infarction   52. a. Aspirin   53. d. Delayed...
          54. d. Cushing's...   55. b. Phenytoin   56. c. Streptokinase   57. b. Abdominal pain...
          58. a. Calcium   59. b. Deafness   60. a. Measles   61. c. Burning...
          62. c. Vitamin B12...   63. b. Hemophilia B

64. Bull neck in diphtheria is due to:
    a. Cellulitis
    b. Laryngeal edema
    c. Retropharyngeal abscess
    d. Lymphadenopathy

65. Spider nevi, palmar erythema, gynecomastia are features of:
    a. Acute amoebic dysentery
    b. Chronic amoebic dysentery
    c. Acute liver disease
    d. Chronic liver disease

66. The complication of enteric fever during second to third week is:
    a. Deafness
    b. Perforation of intestine
    c. Anemia
    d. None of the above

67. One of the following statement is true about primary chancre:
    a. It is caused by *Mycobacterium*
    b. Incubation period is under a week
    c. The red macule is eroded to form an indurated painful ulcer
    d. It resolves within 2–6 weeks without treatment

68. Long-term treatment with overdoses of corticosteroids may result in all the following, *except*:
    a. Osteoporosis
    b. Diabetes mellitus
    c. Blood dyscrasias
    d. Susceptibility to infection

69. Hepatitis A is spreaded by:
    a. Feco-oral route
    b. Vertical transmission
    c. Blood transfusion
    d. Droplet infection

70. Treatment of angular stomatitis and cheilosis is:
    a. Pyridoxine
    b. Riboflavin
    c. Cyanocobalamin
    d. Vitamin C

71. In emergency, treatment of choice for anaphylactic shock is:
    a. Ampicillin
    b. Adrenaline
    c. Amiodarone

72. Which parameter can be used to monitor severity of bronchial asthma at home?
    a. ECG
    b. PEFR
    c. EEG
    d. EMG

73. Which is responsible for rheumatic fever?
    a. *Staphylococcus*
    b. *E. Coli*
    c. *Streptococcus*
    d. *Clostridium*

74. Which drug is useful for prevention of migraine?
    a. Aspirin
    b. Paracetamol
    c. Ergot
    d. Flunarizine

75. ADA criteria for diagnosis of diabetes fasting blood glucose should be equal to or more than
    a. 50 mg/dL
    b. 100 mg/dL
    c. 126 mg/dL
    d. 102 mg/dL

76. In acute LVF (Pulmonary edema), treatment of choice in emergency is:
    a. Furosemide
    b. Ciprofloxacin
    c. Quinidine
    d. Thiazide

77. Exophthalmos is clinical feature of:
    a. Hypothyroidism
    b. Malaria
    c. Thyrotoxicosis
    d. Diabetes

78. A continuous murmur is present in which congenital heart disease:
    a. ASD
    b. VSD
    c. Patent ductus arteriosus (PDA)
    d. CHB

79. Fever, headache, vomiting and neck rigidity is seen in which condition:
    a. Pneumonia
    b. Panic attack
    c. Meningitis
    d. Anxiety

Answers: 64. d. Lymphadenopathy   65. d. Chronic liver disease   66. c. Anemia   67. c. The red macule...
               68. c. Blood dyscrasias   69. a. Feco-oral route   70. b. Riboflavin   71. b. Adrenaline
               72. b. PEFR   73. c. *Streptococcus*   74. c. Ergot   75. c. 126 mg/dL
               76. a. Furosemide   77. c. Thyrotoxicosis   78. c. Patent ductus... 79. c. Meningitis

80. **Postural hypotension is common side effect of which drug:**
    a. Prazosin
    b. Dilantin
    c. Chloroquine
    d. Clopidogrel

81. **Following hepatitis viruses are RNA viruses, *except*:**
    a. Hepatitis A
    b. Hepatitis B
    c. Hepatitis C
    d. Hepatitis D

82. **Liver synthesizes following clotting factors, *except*:**
    a. Factor VIII
    b. Factor VII
    c. Vitamin K
    d. Fibrinogen

83. **Milk is devoid of:**
    a. Iron
    b. Proteins
    c. Fats
    d. Calcium

84. **Steatorrhea is a feature of:**
    a. Amoebic dysentery
    b. Malabsorption syndrome
    c. Bacillary dysentery
    d. Pseudomembranous colitis

85. **Casal's necklace is a feature of deficiency of:**
    a. Thiamine
    b. Riboflavin
    c. Pyridoxine
    d. Niacin

86. **Which of the following malignancy is associated with HIV infection?**
    a. Kaposi's sarcoma
    b. Lymphatic leukemia
    c. Hepatocellular carcinoma
    d. Chronic myeloid leukemia

87. **For labeling, a patient of PUO, the duration of fever should be:**
    a. 1 week
    b. 2 weeks
    c. 3 weeks
    d. 4 weeks

88. **Generalized lymphadenopathy is a feature of:**
    a. Latent syphilis
    b. Secondary syphilis
    c. Primary syphilis
    d. Neurosyphilis

89. **Iron absorption mainly takes place in:**
    a. Stomach
    b. Ileum
    c. Jejunum
    d. Colon

90. **Pernicious anemia is caused by the deficiency of:**
    a. Folic acid
    b. Thiamine
    c. Cyanocobalamine
    d. Ascorbic acid

91. **Chronic smoking is a risk factor for:**
    a. Bronchogenic carcinoma
    b. Pneumonia
    c. PTB
    d. ARDS

92. **During examination of a patient hyper-resonant will be seen in case of:**
    a. Pneumothorax
    b. Pleural effusion
    c. Pneumonia
    d. PTB

93. **Irregularly irregular pulse is seen in a case of:**
    a. CHB
    b. VT
    c. SVT
    d. Atrial fibrillation

94. **Which drug is used for thyrotoxicosis?**
    a. Carbamazepine
    b. Dilantin
    c. Carbimazole
    d. Aspirin

95. **In acute myocardial infarction which drug can be used for reperfusion?**
    a. Ceftriaxone
    b. Streptokinase
    c. Warfarin
    d. Dapsone

96. **Hypoglycemia can be treated in acute stage by:**
    a. Ampicillin
    b. Dexamethasone
    c. Glucagon
    d. GH

97. **Which one is good cholesterol?**
    a. HDL
    b. LDL
    c. VLDL
    d. TG

Answers: 80. a. Prazosin   81. b. Hepatitis B   82. a. Factor VIII   83. a. Iron
84. b. Malabsorption...   85. c. Pyridoxine   86. a. Kaposi's sarcoma   87. c. 3 weeks
88. b. Secondary syphilis   89. c. Jejunum   90. c. Cyanocobalamine   91. a. Bronchogenic...
92. a. Pneumothorax   93. d. Atrial fibrillation   94. c. Carbimazole   95. b. Streptokinase
96. c. Glucagon   97. a. HDL

98. Pulse pressure is wide in which valvular heart disease:
    a. Aortic regurgitation (AR)
    b. MS
    c. AS
    d. PS

99. Cushing's syndrome is due to excess of which hormone:
    a. Glucocorticoids
    b. Insulin
    c. Growth hormone
    d. TSH

100. In SVT of new onset treatment of choice is:
    a. Cardioversion
    b. Digoxin
    c. Beta-blocker
    d. Verapamil

101. TSH is raised in:
    a. Hyperthyroidism
    b. Hypothyroidism
    c. Euthyroidism
    d. All of the above

102. Gait in parkinsonism is:
    a. Hemiplegic
    b. Shuffling
    c. Drunkin
    d. All of the above

103. Mid-diastolic murmur is seen in:
    A. Mitral stenosis
    B. Atrial stenosis
    C. Aortic regurgitation
    D. All of the above

104. ACE inhibitors are contraindicated in:
    a. Adult + hypertension
    b. Diabetic hypertension
    c. Pregnancy hypertension
    d. None of the above

105. Drug of choice in diabetic ketoacidosis is:
    a. Sulfonylurea
    b. Metformin
    c. Insulin
    d. All of the above

106. Normal blood pH is:
    a. 7.4
    b. 7.2
    c. 7.1
    d. None of the above

107. Increase in blood homocysteine level causes:
    a. Pneumonia
    b. Nephritis
    c. Coronary artery disease
    d. All of the above

108. Petechial hemorrhages are seen in:
    a. Tubercular meningitis
    b. Pneumococcal meningitis
    c. Meningococcal meningitis
    d. All of the above

109. Subcutaneous nodules are seen in:
    a. Rheumatic fever
    b. Bacterial endocarditis
    c. Angina pectoris
    d. All of the above

110. Blackish discoloration of buccal mucosa is seen in:
    a. Tetany
    b. Acromegaly
    c. Addison's disease
    d. None of the above

111. T3 is raised in:
    a. Hypothyroidism
    b. Hyperthyroidism
    c. Euthyroid
    d. All of the above

112. Tremors, rigidity and hypokinesia is a feature of:
    a. Meningitis
    b. Encephalitis
    c. Parkinsonism
    d. All of the above

113. Pan systolic murmur is seen in:
    a. Mitral stenosis
    b. Mitral regurgitation
    c. Aortic stenosis
    d. All of the above

114. Drug of choice in pregnancy hypertension is:
    a. ACE inhibitor
    b. ARBs
    c. Methyldopa
    d. All of the above

115. Drug of choice in gestational diabetes is:
    a. Metformin
    b. Insulin
    c. Sulfonylurea
    d. All of the above

Answers:
98. a. Aortic...
99. a. Glucocorticoids
100. d. Verapamil
101. b. Hypothyroidism
102. a. Hemiplegic
103. a. Mitral stenosis
104. d. None of the above
105. c. Insulin
106. a. 7.4
107. c. Coronary artery
108. c. Meningococcal...
109. a. Rheumatic fever
110. c. Addison's disease
111. b. Hyperthyroidism
112. c. Parkinsonism
113. b. Encephalitis
114. c. Methyldopa
115. a. Metformin

116. **Clubbing and chymosin both are seen in:**
    a. Mitral stenosis
    b. Congestive heart failure
    c. Fallot's teratology
    d. None of the above

117. **Exophthalmos is seen in:**
    a. Graves' disease
    b. Acromegaly
    c. Tetany
    d. None of the above

118. **Water hammer pulse is seen in:**
    a. Mitral stenosis
    b. Aortic regurgitation
    c. Aortic stenosis
    d. All of the above

119. **Insulin resistance is seen in:**
    a. Type I-diabetes
    b. Type II-diabetes
    c. Both of the above
    d. None of the above

120. **Smoking is a risk factor for:**
    a. Lung cancer
    b. Myocardial infarction
    c. Chronic obstructive pulmonary disease
    d. All of the above

121. **TSH is decreased in:**
    a. Hypothyroidism
    b. Hyperthyroidism
    c. Euthyroidism
    d. None of the above

122. **Drug of choice in gestational diabetes is:**
    a. Sulfonylurea
    b. Metformin
    c. Insulin
    d. All of the above

123. **ACE inhibitors are contraindicated in:**
    a. Adult hypertension
    b. Diabetic hypertension
    c. Pregnancy hypertension
    d. None of the above

124. **Osler's nodes are found in:**
    a. Rheumatic fever
    b. CCF
    c. Infective endocarditis
    d. All of the above

125. **Tremors, rigidity and hypokinesia is the feature of:**
    a. Parkinsonism
    b. Mitral stenosis
    c. Aortic regurgitation
    d. All of the above

126. **Hypoglycemia can be treated in acute stage by:**
    a. Sulfonylurea
    b. Glucagon
    c. Dexamethasone
    d. Insulin

127. **Drug of choice in thyrotoxicosis:**
    a. Carbimazole
    b. Dilantin
    c. Carbamazepine
    d. Levothyroxine

128. **Water hammer pulse is seen in:**
    a. Aortic regurgitation
    b. Mitral stenosis
    c. CCF
    d. None of the above

129. **Cushing's syndrome is due to excess of which hormone:**
    a. Insulin
    b. TSH
    c. Growth hormone
    d. Glucocorticoids

130. **Which drug is useful for prevention of migraine?**
    a. Aspirin
    b. Paracetamol
    c. ACE inhibitors
    d. Flunarizine

131. **Gum hypertrophy is caused by:**
    a. Phenytoin sodium
    b. Phenobarbitone
    c. Sodium valproate
    d. Carbamazepine

132. **Chronic hepatitis is seen in (most commonly):**
    a. Hepatitis A
    b. Hepatitis B
    c. Hepatitis C
    d. Hepatitis D

133. **Swelling of salivary glands is seen in:**
    a. Infectious mononucleosis
    b. Measles
    c. Mumps
    d. Rubella

Answers: 116. d. None of the above   117. a. Graves' disease   118. b. Aortic regurgitation   119. b. Type II-diabetes
120. d. All of the above   121. b. Hyperthyroidism   122. c. Insulin   123. c. Pregnancy...
124. c. Infective...   125. a. Parkinsonism   126. b. Glucagon   127. a. Carbimazole
128. b. Mitral stenosis   129. d. Glucocorticoids   130. c. ACE inhibitors   131. a. Phenytoin sodium
132. b. Hepatitis B   133. c. Mumps

134. **Xerophthalmia is seen in:**
    a. Vitamin A deficiency
    b. Vitamin B deficiency
    c. Vitamin C deficiency
    d. Vitamin D deficiency

135. *Corynebacterium diphtheriae* **has following features:**
    a. Non-motile
    b. Non-sporing
    c. Gram-positive
    d. All of the above

136. **Ludwig's angina involves spaces,** *except*:
    a. Subarachnoid
    b. Bilateral sublingual
    c. Bilateral submental
    d. Bilateral submandibular

137. **Generalized lymphadenopathy is the feature of:**
    a. Agranulocytosis
    b. Diarrhea
    c. Lymphomas
    d. Renal failure

138. **Von Willebrand disease is caused by deficiency of:**
    a. Factor VII
    b. Subendothelial factor VIII
    c. Factor IX
    d. Factor X

139. **In cases of agranulocytosis:**
    a. Platelet count is increased
    b. RBC count is increased
    c. WBC count is decreased
    d. WBC count is increased

140. **Hemodialysis is done in cases of:**
    a. Congestive cardiac failure
    b. Chronic myeloid leukemia
    c. Chronic renal failure
    d. Chronic obstructive lung disease

141. **Dangerous type of wear:**
    a. Attic granulation
    b. Central perforation
    c. Marginal perforation
    d. Multiple perforation

142. **Ototoxic drug is:**
    a. Gentamicin
    b. Metrogyl
    c. Penicillin
    d. Ampicillin

143. **No hepatic dose adjustment is required in:**
    a. Rifampicin

    b. INH
    c. Ethambutol
    d. PZA

144. **Fatty change in liver is due to accumulation of:**
    a. Cholesterol
    b. VLDL
    c. LDL
    d. Triglyceride

145. **Which inhaled pollutant likely to cause pulmonary fibrosis:**
    a. Silica
    b. Tobacco
    c. Ozone
    d. Carbon dioxide

146. **Not associated with cancer:**
    a. Fragile X syndrome
    b. Fanconi's syndrome
    c. Down's syndrome
    d. Bloom syndrome

147. **Radiofrequency ablation is done for:**
    a. Ventricular tachycardia
    b. PSVT
    c. WPW
    d. Atrial tachycardia

148. **Nosocomial pneumonia is most commonly caused by:**
    a. Gram-negative bacilli
    b. Gram-positive bacilli
    c. Gram-negative cocci
    d. *Mycoplasma*

149. **Electrical alternans is seen in:**
    a. Cardiac tamponade
    b. Restrictive cardiomyopathy
    c. Left atrial myxoma
    d. COPD

150. **In Kartagener syndrome all are seen,** *except*:
    a. Cystic fibrosis
    b. Dextrocardia
    c. Sinusitis
    d. Absence of cilia

151. **Most common cause of superior vena cava obstruction is:**
    a. Thrombosis
    b. Extrinsic compression
    c. Mediastinal lymphoma
    d. Teratoma

Answers: 134. a. Vitamin A...   135. d. All of the above   136. a. Subarachnoid   137. c. Lymphomas
138. b. Subendothelial...   139. c. WBC count is...   140. c. Chronic renal failure   141. b. Central perforation
142. a. Gentamicin   143. c. Ethambutol   144. d. Triglyceride   145. a. Silica
146. c. Down's...   147. b. PSVT   148. a. Gram-negative bacilli 149. a. Cardiac tamponade
150. b. Dextrocardia   151. c. Mediastinal...

152. **Most common sign of aspiration pneumonitis:**
   a. Tachypnea
   b. Bronchospasm
   c. Cyanosis
   d. Crepitation

153. **Aspirin sensitive asthma is associated with:**
   a. Extrinsic asthma
   b. Urticaria
   c. Nasal polyp
   d. Obesity

154. **Ursodeoxycholic acid is a:**
   a. Urinary stone dissolving drug
   b. Thrombolytic drug
   c. Gallstone dissolving drug
   d. Antiplatelet

155. **Highest concentration of K⁺ is seen in:**
   a. Duodenum
   b. Jejunum
   c. Ileum
   d. Colon

156. **Diabetes insipidus is due to lack of:**
   a. ANP
   b. Vasopressin
   c. Aldosterone
   d. Insulin

157. **Elevated glucose level especially in obese may be due to:**
   a. DKA
   b. Glucose intolerance
   c. Insulin resistance
   d. Insulin shock

158. **Which of the following is hypoglycemic drug:**
   a. Atorvastatin
   b. Vildagliptin
   c. Glimepiride
   d. Clopidogrel

159. **"Master gland" of endocrine system located in base of brain:**
   a. Apical gland
   b. Bartholin gland
   c. Pituitary gland
   d. Thyroid gland

160. **Glitazones are used to treat:**
   a. Diabetes insipidus
   b. NIDDM
   c. Infertility
   d. Hypothyroidism

161. **Pernicious anemia is due to failure of production of:**
   a. Bile
   b. Insulin
   c. Intrinsic factor
   d. ACTH

162. **Complication of herpes zoster is:**
   a. Hemolytic uremic syndrome
   b. Toxic mega colon
   c. Progressive multifocal leukoencephalopathy
   d. Ramsay Hunt syndrome

163. **Digoxin is used in:**
   a. NIDDM
   b. Cardiac arrhythmia
   c. Diabetes insipidus
   d. Hypothyroidism

164. **Which of these is a hemolytic anemia:**
   a. Sideroblastic anemia
   b. Aplastic anemia
   c. Hereditary anemia
   d. Aplastic anemia

165. **HAART is used in treatment of following infection:**
   a. HAV
   b. HBV
   c. HCV
   d. HIV

166. **Community acquired pneumonia is most commonly caused by:**
   a. *Pseudomonas aeruginosa*
   b. *Streptococcus pyogenes*
   c. *Streptococcus pneumoniae*
   d. *Mycoplasma*

167. **Autoimmune disease causing oral ulcer is:**
   a. Liver cirrhosis
   b. Diabetes insipidus
   c. Systemic lupus erythematosus
   d. Hypothyroidism

168. **Hepatitis B virus belongs to family called:**
   a. Flaviviridae
   b. Picornavirus
   c. Delta viridae
   d. Hepadnaviridae

169. **Hyperglycemic hyperosmolar state is complication of:**
   a. Hyperthyroidism
   b. Hypothyroidism
   c. Diabetes insipidus
   d. Diabetes mellitus

Answers: 152. a. Tachypnea   153. a. Extrinsic asthma   154. c. Gallstone dissolving... 155. d. Colon
156. b. Vasopressin   157. c. Insulin resistance   158. Both b and c   159. c. Pituitary gland
160. b. NIDDM   161. c. Intrinsic factor   162. d. Ramsay Hunt...   163. b. Cardiac arrhythmia
164. c. Hereditary...   165. d. HIV   166. c. *Streptococcus*...   167. c. Systemic lupus...
168. d. Hepadnaviridae   169. c. Diabetes insipidus

170. **Which of the following is thiazolidinedione:**
    a. Glimepiride
    b. Vildagliptin
    c. Pioglitazone
    d. Metformin

171. **Common causative agent for subacute infective endocarditis:**
    a. *Staphylococcus epidermis*
    b. *Neisseria gonorrhoeae*
    c. Enterococci
    d. *Streptococcus viridians*

172. **Paroxysmal nocturnal dyspnea is a symptom of:**
    a. Liver cirrhosis
    b. Hypertension
    c. Heart failure
    d. Renal failure

173. **Drug used in treatment of CML is:**
    a. Imatinib mesylate
    b. Fludarabine
    c. Rituximab
    d. Cyclophosphamide

174. **Cushing's syndrome is due to:**
    a. Increased insulin
    b. Hypoaldosteronism
    c. Increased mineralocorticoid
    d. Increased glucocorticoid

175. **In nephrotic syndrome there is:**
    a. Hyperalbuminemia
    b. Massive proteinuria
    c. Mild proteinuria
    d. Hypolipidemia

176. **Bell's palsy is a:**
    a. Upper motor neuron type of 5th nerve palsy
    b. Upper motor neuron type of 7th nerve palsy
    c. Lower motor neuron type of 5th nerve palsy
    d. Lower motor neuron type of 7th nerve palsy

177. **Which of the following is an antiplatelet drug:**
    a. Prednisone
    b. Repaglinide
    c. Clopidogrel
    d. Atorvastatin

178. **Second line antitubercular drug is:**
    a. Ethionamide
    b. Isoniazid
    c. Streptomycin
    d. Rifampcin

179. **Status epilepticus refers to:**
    a. Cardiac arrhythmia
    b. Continuous seizures
    c. Continuous fever
    d. Hyperglycemia

180. **β adrenoceptor agonist are used in:**
    a. Diabetes mellitus
    b. Myocardial infarction
    c. Atrial fibrillation
    d. Bronchial asthma

181. **Approximate time interval between HIV infection and manifestation of AIDS is:**
    a. 7.5 years
    b. 10 years
    c. 12 years
    d. 15 years

182. **Tourniquet test is used for monitoring patients with:**
    a. Infectious mononucleosis
    b. Zika virus infection
    c. Dengue fever
    d. Chikungunya

183. **Sinus bradycardia is defined as heart rate of:**
    a. Less than 40/min
    b. Less than 50/min
    c. Less than 60/min
    d. Less than 80/min

184. **What is the treatment of anaphylactic shock:**
    a. 1 mL IV adrenaline 1 in 100000
    b. 0.5 mL IM epinephrine 1 in 1000
    c. 0.5 mL IM epinephrine 1 in 10000
    d. 1 mL IV adrenaline 1 in 10000

185. **Osler's nodes are seen in:**
    a. Rheumatoid arthritis
    b. Rheumatic heart disease
    c. SABE
    d. Typhoid

186. **Most common cause of infective endocarditis is:**
    a. *Staphylococcus aureus*
    b. *Streptococcus pyogenes*
    c. *Streptococcus viridians*
    d. *Streptococcus mutans*

187. **In Glasgow coma scale maximum and minimum scores are:**
    a. 18 and 3
    b. 18 and 0
    c. 15 and 3
    d. 15 and 0

Answers: 170. d. Metformin   171. c. Enterococci   172. a. Liver cirrhosis   173. a. Imatinib mesylate
174. d. Increased...   175. b. Massive proteinuria   176. d. Lower motor...   177. c. Clopidogrel
178. c. Streptomycin   179. b. Continuous seizures   180. d. Bronchial asthma   181. b. 10 years
182. c. Dengue fever   183. c. Less than 60/min   184. b. 0.5 mL IM ...   185. c. SABE
186. c. *Streptococcus* ...   187 c. 15 and 3

188. **Which is the most common cause of death in Type I diabetes mellitus:**
    a. Kidney disease
    b. Myocardial disease
    c. Stroke
    d. Infection

189. **Obesity is not a feature of:**
    a. Hypothyroidism
    b. Hypogonadism
    c. Adrenal insufficiency
    d. Cushing's syndrome

190. **Thyroid storm is seen in:**
    a. Thyroid surgery
    b. Neonatal thyrotoxicosis
    c. Perioperative infection
    d. All of these

191. **All of the following are seen in rickets, *except*:**
    a. Bow legs
    b. Gunstock deformity
    c. Pot belly
    d. Craniotabes

192. **A 65-year-old woman after total knee implant surgery complaint of calf pain and swelling in leg from last 2 days. Later she complaint of breadthlessness and dies suddenly in the ward. Probable cause is:**
    a. Pulmonary embolism
    b. Myocardial infarction
    c. Stroke
    d. ARDS

193. **Maximum chance of spread in accidental needle stick injury is:**
    a. Hepatitis B
    b. Hepatitis C
    c. HIV
    d. EBV

194. **Which is not a characteristic of portal hypertension:**
    a. Splenomegaly
    b. Hypersplenism
    c. Ascites
    d. Gynecomastia

195. **Raised serum amylase levels are used to diagnose:**
    a. Autoimmune disease
    b. Degenerative diseases
    c. Acute cholecystitis
    d. Acute pancreatitis

196. **In rheumatoid arthritis the characteristic joint involvement is:**
    a. Spine
    b. Knee joint
    c. Metacarpophalangeal joint
    d. Hip joint

197. **All of the following are associated with sjogren's syndrome, *except*:**
    a. Dry eyes
    b. Dry mouth
    c. Parotid gland enlargement
    d. Systemic manifestations

198. **HIV does not spread by:**
    a. Infected syringes
    b. Pregnant mother to fetus
    c. Blood products
    d. Mosquito bite

199. **Which is not an antihypertensive drug:**
    a. Minoxidil
    b. Alprazolam
    c. Amlodipine
    d. Furosemide

200. **Which drug should be withheld pre- and post-dental extractions:**
    a. Antibiotic
    b. Antiplatelet
    c. Analgesics
    d. Antihypertensive

201. **Typhoid is treated by all, *except*:**
    a. Erythromycin
    b. Amikacin
    c. Ceftriaxone
    d. Ciprofloxacin

202. **Most common cause of diarrhea in AIDS patient is:**
    a. *Salmonella*
    b. *Cryptosporidium*
    c. *Candida*
    d. Isophora

203. **Investigation for diagnosis of ischemic heart disease is:**
    a. EMG
    b. EEG
    c. ECG
    d. All of the above

204. **Acute rheumatic fever affects all, *except*:**
    a. Joint
    b. Heart
    c. Skin
    d. Brain

Answers:	188. b. Myocardial...	189. c. Adrenal insufficiency	190. d. All of these	191. b. Gunstock deformity
	192. a. Pulmonary...	193. a. Hepatitis B	194. d. Gyanecomastia	195. d. Acute pancreatitis
	196. c. Metacarpo....	197. c. Parotid gland...	198. d. Mosquito bite	199. b. Alprazolam
	200. b. Antiplatelet	201. a. Erythromycin	202. b. *Cryptosporidium*	203. c. ECG
	204. d. Brain			

205. Not a feature of diabetes mellitus:
    a. Polyurea
    b. Polydipsia
    c. Polyphagia
    d. None of the above

206. Microcytic anemia is due to deficiency of:
    a. Iron
    b. Folic acid
    c. Vitamin B12
    d. None of the above

207. Amoebiasis is caused by:
    a. Virus
    b. Bacteria
    c. Fungus
    d. Protozoa

208. Drug not used in treatment of malaria:
    a. Clindamycin
    b. Artesunate
    c. Azithromycin
    d. Quinine

209. Blood transfusion should be completed within ....hours of initiation
    a. 1 to 4 hours
    b. 3 to 6 hours
    c. 4 to 8 hours
    d. 8 to 12 hours

210. Low serum iron and low serum ferritin is seen in:
    a. Iron deficiency anemia
    b. Chronic kidney disease
    c. Fanconi anemia
    d. Megaloblastic anemia

211. Sinus bradycardia is defined as the heart rate of
    a. Less than 40/min
    b. Less than 50/min
    c. Less than 60/min
    d. Less than 70/min

212. Which of the following is not the component of Glasgow coma scale:
    a. Eye opening
    b. Motor response
    c. Pupil size
    d. Verbal response

213. Which of the following represent tertiary syphilis:
    a. Condyloma lata
    b. Gumma formation
    c. Matted lymph nodes
    d. Condyloma acuminate

214. A chronic alcoholic presenting with bleeding gums and petechiae is more likely o have deficiency of:
    a. Vitamin B12
    b. Vitamin C
    c. Thiamine
    d. Pyridoxine

215. Prolonged immobilization leads to:
    a. Hypercalcemia
    b. Hypocalcemia
    c. Hyperkalemia
    d. Hypokalemia

216. Pernicious anemia is associated with all of the following, *except*:
    a. Macrocytosis
    b. Vitamin B12 deficiency
    c. Tingling and numbness
    d. Raised reticulocyte count

217. Iron overload occurs in all, *except*:
    a. Thalassemia
    b. Myelodysplastic syndrome
    c. Polycythemia vera
    d. Sideroblastic anemia

218. All are used in bronchial asthma, *except*:
    a. Salbutamol
    b. Morphine
    c. Aminophylline
    d. Steroid

219. Most common oral infection in diabetes mellitus:
    a. *Candida*
    b. *Aspergillus*
    c. *Streptococcus*
    d. *Staphylococcus*

220. A hypertensive diabetic is having proteinuria, antihypertensive of choice is:
    a. Propranolol
    b. Clonidine
    c. Enalapril
    d. Verapamil

221. Drug of choice to control acute sudden onset supraventricular tachycardia:
    a. Digoxin
    b. Adenosine
    c. Verapamil
    d. Propranolol

222. Cause of wide pulse pressure:
    a. Aortic stenosis
    b. Mitral stenosis
    c. Aortic regurgitation
    d. Tricuspid stenosis

Answers: 205. d. None of the...   206. a. Iron   207. d. Protozoa   208. c. Azithromycin
        209. a. 1 to 4 hours   210. a. Iron deficiency...   211. c. Less than 60/min   212. c. Pupil size
        213. b. Gumma   214. b. Vitamin C   215. b. Hypocalcemia   216. d. Raised...
        217. c. Polycythemia...   218. b. Morphine   219. a. Candida   220. c. Enalapril
        221. c. Verapamil   222. c. Aortic regur...

223. Steroids are contraindicated in all, *except*:
    a. Diabetes mellitus
    b. PTB
    c. Peptic ulcer
    d. Brain tumor

224. Macrocytic anemia occurs in:
    a. Hypothyroidism
    b. CRP
    c. Anemia of chronic disease
    d. Vitamin C deficiency

225. Most common cause of DIC:
    a. Snake bite
    b. Sepsis
    c. Diabetes mellitus
    d. Thyroid disease

226. Drug of choice in influenza A is:
    a. Acyclovir
    b. Retinovir
    c. Oseltamivir
    d. Abacavir

227. The drug of choice for absence seizure is:
    a. Valproate
    b. Gabapentin
    c. Phenytoin
    d. Carbamazepine

228. Most common site of brain hemorrhage is:
    a. Internal capsule
    b. Ventral pons
    c. Putamen
    d. Cerebellar

229. Wheel chair sign is seen in:
    a. Wilson's disease
    b. Thompsen disease
    c. Beckers dystrophy
    d. Parkinsonism

230. Most common oral infection in diabetes mellitus:
    a. *Aspergillus*
    b. *Candida*
    c. *Streptococcus*
    d. *Staphylococcus*

231. Curschmann's spirals in sputum are seen in:
    a. PTB
    b. Asthma
    c. Bronchitis
    d. Bronchiectasis

232. Caplan syndrome is pneumoconiosis with:
    a. CCF
    b. HIV
    c. Rheumatoid arthritis
    d. Lymphadenopathy

233. Which one of the following is transmitted non-parenterally:
    a. HBV
    b. HEV
    c. HDV
    d. HCV

234. Which is not the characteristic of portal hypertension:
    a. Ascitis
    b. Splenomegaly
    c. Caput medusa
    d. Gynecomastia

235. Gray turners sign is seen in:
    a. Myocarditis
    b. Pancreatitis
    c. Cholecystitis
    d. Pleural effusion

236. Which of the following is not an autoimmune disease:
    a. SLE
    b. Grave's disease
    c. Rheumatoid arthritis
    d. Ulcerative colitis

237. Kussmaul breathing is associated with:
    a. High altitude
    b. DKA
    c. Flial chest
    d. ARDS

238. Common cause of pulmonary embolism is:
    a. Atherosclerosis
    b. Fracture fixation
    c. Pelvic surgery
    d. CABG

239. All causes acute renal failure, *except*:
    a. Pyelonephritis
    b. Snake bite
    c. Rhabdomyolysis
    d. Analgesic nephropathy

240. Not spreaded by blood:
    a. HIV
    b. HBV
    c. HAV
    d. None of the above

241. Which is an antiplatelet drug:
    a. Atorvastatin
    b. Vildagliptin
    c. Glimepiride
    d. Clopidogrel

Answers: 223. d. Brain tumor   224. a. Hypothyroidism   225. b. Sepsis   226. c. Oseltamivir
227. a. Valproate   228. c. Putamen   229. d. Parkinsonism   230. b. Candida
231. b. Asthma   232. c. Rheumatoid arthritis   233. b. HEV   234. d. Gynecomastia
235. b. Pancreatitis   236. d. Ulcerative colitis   237. b. DKA   238. c. Pelvic surgery
239. b. Snake venom   240. c. HAV   241. d. Clopidogrel

242. **Relative tachycardia is seen in:**
    a. Malaria
    b. Heart failure
    c. Anemia
    d. Enteric fever

243. **Clubbing is not as sign of:**
    a. COPD
    b. Lung cancer
    c. SABE
    d. CVA

244. **Not an antihypertensive:**
    a. Cilnidipine
    b. Terbutaline
    c. Prazosin
    d. Ramipril

245. **Which is a hypolipidemic drug:**
    a. Tetracycline
    b. Neomycin
    c. Doxycycline
    d. None of the above

246. **Hairy leukoplakia is seen in:**
    a. ARDS
    b. AIDS
    c. Addison's disease
    d. None of the above

247. **Clinical manifestations of diabetic ketoacidosis:**
    a. Nausea
    b. Tachycardia
    c. Polyuria
    d. All of the above

248. **Recurrent oral, ocular and genital ulcerations are a feature of:**
    a. Behcet's syndrome
    b. Gardener's syndrome
    c. Cirrhosis of liver
    d. Cushing's syndrome

249. **Unilateral painful vesicles are seen in:**
    a. Enteric fever
    b. Malaria
    c. Herpes simplex
    d. Herpes zoster

250. **Brown tumor of jaws is an oral manifestation of:**
    a. Rickets
    b. Scurvy
    c. Syphilis
    d. Hyperparathyroidism

251. **Pain in left side of lower jaw can be a manifestation of:**
    a. Angina pectoris
    b. Hepatitis
    c. Diabetes
    d. Nephrotic syndrome

252. **Used in COPD:**
    a. Aspirin
    b. Sorbitrate
    c. Oxygen
    d. Metoprolol

253. **Widal test is done for:**
    a. Thyrotoxicosis
    b. HIV
    c. Enteric fever
    d. None of the above

254. **Gum hypertrophy is seen as a side effect of which drug:**
    a. Telmisartan
    b. Metformin
    c. Phenytoin
    d. Ranitidine

255. **Not a feature of microcytic anemia:**
    a. Low iron level
    b. Low folic acid
    c. Decreased MCV
    d. Decreased WBC

256. **Not a symptom of thyrotoxicosis:**
    a. Palpitation
    b. Polyurea
    c. Diarrhea
    d. Obesity

257. **Drugs can cause seizures:**
    a. Chloroquine
    b. Acyclovir
    c. Anti-psychotics
    d. All of the above

258. **Ischemic heart disease is due to involvement of:**
    a. Heart valves
    b. Coronary arteries
    c. SA node
    d. Bundle of His

259. **Drug used in Bell's palsy:**
    a. Amlodipine
    b. Insulin
    c. Prednisolone
    d. All of the above

Answers: 242. b. Heart failure 243. d. CVA 244. b. Terbutaline 245. d. None of the...
246. b. AIDS 247. d. All of the above 248. a. Bechet's syndrome 249. d. Herpes zoster
250. d. Hyperpara.... 251. a. Angina pectoris 252. d. Metoprolol 253. c. Enteric fever
254. c. Phenytoin 255. b. Low folic acid 256. d. Obesity 257. c. Anti-psychotics
258. b. Coronary arteries 259. c. Prednisolone

FILL IN THE BLANKS

As per DCI and Examination Papers of Various Universities

1 Mark Each

1. Herpes simplex is caused by ....
Ans. HSV-1 and HSV-2

2. Diptheria is caused by ....
Ans. *Corynebacterium diphtheriae*

3. Syphilis is caused by ....
Ans. *Treponema pallidum*

4. Amoebiasis is caused by ....
Ans. *Entamoeba histolytica*

5. The most common cause of pleural effusion is ....
Ans. Pneumonia

6. Pellagra is caused by ....
Ans. Vitamin B3 deficiency

7. Vitamin C deficiency causes ....
Ans. Scurvy

8. TSH level is raised in ....
Ans. Hypothyroidism

9. Syncope is due to ....
Ans. Hypotension

10. Agranulocytosis means decrease of ....
Ans. White blood cells

11. Stomatitis is the feature of deficiency of ....
Ans. Iron

12. Acromegaly occurs due to ....
Ans. Secretion of excess growth hormone

13. Smoking commonly causes cancer of ....
Ans. Lungs

14. Caput Medusae is seen in ....
Ans. Portal hypertension

15. Hypertension means BP above .... mm Hg.
Ans. 140/90

16. Ischemic heart disease is due to occlusion of arteries called ....
Ans. Coronary artery

17. Antiviral drug use in treatment of viral hepatitis B is ....
Ans. Lamivudine

18. Kernig's sign is positive in ....
Ans. Meningitis

19. Addison's disease is due to ....
Ans. Adrenal insufficiency

20. Cushing's syndrome is due to ....
Ans. Excess of ACTH hormone

21. Mumps cause enlargement of glands called ....
Ans. Parotid

22. Full form of AIDS is ....
Ans. Acquired Immunodeficiency Syndrome

23. Enteric fever is caused by ....
Ans. *Salmonella typhi*

24. AIDS is caused by ....
Ans. HIV virus

25. TSH level is decreased in ....
Ans. Hyperthyroidism

26. Water soluble vitamins are .... and ....
Ans. B-Complex and Vitamin C

27. Vitamin B1 deficiency causes ....
Ans. Beriberi

28. Bell's Palsy is paralysis of .... cranial nerve.
Ans. Facial nerve (Seventh)

29. Tachycardia means heart rate more than ....
Ans. 100 beats/min

30. Most common cause of pneumonia is ....
Ans. Bacteria

31. Cause of bacillary dysentery is ....
Ans. *Shigella Bacterium*

32. Viral hepatitis occur due to hepatitis ...., ... and .... virus.
Ans. A, B, C, D and E

33. Night blindness is the feature of vitamin .... deficiency.
Ans. Vitamin A

34. Cretinism occurs due to ....
Ans. Hypothyroidism

35. Neck rigidity is seen in ....
Ans. Meningitis

36. Drugs causing Cushing's syndrome is ....
Ans. Glucocorticoid drugs

37. Full form of HIV is ....
Ans. Human Immunodeficiency Virus

38. Trigeminal neuralgia occur due to involvement of .... Cranial nerve.
Ans. Fifth nerve

39. Full form of ARDS is ....
Ans. Acute respiratory distress syndrome

40. Infectious mononucleosis occurs due to ....
Ans. Epstein-Barr virus

41. **Pneumothorax means...................**
Ans. Collection of air in chest or pleural cavity

42. **Thyrotoxicosis means.................**
Ans. Excess of thyroid hormone in body

43. **Cranial nerves originating from Pons are .... and ....**
Ans. Trigeminal nerve and facial nerve

44. **Hepatitis B causes cancers of ....**
Ans. Liver

45. **Drugs used in treatment of herpes zoster is ....**
Ans. Acyclovir

46. **Meningiococcal meningitis is caused by ....**
Ans. *Bacterium Neisseria* meningitidis

47. **Algid malaria presents with ....**
Ans. Hemodynamic disorders as shock with pronounced metabolic changes and hypothermia.

48. **Acromegaly is caused by ....**
Ans. Excessive secretion of growth hormone

49. **Vitamin A deficiency causes..................**
Ans. Night blindness

50. **Drug used in treatment of trigeminal neuralgia..................**
Ans. Carbamazepine

51. **The most common cause of hyperthyroidism is ....**
Ans. Grave's disease and toxic nodular goiter

52. **Nephrotic syndrome is increased excretion of .... in urine**
Ans. Protein

53. **Good pasture's syndrome is simultaneous involvement of .... and lungs.**
Ans. Kidney

54. **Syphilis is caused by..................**
Ans. *Treponema pallidum*

55. **Drug used in treatment of petit mal epilepsy ....**
Ans. Ethosuximide, valproic acid and clonazepam

56. **The most common cause of hepatitis is..................**
Ans. Virus

57. **Commonest cause of cirrhosis in India is ....**
Ans. Alcohol

58. **Caput medusa is seen in..................**
Ans. Umbilicus

59. **Emphysema is commonly seen in..................**
Ans. Smokers

60. **Clubbing is obliteration of ....**
Ans. Nailbeds

61. **JVP stands for..................**
Ans. Jugular venous pressure

62. **Idiopathic facial palsy is called as..................**
Ans. Bell's palsy

63. **Vitamin D deficiency caused.................. in children.**
Ans. Rickets

64. **ARDS stands for ....**
Ans. Acute respiratory distress syndrome

65. **Peptic ulcer is caused by..................**
Ans. *Helicobacter pylori*

66. **Janeway lesions are seen in..................**
Ans. Palms or soles in infective endocarditis

67. **Bald tongue is the feature of..................**
Ans. Iron deficiency anemia

68. **Tuberculosis is caused by..................**
Ans. *Mycobacterium tuberculosis*

69. **The most common cause of lower motor neuron type of facial palsy is ....**
Ans. Trauma

70. **Single most important etiological factor for COPD is..................**
Ans. Smoking

71. **Pulse rate in hypothyroidism is ....**
Ans. Slow

72. **Hookworm infestation causes .... anemia**
Ans. Nutritional

73. **Viral cause of bilateral parotid enlargement is..................**
Ans. Mumps

74. **Neck stiffness and Kernig's sign is seen in..................**
Ans. Meningitis

75. **The most common organism causing community acquired pneumonia (CAP) is ....**
Ans. *Mycobacterium pneumoniae*

76. **Addison's disease occurs due to deficiency of ....**
Ans. Adrenocorticoids

77. **Arthritis of acute rheumatic fever is..................**
Ans. Polyarthritis

78. **Common infective cause of jaundice is..................**
Ans. Viral

79. **Osler nodes are seen in..................**
Ans. Infective endocarditis

80. **Drug used for trigeminal neuralgia is ....**
Ans. Carbamazepine

81. **Cerebral malaria is caused by..................**
Ans. *Plasmodium falciparum*

82. **Endocrine disorder that causes macroglossia (large tongue) is ....**
Ans. Acromegaly

83. **Common adverse effect of ACE inhibitor is** ....

Ans. Profound hypotension

84. **For diagnosis of nephritic syndrome 24 hours urinary protein should be** ....

Ans. More than 3.5 g/day

85. **Preferred route of drug delivery for treatment of bronchial asthma is** ....

Ans. Inhalation

86. **Pneumothorax is collection of air in** ....

Ans. Pleural cavity

87. **Night blindness is caused by deficiency of** ....

Ans. Vitamin A

88. **Changes in nail in patient with broncheictasis is** ....

Ans. Clubbing

89. **In vitamin B12 deficiency the color of tongue is** ....

Ans. Beefy or fiery red

90. **The infection of measles is spreaded by** .... **method**

Ans. Airborne

91. **The diagnostic feature of diphtheriais** .... **on tonsil**

Ans. Presence of grayish green membrane

92. **The most important etiological factor of cirrhosis liver is** ....

Ans. Alcohol

93. **Enteric fever is caused by** ....

Ans. *Salmonella typhi*

94. **In upper motor neuron type of facial palsy, this** .... **half of the face is spared.**

Ans. Upper

95. **The type of anemia of renal origin is** .... **Type.**

Ans. Normocytic normochromic

96. **The name of first cranial nerve is** ....

Ans. Olfactory

97. **In** .... **air and fluid both are present in pleural cavity.**

Ans. Pleural effusion

98. **In pneumonia (consolidation), the type of breathing is** ....

Ans. Bronchial

99. .... **is an important sign of meningitis.**

Ans. Stiff neck

100. **In jaundice, the level of** .... **is increased.**

Ans. Bilirubin

101. **Black water fever is a complication of** ....

Ans. Malaria

102. **In hypothyroidism, the pulse rate is** ....

Ans. Slow

103. **Beriberi is caused by the deficiency of** ....

Ans. Vitamin B

104. .... **is an important clinical feature of lung abscess and bronchiectasis.**

Ans. Chronic lung sepsis

105. **In thyrotoxicosis, the level of** .... **is decreased.**

Ans. TSH

106. .... **is the most common cause of bleeding gums.**

Ans. Vitamin C deficiency

107. **Retinopathy is a complication of** .... **and is** ....

Ans. Diabetes mellitus and hypertension

108. **The most common complication of mitral stenosis is** ....

Ans. Acute pulmonary edema

109. **Ascites is present in** .... **cavity.**

Ans. Peritoneal

110. **Diphtheria is caused by** ....

Ans. *Bacterium corynebacterium diphtheriae*

111. **Aminoglycoside antibiotics are (name** ....

Ans. Streptomycin, Gentamicin, Tobramycin, Amikacin, Kanamycin, Sisomicin, Neomycin, Framycetin and Netilmicin

112. **Composition of oral rehydration salt/solution is** ....

Ans. Sodium chloride – 2. 6 g
Potassium chloride – 1.5 g
Sodium citrate – 2.9 g
Glucose – 13.5 g
Water – 1 L

113. **Drug of choice for amoebiasis is** ....

Ans. Diloxanide furoate

114. **Write down the common investigation for day-to-day tooth extraction are** ....

Ans. CBC, FBS and PPBS, Rapid HbSAg, Rapid HIV

115. **Write down three salient features of Graves' disease** ....

Ans. Diffuse goiter, sign and symptoms of hypothyroidism, exophthalmosis, pre-tibial myxedema

116. **Three commonly prescribed antimalarials are** ....

Ans. Quinine, chloroquine, artemisinin

117. **Drugs contraindicated in asthma patients are** ....

Ans. NSAIDs and β-blockers

118. **Three clinical features of AIDS are** ....

Ans. Weight loss, anorexia, night sweats

119. **Two clinical features of Stevens-Johnson syndrome are.........................**

Ans. Involvement of oral, genital, ocular and nasal involvement, Nikolsky's sign is positive

120. **Write down five antitubercular medicines of short course therapy.....................**

Ans. Rifampicin, Isoniazid, Pyrazinamide, Ethambutol, Streptomycin

121. **Three common clinical features of migraine ....**

Ans. Unilateral, episodic, throbbing headache associated with nausea, vomiting and visual disturbances; females are more affected as compared to males; frequency of each attack is from hours to days.

122. **Drug of choice, doses and duration of treatment for herpes zoster...............**

Ans. Acyclovir, 800 mg, 5 times a day for a week

123. **Clinical features (any five) of cirrhosis of liver ....**

Ans. Ascites, painless hepatomegaly, palmer erythema, loss of libido, presence of mild-to-moderate jaundice

124. **Three commonly used medicines for acid peptic disease are...............**

Ans. H_2 receptor antagonists, proton-pump inhibitors, mucosal protective agents

125. **Prophylaxis of rheumatic fever is with ....**

Ans. Amoxicillin 50 mg/kg (max, 1 g) orally once daily for 10 days

126. **Three clinical features of acromegaly are...............**

Ans. Macroglossia, arthropathy, myopathy

127. **Complications of recurrent rheumatic fever episodes are...................**

Ans. Atrial fibrillation, mitral stenosis, mitral regurgitation and heart failure

128. **Three clinical features of acute nephritis are..............**

Ans. Hypertension, edema over face, oliguria

129. **Two common causes of agranulocytes are ....**

Ans. Use of cytotoxic drugs, irradiation

130. **Drugs of choice for epilepsy are (any two are ....**

Ans. Carbamazepine, phenytoin

131. **BMI (Body mass index) is calculated by formula is..................**

Ans. Weight + Height (kg/m^2)

132. **Four common causes of cervical lymphadenopathy are ....**

Ans. Syphilis, tuberculosis, herpes simplex infection, lymphoma

133. **Mention causes of strawberry gingivitis is ....**

Ans. Wegner's granulomatosis

134. **Mention causes of strawberry tongue is..................**

Ans. Scarlet fever

135. **Mention causes of bald tongue is..................**

Ans. Pernicious anemia

136. **Mention causes of cobblestoning of buccal mucosa is...............**

Ans. Crohn's disease

137. **Mention causes of diffuse melanin pigmentation is..................**

Ans. Physiologic oral pigmentation

138. **Mention causes of honeycomb plaques is ....**

Ans. Lupus erythematosus

139. **Mention causes of floating teeth is..................**

Ans. Cherubism

140. **The infection of syphilis is caused by..................**

Ans. *Treponema pallidum*

141. **Amoebiasis is caused by..................**

Ans. *Entamoeba histolytica*

142. **The name of fifth cranial nerve is..................**

Ans. trigeminal nerve

143. **In this.................. air and pus both are present in pleural cavity.**

Ans. Pyopneumothorax

144. **HIV infection is caused by..................**

Ans. HIV-1 or HIV-2 viruses

145. **The fluid in peritoneal cavity is called as..................**

Ans. Ascites

146. **Diphtheria is caused by..................**

Ans. *Corynebacterium diphtheriae*

147. **Dysphagia means the difficulty in ....**

Ans. Swallowing

148. **PEM means is..................**

Ans. Protein energy malnutrition

149. **The lower motor neuron type of facial palsy is also known as..................**

Ans. Bell's palsy

150. **The thiamine deficiency causes..................**

Ans. Wet beriberi and dry beriberi

151. **In mitral stenosis, the first heart sound is..................**

Ans. Loud

152. **TSH is.................. in hypothyroidism.**

Ans. Increased

153. **Peripheral neuropathy is the complication of ....**

Ans. Diabetes mellitus

154. **.................. bronchial breathing suggests the presence of cavity in the lung.**

Ans. Tubular

155. **Mumps is the infection of..................**

Ans. Parotid gland

156. **Matted lymph nodes are present in..................**
Ans. Tuberculosis

157. **The most common cause of endocarditis is..................**
Ans. Streptococci

158. **Normal serum creatinine level is less than............ mg.**
Ans. 1.5

159. **Bradycardia means the pulse rate less than .... beats per minute.**
Ans. 60

160. **Cerebral malaria is a complication of..................**
Ans. *Plasmodium falciparum*

161. **Halitosis is present in..................**
Ans. Oral cavity

162. **Megaloblastic anemia is caused by vitamin .... deficiency**
Ans. B_{12}

163. **Name of the 7th cranial nerve is.....................**
Ans. Facial nerve

164. **Presence of blood in urine.....................**
Ans. Hematuria

165. **Aspirin is.....................drug.**
Ans. Antiplatelet

166. **BCG vaccine is given to prevent.........................**
Ans. Tuberculosis

167. **HIV stands for.....................**
Ans. Human immunodeficiency virus

168. **In dengue,.....................(blood component) is decreased**
Ans. Platelet

169. **Diagnostic feature of diphtheria is .... on tonsil.**
Ans. Gray membrane

170. **Increase steroid intake can cause.................. Facies.**
Ans. Moon

171. **Massive proteinuria is found in.................. syndrome.**
Ans. Nephrotic

172. **Heart beat of less than 60 beats/min is called ....**
Ans. Bradycardia

173. **................. is an important sign of meningitis.**
Ans. Brudzinski's sign

174. **Malaria spread by bite of...................**
Ans. Infected *Anopheles* mosquito

175. **Sydenham's chorea is found in..................**
Ans. Rheumatic fever

176. **Erythropoietin is produced by..................**
Ans. Kidney

177. **Most common valve involvement in RHD is.....................**
Ans. Aortic valve

178. **Pellagra is caused by deficiency of vitamin ....**
Ans. B_3 or niacin

179. **Acromegaly is caused by.................... hormone excess.**
Ans. Growth

180. **Retinopathy is complication of............... and...............**
Ans. Diabetes mellitus and hypertension

181. **Warfarin causes prolongation of...................... time.**
Ans. Prothrombin

182. **In leukemia, ...count is decreased.**
Ans. RBC

183. **Cirrhosis is caused by hepatitis............... and .... virus.**
Ans. B and C

184. **To diagnose hypothyroidism, test used is................**
Ans. Thyroid function test

185. **Pulmonary tuberculosis is caused by...................**
Ans. *Mycobacterium tuberculosis*

186. **Three causes of stomatitis are...................**
Ans. Cheek bite, trauma due to dentures, viral infection, i.e., herpes, chemotherapy treatment for cancer

187. **Beriberi is due to deficiency of..................**
Ans. Vitamin B

188. **Causative organism of syphilis is.....................**
Ans. *Treponema pallidum*

189. **Drug of choice in anaphylaxis is.....................**
Ans. Epinephrine

190. **Cause of rheumatic fever is...................**
Ans. *Group A Treptococcus*

191. **Megaloblastic anemia is due to deficiency of ....**
Ans. Vitamin B12

192. **Syncope is due to....................**
Ans. Insuficient flow of blood to brain

193. **Features of nephrotic syndrome are...............**
Ans. Proteinuria, hypoalbuminemia, edema, hypercholes-trolemia

194. **Endocarditis is an inflammation of..................**
Ans. Endocardium

195. **Scurvy is due to deficiency of....................**
Ans. Vitamin C

196. **Three clinical features of portal hypertension** ....
Ans. Ascites, splenomegaly, esophageal varices, hematemesis

197. **Drug of choice in herpes zoster is**......................
Ans. Acyclovir

198. **Agranulocytosis means**................
Ans. Decrease in neutrophil number

199. **CPR means**...................
Ans. Cardiac pulmonary resuscitation

200. **Master of endocrine orchestra is**......................
Ans. Pituitary gland

201. **Three common cardiac arrhythmias are**..................
Ans. Atrial fibrillation, ventricular tachycardia, paroxysmal supraventricular tachycardia

202. **Three common heart diseases are**....................
Ans. Hear failure, heart valvular disease, congenital heart disease

203. **Body temperature is regulated by**.................
Ans. Hypothalamus

204. **Hyperhidrosis means**....................
Ans. Increased sweating

205. **Graves' disease is due to**....................
Ans. Hyperthyroidism

206. **Painful deglutition is known as**.....................
Ans. Dysphagia

207. **Beriberi is caused by deficiency of**..................
Ans. Vitamin B_1

208. **Molluscum contagiosum is a**...................illness.
Ans. Viral

209. **Tarry black stools are known as**..............
Ans. Melena

210. **Hemoptysis is blood in**.................
Ans. Cough

211. **Leprosy is caused by**.....................
Ans. *Mycobacterium lepare*

212. **Vitamin C deficiency causes**..............
Ans. Scurvy

213. **Dengue is caused by bite of**....................mosquito.
Ans. *Aedes*

214. **Peptic ulcer is caused by this organism**.....................
Ans. *H. pylori*

215. **Cholera is** ....borne disease.
Ans. Water

216. **In nephrotic syndrome, this is lost in urine**.................
Ans. Protein

217. **Hemophilia is treated with injection of**.................
Ans. Factor VIII or factor IX

218. **Fluconazole is a**.............. drug.
Ans. Antifungal

219. **Megaloblastic anemia is caused by**....................
Ans. Deficiency of vitamin B12

220. **Inhalational steroids are used in**...................
Ans. Bronchial asthma

221. **Enumerate four first-line antitubercular drugs** ....
Ans. Isoniazid, Rifampin, Ethambutol, Streptomycin

222. **Treadmill test is done to diagnose**....................
Ans. Effects of exercise on heart

223. **EEG is done in the neurological condition**....................
Ans. Seizure disorder

224. **Enteric fever is diagnosed by the test**..................
Ans. Widal

225. **CD4 counts are done for monitoring this disease**..................
Ans. AIDS

226. **Liver transplant is usually indicated for**..................
Ans. Liver failure

227. **Which drug should be avoided in dengue** ....?
Ans. Aspirin

228. **In primary hypothyroidism,**..................... **is increased.**
Ans. TSH

229. **Name of the fifth cranial nerve is**............
Ans. Trigeminal

230. **Malaria is caused by the bite of**....................
Ans. *Anopheles* mosquito

231. **Oral ulcer, cheilosis mainly caused by the deficiency of**..................vitamin.
Ans. B2 (Riboflavin)

232. **Diagnostic feature of diphtheria is**................... **on tonsil.**
Ans. Pseudomembrane

233. **Heparin is**................
Ans. Anticoagulant

234. **Carditis is feature of**...................
Ans. Rheumatic fever

235. **In AIDS,**...............count is decreased.
Ans. Lymphocyte

236. **Difficulty in deglutition is called as**.................
Ans. Dysphagia

237. **Fluid in pleural cavity is known as**...............
Ans. Pleural effusion

238. **Fever, neck rigidity, vomiting, headache are the features of**....................
Ans. Meningitis

239. In cirrhosis which organ is mainly involved ....

Ans. Liver

240. Heart rate >100 is known as.....................

Ans. Tachycardia

241. Gum hypertrophy is side effect of which anti-epileptic drug...................

Ans. Dilantin sodium

242. Swine flu is caused by.......................virus.

Ans. H1N1

243. Painless oral ulcer found in.................connective tissue disease.

Ans. Systemic lupus erythematosus

244. Tetany is caused by deficiency of............................

Ans. Calcium

245. Increase steroid intake can cause......................facies.

Ans. Moon

246. Blood in vomiting is called as....................

Ans. hemoptysis

247. Yellow discoloration of sclera is...............

Ans. Jaundice

248. Koilonychia is found in.....................deficiency anemia.

Ans. Iron

249. Rifampin drug is used in ....

Ans. Tuberculosis.

250. Treatment of choice in chronic renal failure is...........................

Ans. Hemodialysis

251. Complication of dental surgery in diabetes is......................

Ans. Delayed wound healing

252. Most common congenital cyanotic heart disease is.......................

Ans. Tetralogy of Fallot

253. Drug of choice for amoebiasis is..........................

Ans. Metronidazole

254. Exopthalmos is a sign of.................................

Ans. Hyperthyroidism

255. Most common cause of pleural effusion is ....

Ans. Pneumonia

256. Tuberculosis is caused by.........................

Ans. Mycobacterium tuberculosis

257. ....is common valvular heart disease.

Ans. Aortic stenosis

258. HIV epidemic will end up to year...........................

Ans. 2030

259. Herpes zoster is caused by...............................

Ans. Varicella zoster virus

260. Hemophilia is due to deficiency of ....

Ans. Factor VIII

261. Bell's palsy is a............................

Ans. Lower motor neuron facial palsy

262. Drug of choice for falciparum malaria is................. ....

Ans. Quinine

263. PEP drug of HIV is.................................

Ans. Emtricitabine

264. Increased TSH is found in..............................

Ans. Hypothyroidism

265. Fever, neck rigidity, vomiting and headache is features of.....................................

Ans. Meningitis

266. Koilonychia is a sign of.............................

Ans. Iron deficiency anemia

267. Tetany is caused by.......................

Ans. Deficiency of calcium

268. Hypertension is a............................killer.

Ans. Silent

269. Vitamin D deficiency causes...............................

Ans. Rickets

270. Trigeminal neuralgia is...........................

Ans. A disorder characterized by the *paroxysmal attacks of neuralgic pain with affection of one or more division of trigeminal nerve. The pain involves the third and second divisions equally and rarely the first.

271. Hepatitis B is prevented by.............................

Ans. Vaccination

VIVA-VOCE QUESTIONS FOR
PRACTICAL EXAMINATION

1. **Name the route of infection caused by Hepatitis E virus.**
Ans. Feco-oral route

2. **Name the hepatitis virus which spreads by parenteral route.**
Ans. Hepatitis B, C and D

3. **Name the carcinoma by which Epstein-Barr virus is associated with.**
Ans. Nasopharyngeal carcinoma

4. **Name the disease in which transaminase levels get raised.**
Ans. Myocardial infarction

5. **Which type of a virus is herpes virus?**
Ans. DNA virus

6. **Which type of virus is HIV virus?**
Ans. It is a retro virus

7. **What is the incubation period of hepatitis B virus infection?**
Ans. Incubation period is 1 to 6 months

8. **Name the cells which get decreased in AIDS.**
Ans. CD4, i.e., below 200/mm^3

9. **After how much duration of infection; the HIV is positive in the serological test?**
Ans. 8 weeks

10. **What is the most common route of transmission of AIDS?**
Ans. Heterosexual contact

11. **Name the test by which HIV is detected and also get confirmed.**
Ans. Polymerase chain reaction (PCR) method

12. **Name the most common neoplasm which occur in HIV positive homosexual males.**
Ans. Glomus tumor

13. **What do you mean by scrofula?**
Ans. Tuberculosis of lymph nodes

14. **What is the route of spread of tubercle bacilli in the military tuberculosis.**
Ans. Bloodstream

15. **Which physiological system does tertiary syphilis affects?**
Ans. Central nervous system

16. **Which type of ulcer is seen on the male genitalia in primary syphilis?**
Ans. A punched out ulcer

17. **Name the type of ulcers seen in amoebiasis.**
Ans. Flask-shaped

18. **In which disease does Koplik spots appear.**
Ans. Measles

19. **On which day rashes of measles occur.**
Ans. On fourth day

20. **Name the first sensation which becomes lost in leprosy.**
Ans. Temperature

21. **In which diseases does neutropenia occur.**
Ans. Typhoid, viral infection, protozoal infections, agranulocytosis

22. **In which age group does mumps commonly occur.**
Ans. Children

23. **Name the virus which leads to chickenpox.**
Ans. Varicella zoster virus

24. **In which disease, rose spots are seen.**
Ans. Typhoid

25. **Which disease of show bitot spots?**
Ans. Vitamin A deficiency

26. **What is lupus vulgaris?**
Ans. It is the cutaneous tuberculosis

27. **What is Pott's disease?**
Ans. It is the tuberculosis of spine

28. **What is Ghon's focus?**
Ans. It is the presence of subpleural focus in primary tubercular granuloma along with central caseation.

29. **What is Ghon's complex?**
Ans. It is the Ghon's focus along with regional lymph node involvement.

30. **Name the first earliest manifestation of tetanus.**
Ans. Trismus

31. **Name the neurotoxin which is released by *Clostridium tetani*.**
Ans. Tetanospasmin

32. **What is C-reactive protein?**
Ans. It is the acute phase reactant, which is synthesized by the liver, it opsonizes invading pathogens

33. **Name the drug of choice of trigeminal neuralgia.**
Ans. Carbamazepine

34. **What is the other name of trigeminal neuralgia?**
Ans. Tic douloureux, and Fothergill's disease

35. **What is parkinsonism?**
Ans. It is the disease caused by the depletion of pigmented dopaminergic neurons in substantia nigra, Lewy bodies and atropic changes in substantia nigra.

36. **Which is the drug of choice for partial and tonic clonic seizures?**
Ans. Phenytoin

37. **What do you mean by hematuria?**
Ans. It is the presence of RBCs in urine.

38. **Which is the earliest marker appearing in serum in acute hepatitis B infection.**
Ans. HBsAg

39. **What is tetany?**
Ans. It occur due to hypocalcemia and there is stridor due to spasm of glottis and not dysphagia.

40. **Which is the most common bacterial infection in general medical practice?**
Ans. Urinary tract infection

41. **Name the triad of symptoms in portal hypertension.**
Ans. Ascites, splenomegaly and esophageal varices

42. **In which disease, there is increase in level of SGOT.**
Ans. In liver disease

43. **Why icterus is more marked in sclera?**
Ans. It is white

44. **In which disease does dark color urine and clay stool is visible?**
Ans. Obstructive jaundice

45. **In which type of jaundice does conjugated and unconjugated bilirubin get raised?**
Ans. Hepatocellular jaundice

46. **Name the blood coagulation factor whose deficiency leads to classical hemophilia or hemophilia A.**
Ans. Factor VIII

47. **Name the blood coagulation factor whose deficiency leads to Christmas disease or hemophilia B.**
Ans. Factor IX

48. **Name the blood coagulation factor whose deficiency leads to hemophilia C.**
Ans. Factor XI

49. **Name the blood coagulation factor whose deficiency leads to vascular hemophilia or Von Willebrand disease.**
Ans. Von Willebrand factor

50. **Name the blood coagulation factor, whose deficiency leads to parahemophilia.**
Ans. Factor V

51. **As patients of hemophilia get operated what is given them to stop surgical bleeding?**
Ans. Factor VIII concentrate

52. **Name the disease in which bleeding time is prolonged.**
Ans. Thrombocytopenic purpura and Von Willebrand disease

53. **How much is the normal platelet count?**
Ans. It is 1.5 to 4 lakhs/cumm of blood.

54. **What is critical count of platelet?**
Ans. When count of platelet is below 40000/mm^3 it is critical count of platelet.

55. **What is thrombocytopenic purpura?**
Ans. It is the abnormal decrease in the count of platelets.

56. **Name the components, which get destroyed in the blood.**
Ans. WBC, clotting factors and platelets

57. **Name the diseases which constitute hemoglobinopathies.**
Ans. Sickle cell anemia and thalassemia

58. **Name the cardinal features of diabetic ketoacidosis.**
Ans. Hyperglycemia, hyperketonemia and metabolic acidosis

59. **What is osteoporosis?**
Ans. This is a disease which is characterized by decrease in the bone mass, microarchitectural destruction of bone and there is increased risk of fracture.

60. **Name the drugs used in treatment of osteoporosis.**
Ans. Bisphosphonates

61. **What is glycosylated hemoglobin?**
Ans. It gives an accurate and objective measure of glycemic control over period of weeks to months.

62. **What is Philadelphia chromosome?**
Ans. It is the chromosome, which is associated with chronic myeloid leukemia.

63. **What is the hallmark of obstructive lung disease?**
Ans. Decreased expiratory flow rate

64. **What is Kussmaul breathing?**
Ans. It is the increase in both the rate and depth of respiration in diabetic ketoacidosis and anemia.

65. **What is the surfactant?**
Ans. It reduces the surface tension and counteract tendency of alveoli to collapse.

66. **What is asthma?**
Ans. It is the disorder, which is characterized by the chronic airway obstruction as well as increased airway responsiveness which leads to wheeze, breathlessness, cough, chest tightness.

67. **What is emphysema?**
Ans. It is the pathological process in which there is permanent destructive enlargement of spaces distal to the terminal bronchioles.

68. **What is pleural effusion?**
Ans. It is the accumulation of serous fluid in pleural space.

69. **What is Ghon's focus?**
Ans. It is the unilateral solitary area of consolidation of tuberculus inside the pleura in lower part of upper lobe.

70. **Name the most common site for deep vein thrombosis.**
Ans. Calf vein

71. **What is lobar pneumonia?**

Ans. It is the radiological and pathological term which refers to the homogeneous consolidation of one or more lung lobes.

72. **What is bronchiectasis?**

Ans. It is the irreversible dilation of bronchi.

73. **What happens in the clubbing?**

Ans. In clubbing, the normal angle between proximal part of nail and skin become lost.

74. **What is hemoptysis?**

Ans. It is the coughing of the Frank blood.

75. **What is hematemesis?**

Ans. It is the vomiting of the altered blood.

76. **What is epistaxis?**

Ans. It refers to the bleeding from the nose.

77. **What is malena?**

Ans. It refers to the dark tarry colored stools.

78. **What do you mean by stable angina.**

Ans. When there is an imbalance between the myocardial oxygen supply and demand, stable angina occur.

79. **What do you mean by unstable angina.**

Ans. It is the rapidly worsening angina when patient is on rest.

80. **Name the most common congenital heart disease.**

Ans. Ventricular septal defect.

81. **Name the most common congenital cyanotic heart disease.**

Ans. Tetralogy of Fallot

82. **Name the most common cause of acute rheumatic fever.**

Ans. β-hemolytic streptococci

83. **Name the most common complication of subacute bacterial endocarditis.**

Ans. Thromboembolism

84. **What do you mean by tachycardia and bradycardia?**

Ans. When heart beat is more than 100 beats per min, it is known as tachycardia and when heart beat is less than 60 per min, it is known as bradycardia.

85. **What do you mean by cyanosis?**

Ans. Cyanosis is the bluish discoloration of nails because of increased amount of reduced hemoglobin in the capillary blood.

86. **What is coarctation of aorta?**

Ans. It is the narrowing of aorta at isthmus just below the origin of left subclavian artery.

87. **Name the most common heart valve involved in IV drug abuse.**

Ans. Tricuspid valve

88. **What is pulsus paradoxus?**

Ans. It is the dramatic fall in blood pressure due to inspiration.

89. **What do you mean by hypertensive urgency?**

Ans. It is defined as the marked elevation of blood pressure without the end organ damage.

90. **What do you mean by hypertensive emergency?**

Ans. It is defined as the marked elevation of blood pressure with end organ damage.

91. **Name the microorganism which leads to dental caries, infective endocarditis and atherosclerosis?**

Ans. *Streptococcus mutans*

92. **What do you mean by sinus tachycardia?**

Ans. It is the sinus rate of more than 100 beats per min.

93. **What do you mean by hemochromatosis?**

Ans. It is the condition in which total body iron get increased.

94. **What do you mean by bronze diabetes?**

Ans. It is the diabetes mellitus which is associated with hemochromatosis with iron deposit in skin, liver, pancreas and other viscera.

95. **What is gout?**

Ans. It is the condition which is characterized by the recurrent attack of acute inflammatory arthritis.

96. **Which node does act as a pacemaker?**

Ans. SA node

97. **What is pulsus alternans?**

Ans. It is the strong and weak beat which occur alternatively.

98. **What is pulsus bisferiens?**

Ans. It is the rapidly rising amd two time beating pulse whose both the waves are felt at the time of systole.

99. **What is pulsus tardus?**

Ans. It is felt in aortic stenosis.

100. **What is trilogy of Fallot?**

Ans. It is the combination of ventricular septal defect, pulmonary stenosis and overriding of aorta.

ADDITIONAL INFORMATION

Classification of AIDS

Class I	• Primary infection • Fever, arthralgia, myalgia • Occurrence of primary infection 2 to 4 weeks after an exposure. • Appearance of specific, Anti–HIV antibodies in serum (sero conversion) takes place later at 3 to 12 weeks (median 8 weeks)
Class II	Asymptomatic infection
Class III	Persistent generalized lymphadenopathy. It is defined as enlarged glands at more than two inguinal sites.
Class IV	AIDS syndrome • Characterized by opportunistic infection, tumors, etc. • Bacterial, viral and fungal infections • Candidiasis • Pneumocystis carinii pneumonia • Mycobacterium avium • Herpes simplex • Toxoplasmosis • Molluscum contagiosum • Tumors • Kaposi sarcoma • Non-Hodgkin's lymphoma • Oral hairy leukoplakia

CD4 Cell Count in HIV Associated Diseases

CD4 cell count	HIV associated diseases
Greater than 500 cells/mm^3	• Acute primary infection • Persistent generalized lymphadenopathy • Recurrent vaginal candidiasis
Less than 500 cells/mm^3	• Pulmonary tuberculosis • Pneumococcal pneumonia • Herpes zoster • Kaposi sarcoma • Oral hairy leukoplakia • Herpes zoster
Less than 200 cells/mm^3	• *Pneumocystis carinii* • Herpes simplex • Esophageal candidiasis • Miliary tuberculosis • Peripheral neuropathy • Cryptosporidium • Microsporidium
Less than 100 cells/mm^3	• Cerebral toxoplasmosis • Cryptococcal meningitis • Non-Hodgkin's lymphoma • HIV-associated dementia
Less than 50 cells/mm^3	Cytomegalovirus retinitis Disseminated *Mycobacterium avium* intracellulare

Various Serum Markers in Hepatitis–B and their Indications

Marker	Indication
HBsAg	Acute HBV infection
Anti-HBsAg	Previous vaccination
Anti-HBC (IgM)	Acute HBV infection
Anti-HBC (IgG)	Chronic HBV infection
HBeAg	Active replication
Anti-HBS Ag + Anti-HBC	Previous infection

Various Viruses and their Diseases

Name of virus	Name of diseases
Herpes simplex virus Type 1	• Primary stomatitis • Keratoconjunctivitis • Encephalitis • Herpes labialis • Herpetic whitlow
Herpes simplex virus Type 2	Genital infection
Cytomegalovirus	• Congenital infection • Pneumonitis • Retinitis • Disease in immunocompromised patients
Epstein Barr virus	• Infectious mononucleosis • Burkitt's lymphoma • Nasopharyngeal carcinoma • Oral hairy leukoplakia
Varicella zoster virus	• Chickenpox • Shingles
Herpes simplex virus - 8	Kaposi's sarcoma

Incubation Periods of Various Diseases

Infection	Incubation period
Short incubation period	
• Anthrax	2 to 5 days
• Diphtheria	2 to 5 days
• Scarlet fever	1 to 3 days
• Typhoid	5 days
• Cholera	2 to 3 hours
Intermediate incubation period	
• Measles	7 to 14 days
• Mumps	2 to 3 weeks
• Rubella	2 to 3 weeks
• Chickenpox	14 to 21 days
Long incubation period	
• Hepatitis-A	2 to 6 weeks
• Hepatitis-B	6 weeks to 6 months
• Tuberculosis	Months to years
• Leprosy	2 to 5 years

Complications of Various Diseases

Disease	Complications
Measles	Otitis media
Rubella	Polyarthritis
Mumps	Aseptic meningitis in children; Orchitis and Oophoritis
Streptococcal pharyngitis	Rheumatic fever
Typhoid	Paralytic ileus
Tetanus	Obstruction of airway

Various Diseases and their Rashes

Disease	Rash
Bromide poisoning	Presence of acne from rash
Chickenpox	Rash is seen on second day of infection which appears first on trunk. Lesions can be seen during all stages of development.
Eczema	Monk's cowl rash present on face and neck
Erythema infectiosum	Presence of slap cheek rash with circumoral pallor
Kwashiorkor	Presence of crazy pavement epithelium rash
Measles	Presence of maculopapular rash which begin at hairline and behind ears. It spread to neck, chest and over extrimities
Pellagra	Sunburn rash and necklace rash
Rubella	Maculopapular rash which start over face and move to trunk
Scarlet fever	Presence of diffuse erythematous rash which blanch on pressure. Rash disappear under 7 to 10 days
Smallpox	Face is involved and pitting scars are present.
Typhoid	As first week is over, rash is seen on upper abdomen. Rose red spots are present which are sparse, slightly raised and fade on giving pressure

Various Types of Spots in Diseases

Disease	Type of spot
Bitot's spot	Vitamin A deficiency. Seen in eye
Forchheimer spot	Rubella. Seen on soft palate
Koplick's spot	Measles. Seen on buccal mucosa
Rose spot	Typhoid. Seen on abdomen
Roth spot	Infective endocarditis. Seen in eye

Diseases Affecting Various Parts of Spinal Cord

Part of spinal cord affected	Name of disease
Disease affecting central part of spinal cord	Syringomyelia
Disease affecting posterior column	• Tabes dorsalis • Diabetic pseudotabes
Disease affecting posterolateral columns	• Subacute degeneration of spinal cord • Subacute myelo-optic neuropathy
Complete cord transaction	• Trauma • Multiple sclerosis

Various Nerve Lesions and their Effect on Oral Structures

Nerve lesion	Oral structure affected
Trigeminal nerve lesion	On protrusion jaw deviates towards side of lesion
Facial nerve lesion	Deviation of angle of mouth to opposite side
Vagus nerve lesion	On elevating the palate, uvula deviates to opposite side of lesion
Hypoglossal nerve lesion	On protrusion tongue deviates to side of lesion

Difference between Upper Motor Neuron Lesion and Lower Motor Neuron Lesion

Upper motor neuron lesion	Lower motor neuron lesion
This is the lesion of intracranial portion which is proximal to pontine nucleus.	This is the lesion of facial nerve or its nucleus inside the pons.
Etiology • Tumors • Cerebrovascular accidents • Demyelination	**Etiology** • Herpes zoster infection • Parotid tumor • Bell's Palsy • Lesion in cerebellopontine angle
Clinical features • Involvement of opposite side of face, i.e., contralateral side. • Involvement of lower half of face as in lower motor neuron palsy while upper part of face is spared.	**Clinical features** • Involvement of half of the face of same side of lesion. • Loss of muscles of facial expression • Furrowing of face is absent on same side. • Patient is inable to close the eye of same side. • Angle of mouth gets flattened. • Mouth gets deviated towards the opposite side.
Power is decreased	Power is much decreased
Clasp knife spasticity is present	Flaccidity is present
Atrophy is minimum	Atrophy is marked
Deep reflexes are exaggerated/brisk	Deep reflexes are absent or reduced
Clonus is present	Clonus is absent
Fasciculations are absent	Fasciculations are present
Reaction of degeneration in muscle is absent	Reaction of degeneration in muscle is present

Drugs of Choice in Seizures

Type of seizure	Choice of drug
In absence seizure	• Ethosuximide • Sodium valproate
For partial and tonic clonic seizure	Phenytoin
For myoclonic seizure	Piracetam

Various Lobes and their Functions

Name of lobe	Functions
Frontal	• Behavior • Emotional control • Language • Personality
Parietal dominant	• Language • Calculation
Parietal non-dominant	• Construction skill • Spatial orientation
Temporal dominant	• Auditory perception • Balance • Smell • Verbal memory
Temporal non-dominant	• Auditory perception • Balance • Smell • Non-verbal memory
Occipital	Visual processing

Various Blood Disorders with their Laboratory Predictions

Disease	Factor deficient	Bleeding time	Clotting time	Prothrombin time	Partial Thromboplastin time
Hemophilia A	VIII	Remain normal	Increases	Remain normal	Increases
Hemophilia B	IX	Remain normal	Increases	Remain normal	Increases
Hemophilia C	XI	Remain normal	Increases	Remain normal	Slightly prolonged
Para-Hemophilia	V	Remain normal	Increases	Increases	Increases
Von Williebr- and Disease	Von Willie- brand Factor	Increases	Remain normal	Remain normal	Slightly prolonged

Various Disorders and their Presenting Abnormality in Peripheral Blood Film

Name of disorder	Abnormality in peripheral blood film
Aleukemic leukemia	Circulating leukoerythroblasts
Hereditary spherocytosis	Microspherocytes
Infectious mononucleosis	Atypical lymphocytes
Malaria	Schuffner's dots

Megaloblastic anemia	Megaloblasts and hypersegmented neutrophils
After splenectomy	Howell-Jolly bodies, target cells, spur cells, spherocytes
Sepsis	Neutrophilia and Dhol bodies
Thalassemia	Microcytes, tear drops and target cells

Various Types of Breath in Various Diseases

Name of breadth	Name of disease
Acetone breadth	Diabetes mellitus
Alcoholic breadth	Alcoholics
Musty breadth	Hepatic coma
Uremic breadth	Renal disease

Features of Hypothyroidism and Hyperthyroidism

Hypothyroidism	Hyperthyroidism
Cold intolerance	Heat intolerance
Menorrhagia	Amenorrhea/Oligomenorrhea
Weight gain, goiter, hoarseness and tiredness	Loss of weight despite normal apetite, diffuse bruit
Bradycardia, hypertension, congestive heart failure	Tachycardia, dyspnea, atrial fibrillation
Dry skin, alopecia, myxedema	Pretibial myxedema, pigmentation, increased sweating
Depression, ache and pain, Carpal tunnel syndrome	Irritability, nervousness, tremor, emotional lability
Iron deficiency anemia and macrocytosis	Diplopia, Exophthalmos, lid retraction

Various Diseases and their Effect on Serum Calcium, Serum Phosphorus and Alkaline Phosphatase

Name of disease	Serum calcium	Serum phosphorus	Alkaline phosphatase
Chronic renal failure	Decrease	Increase	Normal
Hyperparathyroidism	Increase	Decrease	Increase
Hypoparathyroidism	Decrease	Increase	Normal
Osteoporosis	Normal	Normal	Normal
Rickets	Increase	Decrease	Increase

Diagnosis of Oral Glucose Tolerance Test

Interpretation	Fasting glucose	2 hours after glucose load
Fasting hyperglycemia	110 to 125 mg/dL	<140 mg/dL
Impaired glucose tolerance	<126 mg/dL	140 to 199 mg/dL
Diabetes	>126 mg/dL	>200 mg/dL

Various Volumes and Capacities in Obstructive and Restrictive Respiratory Diseases

Name of volume or capacity	Obstructive respiratory disease	Restrictive respiratory disease
Diffusion capacity	Normal	Decrease
Forced expiratory volume in 1 second/ Forced vital capacity	Decrease	Increase
Lung compliance	Unaffected	Decrease
Residual volume	Increase	Decrease
Total lung capacity	Normal to increase	Decrease
Vital capacity	Decrease	Decrease

Various Chest Deformities

Name of chest deformity	Features
Barrel-shaped chest	• Seen in chronic obstructive pulmonary disease. • In emphysema anteroposterior diameter of chest increase relatively to lateral diameter.
Kyphoscoliosis	• Abnormality in alignment of dorsal spine which is caused by polio, trauma or congenital abnormality. • This restricts and distorts the wall of chest.
Pigeon chest or pectus carinatum	• Seen in severe asthma during childhood • Seen in rickets also
Funnel chest or pectus excavatum	• In this body of sternum mainly lower end is curved backward. • It restrict chest expansion and decreases vital capacity

Various Important Points in Respiratory Diseases

Important point	Answer
Which is the most important cause of community acquired pneumonia	*Streptococcus pneumoniae* or *Pneumococcus pneumoniae*
Which are the microorganisms leading to atypical pneumonia	Chlamydia, mycoplasma, *Pneumocystis carinii*
Which are the most common microorganisms isolated from patients with nosocomial pneumonia	Gram-negative bacilli
Which is the drug of choice for atypical pneumonia which is caused by pneumocystis carini	Cotrimoxazole and Clindamycin
Which is the drug of choice for atypical pneumonia which is caused by mycoplasma	Erythromycin and clarithromycin
Which is the drug of choice for community acquired pneumonia	Clarithromycin and flucloxacillin
Which is the drug of choice for atypical pneumonia which is caused by Chlamydia	Doxycycline and erythromycin

Various Occupational Lung Diseases

Name of the occupational lung disease	Description
Anthracosis	Caused due to deposition of carbon particles
Asbestosis	Asbestos particles deposit in lungs
Bagassosis	Caused due to inhalation of sugarcane dust
Byssinosis	Caused due to deposition of cotton fiber particles
Farmer's lung	Caused due to mouldy hay

Various Diseases and Color of Pleural Fluid

Diseases	Color of pleural fluid
Acute pancreatitis	Blood stained
Malignant disease	Blood stained
Obstruction of thoracic outlet	Milky
Rheumatoid disease	Turbid
Tuberculosis	Amber

Various Diseases and Color of Sputum

Diseases	Color of sputum
Active bronchopulmonary infection	Mucopurulent
Bronchial carcinoma	Red
Bronchiectasis and lung abscess	Purulent
Anthracosis and aspergillosis	Black
Pneumonia	Rusty
Pulmonary edema	Pink frothy

Laennec's Division of Pneumonia Phases

Phases	Description
Stage of congestion	• Numerous bacteria • Dilation and congestion of capillaries in alveolar wall • Alveolar fluid consist of few red cells and neutrophils • In air spaces, there is presence of air spaces
Early consolidation or Red hepatization	• Replacement of edema fluid by fibrin • Marked cellular exudates of neutrophils by red cells • Less prominent alveolar septa
Late consolidation or Gray hepatization	• Dense fibrin strands • Red cells and neutrophils are disintegrated • Cellular exudates often separated from walls by thin clear space
Resolution	• Removal of fluid by expectoration which result in restoration of lung parenchyma • Enzymatic digestion of fibrin strands • Engorged alveolar capillaries

Different Types of Murmur

Systolic murmers	
Ejection systole	It is present in atrial systole, pulmonary systole and atrial septal defect
Pan systolic	It is present in mitral regurgitation, tricuspid regurgitation and ventricular septal defect. This is best heard at the time of expiration
Late systolic	It is present in coarctation of aorta and mitral valve prolapse
Diastolic murmurs	
Mid diastolic	It is present in mitral stenosis, tricuspid stenosis and atrial regurgitation. Its character is rough rumbling, localized, low pitch. It is heard in mitral region with bell placed in left lateral position. Sound increased during expiration and exercise
Early diastolic	It is present in aortic regurgitation and pulmonary regurgitation

Types of Endocarditis and Microorganisms Involved in Them

Name of Endocarditis	Microorganisms present
Subacute endocarditis	Streptococcus viridians group, i.e., S. sanguis, S. mitis, α hemolytic streptococci
Acute endocarditis	Staphylococcus aureus and Streptococcus pneumoniae
Postoperative endocarditis	Staphylococcus epidermidis

Various Markers in Myocardial Infarction

Condition	Markers present
Enzymes which are elevated in plasma during myocardial infarction	CPK-MD, SGOT, LDH
Proteins elevated in plasma during myocardial infarction	Troponin T and Troponin I
Preferred biochemical markers for myocardial infarction	Troponins and CPK-MB
Markers arise first in myocardial infarction	CPK-MB and Troponin T
Marker appear last in myocardial infarction	LDH

Important Questions with Answers in Cardiovascular System

Question	Answer
Which is the common congenital heart disease	Ventricular septal defect
Which is the common cyanotic congenital heart disease	Tetralogy of Fallot
What is the common cause of mitral stenosis, mitral regurgitation, aortic regurgitation and tricuspid regurgitation	Rheumatic valvulitis
Name the common cause of acute rheumatic fever	β hemolytic streptococci
Name the common complication of sub acute bacterial endocarditis	Thromboembolism
Name the valves involved in rheumatic phenomenon	Mitral and aortic valves
Which is the common valvular lesion following myocardial infarction	Mitral regurgitation
Which is the common cause of high output failure	Chronic anemia
Name the common disease complicated by sub acute bacterial endocarditis	Rheumatic mitral regurgitation
Name the common complication of prosthetic valve	Subacute bacterial endocarditis
Name the valve commonly involved in Ebstein anomaly	Tricuspid valve

Types of Fallot and their Features

Name of Fallot	Features
Trilogy of Fallot	Ventricular septal defect + Pulmonary stenosis + Overriding of aorta
Tetrology of Fallot	Ventricular septal defect + Pulmonary stenosis + Overriding of aorta + Right ventricular hypertrophy
Pentalogy of Fallot	Ventricular septal defect + Pulmonary stenosis + Overriding of aorta + Right ventricular hypertrophy + Atrial septal defect

Various Heart Sounds

Name of heart sound	Time	Mechanism	Abnormality
First or S1	Onset of systole	Due to closure of both mitral and tricuspid valves	• Loud sound is heard in anemia, pregnancy, thyrotoxicosis, mitral stenosis • Slow sound is heard in mitral regurgitation and heart failure
Second or S2	End of systole	Due to closure of both aortic and pulmonary valves	• Fixed wide splitting: Atrial septal defect • Variable splitting: Right and left bundle branch block
Third or S3	Early diastole, just after completion of S2	Due to abrupt cessation of rapid filling from ventricular valve	In heart failure and mitral regurgitation
Fourth or S4	End of diastole just before commencement of S1	Ventricular origin	• Absent in atrial fibrillation • Present in left ventricular hypertrophy

Waves or Segments of ECG

Wave or Segment	Onset	Cause
P wave	---------	Due to atrial depolarization
QRS complex	--------	Due to ventricular depolarization
T wave	---------	Due to ventricular repolarization
P-R interval	Onset of P wave to onset of Q wave	Due to atrial depolarization and conduction via AV node
QRS duration	Onset of Q wave and end of S wave	Due to ventricular depolarization
Q-T interval	Onset of Q wave and end of T wave	Due to electrical activity inside ventricles
ST segment	End of S wave and onset of T wave	-----------

Elements and Events of Jugular Venous Pressure

Element	Event
'a' wave	During right atrial contraction
'c' wave	Transmitted carotid impulse during onset of systole
'v' wave	Passive atrial filling against close tricuspid valve in systole
'x' descent	During right atrial relaxation and descent or displacement of tricuspid valve in systole
'y' descent	During opening of tricuspid valve and passive filling of right ventricle during start of diastole

Classification of Bone Density by Misch

Type	Hounsfield units	Type of bone
D1	>1250 units	Dense cortical bone
D2	850 to 1250 units	Thick porous cortical bone on crest and within coarse trabecular bone
D3	350 to 850 units	Thinner porous cortical crest and fine trabecular bone
D4	150 to 350 units	Almost no crestal cortical bone
D5	<150 units	Very soft bone with incomplete mineralization

Various Viruses and Infections Caused by them

Herpes simplex HSV Type I	• Encephalitis • Keratoconjunctivitis • Primary stomatitis • Herpes labialis • Herpetic whitlow
HSV Type II	• Infections of genitals
Cytomegalovirus	• Congenital infection • Retinitis • Pneumonitis • Disease in immunocompromised patients
Epstein barr virus	• Burkitt's lymphoma • Infectious mononucleosis • Oral hairy leukoplakia • Nasopharyngeal carcinoma
Varicella-zoster virus	• Chickenpox • Shingles
Human herpes virus-8	• Kaposi sarcoma

Diabetes Related Compliations

Vascular complications

♦ Microvascular: Retinopathy, neuropathy and nephropathy
♦ Macrovascular: Coronary heart disease, peripheral arterial disease, cerebrovascular disease.

Non-vascular Complications

♦ Gastroparesis
♦ Infections
♦ Skin changes
♦ Hearing loss

Various Signs of Aortic Regurgitation

♦ *Gerhard sign:* Pulsation of spleen in presence of splenomegaly
♦ *Landolfis sign:* systolic contraction and diastolic dilatation of pupil
♦ *Quinckes sign:* Capillary pulsations seen on the light compression of nail bed.
♦ *Becker:* Visible pulsation of retinal arterioles
♦ *Corrigans neck sign:* A rapid and forceful distention of arterial pulse with as quick collapse.
♦ *De mussets sign, duroziez sign:* Bobbing of the head with each heart beat and gradual pressure over the femoral artery leads to systolic and diastolic brut respectively.
♦ *Traubes sign:* Systolic and diastolic sounds heared over the femoral artery.
♦ *Muller sign:* Visible pulsation of uvula.
♦ *Mayne sign:* A decrease in diastolic blood pressure of 15 mm Hg when the arm is held above the head.
♦ *Rosenbch sign:* Presence of hepatic pulsations.
♦ *Hills sign:* Popliteal systolic blood pressure exceeding systolic branchial blood pressure by ≥60 mm Hg.

Various Causes of Pedal Edema

More common
♦ Heart failure
♦ Hypothyroidism
♦ Lymphedema
♦ *Medications:*
  • Calcium channel blockers
  • Steroids
  • NSAID
♦ Obesity

- Pulmonary hypertension
- Venous insufficiency

Less common

- Gastrointestinal disorders
- Anemia
- Liver disease
- *Medications:*
  - Diuretics
  - Estrogens
  - Thiazolidinediones
  - Renal disease
  - Venous outflow obstruction.

Smokers as per CDC National Health Interview Survey

- *Never smoker:* An adult who has never smoked, or who has smoked less than 100 cigarettes in his/her lifetime.
- *Former smoker:* An adult who has smoked atleast 100 cigarettes in his/her lifetime, but who had quit smoking at the time of interview. Previously known as "Past smoker".
- *Current smoker:* An adult who had smoked 100 cigarettes in his/her lifetime and who currently smoke cigarettes.
- *Somedays smoker:* An adult who had smoked 100 cigarettes in his/her lifetime, who smokes now, but does not smoke everyday. Previously called as an "occasional smoker".
- *Every day smoker:* An adult who had smoked 100 cigarettes in his/her lifetime, and who now smokes everyday. Previously called as "regular smoker".

Various Breadth Sounds

Name of the breadth sound	Explanation
Bronchial	• It is characterized by active inspiration because of passage of air into bronchi. Alveolar phase here is absent, expiration is also active which occupy same duration of time as inspiration. No rustling quality of sound. • Heard in patients with cavity, consolidation, partial collapse, pneumothorax and above level of pleural perfusion.
Bronchovesicular	• It is characterized by active inspiration because of passage of air into bronchi and alveoli which gives vesicular type of inspiratory sound. • At the time of expiration, there is increased resistance in airway because of spasm causing expiration to be active and prolonged.
Rales	• These are crackling sounds which originate in smaller bronchi or alveoli because of explosive opening of airways. • Inspiratory rales, e.g., chronic bronchitis, cavity, bronchiectasis, lung abscess and fibrosis.
Rhonchi/Wheeze	It is seen in COPD, asthma and bronchitis.
Stridor	• It is a loud inspiratory sound heard over the airways due to obstruction to respiratory tract. • Obstruction to larynx leads to laryngeal stridor. • Obstruction to trachea leads to tracheal stridor

Vesicular	It is characterized by the active inspiration because of passage of air into bronchi and alveoli followed without pause by passive short expiration. Sound is rustling because of passage of air through alveoli. Normal breadth sounds are vesicular.

Name of the Diseases and their Abnormality in Peripheral Blood Smear

Disease	Abnormality in peripheral blood film
Aleukaemic leukemia	There are circulating leukoerythroblastosis
Hereditary spherocytosis	Presence of microspherocytes
Thalassemia	Presence of microcytosis, tear drops and target cells
Megaloblastic anemia	Presence of megaloblasts and hypersegmented neutrophils
Infectious mononucleosis	Presence of atypical lymphocytes
Malaria	Presence of Schuffner's dots
Post-splenectomy	Howell jolly bodies, target cells, spur cells, spherocytes
Sepsis	Neutrophilia, shift to lift, dhole bodies

Various Smells and Disease Associated with them

Name of the smell	Disease associated
Rotten eggs smell	Indicative of volatile sulfur compounds producing halitosis
Sweet odor of dead mice	Liver insufficiency
Smell of rotten apples	Unbalance insulin dependent diabetes
Fish odor	Kidney insufficiency

Various Lobes and their Functions

Name of the lobe	Function
Frontal	• Behavior • Emotional control • Language • Personality
Parietal dominant	• Calculation • Language
Parietal non-dominant	• Construction skills • Spatial orientation
Temporal dominant	• Auditory perception • Balance • Smell • Verbal memory
Temporal non-dominant	• Auditory perception • Balance • Smell • Non-verbal memory
Occipital	Visual processing

General Surgery

GENERAL SURGERY

1. WOUND, SINUS AND FISTULA

Q.1. Write short note on lacerated wound.

(Sep 2008, 3 Marks)

Ans. Lacerated wound is an open wound.

- Lacerated wounds are caused by the blunt objects like fall on the stone or due to road traffic accident.
- Edges of lacerated wound are *jagged.
- Injury involves skin or subcutaneous tissue or sometimes deeper structures also.
- In the lacerated wound, there is crushing of tissue due to blunt nature of the object, which results in hematoma, bruising, or even necrosis of tissue.

Management

Ideal form of management of incised or lacerated wound is surgical inspection, cleaning, excision and closure, under appropriate anesthesia and *tourniquet in case of a limb.

- Wound must be thoroughly inspected to ensure that there is no damage to deep structure, or where encountered, there must be repaired.
- All dirt and foreign material must be removed.
- Excision of damage skin, wound margins and excision of devitalized tissue, such as muscle and fascia.
- After excision, wound is irrigated with antiseptic agent and then suturing must be done.
- There are precise suture placement technique for nerves, tendons and blood vessels.
- Muscles can be apposed in layer by mattress suture and fascia and subcutaneous fat should be apposed by interrupted absorbable suture to allow a firm platform for skin closure.
- On the face, fine nylon suture should be placed near to the wound margins, to be removed on the 5th day.

- An alternative to suturing is the application of adhesive tape strips.
- Systemic antibiotics should be given
- Injection tetanus toxoid for prophylaxis against tetanus.

Q.2. Enumerate the various types of surgical wounds and describe their management.

(Apr 2010, 15 Marks) (Apr 2008, 15 Marks)

Ans. Surgical wounds are classified into four categories according to possibility of infection occurring in them.

Management of Surgical Wounds

- Airways should be maintained.
- Bleeding of the patient should be controlled.
- IV fluids should be started.
- If it is an incised wound, then primary suturing is done after thorough cleaning.
- If it is a lacerated wound, then it is excised and primary suturing is done.
- If it is a crushed wound, there will be edema and tension in wound. In such cases, debridement of wound is done and all the devitalized tissues are excised, edema should subside in 5–6 days. Afterwards delayed primary suturing is done.
- If the wound is deep devitalized, debridement of wound is done and it is allowed to granulate completely. If wound is small secondary suturing is done. If wound is large, split skin graft is used to cover the defect.
- If wound is with tension, then fasciotomy is done.
- Antibiotics, fluid and electrolytic balance, blood transfusion, tetanus toxoid or anti-tetanus globulin injection.

Classification of Surgical Wounds

See Table below:

Wound class	Definition	Examples of typical procedure	Wound infection rate	Usual organism
Clean	Nontraumatic	Mastectomy	2%	Staphylococcus aureus
	Elective surgery	Vascular procedure		
	Gastrointestinal, respiratory or genitourinary tract not entered			
Clean contaminated	Respiratory Genitourinary or gastrointestinal tracts entered but minimal contamination	Gastrectomy, hysterectomy, cholecystectomy	<10%	Related to viscous entered
Contaminated	Open, fresh, traumatic wounds. Uncontrolled spillage from an unprepared viscous. Minor break in sterile technique.	Ruptured appendix, resection of unprepared bowel	15–30%	Depend upon underlying causes
Dirty	Open, traumatic dirty wounds. Traumatic perforated viscous. Pus in operative field	Resection of gangrene	40–70%	Depend upon underlying causes

---

Q1.   *Jagged = Unevenly cut or torn.

      *Tourniquet = Any constrictor used on an extremity to apply pressure over an artery and thereby control bleeding.

Q.3. Write short note on keloid.

(Feb 2013, 5 Marks) (Apr 2008, 5 Marks)

Ans. Keloid means like a claw.

♦ In keloid, there is defect in maturation and stabilization of collagen fibrils. Normal collagen bundles are absent.
♦ Keloid is common in blacks.
♦ It is more common in females.
♦ It is genetically predisposed, often familial and is very rare in Caucasians.
♦ Keloid continues to grow even after 6 months, may be for many years. It extends into adjacent normal skin. It is brownish black/pinkish black (due to vascularity) in color, painful, tender and sometimes hyperaesthetic; spreads and causes itching.
♦ Keloid may be associated with Ehlers–Danlos syndrome or scleroderma.
♦ When keloid occurs following an unnoticed trauma without scar formation is called as spontaneous keloid, commonly seen in Negroes.
♦ Some keloids occasionally become nonprogressive after initial growth.
♦ Pathologically, keloid contains proliferating immature fibroblasts, proliferating immature blood vessels and type III thick collagen stroma.
♦ Keloid is common over the sternum. Other sites are upper arm, chest wall, lower neck in front.

Precipitating Factors

♦ Negro race
♦ Tuberculosis patient
♦ Vaccination site.

Complications

♦ Ulceration
♦ Infection.

Treatment

♦ *Steroid injection:* Intrakeloidal triamcinolone, is injected at regular intervals, may be once in 7–10 days, of 6–8 injections. Its sequence is steroid injection—excision—steroid injection.
♦ Methotrexate and vitamin A therapy into the keloid.
♦ Compressive dressings with silicone gel sheets reduce the tendency of keloid to recur.
♦ Laser therapy can be given.
♦ Vitamin E/palm oil massage.
♦ Intralesional excision retaining the scar margin may prevent recurrence. It is ideal and better than just excision.
♦ Excision and skin grafting may be done.

Q.4. Classify wound and describes in detail the stage of wound healing. *(Sep 2006, 15 Marks)*

Ans. Wound is discontinuity or break in epithelium.

A wound is break in the integrity of skin or tissues often which may be associated with disruption of the structure and function.

Classification of Wound

♦ **Rank and Wakefield classification**
   • *Tidy wounds:*
      – They are wounds, such as surgical incisions and wounds caused by sharp objects.
      – It is incised, clean, healthy wound without any tissue loss.
      – Usually primary suturing is done. Healing is by primary intention.
   • *Untidy wounds:*
      – They are due to crushing, tearing, avulsion, devitalized injury, vascular injury, multiple irregular wounds, burns.
      – Fracture of the underlying bone may be present.
      – Wound dehiscence, infection, delayed healing are common.
      – Liberal excision of devitalized tissue and allowing to heal by secondary intention is the management.
      – Secondary suturing, skin graft or flap may be needed.
♦ **Classification based on type of wound**
   • Clean incised wound
   • Lacerated wounds
   • Bruising and contusion
   • Hematoma
   • Closed blunt injury
   • Puncture wounds and bites
   • Abrasion
   • Traction and avulsion injury
   • Crush injury
   • War wounds and gunshot injuries
   • Injuries to bones and joints, may be open or closed
   • Injuries to nerves, either clean cut or crush
   • Injuries to arteries and veins (major vessels)
   • Injury to internal organs, may be of penetrating or non-penetrating (blunt) types
   • Penetrating wounds.
♦ **Classification based on thickness of the wound**
   • Superficial wound
   • Partial thickness wound
   • Full thickness wound
   • Deep wounds
   • Complicated wounds
   • Penetrating wound.
♦ **Classification based on involvement of structures**
   • Simple wounds
   • Combined wounds.
♦ **Classification based on the time elapsed**
   • Acute wound
   • Chronic wound.
♦ **Classification of surgical wounds**
   • Clean wound
   • Clean contaminated wound
   • Contaminated wound
   • Dirty infected wound

Stages of Wound Healing

♦ **Epithelialization:** Epithelialization occurs mainly from the edges of wound by process of cell migration and multiplication. This is brought about by marginal basal cells. Thus within 48 hours entire wound is re-epithelialized.

♦ **Wound contraction:** It starts after 4 days and usually complete by 14 days. It is brought about by specialized fibroblasts. Because of their contractile elements, they are called as myofibroblasts. Wound contraction readily occurs when there is loose skin as in back.

♦ **Connective tissue formation:** Formation of granulation tissue is most important and fundamental step in wound healing. Injury results in release of mediators of inflammation. This result in increased capillary permeability, later kinins and prostaglandin act and play chemotactic role for white cells and fibroblasts. In first 48 hours, polymorphonuclear (PMN) leukocytes dominate. They play role of scavengers by removing dead and necrotic tissue. Between 3rd and 5th day, PMN leukocytes diminished but monocytes increases. By 5th or 6th day, fibroblasts appear which proliferate and eventually give rise to protocollagen, which is converted in collagen in presence of enzyme protocollagen hydroxylase; O_2, ferrous ion and ascorbic acid are necessary. The wound is fiber-gel-fluid system.

♦ **Scar formation:** Following changes takes place during scar formation:
  • *Fibroplasia and lying of collagen is increased.
  • Vascularity becomes less.
  • Epithelialization continues.
  • Ingrowth of lymphatics and nerve fiber takes place.
  • Remodeling of collagen takes place with cicatrization result in scar.

Q.5. Write short note on preauricular sinus.

(Sep 2006, 5 Marks) (Mar 2009, 5 Marks)

Ans. It is a congenital entity occurring due to imperfect fusion of the six tubercles which form ear cartilage.

Clinical Features

♦ It is seen since childhood.
♦ It can be unilateral or bilateral.
♦ Often swelling appears and apparently disappears repeatedly.
♦ Pain and discharge is common.
♦ It causes a cosmetic problem in young individual.
♦ Sinus opening may be seen at the root of the helix or on the tragus.
♦ Track is quiet deep running backwards, slightly upwards towards the helix. It usually ends blindly.
♦ Outer opening of the sinus often closed causing formation of a cystic swelling which contains fluid which is often infected.
♦ Preauricular sinus in no instance will communicate with the external auditory meatus.
♦ Bursting of this swelling leads into formation of ulcer like lesion.

Q4.   *Fibroplasia = Developing of fibrous tissue.

♦ Occasionally, multiple sinuses are seen.
♦ Opening of the sinus occurs in a small triangular area in front of the ear at the level of the tragus.
♦ Scarring is common around the opening due to repeated infection.

Investigations

♦ Discharge study should be done.
♦ Sinusogram is done to assess the track.
♦ MR sinusogram is beneficial.

Differential Diagnosis

♦ Cold abscess
♦ Sebaceous cyst

Treatment

♦ If sinus is infected antibiotics and drainage are required followed by excision when infection passes off.
♦ Under general anesthesia complete excision of tract is only recommended.

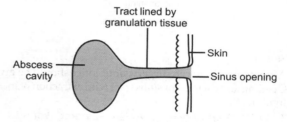

Fig. 1: Sinus.

Q.6. Write short note on mental sinus. *(Sep 2006, 5 Marks)*

Ans. It is a chronic infective acquired condition, wherein there is infection of roots of one or both lower incisor teeth forming root abscess which eventually tracks down between two halves of lower jaw in the midline presenting as discharging sinus on the point of chin at midline.

Clinical Features

♦ Usually painless discharging sinus in the midline on the point of chin.
♦ Often incisor infection may be revealed.
♦ Osteomyelitis of the mandible is the possible complication.
♦ Pus discharges through the sinus in center of chin.
♦ Patient present with recurrent swelling in submental region, which burst, open subcutaneously discharging mucus and seropurulent fluid at times.
♦ There is repeated history of swelling, discharge and healing which are the common presentations.

Investigations

♦ Dental X-ray is diagnostic.
♦ Discharge study should be done.

Differential Diagnosis

- Infected sebaceous cyst
- Tuberculous sinus
- Osteomyelitis

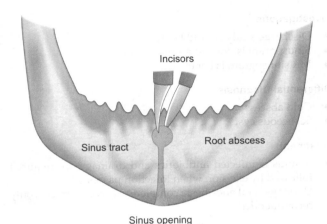

Fig. 2: Mental sinus.

Treatment

- After doing discharge surgery, antibiotics should be given.
- Opening and excision of sinus tract with extraction of incisor tooth/teeth.

Q.7. Write short note on crushed lacerated wound.

(Apr 2007, 10 Marks)

Ans.

- Crushed lacerated wound is caused by road accidents, or a machinery accidents.
- Crushing of the parts with lacerated skin, devitalization or crushing of the musculature is seen. These devitalized tissues must be excised in order to obtain proper healing.
- Damage to blood vessels and nerves with associated profuse bleeding is also observed. The bone or bones are shattered.
- The wound is highly contaminated.
- There can be loss of soft/hard tissue.

Treatment of Crushed Lacerated Wound

- Cleaning of wound
- Removal of foreign bodies
- Debridement
- Hemostasis
- Closure in layers, i.e., primary closure
- Dressing
- Prevention of infection
- Pain control
- Follow up.

Q.8. Write short note on sinus and fistula.

(Jan 2012, 5 Marks) (Dec 2007, 3 Marks)

Or

Write short answer on sinus and fistula.

(June 2018, 3 Marks)

Ans.

Sinus

It is a blind tract leading from the surface down into the tissues. It is lined with a granulation tissue.

Causes

- *Congenital sinus:* Preauricular sinus.
- *Acquired sinus:*
    - *Median mental sinus:* Occurs as a result of tooth abscess.
    - *Pilonidal sinus:* Occurs in the midline in the anal region.
    - *Osteomyelitis:* Gives rise to sinus discharging pus with or without bony spicules.

Fistula

It is an abnormal communication between the lumen of one viscus and the lumen of another (internal) or communication of one hollow viscus with the exterior, i.e., body surface (external fistula).

- *Examples of internal fistula:*
    - Tracheoesophageal fistula
    - Colovesical fistula
- *Examples of external fistula:*
    - Orocutaneous fistula due to carcinoma of the oral cavity infiltrating the skin
    - Branchial fistula
    - Thyroglossal fistula

Clinical Features of Sinus/Fistula

- Discharge from the opening of sinus
- No floor is present
- Raised indurated edge, indurated base and nonmobile
- Often sprouting granulation tissue over sinus opening.
- Bone thickening in osteomyelitis
- Surrounding skin may be erythematous and inflammatory. Bluish in tuberculosis, excoriated in fecal fistula, pigmented in chronic sinuses and fistulas.
- Induration is the feature of all chronic fistulas except tuberculosis.
- Discharge typical of the cause will be evident which will be obvious after applying pressure over surrounding area.
- Thickening of the bone underneath on palpation if sinus is adherent to bone or if there is osteomyelitis.
- Enlargement of regional lymph nodes is present.
- Sinus can be single or multiple.

Investigations

- Fistulogram/Sinusogram using ultra fluid lipiodol or water soluble iodine dye.
- Biopsy from edge for tuberculosis and malignancy
- X-ray of the involved part.
- Proctoscopy of fistula.
- Discharge for C/S, AFB, cytology, staining.
- CT sinusogram
- Probing gently with care
- Digital examination of rectum and proctoscopy in fistula in ano.

Treatment

♦ Cause should be treated
♦ Excision of sinus or fistula and specimen should be sent for histology
♦ Antibiotics, antitubercular drugs, rest and adequate drainage.

Q.9. Write short note on complication of furunculosis.
(Dec 2007, 3 Marks)

Ans. Furunculosis is the reoccurring presence of pus-filled sores, known as boils, on the skin.

Following are the complications of furunculosis:

♦ Carbuncles
♦ Cellulitis
♦ Gangrene
♦ Necrotizing fasciitis
♦ Hidradenitis suppurativa (infection in group of hair follicles)
♦ Lymphadenitis
♦ Cavernous sinus thrombosis.

Q.10. Describe wounds, their classification, wound healing and its treatment. *(Jan 2011, 10 Marks)*

Ans. *For description of wound, its classification and wound healing refer to Ans. 4 of same chapter.*

Treatment

♦ Wound is inspected and classified as per the type of wounds.
♦ If it is in the vital area, then:
  • The airway should be maintained.
  • The bleeding, if present, should be controlled.
  • Intravenous fluids are started.
  • Oxygen, if required, may be given.
  • Deeper communicating injuries and fractures, etc., should be looked for.
♦ If it is an incised wound, then primary suturing is done after thorough cleaning.
♦ If it is a lacerated wound, then the wound is excised and primary suturing is done.
♦ If it is a crushed or devitalized wound, then there will be edema and tension in the wound. So after wound debridement or wound excision by excising all devitalized tissue, the edema is allowed to subside for 2–6 days. Then, delayed primary suturing is done.
♦ If it is a deep devitalized wound, after wound debridement it is allowed to granulate completely. Later, if the wound is small secondary suturing is done.
♦ In a wound with tension, fasciotomy is done so as to prevent the development of compartment syndrome.
♦ Antibiotics, fluid and electrolyte balance, blood transfusion, tetanus toxoid (0.5 mL intramuscular to deltoid muscle), or anti-tetanus globulin (ATG) injection.
♦ Wound debridement (wound toilet, or wound excision) is liberal excision of all devitalized tissue at regular intervals.

Q.11. Write short note on complications of wounds.
(Dec 2007, 5 Marks)

Ans.

Complications of Wounds

♦ **Infection:** It is the most important complication which is responsible for delay in wound healing. Bacteria mainly remain endogenous. Based on pus culture and blood report antibiotics should be prescribed.
♦ **Scar:** Present due to infection.
♦ Hypertrophic scar and keloid formation due to altered collagen synthesis in wound healing process.
♦ Skin pigmentation
♦ **Marjolin ulcer:** As repeated breakdown of hypertrophic scar occur it becomes Marjolin's ulcer.

Q.12. Write short note on general factors affecting wound healing. *(Feb 2013, 5 Marks)*

Ans.

General Factors

General factors affecting wound healing are as follows:
♦ Age
♦ Malnutrition
♦ Vitamin deficiency (vitamin C, vitamin A)
♦ Anemia
♦ Malignancy
♦ Uremia
♦ Jaundice
♦ Diabetes, metabolic diseases
♦ HIV and immunosuppressive diseases
♦ Steroids and cytotoxic drugs

Age: In younger age group, wound healing is faster and better while in elderly healing is delayed due to reduction in collagen synthesis, epithelialization, growth factors and angiogenesis. But final scar will be excellent in old individuals.

Malnutrition and vitamin deficiency: Adequate vitamin, trace elements, fatty acids and proteins are essential for wound healing. Vitamin A deficiency affects monocyte activation, inflammatory phase, collagen synthesis and growth factor actions. Vitamin K deficiency affects synthesis of prothrombin (ll), factors VII, IX and X. vitamin E, being an antioxidant stabilizes the cell membrane. Vitamin C deficiency impairs collagen synthesis, fibroblast proliferation and angiogenesis; increases the capillary fragility and susceptibility for infection. Zinc is an essential cofactor for RNA and DNA polymerase; magnesium is a co-factor for synthesis of proteins and collagen; copper is a required co-factor for cytochrome oxidase.

Anemia: Hemoglobin less than 8% causes poor oxygenation of tissues preventing healing of the wounds.

Diabetes mellitus: In diabetic patients, wound healing is delayed because of several factors, such as microangiopathy, atherosclerosis, decreased phagocytic activity, proliferation of bacteria due to high blood sugar etc.

Metabolic causes: Obesity causes hypoperfusion, reduced microcirculation, increased wound tension, and hence prevents wound healing.

Jaundice and uremia: Jaundiced and uremic patients have poor wound healing because fibroblastic repair is delayed.

HIV and immunosuppressive diseases and malignancy: HIV and immunosuppression of varying causes, malignancy leads into poor wound healing.

Drugs: Steroids interfere with activation of macrophages, fibroblasts and angiogenesis in the early phase of healing (proliferative). Nonsteroidal anti-inflammatory drugs (NSAIDs) decrease collagen production. Chemotherapeutic agents used in oncology inhibit cellular proliferation, protein synthesis. Alcohol consumption decreases the phagocyte response and proinflammatory cytokine release; diminishes host response and thus increasing the infection rate.

Q.13. Write short note on hypertrophic scar.

(May/June 2009, 5 Marks)

Or

Write short answer on hypertrophic scar.

(Sep 2018, 3 Marks)

Ans. In hypertrophic scar, there is hypertrophy of mature fibroblasts. Blood vessels are minimum in this condition.

♦ It can occur anywhere in the body.
♦ Growth limits up to 6 months.
♦ Hypertrophic scar is limited to scar tissue and does not extend to normal skin.
♦ It is pale brown in color and is nontender.
♦ It is self-limiting.
♦ It is common in wounds crossing tension lines, deep dermal burns, wounds heal by secondary intension.

Complications

♦ Scar breaks repeatedly and cause infection and pain.
♦ After repeated breakdown, it may turn into Marjolin's ulcer.

Treatment

♦ It is controlled by pressure garments or often revision excision of scar and closure if required with skin graft.
♦ Triamcinolone injection is second line of therapy.

Q.14. Discuss briefly branchial fistula.

(May/Jun 2009, 5 Marks)

Or

Write in brief on branchial fistula. *(Aug 2011, 5 Marks)*

Or

Write short answer on branchial fistula.

(Apr 2019, 3 Marks)

Ans. Branchial fistula is commonly a congenital lesion.

♦ It is persistent precervical sinus between 2nd branchial cleft and 5th branchial cleft having opening in the skin at lower 1/3rd of neck on the inner margin of sternocleidomastoid muscle, often ends as a sinus just proximal to the posterior pillar of fauces behind tonsil which is also the site of inner opening when presents as a fistula.
♦ Fistula runs between the structures related to second and 3rd branchial arches. From external opening at skin below, it runs in subcutaneous plane to pierce deep fascia at level of thyroid cartilage; to travel between 2nd arch artery and third arch artery behind posterior digastric belly and stylohyoid; outer to stylopharyngeus, hypoglossal and glossopharyngeal nerves; perforates superior constrictor to reach the internal opening.
♦ Occasionally, acquired branchial fistula can occur due to rupture of or after drainage of infected branchial cyst or incomplete excision of the cyst tract. This type of fistula is located outside the skin at the level of upper third of sternomastoid muscle.

Clinical Features

♦ It is a persistent second branchial cleft with a communication outside to the exterior. It is commonly a congenital fistula.
♦ Occasionally, the condition is secondary to incised infected branchial cyst.
♦ Often it is bilateral.
♦ External orifice of the fistula is situated in the lower third of the neck near the anterior border of the sternomastoid muscle.
♦ Internal orifice is located on the anterior aspect of the posterior pillar of the fauces, just behind the tonsils.
♦ Sometimes fistula ends internally as blind end.
♦ It is common in children and early adolescent period. Its occurrence is equal in both sexes.
♦ External orifice is very small with a dimple which becomes more prominent on dysphagia with tuck in appearance.
♦ Discharge is mucoid or mucopurulent.

Treatment

Only surgical treatment is the choice.

♦ Under general anesthesia, methylene blue is injected into the tract. Probe is passed into the fistulous tract. Through circumferential/elliptical incision around the fistula opening, entire length of the tract is dissected until the internal orifice. Care should be taken to safeguard carotids, jugular vein, hypoglossal nerve, glossopharyngeal nerve and spinal accessory nerve. Entire tract should be excised.
♦ Step-ladder dissection is done using two parallel incisions one below at lower part another above at upper part of the neck, will make dissection easier and complete.

Q.15. Describe briefly primary and secondary healing of wounds. *(Jun 2010, 5 Marks)*

Ans.

Primary Healing of Wound

♦ In primary healing of wound, edges are approximated by surgical sutures.
  • In the initial phase, there will be formation of blood clot, which helps to hold the parts of the wound together.
♦ The tissue becomes edematous and an inflammatory process starts, with the infiltration of polymorphonuclear neutrophils (PMN) and lymphocytes into the area.
♦ The tissue debris collected in the wound are cleared either by the process of phagocytosis or by their lysis with the help of proteolytic enzymes, liberated by the inflammatory cells.
♦ Once the tissue debris are cleared, granulation tissue forms that replaces the blood clot in the wound, and it usually consists of young blood capillaries, proliferating fibroblasts, PMN and other leukocytes.
♦ The epithelium at the edge of the wound starts to proliferate and gradually, it covers the entire wound surface.
♦ Finally, the healing process is complete with progressive increase in the amount of dense collagen bundles and decrease in the number of inflammatory cells in the area.

Secondary Healing of Wound

♦ When the opposing margins of the wound cannot be approximated together by suturing, the wound fills in from the base with the formation of a larger amount of granulation tissue, such type of healing of the open wound is known as healing by "secondary intention" or "secondary healing".

- The secondary healing occurs essentially by the same process as seen in the primary healing, the only difference is that a more severe inflammatory reaction and an exuberant fibroblastic and endothelial cell proliferation occur in the later.
- In secondary healing, once the blood clot is removed, the granulation tissue fills up the entire area and the epithelium begins to grow over it, until the wound surface is completely epithelized.
- Later on, the inflammatory exudates disappear slowly and the fibroblasts produce large amounts of collagen.
- Most of the healing processes occurring due to secondary intention, result in scar formation at the healing site.

However, in the oral cavity these are rare.

Q.16. Write briefly on factors influencing wound healing.

(Aug 2011, 5 Marks)

Ans.

General Factors

General factors affecting wound healing are as follows:
- Age
- Malnutrition
- Vitamin deficiency (vitamin C, vitamin A)
- Anemia
- Malignancy
- Uremia
- Jaundice
- Diabetes, metabolic diseases
- HIV and immunosuppressive diseases
- Steroids and cytotoxic drugs

Age: In younger age group, wound healing is faster and better while in elderly healing is delayed due to reduction in collagen synthesis, epithelialization, growth factors and angiogenesis. But final scar will be excellent in old individuals.

Malnutrition and vitamin deficiency: Adequate vitamin, trace elements, fatty acids and proteins are essential for wound healing. Vitamin A deficiency affects monocyte activation, inflammatory phase, collagen synthesis and growth factor actions. Vitamin K deficiency affects synthesis of prothrombin (ll), factors VII, IX and X. Vitamin E, being an antioxidant stabilizes the cell membrane. Vitamin C deficiency impairs collagen synthesis, fibroblast proliferation and angiogenesis; increases the capillary fragility and susceptibility for infection. Zinc is an essential cofactor for RNA and DNA polymerase; magnesium is a cofactor for synthesis of proteins and collagen; copper is a required cofactor for cytochrome oxidase.

Anemia: Hemoglobin <8% causes poor oxygenation of tissues preventing healing of the wounds.

Diabetes mellitus: In diabetic patients, wound healing is delayed because of several factors, such as microangiopathy, atherosclerosis, decreased phagocytic activity, proliferation of bacteria due to high blood sugar, etc.

Metabolic causes: Obesity causes hypoperfusion, reduced microcirculation, increased wound tension, and hence prevents wound healing.

Jaundice and uremia: Jaundiced and uremic patients have poor wound healing because fibroblastic repair is delayed.

HIV and immunosuppressive diseases and malignancy: HIV and immunosuppression of varying causes, malignancy leads into poor wound healing.

Drugs: Steroids interfere with activation of macrophages, fibroblasts and angiogenesis in the early phase of healing (proliferative). Non-steroidal anti-inflammatory drugs (NSAIDs) decrease collagen production. Chemotherapeutic agents used in oncology inhibit cellular proliferation, protein synthesis. Alcohol consumption decreases the phagocyte response and proinflammatory cytokine release; diminishes host response and thus increasing the infection rate.

Local Factors

Local factors affecting wound healing are as follows:
- Infection
- Presence of necrotic tissue and foreign body
- Poor blood supply
- Venous or lymph stasis
- Tissue tension
- Hematoma
- Large defect or poor apposition
- Recurrent trauma
- X-ray irradiated area
- Site of wound
- Underlying diseases, such as osteomyelitis and malignancy
- Mechanism and type of wound-incised/lacerated/crush/avulsion
- Tissue hypoxia locally reduces macrophage and fibroblast activity

Wound infection: Infection prolongs inflammatory phase, releases toxins and utilizes vital nutrients thereby prevents wound epithelialization. The β-hemolytic streptococci more than 105 per gram of tissue prevent wounds healing. Formation of biofilms on the wound surface by microorganisms prevents wound healing.

Presence of necrotic tissue and foreign body: Necrotic tissue and foreign bodies, such as sutures cause intense inflammatory reaction and infection.

Poor blood supply: Improper blood supply to wound delays wound healing.

Tissue tension: It affects quantity, aggregation and orientation of collagen fibers.

Hematoma: It precipitates infection and delays wound healing.

Hypoxia: Hypoxia prevents fibroblast proliferation and collagen synthesis; it also promotes bacterial invasion into the wound.

Site of wound: Movement of wound area delays wound healing. e.g., wound over the joints and back has poor healing.

X-ray irradiated area: Both external radiotherapy or ionizing radiation cause endarteritis, fibrosis and delay in wound healing. Radiation may itself cause local tissue necrosis, sepsis and hypoxia.

Poor apposition: Poor apposition leads to the infection in the wound area which delays healing.

Q.17. Define and describe differentiating features of incised wound and lacerated wound.

(Jan 2012, 5 Marks)

Ans.

Incised wound	Lacerated wound
This wound is caused by sharp objects, such as knife, blade, glass, etc.	They are caused by blunt objects, such as fall on a stone or due to road traffic accidents
Edges of wound are sharp	Edges of wound are jagged
Contamination is less	Contamination is more
Does not involve deeper structures	Involve deeper structures
Crushing of tissue does not occur	Crushing of tissue is present
Only primary suturing is done	Wound excision and primary suturing is done

Q.18. Write short note on causes of delayed wound healing.

(Aug 2012, 5 Marks)

Or

Write short note on delayed wound healing.

(June 2015, 5 Marks)

Ans. *For the causes of delayed wound healing refer to Ans. 16 in detail.*

Q.19. Discuss the etiology, clinical features and management of wounds. *(Dec 2012, 10 Marks)*

Ans. A wound is the break in the integrity of skin or tissues often which may be associated with disruption of structure and function.

Etiology and Clinical Features

- Tidy wounds:
  - They are wounds, such as surgical incisions and wounds caused by sharp objects.
  - It is incised, clean, healthy wound without any tissue loss.
- Untidy wounds:
  - They are due to crushing, tearing, avulsion, devitalized injury, vascular injury, multiple irregular wounds, burns.
  - Fracture of the underlying bone may be present.
  - Wound dehiscence, infection, delayed healing are common.

Classification Based on Type of Wound

- Clean incised wound: It is a clean cut wound with linear edge.

- Lacerated wounds: The lacerated wounds are caused by the blunt objects, such as fall on the stone or due to road traffic accident.
  - The edges of lacerated wound are *jagged.
  - The injury involves skin or subcutaneous tissue or sometimes-deeper structures also.
  - In the lacerated wound there is crushing of tissue due to blunt nature of the object.
- Bruising and contusion: It is a minor soft tissue injury with discoloration and hematoma formation without skin break.
- Hematoma: Caused due to injury. It consist of reddish plasmatic fluid which can be aspirated and if it get infected, then pus is formed.
- Closed blunt injury.
- Puncture wounds and bites.
- Abrasion: Occurs due to shearing of skin where surface is rubbed off.
- Traction and avulsion injury.
- Crush injury: It is caused in wars, road traffic accidents, tourniquet.
  - Muscle ischemia is present.
  - Presence of gangrene and loss of tissue.
- War wounds and gunshot injuries.
- Injuries to bones and joints, may be open or closed.
- Injuries to nerves, either clean cut or crush.
- Injuries to arteries and veins (major vessels).
- Injury to internal organs, may be of penetrating or non-penetrating (blunt) types.
- Penetrating wounds.

Classification Based on Thickness of the Wound

- Superficial wound
- Partial thickness wound
- Full thickness wound
- Deep wounds
- Complicated wounds
- Penetrating wound.

Classification Based on Involvement of Structures

- Simple wounds
- Combined wounds.

Classification Based on the Time Elapsed

- Acute wound
- Chronic wound.

Classification of Surgical Wounds

- Clean wound
- Clean contaminated wound
- Contaminated wound
- Dirty infected wound

Management

- Wound is inspected and classified as per the type of wounds.
- If it is in the vital area, then:
  - The airway should be maintained.
  - The bleeding, if present, should be controlled.

Q19.   *Jagged = Unevenly cut or torn.

- Intravenous fluids are started.
- Oxygen, if required, may be given.
- Deeper communicating injuries and fractures, etc., should be looked for.
♦ If it is an incised wound, then primary suturing is done after thorough cleaning.
♦ If it is a lacerated wound, then the wound is excised and primary suturing is done.
♦ If it is a crushed or devitalized wound, then there will be edema and tension in the wound. So after wound debridement or wound excision by excising all devitalized tissue, the edema is allowed to subside for 2–6 days. Then delayed primary suturing is done.
♦ If it is a deep devitalised wound, after wound debridement it is allowed to granulate completely. Later, if the wound is small secondary suturing is done. If the wound is large a split skin graft (Thiersch graft) is used to cover the defect.
♦ In a wound with tension, fasciotomy is done so as to prevent the development of compartment syndrome.
♦ Vascular or nerve injuries are dealt with accordingly.
♦ Vessels are sutured with 6-zero polypropylene nonabsorbable suture material. If the nerves are having clean-cut wounds then it can be sutured primarily with polypropylene 6-zero or 7-zero suture material. If there is difficulty in identifying the nerve ends, or if there are crushed cut ends of nerves, then marker stitches are placed using silk at the site and later secondary repair of the nerve is done.
♦ Internal injuries has to be dealt with accordingly. Fractured bone is also identified and properly dealt with.
♦ Antibiotics, fluid and electrolyte balance, blood transfusion, tetanus toxoid, antitetanus globulin (ATG) injection.
♦ Wound debridement is liberal excision of all devitalized tissue at regular intervals until healthy, bleeding, vascular tidy wound is created.

Q.20. Enumerate differences between sinus and fistula.

(June 2014, 2 Marks)

Or

Write differences between sinus and fistula.

(Apr 2017, 2 Marks)

Or

Differences between sinus and fistula.

(Jan 2017, 10 Marks)

Or

Write differences between fistula and sinus.

(Feb 2019, 5 Marks)

Ans.

Sinus	Fistula
It is a blind track-lined by granulation tissue leading from an epithelial surface into the surrounding tissues	It is an abnormal communication between the lumen of one viscus to another or the body surface or between the vessels
Congenital cause is preauricular sinus	Congenital cause is branchial fistula, tracheoesophageal fistula, congenital AV fistula and umbilical fistula

Contd…

Contd…

Sinus	Fistula
Acquired causes are actino-mycosis, tuberculosis, pilonidal sinus, chronic osteomyelitis, medial, mental sinus	Acquired causes are traumatic, inflammatory and malignancy
In this a single epithelialized surface is involved	In this, two epithelialized surfaces are involved.
Extension of sinus is from cavity to cavity	Extension of fistula is from cavity to outside.
In oral cavity, sinus is a drainage passage through bone piercing the oral mucosa, e.g., in infections, such as periapical abscess	Fistula is a passage between two hollow cavities, e.g., oroantral fistula.
On inspection the location of various sinus is: • Preauricular sinus is at root of helix of ear • Sinus of TB is located at neck	On inspection the location of fistula is: • *Branchial fistula:* Sternomastoid anterior border • *Parotid fistula:* Parotid region
It cannot be surgically created.	It can be surgically created for therapeutic reasons.

Q.21. Describe pathophysiology of primary and secondary healing. Enumerate their clinical advantages and disadvantages in tabular form. List when assault becomes a cognizable offence. *(June 2014, 10 Marks)*

Ans. *Pathophysiology of primary and secondary healing means primary and secondary healing of wounds. For details, refer to Ans. 15 of same chapter.*

Assault is the act of creating apprehension of an imminent harmful or offensive contact with a person. Generally, cognizable offence means a police officer has the authority to make an arrest without a warrant and the police is also allowed to start an investigation with or without the permission of a court.

Following are the cognizable offences:
♦ All grievous hurts
♦ Simple hurt by dangerous weapon
♦ Murder
♦ Culpable homicide
♦ Causing death by rash or negligence act.
♦ Dowry death
♦ Abetment to suicide
♦ Attempt to murder
♦ Attempt to commit suicide
♦ Rape.

Primary healing	
Advantages	Disadvantages
Easy for the patient to manage the wound	Risk of wound infection
Rapid return of function of the wounded part final cosmetic result is superior	
Tissue heal closer to normal length	
Blood supply is restored soon	

Contd…

Contd…

Secondary healing	
Advantages	**Disadvantages**
Wound infection is virtually impossible	Daily dressing changes are required until the wound is healed, which may take some time, and the final result is a cicatrix that may be unsightly
	Final cosmetic result is poor. Granulation results in a broader scar
	Healing process can be slow due to presence of drainage from infection

Q.22. Enumerate causes for chronicity of sinus and fistula.
(Feb 2014, 3 Marks)

Ans. Following are the causes for chronicity of sinus and fistula:
♦ A foreign body or necrotic tissue underneath., e.g., suture, sequestrum.
♦ Insufficient or nondependent drainage
♦ Persistent obstruction in lumen, e.g., In fecal fistula, biliary fistula
♦ Lack of rest, persistent infection
♦ Wall become lined with epithelium and endothelium
♦ Dense fibrosis prevents contraction and healing
♦ Specific infections: Tuberculosis and actinomycosis
♦ Presence of malignant disease, post–irradiation.

Q.23. What is primary and secondary healing, advantage of one over other? What are the injuries that constitute cognizable offence in IPC? *(Apr 2015, 10 Marks)*

Ans. Primary healing: It occurs in a clean incised or surgical wound. Edges of the wound are approximated by sutures. Epithelial regeneration is more as compared to fibrosis. Wound healing takes place rapidly with complete closure. Scar will be linear, supple and smooth.

Secondary healing: It occurs in a wound with extensive soft tissue loss like in major trauma, burn, wound with sepsis. Healing by secondary intention occur slowly with fibrosis. This also leads to the formation of wide scar which is hypertrophied and contracted. This can also lead to disability.

For primary and secondary healing in details, refer to Ans. 15 of same chapter.

For advantages of one another, refer to Ans. 21 of same chapter.

Injuries that Constitute Cognizable Offence in IPC

Cognizable offence means an offence for which a police officer may arrest without a warrant.

Following are the cognizable offences:
♦ Murder (S.302)
♦ Causing death by rash or negligent act (S. 304A)
♦ Dowry death (S.304B)
♦ Abetment of suicide (S. 306)
♦ Attempt to commit suicide (S. 309)
♦ Causing miscarriage without women's consent (S. 313)

♦ Grievous hurt (S. 325, 326)
♦ Rape (S. 376)
♦ Theft (S. 379).

Q.24. Write short note on granulation tissue.
(Feb 2015, 5 Marks)

Ans. Granulation tissue is the proliferation of newer capillaries along with fibroblasts which are intermingled with RBCs and WBCs with thin fibrin cover over it.

Types of Granulation Tissue

Following are the types of granulation tissue:
♦ **Healthy granulation tissue**
  • It results in an healing ulcer.
  • It has got a sloping edge with serous discharge.
  • It bleeds on manipulation.
  • Skin graft takes well with healthy granulation tissue.
  • Healthy granulation tissue consists of 5Ps, i.e., pink, punctuate hemorrhage, pulseful, painless, pin head
♦ **Unhealthy granulation tissue**
  • This is pale in color with purulent discharge.
  • Floor of granulation tissue is covered with slough.
  • Its edges are inflamed and edematous.
  • It is a type of a spreading ulcer.
♦ **Unhealthy, pale, flat, granulation tissue**
  • It is seen in chronic nonhealing ulcer.
  • Exuberant granulation tissue
  • It occurs in sinus where granulation tissue protrude out of orifice of sinus as proliferating mass.
  • Mostly associated with retained foreign body in sinus cavity.
♦ **Pyogenic granuloma**
  • Here granulation tissue protrudes from an infected wound or ulcer bed and presents a well localized, red swelling which bleed on manipulation.
  • It is treated by surgical excision.

Q.25. Write briefly on cognizable offence.
(Jan 2016, 2 Marks)

Ans. Generally, cognizable offence means a police officer has the authority to make an arrest without a warrant and to start an investigation with or without the permission of a court.
♦ In cognizable offence, police has to record information in writing.
♦ The police can file a First Information Report (FIR) only for cognizable offences.
♦ In cognizable offences, police can start investigation without the order of magistrate.
♦ Cognizable offence is more serious and carry a sentence of 3 years or more.

Q.26. Write difference between hypertrophic scar and keloid. *(Feb 2019, 5 Marks) (Mar 2016, 3 Marks)*

Ans. Following are differences between hypertrophic scar and keloid:

Features	Hypertrophic scar	Keloid
Genetic predisposition	Yes	No
Site of occurrence	Chest wall, upper arm, lower neck, ear	Anywhere in the body, common in flexor surfaces
Growth	Continues to grow without time limit. Extends to normal skin	Growth limits for 6 months. Limited to scar tissue only
Treatment	Poor response	Good response to steroids
Recurrence	Very high	Is uncommon
Collagen synthesis	20 times more than normal skin (Type III thick)	3–6 times more than normal skin (Type III fine collagen)
Relation of size of injury and lesion	No relation. Small healed scar can form large keloid	Related to size of injury and duration of healing
Age	Adolescents, middle age	Children
Sex	Common in females	Equal in both
Race	More in blacks (15 times)	No racial relation
Structure	Thick collagen with increased epidermal hyaluronic acid	Fine collagen with increased alpha actin
Features	Vascular, tender, itching	Not vascular, non-tender, no itching
Natural history	Progressive	Shows regression
Problems	Hyperesthesia, ulceration	Not much

Q.27. Describe differentiating features of ulcer and wound.

(Jan 2017, 4 Marks)

Ans. Following are the differences between ulcer and wound:

Ulcer	Wound
An ulcer is break in the continuity of covering epithelium either skin or mucous membrane due to molecular death.	A wound is a break in the integrity of the skin or tissues often, which may be associated with the disruption of the structure and function
In ulcer, there is disruption or break in continuity of any lining may be skin, mucous membrane and others.	In wound, there is disruption of soft tissues or bone or internal organ
Ulcer is one of the type of a wound	Wound is a break in the integrity of the skin or tissues
In an ulcer, the primary tissue breakdown is internal	In a wound, the primary tissue breakdown is caused by a force originating from the external world
Ulceration on the skin is caused by pressure or circulatory problems that impede the blood flow in the area and the surrounding tissues.	Wound is caused by injury to the skin.

Contd...

Contd...

Ulcer	Wound
Ulcers seem more prone to host biofilms	Wounds seem less prone to host biofilms as compared to ulcer
Ulcers are often dressed once or twice weekly at walk-in clinics with complex dressing techniques.	Major wounds may require daily changes.
Mortality directly from ulcers is rare and therefore ulcers are of less clinical concern	Mortality directly from wounds is more and therefore wounds are of more clinical concern

Q.28. Describe primary and secondary wound healing. Discuss mechanism and various phases of wound healing.

(Apr 2017, 15 Marks)

Ans.

Primary Wound Healing

- It occurs in a clean incised wound or surgical wound.
- Wound edges are approximated with sutures. There is more epithelial regeneration than fibrosis. Wound heals rapidly with complete closure.
- Scar will be linear, smooth and supple.

Secondary Wound Healing

- It occurs in a wound with extensive soft tissue loss like in major trauma, burns and wound with sepsis.
- It heals slowly with fibrosis.
- It leads into a wide scar, often hypertrophied and contracted.
- It may lead into disability.
- Re-epithelialization occurs from remaining dermal elements or wound margins.

Mechanism of Primary Healing of Wound

- In primary healing of wound, edges are approximated by surgical sutures.
- In the initial phase, there will be formation of blood clot, which helps to hold the parts of the wound together.
- Within 10–15 minutes of injury vasodilatation occur and there is increased capillary permeability mediated by vasoactive substances released by damage cells and clot breakdown.
- The tissue becomes edematous and an inflammatory process starts, with the infiltration of polymorphonuclear neutrophils (PMN) and lymphocytes into the area.
- The tissue debris collected in the wound are cleared either by the process of phagocytosis or by their lysis with the help of proteolytic enzymes, liberated by the inflammatory cells.
- Once the tissue debris are cleared, granulation tissue forms that replaces the blood clot in the wound, and it usually consists of young blood capillaries, proliferating fibroblasts, PMN and other leukocytes.
- The epithelium at the edge of the wound starts to proliferate and gradually, it covers the entire wound surface.
- Finally, the healing process is complete with invasion of wound area by fibroblast on 3rd day, progressive increase

in the amount of dense collagen bundles on 5th day and formation of scar tissue with scanty cellular and vascular elements, some inflammatory cells and epithelialized surface by 4th week.

Mechanism of Secondary Healing of Wound

♦ When the opposing margins of the wound cannot be approximated together by suturing, the wound fills in from the base with the formation of a larger amount of granulation tissue, such type of healing of the open wound is known as healing by "secondary intention" or "secondary healing".

♦ The secondary healing occurs essentially by the same process as seen in the primary healing, the only difference is that a more severe inflammatory reaction and an exuberant fibroblastic and endothelial cell proliferation occur in the later.

♦ In secondary healing, once the blood clot is removed, proliferation starts, the granulation tissue fills up the entire area, contraction of wound occur and the epithelium begins to grow over it, until the wound surface is completely epithelized.

♦ Later on, the inflammatory exudates disappear slowly and the fibroblasts produce large amounts of collagen. Most of the healing processes occurring due to secondary intention, result in scar formation at the healing site. However, in the oral cavity scars are very rare.

Phases of Wound Healing

Inflammatory Phase

♦ It begins at the time of injury and lasts 2–4 days.
♦ This phase is characterized by hemostasis and inflammation.
♦ First hemostasis occurs and there is formation of the platelet plug.
♦ Injury to vascular tissue initiates the extrinsic coagulation pathway by releasing intracellular calcium and tissue factor that activate factor VII. Resulting fibrin plug leads to hemostasis which is aided by reflex vasoconstriction.
♦ Now this plug acts as a lattice for aggregation of platelets, this is the indication of early inflammatory phase.
♦ In inflammatory phase, both bacteria and debris are phagocytosed and removed, now the factors are released that cause the migration and division of cells involved in the proliferative phase.
♦ Collagen which were exposed at the time of wound formation causes activation of the clotting cascade (both the intrinsic and extrinsic pathways), initiating the inflammatory phase.
♦ Injured tissues, via activated phospholipase A, catalyze arachidonic acids to produce potent vasoconstrictors thromboxane A2 and prostaglandin 2-alpha, which is collectively known as eicosanoids. This initial response limits hemorrhage.
♦ After a short period of time capillary vasodilatation occurs which is due to local histamine release, and the cells of inflammation migrate to the wound bed.
♦ Chemical mediators, i.e., platelets release platelet-derived growth factor (PDGF) and transforming growth factor beta (TGF-β) from their alpha-granules attract neutrophils and macrophages.

♦ Now, neutrophils scavenge for bacteria and foreign debris and macrophages continue to release growth factors to attract fibroblasts and enter in the next phase of wound healing.

Proliferative Phase

♦ It starts from day 3 and last for 3–6 weeks. It overlaps with the inflammatory phase. This phase is characterized by angiogenesis, collagen deposition, granulation tissue formation, and epithelialization.

♦ Fibroblasts initiate angiogenesis, epithelialization, and collagen formation. Fibroblasts migrate inside from wound margins over the fibrinous matrix which is established during this phase.

♦ During first week, fibroblasts begin secreting glycosaminoglycans and proteoglycans, the ground substance for granulation tissue, as well as collagen, in response to macrophage synthesized FGF and TGF-β, as well as PDGF. Fibroblasts grow and form a new, provisional extracellular matrix (ECM) by excreting collagen and fibronectin.

♦ There is re-epithelialization of the epidermis, in which epithelial cells proliferate and reaches to the wound bed, providing cover for the new tissue. This process starts from the basement membrane, if the basement membrane remains intact, otherwise the process initiates from the wound edges.

♦ Fibroblasts produce mainly type III collagen in this phase.

♦ As fibrin clot and provisional matrix degrades, there is deposition of granulation tissue (ground substance, collagen, capillaries), which continues until the wound is covered. Granulation tissue formed during this phase, is important in secondary wound healing.

Remodeling Phase

♦ Remodeling continues for 6–12 months after injury.
♦ In this, there is maturation of collagen by cross linking and realignment of collagen fibers along the line of tension which is responsible for tensile strength of scar. Vascularity of wound reduces. Fibroblast and myofibroblast leads to wound contraction. Here type III collagen is replaced by type I collagen causing maturity of collagen. Ratio of type I collagen to type III collagen is 4:1.
♦ Early extracellular matrix consists of fibronectin and collagen type III; eventually it consists of glycosaminoglycans and proteoglycans; final matrix consists of type I collagen.
♦ Strength of scar is 3% in one week, 20% in 3 weeks, 80% in 12 weeks. Finally, matured scar is acellular and avascular.

Q.29. Classify wounds and discuss management of different types of wounds. *(Jan 2018, 20 Marks)*

Ans. *For classification of wounds refer to Ans. 4 of same chapter.*

Management of Different Types of Wounds

♦ Wound is inspected and classified as per the type of wounds.
♦ If wound is in the vital area, then:
  • The airway should be maintained.
  • The bleeding, if present, should be controlled.

- Intravenous fluids are started.
- Oxygen, if required, may be given.
- Deeper communicating injuries and fractures, etc., should be looked for.

♦ If it is an incised wound, then primary suturing is done after thorough cleaning.

♦ If it is a lacerated wound, then the wound is excised and primary suturing is done.

♦ If it is a crushed or devitalized wound there will be edema and tension in the wound. So after wound debridement or wound excision by excising all devitalized tissue, the edema is allowed to subside for 2–6 days. Then delayed primary suturing is done.

♦ If it is a deep devitalized wound, after wound debridement it is allowed to granulate completely. Later, if the wound is small secondary suturing is done. If the wound is large a split skin graft (Thiersch graft) is used to cover the defect.

♦ In a wound with tension, fasciotomy is done so as to prevent the development of compartment syndrome.

♦ Vascular or nerve injuries are dealt with accordingly. Vessels are sutured with 6-zero polypropylene nonabsorbable suture material. If the nerves are having clean, cut wounds it can be sutured primarily with polypropylene 6-zero or 7-zero suture material. If there is difficulty in identifying the nerve ends or if there are crushed cut ends of nerves then marker stitches are placed using silk at the site and later secondary repair of the nerve is done.

♦ Internal injuries (intracranial by craniotomy, intrathoracic by intercostal tube drainage, intra-abdominal by laparotomy) has to be dealt with accordingly. Fractured bone is also identified and properly dealt with.

♦ Antibiotics, fluid and electrolyte balance, blood transfusion, tetanus toxoid (0.5 mL intramuscular to deltoid muscle), or antitetanus globulin (ATG) injection.

♦ *Later definitive management is done with:* Wound debridement (wound toilet, or wound excision) is liberal excision of all devitalized tissue at regular intervals (of 48–72 hours) until healthy, bleeding, vascular tidy wound is created.

Q.30. Describe wound healing, factors affecting it and types of dressing. *(Sep 2018, 5 Marks)*

Ans. *For description of wound healing refer to Ans. 4 of same chapter.*

For factors affecting wound healing refer to Ans. 16 of same chapter.

Types of Dressing

Dressings are of two types:

♦ Dry dressings: It is used in clean, sutured operated wound. It should not be changed at regular intervals.

♦ Wet dressings: It is used in ulcers and wounds. Dressings are made wet by using jelly or sofra tulle sheets.

Q.31. Write short answer on sinuses. *(Apr 2019, 3 Marks)*

Ans. *For sinus in detail refer to Ans. 8 of same chapter.*

For preauricular sinus refer to Ans. 5 of same chapter.

For mental sinus refer to Ans. 6 of same chapter.

Q.32. Write short answer on fistula. *(Sep 2018, 3 Marks)*

Ans. It is an abnormal communication between the lumen of one viscus and the lumen of another (internal) or communication of one hollow viscus with the exterior, i.e., body surface (external fistula).

♦ *Examples of internal fistula:*
  - Tracheoesophageal fistula
  - Colovesical fistula
  - Cholecytoduodenal fistula
  - Rectovesical fistula

♦ *Examples of external fistula:*
  - Orocutaneous fistula due to carcinoma of the oral cavity infiltrating the skin
  - Branchial fistula
  - Thyroglossal fistula
  - Enterocutaneous fistula
  - Appendicular fistula

Causes of Fistula

♦ Congenital: Branchial fistula, tracheoesophageal fistula, congenital AV fistula, umbilical fistula.

♦ Acquired:
  - Traumatic
    – Following surgery: Intestinal fistulas
    – Following instrumental delivery or difficult labor
  - Inflammatory: Intestinal actinomycosis and tuberculosis
  - Malignancy: When the growth of one organ penetrates into the nearby organ.

For more details refer to Ans. 8 of same chapter.

2. ACUTE INFECTIONS

Q.1. Describe briefly Ludwig's angina.

(Nov 2008, 5 Marks)

Or

Write short note on Ludwig's angina.

(Aug 2012, 5 Marks) (Aug 2011, 5 Marks)
(June 2010, 5 Marks) (Apr 2010, 5 Marks)
(Dec 2009, 5 Marks) (Sep 2008, 3 Marks)
(Apr 2008, 5 Marks) (Mar 2007, 5 Marks)
(Apr 2007, 5 Marks) (Sep 2006, 6 Marks)
(Feb 2013, 5 Marks) (Apr 2017, 4 Marks)

Or

Define, describe clinical feature and principles of treatment of Ludwig's angina. *(Jan 2017, 5 Marks)*

Or

Write short answer on Ludwig's angina.

(June 2018, 3 Marks)
(Feb 2019, 3 Marks) (Apr 2019, 3 Marks)

Ans.

Ludwig's Angina

It is a rapidly progressive polymicrobial cellulitis of the sublingual and submandibular spaces involving the floor of the mouth and suprahyoid area on both sides of the neck.

The most common cause is dental infection of second or third molar teeth.

Precipitating Factors

- Tooth extraction
- Submandibular sialadenitis
- Trauma
- Peritonsillar abscess
- Upper respiratory infection
- Interventions like endotracheal intubation.

Predisposing Factors

- Diabetes mellitus
- Chemotherapy
- Oral cancer
- Alcohol
- Neutropenia.

Microscopic Organisms

- As Ludwig's angina is of dental origin streptococci or mixed oral flora are the most commonly reported microorganisms.
- Presence of staphylococci, *E. coli*, *Pseudomonas* and anaerobes including bacteroides and *Peptostreptococcus*, *Prevotella* species have also been isolated.
- Role of anaerobes as primary or synergistic organisms should not be omitted in the culture.

Clinical Features

- Presence of diffuse painful swelling with woody brawny induration of the mouth and anterior neck. Swelling is nonfluctuant but with redness and tenderness. Bilateral submandibular edema with marked tenderness on palpation at suprahyoid area with bull's neck appearance.
- Toxic features, such as fever, tachycardia, tachypnea is common.
- Difficulty in speech, earache, drooling of saliva and putrid halitosis.
- Involvement of connective tissues, muscles and fascial spaces but not glandular structures.
- Infection spread via fascial planes in continuity not by lymphatics; no lymph node enlargement.
- Edema of the tongue with pushing against palate (elevation) upwards and backwards causing airway obstruction, dysphagia and odynophagia.
- Stridor, respiratory distress and cyanosis may develop due to edema of tongue and larynx.

Investigations

- CT scan or MRI is useful to identify airway block, fluid collection and presence of gas.
- Ultrasound neck is simpler method to identify same.
- Total count, blood sugar, chest X-ray and often blood gas analysis (in severe cases) is done.

Differential Diagnosis

- Angioneurotic edema
- Sublingual hematoma
- Sialadenitis
- Lymphadenitis.

Complications

- Laryngeal edema can occur due to spread of inflammation to glottis submucosa via stylohyoid tunnel. It may require emergency tracheostomy to maintain the respiration.
- Mediastinitis due to spread of infection into mediastinum; aspiration pneumonia.
- Septicemia.
- Spread of infection into the parapharyngeal space leads to thrombosis of the internal jugular vein which may extend above into the sigmoid sinus which may be fatal.

Management

Main principles of treatment of Ludwig's angina are:
- Airway maintenance
- Parenteral antibiotics
- Surgical decompression of tissues
- Hydration of patient
- Removal of cause

Airway Maintenance

- Edema of the glottis is what leads to airway obstruction and death of the patient, if untreated. Maintaining a patent airway is thus of prime importance.
- Intubation is done by an experienced anesthetist.
- Bulging of the posterior pharyngeal wall makes intubation difficult. Perforation may lead to aspiration of pus, if an endotracheal tube is forced in blindly.
- A tracheotomy or cricothyroidotomy may be advisable. Tracheostomy is usually difficult because the anatomical landmarks on the neck are not easily identifiable with the swelling.

Parenteral Antibiotics

- Penicillin is the antibiotic of choice.
- Others, such as amoxicillin, cloxacillin may also be used.
- Metronidazole is given against anaerobic organisms.
- Gentamicin can also be given along with penicillin for coverage of *Pseudomonas*.

Surgical Decompression

- It is usually preferred under LA instead of GA. The main aim is to relieve the pressure within the tissues for the edema to reduce. Also, the pressure within the tissues compresses the blood vessels preventing the penetration of antibiotics in the area of interest. Thus decompression improves vascularity and potentiates the action of antibiotics.
- If there is pus, it provides a channel for the drainage of pus.
- Pus obtained from a drainage may be sent for culture and sensitivity testing.
- Decrease in edema reduces the respiratory embarrassment.
- Ethyl chloride spray may be used or LA may be injected locally in the area of incision.
- Bilateral submandibular incisions with a midline submental incision may be placed.
- Blunt dissection through the skin, superficial fascia, platysma, deep fascia and mylohyoid muscle is done to reach the sublingual space. The sublingual space may alternatively be drained intraorally by an incision in the floor of the mouth if the mouth opening is adequate.

♦ A drain is inserted through all these layers and stabilized.

♦ There may be no pus at all in most cases of Ludwig's angina. Pus may only be seen at later stages.

♦ A loose dressing is placed which is changed everyday after careful cleaning of the drain.

Hydration of the Patient

♦ Pyrexia and dysphagia may lead to dehydration of the patient.

♦ It is necessary to put the patient on IV fluids.

Removal of Cause

Once the patient is stabilized and the trismus relieved to an extent, the offending tooth may be removed.

Q.2. Write short note on carbuncle.   *(Aug 2012, 5 Marks)*
(Dec 2010, 5 Marks) (Nov 2008, 5 Marks)
(Apr 2007, 5 Marks) (Sep 2007, 2.5 Marks)
(Mar 2007, 2.5 Marks) (June 2015, 5 Marks)
(Apr 2017, 4 Marks)

Or

Write in short about carbuncle.   *(Jan 2018, 5 Marks)*

Or

Write brief notes on carbuncle.   *(Apr 2017, 2 Marks)*

Or

Define, describe clinical features and principles of treatment of carbuncle.   *(Jan 2017, 5 Marks)*

Ans. Word meaning of carbuncle is charcoal. It is caused by extensive infectious gangrene of the adjacent hair follicle and subcutaneous tissue by *Staphylococcus aureus*.

♦ It commonly occur in diabetic patients.

♦ Nape of neck is the most common site followed by back and shoulder region. Skin of the site is coarse and has poor vascularity.

Pathology

Flowchart 1: Pathology of carbuncle.

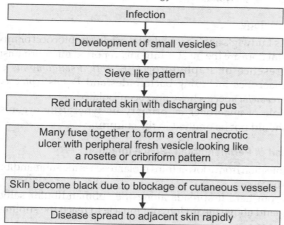

Clinical Features

♦ It is common in diabetics after 40 years of age

♦ Surface is red and looks like a red-hot coal.

♦ Symptom like fever with chills.

♦ Severe pain and swelling in nape of neck and back.

♦ Surrounding area is indurated.

♦ Skin on center of carbuncle softens and peripheral satellite vesicle appears, if rupture, discharge pus and give rise to cribriform appearance.

♦ Later development of large crateriform ulcer with center slough.

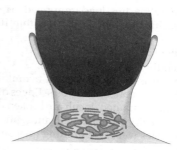

Fig. 3: Carbuncle of neck.

Complications

♦ Worsening in diabetic status resulting in diabetic ketoacidosis

♦ Extensive necrosis of skin overlying carbuncle. Hence, it is included under acute infective gangrene.

♦ Septicemia and toxemia.

Management

Principles of treatment of carbuncle are:

♦ Control of diabetes

♦ Parenteral antibiotics

♦ *Surgical management:*

  • Diabetes control preferably with injectable insulin.

  • Appropriate parenteral antibiotics are given till complete resolution occurs. Most strains of *Staphylococcus aureus* are sensitive to cloxacillin, flucloxacillin, erythromycin and some of the cephalosporins. However, methicillin resistant *Staphylococcus aureus* (MRSA) are resistant to the drugs mentioned above. They are sensitive only to expensive drug vancomycin which has to be given intravenously.

  • Improve general health of the patient

  • If carbuncle does not show any softening or if it shows evidence of healing, it is not incised. It can be left open to the exterior or saline dressings are applied to reduce edema. Complete resolution may take place within 10–15 days.

Q.3. Write the management of carbuncle.
(Dec 2012, 5 Marks)

Or

Discuss the management of carbuncle.
(Jan 2011, 5 Marks)

Ans.

Management of Carbuncle

♦ Diabetes control preferably with injectable insulin.

♦ Appropriate parenteral antibiotics are given till complete resolution occurs. Most strains of staphylococcal aureus are sensitive to cloxacillin, flucloxacillin, erythromycin and some of the cephalosporins. However, methicillin Resistant *Staphylococcus aureus* (MRSA) are resistant to the drugs mentioned above. They are sensitive only to expensive drug vancomycin which has to be given intravenously.

♦ Improve general health of the patient
♦ If carbuncle does not show any softening, or if it shows evidence of healing, it is not incised. It can be left open to the exterior or saline dressings are applied to reduce edema. Complete resolution may take place within 10–15 days.

Surgical Management

♦ Surgery is required when there is pus.
♦ Cruciate incision is preferred because of multiple abscesses and extensive subcutaneous necrosis. Edges of the skin flap are excised, pus is drained, loculi are broken down, slough is excised, and cavity is treated with antiseptic agents. Once wound granulates well, skin grafting may be required.

Q.4. Write short note on cold abscess.

(Feb 2013, 5 Marks) (Jan 2011, 5 Marks)

Or

Write in brief about cold abscess. *(July 2016, 5 Marks)*

Or

Write short answer on cold abscess.

(Sep 2018, 3 Marks)

Ans. Cold abscess is also known as tuberculous abscess.

Abscess shows no signs of acute inflammation, that is why it is known as cold abscess.

It occurs most commonly in the neck, groin, psoas region, paraspinal area.

Areas of Origin

♦ In tuberculous lymphadenitis, cold abscess is commonly seen in anterior triangle of neck.
♦ In tuberculosis of cervical spine, cold abscess occur in posterior triangle of neck.

Clinical Features

♦ It is more common in younger age group and is seen at any age.
♦ There is presence of swelling over the neck which is smooth, soft, fluctuant, nontender, nontransilluminant and have restricting mobility.
♦ With the change in posture when patient is seated, he support his head with hands and forearm. This is known as Rust's sign.
♦ There is also presence of evening fever, loss of weight, and appetite and anemia.
♦ Matted lymph nodes are present adjacent to cold abscess which are palpable.
♦ Abscess shows no signs of acute inflammation.

Investigations

♦ ESR is raised.
♦ Mantoux test is positive.
♦ Presence of anemia and lymphocytosis
♦ Chest X-ray shows pulmonary tuberculosis
♦ On FNAC epithelioid cells are seen.

♦ X-ray of neck in tuberculous cervical spine is done to identify reduced joint space, vertebral destruction and soft tissue shadow.
♦ MRI of cervical spine, US/CT scan of neck are needed for confirming the anatomical location and number of lesions.

Sequelae

♦ Secondary infection occurs in cold abscess, and it become tender.
♦ Collar stud abscess forms, as pressure increases in cold abscess it provide a way through deep fascia to reach subcutaneous plane and adhere to skin.
♦ Formation of sinus.
♦ Disease spread to other lymph nodes and organs.

Differential Diagnosis

♦ Branchial cyst and other cystic swellings of neck.
♦ Secondaries of neck lymph nodes
♦ Secondaries in cervical spine.

Treatment

♦ Antitubercular drugs should be started.
♦ Zig-zag aspiration by wide bore needle in nondependent aspiration of cold abscess.
♦ Excision of affected lymph nodes
♦ Cervical spine should be immobilized by plaster jacket for 4 months.
♦ Drainage using nondependent incision and later closure of wound without placing the drain.

Q.5. Describe the bacteriology of perimandibular space infection, its spread and management.

(Sep 2004, 20 Marks)

Ans. Submandibular, sublingual and submental spaces are collectively called as perimandibular space. When the perimandibular spaces are involved in an infection, it is known as Ludwig's angina.

Bacteriology

♦ As Ludwig's angina is of dental origin streptococci or mixed oral flora are the most commonly reported microorganisms.
♦ Presence of staphylococci, *E. coli, Pseudomonas* and anaerobes including bacteroides and *Peptostreptococcus, Prevotella* species have also been isolated.
♦ Role of anaerobes as primary or synergistic organisms should not be omitted in the culture.

Spread of Perimandibular Space Infection

♦ Infection from a lower third molar reaches the submandibular space.
♦ From here it spreads along the submandibular salivary gland above the mylohyoid muscle to reach the sublingual space.
♦ From one side of the sublingual space, it moves across the genioglossus muscles and reaches the sublingual space on the other side. It can then cross over the mylohyoid muscle and reach the opposite side submandibular space.
♦ The submental space gets involved via the lymphatics.

- Since it is a cellulitis and not an abscess, it does not remain localized but rapidly spreads along the fascial planes and tissue spaces.
- After involving the three spaces, the cellulitis spreads within the substance of the tongue posteriorly along the course of the sublingual artery in the cleft between the genioglossus and geniohyoid muscles. This reaches the region of the epiglottis producing edema and inflammation of the laryngeal inlet. This causes severe airway compromise.
- Also from the submandibular space it can pass along the investing layer of the deep cervical fascia all along the anterior aspect of the neck to the clavicle and continue into the mediastinum.
- Communication of the submandibular space with the pterygomandibular, masseteric and lateral pharyngeal spaces causes trismus and further enhances airway compromise.

Management

The main aspect of management is:
- Airway maintenance
- Parenteral antibiotics
- Surgical decompression of tissues
- Hydration of patient
- Removal of cause

Airway Maintenance

- Edema of the glottis is what leads to airway obstruction and death of the patient, if untreated. Maintaining a patent airway is thus of prime importance.
- Intubation is done by an experienced anesthetist.
- Bulging of the posterior pharyngeal wall makes intubation difficult. Perforation may lead to aspiration of pus, if an endotracheal tube is forced in blindly.
- A tracheotomy or cricothyroidotomy may be advisable. Tracheostomy is usually difficult because the anatomical landmarks on the neck are not easily identifiable with the swelling.

Parenteral Antibiotics

- Penicillin is the antibiotic of choice.
- Others, such as Amoxicillin, cloxacillin may also be used.
- Metronidazole is given against anaerobic organisms.
- Gentamicin can also be given along with penicillin for coverage of *Pseudomonas*.

Surgical Decompression

- It is usually preferred under LA instead of GA. The main aim is to relieve the pressure within the tissues for the edema to reduce. Also, the pressure within the tissues compresses the blood vessels preventing the penetration of antibiotics in the area of interest. Thus decompression improves vascularity and potentiates the action of antibiotics.
- If there is pus, it provides a channel for the drainage of pus.
- Pus obtained from a drainage may be sent for culture and sensitivity testing.
- Decrease in edema reduces the respiratory embarrassment.
- Ethyl chloride spray may be used or LA may be injected locally in the area of incision.

- Bilateral submandibular incisions with a midline submental incision may be placed.
- Blunt dissection through the skin, superficial fascia, platysma, deep fascia and mylohyoid muscle is done to reach the sublingual space. The sublingual space may alternatively be drained intraorally by an incision in the floor of the mouth if the mouth opening is adequate.
- A drain is inserted through all these layers and stabilized.
- There may be no pus at all in most cases of Ludwig's angina. Pus may only be seen at later stages.
- A loose dressing is placed which is changed everyday after careful cleaning of the drain.

Hydration of the Patient

- Pyrexia and dysphagia may lead to dehydration of the patient.
- It is necessary to put the patient on IV fluids.

Removal of Cause

Once the patient is stabilized and the trismus relieved to an extent, the offending tooth may be removed.

Q.6. Write short note on cellulitis. *(June 2015, 5 Marks)*
(May/June 2009, 5 Marks) (Mar 2008, 5 Marks)

Or

Define, describe clinical features and principle of treatment of cellulitis. *(June 2017, 5 Marks)*

Ans. Cellulitis is defined as spreading inflammation of subcutaneous tissues and fascial planes.

When a periapical infection fail to localize as abscess it leads to cellulitis where infection rapidly spreads through facial tissue planes diffusely.

Bacteriology

- Commonly due to *Streptococcus pyogenes* and other Gram-positive organisms. Release of streptokinase and hyaluronidase can cause spread of infection.
- Often gram-negative organisms, such as *Klebsiella, Pseudomonas, E. coli* are also involved.

Source of Infection

- Injuries
- Graze or scratch
- Snake bite.

Clinical Features

- Acute inflammatory lesions, such as cellulitis especially when situated in the dangerous area of the face are prone to spread in cavernous sinus.
- Patient is morbidly ill and may be delirious or semi-conscious.
- High grade fever, headache, nausea, vomiting are common.
- Local signs, such as edema of conjunctiva and eyelids, dilated and sluggishly reacting pupil may be present.
- Also there will be movements of eyeball due to involvement of 3rd, 4th and 6th cranial nerves.
- Proptosis and involvement of opposite side eye in advanced cases

♦ It spreads through loose connective and interstitial tissues of face.

♦ Tender regional lymph nodes may be palpable which signifies severity of infection.

♦ There is no edge, no pus, no fluctuation and no limit.

Complications

♦ Cellulitis can drain into an abscess which needs to be drained.

♦ *Necrotizing fasciitis:* Certain highly invasive strains of *Streptococcus pyogenes* can cause extensive necrosis of skin, subcutaneous tissue and may result in necrotizing fasciitis.

♦ *Toxemia and septicemia:* Streptococcal toxic shock syndrome can result if exotoxins are produced by microorganisms.

♦ Cellulitis can precipitate ketoacidosis, if patient is diabetic.

Treatment

Principles of treatment are:

♦ Bed rest and elevation of limb

♦ Dressing of glycerine magnesium sulfate

♦ Control of diabetes mellitus

♦ Parenteral antibiotic therapy

♦ Treatment of septicemia, if present

♦ Surgical decompression of tissues
  • Bed rest and elevation of limb or part to reduce edema, so as to increase the circulation and bandaging.
  • Glycerine magnesium sulfate dressing should be given which decreases edema of affected part.
  • Diabetes mellitus, if present is treated with insulin therapy.
  • Appropriate antibiotics, such as injection crystalline penicillin 10 lakh units IM or IV 6 hourly for 5–7 days or ciprofloxacin 500 mg BD is given.
  • Often patient may be in septicemia, patient in this condition is treated with higher antibiotics, critical care with fluid management, along with maintaining adequate urine output.

Surgical Management

♦ Since the tissues are tense and stretched, an incision and exploration of that area decompress or relieve pressure within the tissues.

♦ Decompressing the tissues help improve the vascularity, allowing better penetration of IV antibiotics to the area.

Q.7. Write short note on Cellulitis in oral cavity.

(Sep 2009, 5 Marks) (Feb/Mar 2004, 5 Marks)

Ans. Cellulitis is defined as spreading inflammation of subcutaneous tissues and fascial planes.

Etiology

Alpha-hemolytic streptococci is the etiologic agent.

Clinical Features

♦ Presence of widespread swelling, redness and tenderness without proper localization.

♦ Tissues become edematous and there is presence of induration. On palpation, tissues are firm to hard in consistency.

♦ Tissues get discolored and temperature rises up.

♦ Depending on the location and proximity of anatomical structures pus can evacuate on nose, maxillary sinus, vestibule, floor of mouth, infratemporal fossa and fascial spaces.

♦ Infection occurring in maxilla perforate outer cortical layer of bone above buccinators and leads to swelling of upper half of the face, and if infection perforates outer cortical plate in mandible below buccinators, there is swelling in lower half of face.

♦ If maxillary tooth is associated with infection, then redness can be seen in the eye.

Management

♦ *Surgical incision and drainage:* This is done if pus is diagnosed. In large cellulitis, an erythematous area is present which consists of pus near superficial surface. These areas are incised and drained under local anesthesia. Knife is inserted in most inferior portion of fluctuant area. A small sinus forceps is inserted in the wound and is opened in various directions, so that pus is drained. Rubber drain is placed in deepest area of the wound and suturing is done. Dressing is given.

♦ Broad-spectrum antibiotics should be given to the patient. Antibiotics of cephalosporin family are preferred.

♦ Associated tooth should be extracted.

Q.8. Describe pathology, clinical features, treatment and complications of alveolar abscess.

(Sep 2002, 15 Marks)

Or

Write briefly on alveolar abscess. *(Dec 2010, 5 Marks)*

Ans. Alveolar abscess occur due to spread of infection from root of tooth in periapical tissue. Initially it forms periapical abscess which later spreads through cortical part of bone into soft tissues and form an alveolar abscess.

Pathology

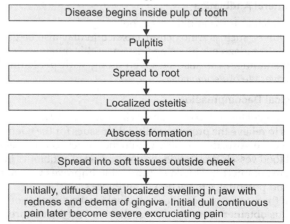

Flowchart 2: Pathology of alveolar abscess.

Clinical Features

♦ It is common odontogenic infection and constitutes 2% of apical radiolucencies.

- Due to acute abscess, there is pain in the affected tooth.
- Localized swelling and an erythematous change in overlying mucosa is present.
- The affected area of jaw may be tendered during palpitation.
- Pain aggravates during percussion and when pressure is applied with the opposing tooth.
- Application of heat intensifies pain, whereas application of cold relieves pain temporarily.
- Pus discharging sinus often develops on alveolar mucosa over the affected root apex and sometimes on skin overlying the jaw bone.
- Infection from acute periapical abscess often spread to facial spaces, leading to space infections.

Treatment

- Rest is given
- Incision and drainage under general anesthesia
- Appropriate antibiotics
- IV fluids to correct dehydration.
- Extraction of tooth at later period
- Extraction of sinus whenever required.

Complications

- Septicemia.
- Spread of infection into other spaces, such as parapharyngeal spaces; sublingual and submandibular spaces causing Ludwig's angina; edema of epiglottis and respiratory distress; spread to pterygoid space and along pterygoid muscles through emissary vein leading to cavernous sinus thrombosis; upper canine tooth abscess spreading to corner of eye causing angular vein thrombophlebitis which further progress to cavernous sinus thrombosis; submasseteric abscess.
- Lower incisor abscess can cause abscess in the chin and median mental sinus; chronic osteomyelitis of the jaw with discharging sinuses. Osteomyelitis is common in mandible —horizontal process near the mentum, presenting with pain, swelling, discharging sinuses, bone thickening, loose tooth and trismus. Sequestrum is commonly seen.

Q.9. Enumerate differences between cellulitis and erysipelas. *(June 2014, 2 Marks)*

Ans.

Cellulitis	Erysipelas
It is a spreading inflammation of subcutaneous and facial planes	It is a spreading inflammation of skin and subcutaneous tissue
It is caused by *S.pyogenes, Klebsiella, pseudomonas* and *E.coli*	It is caused by *S.pyogenes*
Bacteremia, septicemia and pyemia are present	Toxemia is present
Milian's ear sign is negative	Milian's ear sign is positive
Cutaneous lymphangitis with development of rose pink rash with cutaneous lymphatic edema is not seen	Cutaneous lymphangitis with development of rose pink rash with cutaneous lymphatic edema is predominant feature

Q.10. Write short note on erysipelas. *(Dec 2015, 5 Marks)*

Ans. Erysipelas is an acute spreading inflammation of skin and subcutaneous tissues which is caused by *Streptococcus pyogenes* and is associated with severe lymphangitis.

Infection occurs through small scratch or abrasion and spread rapidly causing toxemia.

Clinical Features

- It occurs commonly in children and old people.
- Sites commonly affected are face, eyelids, scrotum in infants and umbilicus.
- There is presence of rose pink rash with raised edge and its consistency is of button hole.
- Features of toxemia are commonly present.
- Redness of the lesion becomes brown and later on yellow with presence of vesicles.
- Discharge from the lesion is serous.
- There is presence of edema of face and orbit.
- When erysipelas occurs on the face it involves pinna since it is a cuticular lymphangitis. This is called as Milian's ear sign positive. This sign differentiate erysipelas from cellulitis.
- Tender, regional lymph nodes are palpable.

Complications

- Toxemia and septicemia.
- Gangrene of skin and subcutaneous tissue.
- Lymphedema of face and eyelids occur due to lymphatic obstruction.
- Abscess pneumonia and meningitis may develop.

Treatment

Injection crystalline penicillin 10 lakh units 6 hourly IM/IV for 5–10 days.

Q.11. Name etiological agent, pathognomic diagnostic feature and treatment (only modalities) of erysipelas.
(Jan 2017, 3 Marks)

Ans.

Etiological Agent

Beta hemolytic *Streptococcus pyogenes*

Pathognomic Diagnostic Feature

When erysipelas occurs on the face, it involves pinna because erysipelas is a cuticular lymphangitis. It is described as Milian's ear sign positive. This sign differentiates cellulitis of face from facial erysipelas. In cellulitis of face, pinna does not get involved because of close adherence of skin to cartilage.

Treatment (Only Modality)

Antibiotic treatment should be given.

Q.12. Describe differentiating features of acute abscess and cold abscess. *(Jan 2017, 4 Marks)*
Ans. See Table below:

Acute abscess	Cold abscess
No previous history of swelling	Soft, cystic fluctuant swelling
Throbbing pain is characteristic	Pain is not present
Extremely tender	No tenderness
Local rise in temperature is present	No local rise in temperature
Redness is present	No redness is seen
Pyogenic bacteria are nonspecific organisms	Tuberculous bacteria
For drainage, dependent incision is used	Nondependent incision is used
Suturing of wound is not done	Wound is sutured
Drain is placed	Drain is not placed.
It contains pus	It contain cheesy caseating material

Q.13. Define, describe clinical features and principles of treatment of cavernous sinus thrombosis.

(Jan 2017, 5 Marks)

Ans. In cavernous sinus thrombosis, the infection from maxillary anterior region is carried via facial, angular and nasofrontal veins to superior ophthalmic vein which enter cavernous sinus via superior orbital fissure. Veins of dangerous area of face are valveless and allow retrograde infection in form of cavernous sinus thrombosis.

Clinical Features

♦ Patient had sinusitis or midfacial infection which was manipulated.
♦ Prior to ocular symptoms, there is presence of headache, fever and malaise.
♦ Patient complaints of orbital fullness and pain along with visual disturbances.
♦ If the complaint remains untreated for long time symptoms get spread to other eye and it can be fatal too.
♦ Signs of venous congestion are present, i.e., chemosis, edema of eyelid, periorbital edema.
♦ Signs of retrobulbar pressure are present, such as exophthalmos, ophthalmoplegia and loss of corneal reflex
♦ Meningeal signs are present, i.e., nuchal rigidity, Brudzinski's sign.
♦ Systemic signs are also present, such as chills, fever, delirium and shock.

Principles of Treatment

♦ Aggressive antibiotic therapy with broad-spectrum antibiotics.
♦ Anticoagulation is done by giving heparin.
♦ Steroids are given to reduce the inflammation.
♦ Primary source of the infection should be eliminated.

Q.14. Describe etiopathogenesis and principle of management of acute pyogenic abscess.

(Apr 2010, 15 Marks)

Q14. *Abscess = An abscess is a localized collection of pus

Ans. Pyogenic *abscess: It is the most common form of an abscess, subcutaneous, deep or it can occur within the viscera, such as liver or kidney.

Etiopathogenesis

♦ It is usually produced by staphylococcal infections.
♦ Organism enters in the soft tissue by an external wound, minor or major.
♦ It can also be due to hematogenous spread from a distant focus like tonsillitis or carious tooth, etc.
♦ Pyogenic abscess can also be due to cellulitis.
♦ Following an injury, there is inflammation of the part brought about by the organisms.
♦ The end result is production of pus, which is composed of dead leukocytes, bacteria and necrotic tissue.
♦ The area around the abscess is encircled by fibrin products and it is infiltrated with leukocytes and bacteria. It is called pyogenic membrane.

Management

♦ *When pus is not localized:* Conservative treatment is needed.
  • Proper antibiotics and anti-inflammatory agents.
♦ *When pus is localized:* There is a golden rule that "Pus should be drained".
  • Incision and drainage (I and D) under general anesthesia.
    – General anesthesia is preferred because of the presence of infection.
  • *Infection:*
    – *Free or liberal incision:*
      » It is made on most prominent part to avoid damage to healthy tissue. Incision should be adequate for easy drainage of pus.
      » In case, if nerve and vessels are present below or surrounding abscess, incision parallel to nerve and vessel is given to avoid these structures.
    – *Incision by Hilton method:*
      » This method is used when there are plenty of nerves and vessels around the abscess cavity, which could be injured.
      » In this method, incision is given on most prominent and most dependent part.
      » A pair of artery forceps or sinus forceps is introduced and then the blades are open. It is swiped in the abscess cavity to break abscess loculi.
      » After removal of forceps, finger is introduced to explore the abscess cavity.
  • *Counter incision:* When prominent part is not the most dependent part, a counter incision is made on most dependent part facilitates pus drainage under gravity. In case of counter incision, sinus forceps is introduced on most dependent part rather than most prominent part.
  • *Drainage:*
    – A corrugated rubber drain is usually used for drainage of pus.
    – It is removed when pus stop coming out.
  • *Follow-up:* Proper antibiotics and analgesics are given.

Q.15. Describe the clinical features and treatment of acute abscess. *(Sep 2009, 5 Marks)*

Ans. *For treatment refer to Ans. 14 of same chapter.*

Clinical Features

- Fever with chills and rigors.
- Localized swelling which is smooth, soft and fluctuant.
- Pus is visible
- Throbbing pain and pointing tenderness
- Brawny induration around
- Redness and warmth with restricted movement around a joint
- Rubor (redness), Dolor (pain), calor (warmness), tumor (swelling) and functio laesa (loss of localized and adjacent tissue/joint function) are quite obvious.

Q.16. Write short note on various types of abscesses and Hilton's method of drainage. *(Jun 2010, 5 Marks)*

Ans. An abscess is a pathological thick-walled tissue cavity filled with necrotic tissue, bacteria and leukocytes caused by localized collection of purulent inflammatory tissue and suppuration from infection in a buried tissue, organ or confined space.

Types of Abscess

- *Pyogenic abscess:* It is produced by staphylococcal bacteria. Organism enter soft tissues by an external wound. It can be subcutaneous, deep or it can be a viscera.
- *Pyemic abscess:* It is due to pus-producing organisms in circulation. It is the systemic effect of sepsis. It commonly occurs in diabetics and patients receiving chemotherapy and radiotherapy.
- *Cold abscess:* It means an abscess with no signs of inflammation. It is caused due to tuberculosis.

Hilton's Method of Drainage

- Initially broad-spectrum antibiotics are started.
- Under general anesthesia or regional block anesthesia after cleaning and draping, abscess is aspirated and presence of pus is confirmed.
- Skin is incised adequately in line parallel to neurovascular bundle.
- Pyogenic membrane is opened using sinus forceps and all loculi are broken up.
- Abscess cavity is cleared of pus and washed with saline.
- A drain is placed
- Wound is not closed, wound is allowed to heal and granulate.

Q.17. Write short answer on Hilton's method of treatment. *(June 2018, 3 Marks)*

Ans. Hilton's method of treatment is the surgical method of draining the abscess.

For Hilton's method in detail refer to Ans. 16 of same chapter.

Q.18. Write difference between carbuncle and furuncle. *(Feb 2019, 5 Marks)*

Ans. Following are the differences between carbuncle and furuncle:

Carbuncle	Furuncle
It is an infective gangrene of skin and subcutaneous tissue caused by *Staphylococcus aureus*	It is an acute staphylococcal infection of a hair follicle with perifolliculitis which proceed to suppuration and central necrosis
It has diameter of several centimeter and its surface is red, angry looking like red hot coal.	It is 1 cm in size, tender, red papule or fluctuant nodule
It occurs at nape of neck and back	It occurs at areas of sweat and abrasion
They affect deep layers and can lead to scarring	They affect hair follicle and surrounding tissue
It starts as painful swelling with surrounding area indurated which results in necrosis of subcutaneous fat which give rise to multiple abscesses. These abscesses intercommunicate and open to exterior by multiple openings which are known as sieve like openings. This appearance is described as cribriform appearance and is pathognomic for carbuncle. Its end result is development of large crateriform ulcer with central slough.	It starts as painful indurated swelling which is surrounded by edema. After 1 to 2 days, it get soften in center and pustule develops which burst spontaneously discharging the pus. Necrosis of subcutaneous tissue produces green slough. Skin overlying boil undergo necrosis.
Cruciate incision is given due to multiple abscesses and extensive subcutaneous necrosis. Edges of skin flap are excised and pus is drained, loculi should be broken down and slough is excised.	Incision and drainage is done with excision of slough.

3. SPECIFIC INFECTIONS

Q.1. Describe clinical features and treatment of gas gangrene. *(Apr 2010, 5 Marks)*

Ans. It is highly fatal spreading infection caused by *Clostridium* organism, which result in "myonecrosis".

- It is also known as clostridial myositis, clostridial myonecrosis, and infective gangrene of muscles.
- The most common causing agent is *Clostridium welchii*.

Clinical Features

- Presence of features of toxemia, fever, tachycardia and pallor.
- Wound is under tension with foul smelling discharge.
- Color of skin is *khaki* brown due to hemolysis.
- Crepitus can be felt.
- Jaundice can be present and oliguria signifies renal failure.
- Most commonly the site affected are adductor region of lower limb and buttocks and subscapular region in upper limb.

Treatment

- Injection benzyl penicillin 20 lakh 4 hourly + injection metronidazole 500 mg 8 hourly + injection aminoglycosides or third generation cephalosporins or metronidazole.
- Fresh blood transfusion.

♦ Polyvalent antiserum 25,000 units given intravenously after a test dose and repeated after 6 hours.

♦ Hyperbaric oxygen is very useful.

♦ Liberal incisions are given. All dead tissues are excised and debridement is done until healthy tissue bleeds.

♦ Rehydration and maintaining optimum urine output.

♦ Electrolyte management is done.

♦ In severe cases, amputation has to be done as a life-saving procedure-stump should never be closed (Guillotine amputation).

♦ Often ventilator support is required.

♦ Once a ward or operation theater is used for a patient with gas gangrene, it should be fumigated for 24–48 hours properly to prevent the risk of spread of infection to other patients especially with open wounds.

♦ Hypotension in gas gangrene is treated with whole blood transfusion.

Q.2. Write short note on gas gangrene. *(Apr 2017, 4 Marks)*
(Dec 2010, 5 Marks) (May/June 2009, 5 Marks)

Or

Write in short about gas gangrene.
(July 2016, 5 Marks)

Or

Describe gas gangrene, etiology and management.
(Jan 2018, 10 Marks)

Or

How to diagnose and manage a case of gas gangrene? *(Aug 2018, 10 Marks)*

Ans.

Definition

This is a spreading infective gangrene of the muscles characterized by collection of gas in the muscles and subcutaneous tissue. As this condition is caused by *Clostridium* infection, it is also called '*Clostridium myonecrosis*'.

Etiology

Gas gangrene is caused by *Clostridium perfringens* which is the most common microorganism. Various other organisms causing gas gangrene are *Clostridium septicum, Clostridium oedematiens, Clostridium histolyticum*.

Predisposing Factors

♦ Contaminated, manured or cultivated soil, intestines are the sources. Fecal flora commonly contains clostridial organisms enters the wound; in presence of calcium from blood clot or silica (silicic acid) of soil, it causes infection.

♦ It is common in crush wounds, following road traffic accidents, after amputations, ischemic limb, gunshot wounds, war wounds. Injury or ischemia or necrosis of the muscle due to trauma predisposes infection.

♦ Anaerobic environments in the wound-initial infection with aerobic organism utilizes existing oxygen in tissues creating anaerobic environment to cause clostridial sepsis.

Types

♦ *Subcutaneous type:* This is a crepitant infection involving necrotic tissue, but healthy muscles are not involved.

Cellulitis is characterized by foul smelling, seropurulent infection of a wound.

♦ *Single muscles type:* The infection is limited to one muscle.

♦ *Group type:* The gas gangrene is limited to one group of muscles.

♦ *Massive type:* The gas gangrene involved almost the whole muscle mass of one limb.

♦ *Fulminating type:* In this condition, the gas gangrene spreads very rapidly even beyond the limb and is often associated with intense toxemia with high fatal rate.

Clinical Features

♦ Presence of features of toxemia, fever, tachycardia and pallor.

♦ Wound is under tension with foul-smelling discharge.

♦ Color of skin is *khaki* brown due to hemolysis.

♦ Crepitus can be felt.

♦ Jaundice can be present and oliguria signifies renal failure.

♦ Most commonly the site affected are adductor region of lower limb and buttocks and subscapular region in upper limb.

Investigations/Diagnosis

♦ X-ray shows gas in muscle plane or under the skin.

♦ Liver function tests, blood urea, serum creatinine, total count, PO_2, PCO_2

♦ CT scan of the part may be useful, especially in chest or abdominal wounds.

♦ Gram stain shows gram-positive bacilli.

♦ Robertson's cooked meat media is used which causes meat to turn pink with sour smell and acid reaction.

♦ *Clostridium welchii* is grown in culture media containing 20% human serum in a plate. Antitoxin is placed in one—half of the bacteria grown plate sparing the other half. Zone of opacity will be seen in that half of the plate where there is no antitoxin. In the other half part of the plate where there is antitoxin there is no opacity—Nagler reaction.

Complications

♦ Septicemia, toxemia

♦ Renal failure, liver failure

♦ Circulatory failure, disseminated intravascular coagulation, secondary infection.

♦ Death occurs in critically-ill patients.

Treatment/Management

♦ Injection benzyl penicillin 20 lakh 4 hourly + injection metronidazole 500 mg 8 hourly + injection aminoglycosides or third generation cephalosporins or metronidazole.

♦ Fresh blood transfusion.

♦ Polyvalent antiserum 25,000 units given intravenously after a test dose and repeated after 6 hours.

♦ Hyperbaric oxygen is very useful.

♦ Liberal incisions are given. All dead tissues are excised and debridement is done until healthy tissue bleeds.

♦ Rehydration and maintaining optimum urine output.

♦ Electrolyte management is done.

♦ In severe cases, amputation has to be done as a life-saving procedure-stump should never be closed (Guillotine amputation).

♦ Often ventilator support is required.

- Once a ward or operation theater is used for a patient with gas gangrene, it should be fumigated for 24–48 hours properly to prevent the risk of spread of infection to other patients especially with open wounds.
- Hypotension in gas gangrene is treated with whole blood transfusion.

Q.3. Write short note on cancrum oris.

(Sep 2006, 6 Marks) (Apr 2017, 5 Marks)

or

Write short answer on cancrum oris.

(Oct 2019, 3 Marks)

Ans. It is also called as NOMA or gangrenous stomatitis.

- It is a rapidly spreading gangrene of oral and facial tissues occurring in deliberated or nutritionally deficient person.
- The disease is caused by *Borrelia vincentii* and fusiformis bacteria.

Predisposing Factors

- *Low socioeconomic status:* It occurs in people of low socioeconomic status or in poverty.
- *Diseases:* In debilitated diseases, such as diphtheria, measles, pneumonia, scarlet fever, etc.
- *Injury:* In cases with mechanical injury.
- *Immunodeficiency state:* In AIDS
- *Poor oral hygiene:* This leads to growth of bacteria causing increase chances of infection.

Clinical Features

- It is seen chiefly in children mainly in malnourished children.
- The common sites are areas of stagnation around fixed bridge or crown.
- The commencement of gangrene is denoted by blenching of skin. Small ulcers of gingival mucosa spread rapidly and involve surrounding tissue of jaws, lips and cheeks by gangrenous necrosis.
- Odor is foul. Patient has high temperature during course of disease, suffers secondary infection and may die from toxemia.
- Overlying skin is inflamed, edematous and finally necrotic which results in formation of line of demarcation between healthy and dead tissue.
- In advanced stage, there is blue black discoloration of skin.
- As gangrenous process advances, slough appears and soon separated, leaving perforating wound in involved area.
- The large masses may be sloughed out leaving jaws exposed.

Treatment

- Systemic antibiotics should be given, i.e., high dose penicillin and metronidazole.
- Thorough nasogatric tube, high protein and vitamin rich diet should be given.
- Blood transfusion is given.
- Parenteral fluid is given.
- Wound irrigation and liberal excision of dead tissue is done.
- Later on patient require flap to cover the defect.

Characteristic	Primary syphilis	Secondary syphilis	Tertiary syphilis
Site	Chancre occurs at the site on entry of treponema. It occurs on lip, oral mucosa, and lateral surface of tongue, soft palate, tonsillary region, pharyngeal region and gingiva.	Mucus patches are present on tongue, buccal mucosa, pharyngeal region and lips. Split papules develop at commissure of lips.	Gumma can occur anywhere in jaw but more frequent site is palate, mandible and tongue.
Appearance	It has narrow copper-colored slightly raised borders with reddish-brown base in centers.	Mucus patches appears as slightly raised grayish white lesions surrounded by erythematous base. The split papules are cracked in middle giving "Split pea appearance".	Gumma manifests as solitary, deep punched out mucosal ulcer. Lesion is sharply demarcated and necrotic tissue at base of ulcer may slough leaving punched out defects.
Symptom	Intraoral chances are slightly painful due to secondary infection and are covered with grayish white film.	Mucus patches are painless but sometime mild-to-moderately painful.	In gumma, the breathing and swallowing difficulty may be encountered by the patient
Signs	White sloughy material is present	Snail tract ulcers and raw bleeding surfaces are present.	Perforation of palatal vault is present.
Tongue	Tongue lesion may be commonly seen on lateral surface of anterior two- thirds- or on dorsal surface and often there is enlargement of folate papilla.	Tongue gets fissured.	• Numerous small healed gumma in tongue results in series of nodules or sparse in deeper area of organ giving tongue an upholstered or tufted appearance. • Luetic glossitis: There is complete atrophy of papillary coating and firm fibrous texture is seen. • Chronic superficial interstitial glossitis: Tongue can involve diffusely with gumma and appear, large, lobulated and irregular shaped.
Lip	Extraoral lip chancre has more typical brown crusted appearance which can be multiple. Lower lip is mainly involved.	Split papule is a raised papular lesion which develops at commissure of lip and with fissure which separates upper lip portion from the lower lip portion.	Lip is not commonly involved.

Q.4. Describe various syphilitic lesion of lip and oral cavity. *(Sep 2002, 5 Marks)*

Or

Write short note on syphilis. *(Nov 2014, 3 Marks)*

Ans. *For syphilitic lesions of lips and oral cavity, refer to the table above.*

Diagnosis

- By blood tests using treponemal or nontreponemal tests.
- Nontreponemal tests are used initially and are VDRL and rapid plasma regain tests.
- Positive confirmation is required by treponemal test, such as *Treponema pallidum* particle agglutination or fluorescent treponemal antibody absorption test.

Treatment

- Primary and secondary syphilis are treated by injection procaine penicillin 10 lakh units IM for 14 days.
- In late syphilis, the above-mentioned treatment should be continued for 21 days.

Q.5. Write short note on actinomycosis.
(Feb 2013, 5 Marks) (Feb 2015, 5 Marks)
(Dec 2015, 5 Marks)

Or

Write short note on actinomycosis of jaw.
(Aug 2012, 5 Marks)

Or

Write brief answer on actinomycosis.
(Apr 2017, 5 Marks)

Ans. It is a chronic granulomatous suppurative disease which is caused by anaerobic or microaerophilic Gram-positive non-acid-fast branched filamentous bacteria.

The most common organism is *Actinomyces israelii, A. naeslundii, A. viscosus, A. odontolyticus* and *A. propionica.*

Clinical Types of Actinomycosis

- *Faciocervical:* It is the most common type. Infection spreads either from tonsil or from adjacent infected tooth. Initially, an induration develops. Nodules form with involvement of skin of face and neck. It softens and bursts through the skin as sinuses which discharge pus which contains sulfur granules (60%).
- *Thorax:* Lungs and pleura get infected by direct spread from pharynx or by aspiration. Empyema develops. Later chest wall nodules appear leading to sinuses with discharge (20%).
- *In right iliac fossa:* It presents as a mass abdomen with discharging sinus.
- Liver is infected through portal vein (honeycomb liver).
- *Pelvic:* Pelvic actinomycosis can occur due to intrauterine devices.

Pathogenesis

Organism enters through deeper plane of the tissue, causes subacute inflammation with induration and nodule formation. Eventually discharging sinus forms at the surface. Pus collected in a swab or sterile tube will show sulfur granules.

Predisposing Factors

- Trauma
- Presence of carious tooth
- Secondary bacterial invasion
- Hypersensitivity reaction.

Clinical Features

Cervicofacial Actinomycosis/Actinomycosis of Jaw/Faciomaxillary

- Its occurrence is more common in males.
- Disease may remain localized to soft tissues or spread to involve salivary glands, bone (maxilla or mandible), skin of face and neck. Most commonly involve area is submandibular region.
- Presence of trismus is there before formation of pus.
- The disease is characterized by presence of palpable mass which is indurated and is painless. Skin surrounding the lesion has wooden indurated area of fibrosis.
- Multiple subcutaneous nodules over bluish-colored skin of jaw.
- Nodules rupture resulting in multiple discharging sinuses.

Abdominal Actinomycosis

- It is more severe form of disease.
- Patient complains of fever with chills and vomiting.
- There is involvement of liver and spleen.
- On palpation, abdominal mass is felt which is the sign in diagnosis of disease.

Thoracic Actinomycosis

- Patient gives history of aspiration.
- Dry or productive cough, occasionally blood-streaked sputum, shortness of breath and chest pain.
- Sinus tracts are present with drainage from chest wall.

Pelvic Actinomycosis

- History of IUCD is present.
- Presence of lower abdominal discomfort, abnormal vaginal bleeding or discharge.

Investigations

- Pus under microscopy shows branching filaments.
- Gram's staining shows Gram-positive mycelia in center with Gram-negative radiating peripheral filaments. These clubs are due to host reaction which are lipoid material (antigen-antibody complex).
- Cultured in brain heart infusion agar and thioglycolate media.

Differential Diagnosis

- Chronic pyogenic osteomyelitis.
- Carcinomas at the site.
- Tuberculous disease

Management

- Penicillins are the drug of choice and should be given for longer period (6–12 weeks). If patient is allergic to penicillin doxycycline can be given.
- Antifungals are often given because it is fungal-like bacterium.
- Surgical debridement is occasionally required. Surgical therapy include incision and drainage of abscess, excision of sinus tracts and recalcitrant fibrotic lesions, decompression of closed space infections and the interventions which are aimed for relieving the obstruction.
- *Welsh regimen:* Injection amikacin 15 mg/kg IV daily for 21 days; such cycle is repeated 3 times at a gap of 15 days along with tablet trimethoprim (7 mg/kg)—sulfamethoxazole (35 mg/kg) daily for 6 months.

Q.6. Write the clinical features of faciomaxillary actino-mycosis. *(Sep 2000, 5 Marks)*

Ans. It is caused by the *Actinomycosis israelii.*

Clinical Features

- **Age:** Commonly seen in adult male.
- **Cause:** Dental plaque, calculus, gingival debris, bad carious tooth.
- **Location:** Submandibular region is the most frequent site of infection. Cheek, masseter region and parotid gland may also involve.
- **Symptoms:** Trismus is a common feature, before pus formation.

Signs

- The first sign of infection is the presence of palpable mass.
- Mass is painful and indurated.
- Multiple subcutaneous nodules over bluish-colored skin of jaw.
- The nodules rupture resulting in multiple discharging sinuses.
- The discharge contains sulfur granules.
- Lymph nodes are not involved.

Q.7. Write short note on candidal infection of oral cavity.
(Sep 1997, 6 Marks)

Ans. Oral candidiasis is most commonly associated with *Candida albicans.*

Oral Candidal Infection

- **Thrush (pseudomembranous candidiasis):**
  - It is superficial infection of upper layer of mucous membrane.
  - Characterized as creamy white removable plaque on the oral mucosa and caused by overgrowth of fungal hyphae mixed with desquamated epithelium and inflammatory cells.
  - This type of candidiasis may involve any part of the mouth or pharynx.
- **Acute atrophic candidiasis:**
  - It is also called as "Antibiotics sore mouth".
  - It appears as flat, red patches of varying size.

- It commonly occurs on the palate and the dorsal surface of the tongue.
- **Chronic hyperplastic candidiasis:**
  - It is called as "candidal leukoplakia".
  - It present as firm and adherent white patches in the oral mucosa.
  - It occurs on cheek, lip and tongue.
    Symptoms of oral candidal infection: Including burning mouth, problem in eating spicy food and change in taste.

Treatment

- Removal of the cause.
- *Topical treatment:* Clotrimazole, nystatin, ketoconazole or amphotericin in ointment or cream base, suspension.
- Systemic treatment:
  - Nystatin 250 mg TDS for 3 weeks.
  - Ketoconazole 200 mg once daily.
  - Fluconazole 100 mg once daily.
  - Itraconazole 100 mg may be used.

Q.8. Discuss etiology, clinical features, differential diagnosis and treatment of tetanus.
(Sep 2009, 15 Marks)

Or

Discuss the clinical features and management of tetanus. *(Dec 2010, 8 Marks)*

Or

Discuss etiology, clinical features and management of tetanus. *(July 2016, 10 Marks)*

Or

Discuss the management of tetanus.
(Dec 2012, 10 Marks)

Ans. Tetanus is also called as lockjaw.

It is a disease of nervous system characterized by intensive activity of motor neuron and resulting in severe muscle spasm.

Etiology

It is caused by anaerobic, gram-positive *Bacillus Clostridium tetani.*

Clinical Features

Symptoms

- Trismus is common.
- Presence of jaw stiffness and pain.
- Sweating is present and patient is anxious.
- Presence of headache, delirium and sleeplessness.
- Presence of dysphagia and dyspnea.

Signs

- Spasm and rigidity of all muscles.
- Hyperreflexia
- Respiratory changes due to laryngeal muscle spasm, infection, aspiration.
- Tonic-clonic convulsions.
- Abdominal wall rigidity often with hematoma formation.
- Severe convulsion may often lead to fractures, joint dislocations and tendon ruptures.

♦ Fever and tachycardia.
♦ Retention of urine (due to spasm of urinary sphincter), constipation (due to rectal spasm).
♦ Rarely features of carditis are seen due to involvement of the cardiac muscle, which is dangerous, as it often leads to cardiac arrest and death.
♦ Symptoms will be aggravated by stimuli-like light and noise.

Differential Diagnosis

♦ Strychnine poisoning
♦ Trismus due to various causes, such as dental, oral, tonsillar sepsis, oral malignancy.
♦ Meningitis
♦ Hydrophobia
♦ Convulsive disorders
♦ Epilepsy
♦ Symptomatic hyperactivity.

Treatment/Management

♦ Patient is admitted and isolated in a dark, quiet room.
♦ Antitetanus globulin (ATG), 3,000 units IM single dose is given.
♦ *Antitetanus serum (ATS):* When ATG is not available or when patient cannot afford, after IV test dose (1,000 units of ATS), full dose is given, i.e., 1,00,000 units, half of it is given IM and half of it is given IV.
♦ Wound debridement, drainage of pus, injection of ATG 250–500 units locally to reduce the toxin effect.
♦ Ryle's tube has to be passed, initially to decompress, so as to prevent aspiration, but later for feeding purpose.
♦ Catheterization should be done.
♦ IV fluids and electrolyte balance has to be maintained.
♦ Tetanus toxoid should be given as disease will not give immunity against further infections. To start first dose, second dose after one month, third dose after six months. Aluminum phosphate absorbed tetanus toxoid 0.5 mL is injected into deltoid muscle. Booster dose should be given every 4 years or after any significant trauma. In patients who have not been immunized earlier it needs 30 days to to develop antibody after tetanus toxoid injection.
♦ IV diazepam 20 mg 4th or 6th hourly. Dose is adjusted depending on severity and convulsions.
♦ IV phenobarbitone 30 mg 6th hourly.
♦ IV chlorpromazine 25 mg 6th hourly.
♦ Injection crystalline penicillin 20 lakh 6th hourly and injection gentamicin and metronidazole to prevent secondary infection.
♦ Regular suction and clearance of respiratory tract.
♦ Nasal oxygen is given.
♦ In severe cases, patient is curarised and placed in ventilator.
♦ Endotracheal intubation or tracheostomy are often life-saving procedures.
♦ *Good nursing care:* Change of position, prevention of bedsores, prevention of DPT.
♦ Chest (respiratory) physiotherapy during recovery period.
♦ Steroids are given when carditis is suspected.
♦ Cardiac pacemaker may be useful in refractory bradycardia and arrhythmias.

♦ Following treatment patient often gets spasm of different muscles (tics) for a long period which can be prevented by giving methocarbamol for 6 months to one year.

Q.9. **Write short note on tetanus prophylaxis.**

(Sep 2006, 6 Marks)

Or

Discuss about prophylaxis of tetanus.

(Sep 2009, 5 Marks) (Mar 2008, 5 Marks)

Or

Write short note on prophylaxis against tetanus.

(Feb 2013, 5 Marks)

Ans.

Tetanus Prophylaxis

♦ In adults in which fresh immunization to start second in one month, next in 6 month period. Tetanus toxoid 0.5 mL IM Booster dose should be given once in every 4 years or after any significant trauma.
♦ Tetanus neonatorum can be prevented by immunization of the mother with two tetanus toxoid injection, ½ mL IM in third trimester of pregnancy.
♦ Infants and children are immunized with tetanus toxoid, diphtheria and pertussis vaccine (DPT) three dose at 6, 10, 14 weeks of age. This is called "Triple antigen". A booster dose is given at 18 months and once in five years, 1 mL of tetanus toxoid is given to achieve active immunity.
♦ ATG—500–1000 units IM given as prophylaxis in road accident, severe burns, crush injuries, war wounds, penetrating wounds and wounds of head and face.

Q.10. **Write short note on tetanus.**

(Mar 2006, 10 Marks) (Mar 2007, 2.5 Marks)
(Dec 2015, 5 Marks) (Feb 2013, 5 Marks)

Ans. *Refer to Ans. 8 of same chapter.*

Q.11. **Write short note on AIDS.**

(Nov 2008, 5 Marks) (Apr 2008, 5 Marks)

Ans. AIDS—Acquired immunodeficiency syndrome.

AIDS is the end stage of a progressive state of immunodeficiency.

Causative organism: Human immunodeficiency virus (HIV).

Mode of Transmission

♦ Sexual intercourse
♦ Mother to fetus
♦ Through contaminated needles
♦ Through contaminated blood transfusion.

General Features

♦ Weight loss more than 10%.
♦ Fever more than 1 month.
♦ Diarrhea more than 1 month.
♦ Neuralgia, arthralgia, headache.
♦ Generalized lymphadenopathy.
♦ Cutaneous rashes, dermatitis, fungal, bacterial, viral (herpes simplex 1 and 2) infection.
♦ Dental infection, gingivitis, candidiasis of oral cavity and esophagus.
♦ Varicella zoster infection.

◆ Opportunistic infections
◆ Poor healing after surgery, trauma, infection with more complications.

Investigations

◆ ELISA test is the screening test
◆ Western blot is the confirmatory test
◆ Polymerase chain reaction
◆ Anti-HIV detection
◆ CD4+ count
  • Normal value is >500/mm^3
  • Values between 200 to 500/mm^3 is seen in Kaposi's sarcoma and candidiasis
  • Values between 50 to 200/mm^3 is seen in *Pneumocystis carinii* and *Toxoplasma* infection.
  • Values <50/mm^3 is seen in atypical mycobacteria, cytomegalovirus, lymphomas.

As patient is HIV infected, a time gap occurs for these tests to become reactive. This time gap is known as window period. During this period, person in infected.

Treatment

◆ Antiviral therapy or HAART therapy
  • *Nucleoside reverse transcriptase inhibitor (NRTI):* Zidovudine, didanosine, abacavir, lamivudine, stavudine.
  • *Non-nucleoside reverse transcriptase inhibitor (NNRTI):* Nevirapine, delavirdine.
  • *Protease inhibitors:* Ritonavir, indinavir, amprenavir.
◆ Treatment of opportunistic infections.
◆ Treatment of tumors.
◆ *Immunotherapy:*
  • Alpha and gamma interferons.
  • Interleukins.
◆ Bone marrow transplantation.
◆ Anti-CD3 or IL-2 after HAART (Highly Active Anti-Retroviral Therapy).
◆ Psychotherapy
◆ Counseling of HIV patients and their families.
◆ Life-expectancy after initial HIV infection is 8–10 years.

Prevention and Control

◆ Safe sexual contact (use of condom)
◆ Prevent sharing of needles among drug abusers.
◆ Separate and sterilized needle should be used for each patient.
◆ Blood transfusion should be done after HIV testing.
◆ Health education.

Q.12. Describe etiology, epidemiology, pathology and prevention of AIDS in dental practice.
(Feb 2002, 10 Marks)

Ans.

Etiology (in Dental Clinic)

◆ Due to infected instruments.
◆ Uses of infected needles.
◆ Infected blood transfusion during dental procedures.
◆ Contaminated gloves and dressing materials.

Epidemiology

◆ AIDS was first describe in US the disease has now attained high proportions involving all continents.
◆ Africa constitutes 50% of all positive cases globally
◆ 1 in every 100 sexually active adult worldwide is infected with HIV.
◆ In India epicenter of epidemic lies in states of Maharashtra or Tamil Nadu which together compromise about 50% HIV

Pathology

Flowchart 3: Pathology of AIDS in dental practice.

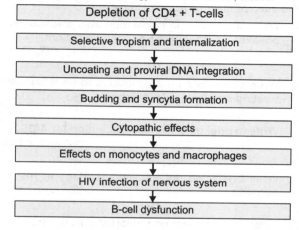

Prevention in Dental Clinic

◆ Needle sharing among patients is avoided.
◆ Instruments are properly sterilized by autoclave or proper use of chemical sterilization.
◆ Before commencement of surgery dentist should use proper asepsis measures.
◆ Patient should be educated about AIDS.

Q.13. Write in brief about the HIV and dental surgeon.
(Feb 2013, 5 Marks) (Mar 2007, 5 Marks)

Ans. The HIV is the virus which results in the causation of the AIDS.

Prophylactic measures to be adopted by dental surgeon while treating AIDS patient.

In OPD

◆ Any patient with open wound, gloves are worn when examining a patient.
◆ During dental diagnostic procedure gloves should be worn.
◆ Use disposable instruments.
◆ Reusable instruments are cleaned in soap and water and emerged in glutaraldehyde.
◆ No surgical procedure involving sharp instrument should be performed in OPD.

In Operating Room

◆ Dental chair is covered with a single sheet of polythene.
◆ The number of personnel in dental operating room should be reduced to minimum.

- The staff with abrasion or lacerations on their hands is not allowed inside the operating room.
- Staff who enter the theater wear overshoes, gloves and disposable water-resistant gowns and eye protectors.

Surgical Technique

- Avoid sharp injury.
- Avoid "needlestick" injuries
- Proper autoclaving at the end of surgery.

AZT—zidovudine, lamivudine and indinavir should be given for the health workers following exposure of susceptible area to infected material from AIDS patient.

Q.14. **Write short note on prevention and precautions to be taken on treating a HIV positive patient.**
(Jan 2012, 5 Marks)

Or

Write short note on precautions to be taken while treating surgical patient with HIV. *(Aug 2012, 5 Marks)*

Or

Write in brief on universal precaution for AIDS.
(Dec 2010, 5 Marks)

Or

Write briefly on universal precautions in HIV and hepatitis. *(Jan 2016, 2 Marks)*

Or

Write short answer on universal precaution.
(Oct 2019, 3 Marks)

Ans.

Preventions and Precautions to be Taken While Treating a HIV Positive or Hepatitis B Patient

- Care in handling sharp objects, such as needles, blades.
- All cuts and abrasions in an HIV or hepatitis B patient should be covered with a waterproof dressing
- Minimal parenteral injections
- Equipment and areas which are contaminated with secretions should be wiped with sodium hypochlorite solution or 2% glutaraldehyde.
- Contaminated gloves, cottons should be incinerated.
- Equipment should be disinfected with glutaraldehyde.
- Disposable equipment (drapes, scalpels, etc.) should be used, whenever possible.
- Walls and floor should be cleaned properly with soap water.
- Separate operation theatre and staff to do surgeries to HIV or hepatitis B patients is justifiable
- Avoid shaving whenever possible before surgery in HIV or hepatitis B patients.
- All people inside the theater should wear disposable gowns, plastic aprons, goggles, overshoes and gloves.
- Surgeons, assistants and scrub nurse should wear in addition double gloves.
- Suction bottle should be half-filled with freshly prepared glutaraldehyde solution.
- Soiled body fluids should be diluted with glutaraldehyde.

- Accidental puncture area in surgeon or scrub nurse should immediately washed with soap and water thoroughly
- Theater should be fumigated after surgery to HIV or hepatitis B patient.

Q.15. **Write briefly on necrotizing fasciitis or subdermal gangrene.** *(Aug 2011, 5 Marks)*

Ans. It is defined as rapidly progressing necrosis of subcutaneous tissue and fascia usually sparing the muscles and accompanied by toxicity, high fever and apathy.

Etiology

Bacteria, such as *Streptococcus pyogenes*, anaerobes, coliforms, Gram-negative organisms

Types

- *Type I: Polymicrobial (80%):* Mixed infection; by non-group A streptococci with anaerobes or clostridial or enterobacteriaceae (*E coli, Pseudomonas*). It is common in perineum, trunk and postoperative wounds; common in diabetics and immunosuppressed people.
- *Type II: Monomicrobial:* It is due to group A hemolytic streptococci or methicillin-resistant *Staphylococcus aureus* (MRSA). It is common in young individual; common in extremities without any comorbid status.
- *Type III:* It is Gram-negative rod (*Vibrio vulficus*) after a minor trauma; associated with chronic liver disease, diabetes, steroid therapy, chronic kidney disease. It is rare.
- *Type IV:* It is due to fungal infection commonly, Aspergillus zygomycetes. it is also rare.

Predisposing Factors

- In old age
- In smokers
- Diabetics
- Immunosuppressed individuals
- Malnourished
- Obesity
- Patients on steroid therapy
- HIV patients.

Clinical Features

- Lesion occurs in limbs, lower abdomen, groin and perineum.
- Presence of sudden swelling and pain in part with edema, discoloration, necrotic areas and ulceration.
- Presence of foul-smell discharge
- Presence of high-grade fever with chills and hypotension
- Oliguria with acute renal failure due to tubular necrosis.
- Jaundice.
- Rapid spread in short period (in few hours).
- Features of multiple organ dysfunction syndrome with drowsy, ill-patient.
- Condition, if not treated properly may be life-threatening.
- The subdermal spread of gangrene is always much more extensive than appears from initial examination.

Management

- IV fluids, fresh blood transfusion.
- Antibiotics depend on culture and sensitivity or broad-spectrum antibiotics. High-dose penicillins are very effective. Clindamycin, third generation cephalosporins, aminoglycosides are also often needed.
- Catheterization and monitoring of hourly urine output.
- Electrolyte management and monitoring.
- Control of diabetes, if patient is diabetic.
- Oxygen, ventilator support, dopamine, dobutamine supplements, whenever required.
- Radical wound excision of gangrenous skin and necrosed tissues at repeated intervals.
- Vacuum-assisted dressing is given.
- Once patient recovers and healthy granulation tissue appears split skin grafting is done. Mesh graft is needed.

Q.16. Define and describe differentiating features of tetanus and gas gangrene. *(Jan 2012, 5 Marks)*

Ans.

Features	Tetanus	Gas gangrene
Definition	It is an infective condition leading to reflex muscle spasm and is often associated with tonic clonic convulsions.	It is an infective gangrene caused by clostridial organisms involving mainly skeletal muscles as edematous myonecrosis.
Etiology	*Clostridium tetani*	*Clostridium welchii* (perfringens)
Incubation period	7–10 days	1–2 days
Toxins	Tetanospasmin and Tetanolysin	Lecithinase (alpha toxin), beta-toxin, Epsilon toxin
Symptoms	Trismus is most common	Extensive necrosis of muscle with production of gas which stains muscle brown
System affected	Affect central nervous system	Affects muscular system
Treatment	Tracheostomy is the live-saving procedure	Amputation of involved organ is the life-saving procedure
Prophylaxis	Inj. Antitetanus globulin	Penicillin should be given as prophylactic antibiotic

Q.17. Enumerate differences between virus of Hepatitis B and HIV. *(June 2014, 2 Marks)*

Ans.

Features	Virus of Hepatitis B	HIV
Diameter	42 nm	90–120 nm
Genome	DNA	RNA
Symmetry	Icosahedral	Spherical
Laboratory diagnosis	HBsAg is present	ELISA is positive and confirmation is done by western blot

Q.18. Enumerate differences between tetanus and strychnine poisoning. *(June 2014, 2 Marks)*

Ans.

Tetanus	Strychnine poisoning
Tetanus is a bacterial infection caused by *Clostridium tetani*	Strychnine poisoning is caused due to the overdosage of chemical known as strychnine. Strychnine is used to kill rats
Predisposing Features • Absence of tetanus toxoid immunization • Chronic otitis media with perforation • Improper sterilization in ward • Tattooing and rusted nails	**Predisposing Features** • Release of strychnine into drinking water • Contamination of food with strychnine • Strychnine is absorbed through the membranes in the nose, eyes, or mouth • Strychnine could be smoked or snorted as a component of street drugs

Contd...

Contd...

Tetanus	Strychnine poisoning
Mechanism of Action Tetanus release exotoxin, i.e., Tetanospasmin and tetanolysin. Tetanospasmin through lymphatic and perineural sheath enters CNS and block cholinesterase enzyme at anterior horn cells. This leads to hyperexcitability and reflex spasm of muscles often with tonic-clonic convulsions	**Mechanism of Action** Strychnine prevents the proper operation of the chemical that controls nerve signals to the muscles. The chemical controlling nerve signals works like the body's "off-switch" for muscles. When this "off-switch" does not work correctly, muscles throughout the body have severe, painful spasms. Eventually, the muscles tire and the person cannot breathe
Time between entry of spore and appearance of first symptom is 7–10 days	It acts within 10–20 min after exposure.

Q.19. Write short note on candidiasis. *(Feb 2013, 5 Marks)*

Ans. Candidiasis is the fungal infection caused by yeast-like fungus, i.e., *Candida albicans*.

Types of Candidiasis

- *Primary candidiasis:*
  - *Acute form:*
    - Pseudomembranous
    - Erythematous
  - *Chronic form:*
    - Hyperplastic
    - Erythematous
    - Pseudomembranous
  - *Candida-associated lesion:*
    - Denture stomatitis
    - Angular stomatitis
    - Median rhomboid glossitis
  - *Keratinized primary lesion super-infected with Candida:*
    - Leukoplakia
    - Lichen planus
    - Lupus erythematosus
- *Secondary candidiasis*

Predisposing Factors

- *Changes in oral microbial flora:* Marked changes in oral microbial flora can be seen during administration of systemic antibiotics, due to chronic use of mouthrinses, xerostomia due to anticholinergic agent. These all lead to candidiasis.
- *Local irritant:* Local irritants, such as denture, due to heavy smoking, orthodontic appliances can lead to candidiasis.
- *Drug therapy:* Administration of immunosuppressive agents, corticosteroids, head and neck radiotherapy can cause candidiasis.
- *Acute and chronic diseases:* Various acute and chronic diseases, such as leukemia, diabetes, tuberculosis can cause candidiasis.
- *Malnutrition state:* Low serum vitamin A, low iron level and low pyridoxine levels may lead to candidiasis.
- *Endocrinopathy:* Endocrinopathies, such as hyperparathyroidism, hypothyroidism and Addison's disease can cause candidiasis.

Clinical Features

- It is more common in females as compared to males.
- Commonly affected sites are roof of mouth, retromolar area, mucobuccal fold and tongue.

- Patient complaints of bad taste and spicy food can cause discomfort.
- Pearly white or bluish white plaques are seen on mucosa. Mucosa adjacent to these plaques appears red and moderately swollen.
- White patches are easily wiped off with wet gauge which leaves normal or erythematous area.
- *Candida* in chronic form does not rub off by lateral pressure. Lesions are slightly white to dense white with cracks and fissures occasionally present. Borders are often vague, which produces appearance of epithelial dysplasia.

Diagnosis

Clinically, pseudomembranous lesion is scrapped off which is diagnostic of candidiasis.

Treatment

- *Removal of cause:*
  - Any of the local irritant should be removed.
  - Withdrawal of antibiotics is done.
- *Topical treatment:*
  - Cotrimazole, one troche 10 mg is dissolved in mouth for 5 times a day.
  - Nystatin oral pastilles can be given, i.e., one or two pastilles five times a day.
  - Amphotericin B 5–10 mL of oral solution used as rinse and then expectorated 3–4 times a day.
- *Systemic treatment:*
  - Nystatin 250 mg TDS for 2 weeks followed by 1 troche per day for third week.
  - Ketoconazole 200 mg tablet with food once daily.
  - Fluconazole 100 mg tablet OD for 2 weeks
  - Itraconazole 200 mg tablet OD for 2 weeks

Q.20. Describe etiopathogenesis, clinical features and management of tetanus. *(Nov 2014, 8 Marks)*

Ans. *For clinical features and management, refer to Ans. 8 of same chapter.*

Etiopathogenesis

Tetanus is caused by Gram-positive, anaerobic, motile, non-capsulated, organism with peritrichous flagella with terminal spores, i.e., bacillus *Clostridium tetani*. Spore is the infective agent and is found in soil, dust, manure, etc. Spore enters the wound through prick injuries which result from road-traffic accidents, penetrating injuries, foreign body, etc.

Flowchart 4: Etiopathogenesis of tetanus.

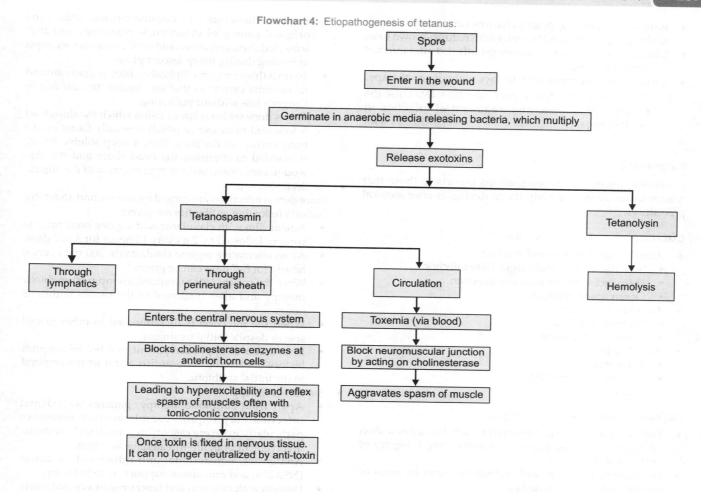

Q.21. **Write short note on prophylaxis of hepatitis B.**
(Apr 2015, 3 Marks)

Ans. Following is the prophylaxis of hepatitis B:

♦ Recombinant hepatitis B vaccine having HBsAg capable of producing active immunization.

♦ Usually three injections of vaccine should be given IM during current, first and sixth month. These vaccinations provide 90% of prophylaxis from hepatitis B virus.

♦ If patient is immunocompromised larger doses of vaccination should be given.

♦ Passive immunization is provided by IM injection of hyperimmune serum globulins which is given within 24 hours or almost within a week of exposure to infected blood.

♦ Active along with passive immunization is provided to the paramedicos who has undergone needle stick injury, to newborn babies of hepatitis B positive mothers and to regular sexual partner of hepatitis B positive patient. Dosage is 500 IU for adults and 200 IU for babies.

Following precautions are to be taken for prevention from hepatitis B:

♦ Avoid infected blood transfusion, body organs, sperms and other tissues. Blood should be screened before transfusion.

♦ Strict sterilization process should be ensured in clinics.

♦ Presterilized needles and syringe should be used.

♦ Avoid injections unless they are absolutely necessary.

♦ Carrier should be told not to share razors or tooth brushes, use barrier methods of contraception, avoid blood donation.

Q.22. **Write briefly on primary chancre.** *(Jan 2016, 2 Marks)*

Or

Write short note on primary chancre.

(Aug 2012, 5 Marks)

Ans.

♦ Primary chancre is the hallmark sign of primary syphilis caused due to *Treponema pallidum*.

♦ Primary chancre is also known as Hunterian chancre or hard chancre.

♦ Primary chancre occurs on penis of males and cervix of females. It can also be seen over extragenital sites, such as fingers, perianal region, nipples, lips tonsils, tongue and palate.

♦ Chancre is slightly raised, ulcerated, nontender, non-bleeding and firm plaque which is round, indurated along with rolled raised edges.

♦ It starts as a papule, then enlarges to various centimeters and converted to ulcer.

♦ Intraorally chancre appears as narrow copper colored with slight raised borders and in center with reddish-brown base.

♦ Chancre remains painless before get infected after infected it becomes tender.

♦ Chancre can disappear after 10 days without any therapy.

Q.23. Define and classify surgical infection. Describe the surgical principles, and treatment of infection in dental surgery. *(Mar 1997, 15 Marks)*

Ans.

Surgical Infections

A disease caused by microorganisms especially those that release toxins or invade body tissue during or after surgical procedures.

Classification of Surgical Infections

♦ *According to depth of wound infection:*
  • Superficial incisional surgical site infection
  • Deep incisional surgical site infection
  • Organ space infection.

♦ *According to etiology:*
  • Primary infection
  • Secondary infection.

♦ *According to the time:*
  • Early infection
  • Intermediate infection
  • Late infection.

Surgical Principles in Dental Surgery

♦ Follow the shortest and most direct route to the accumulation of exudates or pus, but always preserving integrity of anatomical structures.

♦ Performing incisions with esthetic criteria in areas of minimal impact as on the face.

♦ Place the incisions in areas of healthy mucosa or skin, avoiding areas with fluctuation and atrophic alterations.

♦ Perform strictly cutaneous or mucosal incisions (with a No. 11 blade)

♦ The incision is penetrated using hemostat or sinus forceps in closed position, advanced into the pus locules, by blunt dissection in open position of the sinus forceps. The hemostat is withdrawn in the same position in open state to avoid damage to anatomical structures, such as nerves, vessels.

♦ Choice of appropriate drainage material is according to the site of infection. Avoid using gauze as drainage material, since secretions would be retained and coagulate, thereby creating a tamponade that would cause the infection to persist.

Treatment of Infection in Dental Surgery

♦ *Excision of sinus:*
  • In most of the cases, the abscess escapes the tissue spaces spontaneously, through a sinus if left without any treatment for sufficient period of time.
  • Pus discharge through the skin in a location unfavorable for drainage follows and the resulting scar is always puckered, thickened and depressed.

• Further, the sinus will become chronic unless the original source of infection is removed, and it is subjected to exacerbations and remissions with attempts at healing during the quiescent phase.

• To treat this sinus, an elliptical incision is made around its external orifice so that on closure the scar lies in Langer's line without puckering.

• This is done with a scissors, using which the sinus tract is followed to its source which is usually found on the bony surface of the jaws. Then a deep soluble suture is inserted to eliminate the dead space and the skin wounds are closed with careful eversion of the edges.

♦ *Antibiotic therapy:*
Since dental infections are caused by aerobic and anaerobic bacteria following antibiotics are given:
  • Amoxicillin with clavulanic acid 2 g one hour prior to surgery followed by 2 g every 12 hours for 5 to 7 days.
  • As an alternative regime clindamycin 300 mg every 6 hourly for 5–7 days can be given.
  • When the patient fails to respond to empirical antibiotic therapy and after treatment of the causes within 48 hours.
  • When the infection is disseminated to other fascial spaces despite initial treatment.
  • In an immunosuppressed patient, or if he/she has prior history of bacterial endocarditis and does not respond to the initial antibiotic.

♦ *Supportive therapy:*
  • Apart from antibiotic therapy, patients with dental infection may require complementary measures particularly in severe cases with considerable systemic involvement or in life-threatening situation.
  • Analgesics, nonsteroidal anti-inflammatory drugs (NSAIDs) and nutritional support are mandatory.
  • Patients with infection and fever present a considerable loss of body fluids—250 mL for every degree (centigrade) temperature rise.
  • Ambulatory patients must drink 8–10 glasses of water or any other liquid.
  • Intravenous fluids can be given to those patients who are hospitalized to improve hydration.
  • The daily calorie requirement also increases by 13% for each degree (centigrade) above normal body temperature.
  • Thermal agents should be used to aid the body defenses.
  • Heat produces vasodilatation and increased circulation, more rapid removal of tissue breakdown products and greater influx of defensive cells and antibodies.
  • A crucial aspect to be considered in these patients is the potential risk onset of respiratory impairment, requiring airway monitoring, perhaps even on an emergency basis, by means of endotracheal intubation, cricothyrotomy or tracheotomy.

Q.24. Write short note on AIDS and surgeon.

(Apr 2007, 5 Marks)

Or

Write in brief about HIV and surgeons.

(Dec 2012, 5 Marks)

Ans. The HIV is the virus which results in the causation of the AIDS.

Prophylactic measures to be adopted by surgeon while treating AIDS patient.

In OPD

♦ Any patient with open wound, gloves are worn when examining a patient.
♦ During proctoscopy or sigmoidoscopy, gloves should be worn.
♦ Hand gloves and eye protection during flexible endoscopy.
♦ Use disposable instruments.
♦ Reusable instruments are cleaned in soap and water and emerged in glutaraldehyde.
♦ No surgical procedure involving sharp instruments is performed in OPD.

In Operating Room

♦ Operating table is covered with a single sheet of polythene.
♦ The number of personnel in operating room should be reduced to minimum.
♦ The staff with abrasion or lacerations on their hands is not allowed inside the operating room.
♦ Staff who enter the theater wear over-shoes, gloves and disposable water-resistant gowns and eye protectors.

Surgical Technique

♦ Avoid sharp injury.
♦ Prefer scissors or diathermy to scalpel
♦ Use of skin clips
♦ Avoid "needle-stick" injuries
♦ Proper autoclaving at the end of surgery.
♦ AZT—zidovudine, lamivudine and indinavir should be given for the health workers following exposure of susceptible area to infected material from AIDS patient.

Q.25. Write short note on HIV.

(Feb 2015, 5 Marks) (Feb 2014, 3 Marks)

Or

Write briefly on HIV.　　*(June 2015, 2.5 Marks)*

Ans. HIV means human immunodeficiency virus.

♦ HIV was discovered in 1983 and first case was detected in UK.
♦ It was discovered by Barre–Sinoussi and Montagnier.
♦ HIV virus is classified under HTLV-III.
♦ HIV is of two types, i.e., HIV-1 and HIV-2 which are the retroviruses.

Mode of Transmission of HIV

♦ Sexual intercourse either vaginal or anal.
♦ Needle pricks, i.e., using unsterilized needles for injections, in IV drug abusers, careless handling
♦ *Mother to child:* During birth through vaginal secretion, transplacental, through breast milk
♦ Through blood transfusions and organ transplantations

Pathogenesis

Envelope glycoprotein of HIV binds with surface molecules of CD4 cells of T-lymphocytes, monocytes, macrophages, Langerhans cells and dendritic cells of all tissues.

CD4 of lymphocytes and T helper cells control normal immune response. HIV suppresses immune response completely suppressing B-cell. Finally, it dismantles and destroy immune system making the individual prone to opportunistic infections.

Clinical Classification of HIV

♦ Acute infections
♦ Asymptomatic but positive HIV.
♦ Persistent generalized lymphadenopathy
♦ *AIDS (HIV-related diseases):*
  • Constitutional diseases, such as weight loss, fever, diarrhea
  • Neurological diseases, such as dementia, neuropathy, myelopathy
  • Opportunistic infections
  • *Malignancies:* Kaposi's sarcoma, non-Hodgkin's lymphoma
  • Other diseases attributable to HIV infection.

Test for HIV

♦ ELISA test (screening test)
♦ Western blot (diagnostic test)
♦ Polymerase chain reaction
♦ Anti-HIV antibody reaction
♦ Viremia quantification—to start the treatment and to see the response of antiviral drugs.
♦ *CD4 cell count:*
  • Normal value >500/mm^3
  • Values between 200 to 500/mm^3 is seen in Kaposi's sarcoma, *Candida* infection and *M. tuberculosis*
  • Values between 50 to 200/mm^3 is seen in *Pneumocystis carinii* and *Toxoplasma* infection
  • Values <50/mm^3 is seen in atypical mycobacteria, cytomegalovirus and lymphomas.

After the HIV infection, there is time gap for the patient to become reactive to tests. This time is known as "Window period". This period is variable and during this period an individual is infective.

Treatment of HIV

♦ Antiviral therapy or HAART therapy
  Nucleoside reverse transcriptase inhibitor (NRTI): Zidovudine, didanosine, abacavir, lamivudine, stavudine.
  Non-nucleoside reverse transcriptase inhibitor (NNRTI): Nevirapine, delavirdine.
  Protease inhibitors: Ritonavir, indinavir, amprenavir.
♦ Treatment of opportunistic infections.
♦ Treatment of tumors.
♦ *Immunotherapy:*
  • Alpha and gamma interferons.
  • Interleukins.

- Bone marrow transplantation.
- Anti-CD3 or IL-2 after highly active antiretroviral therapy (HAART).
- Psychotherapy
- Counseling of HIV patients and their families.
- Life-expectancy after initial HIV infection is 8–10 years.

Q.26. Describe the mode of spread of HIV. Describe treatment. *(Jan 2017, 10 Marks)*

Ans.

Mode of Spread of HIV

- Sexual intercourse either vaginal or anal.
- Needle pricks, i.e., using unsterilized needles for injections, in IV drug abusers, careless handling
- *Mother to child:* During birth through vaginal secretion, transplacental, through breast milk
- Through blood transfusions and organ transplantations

Treatment of HIV

For details refer to Ans. 25 of same chapter.

Q.27. Describe the nosocomial infection.
(Jan 2017, 10 Marks)

Ans. It is an infection acquired due to hospital stay.

Sources

- Contaminated infected wounds.
- Urinary tract infections.
- Respiratory tract infections.
- Opportunistic infections.
- Abdominal wounds with severe sepsis.
- Spread can occur from one patient to another, through nurses or hospital staff who fail to practice strict asepsis.
- It is more common in:
  - Diabetics
  - Immunosuppressed individuals
  - Patients on steroid therapy and life-supporting machines
  - Instrumentations (including catheter, IV cannula, tracheostomy tube)
  - Patients with artificial prosthesis

Organisms

- *Staphylococcus aureus* is the most common organism causing hospital-acquired wound infection. Others are *Pseudomonas, Klebsiella, E. coli, Proteus.*
- *Streptococcus pneumoniae, Haemophilus,* Herpes, Varicella, Aspergillus, *Pneumocystis carinii* are the most common pathogens involved in hospital-acquired respiratory tract infection which spreads through droplets.
- *Klebsiella* is the most common pathogen involved in hospital acquired UTI which is highly resistant to drugs.

Management

Most of the time, organisms involved are multidrug resistant, virulent and hence, cause severe sepsis.

- Antibiotics.
- Isolation.

- Blood, urine, pus for culture and sensitivity to isolate the organisms.
- Blood transfusion, plasma or albumin therapy.
- Ventilator support.
- Maintaining optimum urine output.
- Nutritional support.

Prevention

- Isolation of patients with badly infected open wounds.
- Severe RTI/UTI.
- Following strict aseptic measures in OT and in ward by hospital attendants.
- Proper cleaning and use of disinfectant lotions and sprays for bedpans, toilets and floor.
- The precipitating causes have to be treated, along with caring for proper nutrition and improving the anemic status by blood transfusion.

Q.28. Name etiological agent, pathognomic diagnostic feature and treatment (only modalities) of actinomycosis. *(Jan 2017, 3 Marks)*

Ans.

Etiological Agent

It is caused by *Actinomyces israelii.*

Pathognomic Diagnostic Feature

Multiple discharging sinuses which discharge sulfur granules and there is no lymph node enlargement present.

Treatment (Only modalities)

- Antibiotic therapy
- Excision of sinuses
- Actinomycosis of right iliac fossa should undergo hemicolectomy

Q.29. Name etiological agent, pathognomic diagnostic feature and treatment (only modalities) of anthrax.
(Jan 2017, 3 Marks)

Ans.

Etiological Agent

Anthrax is caused by Bacillus anthracis.

Pathognomic Diagnostic Feature

After 3–4 days of incubation an itching *erythematous papule* develop on exposed portion of body, i.e., hand, forearm, etc. The papules suppurate and form black slough. This lesion is surrounded by vesicles known as malignant pustule.

Treatment (Only Modality)

Antibiotic therapy is given.

Q.30. Name etiological agent, pathognomic diagnostic feature and treatment (only modalities) of chancre.
(Jan 2017, 3 Marks)

Ans.

Etiological Agent

It is caused by *Treponema pallidum*.

Pathognomic Diagnostic Feature

A shallow, painless, indurated, non-bleeding ulcer seen on genitalia, lips, breasts and anal region, this is known as Hunterian chancre. This is confirmed by dark-field microscopic study of discharge for organism.

Treatment (Modality only)

Antibiotic therapy should be given.

Q.31. Write short note on septicemia.

(Feb 2013, 5 Marks) (Apr 2007, 10 Marks)

Ans. Presence of overwhelming and multiplying bacteria in blood with toxins causing systemic inflammatory response syndrome or multiorgan dysfunction syndrome.

Clinical Features

♦ Intermittent high-grade pyrexia (fever)
♦ Rigors and chills.
♦ Jaundice due to liver damage.
♦ Peripheral circulatory failure.
♦ Intravascular coagulation.
♦ Patient may go into septic shock.
♦ Septic shock is secondary to sepsis; it is characterized by inadequate perfusion of tissue.
♦ The septic shock differs from all other forms of shock by having hot stage before cold stage.

Types

♦ *Gram-positive septicemia:* It is due to staphylococci, streptococci, pneumococci, etc. It is common in children, old age. diabetics and after splenectomy. Common origin is skin, respiratory infection
♦ *Gram-negative septicemia* is common in acute abdomen, such as peritonitis, abscess, urinary infections, biliary infections, postoperative sepsis. It is commonly seen in malnutrition, old age, diabetics, immunosuppressed people. Common focus of infection is gram-negative infection is urinary infection, abscess or infected wounds, biliary sepsis, postoperative wounds.

Investigations

♦ Urine/pus/discharge culture
♦ Blood culture
♦ Hematocrit
♦ Electrolyte assessment
♦ PO_2 and CO_2 analysis
♦ Blood urea, serum creatinine, liver function test

Complications

♦ Disseminated intravascular coagulation
♦ Acute respiratory distress syndrome
♦ Liver dysfunction
♦ Renal failure
♦ Bone marrow suppression—thrombocytopenia
♦ Multiorgan failure

Treatment

♦ Antibiotics, such as cefoperazone, ceftazidime, cefotaxime, amikacin, tobramycin, metronidazole.
♦ Fresh blood transfusion.
♦ Adequate hydration.
♦ Oxygen supplementation.
♦ Ventilatory support.
♦ Electrolyte management.
♦ Parenteral nutrition
♦ CVP line for monitoring and perfusion.
♦ Fresh-frozen plasma or platelets in disseminated intravascular coagulation

Q.32. Write short note on septicemia, toxemia and pyemia.

(Jun 2010, 5 Marks)

Or

Describe toxemia.　*(Sep 2018, 5 Marks)*

Ans. *For septicemia, refer to Ans. 31 of same chapter.*

Toxemia

Distribution throughout the body of poisonous product of bacteria growing in a focal or local site, thus producing generalized symptoms, such as fever, diarrhea, vomiting.

Clinical Features

♦ Intermittent high-grade pyrexia (fever)
♦ Rigors and chills.
♦ Jaundice due to liver damage.
♦ Peripheral circulatory failure.
♦ Intravascular coagulation.
♦ Patient may go into septic shock.
♦ *Septic shock is secondary to sepsis;* it is characterized by inadequate perfusion of tissue.
♦ The septic shock differs from all other forms of shock by having hot stage before cold stage.

Treatment

♦ Management of primary focus of infection.
♦ Broad-spectrum antibodies are given.
♦ Blood and fluid transfusion to correct septic shock.
♦ Injection of hydrocortisone in case of septic shock may be useful.

Pyemia

Presence of multiplying bacteria in blood as emboli which spread and lodge in different organs in the body like liver, lungs, kidneys, spleen, brain causing pyemic abscess. This may lead to multiorgan dysfunction syndrome (MODS). It may endanger life, if not treated properly.

Clinical Features

♦ Fever with chills and rigors
♦ Jaundice, oliguria, drowsiness
♦ Hypotension, peripheral circulatory collapse and later coma with MODS

Common Causes

♦ Urinary infection (most common)
♦ Biliary tract infection.

- Lower respiratory tract infection.
- Abdominal sepsis of any cause.
- Sepsis in diabetics and immunosuppressed individuals, such as HIV, steroid therapy.

Investigations

- Total leukocyte count, platelet count
- Biliary tract infection
- Pus, blood and urine culture depending on the need.
- Blood urea, serum creatinine
- Liver function tests, prothrombin time
- Chest X-ray, USG abdomen
- CT chest/abdomen/brain as needed
- Arterial blood gas analysis, if needed

Treatment

- Monitoring of vital parameters
- Antibiotics mainly cephalosporins
- IV fluids and maintenance of urine output.
- Hydrocortisone
- Blood and plasma transfusion
- Nasal oxygen, ventilator support, monitoring of pulmonary function.

Q.33. Describe differentiating features of septicemia and pyemia. *(Jan 2017, 4 Marks)*

Ans. Following are the differentiating features of septicemia and pyemia:

Septicemia	Pyemia
Septicemia is a disease	Pyemia is the type of septicemia
In septicemia actual "putrid" matter (of unknown character) was supposed to be present in the blood	In pyemia, the pus cells were floating with blood
Presence of overwhelming and multiplying bacteria in blood with toxins causing systemic inflammatory response syndrome or multiorgan dysfunction syndrome.	Presence of multiplying bacteria in blood as emboli which spread and lodge in different organs in the body like liver, lungs, kidneys, spleen, brain causing pyemic abscess.
It is differentiated into two types, i.e., Gram-positive and Gram-negative	It is of various types, i.e., arterial, cryptogenic, metastatic, portal
Gram-positive or Gram-negative bacteria are the etiological agents.	Mainly Gram-negative bacteria are the etiological agents
Septicemia comprehends systemic infection from various causes; the original infection is not always to be determined, and it is so often of a mixed character that its real nature is difficult of determination.	Pyemia in its present acceptance comprehends a focus of necrotic tissue, caused by the peculiar organisms of pus development with pus cells present in greater or less quantities.

Q.34. Describe differentiating features of bacteremia and septicemia. *(Jan 2017, 4 Marks)*

Ans. Following are the differentiating features of bacteremia and septicemia:

Bacteremia	Septicemia
Bacteremia is the simple presence of bacteria in the blood.	Septicemia is the presence and multiplication of bacteria in the blood.
Bacteremia is not as dangerous as septicemia.	Septicemia is a potentially life-threatening infection.
Less amount of bacteria are present in blood.	Large amounts of bacteria are present in the blood.
This may occur through a wound or infection, or through a surgical procedure or injection.	It can arise from infections throughout the body, including infections in the lungs, abdomen, and urinary tract.
Toxins are not produced.	Toxins may be produced by bacteria.
Bacteremia usually causes no symptoms or it may produce mild fever.	It shows symptoms, such as chills, fever, prostration, very fast respiration and/or heart rate.
It can resolve without treatment.	Untreated septicemia can quickly progress to sepsis.
Rapidly removed from the bloodstream by the immune system.	Antibiotics will be used to treat the bacterial infection that is causing septicemia.
Caused by Staphylococcus, Streptococcus, Pseudomonas, Haemophilus, E. coli, dental procedures, herpes (including herpetic whitlow), urinary tract infections, peritonitis, *Clostridium difficile* colitis, intravenous drug use, and colorectal cancer.	*Staphylococci,* are thought to cause more than 50% of cases of sepsis. Other commonly implicated bacteria include *Streptococcus pyogenes, Escherichia coli, Pseudomonas aeruginosa, Klebsiella* species and even *Candida spp.*

Q.35. Differentiate between Gram-negative and Gram-positive septicemia and management. *(Jan 2018, 10 Marks)*

Ans.

Gram-positive septicemia	Gram-negative septicemia
It is caused by staphylococci, streptococci, pneumococci, etc.	It is caused by *E. coli, Klebsiella, Pseudomonas* and *Proteus*
Overwhelming post-splenectomy infection is the classical example.	It leads to urinary infection, biliary sepsis, peritonitis, abdominal infection, postoperative sepsis.
It is common in children, old age, diabetics and after splenectomy.	It is commonly seen in malnourished, old age, diabetics and immunocompromised people.
Common origin is skin and respiratory infection	Commonly occur in urinary tract and wounds
Leads to gram-positive septic shock	Leads to Gram-negative septic shock
Gram-positive septicemia is caused by exotoxin	Gram-negative septicemia is caused by endotoxin
In this fluid loss, hypotension is common with normal cardiac output	Urinary/gastrointestinal/biliary and respiratory foci is common.

Management of Gram-Positive and Gram-Negative septicemia

♦ Correction of fluid and electrolyte by crystalloids, blood transfusion. Perfusion is very/most important.
♦ Appropriate antibiotics—third generation cephalosporins/aminoglycosides.
♦ Treat the cause or focus—drainage of an abscess; laparotomy for peritonitis; resection of gangrenous bowel; wound excision.
♦ Pus/urine/discharge/bile/blood culture and sensitivity for antibiotics.
♦ Critical care, oxygen, ventilator support, dobutamine/dopamine/noradrenaline to maintain blood pressure and urine output.
♦ Activated C protein prevents the release of inflammatory mediators and blocks the effects of these mediators on cellular function.
♦ Monitoring the patient by pulse oximetry, cardiac status, urine output, arterial blood gas analysis.
♦ Short-term (one or two doses) high-dose steroid therapy to control and protect cells from effects of endotoxemia. It improves cardiac, renal and lung functions. Single dose of methylprednisolone or dexamethasone which often may be repeated again after 4 hours is said to be effective in Gram-negative septicemia.

Q.36. Write short answer on Australian antigen.

(Apr 2018, 3 Marks)

Ans. A scientist named Blumberg and his coworkers in 1965 describe a protein antigen in serum of an Australian aborigine which gave positive precipitation reaction with sera from two hemophiliacs who had received multiple transfusions. This antigen was named as Australian antigen.

♦ HBsAg is known as Australia antigen and was established to be the surface component of hepatitis B virus.
♦ Australian antigen consists of two different antigenic determinants i.e.,
  • A group specific antigenic determinant – a
  • Two pairs of type – specific antigens – d – y and w – r. In these only one member of each pair is present at a time.
♦ Australia antigen on the basis of type specific pairing is divided in four types:
  • adw is worldwide in distribution
  • adr in Asia
  • ayw in Africa, India, Russia
  • ayr in Africa, India, Russia
♦ Various additional surface antigens, i.e., q, x, f, t, j, n and g are described, but their characterization is not done.
  • Electron microscopy of serum of hepatitis B patients show three types of particles, i.e.
    – Spherical particle: It is most abundant and is 22 nm in diameter.
    – Tubular particle: It is of varying length and is 22 nm in diameter.
    – Dane particle: It is double shielded spherical structure which is 42 nm in diameter. This particle is complete hepatitis B virus.

♦ The spherical and tubular particles are antigenically identical and are surface subunits of hepatitis B virus Australia antigen (HBsAg).

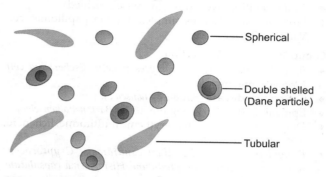

Fig. 4: Structure of Australian antigen.

Q.37. Write difference between pyemia and toxemia.

(Feb 2019, 5 Marks)

Ans. Following are the differences between pyemia and toxemia:

Pyemia	Toxemia
Presence of multiplying bacteria in blood as emboli which spread and lodge in different organs in the body, such as liver, lungs, kidneys, spleen, brain causing pyemic abscess.	Toxemia is the formation of toxic products in the blood.
In pyemia, the pus cells were floating with blood	In toxemia, the toxins were floating with blood
It is of various types, i.e., arterial, cryptogenic, metastatic, portal	It is acute and chronic.
Mainly Gram-negative bacteria are the etiological agents	Etiologically, it is can be antigenic and metabolic

Q.38. Write short answer on oral manifestations of HIV.

(Oct 2019, 3 Marks)

Ans. Following are the oral manifestations of AIDS/HIV infection:

Classification of Oral Manifestations by EC-Clearing House

Group 1: Strongly associated with HIV infection

♦ *Candidiasis:* Erythematous, pseudomembranous, angular cheilitis
♦ Hairy leukoplakia
♦ Kaposi's sarcoma
♦ Non-Hodgkin's lymphoma
♦ *Periodontal diseases:* Linear gingival erythema, necrotizing gingivitis, necrotizing periodontitis

Group 2: Less commonly associated with HIV infection

♦ *Bacterial infections: Mycobacterium avium*—intracellular, *Mycobacterium tuberculosis*
♦ Melanotic hyperpigmentation
♦ Necrotizing ulcerative stomatitis

- *Salivary gland disease:* Dry mouth, unilateral or bilateral swelling of major salivary glands.
- Thrombocytopenia purpura
- Oral ulcerations NOS (not otherwise specified)
- *Viral infections:* Herpes simplex, human papillomavirus, Varicella-Zoster

Group 3: Seen in HIV infection

- *Bacterial infections: Actinomyces israelii, Escherichia coli, Klebsiella,* pneumonia.
- Cat-scratch disease (*Bartonella henselae*).
- Epithelioid (bacillary) angiomatosis (*Bartonella henselae*)
- *Drug reactions:* Ulcerative, erythema multiforme, lichenoid, toxic epidermolysis.
- *Fungal infections other than candidiasis: Cryptococcus neoformans, Geotrichum candidum, Histoplasma capsulatum, Mucoraceae* (Mucormycosis/Zygomycosis), *Aspergillus flavus.*
- *Neurologic disturbances:* Facial palsy, trigeminal neuralgia
- Recurrent aphthous stomatitis.
- *Viral infections: Cytomegalovirus,* Molluscum contagiosum.

Description of Oral Manifestations

- Candidiasis is the most common oral manifestation of HIV infection. All the three types, i.e., erythematous, pseudomembranous and hyperplastic forms are seen. Erythematous candidiasis is seen when the CD4 count drops below 400 cells/mm^3 and pseudomembranous develop when CD4 count drop below 200 cells/mm^3.
- *Hairy leukoplakia:* Presence of soft painless plaque on the lateral border of tongue with corrugated surface.
- *Kaposi's sarcoma:* Single or multiple bluish swellings are seen with or without ulceration over gingiva and palate.
- *Angular cheilitis:* Linear fissures or linear ulcers are seen at the angle of mouth.
- *Linear gingival erythema:* It is fiery red band along the gingival margin and attached gingiva with profuse bleeding.
- *Necrotizing ulcerative gingivitis:* Destruction of interdental papillae is seen.
- *Necrotizing ulcerative periodontitis:* There is advanced necrotic destruction of periodontium, rapid bone loss, loss of periodontal ligament and sequestration.
- *Oral ulcerations:* Single or multiple major recurrent aphthous ulcers are seen with white pseudomembrane surrounding the erythematous halo.
- *Non-Hodgkin's lymphoma:* It is the malignancy of HIV infected individuals. It occurs in extranodal locations and CNS is the common site. Intraosseous involvement is also seen.
- *Mycobacterial infection:* Mycobacterial infection in form of tuberculosis is seen. When present tongue is affected most commonly. Affected areas show common ulcerations.
- *Herpes simplex virus:* Recurrent or secondary herpes simplex infection is seen in the patients. Herpes simplex lesions increase when CD4 cell count drops below 50 cells/mm^3.
- *Herpes zoster:* It is common in HIV infected individuals. Orally, involvement is severe and leads to sequestration of bone as well as loss of teeth.

- *Histoplasmosis:* It is the fungal infection caused by *Histoplasma capsulatum.* Sign and symptoms of disease are fever, weight loss, splenomegaly and pulmonary infiltrate.
- *Molluscum contagiosum:* It is caused by poxvirus. Lesions are small, waxy, dome-shaped papules which demonstrate central depressed crater.

Q.39. Write short note on dog bite and its management.
(Sep 2018, 5 Marks)

Ans. Dog bite in humans lead to a zoonotic disease known as rabies.

It is an acute fatal encephalomyelitis caused by a single stranded RNA virus Lyssa virus type 1.

Pathogenesis

- There is no predilection for age or sex even though, it is observed more in children and adult males.
- About 95% percent of rabies develops due to bite of rabid dog.
- Asymptomatic carrier stage occurs only in animals, but they are unlikely to be infective. Only symptomatic animals are considered to be infective.
- Rabies virus is bullet shaped envelop virus (75 nm x 180 nm) with numerous glycoprotein spikes to help in attachment of virus and also to induce antibodies. Natural occurring rabies virus is called as street virus which shows long incubation period of 20–60 days. Serial passage of this virus to brain of rabbits creates fixed virus which has got short incubation period of 4–6 days which does not show Negri bodies. This fixed virus which cannot multiply in extraneural tissues is inactivated to prepare vaccine.
- Infection commonly occurs by animal bite, often by licks, scratches. Licks on abraded skin and licks on abraded or unabraded mucosa can cause infection. Licks are often ignored dangerously. Severity of infection depends on viral load in the animal saliva and class of wound.
- Virus multiplies at the site of infection and passes (ascends) through the peripheral nerves into the CNS to develop Negra bodies in the brain leading into fatal encephalomyelitis. From the brain virus descends into different tissues like salivary glands, muscles, heart, adrenals and skin. It also involves salivary glands to get secreted in the saliva to cause infection.

Clinical Features

- Its incubation period is 3–6 weeks; but rarely can be up to many years.
- Prodromal symptoms, such as fever, headache are present.
- Pain, tingling sensation at the site of bite.
- Hyperexcitability and irritability; increased muscle reflexes and spasms.
- Increased salivation, sweating, lacrimation.
- Hydrophobia (fear of water) and aerophobia (fear of air) is pathognomonic.
- Mental instability, dilatation of pupils.
- Symptoms are aggravated by swallowing water or blowing air on them.
- Once disease starts, patient die in 72 hours.

Classification of Dog Bite

Class I: Touching or feeding the diseased animal, lick over intact skin or scratches without oozing of blood.

Class II: Licks on broken skin, scratches with blood ooze, and all bites except over head, face, palms and fingers. Minor wounds less than five in number.

Class III: All bites overhead, face, palms and fingers, lacerated wounds, wounds more than five in number, wild animal bites, and contamination of mucous membrane with saliva.

Wound Treatment

♦ Proper local wound care reduces the chances of rabies infection by 80%. Immediate cleaning and washing of the wound with running water for 15 minutes is essential to reduce the viral load at the wound site. It soap is available soap water is also used. It is better to wash with warm water if available.

♦ Wound should be cleaned with virucidal agents, such as alcohol, tincture, povidone iodine. Savlon or carbolic acid or nitric acid should not be used.

♦ Wounds should not be closed. ARS should be injected locally. In deep wounds it may be closed only after 48 hours with loose sutures after thorough washing.

♦ ARS (horse or human) should be injected to all wounds locally.

♦ One should not scrub the wound.

♦ One should not touch the wound with bare hands. One should wear gloves to touch the wound.

Passive Immunity

It is used in all severe exposures, class II and class III and in all wild animal exposure. Present recommendation is injection of ARS with vaccine in all exposed patient irrespective of the class.

Types of ARS

♦ Horse anti-rabies serum: It is given on first day with a dose of 40 IU/kg body weight. Half is given into the wound and another half is given into the gluteal muscle (IM) single dose.

♦ Human rabies immunoglobulin (HRIG): Dose is 20 units/kg body weight. Part is injected into the wound remaining part into the gluteal muscle (IM)—single dose. Patient should be immunized actively along with serum with additional booster doses. Side effects are rare here.

Postexposure prophylaxis

Cell culture and purified duck embryo vaccines are used as they are safe and efficacious.

All vaccines should be given to deltoid region. Vaccine should be stored at 4–8°C after reconstitution and should be used immediately.

Mode of Injection

a. **Intramuscular into deltoid region**—Essen regimen: It is commonly used and technically easier but higher dose is required compared to intradermal. It is injected at a schedule of 0, 3, 7, 14, and 28 days and booster at 90 days. First dose should be combined with ARS preferably HRIG. Multisite IM regime is often used as follows—first dose on day 0 two doses of IM vaccine is injected one on each side deltoid. Later single doses on 7 and 21 days [as 0 (2), 7 (1). 21 (1)].

b. **Intradermal route:**
   • Two site intradermal method is used. 1/5th of the IM dose of selected vaccine is used. Two sites on the day 0, 3, 7 and one site on the days 28 and 90. Purified vero cell rabies vaccine (PVRV) 0.1 mL; Purified chick embryo cell culture vaccine (PCECV) 0.2 mL; Purified duck embryo vaccine (PDEV) 0.2 mL.
   • Eight site intradermal method is used. On day 0, eight sites intradermal injections at both deltoids, both suprascapular, both thighs, both lower quadrants of abdomen are given. On day 7, on 4 sites—both deltoids, both thighs intradermal injections are given. On days 28 and 90 one dose on each day intradermal vaccine is injected at one site. Human diploid cell vaccine (HDCV) 0.2 mL is used. It is like 0 (8); 7 (4); 28 (1); 90 (1). In whatevertype, on first day (0) rabies immunoglobulin should be injected locally as well as IM.

Postexposure Vaccination

If individual has been vaccinated earlier. Doses on days 0, 3, and 7 are given. But ideally assessed by serum antibody level (should be more than 0.5 IU/mL). Passive immunity is not given in individuals who had vaccination earlier.

Pre-exposure Prophylaxis

It is given to veterinarians, animal handlers. Dose: 1 mL of cell culture vaccine IM or 0.1 mL intradermally on days 0, 7, 28. Serum titer for antibodies should be assessed after 1 month. It is less than 0.5 IU/mL then one booster dose is injected. Booster doses are given once in every 2 years.

---

4. ULCER

Q.1. Write note on nonhealing ulcer. *(Sep 1997, 6 Marks)*

Ans. Nonhealing ulcer is classified under clinical classification of ulcers.

Nonhealing ulcer is also known as chronic ulcer depending on cause of ulcer.

♦ Chronic ulcer has no tendency to heal by itself.

♦ The bases of ulcer are indurated (hard).

♦ Floor of ulcer contain unhealthy granulation tissue and slough.

♦ Here edges depend on the cause, i.e., punched out, undermined, rolled out and beaded.

♦ Regional draining lymph nodes may be enlarged but nontender.

Causes of Chronic or Nonhealing Ulcer

Local Causes

♦ Recurrent infection

♦ Trauma, presence of foreign body or sequestrum

- Absence of rest and immobilization
- Poor blood supply, hypoxia
- Edema of the part
- Loss of sensation
- Periostitis or osteomyelitis of the underlying bone
- Fibrosis of the surrounding soft tissues
- Lymphatic diseases

General/Specific Causes

- Anemia, hypoproteinemia
- Vitamin deficiencies
- Tuberculosis, leprosy
- Diabetes mellitus, hypertension
- Chronic liver or kidney diseases
- Steroid therapy locally or systemically
- Cytotoxic chemotherapy or radiotherapy
- Malignancy

For Example

- Diabetic ulcer
- Malignant ulcer
- Carcinomatous ulcer
- Ulcer of squamous cell carcinoma
- Rodent ulcer.

Q.2. Write short note on differential diagnosis of ulcer on the lateral border of tongue. *(Sep 2004, 10 Marks)*

Ans. The various types of ulcer on the lateral border of tongue are as follows:

- Aphthous ulcer
- Traumatic or dental ulcer
- Chronic nonspecific ulcer
- Post-pertussis ulcer
- Syphilitic ulcer
- Tuberculous ulcer
- Carcinomatous ulcer
- Herpetic ulcer
- Ulcer due to glossitis.

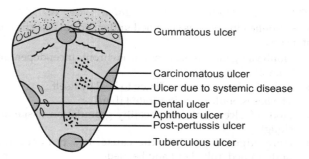

Fig. 5: Ulcers on tongue.

- **Aphthous ulcer:**
  - *Minor aphthous ulcer:*
    - It is small painful ulcer seen on the tip, undersurface and side of the tongue.
    - The ulcer is small, superficial with white floor, yellowish border and surrounded by a hyperemic zone.

- It can occur at any age group, more common in females at the time of menstruation.
  - *Major aphthous ulcer:*
    - When they are larger, deeper, painful, they are called major aphthous ulcer.
    - They subside within a few days.
    - Temporary relief can be obtained by applying salicylate gel.
    - Vitamin B complex is usually given.
- **Traumatic or dental ulcer:**
  - This ulcer occurs due to broken, sharp tooth, ill-fitting dentures, prosthesis, etc.
  - These ulcers occur at the lateral border or under surface of tongue.
  - It often presents a slough at its base and surrounded by a zone of erythema and induration.
  - This ulcer is quit painful.
- **Chronic nonspecific ulcer:**
  - Usually occur in the anterior two-thirds of the tongue.
  - Its etiology is unknown.
  - It is moderately indurated and not very painful.
- **Post-pertussis ulcer:**
  - Occurs only in children with whooping cough.
  - Usually seen on the upper part of frenum lingulae and in the undersurface of tongue.
- **Syphilitic ulcer:**
  - Primary ulcer, i.e., chancre found on the tip of the tongue.
  - Mainly snail-track ulcers are seen in oral cavity in second stage of syphilis.
  - In tertiary syphilis, the gummatous ulcers are found on the midline in the anterior two-thirds of the tongue
  - The gumma found on the dorsum of tongue.
- **Tuberculous ulcer:**
  - Young adults are usually involved.
  - Such ulcers are shallow, often multiple and grayish yellow with slightly red undermining edges.
  - These ulcers are seen at the margin (lateral border), tip or dorsum of tongue.
  - These ulcers are very painful with enlargement of regional lymph nodes.
- **Carcinomatous ulcer:**
  - It usually occur in elderly individual above the age of 50 year.
  - Common site is the margins of tongue.
  - It may occur at the dorsum of tongue.
  - It is usually single, but may be multiple.
  - It is usually painless to start.
  - The ulcer is irregular in shape, has a raised and everted edges with indurated base.
  - The floor of such ulcer is covered with necrotic debris.
  - It bleeds on touch.
  - It is fixed with underlying structures.

Q.3. Write short note on lesion on anterior 2/3rd of tongue. *(Mar 2009, 5 Marks) (Sep 2006, 5 Marks)*

Ans. Lesions on the anterior 2/3rd of tongue are:

Ulcers

- Aphthous ulcer
- Tubercular ulcer
- Traumatic ulcer
- Carcinomatous ulcer
- Gummatous ulcer.

For details of above ulcers refer to Ans. 2 of same chapter.

Q.4. Classify ulcers of tongue. *(Mar 2011, 3 Marks)*

Ans. Classification of ulcers of tongue

- **Nonspecific:**
  - Traumatic or dental ulcer due to sharp tooth or dentures
  - Infective:
    - Simple ulcer due to glossitis
    - Herpetic ulcer
    - Post-pertussis ulcer.
  - Aphthous ulcer.
- **Specific:**
  - Tubercular ulcer
  - Syphilitic ulcer
  - Malignant ulcer.

Q.5. Write short note on trophic ulcer. *(Aug 2011, 5 Marks)*

Ans. It is also called as decubitus ulcer or pressure sore.

Trophic ulcer is tissue necrosis and ulceration due to prolonged pressure. Blood flow to the skin stops once external pressure becomes more than 30 mm Hg and this causes tissue hypoxia, necrosis and ulceration. It is more prominent between bony prominence and an external surface.

Etiology

It is due to:

- Impaired nutrition.
- Defective blood supply.
- *Neurological deficit:* Due to the presence of neurological deficit, trophic ulcer is also called as neurogenic ulcer/ neuropathic ulcer. Initially, it begins as callosity due to repeated trauma and pressure, under which suppuration occurs and gives way through a central hole which extends down into the deeper plane up to the underlying bone as perforating ulcer.

Sites

- Over ischial tuberosity
- Sacrum
- In the heel
- In relation to head of metatarsals
- Buttocks
- Over the shoulder
- Occiput

Clinical Features

- It occurs in 5% of hospitalized patients.
- Ulcer is painless and is punched out.
- Ulcer is nonmobile and base of the ulcer is formed by bone.

Management

- Cause should be treated.
- Nutritional supplementation is given.
- Rest, antibiotics, slough excision, regular dressings.
- *Vacuum-assisted closure:* It is the creation of intermittent negative pressure of minus 125 mm Hg to promote formation of healthy granulation tissue. A perforated drain is kept over the foam dressing covered over the pressure sore. It is sealed with a transparent adhesive sheet. Drain is connected to required vacuum apparatus. Once ulcer granulates well. Flap cover or skin grafting is done.
- Excision of the ulcer and skin grafting is done.
- *Flaps:* Local rotation or other flaps (transposition flaps).
- *Proper care:* Change in position once in 2 hours; lifting the limb upwards for 10 seconds once in 10 minutes; nutrition; use of water bed/air bed/air-fluid floatation bed and pressure dispersion cushions to the affected area; urinary and fecal care; hygiene; psychological counseling. Regular skin observation; keeping skin clean and dry (using regular use of talcum powder); oil massaging of the skin and soft tissues using clean, absorbent porous clothing; control and prevention of sepsis helps in the management.

Q.6. Define and describe differentiating features of Curling ulcer and Cushing ulcer. *(Jan 2012, 5 Marks)*

Ans.

Features	Curling ulcer	Cushing's ulcer
Definition	Acute ulcers which develop after major burns	Acute ulcers which develop after cerebral trauma or after neurological operations
Type	True stress ulcer	Not the true stress ulcer
Number	Multiple	Single ulcer
Symptoms	Pain in epigastric region, vomiting, hematemesis	No symptoms present
Area of occurrence	Body and fundus	Esophagus and duodenum
Treatment	It is conservative, by giving IV ranitidine, IV pantoprazole 80 mg in 100 mL DNS—slow	Treatment is by IV ranitidine
Transfer to malignancy	Commonly transferred to malignancy	Not commonly transferred to malignancy

Q.7. Write short note on ulcer. *(Aug 2012, 5 Marks)*

Ans. An ulcer is the break in the continuity of the covering epithelium either skin or mucus membrane due to molecular death.

Classification of Ulcer

Classification I (Clinical)

- Spreading ulcer
- Healing ulcer

- Nonhealing ulcer
- Callous ulcer

Classification II (Based on Duration)

- *Acute ulcer:* Duration <2 weeks
- *Chronic ulcer:* Duration >2 weeks

Classification III (Pathological)

- *Specific ulcers:*
  - Tuberculous ulcer
  - Syphilitic ulcer
  - Actinomycosis
  - Meleney's ulcer
- *Malignant ulcers:*
  - Carcinomatous ulcer
  - Rodent ulcer
  - Melanotic ulcer
- *Nonspecific ulcers:*
  - Traumatic ulcers
  - Arterial ulcer
  - Venous ulcer
  - Trophic ulcer
  - Infective ulcer
  - Tropical ulcer
  - Ulcers due to chilblain and frostbite
  - Martorell's hypertensive ulcer
  - Bazin's ulcer
  - Diabetic ulcer
  - Ulcers due to leukemia, polycythemia, jaundice, collagen diseases, lymphedema
  - Cortisol ulcers

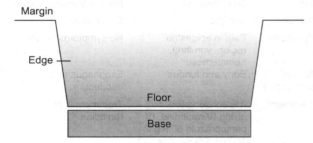

Fig. 6: Parts of an ulcer.

Parts of an Ulcer

- *Margin:* It may be regular or irregular. It may be rounded or oval.
- *Edge:* Edge is the one which connects floor of the ulcer to the margin. Different edges are:
  - *Sloping edge:* It is seen in a healing ulcer. Its inner part is red because of red, healthy granulation tissue. Its outer part is white due to scar/fibrous tissue. Its middle part is blue due to epithelial proliferation.

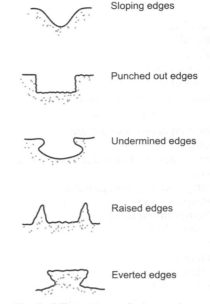

Fig. 7: Different types of edges—ulcers.

- *Undermined edge* is seen in a tuberculous ulcer. Disease process advances in deeper plane (in subcutaneous tissue) whereas (skin) epidermis proliferates inwards.
- *Punched out edge* is seen in a gummatous (syphilitic) ulcer and trophic ulcer. It is due to endarteritis.
- *Raised and beaded edge* (pearly white) is seen in a rodent ulcer (basal cell carcinoma). Beads are due to proliferating active cells.
- *Everted edge (rolled out edge):* It is seen in a carcinomatous ulcer due to spill of the proliferating malignant tissues over the normal skin.
- *Floor:* It is the one which is seen. Floor may contain discharge, granulation tissue or slough.
- *Base:* Base is the one on which ulcer rests. It may be bone or soft tissue.

Induration of ulcer: It is the clinical palpatory sign which means a specific type of hardness in a diseased tissue. It is seen in carcinomatous ulcers.

Investigations for Ulcer

- *Study of discharge:* Culture and sensitivity, acid fast bacilli study and cytology.
- *Edge biopsy:* Biopsy is taken from the edge because edge contains multiplying cells. Usually, two biopsies are taken. Biopsy taken from the center may be inadequate because of central necrosis.
- X-ray of the part to look for periostitis/osteomyelitis.
- FNAC of the lymph node.
- Chest X-ray, Mantoux test in suspected case of tuberculous ulcer.

♦ Hemoglobin, ESR, total WBC count, serum protein estimation.

Management of an Ulcer

♦ Cause should be found and treated
♦ Correct the deficiencies, such as anemia, protein and vitamins deficiencies
♦ Transfuse blood, if required
♦ Control the pain and infection
♦ Investigate properly
♦ Control the infection and give rest to the part
♦ Care of the ulcer by debridement, ulcer cleaning and dressing is done daily or twice daily.
♦ Remove the exuberant granulation tissue
♦ Topical antibiotics for infected ulcers only like, silver sulfadiazine, mupirocin.
♦ Antibiotics are not required once healthy granulation tissues, if are formed
♦ Once granulates, defect is closed with secondary suturing, skin graft, flaps

Q.8. Describe briefly diabetic ulcer. *(Apr 2017, 5 Marks)*

Ans. Diabetic ulcer is most common in foot. It can cause abscess, ulcer, osteomyelitis, gangrene, septicemia. Initially, patient undergo toe amputation but later eventually land with below knee or above knee amputation.

Causes

♦ Increased glucose in the tissue precipitates infection.
♦ Diabetic microangiopathy which affects microcirculation.
♦ Increased glycosylated hemoglobin decreases the oxygen dissociation.
♦ Increased glycosylated tissue protein decreases the oxygen utilization.
♦ Diabetic neuropathy involving all sensory, motor and autonomous components.
♦ Associated atherosclerosis.

Sites

♦ Foot-plantar aspect is the most common site
♦ Leg
♦ Upper limb, back, scrotum, perineum
♦ Diabetic ulcer may be associated with ischemia
♦ Ulcer is usually spreading and deep

Investigations

♦ Blood sugar both random and fasting.
♦ Urine ketone bodies.
♦ Discharge for culture and sensitivity.
♦ X-ray of the part to see osteomyelitis.
♦ Arterial Doppler of the limb; glycosylated hemoglobin estimation.

Problems with Diabetic Ulcer

♦ Neuropathy, in foot—clawing of toes, hammer toe (due to intrinsic muscle paralysis)
♦ Multiple deeper abscesses; osteomyelitis of deeper bones are common.

♦ Reduced leukocyte function; resistant infection; spreading cellulitis
♦ Arterial Insufficiency
♦ Septicemia; diabetic ketoacidosis
♦ Associated cardiac diseases like ischemic heart disease

Treatment

♦ Control of diabetes by using insulin.
♦ Proper antibiotics should be started after culture and sensitivity report
♦ Nutritional supplements.
♦ Regular cleaning, debridement, dressing.
♦ Once granulates, the ulcer is covered with skin graft or flap.
♦ Revascularization procedure is done by endarterectomy or thrombectomy or balloon angioplasty or arterial bypass graft. But if distal vessels are involved, then success rate is less.
♦ Toe foot/leg amputation.
♦ Microcellular rubber (MCR) shoes to prevent injuries; care of foot.

Q.9. Define ulcer. Describe different types of ulcer.
(June 2018, 3 Marks)

Or

Write short answer on ulcer and its types.
(Feb 2019, 3 Marks)

Ans. An ulcer is the break in the continuity of the covering epithelium either skin or mucus membrane due to molecular death.

Different Types of Ulcer

Classification I (Clinical)

♦ *Spreading ulcer:* In this edge is inflamed, irregular and edematous. It is an acute painful ulcer, floor consists of profuse purulent discharge and slough. Surrounding area is red and edematous
♦ *Healing ulcer:* Edge is sloping with healthy pink/red granulation tissue with scanty/minimal serous discharge on the floor, slough is absent. Surrounding area does not show any signs of inflammation or induration. Base is not indurated. Three zones are seen, i.e., innermost red zone of healthy granulation tissue, middle bluish zone of growing epithelium, outer white zone of fibrosis and scar formation.
♦ *Nonhealing ulcer:* In this ulcer, edge of the ulcer depend on the cause punched out (trophic), undermined (tuberculosis), rolled out (carcinomatous ulcer), beaded (rodent ulcer); floor consists of unhealthy granulation tissue and slough, and serosanguineous/purulent/bloody discharge, regional draining lymph nodes are enlarged but nontender.
♦ *Callous ulcer:* This is a chronic nonhealing ulcer, floor consists of pale, unhealthy, flabby, whitish yellow granulation tissue and thin scanty serous discharge or rarely with copious serosanguinous discharge, with indurated nontender edge, base is indurated, nontender and is often fixed. Ulcer does not show any tendency to heal. It lasts for months to years. Induration and pigmentation can be seen.

Classification II (Based on Duration)

- *Acute ulcer:* Duration <2 weeks
- *Chronic ulcer:* Duration >2 weeks

Classification III (Pathological)

- *Specific ulcers:*
  - Tuberculous ulcer: Ulcer can be single or multiple; oval or rounded with undermined edge, painless with caseous material on the floor. Ulcer is not deep
  - Syphilitic ulcer: It has punched out edge, deep with wash leather slough in the floor and indurated base.
  - Actinomycosis: In this initially an induration develops. It softens and bursts via skin as sinuses which discharge pus and have sulfur granules.
  - Meleney's ulcer: It is seen in postoperative wounds in abdomen and chest wall. This is a acute rapidly spreading ulcer with destruction and deep burrowing of subcutaneous tissues.
- *Malignant ulcers:*
  - Carcinomatous ulcer: This ulcer arises from prickle cell layer of skin. It has rolled out/everted edge. Floor consists of necrotic content, unhealthy granulation tissue and blood. Ulcer bleeds on touch and is vascular or friable. Induration is felt at base and edge. It is circular or irregular in shape.
  - Rodent ulcer: It is seen in basal cell carcinoma. Ulcer shows central area of dry scab with peripheral, raised active and beaded edge. Often floor is pigmented. It erodes in deeper planes, such as soft tissue, cartilage and bones
  - Melanotic ulcer: It is the ulcerative form of melanoma. Ulcer is pigmented often with halo around. Ulcer is rapidly growing often with satellite nodules.
- *Nonspecific ulcers:*
  - Traumatic ulcers: It occurs after trauma. Ulcer is superficial, painful and tender.
  - Arterial ulcer: This ulcer occurs after trauma and soon become non – healing. Ulcer is usually deep, destruct deep fascia, exposing tendons, muscles and underlying bone. Ulcer is very painful, tender and often hyperaesthetic
  - Venous ulcer: It is common around ankle due to ambulatory chronic venous hypertension. Ulcer is initially painful but once it become chronic, it is painless. It is vertically oval in shape. Floor is covered with pale or often without any granulation tissue. Edge is sloping. Induration and tenderness is seen often at base of an ulcer.
  - Trophic ulcer: It is the ulcer due to prolonged pressure. Blood flow to skin stops once external pressure becomes more than 30 mm of Hg and this leads to tissue hypoxia, necrosis and ulceration.
  - Infective ulcer
  - Tropical ulcer: It is an acute ulcerative lesion of skin seen in tropical countries. Pustule formation occur which bursts in three days with necrobiosis and phagedena causing spreading painful ulcer with an undermined edge, brownish floor and serosanguineous discharge

- Ulcers due to chilblain and frostbite: This is due to exposure of a part to wet cold below freezing point. Ulcers here are deep
- Martorell's hypertensive ulcer: It is seen in hypertensive patients often with atherosclerosis. In this necrosis of calf skin occur with sloughing away and formation of deep, punched out ulcers extending to deep fascia.
- Bazin's ulcer
- Diabetic ulcer: Diabetic ulcer is most common in foot. It can cause abscess, ulcer, osteomyelitis, gangrene, septicemia. Initially, patient undergo toe amputation but later eventually land with below knee or above knee amputation.
- Ulcers due to leukemia, polycythemia, jaundice, collagen diseases, lymphedema
- Cortisol ulcers: They are due to long time application of cortisol creams to certain skin diseases.

Q.10. Write difference between healing and nonhealing ulcer. *(Feb 2019, 5 Marks)*

Ans. Following are the differences between healing and nonhealing ulcer:

Healing ulcer	Nonhealing ulcer
It is an acute form of ulcer	It is a chronic form of an ulcer
It is severely painful	It is less painful
It does not bleed on manipulation	It bleeds on manipulation
Floor of the ulcer has healthy granulation tissue.	Floor of the ulcer has unhealthy granulation tissue
Healing ulcer has yellowish gray base and is nonindurated	Base of the nonhealing ulcer is indurated
Healing ulcer has sloping edge. Its inner part is red due to red healthy granulation tissue. Outer part is white due to fibrous tissue and middle part is blue due to epithelial proliferation.	Here edges depend on the cause, i.e., punched out, undermined, rolled out and beaded.
Regional draining lymph nodes become enlarged and are tender.	Regional draining lymph nodes may be enlarged but nontender.

Q.11. Enumerate causes of ulcer on tongue. Describe tubercular ulcer of tongue. *(Oct 2019, 5 Marks)*

Ans.

Enumeration of Causes of Ulcer on Tongue

Name of the ulcer of tongue	Causes
Aphthous ulcer	• Due to immunological abnormalities • Because of genetic predilection • Due to α hemolytic streptococcus and *Streptococcus sanguis* • Patients with deficiency of vitamin B12 or folic acid or iron • Due to endocrine conditions • Due to stress • Because of allergy • Patient's having anemia

Contd...

Contd...

Name of the ulcer of tongue	Causes
Dental ulcer	Due to broken tooth, ill fitting denture, prosthesis, etc.
Tubercular ulcer	Tuberculous bacteria
Gummatous ulcer	Syphilis
Autoimmune ulcers	Due to autoimmune diseases, such as pemphigus, SLE and lichen planus
Post-pertussis ulcer	Because of repeated coughing in pertussis
Herpetic ulcer	Due to herpes infection
Nonhealing ulcer or carcinomatous ulcer	• Because of physical trauma • Alcohol • Tobacco smoking or chewing • Candidiasis • Syphilis • Sepsis • Chronic dental trauma • Chronic superficial glossitis

Tubercular Ulcer of Tongue

♦ It affects the tip of tongue, margin and anterior two-thirds of tongue.
♦ Lesion may be preceded by an opalescent vesicle or nodule, a result of caseous necrosis.
♦ The ulcer is painful with enlargement of regional lymph nodes.
♦ The ulcer has undermined edges and is shallow with minimum induration.
♦ Mucosa surrounding the ulcer is inflamed and edematous.
♦ Base of the ulcer is yellowish and granular.
♦ Ulcers are sometimes multiple with serous discharge.

5. LYMPHATICS AND LYMPH NODE ENLARGEMENT

Q.1. Enumerate the causes of lymph node enlargement in neck and describe the clinical features and management of tubercular lymphadenitis. *(Mar 1997, 15 Marks)*

Or

Write in brief about clinical features and management of tuberculous lymphadenitis. *(Mar 2001, 15 Marks)*

Or

Describe the clinical features and treatment of tubercular sinus in neck. *(Mar 2008, 10 Marks)*

Or

Write in brief management of tubercular cervical lymphadenopathy. *(Sep 2007, 5 Marks)*

Ans.

Causes of Enlargement of Lymph Node in Neck

♦ *Inflammatory:* Due to microorganism.
  • Bacterial as: *Streptococcus, Mycobacterium, Treponema pallidum*, Actinomycosis.
  • Viral as: Lymphogranuloma venereum, infectious mononucleosis, HIV
  • Parasite as: *Wuchereria bancrofti*
  • Fungus as: Blastomycosis.
♦ Lymphatic leukemia.
♦ *Autoimmune disorders:*
  • Systemic lupus erythematous
  • Rheumatoid arthritis
  • Sclerosis.
♦ *Neoplasms:* Malignant neoplasm involves lymph node like.
  • Malignant lymphoma
  • Hodgkin's disease
  • Lymphosarcoma
  • Malignant melanoma.
♦ Secondaries in lymph nodes.

Clinical Features of Tubercular Lymphadenitis

♦ Swelling in the neck is present, which is firm and matted.
♦ Cold abscess is soft, smooth, nontender, fluctuant, without involvement of the skin. It is not warm.
♦ As a result of increased pressure, cold abscess ruptures out of the deep fascia to form collar stud abscess which is adherent to the overlying skin.
♦ Once collar stud abscess bursts open, discharging sinus is formed. It can be multiple, wide open mouth, often undermined, nonmobile with bluish color around the edge. It is usually not indurated.
♦ Tonsils may be studded with tubercles and so clinically should always be examined.
♦ Associated pulmonary tuberculosis should also be looked for. In 20% cases of tuberculous lymphadenitis, there may be associated pulmonary tuberculosis or it may be a primary focus.
♦ Cervical spine is examined for tuberculosis.
♦ Axillary nodes, when involved are due to retrograde lymphatic spread from neck nodes or blood spread.
♦ Inguinal lymph nodes are involved occasionally through blood.
♦ Bluish hyperpigmented involved overlying skin is called as scrofuloderma.
♦ Tuberculous pus with caseating cheesy creamy material is infective as it contains multiplying organisms.
♦ Atypical mycobacterial tuberculosis can occur occasionally. Such disease may be resistant to drug therapy.
♦ Sinus may persist due to fibrosis, calcification, secondary infection inadequate reach of drug to maintain optimum concentration in caseation.

Management of Tubercular Lymphadenitis

♦ **Drugs:** Antitubercular drugs have to be started—
  • Rifampicin 450 mg OD on empty stomach. It is bactericidal.

- INH: 300 mg OD. It is bactericidal.
- Ethambutol 800 mg OD. It is bacteriostatic.
- Pyrazinamide 1500 mg OD (or 750 mg BD). It is bactericidal.

Duration of treatment is usually 6–9 months.

♦ **Aspiration:** When there is cold abscess, initially it is aspirated. Wide bore needle is introduced into the cold abscess in a nondependent site along a "Z" track (in zig-zag pathway) so as to prevent sinus formation.

♦ **Incision and drainage:** If cold abscess recurs, then it should be drained. Drainage is done through a nondependent incision. After draining the caseating material, wound is closed without placing a drain.

♦ **Surgical removal:** Surgical removal of tubercular lymph nodes are indicated when
  - There is no local response to drugs
  - When sinus persists.

It is done by raising skin flaps and removing all caseating material and lymph nodes. Care is taken not to injure major structures.

Excision of the sinus tract is often essential when sinus develops.

Q.2. Write in brief about etiology, pathology, clinical features and treatment of cervical tuberculous lymphadenitis. *(Feb 2013, 10 Marks)*

Or

Discuss etiology, pathology, clinical features and treatment of tuberculous lymphadenitis.
(Mar 2003, 15 Marks)

Ans. *For clinical features and treatment of tuberculous lymphadenitis, refer to Ans. 1 of same chapter.*

Etiology

♦ Tuberculous bacillus, i.e., *Mycobacterium tuberculosis* is the bacteria which leads to tuberculosis.

♦ Disease is caused in people of low socioeconomic status, unhygienic living conditions and malnutrition.

♦ In 20% of cases, lymph nodes are affected in posterior triangle due to involvement of adenoid.

Pathology

When the tubercle bacilli are introduced into the tissue.

♦ Initial response of neutrophils
♦ There is progressive infiltration by macrophages
♦ Macrophages start phagocytosing the tubercle bacilli.
♦ Activated CD4 + T-cells develop.
♦ In 2–3 days, the macrophages undergo structural changes and form epithelioid cells.
♦ The epithelioid cells aggregated into tight clusters or granulomas.
♦ Some macrophages form multinucleated giant cells.
♦ Hard tubercles form by the mass of epithelioid cells and the giant cells in a zone of lymphocytes, plasma cells and fibroblasts.
♦ Center of the cellular mass undergoes caseous necrosis, characterized by cheesy appearance called as soft tubercle.

Q.3. Write short note on tuberculous lymphadenitis.
(Mar 2006, 5 Marks) (Sep 2005, 8 Marks)

Or

Discuss briefly tubercular lymphadenitis.
(Aug 2012, 5 Marks)

Or

Write brief notes on tubercular lymphadenitis.
(Apr 2017, 2 Marks)

Or

Write in brief about tubercular cervical lympha-denitis. *(Mar 2007, 5 Marks)*

Ans. Tubercular lymphadenitis is defined as chronic specific granulomatous inflammation with caseation necrosis of lymph node.

Clinical features

Refer to Ans. 1 of same chapter.

Staging

Stage of Lymphadenitis

♦ Common in young adult between 20–30 years.
♦ Upper anterior deep cervical nodes are enlarged.
♦ Nontender, discrete, mobile, firm lymph node is palpable.

Stage of Matting

♦ Results due to involvement of capsule of lymph node.
♦ Nodes moves together
♦ Firm, nontender.

Stage of Cold Abscess

♦ It occurs due to caseation necrosis of lymph node.
♦ No local rise in temperature.
♦ No tenderness.
♦ No redness.
♦ Soft, cystic and fluctuant swelling.
♦ Transillumination is negative.
♦ On sternomastoid contraction test, it becomes less prominent indicating that it is deep-to-deep fascia.

Stage of Collar Stud Abscess

It results when a cold abscess rupture through the deep fascia and form another swelling in the subcutaneous plane which is fluctuant.

Stage of Sinus

♦ Collar stud abscess burst and form tubercular sinus.
♦ Common in young female.
♦ It can be multiple.
♦ Resemble an ulcer with undermined edge.
♦ No indurations.
♦ Skin surrounding the sinus shows pigmentation and sometimes bluish in color.

Differential Diagnosis

♦ Nonspecific lymphadenitis
♦ Secondaries in neck
♦ Lymphomas and chronic lymphatic leukemia
♦ Branchial cyst and lymphatic cyst mimic cold abscess
♦ HIV with lymph node involvement

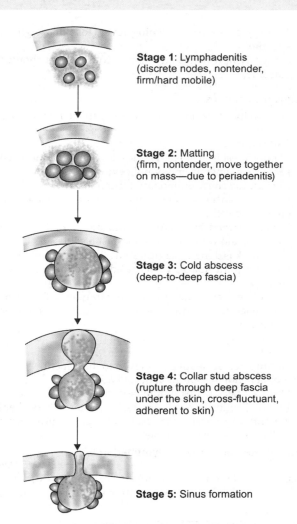

Stage 1: Lymphadenitis (discrete nodes, nontender, firm/hard mobile)

Stage 2: Matting (firm, nontender, move together on mass—due to periadenitis)

Stage 3: Cold abscess (deep-to-deep fascia)

Stage 4: Collar stud abscess (rupture through deep fascia under the skin, cross-fluctuant, adherent to skin)

Stage 5: Sinus formation

Fig. 8: Tubercular lymphadenitis.

Investigations

- Hematocrit, ESR, peripheral smear.
- *FNAC of lymph node and smear for AFB and culture:* FNAC is very useful but not as superior as open node biopsy. False negative, false positive results and altering the node architecture, and so eventual need of open biopsy are the problems. Epithelioid cells (modified histiocytes/macrophages) are diagnostic. Langhans giant cells, lymphocytes, plasma cells are other features.
- *Open biopsy:* Open biopsy is more reliable for tuberculosis (and also in lymphoma; but it is contraindicated in node secondaries); entire node ideally two nodes if possible has to be taken intact; one in formalin for pathology, other in normal saline for microbiology (AFB).
- HIV test (ELISA and western blot).
- Lowenstein–Jensen media is used for culture which takes 6 weeks to give result; so selenite media is often used which shows growth in 5 days.

- Mantoux test may be useful; but not very reliable.
- Chest X-ray to look for pulmonary tuberculosis.
- Polymerase chain reaction (PCR) is very useful method.

Management

Refer to Ans. 1 of same chapter.

Q.4. Write short note on: Collar stud abscess.
(Dec 2010, 5 Marks)
(Sep 2007, 5 Marks) (Sep 2005, 5 Marks)

Ans. Collar stud abscess is an acute suppurative infection of a digit which present stud-like blister.

- It is bilocular abscess with one lobule deep to the deep fascia and another lobule is superficial to fascia.
  Both the locule intercommunicates with each other through a small perforation in the deep fascia.
  Such an abscess can occur anywhere in the body.

Types

- **Pyogenic:** When pyogenic abscess develops deep to deep fascia and gradually pressure mouth so that the deep fascia perforates, the pus comes out into superficial fascia.

  So, pyogenic collar stud abscess is more commonly seen in hand where deep fascia is in the palmer fascia.
- **Tuberculous:** This is more often seen in the neck from caseation tubercular lymph node. The cold abscess beneath the deep fascia ruptures and forms another swelling in subcutaneous plane which is fluctuant. It remains adhere to skin.

Treatment

Pyogenic Collar Stud Abscess

- Drainage of terminal pulp space by an oblique deep incision.
- Systemic antibiotics should be given.

Tuberculous Collar Stud Abscess

It should be treated like as cold abscess, i.e.

- Antitubercular treatment is given.
- Zig-zag aspiration by wide bore needle in nondependent area for prevention of sinus perforation.
- Drainage can be done by using nondependent incision and later on closure of wound is done without placing a drain.

Q.5. Describe the causes of generalized lymphadenopathy and management of Hodgkin's lymphoma.
(Oct 2007, 15 Marks)

Ans. Enlargement of lymph gland is called as lymphadenopathy.

Causes of Generalized Lymphadenopathy

- *Acute infection process:* Glandular fever.
- Tuberculosis
- *Syphilis:* In secondary stage
- Disseminated lupus erythematosus
- *Blood disease:* Acute lymphatic leukemia, chronic lymphatic leukemia

- *Neoplasm:* Secondary carcinoma
- HIV infection and AIDS
- Sarcoidosis.

Management of Hodgkin's Lymphoma

- **Stage I and II:**
  - Mainly radiotherapy, i.e., external high cobalt radiotherapy
  - *Above the diaphragm:* Y-field therapy, covering cervical, axillary, mediastinal lymph nodes.
  - Below the diaphragm: Mantle or inverted-Y field therapy covering para-aortic and iliac nodes.
  - Chemotherapy is also given.
- **Stage III and IV:**
  - In this, mainly chemotherapy is given.
  - Regimens used are:

  MOPP Regimen
  - *Mechlorethamine:* 6 mg/sqm on 1st and 8th day
  - *Oncovine:* 1.4 mg/sqm on 1st and 10th day
  - *Procarbazine:* 100 mg orally daily for 10 days
  - *Prednisolone:* 45 mg orally daily for 10 days
    MOPP combination is given in 6 courses with no drugs given from 15th to 28th day.

  ABVD Regimen
  - *Adriamycin:* 30 mg/sqm
  - *Bleomycin:* 10 mg/sqm
  - *Vinblastine:* 6 mg/sqm
  - *Dacarbazine:* 350 mg/sqm
  - The cycle is repeated on 20th day.
    Splenectomy is done in many patients except with stage IV disease.

Q.6. Write in brief cold abscess in neck.

(Apr 2008, 5 Marks)

Or

Write short note on cold abscess in neck.

(Dec 2009, 5 Marks) (Nov 2008, 5 Marks)

Or

Describe diagnostic features and treatment of cold abscess. *(Jan 2012, 5 Marks)*

Ans. Cold abscess is common in neck.

Etiology

- *Tuberculous lymphadenitis:* Cold abscess is seen commonly in anterior triangle of neck
- *Tuberculosis of cervical spine:* Cold abscess is seen commonly in posterior triangle of neck.

Clinical Features

- It is commonly seen in young individuals but can occur in any age group.
- Swelling in neck is smooth, nontender, soft, fluctuating, nontransilluminant, nonmobile and is not adherent to skin.
- There is presence of neck pain, neck rigidity and restricted movements of cervical spine.
- *Rust sign:* With change in position and often when patient is seated, he support his head with hands and forearm.

- There is presence of evening fever, loss of weight and appetite.
- Matted lymph nodes adjacent to cold abscess should be palpable.

Diagnostic Features

- Oral cavity, chest and tonsils of the patient are thoroughly examined.
- ESR is raised
- Mantoux test is positive. This test is useful but not reliable.
- Presence of anemia and lymphocytosis
- Chest X-ray show pulmonary tuberculosis
- FNAC of cold abscess under microscopic examination show epithelioid cells.
- Fluid obtained by FNAC should be stained by Ziehl–Neelsen stain which reveals acid-fast bacilli
- X-ray neck is done in cervical spine tuberculosis to identify reduced joint space, vertebral destruction, soft tissue shadow.
- MRI of cervical spine, ultrasonography or CT scan neck are needed to confirm anatomical location and number of lesions.

Treatment

- Antitubercular treatment is given to the patient.
- Nondependent aspiration of cold abscess.
- Diseased neck nodes should be excised.
- Immobilization of cervical spine by plaster jacket/collar for 4 months. Cervical spine fusion by open surgical method, if diseased spine is unstable.

Q.7. Write short note on lymphedema.

(May/June 2009, 5 Marks)

Ans. Lymphedema is the accumulation of lymph in extracellular and extravascular fluid compartment commonly in subcutaneous tissue.

It is due to defective lymphatic drainage.

Classification

- Primary without any identifiable lymphatic disease.
- Secondary is acquired.

Pathophysiology

Decreased lymphatic contractility, lymphatic valvular insufficiency, lymphatic obliteration by infection, tumor or surgery causes all effects and pathology of lymphedema. This leads to lymphatic hypertension and dilatation causing lymph stasis, accumulation of proteins, glycosamines, growth factors, and bacteria. There is more collagen formation, deposition of proteins, fibroblasts, ground substance causing fibrosis in subcutaneous and outside deep fascia. Muscles are normal without any edema but may get hypertrophied.

Clinical Features

- Most commonly lower limb is involved.
- Presence of swelling in the foot which extends progressively in the neck and show tree-trunk pattern leg.
- Presence of buffalo hump in dorsum of foot.

♦ Athlete's foot with joint pain and disability
♦ Fever, malaise and headache
♦ Initially pitting edema occurs which later on become non-pitting.
♦ Stemmer's sign is positive, i.e., skin over dorsum of foot cannot be pinched because of subcutaneous fibrosis.

Grading of Lymphedema

This is given by Brunner:

♦ *Latent:* No clinically apparent lymphedema
♦ *Grade I:* Pitting edema which more or less disappears on elevation of the limb.
♦ *Grade II:* Non-pitting edema occur which does not reduce on elevation
♦ *Grade III:* Edema with irreversible skin changes, such as fibrosis, papillae, fissuring.

Treatment

♦ **Conservative:**
  • Elevation of limb, exercise and weight reduction.
  • Static isometric activities should be stopped, such as prolong standing or carrying heavy weight. Rhythmic movements should be encouraged, such as swimming, massaging
  • Daily wearing of below knee stockings
  • Trauma and infection should be avoided.
  • Complex decongestive therapy should be given. It occurs in two phases, i.e., intensive therapy and maintenance therapy.
♦ **Surgeries:**
  • Excision of lesion can be done by Charle's or Homan's operation.
  • *Physiological:* Omentoplasty can be done.
  • *Combination of excision and physiological:* Both excision and creation of communication between superficial and deep lymphatics. Sistrunk and Thompson's operation can be done.
  • Bypass procedures can be done
  • Limb reduction surgeries can be done.

Q.8. Write short note on clinical features of TB and its management, especially "DOTS regime".

(Jun 2010, 5 Marks)

Ans. TB is a granulomatous disease caused by *Mycobacterium tuberculosis.*

Clinical Features

♦ Seen commonly in middle aged and older individuals.
♦ Patient complains of episodes of fever with chills with evening rise of temperature. Patient becomes tired early.
♦ Presence of gradual loss of weight.
♦ Patient has persistent cough with or without hemoptysis.
♦ Swelling on neck is present which is firm and tender on palpation. When abscess is formed swelling perforates and pus drains out.
♦ Scrofula is the condition in which there is marked enlargement of cervical lymph nodes with caseation necrosis and frequent breakdown of gland.
♦ As skin is involved by tuberculosis, this is known as lupus vulgaris.
♦ Tubercular involvement of spine is called as Pott's disease.
♦ When tuberculosis spreads through bloodstream it involves organs, such as liver, kidney the disease is known as miliary tuberculosis.

Management—DOTS Regimen

♦ Directly observed treatment strategy adopted by WHO is followed all over the World including India.
♦ Directly observed treatment means that an observer watches the patient swallowing their tablets.
♦ DOT ensures accountability of TB services and helps to prevent emergence of drug resistance.

Components of DOTS

♦ Political and administrative commitment at all levels.
♦ Diagnosis through sputum microscopy
♦ Uninterrupted supply of short course chemotherapy drugs.
♦ Direct observation of drug intake (DOTS)
♦ Systematic monitoring, evaluation and supervision at all levels.

DOTS Regimen

Category	Features of TB case	Treatment regimen	
		Intensive phase	**Continuation phase**
I	New smear positive primary tuberculosis	$2\ H_3R_3Z_3E_3$	4 (HR)
	Seriously ill sputum smear negative cases.		
	Seriously ill extrapulmonary involvement		
II	Relapse/Failure of treatment cases Others	$2\ S_3H_3R_3Z_3E_3$ followed by $1\ H_3R_3Z_3E_3$	5 (HRE)
III	New sputum smear negative primary tuberculosis New less severe form of extrapulmonary tuberculosis	$2\ H_3R_3Z_3$	$4\ H_3R_3$

H: Isoniazid (300 mg), R: Rifampicin (450 mg), Z: Pyrazinamide (1500 mg), E: Ethambutol (1200 mg), S: Streptomycin (750 mg)

Note: Initial numeral before each regimen indicates the duration of therapy of that regimen. Numeral in subscript refer to thrice weekly schedule for the drugs.

Q.9. Give causes of cervical lymphadenopathy and describe tubercular adenitis. *(Aug 2011, 10 Marks)*

Ans.

Causes of Cervical Lymphadenopathy

- *Inflammation and infection:*
  - *Bacterial infections:*
    - Specific bacterial infection
      - » Tuberculosis
        - Syphilis.
    - Nonspecific bacterial infection
      - » Pericoronitis
      - » Periodontal disease
      - » Peri-apical infections.
  - *Viral infections:*
    - Infection mononucleosis
    - AIDS
    - Herpes simplex
    - Cat-scratch disease.
  - *Fungal infections:*
    - Oral candidiasis
    - Histoplasmosis.
  - *Parasitic infections:*
    - Rickettsial infection.
- *Allergic conditions:*
  - Serum sickness.
- *Primary neoplasms:*
  - Lymphoma.
- *Metastatic tumors:*
  - Oral squamous cell carcinoma
  - Metastasis of carcinoma of breast.
- *Miscellaneous conditions:*
  - Leukemia
  - Collagen diseases
  - Sarcoidosis
  - Nontender lymphoid hyperplasia.

Tubercular Adenitis

For tubercular adenitis in detail, refer to Ans. 2 and Ans. 3 of same chapter.

Q.10. Enumerate causes of cervical lymphadenopathy. Describe etiopathogenesis, clinical features and management of tubercular lymphadenopathy of neck. *(Aug 2012, 10 Marks)*

Ans. For causes of cervical lymphadenopathy, refer to Ans. 9 of same chapter.

Etiopathogenesis

Mycobacterium tuberculosis is the bacteria which lead to tuberculosis. When the tubercle bacilli are introduced into the tissue.

- Initial response of neutrophils
- There is progressive infiltration by macrophages
- Macrophages start phagocytosing the tubercle bacilli
- Activated CD4+ T cells develop

- In 2–3 days, the macrophages undergo structural changes and form epithelioid cells.
- The epithelioid cells aggregated into tight clusters or granulomas.
- Some macrophages form multinucleated giant cells.
- Hard tubercles form by the mass of epithelioid cells and the giant cells in a zone of lymphocytes, plasma cells and fibroblasts.
- Center of the cellular mass undergoes caseous necrosis, characterized by cheesy appearance called as soft tubercle.

For clinical features and management, refer to Ans. 1 of same chapter.

Q.11. Write short note on lymphangitis. *(Aug 2011, 5 Marks)*

Ans. It is an acute nonsuppurative infection and spreading inflammation of lymphatics of skin and subcutaneous tissues due to beta hemolytic streptococci, staphylococci, clostridial organisms.

- It is commonly associated with cellulitis.
- Erysipelas is a type of lymphangitis.
- In endemic areas, filariasis is the most common cause (coastal India). It is caused by *Wulchereria bancrofti.*

Clinical Features

- Streaky redness which is spreading is typical.
- On pressure, area blanches; on release redness reappears.
- Edema of the part, palpable tender regional lymph nodes are obvious.
- Fever, tachycardia, features of toxemia.
- Groin lymph nodes are enlarged and tender in lower limb lymphangitis.
- In upper limb, as lymphatics are mainly located on the dorsum of hand, edema and redness develops on the dorsum. Infection in thumb and index finger causes palpable tender axillary nodes; infection in little and ring finger causes first tender palpable epitrochlear nodes infection to appear; infection in middle finger causes first deltopectoral nodes to enlarge.
- Toxemia, septicamia may occur.
- Rapidity may be more in diabetics and immunosuppressed.
- Chronic lymphangitis occurs due to repeated attacks of acute recurrent lymphangitis leading into acquired lymphedema.

Investigations

- Blood cell count
- Platelet count
- Renal and liver function tests
- Peripheral smear and blood culture

Management

- Antibiotics, such as penicillin, cloxacillin.
- Elevation, rest, glycerine magnesium sulfa dressing.
- Management of toxemia or septicemia with critical care.

Q.12. Enumerate differences between sinus of tuberculosis and actinomycosis. *(June 2014, 2 Marks)*

Ans.

Sinus of tuberculosis	Sinus of actinomycosis
Sinus of tuberculosis occurs when collar stud abscess ruptures through the skin	Nodules form with involvement of skin. Nodule softens and burst through the skin as sinuses
Occurs at the neck	Occurs in face and neck
Induration is not present	Induration is present
Group of lymph nodes is palpable underneath the sinus	No lymph nodes are palpable
Discharge from sinus contains *M. tuberculosis*	Discharge from sinus contains sulfur granules which are gram-positive mycelia surrounded by gram-negative clubs

Q.13. Enumerate causes of cervical lymphadenopathy. How will you manage this? *(Feb 2014, 8 Marks)*

Ans. *For causes refer to Ans. 9 of same chapter.*

Management

Acute Cervical Lymphadenopathy

- In a situation, where a self-limited infection is thought to be the etiology of acute cervical lymphadenitis, it is reasonable to observe and provide reassurance.
- Unilateral lymphadenopathy that has a history of a rapid onset and overlying erythema of the skin and is accompanied by a fever suggests a bacterial infection. In this case, oral antibiotic therapy for 10–14 days and close follow-up is the appropriate management.
- An ultrasound may be indicated to evaluate for the presence and extent of suppuration. If confirmed surgical drainage is required with the presence of a fluctuant mass, suggesting an abscess.
- On follow-up of adenopathy, further evaluation should be considered, if there is not a decrease in size after 2 weeks.
- Laboratory evaluation may include the following: CBC with differential, ESR, titers for Ebstein–Barr virus/cytomegalovirus/toxoplasmosis/cat-scratch disease, antistreptolysin O or anti-DNase serologic tests, PPD, and chest radiograph.
- Noninfectious causes of cervical lymphadenopathy include Kawasaki disease, PFAPA (periodic fever, aphthous stomatitis, pharyngitis, and cervical adenitis), and sarcoidosis. Cervical lymphadenopathy is accompanied by a number of other signs and symptoms in each of these noninfectious disorders, and evaluation and management is individualized based on the disease.

Chronic Cervical Lymphadenopathy

- Laboratory evaluation includes CBC, ESR, PPD, *B. henselae* serology, and titers for Ebstein–Barr virus/cytomegalovirus/toxoplasma among other tests based on history and physical examination.

- Children who have chronic cervical lymphadenopathy often undergo extensive diagnostic evaluation before an etiology is determined.
- Special attention should be given to the possibility of TB and HIV disease; the hematologic and serologic testing noted previously can be helpful.
- Urine antigen tests for *Histoplasma capsulatum* occasionally can be helpful.
- If there is an increase in lymph node size over 2 weeks, lack of decrease in size over 4–6 weeks, lack of regression to normal within 8–12 weeks, or the presence of persistent fever, weight loss, fatigue, night sweats, hard nodes, or fixation of nodes to surrounding tissues, a biopsy should be performed for further evaluation.
- Biopsy can be in the form of open biopsy or fine needle aspiration to further investigate for certain pathology, including infectious and noninfectious causes, specifically malignancy. Because lymphadenitis caused by non-tuberculous mycobacterium (NTM) evolves to draining skin fistulas associated with scarring, the safety of needle aspiration when this infection is suspected has been questioned.
- Needle aspiration may not lead to increased risk for this complication because the treatment of a node found to be infected with NTM is surgical excision—a cure for skin fistulas.
- NTM and *Bartonella* infection are diagnosed best using material obtained from a suppurative lymph node, which can be stained and cultured for acid-fast organisms and sent for polymerase chain reaction (PCR) examination to detect *B. henselae* infection. Importantly, PCR analysis for Bartonella can be performed on material that was obtained recently and preserved by freezing. It is sensible to freeze extra material obtained by needle aspiration so PCR studies can be performed, if bacterial studies are unexpectedly negative.

Q.14. Write briefly on Burkitt's tumor. *(Feb 2013, 5 Marks)*

Or

Write short on Burkitt's jaw tumor.

(Sep 2009, 5 Marks)

Ans. It is also known as African jaw lymphoma.

Etiology

Epstein–Barr virus is considered to be the etiological factor.

Types

- *Endemic (African):* Occurs commonly in jaw.
- *Nonendemic (Sporadic):* Occurs commonly in abdomen
- *Aggressive lymphoma:* In HIV patients.

Clinical Features

- It is commonly seen in children during the age of 6–9 years.
- Males are commonly affected as compared to females. Male to female ratio is 2:1.

- Lesion is found most commonly in maxilla and spreads towards floor of the orbit.
- In African form jaw is more involved while in American form abdominal involvement is common.
- Lesion has very fast growth and it doubles in size within a day.
- Patient complaints swelling of jaw, abdomen and paraplegia.
- Peripheral lymphadenopathy is commonly seen.
- Renal involvement is present which can be bilateral.
- In females, ovaries are also affected.

Oral Manifestations

- Tumor is rapidly growing and involves maxillary, ethmoidal and sphenoidal sinus along with orbit.
- Presence of loosening and mobility of permanent teeth.
- Presence of paresthesia of inferior alveolar canals and other sensory facial nerves.
- Gingiva adjacent to affected teeth become swollen, ulcerated and necrotic.
- There can be presence of large amount of mass in the mouth on the surface of which present the rootless developing permanent teeth.

Investigations

- *Radiograph:* It shows moth-eaten appearance with loss of lamina dura.
- *Biopsy:* Starry sky appearance is characteristic for Burkitt's lymphoma.
- *USG:* This done for abdomen so that kidneys should be evaluated.
- *Blood urea* and serum creatinine estimation is done.

Treatment

- Radiotherapy.
- Chemotherapy, i.e., cyclophosphamide, methotrexate, orthomelphalan.
- Surgery is usually not indicated unless it is localized or in case of involvement of ovaries.

Q.15. Write briefly on Hodgkin's lymphoma.

(Nov 2014, 3 Marks)

Ans. Hodgkin's lymphoma is a lymphoproliferative disorder which arises from lymph nodes and from lymphoid components of various organs.

Clinical Features

- The tumor is seen in young adults, i.e., during 20–30 years or in elderly people during 5th decade of life.
- Onset of the tumor is insidious with enlargement of one group of superficial nodes.
- Associated lymph nodes are painless. There is presence of generalized weakness, cough, dyspnea and anorexia.
- Lymph nodes are discrete and rubbery in consistency with overlying skin is purely mobile.
- Pel–Ebstein fever is present, i.e., presence of cyclic fever with generalized severe pruritus which is of unknown etiology.

- In oral cavity, the lesion appears as an ulcer or swelling. It can also be present as intrabony lesion which appears as hard swelling.

Ann Arbor Clinical Staging

Stage I (A or B)	I	Involvement of a single lymph node region
	I_E	Involvement of a single extralymphatic organ or site
Stage II (A or B)	II	Involvement of two or more lymph node regions on the same side of the diaphragm
	II_E	(or) with localized contiguous involvement of an extranodal organ of site
Stage III (A or B)	III	Involvement of lymph node regions on both sides of the diaphragm
	III_E	(or) with localized contiguous involvement of an extranodal organ or site.
	III_S	(or) with involvement of spleen
	III_{ES}	(or) both features of IIIE and IIIs
Stage IV (A or B)	IV	Multiple or disseminated involvement of one or More extralymphatic organs of tissues with or without lymphatic involvement

(A: Asymptomatic; B: Presence of constitutional symptoms; E: Extranodal involvement; S: Splenomegaly)

Investigations

- **Blood test:**
  - Nonspecific anemia of chronic disease is common
  - Lymphopenia is present.
  - ESR is elevated.
- **Lymph node biopsy:**
  Show presence of Reed–Sternberg cells.
- **Imaging:**
  - Chest X-ray to look for mediastinal lymph nodes and pleural effusion
  - CT is valuable in detecting intrathoracic and abdominal lymphadenopathy.
- **USG:** To look for liver, spleen and abdominal lymph node.

Management

- **Stage I and II:**
  - Mainly radiotherapy, i.e., external high cobalt radiotherapy
  - *Above the diaphragm:* Y field therapy, covering cervical, axillary, mediastinal lymph nodes.
  - *Below the diaphragm:* Mantle or inverted Y field therapy covering para-aortic and iliac nodes.
  - Chemotherapy is also given.
- **Stage III and IV:**
  - In this, mainly chemotherapy is given.
- **Regimens used are:**
  - **MOPP Regimen**
    - *Mechlorethamine:* 6 mg/sqm on 1st and 8th day.
    - *Oncovine:* 1.4 mg/sqm on 1st and 10th day.
    - *Procarbazine:* 100 mg orally daily for 10 days.
    - *Prednisolone:* 45 mg orally daily for 10 days.
    MOPP combination is given in 6 courses with no drugs given from 15th to 28th day.

- **ABVD Regimen**
  - *Adriamycin:* 30 mg/sqm
  - *Bleomycin:* 10 mg/sqm
  - *Vinblastine:* 6 mg/sqm
  - *Dacarbazine:* 350 mg/sqm

The cycle is repeated on 20th day.

Splenectomy is done in many patients except with stage IV disease.

Q.16. Write short note on lymphoma. *(Apr 2015, 3 Marks)*

Ans. Lymphomas are the progressive neoplastic condition of lymphoreticular system which arises from stem cells.

Lymphoma is the third most common malignancy among the children.

Classification of Lymphoma

WHO modified REAL (Revised European American Lymphoma) classification of lymphoma.

- B-cell neoplasms:
  - *Precursor B-cell neoplasm:* ALL, LBL.
  - *Precursor B-cell neoplasm:* It includes all B-cell-related non-Hodgkin's lymphomas.
- T-cell and putative NK cell neoplasms:
  - *Precursor B-cell neoplasm:* ALL, LBL T cell related.
  - *Precursor T-cell and NK cell neoplasm:* It includes all T-cell related non-Hodgkin's lymphomas.
- *Hodgkin's lymphoma:*
  - *Predominant Hodgkin's lymphoma:* Nodular lymphocyte type.
  - *Classical Hodgkin's lymphoma:*
    - Nodular sclerosis
    - Lymphocyte rich
    - Mixed cellularity
    - Lymphocyte depletion.
- Precursor lymphoid neoplasms
- Immunodeficiency associated lymphoproliferative disorders.

ALL is acute lymphoblastic leukemia.

LBL is lymphoblastic lymphoma.

Etiology

- Genetic predisposition
- Sjogren's syndrome
- HIV infection
- Virus etiology, i.e., Epstein–Barr virus infection
- *Occupational causes:* Hair dye workers, herbicide exposure
- Ionizing radiation
- Celiac sprue—intestinal T-cell lymphoma
- Bloom's syndrome.

Types of Lymphoma

- Hodgkin's lymphoma
- Non-Hodgkin's lymphoma

Q.17. Discuss differential diagnosis of cervical lymphadenopathy. *(June 2015, 20 Marks)*

Ans. Following is the differential diagnosis of cervicofacial lymphadenopathy:

Infective Causes

- Acute lymphadenitis
- Chronic nonspecific lymphadenitis
- Tuberculous lymphadenitis
- Infectious mononucleosis
- Toxoplasmosis
- Cat scratch fever.

Neoplastic Causes

- Metastatic lymph node enlargement
- Lymphomas, i.e., Hodgkin's lymphoma, non-Hodgkin's lymphoma, Burkitt's lymphoma
- Chronic lymphatic leukemia.

Other Causes

- Autoimmune diseases, i.e., systemic lupus erythematosus, rheumatoid arthritis
- HIV infection, immunosuppression.

Acute Suppurative Lymphadenitis

- It is a bacterial infection leading to acute inflammation and suppuration of lymph nodes caused by group A streptococci or staphylococci.
- There is presence of tender, enlarged, firm or soft palpable neck lymph nodes.

Chronic Nonspecific Lymphadenitis

- Infections, such as chronic tonsillitis, recurrent dental infection can lead to chronic nonspecific lymphadenitis.
- There is presence of firm, nontender, multiple, bilateral lymph node enlargement in neck.
- Tuberculous lymphadenitis
- It is caused by *Mycobacterium tuberculosis* infection.
- Lymph nodes are matted, enlarged with cold abscess or sinus formation.

Infectious Mononucleosis

- Caused by Epstein–Barr virus.
- There is presence of generalized lymphadenopathy.
- Monospot test is positive.

Toxoplasmosis

- Caused by *Toxoplasma gondii*, protozoa through meat.
- Cervical lymphadenopathy is most common.
- Diagnosed by Sabin Feldman dye test.

Cat Scratch Disease

- Caused by *Bartonella henselae*.
- Lymphadenopathy is present.
- Diagnosed by lymph node biopsy with Warthin–Starry staining.

Lymphomas

♦ In Hodgkin's lymphoma, there is painless progressive enlargement of lymph nodes. Lymph nodes are smooth, firm, nontender. In this cervical lymph nodes, i.e., lower deep cervical group in posterior triangle are commonly enlarged. In this type, peripheral lymph node involvement is not common.

♦ In non-Hodgkin's lymphoma any group of lymph node is involved. In this type, peripheral lymph node involvement is common.

Q.18. Write briefly on chemotherapy of tuberculosis.
(Jan 2016, 2 Marks)

Ans. **Category-wise Alternative Treatment Regimens for Tuberculosis (WHO-1997)**

TB category	Patient type	Initial phase (daily 3 × per-week)	Continuation phase	Duration
I	New sputum positive or new smear negative or new case with severe from of extrapulmonary tuberculosis	2 HRZE (S)	4HR/4H3R3 or 6HE	6 months 8 months
II	Smear positive failure or smear positive relapse or sputum positive treatment after default	2 HRZES	5 HRE or 5H3R3E3	8 months 8 months
III	Smear negative pulmonary TB with limited parenchymal involvement or less severe from of extrapulmonary TB	2 HRZ	4HR/4H3R3 or 6HE	6 months 8 months
IV	Chronic cases or suspected MDR-TB cases	For H resistance for H + R resistance	RZE ZE + S/Ethionamide + Ciprofloxacin/ofloxacin	12 months

Explanation of Standard Code

♦ Each antitubercular drug has standard abbreviation, i.e.
  • Isoniazid (H)
  • Rifampicin (R)
  • Pyrazinamide (Z)
  • Ethambutol (E)
  • Streptomycin (S).
♦ Numerical before a phase is the duration of that phase in months.
♦ Numerical in subscript is the number of doses of that drug per week. If there is no subscript numerical, then the drug is given daily.

Q.19. Name etiological agent, pathognomic diagnostic feature and treatment (only modalities) of matted lymph nodes in neck. *(Jan 2017, 3 Marks)*

Ans.

Etiological Agent

Since matted lymph nodes in neck are seen in tuberculosis, the etiological agent is *Mycobacterium tuberculosis*.

Pathognomic Diagnostic Feature

Matting of lymph nodes in neck is itself a pathognomic diagnostic feature of tuberculosis. Matting is due to involvement of capsule. Nodes are firm and nontender.

Treatment (Only Modality)

Antitubercular treatment should be given to the patient.

6. SKIN TUMORS

Q.1. Write short note on basal cell carcinoma.
(May/June 2009, 5 Marks) (Sep 2005, 5 Marks)

Ans. It is the most common malignant skin tumor.

♦ It is a slow growing neoplasm.
♦ It arises from basal cell of the pilosebaceous adnexa and occurs only on the skin.

Common Sites

♦ Majority of lesions are found on the face, inner canthus and outer canthus of eyes, eyelids, bridge of the nose, and around nasolabial fold.
♦ These sites are the area where the tears roll down; hence, it is also called 'Tear cancer'.
♦ *Nodular:* Common on face.
♦ Cystic/nodulocystic
♦ Ulcerative
♦ *Multiple:* Associated with syndromes and other malignancies.
♦ *Pigmented basal cell carcinoma:* It mimics melanoma.
♦ Geographical or forest fire basal cell carcinoma: Involve wide area with central scabbing and peripheral active proliferating edge.
♦ *Basio-squamous:* Behave-like squamous cell carcinoma and spread in lymph nodes

Etiology

♦ Ultraviolet rays are the main factor for its development.
♦ Fair skin is vulnerable for development of it.
♦ Prolonged administration of arsenic in the form of arsenical ointments.

Clinical Features

♦ It is common in males in middle aged and elderly
♦ The most common clinical presentation is an ulcer that never heals.
♦ It is common on the region of face, i.e., above the line drawn between angle of mouth and ear lobe.
♦ It can also present as a painless, firm, nodule.
♦ It is pigmented with fine blood vessels on its surface.

♦ The ulcer has raised and *beaded edge, induration may be present, and bleed on touch.

Spread

♦ It spread by local invasion.
♦ It slowly penetrates deep inside, destroying the underlying tissue-like bone, cartilage or even eyeball, hence, the name "rodent ulcer".

Treatment

♦ It is radiosensitive. If lesion is away from vital structure then curative radiotherapy can be given. Radiotherapy is not given, once it erodes cartilage or bone.
♦ *Surgery:* Wide excision (l cm clearance) with skin grafting, primary suturing or flap (Z plasty, rhomboid flap, rotation flap) is the procedure of choice.
♦ Laser surgery, photodynamic therapy, 5-fluorouracil local application.
♦ Cryosurgery.
♦ Microscopically oriented histographic surgery (MOHS): It is useful to get a clearance margin and in conditions, such as basal cell carcinoma close to eyes, nose or ear, to preserve more tissues. MOHS is becoming popular in basal cell carcinoma. Procedure is done by dermatological surgeon along with a histotechnician/histologist. Under local anesthesia, a saucerized excision of the primary tumor is done and quadrants of the specimen are mapped with different colors. Specimen is sectioned by histotechnician from margin and depth and it is stained using eosin and hematoxylin. It is studied by MOHS surgeon or histologist. Residual tumor from relevant mapped area is excised and procedure is repeated until clear margin and clear depth are achieved. Clearance must be complete and proper in basal cell carcinoma.

Q.2. Write short note on epithelioma. *(Mar 1997, 5 Marks)*

Ans. It is also called "squamous cell carcinoma".

♦ It is the second common malignant tumor of skin after basal cell carcinoma.
♦ It arises from prickle cell layer of the skin.
♦ It usually affects elderly males.

Clinical Features

♦ It is an ulcerative or cauliflower-like lesion.
♦ Edges are *everted and *indurated.
♦ Base is indurated and it may be subcutaneous tissue, muscle or bone.
♦ Floor contains cancerous tissue, which look like granulation tissue.
♦ It is pale, *friable, bleed easily on touch.
♦ Surrounding area is also indurated
♦ Mobility is usually restricted.

Investigations

♦ Wedge biopsy from edge.
♦ FNAC from lymph node

♦ USG/CT scan to identify the nodal disease
♦ MRI to identify local extension.

Treatment

♦ Radiotherapy using radiation needles, moulds, etc., is given.
♦ Wide excision, 2 cm clearance followed by skin grafting or flaps. Wide excision should show clearance both at margin as well as in the depth. If muscle, fascia, cartilage are involved, it should be cleared. Reconstruction is usually done by primary split skin grafting. Delayed skin grafting can also be done once wound granulates well. Often flaps of different type are needed depending on the site of lesion.
♦ Amputation with one joint above.
♦ For lymph nodes, block dissection of the regional lymph nodes is done.
♦ Curative radiotherapy is also useful in tumors which are not adherent to deeper planes or cartilage as squamous cell carcinoma is radiosensitive. It is also useful in recurrent squamous cell carcinoma and in patients who are not fit for surgery. A dose of 6,000 cGy units over 6 weeks; 200 units/day is used. Recurrence after radiotherapy is treated by surgical wide excision.
♦ In advanced cases with fixed lymph nodes, palliative external radiotherapy is given to palliate pain, fungation and bleeding.
♦ Chemotherapy is given using methotrexate, vincristine, bleomycin.
♦ Field therapy using cryoprobe or topical fluorouracil or electrodessication.

Q.3. Write short note on neurofibroma.
(May/June 2009, 5 Marks) (Aug 2011, 5 Marks)

Ans. Neurofibroma is a benign tumor arising from connective tissue of nerve containing ectodermal neural and mesodermal connective tissue components.

Types of Neurofibroma

♦ *Nodular:*
  • Single, smooth, firm, tender swelling which moves horizontally or perpendicular to direction of nerve.
♦ *Plexiform:*
  • Occurs along distribution of trigeminal nerve in skin of face.
  • Attain enormous size with thickening of skin which hang downwards.
♦ *Von-Recklinghausen's disease:*
  • Inherited disease with multiple neurofibromas in body.
  • It can be cranial, spinal or peripheral
  • Associated with pigmented spots on skin, i.e., Café-au-lait spots.
♦ *Elephantiatic:*
  • Origin is congenital and involve limbs.
  • Skin of limb is thickened, dry and coarse.
♦ *Cutaneous:*
  • Small, multiple, firm/hard nodules arising from terminal ends of dermal nerves
  • It can be pedunculated or sessile.

Clinical Features

- Mild pain or painless swellings seen in subcutaneous and cutaneous plane with tingling, numbness and paresthesia.
- Most commonly affected sites are trunk, face and extremities
- Sessile or pedunculated elevated small nodules of various sizes
- Majority of patients have asymmetric areas of pigmentation known as Café-au-lait spots. They are smooth edge dark brown macules.
- Lisch nodules are present which are translucent brown pigmentation on iris.
- Crowe's sign is present, i.e., axillary freckling, brown spot on skin.

Complications

- Cystic degeneration is present.
- Spinal and cranial neurofibromas can cause neurological deficits.
- Spine dumb-bell tumor lead to compression of spinal cord and paralysis of limb.
- Hemorrhage in tissues.

Treatment

Excision is done.

Q.4. Describe features of mole turning into melanocarcinoma. *(Jan 2012, 5 Marks)*

Ans.

Features

- Lesion show superficial radial growth pattern.
- Lesion becomes ulcerated and growing day by day in size.
- Fungating growth is present associated with the bleeding.
- It leads to destruction of the underlying bone
- Lesion is firm on palpation
- Borders of lesion are erythematous.

Q.5. Write difference between squamous cell carcinoma and basal cell carcinoma. *(Mar 2016, 3 Marks)*

Ans. Following are the differences between squamous cell carcinoma and basal cell carcinoma:

Squamous cell carcinoma	Basal cell carcinoma
It is also known as epithelioma	It is also known as rodent ulcer
It spreads commonly	It spreads rarely
It can occur anywhere on skin or mucous membrane	It is found on upper part of face
It arises from squamous cell layer of epidermis	It arises from basal cell layer of epidermis
Edge of the lesion is raised and everted	Edge of the lesion is raised and rolled up
Base is indurated	Base is non-indurated
Microscopically, it shows cell nests or epithelial pearls	Microscopically, cells are arranged in palisaded pattern

7. BLEEDING DISORDERS

Q.1. Write short note on hemophilia. *(Feb 2013, 5 Marks)*
(Feb 2015, 5 Marks) (Aug 2012, 5 Marks)
(Jan 2012, 5 Marks) (Dec 2015, 5 Marks)

Or

Write briefly on hemophilia. *(June 2015, 2.5 Marks)*

Or

Answer briefly on hemophilia. *(Mar 2016, 3 Marks)*

Or

Write short answer on hemophilia. *(Oct 2019, 3 Marks)*

Ans. It is a hereditary disorder of blood coagulation, characterized by excessive hemorrhage due to prolonged bleeding time.

It is the X-linked genetic disorder of coagulation.

Types

Following are the types of hemophilia:

- *Hemophilia A or classic hemophilia:* Deficiency of factor VIII or antihemophilic factor is the cause of hemophilia A. It is recessive X-linked. Females are always carrier and males are sufferer.
- *Hemophilia B or Christmas disease:* Deficiency of factor IX is the cause of hemophilia B.

Clinical Features

- The most common manifestation is hemorrhage into joint.
- Because of repeated hemorrhage knee joint becomes non-functional hemarthroses takes place.
- Bleeding in muscles take place.
- Bleeding from GIT occurs in form of esophageal varices.
- Bleeding from genitourinary tract occurs in form of hematuria.
- A simple cut or injury may lead to profuse bleeding.
- First symptom is seen in form of large bruises and hematomas on hips which regresses as the child learn to walk.

Laboratory Diagnosis

Bleeding time is normal but coagulation time is prolonged.

Treatment

Hemophilia A

The main aim is to raise the factor VIII level, which can arrest bleeding.

- *Replacement therapy:* Various form of replacement therapy are available like plasma, cryoprecipitate and factor VIII concentrates.
- Give 30% amount of factor VIII, because it is very expensive.
- Any major operation or tooth extraction requires 100% concentration of factor VIII.
- Hypovolemia, allergic reaction and development of factor VIII antibodies are complication of factor VIII concentrate.

To avoid this complication, cryoprecipitate from animal origin should be given in between human cryoprecipitate.

Hemophilia B

Fresh frozen plasma or Factor IX concentrates should be given to the patient.

Q.2. Describe different types of hemorrhage and management of hemorrhage.
(Mar 2003, 15 Marks) (Mar 2001, 15 Marks)

Ans. Hemorrhage is the escape of blood from a blood vessel.

Types of Hemorrhage

- *Depending upon the nature of the vessel involve:*
  - *Arterial hemorrhage:*
    - Bright red in color, jet out.
    - Pulsation of the artery can be seen.
    - It can be easily controlled as, it is visible.
  - *Venous hemorrhage:*
    - Dark red in color.
    - It never jet out but oozes out.
    - Difficult in control because vein gets retracted, non pulsatile.
  - *Capillary hemorrhage:*
    - Red color, never jet out, slowly oozes out.
    - It becomes significant, if there are bleeding tendencies.
- *Depending upon the timing of hemorrhage:*
  - *Primary hemorrhage:* Occurs at the time of surgery.
  - *Reactionary hemorrhage:* Occurs after 6–12 hours of surgery. Hypertension in postoperative period, violent sneezing, coughing or retching are the usual causes.
  - *Secondary hemorrhage:* Occurs after 5–7 days of surgery. It is due to infection which eats away the suture material, causing sloughing of vessel wall.
- *Depending upon the duration of hemorrhage:*
  - *Acute hemorrhage:* Occurs suddenly, e.g., esophageal varices bleeding.
  - *Chronic hemorrhage:* Occurs over a period of time, e.g., hemorrhoids/piles.
  - *Acute or chromic hemorrhage:* It is more dangerous as bleeding occur in individuals who are already hypoxic, which may get worsened faster.
- *Depending upon the nature of bleeding:*
  - External hemorrhage or reversal hemorrhage, e.g., epistaxis, hematemesis.
  - Internal hemorrhage or concealed hemorrhage, e.g., splenic rupture following injury.
- *Based on the possible intervention:*
  - *Surgical hemorrhage:* Can be corrected by surgical intervention
  - *Nonsurgical hemorrhage:* It is diffuse and ooze due to coagulation abnormalities and disseminated intravascular coagulation.

Management of Hemorrhage

- General management:
  - Hospitalization
  - Care of critically ill patients start with A, B, C (Airways, breathing, circulation).
  - Oxygen should be administered.
  - Intravenous line: Urgent intravenous administration of isotonic saline to restore the blood volume to normal.
  - Colloids, such as gelatins or hetastarch have also been used.
- *Specific measures:*
  - *Conservative:*
    - By local pressure and packing:
      » Pressure applied with tight dressing, applying digital pressure, or a cloth pegs for epistaxis. Use of double balloon in the esophagus and stomach to control the bleeding from esophageal varices.
      » Packing by means of rolls of wide gauge is an important stand by in operative surgery.
    - Elevation of part: As in bleeding varicose ulcer.
      » *Rest:* Absolute rest.
      » *Sedation:* With diazepam.
      » *Treatment of shock:* Treatment of hypovolemia by restoration of blood volume by blood transfusion and or saline, dextrose, etc.
  - *Operative:*
    - Clamping the bleeding vessels with catgut, thread or silk.
    - Coagulation by thermocautery or diathermy.
    - By local application of adrenaline swabs.
    - Application of silver clips as in neurosurgery.
    - Under running or transfusion of vessels by needle and suture.
    - Application of crushed piece of muscle at the site of bleeding.
    - Bone wax or bismuth iodoform paraffin paste (BIPP) is used for oozing from bone.
    - Repair of vascular defect by patches of vein or Dacron mash.
    - Excision of bleeding organ: Splenectomy.
  - Restoration of blood volume after hemorrhage
  - Resuscitation from hemorrhage includes restoration of the circulating volume. So Ringer lactate is preferred over the normal saline. Isotonic crystalloid or colloid solutions can be used for volume replacement in hemorrhage.
  - Blood transfusion: For restoring the circulating volume and replace coagulation factors and oxygen carrying capacity many blood products are available. By crystalloid solution hypovolemia is corrected. Packed RBCs restore intravascular volume and oxygen carrying capacity. Platelet transfusions can be done in significant thrombocytopenia and continued hemorrhage.

Q.3. Enumerate difference between capillary, venous and arterial bleeding. *(June 2014, 2 Marks)*

Ans.

Features	Capillary bleeding	Venous bleeding	Arterial bleeding
Color	Intermediate red	Dark red	Bright red
Pulsating character	Capillary bleeding may be quite aggressive	Negative	Positive
Vigour of flow	Oozing type	Less rapid flow	Increased
Spurt	Ooze from raw surface	It does not spurt	Blood will spurt with each heart beat from cut end of artery

Q.4. Give a brief account of bleeding disorders, their etiology, and management in dental practice.

(Sep 1999, 15 Marks)

Ans. Bleeding disorders: Bleeding disorder or hemorrhagic diatheses are a group of disorders characterized by defective hemostasis with abnormal bleeding.

Etiology of Bleeding Disorders

♦ **Vascular defects:** Bleeding disorders caused by vascular defects may be caused by structural malformation of vessels. Hereditary disorders of connective tissue and acquired connective tissue disorders. Vascular defects rarely cause serious bleeding. Bleeding into skin or mucous membrane starts immediately alter trauma but ceases within 24–48 hours. The vascular defects are hereditary hemorrhagic telangectasia, Henoch–Schönlein purpura.

♦ **Platelet disorder:** It can be of two types:
  • *Reduction in number:* Thrombocytopenic purpura. If the total number of circulating platelets falls below 50,000 per mm³ of blood the patient can have bleeding. In some cases the total platelet count is reduced by unknown mechanism, this is called primary or idiopathic thrombocytopenic purpura (ITP). Chemicals, radiation and various systemic disease, (e.g., leukemia) may have direct effect on the bone marrow and may result in secondary thrombocytopenia.
  • *Defect in quality:*Non-thrombocytopenic purpura, e.g., von Willebrand's disease, Bernard–Soulier disease, Glanzmanns thrombasthenia.

Von-Willebrand's disease (pseudohemophilia) is the most common inherited bleeding disorder. Unlike hemophilia it can occur in females. This is a disease of both coagulation factors and platelets. It is caused by an inherited defect involving platelet adhesion. Platelet adhesion is affected because of a deficiency of Von Willebrand`s factor.

Various drugs, such as carbamazepine, aspirin, methyldopa, phenytoin can also lead to platelet disorders.

♦ **Coagulation defects:**
  • *Hemophilia A:* It is the most common coagulation defect. It is inherited as X-linked recessive trait. The hemostatic abnormality in hemophilla A is caused by a deficiency/ defect of factor VIII. Until recently, factor VIII was thought to be produced by endothelial cells and not by the liver as most of coagulation factors. The defective gene is located on the X chromosome.
  • *Hemophilia B (Christmas disease):* Factor IX is deficient or defective. It is inherited as X- linked recessive trait. Like Hemophilia A, the disease primarily affects males and the clinical manifestations of the two are identical.
  • *Disseminated intravascular coagulation (DIC):* It is a condition that results when the clotting system is activated in all or a major part of vascular system. Despite wide spread fibrin production, the major clinical problem is bleeding not thrombosis. DIC is associated with a number of disorders, such as infection, obstetric complications, cancer and snake bite.

Management of Bleeding Disorders

I. Hereditary Hemorrhagic Telangiectasia

It is transmitted as autosomal dominant trait and is characterized by bleeding from mucous membrane.

Management

♦ In patient having repeated attacks of epistaxis septal dermoplasty should be done. In septal dermoplasty involved mucosa get removed and skin grafting is done.

♦ If spontaneous hemorrhages are present or nasal bleeding is present, it is controlled by giving pressure packs.

♦ Sclerosing agents, i.e., sodium tetradecyl sulfate, if injected intralesionally stop bleeding.

♦ Electrocautery is done. It helps in arresting bleeding.

II. Idiopathic Thrombocytopenic Purpua (ITP)

Steroid Treatment Protocol

Initial steroid treatment protocol for ITP: Initial steroid treatment protocol 1 mg/kg/day prednisolone, PO for 2–6 weeks. subsequent steroid treatment protocol for ITP: Prednisolone dose is individualized for every patient. Usually the dose of prednisolone is tapered to less than 10 mg per day for 3 months and then withdrawn. Splenectomy is done, if discontinuation of prednisolone causes a relapse. Follow the 'rule of two's for major dental treatment and provide extra steroids prior to surgery, if the patient is currently on steroids or has used steroids for 2 weeks longer within the past 2 years.

Minor Surgery

♦ Hemostasis after minor surgery is usually adequate, if platelet levels are above 50,000 cells/mm³.

♦ Platelets can be replaced or supplemented by platelet transfusions; though sequestration of platelets occurs rapidly. Platelet transfusion is indicated for established thrombocytopenic bleeding.

♦ When given prophylactically platelets should be given half before surgery to control capillary bleeding and half at the end of the operation to facilitate the placement of adequate sutures.

♦ Platelets should be used within 6–24 hours after collection and suitable preparations include platelet-rich plasma (PRP), which contains about 90% of the platelets from a unit of fresh blood and platelet-rich concentrate (PRC), which contains about 50% of the platelets from a unit of fresh whole blood.

♦ PRC is thus the best source of platelets. Platelet infusions carry the risk of isoimmunization, infection with blood-borne viruses and, rarely, graft-versus-host disease.

♦ Where there is immune destruction of platelets (e.g., in ITP), platelet infusions are less effective.

♦ The need for platelet transfusions can be reduced by local hemostatic measures and the use of desmopressin or tranexamic acid or topical administration of platelet concentrates.

♦ Absorbable hemostatic agents, such as oxidized regenerated cellulose (Surgicel), synthetic collagen (Instat) or microcrystalline collagen (Avitene) may be put in the socket to assist clotting in postextraction socket.

♦ Drugs that affect platelet function, such as gentamicin, antihistamines and aspirin should be avoided.

Major Surgery

For major surgery, platelet levels over 75,000 cells/mm³ are desirable.

III. Hemophilia

It is a hereditary disorder of blood coagulation characterized by excessive hemorrhage due to increased coagulation time. It is of two types, i.e., Hemophilia A and hemophilia B.

Management

♦ Local anesthesia is contraindicated. So intrapulpal anesthesia, intraligamentary anesthesia should be used. Sedation with diazepam or NO_2–O_2 sedation can be given.

♦ Endodontic procedures should be carried out and care is taken not to do instrumentation beyond apex. If hemorrhage is present it should be controlled by 1:1,000 aqueous epinephrine on paper point.

♦ Restorative treatments can be carried out by proper application of rubber dam for avoiding trauma to gingiva and other soft tissues. In case, if rubber dam is not present an epinephrine impregnated hemostatic cord is kept in gingival sulcus before preparation of crown or inlay margin.

♦ Complete dentures and removable partial dentures can be given to hemophilic patients and are well tolerated by them. Patient has to take care for proper maintenance of hygiene of prosthesis.

♦ Conservative periodontal treatment should be done rather than attempting for periodontal surgeries.

♦ In case, if oral surgical procedures are to be done local hemostatic agents should be used, pressure surgical packs should be employed, sutures, topical thrombin is used. After removal of tooth socket, is packed with mechanical splint. Postoperative use of antifibrinolytic agent is used to support clot maintenance.

♦ In cases of hemophilia A, human freeze-dried factor VIII concentrate or new recombinant factor VIII is used.

♦ In hemophilia B, human dried factor IX concentrate is supplied as powder which is to be mixed with distill water and administer IV (intravenously).

IV. Von Willebrand Disease

♦ It is the most common inherited bleeding disorder. It is inherited as autosomal dominant but a severe form of disease may be inherited as a sex-linked recessive trait.

♦ It is caused due to the deficiency or defect in Von Willebrand factor.

♦ Types of Von–Willebrand diseases are: Type I, Type II A and II B, Type III.

Management

♦ Surgical procedures can be performed in patients with mild Von Willebrand disease by using DDAVP and EACA. Patients with severe Von Willebrand disease requires cryoprecipitate and factor VIII concentrate.

♦ Bleeding should be controlled by using local measures, such as pressure packs, gelfoam with thrombin, tranexamic acid etc.

♦ Aspirin and NSAIDs are avoided and acetaminophen can be given to patients.

♦ In majority of patients with Von Willebrand disease, hemostatic defect is controlled with desmopressin via nasal spray.

♦ Type I Von Willebrand disease is treated with desmopressin while Type II A and B, and Type III require clotting factor replacement.

V. Disseminated Intravascular Coagulation

♦ Correction of hemodynamic instability by fluid therapy, transfusion of packed cells or whole blood.

♦ *Factor replacement:* This is the specific therapy, in this fresh frozen plasma, cryoprecipitate, platelet concentrate transfusions are essential. Fresh-frozen plasma is given at the dose of 15 mL/kg. Platelet is transfused at the dosage of 0.1 unit/kg.

Q.5. Write short note on treatment of hemangioma.

(Sep 2009, 3 Marks)

Ans. Hemangioma is a benign tumor containing hyperplastic endothelium with cellular proliferation with increased mast cells.

Treatment of Capillary Hemangioma

♦ They are treated by wait and watch policy commonly allowed for spontaneous regression.

♦ Diode laser, surgical excision and reconstruction may need to be ligated after wide exposure before achieving complete extirpation. Sclerotherapy/cryotherapy/CO_2 snow therapy cause unpleasant scarring.

♦ Preoperative embolization facilitates surgical excision and reduces the operative blood loss. When once embolization done surgery should be done as early as possible otherwise recurrence occurs and much more worried formation of enlarged collaterals can occur.

♦ Rapidly growing hemangioma may need systemic/oral and intralesional steroid therapy.

♦ Antiangiogenic interferon 2α may be useful.

♦ Life-threatening platelet trapping may be controlled by cyclophosphamide chemotherapy.

♦ Hemangioma with drug resistant CCF can be treated with radiotherapy.

Treatment of Cavernous Hemangioma

♦ *Sclerosant therapy:* It is the initial first line therapy. It causes aseptic thrombosis and fibrosis of the cavernous hemangioma with less vascularity and smaller size. It is directly injected into the lesion. Sodium tetradecyl Sulfate hypertonic saline are used. Often multiple injections are needed to achieve complete required effect. Later excision of the lesion is done.

♦ Ligation of feeding artery and often at later stage excision is done once hemangioma shrinks.

♦ Therapeutic embolization.

♦ If small and located in accessible area, excision is the initial therapy.

♦ **LASER ablation:** Diode-pulsed LASER is becoming popular because of good control of bleeding.

Q.6. Describe hemorrhage—its types, causes, clinical features and management. *(Jan 2012, 10 Marks)*

Or

Write a long answer on cause of hemorrhage and its management. *(June 2018, 5 Marks)*

Ans. Hemorrhage is the escape of blood from the blood vessel.

For types and management refer to Ans. 2 of same chapter.

Causes

♦ Hemorrhage occurs due to road accidents and injuries

♦ Gun shot wounds

♦ During surgeries, such as thyroid surgery, circumcision and hydrocele surgery.

♦ Due to erosion of carotid artery by cancer.

♦ During inguinal block dissection.

♦ In bleeding disorders, such as hemophilia.

Clinical Features

♦ Patient becomes pallor and thirsty. At times, cyanosis is also present.

♦ There is presence of tachycardia and tachypenia

♦ Patient feels air hunger.

♦ Skin is cold and clammy due to vasoconstriction.

♦ Patient has dry face, dry mouth and goose skin appearance.

♦ There is presence of rapid thready pulse and hypotension

♦ Oliguria is present.

Signs of Hemorrhage

♦ Pulse >100/min

♦ Systolic blood pressure <100 mm Hg

♦ Diastolic blood pressure drop on sitting or standing >10 mm Hg

♦ Pallor/sweating

♦ Shock index, i.e., ratio of pulse rate to blood pressure >1

Q.7. Discuss briefly hemangioma. *(Nov 2008, 5 Marks)*

Or

Write short answer on hemangioma.

(Feb 2019, 3 Marks)

Ans. Hemangioma is a benign tumor containing hyperplastic endothelium with cellular proliferation with increased mast cells.

Classification

♦ *Capillary hemangioma:*
  • Salmon patch
  • Strawberry hemangioma
  • Port-wine stain.

♦ Cavernous hemangioma.

Clinical Features

♦ It is a most common tumor in children.

♦ It has biphasic growth showing initial rapid growth with gradual involution over 5–7 years.

♦ It is more common in girls.

♦ It is commonly seen in skin and subcutaneous tissue but can occur anywhere in the body like liver, brain, lungs and other organs.

♦ It grows rapidly in first year and 70% involutes in 7 years.

♦ Early proliferative lesion is bright red, irregular; deep lesion is bluish colored. Involution causes color fading, softness, shrinkage leaving crepe paper like area.

♦ Commonly it is central; common in head and neck region.

♦ Often large hemangiomas may be associated with visceral anomalies. Head and neck hemangioma is associated with ocular and intracranial anomalies; sacral with spinal dysraphism.

♦ Multiple cutaneous hemangiomas may be associated with hemangioma of liver causing hepatomegaly, cardiac failure (CCF), anemia.

♦ Ulceration, bleeding, airway block and visual disturbances are common complications.

♦ A definitive even though rare, but important life-threatening complication is platelet trapping and severe thrombocytopenia presenting as ecchymosis, petechiae, intracranial hemorrhage and massive gastrointestinal bleed.

Treatment

Refer to Ans. 5 of same chapter.

Q.8. Define hemorrhage, its types, causes, investigations and measures to control hemorrhage.

(Jun 2010, 15 Marks)

Ans. Hemorrhage is defined as the escape of blood from cardiovascular system to the surface of body or into the body tissues or cavities.

Types

Refer to Ans. 2 of same chapter.

Causes

♦ Trauma
♦ Infections
♦ Local irritants
♦ Congenital malformations
♦ Surgical (intraoperative/postoperative)
♦ Hemorrhage due to abnormalities in clotting factors:
  • *Clotting factor deficiencies*
    – Hereditary: Hemophilia A, Hemophilia B, Thrombocytopenia.
    – Anticoagulant, antiplatelet or fibrinolytic therapy: Warfarin, coumarin, heparin, enoxaparin, aspirin, clopidogrel, etc.
    – Liver disease.
  • *Dysfunction of clotting—multiple myeloma:*
    – Hemorrhage due to abnormalities in platelets
      » *Deficiencies:*
        ▪ Idiopathic thrombocytopenia purpura
        ▪ Secondary thrombocytopenia purpura
        ▪ Leukemia.
      » Thrombocytosis
      » Dysfunction: Thrombocytopenia.
    – Hemorrhage due to systemic disease
      » Viral infection
      » Scurvy
      » Allergy.

Investigations

Patients with the above mentioned causes may be advised to be subjected to an investigation before any oral surgical procedure.

Investigations are:

♦ Clotting time
♦ Bleeding time
♦ Prothrombin time and International normalized ratio (INR)
♦ Activated partial thromboplastin time
♦ Factors assay.

Investigations for Measuring the Blood Loss

♦ Hb% and PCV estimation
♦ Blood volume estimation using radioiodine technique or microhematocrit method
♦ Measurement of CVP or PCWP
♦ Investigations specific for cause, i.e., ultrasonography of abdomen, Doppler and often angiogram in vascular injury, Chest X-ray in hemothorax, CT scan in major injuries, CT scan head in head injuries.

Measures to Control Hemorrhage

Mechanical Methods

♦ *Pressure:* Firm pressure is applied over bleeding site for 5 minutes.

♦ *Hemostat:* It is applied at bleeding points and leads to direct occlusion of bleeding vessel
♦ *Sutures and ligation:* For severed blood vessels ligature is done. For large pulsating artery suturing is done.

Chemical Methods

♦ Adrenaline: It leads to vasoconstriction of bleeding capillaries
♦ Thrombin: Converts fibrinogen into fibrous clot
♦ Surgicel: Acts by forming acid products from partial dissolution which coagulate plasma protein
♦ Surgicel fibrillar: It is modified surgical and is used in irregular surfaces and inaccessible areas
♦ Oxycel: Platelet plug in its meshwork and forms the clot
♦ Gelatine sponge Or Gelfoam/surgifoam
♦ Microfibrillar collagen (Avitene)
♦ Fibrous glue
♦ Styptics and astringents: They precipitate protein and arrest bleeding
♦ Alginic acid
♦ Natural collagen sponge: It activates coagulation factors XI and XIII and helps in clotting
♦ Fibrin sponge: It stimulates coagulation forming normal clot and also act as temporary plug over small injured blood vessels
♦ Bone wax: It is used in cases of bleeding from bone or chipped edges of bone. It is softened with fingers and is applied to bleeding site
♦ Ostene: a new water-soluble bone hemostatic agent.

Thermal Agents

♦ *Eletrocautery/surgical diathermy:* Small capillaries and bleeding vessels are coagulated by diathermy.
♦ Monopolar diathermy
♦ Bipolar diathermy
♦ Cryosurgery
♦ *Lasers:* Coagulate small blood vessels.

Q.9. Write short note on hemophilia—its types and management. *(Jun 2010, 5 Marks)*

Ans.

Types of Hemophilia

Types of hemophilia	Another name	Deficiency of clotting factor
Hemophilia A	Classic hemophilia	Factor VIII or plasma thromboplastinogen
Hemophilia B	Christmas disease	Factor IX or plasma thromboplastin component
Hemophilia C	–	Factor XI or plasma thromboplastin antecedent

Management

For management, refer to Ans. 4 of same chapter.

Q.10. Define and describe differentiating features of cirsoid aneurysm and strawberry hemangioma.

(Jan 2012, 5 Marks)

Ans.

Features	Cirsoid aneurysm	Strawberry hemangioma
Definition	It is a rare variant of capillary hemangioma occurring in skin beneath which abnormal artery communicates with the distended veins	It may start at birth in between one to three weeks it appears as red mark which increases in size within 3 months and form strawberry hemangioma
Type	Variant of capillary hemangioma	True capillary hemangioma
Swelling	Pulsatile swelling	Cystic swelling
Bony involvement	Involves bone	Does not involve bone
Treatment	Ligation of feeding artery and excision of lesion	Wait and watch policy as the lesion disappears till age of 7–8 years

Q.11. Enumerate differences between primary, reactionary and secondary hemorrhage. *(Jun 2014, 2 Marks)*

Ans.

Primary hemorrhage	Reactionary hemorrhage	Secondary hemorrhage
Occurs during surgery	Occurs after 6–12 hours of surgery	Occur after 5–7 days of surgery
Occurs due to accidental cut of vessel during surgery	Hypertension in postoperative period, violent sneezing, coughing or retching are the causes	Occurs due to infection which eats away the suture material causing sloughing of vessel wall

Q.12. Write short note on capillary hemangioma.

(June 2015, 5 Marks)

Ans. Capillary hemangioma is of three types:
- Salmon patch
- Strawberry hemangioma
- Port-wine stain

Salmon Patch

- It is present at the time of birth.
- It commonly occurs at the nape of neck, face, scalp and limbs.
- Lesion involves the wide area of skin.
- It is caused due to the area of persistent fetal dermal circulation.
- It regresses with the age and disappear completely.

Strawberry Hemangioma

- Child is normal at birth, but between 1 to 3 weeks lesion appear as red mark which increases in size to 3 months.
- This is a true capillary hemangioma.
- Lesion is 20 times more common than port-wine stain.
- Lesion is seen more commonly in white girls
- Its male to female ratio is 1:3.

- Lesion occurs most commonly in head and neck region.
- On palpation lesion is compressible and is warm with bluish surface.
- Lesion involves skin, muscles and subcutaneous tissues.
- Lesion begins to disappear one year of age and it completely regresses in 7 to 8 years.

Port-wine Stain

- It occurs at birth and persists throughout the life.
- It presents as smooth, flat, reddish blue or purplish.
- Lesion is common in head, neck and face.
- Eventually surface of lesion become nodular and keratotic.
- It results due to defect in maturation of sympathetic innervations of skin causing localized vasodilatation of intradermal capillaries.
- It requires cosmetic coverage. Excision, grafting or LASER ablation.

Treatment of Capillary Hemangioma

- They are treated by wait and watch policy commonly allowed for spontaneous regression. Diode laser, surgical excision and reconstruction may need to be ligated after wide exposure before achieving complete extirpation. Sclerotherapy/Cryotherapy/CO_2 snow therapy cause unpleasant scarring.
- Preoperative embolization facilitates surgical excision and reduces the operative blood loss. When once embolization done surgery should be done as early as possible otherwise recurrence occurs and much more worried formation of enlarged collaterals can occur.
- Rapidly growing hemangioma may need systemic/oral and intralesional steroid therapy.
- Antiangiogenic interferon 2a may be useful.
- Life-threatening platelet trapping may be controlled by cyclophosphamide chemotherapy.
- Hemangioma with drug resistant CCF can be treated with radiotherapy.

Q.13. Write short note on coagulation. *(June 2015, 5 Marks)*

Ans. It is the spontaneous arrest of the bleeding.

Following are the factors which are involved in the mechanism of coagulation of blood:
- Factor I—Fibrinogen
- Factor II—Prothrombin
- Factor III—Thromboplastin (tissue factor)
- Factor IV—Calcium ions
- Factor V—Labile factor
- Factor VI—Presence not approved
- Factor VII—Stable factor
- Factor VIII—Antihemophilic factor
- Factor IX—Christmas factor
- Factor X—Stuart–Prower factor
- Factor XI—Plasma thromboplastin antecedent
- Factor XII—Hageman factor
- Factor XIII—Fibrin-stabilizing factor
- Factor XIV—Prekallikrein
- Factor XV—Kallikrein
- Factor XVI—Platelet factor

Clotting Occurs in Three Stages

1. Formation of prothrombin activator.
2. Conversion of prothrombin into thrombin.
3. Conversion of fibrinogen to fibrin.

Formation of Prothrombin Activator

The prothrombin activator is formed into two ways:

♦ **Extrinsic pathway:**
  • Factor III initiates this pathway after injury to damage tissues. After injury, these tissues release thromboplastin which contains protein, phospholipid and glycoprotein which act as proteolytic enzymes.
  • The glycoprotein and phospholipid component of thromboplastin convert factor X into activated factor X, in presence of factor VIII.
  • Activated factor X reacts with factor V and phospholipid content of tissue thromboplastin to form prothrombin activator in presence of calcium.
  • Factor V is activated by thrombin formed from prothrombin. This factor V now accelerates formation of prothrombin activator.

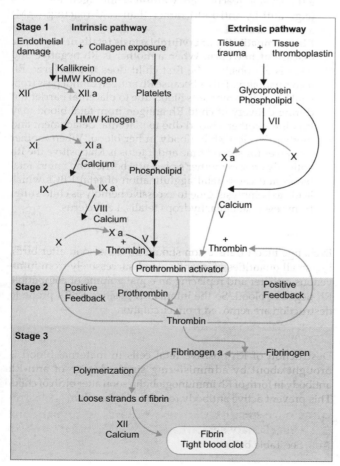

a: activated; + : thrombin induces formation of more thrombin (positive feedback)

Fig. 9: Coagulation pathway.

♦ **Intrinsic pathway:** It occurs in the following sequence:
  • During injury, the blood vessel is ruptured, endothelium is damaged and collagen beneath endothelium is exposed.
  • When factor XII comes in contact with collagen, it is converted to active factor XII.
  • The active factor XII converts inactive factor XI to active factor XI in presence of kininogen.
  • The activated factor XI activates factor IX in presence of calcium ions.
  • Activated factor IX activates factor X in presence of factor VIII and calcium.
  • When platelet comes in contact with collagen of damaged blood vessel, it releases phospholipids.
  • Now, active factor X reacts with platelet phospholipid and factor V to form prothrombin activation in presence of calcium ions.
  • Factor V is activated by positive feedback method.

Conversion of Prothrombin into Thrombin

Prothrombin activator converts prothrombin into thrombin in presence of calcium by positive feedback mechanism. This accelerates formation of extrinsic and intrinsic prothrombin activator.

Conversion of Fibrinogen to Fibrin

During this, the soluble fibrinogen is converted to fibrin by thrombin. The fibrinogen is converted to activated fibrinogen due to loss of two pairs of polypeptides. The first form fibrin contains loosely arranged strands which are modified later into tight aggregate by factor XIII in presence of calcium ions.

Q.14. Classify hemorrhages. Management of hypovolemic shock. Complications of blood transfusion.

(Dec 2015, 10 Marks)

Or

Describe various blood transfusion reactions.

(Oct 2019, 5 Marks)

Ans.

Classification of Hemorrhage

♦ **Depending upon the nature of the vessel involve:**
  • *Arterial hemorrhage:*
    – Bright red in color, jet out.
    – Pulsation of the artery can be seen.
    – It can be easily controlled as, it is visible.
  • *Venous hemorrhage:*
    – Dark red in color.
    – It never jet out but oozes out.
    – Difficult in control because vein gets retracted, non-pulsatile.
  • *Capillary hemorrhage:*
    – Red color, never jet out, slowly oozes out.
    – It becomes significant if there are bleeding tendencies.

♦ **Depending upon the timing of hemorrhage:**
  • *Primary hemorrhage:* Occurs at the time of surgery.
  • *Reactionary hemorrhage:* Occurs after 6–12 hours of surgery. Hypertension in postoperative period, violent sneezing, coughing or retching are the usual causes.

- *Secondary hemorrhage:* Occurs after 5–7 days of surgery. It is due to infection which eats away the suture material, causing sloughing of vessel wall.

♦ **Depending upon the duration of hemorrhage:**
  - Acute hemorrhage: Occurs suddenly, e.g., esophageal varices bleeding.
  - Chronic hemorrhage: Occurs over a period of time, e.g., hemorrhoids/piles.

♦ **Depending upon the nature of bleeding:**
  - External hemorrhage or reversal hemorrhage, e.g., epistaxis, hematemesis.
  - Internal hemorrhage or concealed hemorrhage, e.g., splenic rupture following injury.

♦ **Based on the possible intervention:**
  - *Surgical hemorrhage:* Can be corrected by surgical intervention
  - *Nonsurgical hemorrhage:* It is diffuse and ooze due to coagulation abnormalities and disseminated intravascular coagulation.

Complications of Blood Transfusion/Blood Transfusion Reactions

♦ **Febrile reactions:** It is the most common complication due to impurities like pyrogens in the blood or in infusion set. Headaches, fever, chills and rigors, tachycardia, nausea are the features. Transfusion is temporarily stopped or the flow is slowed down with administration of antipyretic drug to reduce fever. Often transfusion of that unit needs to be discontinued.

♦ **Allergic reaction:** Urticaria and allergy to specific proteins in the donor's plasma can occur. Usually, it is mild and is treated with steroid and antihistaminics. In severe urticaria that unit of blood is discarded; new washed RBC's and platelets are used.

♦ **Acute hemolytic reactions:** It is the most dangerous complication. It is due to ABO incompatibility. Usually it is nonfatal but occasionally can be fatal. It is commonly due to technical error at different levels. It amounts for criminal negligence in court of law.

♦ **Transfusion-related graft versus host disease:** This very serious, very rare complication occurs due to recognition and reaction against host tissues by infused donor lymphocytes. It is common in immunosuppressed, lymphoma, leukemic patients. Any type of blood products including leukocyte reduced blood can cause the condition. Features are pancytopenia, toxic epidermal necrosis, liver dysfunction with more than 90% mortality. It is difficult to treat.

♦ **Congestive cardiac failure:** It occurs if especially large quantities of whole blood are transfused in chronic severe anemia, pregnancy, elderly patients, in patients who have cardiac problems.

For management of hypovolemic shock refer to Ans. 2 of chapter SHOCK.

Q.15. Write briefly on Rhesus (Rh) blood group.
(Jan 2016, 2 Marks)

Ans. Rhesus blood group was discovered by Landsteiner and Weiner in 1940.

♦ Rh antigen system has three closely linked gene loci, coding for D antigen (there is no d antigen), C and/or c antigen and E and/or e antigen. Thus, the antigens produced are C, D, E. c and e.

♦ An individual may have similar or different sets of these three Rh antigens on each chromosome; for example, CDE/cde, cde/cde, or CdE/cdE (each person inherits one trio gene from each parent).

♦ Individuals who are positive for D antigen are considered Rh-positive (85% of the population) and those who lack it are Rh-negative.

♦ Individuals with a weak variant of D antigen, called the Du variant, are also considered Rh-positive.

♦ Alloimmunization, i.e., formation of an antibody against an antigen occurs if a person is exposed to an Rh antigen that is not on the patients RBCs.

♦ The majority of clinically important antibodies that produce a transfusion reaction are warm-reacting (IgG) antibodies (e.g., anti-D, anti-Kell) rather than cold-reacting (IgM) antibodies.

Rh incompatibility or erythroblastosis fetalis or hemolytic disease of newborn: When a mother is Rh negative and fetus is Rh positive the first child does not undergo Rh incompatibility. This is because Rh antigen cannot pass from fetal blood into mother's blood due to placental barrier but during delivery of child Rh antigen from fetal blood may leak into mother's blood due to placental detachment and mother develop Rh antibody in her blood. When mother conceives for second time and if fetus is Rh positive the Rh antibody crosses mother's placental barrier and enters fetal blood and cause fetal agglutination of fetal RBCs which leads to hemolysis. Due to excessive hemolysis child suffer from severe anemia, hydrops fetalis, kernicterus.

Treatment

Exchange blood transfusion should be done soon after birth, i.e., small quantities of infant's blood successively from intravenous catheter and replacing an equal volume of compatible Rh negative blood. So the infants Rh positive RBCs prone to destruction are removed from circulation.

Prevention

Destruction of Rh positive fetal cells in maternal blood is brought about by administering single dosage of anti-Rh antibody in form of Rh immunoglobulin soon after birth of child. This prevent active antibody formation by mother.

Q.16. Describe differentiating features of primary and reactionary hemorrhage. *(Jan 2017, 4 Marks)*

Ans. See Table below:

Primary hemorrhage	Reactionary hemorrhage
It occur during the surgery	It occurs after 6–12 hours of surgery
It is due to the accidental cut of vessel during surgery. This bleeding is more common in surgery on malignancy	Causes of reactionary hemorrhage are: Slipping away of ligatures Dislodgement of clots Cessation of reflex vasospasm normalization of blood pressure
This should be resolved during the operation, with any major hemorrhages recorded in the operative notes and the patient monitored closely postoperatively.	As the causing factor is corrected the hemorrhage stops
Primary hemorrhage can be arterial, venous or capillary	Reactionary hemorrhage can be arterial or venous. Bleeding starts when there is rise in arterial or venous pressure

Q.17. How to control the bleeding during operations?

(Aug 2018, 10 Marks)

Ans. Following are the methods to control bleeding during operations:

Pressure and Packing

- It is the method of choice to stop the bleeding when bleeding site is inaccessible.
- For controlling the bleeding from nose and scalp. Packing of the wound is done by roller gauze with or without adrenaline to control bleeding from nose.
- Bleeding from the vein: During thyroidectomy middle thyroid vein, during lumbar sympathectomy the lumbar vein bleeding is controlled by using the pressure pack for few minutes.
- Sengstaken tube is indicated in controlling the bleeding from esophageal varices.

Surgical Methods to Stop Hemorrhage

- Application of artery forceps is done to control bleeding from veins, arteries and capillaries.
- Application of ligatures for the bleeding vessels
- By cauterization
- By application of bone wax to control the bleeding from cut edges of the bone.
- Silver clips are used to control bleeding from cerebral vessels.
- Various surgical procedures are done to stop the bleeding, i.e., laparotomy and splenectomy for splenic rupture, hysterectomy for uncontrollable postpartum hemorrhage, laparotomy for controlling the bleeding from the ruptured ectopic pregnancy.

Position and Rest

- Elevation of legs controls bleeding from varicose veins.
- Elevation of head end decreases venous bleeding in thyroidectomy, i.e., anti-trendelenburg position.

Tourniquet

Tourniquet is often used in operation theatr for control of hemorrhage in limbs. But this is not advisable as first aid measure. It is of two types, i.e., pneumatic cuffs with pressure gauge and rubber bandage. If tourniquet is too loose it does not serve the purpose, too tight tourniquet causes arterial thrombosis can occur which result in gangrene, too long application leads to gangrene of limb.

Control of Hemorrhage from External and Internal Hemorrhage

- If external hemorrhage is present ligation of small vessel, suturing the wound part, vessel suturing, topical application for local ooze—oxycel, gauze soaked with adrenaline, bone wax for oozing from bone and local hemostatic agent.
- If internal hemorrhage is present intercostals tube is placed for hemothorax; laparotomy for liver or spleen or mesentry or bowel injuries, suturing, splenectomy. Just placing intra-abdominal pack to control bleeding mainly in liver injury as damage control surgery is very useful. Upper and lower gastrointestinal bleeding is managed differently after initial resuscitation—endoscopic control or angiographic control, etc.

Q.18. Write short answer on Rh incompatibility.

(Sep 2018, 3 Marks)

Ans. Rh incompatibility occurs when an Rh negative individual receives Rh positive blood.

- Normally, when an Rh negative person receive Rh positive blood, there will be no immediate reactions as Rh negative individual does not normally has anti-Rh antibody.
- However, the donor's red cells induce an immune response in the recipient to synthesize anti-Rh antibodies, which takes about two to four months to reach a significant titer. However, by that time the donor's red cells die their natural death within 120 days. The anti-Rh antibody cannot produce any harm to the recipient's red cells because the Rh negative recipient's red cells contain no Rh antigens.
- But, if the same Rh negative person who has already received a Rh positive blood before, receives a second Rh positive transfusion later, the anti-Rh antibodies are synthesized in large amount immediately by the memory cells. This antibody reacts against the donor cells and causes reactions of mismatch transfusion.
- Thus, the Rh negative individual can safely receive positive blood once in life time.
- Similar Rh incompatibility occurs in pregnancies when Rh negative mother bears Rh positive fetus, which leads to erythroblastosis fetalis. The first child does not suffer. However, subsequent pregnancies carry risk for the fetus. The disorder is called erythroblastosis fetalis.

For more details refer to Ans. 15 of same chapter.

8. SHOCK

Q.1. Discuss shock.   *(Apr 2010, 15 Marks)*

Or

Discuss briefly shock. *(Aug 2012, 5 Marks)*

Or

What is shock? Describe its classification, causes, clinical features and management.

(Jan 2012, 10 Marks)

Or

Write on classification, causes, clinical features and management of shock. *(Nov 2014, 8 Marks)*

Ans. Shock is defined as an acute clinical syndrome characterized by a significant, systemic reduction in tissue perfusion, resulting in decreased tissue oxygen delivery and insufficient removal of cellular metabolic products, resulting in tissue injury and severe dysfunction of vital organs.

Classification of Shock

Following is the classification of shock:
- Hypovolemic shock
- Cardiogenic shock
- *Distributive shock:*
  - Septic shock
  - Anaphylactic shock
  - Neurogenic shock
- Obstructive shock

Hypovolemic Shock

- Hypovolemic shock occurs due to loss of blood plasma or body fluid and electrolytes, usually caused by massive hemorrhage, vomiting, diarrhea, and dehydration.
- Hypovolemic shock is the most common type of shock which is characterized by a loss in circulatory volume, which leads to decreased venous return, decreased filling of the cardiac chambers, and so there is decrease in cardiac output which leads to increase in the systemic vascular resistance.

Cardiogenic Shock

- Cardiogenic shock occurs due to the dysfunction of one ventricle or other.
- This type of shock is seen in myocardial infarction, chronic congestive cardiac failure, cardiac arrhythmias, pulmonary embolism, etc., resulting in inability of the heart to pump the adequate amount of blood into the lungs and decreased cardiac output.
- Myocardial infarction is the most common cause of cardiogenic shock.

Distributive Shock

Distributive shock occurs when the afterload is excessively reduced due to extensive vasodilatation and is associated not only with poor vascular tone in the peripheral circulation but maldistribution of blood flow to organs within the body also.

- **Septic shock:** This type of shock is mostly due to release of endotoxins in blood, which causes wide spread vasodilation of blood vessels resulting in fall in the cardiac output. Bacteria responsible for release of endotoxins are *E. coli*, *Pseudomonas proteus*, etc. It is most common shock among all the distributive shocks.

- **Neurogenic shock:** This type of distributive shock is caused by the suppression or loss of sympathetic tone caused any disruption of the sympathetic nervous system like spinal injury, spinal anesthesia, and drugs.
- **Anaphylactic shock:** This type of shock is a result of type I hypersensitivity reaction and is caused when the body's antibody—antigen response is triggered by something the person is allergic to drugs, like penicillin, cephalosporins, iodinated contrast media, serum, etc., are common causes of this type of shock.

Obstructive Shock

- This type of shock is associated with physical obstruction of the great vessels or the heart itself.
- Most commonly obstructive shock is due to cardiac tamponade, due to tension pneumothorax and pulmonary embolus.

Causes of Shock

- *Hypovolemic shock—due to reduction in total blood volume. It may be due to:*
  - *Hemorrhage:*
    - External from wounds, open fractures
    - Internal from injury to spleen, liver, mesentery or pelvis.
  - Severe burns, which results in loss of plasma
  - Peritonitis, intestinal obstruction
  - Vomiting and diarrhea of any cause
- *Cardiac causes:*
  - Acute myocardial infarction, acute carditis
  - Acute pulmonary embolism wherein embolus blocks the pulmonary artery at bifurcation or one of the major branches
  - Drug induced
  - Toxemia of any causes
  - Cardiac surgical conditions, such as valvular diseases, congenital heart diseases
  - *Cardiac compression causes:*
    - Cardiac tamponade due to collection of blood, pus, fluid in the pericardial space which prevents the heart to expand leading to shock.
    - Trauma to heart.
- Septic shock is due to bacterial infections which release toxins leading to shock.
- Neurogenic shock—due to sudden anxious or painful stimuli causing severe splanchnic vessel vasodilatation. Here patient either goes for cardiac arrest and dies or recovers fully spontaneously—spinal cord injury/anesthesia can cause neurogenic shock.
- Anaphylactic shock is due to type I hypersensitivity reaction
- *Respiratory causes:*
  - Atelectasis (collapse) of lung
  - Thoracic injuries
  - Tension pneumothorax
  - Anesthetic complications.
- *Other causes:*
  - Acute adrenal insufficiency (Addison's disease)
  - Myxedema.

Pathophysiology of Shock

Flowchart 5: Pathophysiology of shock.

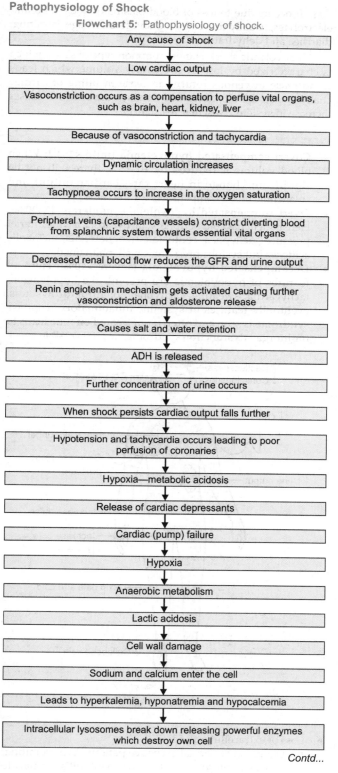

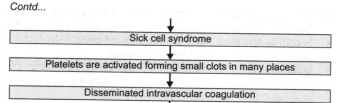

Contd...

| Sick cell syndrome |
| Platelets are activated forming small clots in many places |
| Disseminated intravascular coagulation |
| Further bleeding |

Stages of Shock

Stage 1: Stage of compensatory shock—by neuroendocrine response to maintain the perfusion of the vital organs, such as brain, heart, kidney, liver.

Stage 2: Stage of decompensatory shock—where there is progressive shock causing persistent shock with severe hypotension (with mean arterial pressure <65 mm Hg); oliguria, tachycardia.

Stage 3: Stage of irreversible shock—with severe hypoxia and multiorgan dysfunction syndrome (MODS).

Clinical Features of Shock

♦ Presence of anxiety, restlessness, altered mental state due to decreased cerebral perfusion and subsequent hypoxia.
♦ Hypotension because of decrease in circulatory volume.
♦ Due to decreased blood flow there is tachycardia and weak thready pulse.
♦ Cold and clammy skin due to vasoconstriction and stimulation of vasoconstriction.
♦ Rapid and shallow respirations (tachypnea) due to sympathetic nervous system stimulation and acidosis.
♦ Hypothermia due to decreased perfusion and evaporation of sweat.
♦ Thirst and dry mouth due to fluid depletion.
♦ Fatigue due to inadequate oxygenation.
♦ Cold and mottled skin, especially extremities, due to insufficient perfusion of the skin.
♦ Pallor is present
♦ Fainting
♦ Oliguria/anuria due to decreased renal perfusion and afferent arteriolar vasoconstriction.

Investigations and Monitoring of Shock

♦ Regular monitoring with blood pressure, pulse, heart rate, respiratory rate, urine output measurement (hourly) should be done. Urine output should be >0.5 mL/kg/hour. Pulse oximetry should be used.
♦ Central venous pressure (CVP), pulmonary capillary wedge pressure (PCWP—an accurate assessment of left ventricular/ function) monitoring should be done. ICU care is needed during monitor period. But both CVP and PCWP are not accurate method of assessing tissue perfusion.
♦ Complete blood count, ESR, pH assessment, serum electrolyte estimation, chest X-ray (to rule out acute respiratory distress syndrome/pulmonary problems).

Contd...

♦ Pus/urine/blood/bile/sputum cultures depending on the focus and need in sepsis.

♦ Serum lactate estimation is an important prognostic factor. Level >2 mEq/L suggest tissue ischemia.

♦ USG of a part, CT/MRI of the location of pathology of standard focus should be done; often may require repetition of these imaging to assess progress.

♦ Blood urea, serum creatinine, liver function tests, prothrombin time (PT), activated partial thromboplastin time (APTT), ECG monitoring are also should be done.

♦ All these tests including platelet count and arterial blood gas (ABG) should be repeated at regular intervals.

Treatment of Shock

♦ Treat the cause, e.g., arrest hemorrhage, drain pus.

♦ *Fluid replacement:* Plasma, normal saline, dextrose, Ringer's lactate, plasma expander (haemaccel). Dosage is maximum 1 L can be given in 24 hours. Initially crystalloids then colloids are given. Blood transfusion is done whenever required.

♦ *Ionotropic agents:* Dopamine, dobutamine, adrenaline infusions—mainly in distributive shock like septic shock.

♦ *Correction of acid–base balance:* Acidosis is corrected by using 8.4% sodium bicarbonate intravenously.

♦ Steroid is often lifesaving. 500–1,000 mg of hydrocortisone can be given. It improves the perfusion, reduces the capillary leakage and systemic inflammatory effects.

♦ Antibiotics in patients with sepsis; proper control of blood sugar and ketosis in diabetic patients.

♦ Catheterization to measure urine output (30–50 mL/hour or >0.5 mL/kg/hour should be maintained).

♦ Nasal oxygen to improve oxygenation or ventilator support with intensive care unit monitoring has to be done.

♦ Central venous pressure line to perfuse adequately and to monitor fluid balance. Total parentral nutrition is given when required.

♦ Pulmonary capillary wedge pressure to monitor very critical patient.

♦ Hemodialysis may be necessary when kidneys are not functioning.

♦ Control pain—using morphine (4 mg IV).

♦ Ventilator and ICU/critical care management.

♦ Injection ranitidine IV or omeprazole IV or pantoprazole IV.

♦ Activated protein even though costly is beneficial as it prevents the release and action of inflammatory response.

♦ Military antishock trouser (MAST) provides circumferential external pressure of 40 mm Hg. It is wrapped around lower limbs and abdomen, and inflated with required pressure. It redistributes the existing blood and fluid towards center. It should be deflated carefully and gradually.

Q.2. Describe clinical feature and management of hypovolemic shock.

(Apr 2019, 5 Marks) (Jan 2018, 20 Marks)

Or

Write a short note on hypovolemic shock.

(Apr 2017, 4 Marks)

Ans. It occurs due to loss of blood plasma or body fluid and electrolytes, usually caused by massive hemorrhage, vomiting, diarrhea and dehydration.

Hypovolemic shock is most common type of shock which is characterized by loss in circulatory volume which leads to decrease in venous return, decrease in filling of cardiac chambers, so there is decreased cardiac output which causes increase in systemic vascular resistance.

Types of Hypovolemia

♦ **Covert compensated hypovolemia (mild <15%):** When blood volume is reduced by 10–15%, there will not be significant change in heart rate, cardiac output and splanchnic blood compensates for the same.

♦ **Overt compensated hypovolemia (moderate 15–40%):** Here patient has cold periphery, tachycardia, a wide arterial pressure, tachypnea, confusion, hyponatremia, metabolic acidosis, but systolic pressure is well maintained.

♦ **Decompensated hypovolemia (severe >40%):** Here all features of hypovolemia are present like hypotension, tachycardia, sweating, tachypnea, oliguria, drowsiness, eventually features of systemic inflammatory response syndrome is seen and often if not treated on time leads to multiorgan dysfunction syndrome, i.e., irreversible shock

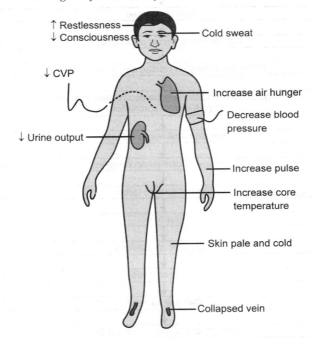

Fig. 10: Hypovolemic shock.

Causes

♦ Loss of extracellular fluid:
  • Deviation of normal exchange pattern: As in vomiting, diarrhea, intestinal obstruction, peritonitis, and acute pancreatitis.

- Increased sweating without replacement in a non-acclimatized individual.
- Third space shift to sodium from extracellular to intracellular compartment due to failure of sodium pump caused by hypoxia.
♦ *Plasma loss:* Due to burn.
♦ *Hemorrhage:* Due to whole blood loss like.
  - *Surgical:* During and following any major surgery especially cardiopulmonary bypass, pelvic surgery or major abdominal surgery.
  - *Traumatic:* As a result of any type of major accident, warfare injuries, homicidal or following suicidal injury as by knife, bullet, etc.
  - *GI bleeding:* Bleeding from peptic ulcer, perforation of intestine, bleeding from esophageal varices, etc.
  - *Obstructive bleeding:* Incomplete abortion, placenta previa, etc.

Clinical Features

- Anxiety, restless, excitation and disorientation
- Pallor
- Thirst and hunger
- Cold and clammy skin
- Faint in upright position
- Tachycardia with rapid, thready pulse
- Hypotension
- Oliguria or anuria

Management

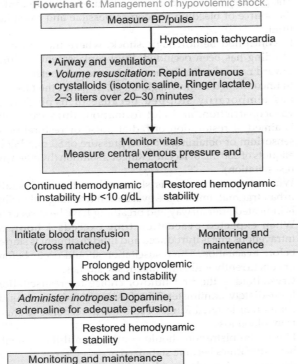

Flowchart 6: Management of hypovolemic shock.

Q.3. Describe briefly anaphylactic shock.
(Apr 2008, 5 Marks)

Ans. This type of shock is a result of type I hypersensitivity reaction.

Anaphylactic shock can occur when a previously sensitized individual is exposed to a specific antigen, iv. Drug, especially penicillin, cephalosporins and iodinated contrast media are common offenders.

Pathophysiology

Injections—penicillins, anesthetics, stings, venom, shellfish may be having antigens which will combine with IgE of mast cells and basophils, releasing histamine and large amount of SRS—A (slow releasing substance of anaphylaxis). They cause bronchospasm, laryngeal edema, respiratory distress, hypotension and shock. Mortality is 10%.

Clinical Features

- Due to reduced cerebral perfusion, there is change in mental status.
- Due to reduced preload and cardiac contractility, there is hypotension.
- Due to release of histamine and other chemical mediators there is urticaria.
- Due to hypoxia the cyanosis is caused.
- Due to anaerobic metabolism and hepatic dysfunction the lactic acidosis is caused.
- Due to coronary ischemia other dysrhythmias are caused.

Treatment

- Summon ambulance
- Always check whether respiratory distress is due to other causes.
- Assess the degree of cardiovascular collapse by checking pulse and blood pressure.
- Assess the degree of airway obstruction
- Stop administration of drug
- Patient should be kept supine
- Assess breathing difficulty by checking for stridor, wheeze
- Administer oxygen to patient by face mask
- Give antihistamine chlorpheniramine maleate 10 mg
- Administer hydrocortisone 20 mg
- Monitor consciousness, airway, breathing, circulation, pulse, blood pressure
- Raise legs if blood pressure is low
- Adrenaline 1:1,000, 0.5 mL IM is given immediately.
- Repeat IM adrenaline every 5 minutes while waiting for ambulance
- Administer 100% oxygen.
- CPR if cardiac arrest occurs.
- If BP fall is rapid, 1:10,000 adrenalin may be infused IV slowly.

Q.4. Describe management of a patient in state of shock.
(Sep 2010, 15 Marks)

Ans. Shock is defined as an acute clinical syndrome characterized by a significant, systemic reduction in tissue perfusion, resulting in decreased tissue oxygen delivery and insufficient removal of cellular metabolic products, resulting in tissue injury and severe dysfunction of vital organs.

Management

- Treat the cause, e.g., arrest hemorrhage, drain pus.
- *Fluid replacement:* Plasma, normal saline, dextrose, Ringer's lactate, plasma expander (haemaccel). Dosage is maximum l liter can be given in 24 hours. Initially crystalloids then colloids are given. Blood transfusion is done whenever required.
- *Ionotropic agents:* Dopamine, dobutamine, adrenaline infusions—mainly in distributive shock like septic shock.
- *Correction of acid-base balance:* Acidosis is corrected by using 8.4% sodium bicarbonate intravenously.
- Steroid is often lifesaving. 500–1,000 mg of hydrocortisone can be given. It improves the perfusion, reduces the capillary leakage and systemic inflammatory effects.
- Antibiotics in patients with sepsis; proper control of blood sugar and ketosis in diabetic patients.
- Catheterization to measure urine output (30–50 mL/hour or >0.5 mL/kg/hour should be maintained).
- Nasal oxygen to improve oxygenation or ventilator support with intensive care unit monitoring has to be done.
- Central venous pressure line to perfuse adequately and to monitor fluid balance. Total parenteral nutrition is given when required.
- Pulmonary capillary wedge pressure to monitor very critical patient.
- Hemodialysis may be necessary when kidneys are not functioning.
- Control pain—using morphine (4 mg IV).
- Ventilator and ICU/critical care management.
- Injection ranitidine IV or omeprazole IV or pantoprazole IV.
- Activated C protein even though costly is beneficial as it prevents the release and action of inflammatory response.
- Military antishock trouser (MAST) provides circumferential external pressure of`40 mm Hg. lt is wrapped around lower limbs and abdomen, and inflated with required pressure. It redistributes the existing blood and fluid towards center. It should be deflated carefully and gradually.

Q.5. Discuss the etiopathology, clinical feature and management of hemorrhage shock.

(Sep 2008, 5 Marks)

Or

Describe hemorrhagic shock and management.

(Jan 2018, 10 Marks)

Or

Enumerate the etiopathogenesis of hemorrhagic shock and its management. *(Sep 2018, 5 Marks)*

Or

Write short answer on hemorrhagic shock.

(Oct 2019, 3 Marks)

Or

Write short note on management of hemorrhagic shock. *(Apr 2007, 5 Marks)*

Or

Write in brief about hemorrhagic shock.

(Sep 2007, 5 Marks)

Or

Write short note on treatment of hemorrhagic shock.

(Sep 2008, 5 Marks)

Ans.

Hemorrhagic Shock

Etiopathology: Due to whole blood loss like.

- Surgical: During and following any major surgery especially cardiopulmonary bypass, pelvic surgery or major abdominal surgery.
- Traumatic: As a result of any type of major accident, warfare injuries, homicidal or following suicidal injury as by knife, bullet, etc.
- GI bleeding: Bleeding from peptic ulcer, perforation of intestine, bleeding from esophageal varices, etc.
- Obstructive bleeding: Incomplete abortion, placenta previa, etc.

Clinical Features

- Anxiety, restless, excitation and disorientation. Pallor
- Thirst and hunger
- Cold and clammy skin
- Faint in upright position
- Tachycardia with rapid, thready pulse
- Hypotension
- Oliguria or anuria.

Management of Hemorrhage Shock

- The primary treatment of hemorrhagic shock is to control the source of bleeding as soon as possible and to replace fluid.
- In controlled hemorrhagic shock, where the source of bleeding has been occluded, fluid replacement is aimed toward normalization of hemodynamic parameters.
- In uncontrolled hemorrhagic shock, in which the bleeding has temporarily stopped because of hypotension, vasoconstriction, and clot formation, fluid treatment is aimed at restoration of radial pulse or restoration of sensorium or obtaining a blood pressure of 80 mm Hg by aliquots of 250 mL of lactated Ringer's solution (hypotensive resuscitation).
- When evacuation time is shorter than 1 hour (usually urban trauma), immediate evacuation to a surgical facility is indicated after airway and breathing have been secured.
- When expected evacuation time exceeds 1 hour, an intravenous line is introduced and fluid treatment is started before evacuation. The resuscitation should occur before, or concurrently with, any diagnostic studies.
- Crystalloid is the first fluid of choice for resuscitation. Immediately administer 2 L of isotonic sodium chloride solution or lactated Ringer's solution in response to shock from blood loss.
- Fluid administration should continue until the patient's hemodynamics become stabilized.
- Because crystalloids quickly leak from the vascular space, each liter of fluid expands the blood volume by 20–30%;

therefore, 3 L of fluid need to be administered to raise the intravascular volume by 1 L.

♦ Alternatively, colloids restore volume in a 1:1 ratio. Currently available colloids include human albumin, hydroxyethyl starch products (mixed in either 0.9% isotonic sodium chloride solution or lactated Ringer's solution), or hypertonic saline-dextran combinations.

♦ Packed red blood cells (PRBCs) should be transfused if the patient remains unstable after 2,000 mL of crystalloid resuscitation. For acute situations, O-negative noncross matched blood should be administered. Administer 2 U rapidly, and note the response. For patients with active bleeding, several units of blood may be necessary.

Q.6. Write short note on syncope. *(Sep 2002, 5 Marks)*

Ans. Syncope may be defined as transient loss of consciousness which comes suddenly, lasts for a short-time and is due to diminished blood supply to the brain.

The symptoms are fainting and vasovagal attack.

Etiology

♦ Simple faint
♦ Decreased cardiac output in various heart diseases.
♦ Fear and sudden anxiety.
♦ Trauma to the deep lying structures.
♦ Hypoglycemia
♦ Bouts of coughing, etc.

Clinical Features

♦ Syncopal attack is sudden.
♦ *Prodromal symptoms:* Tingling or numbness in limbs, sudden darkness before eyes and patient may have a feeling blacking out.
♦ Person is cold and sweating fall in ground suddenly becoming unconscious.

Treatment

♦ All the dental procedure or treatment is stopped.
♦ Remove instruments from oral cavity, such as rubber dam, gauze, cotton, etc.
♦ Patient is kept in Trendelenburg position, i.e., patient is kept in a head low and feet up position.
♦ Loose tighten clothing of patient.
♦ Aromatic fumes inhalation is given or sprinkle cold water on face of patient for reflex stimulation.
♦ If recovery is gained escort patient home.
♦ If recovery is not gained Injection atropine 0.6 mg IM or IV is given.
♦ If still recovery is not gained look for hypoglycemia and Addison's crisis.
♦ Start basic life support
♦ Summon medical help.

Q.7. How will you manage a patient in shock from road side accident having fracture of mandible and maxilla? *(Feb 2013, 10 Marks)*

Ans. In such case, there following shock occurs:
♦ Neurogenic or vasovagal shock

♦ This is a response to sudden fear or severe pain and the effects from slight fainting fit to death.
♦ This type of shock is also known as neurogenic or psychogenic shock.
♦ There is sudden pooling of blood in the capacitance vessels of legs and splanchnic arterial bed. This causes reduced cardiac output and shock. It can be life-threatening due to hypoxia.

Pathophysiology

♦ Nucleus tractus solitarius of the brainstem is activated directly or indirectly by the triggering stimulus.
♦ Simultaneous enhancement of parasympathetic nervous system, i.e., vagal tone and withdrawal of sympathetic nervous system tone, which causes either cardioinhibitory response or vasodepressor response.
♦ Cardioinhibitory response is characterized by a drop in heart rate, i.e., negative chronotropic effect and in contractility, i.e., negative ianotropic effect which causes decrease in cardiac output.
♦ Unconsciousness or vasodepressor response is caused by a drop in blood pressure as low as 80/20 without much change in heart rate.

Clinical Features

♦ History of emotional stress or pain of a sudden nature.
♦ Bradycardia or pallor.
♦ Tachypnea
♦ Fainting
♦ Reflexes are usually intact.

Management

♦ Place the patient flat or in head low position.
♦ Ensure potency of airway
♦ IV atropine may be needed for persistent or increasing bradycardia.

Hypovolemic Shock, i.e., Hemorrhagic Shock

For management refer to Ans. 2 of same chapter.

Q.8. Write in short on septic shock. *(Oct 2007, 5 Marks)*

Or

Write short note on septic shock. *(Apr 2015, 3 Marks)*

Or

Write short note on septicemic shock.
(June 2015, 5 Marks)

Or

Write short answer on septic shock.
(Sep 2018, 3 Marks)

Ans. Septic shock is a vasodilator shock wherein there is peripheral vasodilation causing hypotension which is resistant to vasopressors.

Etiology

Septic shock may be due to gram-positive organisms, gram-negative organisms, fungi, viruses or protozoal origin.

Pathophysiology of Septic Shock

Flowchart 7: Pathophysiology of septic shock.

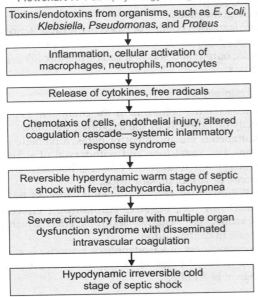

Toxins/endotoxins from organisms, such as *E. Coli, Klebsiella, Pseudomonas,* and *Proteus*

↓

Inflammation, cellular activation of macrophages, neutrophils, monocytes

↓

Release of cytokines, free radicals

↓

Chemotaxis of cells, endothelial injury, altered coagulation cascade—systemic inlammatory response syndrome

↓

Reversible hyperdynamic warm stage of septic shock with fever, tachycardia, tachypnea

↓

Severe circulatory failure with multiple organ dysfunction syndrome with disseminated intravascular coagulation

↓

Hypodynamic irreversible cold stage of septic shock

Clinical Features

Based on stages of septic shock.

♦ *Hyperdynamic or warm shock:*
  • It is a reversible stage.
  • Patient has fever, tachycardia and tachypnea
  • Pyogenic response is intact
♦ *Hypodynamic or cold septic shock:*
  • Pyogenic response is lost.
  • Patient is in decompensated shock.
  • Presence of anuria, cyanosis, jaundice, cardiac depression, pulmonary edema, hypoxia, drowsiness, coma and death.

Treatment/Management

♦ Correction of fluid and electrolyte by crystalloids, blood transfusion. Perfusion is very/most important.
♦ Appropriate antibiotics—third generation cephalosporins and aminoglycosides.
♦ Treat the cause or focus—drainage of an abscess; laparotomy for peritonitis; resection of gangrenous bowel; wound excision.
♦ Pus/urine/discharge/bile/blood culture and sensitivity for antibiotics.
♦ Critical care, oxygen, ventilator support, dobutamine dopamine/noradrenaline to maintain blood pressure and urine output.
♦ Activated C protein prevents the release of inflammatory mediators and blocks the effects of these mediators on cellular function.
♦ Monitoring the patient by pulse oximetry, cardiac status, urine output, arterial blood gas analysis.
♦ Short-term (one or two doses) high dose steroid therapy to control and protect cells from effects of endotoxemia. It

improves cardiac, renal and lung functions. Single dose of methylprednisolone or dexamethasone which often may be repeated again after 4 hours is said to be effective in endotoxic shock.

Q.9. Describe various causes of shock. Discuss in detail management of septic shock.

(Nov 2008, 15 Marks)

Ans. *For various causes of shock refer to Ans. 1 of same chapter.*

For management of septic shock refer to Ans. 8 of same chapter.

Q.10. Enumerate the complications of blood transfusion and describe the management of hypovolemic shock. *(Dec 2010, 10 Marks)*

Ans.

Complications of Blood Transfusion

♦ Congestive cardiac failure
♦ *Transfusion reactions HBV, HCV:*
  • Incompatibility. Major and minor reactions with fever, rigors, pain, hypotension
  • Pyrexial reactions due to pyrogenic ingredients in the blood.
  • Allergic reactions
  • Sensitization to leukocytes and platelets
  • Immunological sensitization.
♦ *Infections:*
  • Serum hepatitis
  • HIV infection
  • Bacterial infection
  • Malaria transmission
  • Epstein–Barr virus infection
  • Cytomegalovirus infection
  • SyphiIis, Yersinia
  • *Babesia microti* infection
  • *Trypanosoma cruzi* infection.
♦ Air embolism
♦ Thrombophlebitis
♦ *Coagulation failure:*
  • Dilution of clotting factors
  • Disseminated intravascular coagulation
  • Dilutional thrombocytopenia occurs in patients with massive blood transfusion.
♦ Circulatory overload causing heart failure
♦ Hemochromatosis in patients with CRF receiving repeated blood transfusions
♦ Citrate intoxication causes bradycardia and hypocalcemia.
♦ Iron overload.

Management

Refer to Ans. 2 of same chapter.

Q.11. Define and classify shock. In your practice local anesthetic is used, which type of shock it can produce? How will you recognize and treat? What precautions should be taken to prevent?

(Jan 2012, 15 Marks)

Ans. Shock is a clinical condition characterized by inadequate tissue perfusion and hence cellular hypoxia.

Classification of Shock

♦ Hypovolemic shock
♦ Cardiogenic shock
♦ Distributive shock
  • Septic shock
  • Anaphylactic shock
  • Neurogenic shock
♦ Obstructive shock

In clinical practice local anesthetic leads to anaphylactic shock.

Recognition of Anaphylactic Shock

♦ Patient has asthma like symptoms, i.e., sneezing and breathing.
♦ Urticaria and angioedema are present.
♦ Presence of bronchospasm and tachycardia
♦ Patient can undergo circulatory collapse.
♦ Due to rapid fall in blood pressure cardiac arrest may occur.

Treatment of Anaphylactic Shock

♦ Summon ambulance
♦ Always check whether respiratory distress is due to other causes.
♦ Assess the degree of cardiovascular collapse by checking pulse and blood pressure.
♦ Assess the degree of airway obstruction
♦ Stop administration of drug
♦ Patient should be kept supine
♦ Assess breathing difficulty by checking for stridor, wheeze
♦ Administer oxygen to patient by face mask
♦ Give antihistamine chlorpheniramine maleate 10 mg
♦ Administer hydrocortisone 20 mg
♦ Monitor consciousness, airway, breathing, circulation, pulse, blood pressure
♦ Raise legs if blood pressure is low
♦ Adrenaline 1:1,000, 0.5 mL IM is given immediately.
♦ Repeat IM adrenaline every 5 minutes while waiting for ambulance
♦ Administer 100% oxygen.
♦ CPR if cardiac arrest occurs.
♦ If BP fall is rapid, 1:10,000 adrenalin may be infused IV slowly.

Precautions Taken to Prevent the Anaphylactic Shock

♦ Intradermal test should be done before administering local anesthetic solution.
♦ Proper medical history of the patient is taken, if patient gives history of allergy from local anesthetic solution, drug should not be administered.

Q.12. What are the different type of hemorrhages? Discuss clinical features and management of hypovolemic shock. *(Aug 2012, 10 Marks)*

Ans. For *different types of hemorrhages refer to Ans. 2 of chapter Bleeding Disorders.*

For clinical features and management of hypovolemic shock refer to Ans. 2 of same chapter.

Q.13. Write in brief about complications of blood transfusion. *(Dec 2012, 5 Marks)*
Ans.

Complications of Blood Transfusion

♦ *Febrile reactions:* It is the most common complication due to impurities like pyrogens in the blood or in infusion set. Headaches, fever, chills and rigors, tachycardia, nausea are the features. Transfusion is temporarily stopped or the flow is slowed down with administration of antipyretic drug to reduce fever. Often transfusion of that unit needs to be discontinued.
♦ *Allergic reaction:* Utrticaria and allergy to specific proteins in the donor's plasma can occur. Usually, it is mild and is treated with steroid and antihistaminics. In severe urticaria that unit of blood is discarded; new washed RBC's and platelets are used.
♦ *Acute hemolytic reactions:* It is the most dangerous complication. It is due to ABO incompatibility. Usually it is nonfatal but occasionally can be fatal. It is commonly due to technical error at different levels. It amounts for criminal negligence in court of law.
♦ *Transfusion related graft versus host disease:* This very serious, very rare complication occurs due to recognition and reaction against host tissues by infused donor lymphocytes. It is common in immunosuppressed, lymphoma, leukemic patients. Any type of blood products including leukocyte reduced blood can cause the condition. Features are pancytopenia, toxic epidermal necrosis, liver dysfunction with more than 90% mortality. It is difficult to treat.
♦ *Congestive cardiac failure:* It occurs if especially large quantities of whole blood are transfused in chronic severe anemia, pregnancy, elderly patients, in patients who have cardiac problems.

Q.14. Enumerate differences between hypovolemic and septic shock. *(June 2014, 2 Marks)*

Or

Write difference between septic and hypovolemic shock. *(Jan 2016, 2 Marks)*
Ans.

Hypovolemic shock	Septic shock
It is due to reduction in total blood volume	It is due to bacterial infections which release toxins leading to shock
Causes are hemorrhage due to trauma, severe burns, peritonitis etc.	Causes are Gram-positive and Gram-negative organisms, fungi, viruses and protozoa
Fluid replacement should be done	Antibiotics are to be given

Q.15. Describe etiopathogenesis and classification of shock. How will you manage hemorrhagic shock? *(Feb 2014, 8 Marks)*

Ans.

Etiopathogenesis

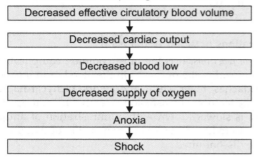

Flowchart 8: Etiopathogenesis of shock.

Classification

- Hypovolemic shock
- Cardiogenic shock
- *Distributive shock:*
  - Septic shock
  - Anaphylactic shock
  - Neurogenic shock
- Obstructive shock

Management of Hemorrhagic Shock

- The primary treatment of hemorrhagic shock is to control the source of bleeding as soon as possible and to replace fluid.
- In controlled hemorrhagic shock, where the source of bleeding has been occluded, fluid replacement is aimed toward normalization of hemodynamic parameters.
- In uncontrolled hemorrhagic shock, in which the bleeding has temporarily stopped because of hypotension, vasoconstriction, and clot formation, fluid treatment is aimed at restoration of radial pulse or restoration of sensorium or obtaining a blood pressure of 80 mm Hg by aliquots of 250 mL of lactated Ringer's solution (hypotensive resuscitation).
- When evacuation time is shorter than 1 hour (usually urban trauma), immediate evacuation to a surgical facility is indicated after airway and breathing have been secured.
- When expected evacuation time exceeds 1 hour, an intravenous line is introduced and fluid treatment is started before evacuation. The resuscitation should occur before, or concurrently with, any diagnostic studies.
- Crystalloid is the first fluid of choice for resuscitation. Immediately administer 2 L of isotonic sodium chloride solution or lactated Ringer's solution in response to shock from blood loss.
- Fluid administration should continue until the patient's hemodynamics become stabilized.
- Because crystalloids quickly leak from the vascular space, each liter of fluid expands the blood volume by 20–30%; therefore, 3 L of fluid need to be administered to raise the intravascular volume by 1 L.

- Alternatively, colloids restore volume in a 1:1 ratio. Currently available colloids include human albumin, hydroxyethyl starch products (mixed in either 0.9% isotonic sodium chloride solution or lactated Ringer's solution), or hypertonic saline-dextran combinations.
- Packed red blood cells (PRBCs) should be transfused if the patient remains unstable after 2,000 mL of crystalloid resuscitation. For acute situations, O-negative noncrossmatched blood should be administered. Administer 2 U rapidly, and note the response. For patients with active bleeding, several units of blood may be necessary.

Q.16. Describe different types of shock. How to manage hemorrhagic shock? *(Jan 2017, 10 Marks)*

Or

Define shock, clinical feature and management of various type of shock. *(Apr 2018, 5 Marks)*

Or

Define shock, its type, clinical feature and management. *(Feb 2019, 5 Marks)*

Ans. Shock is defined as an acute clinical syndrome characterized by a significant, systemic reduction in tissue perfusion, resulting in decreased tissue oxygen delivery and insufficient removal of cellular metabolic products, resulting in tissue injury and severe dysfunction of vital organs.

Description of Different Types of Shock

Classification of Shock

- Hypovolemic shock
- Cardiogenic shock
- *Distributive shock:*
  - Septic shock
  - Anaphylactic shock
  - Neurogenic shock
- Obstructive shock

Hypovolemic shock

- It occurs due to loss of blood plasma or body fluid and electrolytes, usually caused by massive hemorrhage, vomiting, diarrhea and dehydration.
- Hypovolemic shock is most common type of shock which is characterized by loss in circulatory volume which leads to decrease in venous return, decrease in filling of cardiac chambers, so there is decreased cardiac output which causes increase in systemic vascular resistance.

Causes

- *Loss of extracellular fluid:*
  - *Deviation of normal exchange pattern:* As in vomiting, diarrhea, intestinal obstruction, peritonitis, and acute pancreatitis.
  - Increased sweating without replacement in a non-acclimatized individual.
  - Third space shift to sodium from extracellular to intracellular compartment due to failure of sodium pump caused by hypoxia.
- *Plasma loss:* Due to burn.
- *Hemorrhage:* Due to whole blood loss like.

- *Surgical:* During and following any major surgery especially cardiopulmonary bypass, pelvic surgery or major abdominal surgery.
- *Traumatic:* As a result of any type of major accident, warfare injuries, homicidal or following suicidal injury as by knife, bullet, etc.
- *GI bleeding:* Bleeding from peptic ulcer, perforation of intestine, bleeding from esophageal varices, etc.
- *Obstructive bleeding:* Incomplete abortion, placenta previa, etc.

Clinical Features

- Anxiety, restless, excitation and disorientation.
- Pallor
- Thirst and hunger
- Cold and clammy skin
- Faint in upright position
- Tachycardia with rapid, thready pulse
- Hypotension
- Oliguria or anuria

Management

Flowchart 9: Management of hypovolemic shock.

Measure BP/pulse
↓ Hypotension tachycardia
- Airway and ventilation
- *Volume resuscitation:* Repid intravenous crystalloids (isotonic saline, Ringer lactate) 2–3 liters over 20–30 minutes
↓
Monitor vitals
Measure central venous pressure and hematocrit

Continued hemodynamic instability Hb <10 g/dL → Initiate blood transfusion (cross matched)

Restored hemodynamic stability → Monitoring and maintenance

Prolonged hypovolemic shock and instability ↓

Administer inotropes: Dopamine, adrenaline for adequate perfusion
↓ Restored hemodynamic stability
Monitoring and maintenance

Cardiogenic shock

- Myocardial infection is the most common cause of cardiogenic shock.
- Cardiogenic shock occurs if >40% of left ventricle is involved in acute infection.
- Elevated cardiac chamber filling procedure is hallmark of cardiogenic shock.

Clinical Features of Cardiogenic Shock

- The primary problem is decrease in contractility of heart, due to decrease contractility, there is decrease in stroke volume.
- Patient present with tachycardia, low blood pressure and decrease urinary output.
- Jugular venous pressure may be raised.
- Peripheries are cold and patient may be confuse or *moribund.

Treatment

- Proper oxygenation with intubation, ventilator support, cardiac version, pacing, antiarrhythmic drugs, correction of electrolytes, avoiding fluid overload and prevention of pulmonary edema as immediate measures.
- Dobutamine is used to raise cardiac output provided there is adequate preload and intravascular volume. Dopamine is preferred in patients with hypotension. But it may increase peripheral resistance and heart rate worsening cardiac ischemia. Often both dopamine and dobutamine combination may be required.
- Careful judicial use of epinephrine, norepinephrine, phosphodiesterase inhibitors (amrinone, milrinone) are often needed. Anticoagulants and aspirin are given. Thrombolytics can be used β blockers, nitrates (nitroglycerine causes coronary arterial dilatation). ACE inhibitors are also used.
- *Intra-aortic balloon pump:* May need to be introduce; transfemorally as a mechanical circulatory support to raise cardiac output and coronary blood flow.
- Relief of pain, preserving of remaining myocardium and its function, maintaining adequate preload, oxygenation, minimizing sympathetic stimulation, correction of electrolytes should be the priorities.
- Percutaneous transluminal coronary angioplasty (PTCA) and coronary artery bypass graft (CABG) are the final choices.

Distributive Shock

This occurs when the after load is excessively reduced.
Distributive shock occurs in following situations:
- Septic shock
- Anaphylactic shock
- Neurogenic shock

Septic Shock

- This type of shock is mostly due to release of endotoxins in blood, which causes wide spread vasodilation of blood vessels resulting in fall in the cardiac output. Fall in the cardiac output is not initial feature and vasoconstriction is not observed.
- Bacteria responsible for release of endotoxins are *E. coli, Pseudomonas, Proteus,* etc.

Clinical Features

- Restlessness, anxiety
- Cyanosis
- Cold and clammy skin
- Tachycardia

- Oliguria or anuria
- Acidotic breathing

Management

- Sedation with diazepam
- IV fluids
- Blood culture and sensitivity
- *Antimicrobial agents:* Combination of penicillin or cephalosporins and aminoglycosides and metronidazole.
- Injection hydrocortisone

Anaphylactic Shock

Anaphylactic shock can occur when a previously sensitized individual is exposed to a specific antigen, IV drug, especially penicillin, cephalosporins and iodinated contrast media are common offenders.

Clinical Features

- Due to reduced cerebral perfusion, there is change in mental status.
- Due to reduced preload and cardiac contractility, there is hypotension.
- Due to release of histamine and other chemical mediators there is urticaria.
- Due to hypoxia the cyanosis is caused.
- Due to anaerobic metabolism and hepatic dysfunction the lactic acidosis is caused.
- Due to coronary ischemia other dysrhythmias are caused.

Treatment

- Summon ambulance
- Always check whether respiratory distress is due to other causes.
- Assess the degree of cardiovascular collapse by checking pulse and blood pressure.
- Assess the degree of airway obstruction
- Stop administration of drug
- Patient should be kept supine
- Assess breathing difficulty by checking for stridor, wheeze
- Administer oxygen to patient by face mask
- Give antihistamine chlorpheniramine maleate 10 mg
- Administer hydrocortisone 20 mg
- Monitor consciousness, airway, breathing, circulation, pulse, blood pressure
- Raise legs if blood pressure is low
- Adrenaline 1:1,000, 0.5 mL IM is given immediately.
- Repeat IM adrenaline every 5 minutes while waiting for ambulance
- Administer 100% oxygen
- CPR if cardiac arrest occurs
- If BP fall is rapid, 1:10,000 adrenalin may be infused IV slowly.

Neurogenic Shock

- It occurs due to spinal cord injury which leads to dilatation of splanchnic vessels
- There will be bradycardia, hypotension, arrhythmias and decreased cardiac output.

Clinical Features

- History of emotional stress or pain of a sudden nature.
- Bradycardia or pallor
- Tachypnea
- Fainting
- Reflexes are usually intact

Treatment

- Blood pressure should be controlled by giving vasoconstrictors.
- Oxygen is administered
- Hemodynamics should be maintained.
- Airways are cleared.
- Fluid therapy should be given
- Intravenous methylprednisolone therapy is done.
- Dopamine and phenylephrine can be used.

Obstructive Shock

- The obstructive shock is due to cardiac tamponade, due to tension pneumothorax and pulmonary embolus.
- In cardiac tamponade, there is compression of all chambers of heart with reduce cardiac output. The filling pressure of left- and right-sided chambers equalizes. The central venous pressure is high and the BP is low.

Treatment

- To maintain preload with fluid or blood.
- Relief of obstructions, drain pericardial cavity as early as possible.

For management of hemorrhagic shock refer to Ans. 19 of same chapter.

Q.17. Define shock. Name types of shock which can be met within your practice. How will you manage them?

(Jan 2017, 20 Marks)

Ans. Shock is defined as an acute clinical syndrome characterized by a significant, systemic reduction in tissue perfusion, resulting in decreased tissue oxygen delivery and insufficient removal of cellular metabolic products, resulting in tissue injury and severe dysfunction of vital organs.

Types of shock which can be met in my dental practice and management of the same

Following are the shocks which can be in my dental practice:

- *Anaphylactic shock:* It occurs due to the allergy caused by local anesthetic agent. *For details refer to Ans. 11 of same chapter*
- *Hypovolemic shock:* It occur during and following any major dental surgery. *For details refer to Ans. 16 of same chapter.*

Q.18. Hazards of blood transfusion. *(Jan 2017, 10 Marks)*

Or

Blood transfusion hazards. *(Sep 2018, 5 Marks)*

Ans. Following are the hazards of blood transfusion:

Transfusion Reactions—Incompatibility

Causes

- *Mistake in crossmatching:* This is a technical error, if the serum is old or labeling is wrong.

♦ Due to transfusion of blood which is already hemolyzed by warming, over freezing or shaking.

♦ Due to transfusion of blood after expiry date.

Clinical Features of Mismatched Blood Transfusion

♦ Presence of rigors and fever. Patient may complain of nausea, vomiting, headache, pain in the loins, tingling sensation in the extremities.

♦ There can be chest pain and dyspnea.

♦ If the patient is already in shock, it may become more pronounced instead of curing it. Gradually, he will lose consciousness.

♦ Urine output decreases and hemoglobinuria may occur within 2–3 hours.

♦ Jaundice may appear within 24–36 hours, this is the confirmatory evidence of mismatching.

♦ Ultimately renal failure sets in due to the blockage of renal tubules by hematin pigment.

Treatment

♦ Transfusion should be stopped immediately.

♦ Fresh blood specimen of venous blood and urine from the patient should be sent to laboratory for rechecking along with the rejected blood pack.

♦ IV fluids should be started instead of blood.

♦ Alkalization of blood to be done by isotonic solution of sodium lactate and 10 mL of sodium bicarbonate to facilitate precipitation of hematin pigments.

♦ Frusemide 80–120 mg IV should be given for forced diuresis. This may be repeated, if urine output is increased to 30 mL/h.

♦ Antihistamine and hydrocortisones should be given.

♦ In very severe cases, hemodialysis should be undertaken.

Pyrexial Reactions

It is common to see simple reactions, such as pyrexia, chills, rigors, restlessness, headache, tachycardia, nausea and vomiting.

Causes

♦ Improperly sterilized drip sets.

♦ Presence of pyrogens in the donor set.

♦ Transfusion of infected blood.

♦ Very rapid transfusion

Prevention

These reactions can be prevented by using sterilized plastic disposable sets.

Treatment

Transfusion should be stopped immediately though temporarily. Antihistaminics and antipyretics should be given. After his condition returns to normal, blood transfusion can be restarted.

Allergic Reactions

Usually, within few hours of transfusion, patients may get mild urticaria, tachycardia, fever and dyspnea. He may even go into severe anaphylactic shock.

Treatment

Transfusion should be stopped. Antihistamines and cortisones should be given. Shock should be treated.

Transmission of Diseases

♦ *Serum hepatitis:* Hepatitis B is a common disease which can be transmitted during blood transfusion. The symptoms usually appear within 3 months.

♦ *AIDS:* HIV can be transmitted from the donor's blood to the recipient.

♦ *Bacterial infection:* This occurs due to faulty storage technique. This should be treated with higher antibiotics otherwise patient may go into septicemia.

Reaction due to Massive Blood Transfusion

"Massive blood transfusion implies single transfusion of 8–10 units of blood in 24 hours."

♦ Acid–base imbalance results in significant metabolic alkalosis.

♦ Hyperkalemia

♦ *Citrate toxicity:* After massive blood transfusion, increased citrate level consumes ionized calcium from patient's body. The body compensates it by rapidly mobilizing calcium from the bones. Rarely when hypocalcemia is recognized calcium can be infused.

♦ *Hypothermia:* During massive blood transfusion, cold blood is rapidly infused from the refrigerator to the patient. His temperature may drop by 3–4°C.

♦ *Failure of coagulation:* After massive blood transfusion, the natural process of coagulation may fail due to dilution of platelets and various clotting factors. .

♦ *Disseminated intravascular coagulation (DIC):* This may occur after a massive blood transfusion. Actually, it occurs after mismatched blood transfusion.

Complications of Over Transfusion

These complications may be seen in patients with chronic anemia, in children and elderly patients. They should receive packed cells rather whole blood. Transfusions should be given slowly for 4–6 hours and after some intervals. Elderly patients should be given packed cells with diuretics.

Complications of Intravenous Transfusions

Thrombophlebitis and air embolism.

Pulmonary Complications

Syndrome of transfusion—related acute lung injury is defined as noncardiogenic pulmonary edema related to transfusion.

Q.19. Write short note on indications of blood transfusion.

(Apr 2017, 4 Marks)

Ans. Following are the indications of blood transfusion:

♦ Acute blood loss following trauma ≥15% of total body volume in otherwise healthy individuals (liver, spleen, kidney, GIT injuries, fractures, hemothorax, perineal injuries).

- During major surgeries—abdominoperineal surgery, thoracic surgery, hepatobiliary surgery.
- Following burns.
- In septicemia.
- As a prophylactic measure prior to surgery.
- Whole blood is given in acute blood loss.
- Packed cells are given in chronic anemia.
- Blood fractions are given in idiopathic thrombocytopenic purpura, hemophilias.

Q.20. Enumerate the gram-negative and gram-positive bacteria. *(Aug 2018, 10 Marks)*

Ans.

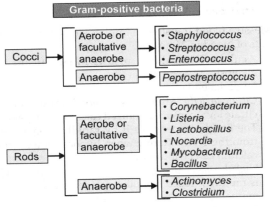

Flowchart 10: Gram-positive bacteria.

Flowchart 11: Gram-negative bacteria.

9. BURN

Q.1. What is Wallace's rule of nine? Calculate the amount of fluid that should be ideally transfused to an adult weighing 60 kg and having 50% deep burns in the first 24 hours. *(Sep 2004, 15 Marks)*

Ans. Wallace's rule of nine is given by Wallace for early assessment of extent of burn in terms of body surface area.

Burn: A burn is a wound in which there is coagulative necrosis of tissue.

Rule of Nine (Wallace's Rule of "9")			
	Adults	**Children**	**Infants**
Head and neck	9%	18%	20%
Front of chest and abdominal wall	9 × 2 = 18%	18%	10 × 2 = 20%
Back of chest and abdominal wall	9 × 2 = 18%	18%	10 × 2 = 20%
Lower limb	18 × 2 = 36%	13.5 × = 27%	10 × 2 = 20%
Upper limb	9 × 2 = 18%	18%	10 × 2 = 20%
Perineum	01%	01%	
Total	100%	100%	100%

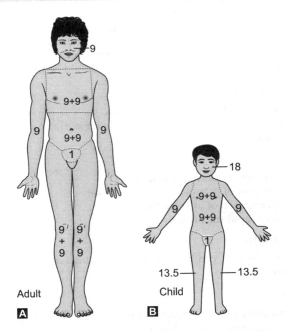

Percentage of burns in (A) Adults; (B) Children

Figs. 11A and B: Extent of burn.

The amount of fluid that should be ideally transfused in case of burn is calculated by:

Muir and Barclay Formula

$$1 \text{ ration} = \frac{\% \text{ of burn} \times \text{Body weight (kg)}}{2}$$

3 ration in 12 hours, 2 ration in next 12 hours and 1 ration in next 12 hours.

50% burns patient weighting 60 kg

$$1 \text{ ration} = \frac{50 \times 60}{2} = 1,500 \text{ mL}$$

1st 12 hours: 1,500 × 3 = 4,500 mL
2nd 12 hours: 1,500 × 2 = 3,000 mL
Total 7,500 mL fluid in 24 hours.

Q.2. Describe the causes of burn and management of face and neck burn. *(Mar 2007, 10 Marks)*
Ans.

Burn

A burn is a wound in which there is coagulative necrosis of tissue.

Causes of Burn

- *Ordinary causes:* Dry heat, fire, hot metal, aeroplane crash.
- Due to moist heat, e.g., boiling liquid or lipids, it is called as scald.
- *Electric burn:* Due to high voltage current.
- *Chemical burns:* Due to strong acid and alkali
- *Radiation burn:* Due to X-ray and radiation
- *Cold burn:* It is caused by prolonged exposure to cold.

Management of Face and Neck Burn
First Aid

- Stop the burning process and keep patient away from burning area.
- Cool the area with tap water by continuous irrigation for 20 minutes.

Definitive Treatment

- Patient should be admitted.
- Airway, breathing and circulation is maintained.
- Percentage, degree and type of burn is assessed.
- Patient should be kept in clean environment.
- Patient is sedated and proper analgesia is given.

Fluid Resuscitation

- Fluid replacement is done by calculating with various formulas, such as Parkland regime, Muir and Buckley regime, etc.
- Fluids used are normal saline, Ringer lactate, Hartmanns fluid. Ringer lactate is the choice of fluid.
- Blood is transfused in later period after 48 hours.

General Treatment

- For first 24 hours only crystalloids should be given.
- After 24 hours up to 30–48 hours, colloids should be given to compensate plasma loss. Plasma, haemaccel (gelatin), dextrans, hetastarch are used. Usually at a rate of 0.35–0.5 mL/kg% burns is used in 24 hours.
- Urinary catheterization to monitor output; 30–50 mL/hour should be the urine output.

- Tetanus toxoid.
- *Monitoring the patient:* Hourly pulse, BP, PO_2, PCO_2 electrolyte analysis, blood urea, nasal oxygen, often intubation is required. Endotracheal intubation is secured in such a way to minimize pressure necrosis of lip.
- IV ranitidine 50 mg 8th hourly is given.
- Ryle's tube insertion initially for aspiration purpose later for feeding.
- *Antibiotics:* Penicillins, aminoglycosides, cephalosporins, metronidazole should be given.
- Culture of the discharge; total white cell count and platelet count at regular intervals are essential to identify the sepsis along with fever, tachycardia and tachypnea.
- In burns of oral cavity tracheostomy may be required to maintain the airway.
- Total parenteral nutrition (TPN) is required for faster recovery, using carbohydrates, lipids, vitamins.
- Tracheostomy/intubation tube may be required in impending respiratory failure or upper airway block.
- Intensive nursing care.

Local Management

- Dressing at regular intervals under general anesthesia using paraffin gauze, hydrocolloids, plastic films, vaseline impregnated gauze or fenestrated silicone sheet or biological dressings, such as amniotic membrane or synthetic Biobrane.
- Open method with application of silver sulfadiazine without any dressings, used commonly in burns of face and neck.
- Closed method is with dressings done to soothen and to protect the wound, to reduce the pain, as an absorbent.
- Tangential excision of burn wound with skin grafting can be done within 48 hours in patients with <25% burns. It is usually done in deep dermal burn wherein dead dermis is removed layer by layer until fresh bleeding occurs. Later skin grafting is done.
- In burns of head and neck region, exposure treatment is advised.
- Slough excision is done regularly.
- After cleaning with povidone iodine solution silver sulfadiazine ointment is used. It is an antiseptic and soothening agent.

Wound Coverage

- Better outcomes can be achieved if the nonhealing areas are excised (likely to take 3 weeks or more) and then skin grafted.
- The donor skin needs to be taken from area above the nipple for the best color match. Many surgeons favor the scalp skin but, alopecia and hair growth from transplanted skin is of concern whereas the upper part of back has thick skin.
- Facial excision is carried out using Goulian knives or Versajet water dissector. Exposed cartilage needs excision with closure of skin.
- Sheet of autografts are used as the meshed grafts are cosmetically unacceptable.
- Epinephrine lysis is essential to limit hemorrhage.
- A face mask should be placed to help immobilization of skin graft.
- Graft should be placed in such a fashion as to mimic the esthetic units. Fibrin glue can be used to enhance the graft adherence.

♦ Postoperative facial elastic mask compression helps in avoiding hypertrophic scar.

Q.3. Describe briefly "rule of nine" and management of burn patient. *(Jun 2010, 5 Marks)*

Or

Describe briefly Wallace's "rule of nine" *(Apr 2017, 5 Marks)*

Ans. *For rule of nine, refer to Ans. 1 and for management of burn patient refer to Ans. 2 of same chapter.*

Q.4. Classify the types of burns and describe the management of a case of 30% burns. *(Mar 2006, 15 Marks)*

Ans.

Classification of Types of Burns

Depending on Percentage of Burns

♦ *Mild:*
- Partial thickness burns <15% in adult or <10% in children
- Full thickness burns <2%
- Can be treated on outpatient basis.

♦ *Moderate:*
- Second degree of 15–25% burns
- Third degree between 2–10% burns
- Burns which do not involve eyes, ears, face, hand, feet.

♦ *Major:*
- Second degree burns >25% in adults and >20% in children.
- All third degree burns of 10% or more
- Burns involving eyes, ears, feet, hands, perineum
- All inhalation and electric burns
- Burns with fractures or major mechanical trauma.

Depending on Thickness of Skin Involved

♦ *First degree:* Epidermis look red and painful, no blisters, heal rapidly in 5–7 days by epithelialization without scaring.
♦ *Second degree:* Affected area is mottled, red, painful with blisters, heals by epithelialization in 14–21 days.
- Superficial second degree burn heals causing pigmentation
- Deep second degree burn heals causing scarring and pigmentation.
♦ *Third degree:* Affected area is charred, parchment, such as painless and insensitive with thrombosis of superficial vessels. It needs grafting. Charred, denatured, insensitive, contracted full thickness burn is known as eschar.
♦ *Fourth degree:* It involve deeper structures, i.e., muscles and bones.

Depending on Thickness of Skin Involved

♦ *Partial thickness burns:* It is a first or second degree burn which is red and painful often with blisters.
♦ *Full thickness burns:* It is a third degree burn which is charred, insensitive, deep involving all layers of skin.

Management of Case of 30% Burn

Case of 30% burn comes under the major burn.
For management in detail refer to Ans. 2 of same chapter.

Q.5. Describe the rule of nine and management of first degree burn. *(Apr 2019, 5 Marks)*

Ans. *For rule of nine refer to Ans. 1 of same chapter.*

Management of First Degree Burn

In first degree burn the epidermis looks red and painful, no blisters, heals rapidly in 5–7 days by epithelialization without scarring. It shows capillary filling.

10. ARTERIAL DISEASES

Q.1. Write in short on Burger's disease. *(Oct 2007, 10 Marks)*

Ans. It is also known as thromboangiitis obliterans or smoker' disease.

A chronic recurring, inflammatory, vascular occlusive disease, chiefly of the peripheral arteries and veins of the extremities.

Classification

♦ Type I: Upper limb thromboangiitis obliterans.
♦ Type II: Involving leg and feet—crural/infrapopliteal
♦ Type III: Femoropopliteal
♦ Type IV: Aortoiliofemoral
♦ Type V: Generalized

Pathogenesis

Flowchart 12: Pathogenesis of Burger's diseases.

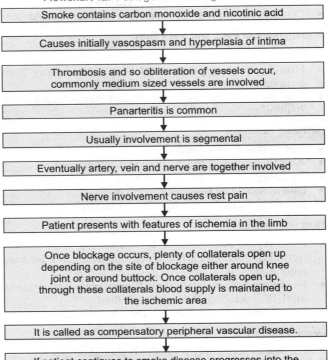

Smoke contains carbon monoxide and nicotinic acid
↓
Causes initially vasospasm and hyperplasia of intima
↓
Thrombosis and so obliteration of vessels occur, commonly medium sized vessels are involved
↓
Panarteritis is common
↓
Usually involvement is segmental
↓
Eventually artery, vein and nerve are together involved
↓
Nerve involvement causes rest pain
↓
Patient presents with features of ischemia in the limb
↓
Once blockage occurs, plenty of collaterals open up depending on the site of blockage either around knee joint or around buttock. Once collaterals open up, through these collaterals blood supply is maintained to the ischemic area
↓
It is called as compensatory peripheral vascular disease.
↓
If patient continues to smoke disease progresses into the collaterals blocking them eventually, leading to severe ischemia and is called as decompensatory peripheral vascular disease. It is presently called as critical limb ischemia. It causes rest pain, ulceration and gangrene

Clinical Features

♦ It is common in male smokers between 20–40 years of age.
♦ Intermittent claudication in foot and calf progressing to rest pain, ulceration and gangrene.
♦ It includes paresthesia of the foot or pain confined to one toe.
♦ Easy fatiguability and leg cramps. The leg fatigue quickly especially during walking.
♦ Ulceration or moist gangrene of hands and feet; amputation may be necessary.
♦ Recurrent migratory superficial thrombophlebitis
♦ Absence/feeble pulses distal to proximal; dorsalis pedis, popliteal and femoral arteries.

Diagnosis

Criteria of Olin (2000)

♦ It occurs typically between 20 and 40 years of age in male, although females are also diagnosed.
♦ History of tobacco use.
♦ Presence of distal extremity ischemia indicated by claudication, pain at rest, ischemic ulcers or gangrene. This is documented by noninvasive vascular testing, i.e., ultrasound.
♦ Exclusion of other autoimmune diseases, such as hypercoagulable states and diabetes mellitus by laboratory tests.
♦ Exclusion of proximal source of emboli by echocardiography and arteriography.
♦ Consistent arteriographic findings in clinically involved and non-involved limbs.

No laboratory test should confirm the diagnosis of Burger's disease. Main goal of various investigations is to exclude other diseases in differential diagnosis.

Treatment

Smoking is strictly stopped.

Drugs

♦ Vasodilators, i.e., nifedipine should be given.
♦ Pentoxifylline should be given since it increases flexibility of RBCs so they reach easily in microcirculation.
♦ Aspirin 75 mg OD is given.
♦ Analgesics, often sedatives, antilipid drugs like atorvastatin may be needed.

Care of the Limbs

Buerger's position and exercise: Regular graded exercises up to the point of claudication improves the collateral circulation. In Buerger's position, head end of bed is raised; foot end of bed is lowered to improve circulation. In Buerger's exercise leg is elevated and lowered alternatively, each for 2 minutes for several times at time.

Care of feet: It is better to wear socks with footwear. Heel raise by raising the heels of shoes by 2 cm decreases the calf muscle work to improve claudication.

Chemical Sympathectomy

Sympathetic chain is blocked to achieve vasodilatation by injecting local anesthetic agent (xylocaine 1%) paravertebrally beside bodies of L 2, 3 and 4 vertebrae in front of lumbar fascia, to achieve temporary benefit. Long time efficacy can be achieved by using 5 mL phenol in water. It is done under C-Arm guidance. Feet will become warm immediately after injection.

Surgery

♦ Omentoplasty to revascularize the affected limb.
♦ Profundaplasty is done for blockage in profunda femoris artery so as to open more collaterals across the knee joint.
♦ Lumbar sympathectomy to increase the cutaneous perfusion so as to promote ulcer healing. But it may divert blood from muscles towards skin causing muscle more ischemic.
♦ Amputations are done at different levels depending on site, severity and extent of vessel occlusion. Usually either below-knee or above-knee amputations are done.
♦ Ilzarov method of bone lengthening helps in improving the rest pain and claudication by creating neo-osteogenesis and improving the overall blood supply to the limb.

Q.2. Discuss briefly pressure sores.

(May/Jun 2009, 5 Marks)

Or

Discuss briefly bed (pressure) sores.

(Aug 2012, 5 Marks)

Ans. It is also known as decubitus ulcer or pressure sores or bedsores.

Pathophysiology

Pressure sore occurs due to compression of tissues by an external force. Blood flow to skin stops as external pressure becomes more than 30 mm of Hg which causes ischemia. Ischemia causes inflammation and tissue anoxia. Tissue anoxia leads to cell death, necrosis and ulceration.

Clinical Features

♦ It is a trophic ulcer with bone as a base.
♦ It is nonmobile, deep, punched out ulcer.
♦ It is commonly seen in old age bed ridden patients, tetanus, orthopedic patients, In diabetics and patients with head injuries.

Sites Affected

♦ Over the ischial tuberosity
♦ Sacrum
♦ In the heel
♦ In relation to head of metatarsal
♦ Buttocks
♦ Over the shoulder
♦ Occiput

Factors Causing Pressure Sore

♦ Normal stimulus to relieve pressure is absent in anesthetized patient.
♦ Nutritional deficiencies worsen the necrosis
♦ Inadequate padding over bony prominences in malnourished patients
♦ Urinary incontinence in paraplegia patient causes skin soiling—maceration—infection—necrosis.

Staging of Pressure Sore

♦ Non-blanching erythema—early superficial ulcer
♦ Partial thickness skin loss—late superficial ulcer

♦ Full thickness skin loss extending into subcutaneous tissue but not through fascia—early deep ulcer
♦ Full thickness skin loss with fascia and underlying structures, such as muscle, tendon, bone, etc.—late deep ulcer

Treatment

♦ Cause for pressure sore should be treated.
♦ Adequate nutritional supplementation should be done.
♦ Proper rest, antibiotics, slough excision, regular dressings should be given.
♦ *Vacuum-assisted closure:* It is the creation of intermittent negative pressure of minus 125 mm Hg to promote formation of healthy granulation tissue. Negative pressure reduces tissue edema, clears the interstitial fluid and improves the perfusion, increases the cell proliferation and so promotes the healing. A perforated drain is kept over the foam dressing covered over the pressure sore. It is sealed with a transparent adhesive sheet. Drain is connected to required vacuum apparatus.
♦ Once ulcer granulates well, flap cover or skin grafting is done.
♦ Excision of the ulcer and skin grafting can also be done.
♦ Flaps—local rotation or other flaps (transposition flaps).
♦ Cultured muscle interposition should be done.
♦ Proper care should be given to the patient, i.e.
   • Change in position once in 2 hours; lifting the limb upwards for 10 seconds once in 10 minutes
   • Use of water bed/air bed/air-fluid floatation bed and pressure dispersion cushions to the affected area.
   • Urinary and fecal care
   • Hygiene should be maintained
   • Psychological counseling should be done.
   • Regular skin observation; keeping skin clean and dry (using regular use of talcum powder); oil massaging of the skin and soft tissues using clean, absorbent porous clothing; control and prevention of sepsis helps in the management.

Q.3. Write short note on gangrene.
(Dec 2007, 3 Marks) (Apr 2007, 10 Marks)
Or
Write short answer on gangrene. *(Sep 2018, 3 Marks)*

Ans. Gangrene is a form of necrosis of tissue with superadded putrefaction.

Etiology

♦ *Trauma:* Direct or indirect
♦ *Infection:* Boil, carbuncle, gas gangrene, Fournier's gangrene, cancrum oris
♦ *Physical:* Burns, scald, frostbite, chemicals, irradiation and electrical
♦ Venous gangrene
♦ Secondary to arterial occlusion, such as atherosclerosis, emboli, diabetes, Raynaud's disease, ergot.

Clinical Features

♦ In gangrene, the organ involved is pale, gray, purple, brownish black. This is due to disintegration of hemoglobin to sulfide
♦ Pulse is absent.

♦ There is loss of sensation and function
♦ There is presence of line of demarcation between vital and dead tissue. A band of hyperemia and hyperesthesia is present along with developmental layer of granulation tissue.

Types of Gangrene

Gangrene is of three types, i.e., dry, wet and gas gangrene.
♦ **Dry gangrene:** It is a condition which results when one or more arteries become obstructed. In this type of gangrene, the tissue slowly dies because of inadequate or no blood supply. It happens mostly in the extremities and it develops in people with diabetes or arteriosclerosis.
♦ **Wet gangrene:** It is a gangrene which develops as a complication of an untreated infected wound, caused by various bacterial infection. The tissue is infected by saprogenic microorganisms, i.e., (*C. perfringens*, fusiformis, etc.) which cause tissue to swell and emit a fetid smell.
♦ **Gas gangrene:** It is is a bacterial infection that produces gas within tissues. It is caused by bacterial exotoxins produced by *Clostridium perfringens* which are mostly found in soil and other anaerobes. Infection spreads rapidly as the gases produced by bacteria expand and infiltrate healthy tissue in the vicinity.
♦ **Other gangrenes:**
   • Noma or cancrum oris is a gangrene of the face.
   • Necrotizing fasciitis affects the deeper layers of the skin.
   • Fournier gangrene usually affects the male genitals and groin.

Investigations

♦ CBC, hemoglobin and blood sugar
♦ Arterial Doppler, angiogram
♦ Ultrasonography of abdomen to find out status of aorta

Treatment of Gangrene

Limb-saving Method
♦ Drugs, such as antibiotics, vasodilators, small dose of as pirin, praxilene are started.
♦ *Care of feet and toes:* Part of the feet or toe should be kept dry.
   • Any injury has to be avoided
   • Proper footwear is advised to patient
   • Pressure areas should be protected.
   • If pus is present, it has to be drained.
   • Limb should not be warmed.
   • Diabetes should be controlled.
   • Surgeries, such as omentoplasty, profundaplasty, arterial bypass graft are done to improve limb perfusion.

Lifesaving Procedures

Amputations can be done as lifesaving procedure.
♦ Below knee amputation is better option as fit of prosthesis is better and movements of knee joint are retained.
♦ In above knee amputation range of movement is less and third support is required to walk.

Q.4. Write short note on dry and wet gangrene.
(Jan 2012, 5 Marks)
Or
Write briefly on wet gangrene. *(Jan 2016, 2 Marks)*
Or

Write short note on dry wet and gas gangrene.
(June 2010, 5 Marks)

Or

Write short answer on dry, wet and gas gangrene.
(June 2018, 3 Marks)

Ans.

Dry Gangrene

♦ It is a condition which results when one or more arteries become obstructed.

♦ In this gangrene, the tissue slowly dies because of inadequate or no blood supply.

♦ It happens mostly in the extremities and it occurs in people with diabetes or arteriosclerosis. It can also develop after prolonged exposure to freezing temperatures.

♦ In dry gangrene tissue first becomes bluish and patient feel cold to the touch, As time progresses, a line of demarcation appears between the healthy and devitalized tissue, which becomes dry and dark black.

♦ Eventually, there may be a separation of the dead tissue from the living tissue; with spontaneous amputation (autoamputation) of the involved extremity.

♦ Treatment of this type of gangrene is aimed at improving circulation, revascularization (i.e. restoration of blood to flow) to the affected area. This may be accomplished with drugs or through the surgical removal of the obstruction.

Wet Gangrene

♦ Wet gangrene is gangrene which develops as a complication of an untreated infected wound, caused by certain bacterial infection.

♦ The tissue is infected by saprogenic microorganisms (*C. perfringens*, fusiformis, etc.) which cause tissue to swell and produces a fetid smell.

♦ This gangrene develops rapidly due to blockage of venous and/or arterial blood flow.

♦ In this affected part is saturated with stagnant blood, which promotes the rapid growth of bacteria.

♦ Toxic products formed by bacteria are absorbed causing systemic manifestation of septicemia and finally death.

♦ Wet gangrene occurs in naturally moist tissue and organs, such as the mouth, bowel, lungs, cervix, and vulva.

♦ Bedsores occurring on body parts, such as the sacrum, buttocks, and heels—although not necessarily moist areas —are also categorized as wet gangrene infections.

♦ The affected part is edematous, soft, putrid, rotten and dark. The darkness in wet gangrene occurs due to the same mechanism as in dry gangrene.

♦ Administration of antibiotics and sometimes the surgical removal of the dead tissue to keep the infection from spreading is the treatment.

Gas Gangrene

♦ Gas gangrene is a bacterial infection that produces gas within tissues. It is caused by bacterial exotoxins produced by *Clostridium perfringens* which are mostly found in soil and other anaerobes (e.g., *Bacteroides* and anaerobic streptococci).

♦ Infection spreads rapidly as the gases produced by bacteria expand and infiltrate healthy tissue in the vicinity.

♦ After an incubation period of one to four or five days, the affected tissue is swollen, painful and cold. A watery, brownish, foul-smelling fluid drains from the wound, and little bubbles of gas develop in the tissues.

♦ Gas gangrene can cause necrosis, gas production, and sepsis. Progression to toxemia and shock is often very rapid.

♦ Gas gangrene is often treated with the antitoxin for Clostridium. In a number of cases. amputation may have to be used to keep the infection under control.

♦ Severe cases have been treated by keeping the patient in an oxygen-rich atmosphere, as in a hyperbaric chamber.

Q.5. Enumerate differences between dry and wet gangrene.
(June 2014, 2 Marks)

Or

Write differences between wet and dry gangrene.
(Sep 2018, 5 Marks)

Ans.

Features	Dry gangrene	Wet gangrene
Cause	Slow occlusion of arteries	Sudden occlusion of arteries
Involvement of part	Small area is gangrenous due to presence of collaterals	Large area is affected due to absence of collaterals
Local findings	Dry, shrivelled and mummified	Wet, turgid, swollen, edematous
Line of demarcation	Present	Absent
Crepitus	Absent	May be present
Odor	Absent	Foul odor
Infection	Not present	Present
Diseases	TAD: Atherosclerosis	Emboli, crush injuries, etc
Treatment	Conservative amputation	Major amputation is necessary

Q.6. Define gangrene. Describe various causes of gangrene and management of diabetic gangrene foot.
(Nov 2008, 15 Marks)

Ans. Gangrene is the death of body tissue associated with loss of vascular supply and followed by bacterial invasion and putrefaction.

Causes

♦ Secondary to arterial occlusion, such as atherosclerosis, emboli, diabetes, Raynaud's disease.

♦ *Infective:* Boil, carbuncle, gas gangrene, Fournier's gangrene, cancrum oris

♦ *Traumatic:* Either direct trauma or indirect trauma

♦ *Physical:* Burns, scalds, frostbite, chemicals, irradiation, electrical

♦ Venous gangrene.

Management of Diabetic Gangrene Foot

Foot can only be saved if good blood supply is present.

♦ Antibiotics should be started based on culture and sensitivity test.

♦ Regular dressings should be given to patient

♦ Drugs, such as vasodilators, pentoxifylline, dipyridamole and low dose aspirin is given.
♦ Diabetes is controlled by insulin
♦ Diet should be controlled
♦ Surgical debridement of the wound is carried out.

Lifesaving Procedures

Amputations of diabetic foot should be done occasionally.
♦ Level of amputation is decided based on skin changes, temperature, line of demarcation and Doppler study.
♦ Below knee amputation is done, in this BK prosthesis is fitted better and also the movements of knee joint are retained.
♦ In above knee amputation range of movements are less, limb is present and require third support to walk.

Care of Feet and Toes

♦ Part of the foot should be kept dry.
♦ Injury to the foot and toes is avoided
♦ Proper footwear is advised to patient, i.e., microcellular rubber footwear
♦ Measures for pain relief are to be taken
♦ Nutritional supplementation is given
♦ Hyperkeratosis is avoided
♦ Localized pus should be drained
♦ Limb should not be warmed.

Q.7. Write short note on diabetic foot. *(Jan 2018, 5 Marks)*

Ans. Diabetic foot consists of callosities, ulceration, abscess, cellulitis of foot, osteomyelitis of different bones, diabetic gangrene and arthritis of joints.

Meggitt's Classification of Diabetic Foot

♦ Grade 0: Foot symptoms like pain, only
♦ Grade 1: Superficial ulcers
♦ Grade 2: Deep ulcers
♦ Grade 3: Ulcer with bone involvement
♦ Grade 4: Forefoot gangrene
♦ Grade 5: Full foot gangrene.

Pathogenesis of Diabetic Foot

♦ High glucose level in tissues is a good culture media for bacteria. So infection is common.
♦ *Diabetic microangiopathy* causes blockade of microcirculation leading to hypoxia.
♦ *Diabetic neuropathy:* Due to sensory neuropathy, minor injuries are not noticed and so infection occurs. Due to motor neuropathy, dysfunction of muscles, arches of foot and joints occur. And loss of reflexes of foot occurs causing more prone to trauma and abscess. Due to autonomic neuropathy, skin will be dry causing defective skin barrier and so more prone for infection.
♦ *Diabetic atherosclerosis:* It itself reduces the blood supply and causes gangrene. Thrombosis can be precipitated by infection causing infective gangrene. Blockage occurs at plantar, tibial and dorsalis pedis vessels.
♦ Increased glycosylated hemoglobin in blood causes defective oxygen dissociation leading to more hypoxia. At tissue level, there will be increased glycosylated tissue proteins, which prevents proper oxygen utilization and so aggravates hypoxia.

Clinical Features

♦ Pain in the foot
♦ Ulceration
♦ Absence of sensation
♦ Absence of pulsations in the foot (posterior tibia and dorsalis pedis arteries).
♦ Loss of joint movements.
♦ Abscess formation
♦ Changes in temperature and color when gangrene sets in.
♦ Patient may succumb to ketoacidosis, septicemia or myocardial infarction.

Investigations

♦ Blood sugar, urine ketone bodies.
♦ Blood urea and serum creatinine.
♦ X-ray of a part to look for osteomyelitis.
♦ Pus for culture and sensitivity.
♦ Doppler study of lower limb to assess arterial patency.
♦ Angiogram to look for proximal blockage.
♦ Ultrasound of abdomen to see the status of abdominal aorta.
♦ Glycosylated hemoglobin estimation.

Treatment

♦ *Foot can be saved if only there is good blood supply:*
  • Antibiotics—decided by pus culture and sensitivity
  • Regular dressing
  • *Drugs:* Vasodilators, pentoxifylline, dipyridamole, low dose aspirin.
  • Diabetes is controlled by insulin only.
  • Diet control, control of obesity.
  • Surgical debridement of wound.
  • Amputations of the gangrenous area. Level of amputation has to be decided by skin changes and temperature changes or Doppler study.
  • Care of feet in diabetic:
♦ Any injury has to be avoided.
♦ Microcellular rubber (MCR) footwears must be used.
♦ Feet has to be kept clean and dry, especially toes and clefts
♦ Hyperkeratosis should be avoided.

11. VENOUS DISEASES

Q.1. Write short note on complications of varicose veins with reasons. *(Mar 2008, 3 Marks)*

Ans. Varicose veins are dilated and tortuous, superficial veins predominantly in lower limbs. Varicose veins are the price that man has to pay for erect posture.

Complications

♦ **Eczema and dermatitis:** This occurs because of extravasation and break down of RBCs in the lower leg. It leads to itching which precipitates varicose ulcer. This condition is treated by application of zinc oxide cream or silver sulfadiazine cream (stasis dermatitis).
♦ **Lipodermatosclerosis:** It refers to various skin changes in the lower leg associated with varicose veins, such as thickening of subcutaneous tissue, indurated feel like wood,

pigmentation, etc. It occurs because of increased venous pressure resulting in capillary leakage with extravasation of blood and fibrin into surrounding tissues. Blood is broken down and heme is released. This combines with iron giving rise to hemosiderin which is responsible for pigmentation. Classically, this affects gaiter area of leg just above the malleoli.

♦ **Hemorrhage:** It occurs due to trauma or eczema. This is controlled by elevation of the leg and crepe bandage.

♦ **Thrombophlebitis:** It refers to the inflammation of superficial vein. In this vein is tender, hard and cord like. Here skin is inflamed and pyrexia is usually present. It is treated by bed rest, elevation, crepe bandage, antibiotics and anti-inflammatory drugs.

♦ **Venous ulcer:** It is also called gravitational ulcer. Precipitating factors are venous stasis and tissue anoxia. Deep vein thrombosis is also an important cause of venous ulcer where in valves is either destroyed or incompetent due to damage. Sustained venous pressure results in extravasation of cells, activation of capillary endothelium resulting in release of free radicals. These free radicals cause tissue destruction and ulceration.

♦ **Calcification:** This is seen inside the walls of vein.

♦ **Periostitis:** It may occur in tibia because of the ulcer present on the medial surface of leg. Due to involvement of periosteum ulcer leads to severe pain.

♦ **Equinovarus deformity:** It occurs due to improper habit of walking on toes which leads to shortening of tendo Achilles.

♦ **Marjolin's ulcer:** It is the squamous cell carcinoma which arises from healed varicose ulcer with scarring.

Q.2. Write short note on varicose veins of lower leg.

(Sep 2008, 3 Marks)

Ans. Dilated, tortuous and elongated superficial veins of limb are called as varicose veins.

Symptoms

♦ Majority of the patients come, with dilated veins in the leg. They are minimal to start with and at the end of the day they are sufficiently large because of the venous engorgement.

♦ Dragging pain in the leg or dull ache is due to heaviness.

♦ Night cramps occur due to change in the diameter of veins.

♦ Aching pain is relieved at night on taking rest or elevation of limbs.

♦ Sudden pain in the calf region with fever and edema of the ankle region suggests deep vein thrombosis.

♦ Patients can present with ulceration, eczema, dermatitis, bleeding, etc. Symptoms of pruritis/itching and skin thickening are also seen.

Signs

♦ Dilated veins are present in the medial aspect of leg and the knee. Sometimes they are visible in the thigh also.

♦ Single dilated varix at SF junction is called saphena varix. It is due to saccular dilatation of the upper end of long saphenous vein at the saphenous opening.

♦ Veins are tortuous and dilated

♦ Ankle flare is a group of veins nearer the medial malleolus.

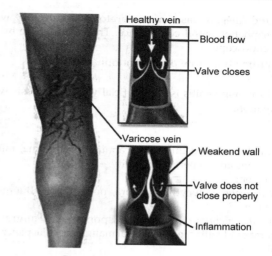

Fig. 12: Varicose vein of lower leg.

Diagnosis

♦ *Venous Doppler:* With the patient standing, Doppler probe is placed at saphenofemoral junction and later wherever required. Basically by hearing the changes in sound, venous flow, venous patency, venous reflux can be well identified.

♦ *Duplex scan:* It is a ultrasonographic Doppler imaging technique which along with direct visualization of veins, gives functional or anatomical information and also the color map.

♦ *Venography:* Before introduction of venous Doppler, venography is the common method of diagnosis.

♦ *Plethysmography:* This is a noninvasive method which measures the volume change in leg.

♦ *Arm foot venous pressure:* Foot pressure is not more than 4 mm Hg above arm pressure.

♦ *Varicography:* In this non-ionic, iso-osmolar, non-thrombogenic contrast is injected directly in variceal vein to get detailed anatomical mapping of varicose veins. This is used in recurrent varicose veins.

Surgical Treatment

♦ *Trendelenburg's operation:*
  • An inguinal incision is made, long saphenous vein identified and the three tributaries are ligated.
  • Long saphenous vein is ligated close to the femoral vein juxta femoral flush ligation.
  • An incision is given in front of the medial malleolus and long saphenous is isolated.
  • The lower end is ligated and the vein incised.
  • A long metallic stripper is introduced within the vein and brought out from the long saphenous vein in the inguinal incision.
  • A metallic head is connected to the stripper and the vein is avulsed.
  • Tight crepe bandage is applied, inguinal incision is sutured and the limb is elevated.

♦ *Subfascial ligation of Cockett and Dodd:*
  • In this operation, perforators are identified deep to deep fascia and they are ligated subfascially. This is

indicated in cases of perforator incompetence with saphenofemoral competence. This is also done by an endoscope.

Q.3. Write short note on thrombophlebitis.
(May/Jun 2009, 5 Marks)

Ans. Thrombophlebitis is a superficial vein thrombosis with inflammation.

Types

- *Acute:* It is caused due to IV cannulation, trauma, minor infections and hypercoagulability.
- Recurrent
- *Spontaneous:* Polycythemia vera, polyarteritis, Buerger's disease
- *Thrombophlebitis migrans:* It is spontaneous migrating thrombophlebitis seen in visceral malignancy like pancreas, stomach.
- Mondor's disease

Clinical Features

- Pain, redness, tenderness, cord like thickening of veins
- Fever is present
- It is seen in upper limb or lower limb.

Investigations

Duplex ultrasound Doppler of both limbs is must.

Complications

- Destruction of venous valves lead to varicose veins
- Embolism, infection.

Treatment

- Elevation of the limb.
- Anti-inflammatory drugs and antibiotics should be given
- Application of crepe bandage—compression therapy
- *Anticoagulation:* Low molecular weight heparin for superficial venous thrombosis >3 cm in length.

12. RECONSTRUCTION

Q.1. Skin grafting, indication and contraindication. Explain partial thickness graft. *(Aug 2018, 10 Marks)*

Ans. Skin grafting is the most common method of achieving the wound cover.

Indications of Skin Grafting

1. **Skin loss:**
   - Post-traumatically: In avulsion and degloving injury.
   - In post-surgical cases: For excision of tumors and excision of burn wounds
   - As a result of pathological process., e.g., venous ulcer and diabetic ulcer.
2. **Mucosa loss:**
   - After the excision of lesion of oral cavity, tongue.
   - For resurfacing reconstructed vagina in vaginal agenesis.

Contraindications of Skin Grafting

- In the infections which are caused by beta hemolytic streptococcus which secretes fibrinolysin and dissolves fibrin.
- Presence of any of the nearby infected wound with copious discharge.
- In avascular wounds with exposed bare bone without periosteum, exposed tendon without paratenon and exposed cartilage without perichondrium.

Partial Thickness Graft

- It is also known as split thickness skin graft or Thiersch graft.
- There is removal of full epidermis along with part of the dermis from the donor area.
- Depending on the amount of thickness of dermis taken, it may be: (1) Thin split thickness skin graft; (2) Intermediate split thickness skin graft; (3) Thick split thickness skin graft.

Indications of Partial Thickness Graft

- In well-granulated ulcer.
- In clean wound or defect which cannot be apposed.
- After surgery to cover and close the defect created.

For example:

- After wide excision in malignancy
- After mastectomy
- After wide excision in squamous cell carcinoma
- Graft can survive over periosteum or paratenon or perichondrium

Contraindications of Partial Thickness Graft

Split thickness skin graft cannot be done over bone, tendon, cartilage, joint.

Technique

- Donor area: Commonly thigh, occasionally arm, leg, forearm; Knife used is Humby's knife; Blade is Eschmann blade, Down's blade; Using Humby's knife graft is taken, punctate bleeding is observed which says that proper graft has been obtained.
- Donor area is dressed and dressing is opened after 10 days, not earlier.
- Recipient area is scraped well and the graft is placed after making window cuts in the graft to prevent the development of seroma. Graft is fixed and tie-overdressing is placed. If graft is placed near the joint, then the part is immobilized to prevent friction which may separate the graft. On 5th day, dressing is opened and observed for graft take up. Mercurochrome is applied over the recipient margin to promote epithelialization.

Stages of Graft Intake

1. **Stage of plasmatic inhibition:** Thin, uniform, layer of plasma forms between recipient bed and graft.
2. **Stage of inoculation:** Linking of host and graft which is temporary.
3. **Stage of neovascularization:** New capillaries proliferate into graft from the recipient bed which attains circulation later.

Note: Graft is stored at low temperature of 4°C for not more than 21 days.

Disadvantages of Partial Thickness Graft

- Contracture of graft: It is of two types:
  1. Primary contracture means spilt thickness skin graft contracts significantly once graft is taken from donor area (20–30%). Thicker the graft more the primary contracture.
  2. Secondary contracture occurs after graft has taken up to recipient bed during healing period, due to fibrosis. Thinner the graft more the secondary contracture.
- Seroma and hematoma formation will prevent graft take up.
- Infection leads to graft failure.
- It causes loss of hair growth and blunting of sensation.
- It produces dry, scaling or skin due to nonfunctioning of sebaceous glands. So after healing, oil (coconut oil) should be applied over the area.

Advantages of Split Thickness Skin Graft

- It is technically easier.
- Wide area of recipient can be covered. To cover large area like burn wound, graft size is increased by passing the graft through a mesher which gives multiple openings to the graft, which can be stretched on the wider area like a net. It can cause expansion up to 6 times.
- Graft take up is better and donor area heals on its own.

Q.2. Write short answer on skin graft. *(Apr 2019, 3 Marks)*

Ans. Skin grafting is the transfer of skin from donor area to the required defective area (recipient area).

Type of Skin grafts

1. Partial thickness graft
2. Full thickness graft

Partial Thickness Graft

For details refer to Ans. 1 of same chapter.

Full Thickness Graft

It is also known as Wolfe graft.

It is used over the face, eyelid, hands, fingers and over the joints. It is removed using scalpel blade. Underlying fat should be cleared off properly. Deeper raw donor area is closed by primary suturing. If large area of graft is taken, then that donor area has to be covered with split skin graft which is a disadvantage in full thickness graft.

Common sites for donor area are post-auricular, supraclavicular and groin crease.

Advantages

- Color match is good. Especially for face. No contracture.
- Sensation, functions of sebaceous glands, hair follicles are retained better compared to split skin graft.
- Functional and cosmetic results are better.

Disadvantages

- It can be used only for small areas.
- Wider donor area has to be covered with split skin graft to close the defect.

Some other Grafts

- Composite graft which includes skin + fat + other tissues like cartilage.
- Tendon graft; bone graft; nerve graft; venous graft; corneal graft
- Combined graft (allograft + autograft)
- Reverdin graft (Jacques–Louis Reverdin, Swiss surgeon): It is a pinch graft taken from the skin and seeded into the needed raw area.

Q.3. Write briefly on types of skin grafts.

(Jan 2016, 2 Marks)

Ans. Skin grafts are of two types:
1. Partial thickness graft
2. Full thickness graft.

Partial Thickness Graft

- It is also known as Thiersch graft or split thickness skin graft
- In it, there is removal of full epidermis and part of dermis from donor area.
- It can be thin, intermediate and thick.
- It is indicated in well-granulated ulcer, clean wound or defect which is not apposed and after the surgery to close and cover the created defect.
- It should not be done over bone, tendon, cartilage and joint.

Full Thickness Graft

- It includes both epidermis and full dermis.
- It should be done over face, eyelid, hand, fingers and over the joints.
- It is used only for small areas.
- Its functional and cosmetic results are excellent.

13. TRANSPLANTATION

Q.1. Write short note on organ transplantation.

(Sep 2018, 5 Marks)

Ans.

Principles of Organ Transplantation

Once brain death has been confirmed in cadaver donor, after giving inotropic support drugs (T3 and argipressin) various organs are surgically removed carefully with preservation of their vessels. After removal, organs are flushed with chilled preservative solution and placed in sterile bags containing saline and organ preservative solutions which are then immersed in 0 to 4°C box containing ice. Donor specimens are transported to the site of the recipient center. Wisconsin and Euro–Collins solutions are commonly used.

- Non-heart beating donors (NHBDs): Here organs are procured from individuals who are just dead on arrival to the hospital or who have died in the hospital in spite of resuscitation. Category I: Dead on arrival; Category II: Unsuccessful resuscitation; Category III: 'Awaiting cardiac arrest' after support withdrawal; Category IV: Cardiac arrest with brain death.

- University of Wisconsin solution contains: Potassium lactobionate; sodium phosphate; magnesium sulfate; adenosine; allopurinol; glutathione; raffinose; hydroxyethyl starch; insulin; dexamethasone; potassium; sodium; with 320 mosmol/L osmolality and pH of 7.4.
- Living donor's organs are used commonly in kidney transplantation from genetically related individuals. It can be used from genetically unrelated donors after proper MHC match. Donor nephrectomy is done through loin incision. Laparoscopic donor nephrectomy has become popular and safe.

Technique of Organ Transplantation

- Positioning the donor on the operating table: Supine position, with arms abducted on boards and legs laid flat and uncrossed. The neck is extended by placing a sandbag under the shoulders (as during thyroidectomy).
- Midline sternotomy incision is used extending up to the pubic symphysis with a supraumbilical horizontal part. Abdomen and thorax are exposed properly. Retroperitoneal right-sided mobilization is done. Cannulation of inferior mesenteric vein is done. Aortic cannulation is done. Perfusion of preservative solution is done.
- Sequence of the thoracic organ procurement: First the heart then the lungs separately or together are procured. Cooling of the abdominal organ has to be continued until the last thoracic organ is procured.
- Sequence of abdominal organ procurement: The small bowel is the most sensitive organ for ischemia; therefore, it is retrieved first. The second organ to be procured is the pancreas followed by the liver. Liver and the pancreas could also be retrieved en block and split on the back table. Finally, the kidneys are the last organs to be procured.
- The most popular tool kit comprises the iliac vessels, which consists of common, external and internal artery and the vein.

---

14. CYST

Q.1. Write short note on sebaceous cyst.

(Feb 2013, 5 Marks) (Aug 2012, 5 Marks)
(Sep 2009, 5 Marks) (Nov 2008, 5 Marks)

Or

Write short answer on sebaceous cyst.

(Apr 2018, 5 Marks)

Ans. Sebaceous cyst is also called as epidermoid cyst.

- This occurs due to obstruction of sebaceous ducts, resulting in accumulation of sebaceous material.
- The sebaceous material becomes enlarged due to retention of its sebum. So it is also called retention cyst.
- The cyst is lined by squamous epithelium material with an unpleasant smell.
- In the center of cyst a black spot is found, it is keratin filled punctum.
- Site: Scalp, face, back, scrotum, etc. The sebaceous cyst may occur anywhere in the body where there are sebaceous glands.

Clinical Features

- It is a painless swelling which is smooth, soft, nontender, freely mobile, adherent to skin especially over the summit, fluctuant, non-transilluminating with punctum over the summit.
- Cyst moulds on finger indentation.
- Punctum is present over the summit in 70% of cases because sebaceous duct opens directly in skin which gets blocked. Punctum is the black colored spot over summit of sebaceous cyst.
- Hair loss over the surface is common because of constant pressure over the roots of hair follicle.
- Unpleasant odor of sebum content is typical.

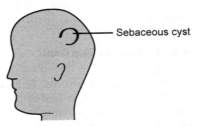

Fig. 13: Sebaceous cyst.

Complication

- Infection and abscess formation
- Surface get ulcerated leading to formation of painful fungating mass with discharge known as Cock's peculiar tumor which resembles epithelioma. Cock's peculiar tumor is not a tumor but a chronic granuloma on ulcerated surface of sebaceous cyst.
- Sebaceous horn results from hardening of slowly discharged sebum through the punctum.

Treatment

- Excision including skin adjacent to punctum using elliptical incision also known as dissection method.
- Incision and avulsion of cystic wall.
- If abscess is formed, then drainage initially and later excision is done.
- If capsule is not removed properly cyst will recur.

Q.2. Describe briefly sublingual dermoid cyst.

(Sep 2008, 3 Marks)

Ans. It is a type of congenital sequestration dermoid cyst.

The cyst is formed by inclusion of the surface ectoderm at the fusion line of two mandibular arches.

Pathology

- The cyst is lined by squamous epithelium.
- The wall of cyst contains hair follicle, sweat and sebaceous glands.
- Cyst contains the cheesy material.
- It never contains hair.

Types

It may be:

- **Median variety:** It is derived from epithelial cell rests at the level of fusion of two mandibular arches. It may be supramylohyoid or inframylohyoid. It is located between two genial muscles, in relation to mylohyoid muscle. It is a midline swelling which is smooth, soft, cystic, nontransilluminant.

♦ **Lateral variety:** It develops in relation to submandibular duct, lingual nerve and stylohyoid ligament. It is derived from first branchial arch. It forms a swelling in the lateral aspect of the floor of mouth.

It also may be:

♦ Supramylohyoid type.
♦ Inframylohyoid type.

Clinical Features

♦ It occurs in young children between the ages of 10–12 years.
♦ Congenital, painless and bidigitally palpable swelling in the floor of mouth.
♦ Swelling is soft and cystic
♦ Fluctuation test is positive.
♦ Transillumination test is negative as it contains thick, cheesy, sebaceous material.
♦ Swelling may often attain large size presenting both sublingually, intraorally and midline submentally on external side.
♦ Occasionally, it can lead to trismus, dysphagia, pain and odynophagia.

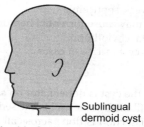

Sublingual dermoid cyst

Fig. 14: Sublingual dermoid cyst.

Differential Diagnosis

♦ *Ranula:* When sublingual dermoid cyst is in midline at floor of the mouth and above mylohyoid muscle ranula is considered as differential diagnosis. Ranula is blue in color and is brilliantly translucent.
♦ *Thyroglossal cyst:* It is to be taken in differential diagnosis when sublingual dermoid cyst is below mylohyoid muscle. Thyroglossal cyst moves up with deglutition whereas sublingual dermoid cyst does not.

Treatment

Excision is done through intraoral approach usually; large cyst extending under geniohyoid muscle may require external approach.

Q.3. Write short note on thyroglossal cyst.
(Feb 2013, 3 Marks) (Jan 2012, 5 Marks)
(Dec 2010, 5 Marks) (June 2010, 5 Marks)

Or

Describe briefly thyroglossal cyst.
(Nov 2008, 5 Marks)

Or

Write brief note on thyroglossal cyst.
(Apr 2017, 2 Marks)

Or

Write in short about thyroglossal cyst.
(Jan 2018, 5 Marks)

Or

Write about thyroglossal cyst.   *(June 2018, 5 Marks)*

Or

Write short answer on thyroglossal cyst and its management.   *(Feb 2019, 3 Marks)*

Ans. It is a congenital tubular dermoid cyst.

♦ It arises from thyroglossal duct, which extends from foramen cecum at the base of tongue to the isthmus of the thyroid gland.
♦ It is lined by pseudostratified, ciliated and columnar or squamous epithelium which produces desquamated epithelial cells or mucus at times.

Sites

♦ Subhyoid is the most common site
♦ At the level of thyroid cartilage
♦ *Suprahyoid:* Double chin appears
♦ At the foramen cecum
♦ At the level of cricoid cartilage
♦ At the floor of the mouth.

Clinical Features

♦ Swelling is present in midline towards the left side.
♦ Moves with deglutition as well as with the protrusion of tongue.
♦ Patient is asked to open the mouth and keep the lower jaw still. Examiner holds the cyst between the thumb and forefinger. When the patient is asked to protrude the tongue, a "tugging sensation" can be felt.
♦ Swelling is smooth, soft, fluctuant (cystic), nontender, mobile, often transilluminant.
♦ Thyroid fossa is empty if there is no thyroid in normal location.
♦ Thyroglossal cyst can get infected and may form an abscess. Cyst wall contains lymphatic tissue and so infection is common.
♦ Malignancy can develop in papillary carcinoma.

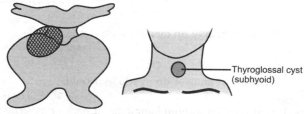

Thyroglossal cyst (subhyoid)

Fig. 15: Thyroglossal cyst.

Differential Diagnosis

♦ Subhyoid bursa
♦ Pretracheal lymph node

- Dermoid cyst
- Solitary nodule of thyroid
- Submental lymph node
- Collar stud abscess

Investigations

- Radioisotope study
- Ultrasound of neck; T3, T4 and TSH estimation
- FNAC from the cyst

Treatment

Sistrunk Operation

Excision of cyst and also full tract up to the foramen cecum is done along with removal of central part of the hyoid bone as the tract passes through it.

Technique

- Thorough transverse neck incision placed over the cyst, skin flap is raised above along with platysma. Care should be taken not to open the cyst.
- Cyst with surrounding tissues is dissected up to the hyoid bone. Sternohyoid and thyrohyoid muscles are divided.
- Central part of the hyoid bone of 1 cm width is resected along with intact tract within it.
- Geniohyoid and mylohyoid muscles are divided off from the hyoid.
- Track with adjacent tissues is dissected above up to the foramen cecum.
- Adjacent tissues also should be removed because of possibility of multiple tracts which otherwise lead to recurrence or fistula formation.
- After this, anesthetist is asked to apply digital pressure over the base of tongue near foramen cecum to facilitate the dissection and to confirm the reach up to the foramen cecum.
- Track is ligated at foramen cecum and removed.
- If there is no normal thyroid gland after the surgery maintenance dose of L-thyroxine 0.1 mg OD is given lifelong.

Complications

- Recurrent thyroglossal fistula formation
- Hemorrhage/hematoma formation
- Infection

Q.4. Write short note on cystic hygroma.

(June 2010, 5 Marks) (Nov 2008, 5 Marks)

Or

Describe briefly on cystic hygroma.

(Apr 2017, 2 Marks)

Or

Write short answer on cystic hygroma.

(June 2018, 3 Marks)

Ans. It is also called as lymphangioma of neck or cavernous lymphangioma or hydrocele of neck.

It is a congenital cystic swelling, which contains multiple lobules of clear lymph.

- It gets filled up with lymph in early week of childhood and present as a large cyst in the lower part of the neck.

- The cyst is not a single cavity but it is a collection of numerous small cysts.
- Their lobules may intercommunicate with one another.
- Each lobule is lined by a single layer of endothelium.
- Cystic hygroma may infiltrate into the muscular plane.

Clinical Features

- Swelling is present at birth in the posterior triangle of neck causing obstructed labor.
- Swelling is smooth, soft, fluctuant (cystic), partially compressible, brilliantly transilluminant. It is not reducible completely.
- During crying swelling often increases in size.
- Disfigurement of face of child which is more worrying factor for the parents.
- Swelling may rapidly increase in size causing respiratory obstruction which is a dangerous sign.
- It may get infected forming an abscess which is a tender, warm, soft swelling. It may cause septicemia which may be life-threatening.
- Rupture with lymph ooze can occur.

Complication

- Too much enlargement of cystic hygroma may cause respiratory distress.
- Infection, abscess, septicemia
- Surgery itself may cause torrential hemorrhage
- Chylous fistula, chylothorax
- Recurrence of cyst in 15% of cases

Treatment

- Aspiration of the cyst is done. Later on sac and capsule is thickened by fibrous tissue and is excised.
- Meticulous dissection is done across all planes including deeper muscular one to clear entire cyst wall. If it is not done properly chances of recurrence are present.
- If respiratory obstruction is present then tracheostomy is done.
- Under antibiotic coverage drainage of abscess is done and later on sac is excised.
- Preoperative injection of sclerosants is given and later on fibrosis develops then excision of entire aggregation of cyst is done. In past days boiling water injection is given at 7 days interval.

Q.5. Write briefly on ranula.

(Jan 2011, 5 Marks) (Dec 2010, 3 Marks)

Or

Write short note on ranula.

(Feb 2013, 5 Marks) (Aug 2012, 5 Marks)
(Dec 2010, 5 Marks) (Dec 2009, 5 Marks)
(Apr 2017, 4 Marks) (Mar 2006, 5 Marks)

Or

Write in short about ranula.

(Jan 2018, 5 Marks)

Or

Write short answer on ranula. *(Apr 2018, 3 Marks)*

Ans. Ranula is a cystic swelling occurs in the floor of the mouth and involves mainly sublingual salivary glands duct.

- It also arises from accessory salivary glands.
- The word ranula is derived from the resemblance of the swellings to the belly of frog.

Etiology

- Ranula occurs due to obstruction to the duct, secreting mucosa.
- Artesia (Obstruction of duct)
- *Stricture of duct due to surgery
- Perforation of duct.

Types

There are two types of ranulas:
1. Oral ranula
2. Plunging ranula or cervical ranula.

Oral ranula occur secondary to mucus extravasation where mucus pool superior to mylohyoid muscle which in plunging ranula mucus extravasation is along the facial planes of neck.

Clinical Features

Oral Ranula

- Seen in young children and adults
- Swelling is typically located in the floor of the mouth to one side of the midline.
- Its surface is smooth with diffuse borders.
- On palpation, it is soft, cystic, nontender and fluctuant swelling which gives brilliant transillumination.
- It is covered by thin mucosa containing clear, serous fluid. Hence, it is bluish in color and resembles like a belly of frog.
- The lesion can cross midline when it is large, this makes offending salivary gland difficult to locate.
- Large oral ranulas displace the tongue and interfere with functions of tongue.
- If the mass is located deep, it looses its bluish translucent color.

Plunging Ranula

- Ranula often extends in submandibular region through deep part of posterior margin of mylohyoid muscle and is known as plunging ranula.
- Plunging ranula is also an intraoral ranula but with cervical extension.
- It remains asymptomatic but enlarges continuously. Overlying skin remains intact.
- The swelling is fluctuant, freely mobile and is nontender.
- It is bidigitally palpable.

Investigations

Ultrasound of neck or MRI neck should be done.

Treatment

Oral Ranula

- Marsupialization can be done initially, in marsupialization major part of the cyst along with mucus membrane of floor

of mouth is excised. Cut edges of cyst wall are sutured to cut mucus membrane and later as the wall of ranula is thickened it should be excised completely.

- If ranula is small, it can be excised without marsupialization.
- Laser ablation and cryosurgery alone or after completion of marsupialization can be done for some patients of oral ranula.

Plunging Ranula

- Plunging ranula often requires approach from neck for complete excision. Excision of submandibular and sublingual salivary gland is often needed in plunging ranula.
- For small plunging ranula excision is done orally along with excision of sublingual salivary gland.

Complications

Rupture for the cyst decreases the size but it can appear at a later date.

When the swelling is big, the tongue is pushed upwards and may cause difficulty in speech and swallowing.

Q.6. Write in brief about dental cyst. *(July 2016, 5 Marks)*

Ans. Dental cyst is also called as radicular cyst or periapical cyst.

It is the most common type of inflammatory cystic lesion, which occurs in relation to the apex of nonvital tooth.

In this case, if the involved tooth is extracted the remaining cystic cavity within the bone is known as residual cyst.

Pathogenesis

The radicular cyst develops due to the proliferation and subsequent cystic degeneration of the "epithelial cell rests of Malassez", in the periapical region of a nonvital tooth.

The process of development of this cyst occurs in various stages:

- Phase of initiation.
- Phase of proliferation.
- Phase of cystification.
- Phase of enlargement.

Phase of initiation: During this phase, the bacterial infection of the dental pulp or direct inflammatory effect of necrotic pulpal tissue, in a nonvital tooth causes stimulation of the "cell rest of Malassez" which are present within the bone near the root apex of teeth.

Phase of proliferation: The stimulation to the cell rests of Malassez leads to excessive proliferation of these cells, which leads to the formation of a large mass or island of immature proliferating epithelial cells at the periapical region of the affected tooth.

Phase of cystification: Once a large bulk of the cell rest of Malassez is produced, its peripheral cells get adequate nutritional supply but its centrally located cells are often deprived of proper nutritional supply. As a result the central group of cells undergo ischemic liquefactive necrosis while the peripheral group of cells survive. This eventually gives rise to the formation of a cavity that contains a hollow space or lumen

---

Q5.   *Stricture = Restriction.

inside the mass of the proliferating cell rest of Malassez and a peripheral lining of epithelial cells around it.

Phase of enlargement: Once a small cyst is formed, it enlarges gradually by the following mechanisms:

♦ Higher osmotic tension of the cystic fluid causes progressive increase in the amount of fluid inside its lumen and this causes increased internal hydrostatic tension within the cyst. The process results in cyst expansion due to resorption of the surrounding bone.

♦ The epithelial cells of the cystic lining release some bone resorbing factors, such as prostaglandins and collagenase, etc., which destroy the bone and facilitate expansion of the cyst.

Clinical Features

♦ It is common in woman around third and fourth decade.
♦ Upper anterior teeth are more affected
♦ The involved tooth shows presence of caries, fracture or discoloration.
♦ Slow enlarging bony hard swelling of jaw with expansion and distortion of cortical plates.
♦ Cyst remain asymptomatic if uninfected
♦ Severe bone destruction by the cystic lesion may produce springiness.
♦ If the cyst is secondary infected, it leads to the formation of abscess then it is called as cyst abscess.

Radiological Features

♦ It appears as a rounded or pear-shaped radiolucency at the apex of nonsensitive tooth or with nonvital tooth.
♦ Radiolucency is more than 1.5 cm in diameter but usually <3 cm in diameter. It has got well-defined outline with thin hyperostotic borders.
♦ *Margins:* In uncomplicated cases margins are smooth, corticated and cortex is usually well-defined, well-etched and continuous, except in some cases, there may be window formation. There is also thin white line surrounding the margins of bone cavity. This thin layer of cortical bone is almost always present unless suppuration supervenes in the cyst.
♦ Image of radiopaque borders is continuous with lamina dura around the associated tooth. Infection may cause the borders to become less distinct.
♦ Radicular cysts of long duration may cause resorption of roots.
♦ Adjacent teeth are usually displaced and rarely resorbed. There is also buccal expansion and involves maxillary area than displacement of antrum occurs.

Differential Diagnosis

♦ *Periapical granuloma:* If radiolucency which appear on the radiograph is smaller than 1.5 cm, it is considered to be periapical granuloma.
♦ *Periapical scar:* It is ruled out on basis of history and location.
♦ *Lateral periodontal cyst:* Radicular cyst originates from maxillary lateral incisor and is positioned in between

root of lateral incisor and canine and is confused with the lateral periodontal cyst. In this case tooth vitality should be checked, tooth associated with lateral periodontal cyst is vital and with radicular cyst is nonvital.

♦ *Periapical cementoma:* In case of radicular cyst tooth is non-vital while in case of periapical cementoma tooth is vital.

Treatment

♦ Nonvital teeth are associated with the cyst can either be extracted or they can be retained by endodontic treatment, i.e., apicoectomy.
♦ External sinus tracts should always be excised to prevent epithelial ingrowth.
♦ Commonly employed surgical procedure for radicular cyst is enucleation.
♦ Very small cysts can be removed through tooth socket.
♦ Large cysts that encroach upon maxillary sinus or inferior alveolar neurovascular bundle may be treated by marsupialization.

Q.7. Write short note on dentigerous cyst.
(Feb 2013, 5 Marks) (Apr 2008, 5 Marks)
(Sep 2008, 5 Marks) (Nov 2008, 5 Marks)

Or

Write brief note on dentigerous cyst.
(Apr 2017, 2 Marks)

Or

Write in short about dentigerous cyst.
(Jan 2018, 5 Marks)

Or

Write short answer on dentigerous cyst.
(Feb 2019, 3 Marks) (Oct 2019, 3 Marks)

Ans. It is also known as follicular odontoma.

It is a common odontogenic cyst of epithelial origin, which encloses the crown of an impacted tooth at its neck portion.

The cyst is lined by squamous epithelium, surrounded by connective tissue.

Within the cyst, the tooth lies obliquely or sometimes embedded in the wall of the cyst.

As cyst grows, it displace the teeth deeper and deeper and prevent from eruption.

Clinical Features

♦ *Age and sex:* It is usually found in children, equal in both the sex.
♦ *Site:* Most common site is mandibular third molar and maxillary canine which are most commonly impacted.
♦ *Symptoms:* Cyst remains asymptomatic, if uninfected. On infection inflammatory signs are present.
♦ *Expansion of mandible:* Since the inner table of mandible is strong the expansion mainly occurs in the outer aspect of the mandible. The bone gets thinned out resulting in egg shell cracking.
♦ *Blue domed cyst:* When it contains blood then it is called as blue domed cyst.

◆ Dentigerous cyst has potential to become an aggressive lesion with expansion of bone and subsequent facial asymmetry.

◆ There is extreme displacement of teeth, severe root resorption of adjacent teeth and pain.

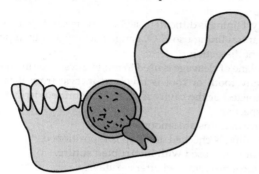

Fig. 16: Dentigerous cyst.

Radiographic Features

◆ It is a well-defined radiolucency usually associated with hyperostotic borders unless it is secondarily infected.

◆ Bony margins are well-defined and sharp.

◆ It may involve the crown symmetrically; it may expand from the crown.

◆ Large cysts are confined to mandible. There may be resorption of roots.

Differential Diagnosis

◆ *Ameloblastoma or ameloblastic fibroma:* They are multilocular and not associated with crown of an unerupted teeth.

◆ *Adenomatoid odontogenic tumor:* They are rare and occur in maxillary anterior region.

◆ *Calcifying odontogenic cyst:* It occurs as pericoronal radiolucency and contains evidences of calcification.

◆ *Developmental primordial and follicular primordial cyst:* It occurs in the crown of unerupted tooth and superimposition of image which may cause cyst like radiolucency to appear as dentigerous cyst on radiograph.

Treatment

◆ Treatment via an intraoral approach or extraoral is decided by the size of cyst, adequate access and whether it desirable to save the involved tooth.

◆ *Marsupialization:* It is indicated in children if the cyst is very large in the size and involved tooth/teeth are to be maintained. Tooth may erupt in occlusion as defect heals with normal bone or orthodontic forces may be used to bring tooth in occlusion.

◆ *Enucleation:* Alternatively cyst can be enucleated together with involved tooth in adults as possibility of tooth eruption is low.

Q.8. Describe the cysts of jaw and their management.

(Oct 2007, 10 Marks)

Ans. Cyst is defined as "A pathological cavity having fluid, semifluid or gaseous contents and which is not created by accumulation of pus."   **—Kramer (1974)**

Classification of Cyst of Jaw by Mervin Shear

◆ **Cysts of the Jaws:**
  • Epithelial:
    – *Developmental*:
      » Odontogenic
        ▪ Gingival cyst of infants
        ▪ Odontogenic keratocyst (neoplasm)
        ▪ Dentigerous cyst
        ▪ Eruption cyst
        ▪ Lateral periodontal cyst
        ▪ Gingival cyst of adults
        ▪ Botryoid odontogenic cyst
        ▪ Glandular odontogenic cyst
        ▪ Calcifying odontogenic cyst (neoplasm).
      » Non-odontogenic
        ▪ Nasopalatine duct cyst
        ▪ Nasolabial cyst
        ▪ Midpalatal raphe cyst of infants
        ▪ Median palatine, median alveolar
        ▪ Median mandibular cyst
        ▪ Globulomaxillary cyst.
    – *Inflammatory*:
      » Radicular cyst, apical and lateral
      » Residual cyst
      » Paradental cyst and mandibular infected buccal cyst
      » Inflammatory collateral cyst.
  • Nonepithelial (pseudocysts)
    – Solitary bone cyst
    – Aneurysmal bone cyst.

◆ **Cyst associated with maxillary antrum:**
  • Benign mucosal cyst of the maxillary antrum
  • Postoperative maxillary cyst.

◆ **Cyst of the soft tissues of mouth, face and neck:**
  • Dermoid and epidermoid cyst
  • Lymphoepithelial cyst (brachial cyst)
  • Thyroglossal duct cyst.
  • Anterior medial lingual cyst (intralingual cyst of foregut origin)
  • Oral cyst with gastric or intestinal epithelium
  • Cystic hygroma
  • Nasopharyngeal cyst
  • Thymic cyst.

◆ **Cyst of salivary glands:** Mucous extravasation cyst, mucous retention cyst, ranula, polycystic disease of the parotid.

◆ **Parasitic cyst:** Hydatid cyst, cysticercus cellulosae, trichinosis.

For description of various types of jaw refer to Table in Ans. 10 of same chapter.

Management of Cysts

It is also known as Partsch operation.

Principle

◆ Marsupialization or decompression, refers to creating a surgical window in the wall of the cyst and evaluation of the cystic contents.

◆ This process decreases intracystic pressure and promotes shrinkage of the cyst and bone fill.

Method

♦ Area is anesthetized with local anesthesia.
♦ Incision should be long enough to provide good exposure (circular/oval).
♦ In edentulous patient, incision is given along the crest of ridge and in dentulous patient, the incision is given around the neck of teeth.
♦ Incision is given bucally or lingually depending on location of cyst.
♦ Mucoperiosteal flap is raised.
♦ The character of underlying bone is determined. If this layer of bone is present on cyst, it is carefully peeled off with periosteal elevator. If the bone over cyst is intact, a window is made with bur/chisel in postage stamp method.
♦ Window is enlarged with rongeurs.
♦ An incision shaped like St Andrew and cross is made on cyst lining.
♦ Fluid content of cyst is evaluated with suction.
♦ Four triangular flaps created are turned outwards and sutured with mucoperiosteum.
♦ Cavity is packed with gauge in iodoform or white heads varnish.
♦ If the cyst lining is friable as in infected cyst, be sutured with mucoperiosteum the gauge is used to hold the cyst lining and mucoperiosteum together.
♦ One week later, the gauge is removed. Sutures also, by new union occur between lining and new periosteum.
♦ Now a plug is made to maintain the opening of cavity patent and prevent food from entering the cavity.
♦ The plug is worn continuous by but removed after meals.
♦ The cavity is irrigated with syringe.
♦ The plug is never made of full cavity depth because it interferes with bone regeneration of cavity.
♦ The size of plug (depth) is decreased gradually as the cavity is filled with bone.
♦ Finally the mucoperiosteum is closed with sutures.

Enucleation

Method

♦ Area is anesthetized by local anesthesia.
♦ Incision should be long enough to provide good exposure and at the end of operation flap edge must rest on healthy bone.
♦ In edentulous patient incision is given along the crest of ridge and in edentulous patient, it is given around the neck of the teeth.
♦ Incision is given facially or lingually depending on location of cyst.
♦ Mucoperiosteal flap is raised.
♦ The character of underlying bone is determined. If thin layer of bone is present on cyst, it is carefully peeled off with periosteal elevator. If the bone over a cyst is intact, a window is made with bur or chisel in postage stamp method.
♦ The window is enlarged with rongeurs forcep to allow complete enucleation.

♦ Care is taken not to puncture cyst wall because the intact cyst is removed easily.
♦ The cyst lining is gently separated from cavity wall using periosteal elevator or curette/Mitchell trimmer/spoon excavator. The convex surface of blade is kept facing the lining of cyst.
♦ If cyst lining is difficult to separate from cavity wall or nasal or antral lining use H_2O_2 gauge packing and then perform blunt dissection.
♦ A plane of cleavage is used to remove cystic sac in one piece.
♦ If any tooth or root is involved in cyst from it is either extracted or the cavity is cleaned, debrided, irrigated and inspected.
♦ Bony margins are smoothened.
♦ Bleeding is checked and flap is repositioned.
♦ Wound is closed with interrupted suture.
♦ Sutures are removed after 6–7 days.
♦ Routine analgesics and antibiotics are prescribed to prevent postoperatory pain and infection.

Decompression Followed by Enucleation

♦ Decompression of a cyst relieves the pressure within the cyst and causes it to grow.
♦ It is performed by making a small opening in the cyst and keeping it open with drain.
♦ Cyst is kept open initially by medicated gauze pack and an acrylic plug.
♦ Bone regeneration occur and cavity reduces in size
♦ This technique is not a definitive treatment but allows a second stage of enucleation to be undertaken on much smaller lesion which would have been impossible.

Q.9. Write short note on thyroglossal sinus.

(Apr 2015, 3 Marks)

Ans. Thyroglossal fistula or sinus is never congenital. It is always acquired due to following reasons:
♦ Infected thyroglossal cyst rupturing into the skin.
♦ Inadequate drained infected thyroglossal cyst.
♦ Incompletely excised thyroglossal cyst.

Clinical Features

♦ It occurs during 10–20 years.
♦ Patient gives history of previous swelling in neck (thyroglossal cyst), which becomes infected, burst forms a fistula.
♦ The fistula or sinus discharges mucus and after sometime fistula closes by itself.
♦ After few days, it again starts discharging mucus and closes by itself again.
♦ The normal position of fistula or sinus remains in midline in front of thyroid cartilage.
♦ Its internal opening is on foramen cecum of tongue.
♦ If fistula becomes infected than surrounding skin becomes red, warm and tender and fistula secrete pus.
♦ A fistulous opening in center of neck which is covered by hood of skin can occur due to increased growth of neck

when compared to that of fistula. This is known as semilunar sign or hood sign.

Investigations

Radioisotope study and fistulogram.

Treatment

♦ Infection is controlled with antibiotics
♦ *Sistrunk's operation is usually performed: For details, refer to Ans. 3 of same chapter.*

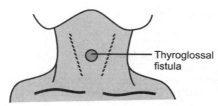

Fig. 17: Thyroglossal fistula.

Q.10. What are different types of cysts in an oral cavity? Describe etiology, pathogenesis and management.
(Mar 2003, 15 Marks)

Ans. Cyst is defined as "A pathological cavity having fluid, semifluid or gaseous contents and which is not created by accumulation of pus." **—Kramer (1974).**

Classification of Cyst in Oral Cavity by Mervin Shear

♦ **Cysts of the jaws:**
  • Epithelial:
    – *Developmental:*
      » Odontogenic
        ▪ Gingival cyst of infants
        ▪ Odontogenic keratocyst (neoplasm)
        ▪ Dentigerous cyst
        ▪ Eruption cyst
        ▪ Lateral periodontal cyst

        ▪ Gingival cyst of adults
        ▪ Botryoid odontogenic cyst
        ▪ Glandular odontogenic cyst
        ▪ Calcifying odontogenic cyst (neoplasm).
      » Nonodontogenic
        ▪ Nasopalatine duct cyst
        ▪ Nasolabial cyst
        ▪ Midpalatal raphe cyst of infants
        ▪ Median palatine, median alveolar
        ▪ Median mandibular cyst
        ▪ Globulomaxillary cyst.
    – *Inflammatory:*
      » Radicular cyst, apical and lateral
      » Residual cyst
      » Paradental cyst and mandibular infected buccal cyst
      » Inflammatory collateral cyst.
  • Nonepithelial (pseudocysts)
    – Solitary bone cyst
    – Aneurysmal bone cyst.
♦ **Cyst associated with maxillary antrum:**
  • Benign mucosal cyst of the maxillary antrum
  • Postoperative maxillary cyst.
♦ **Cyst of the soft tissues of mouth, face and neck:**
  • Dermoid and epidermoid cyst
  • Lymphoepithelial cyst (Brachial cyst)
  • Thyroglossal duct cyst.
  • Anterior medial lingual cyst (Intra lingual cyst of foregut origin)
  • Oral cyst with gastric or intestinal epithelium
  • Cystic hygroma
  • Nasopharyngeal cyst
  • Thymic cyst
♦ **Cyst of salivary glands:** Mucous extravasation cyst, mucous retention cyst, ranula, polycystic disease of the parotid.
♦ **Parasitic cyst:** Hydatid cyst, cysticercus cellulosae, trichinosis.

Etiology, Pathogenesis and Management of Various Cyst of Oral Cavity

Cyst	Etiology	Pathogenesis	Management
Dentigerous cyst	Impacted tooth, i.e., third molars or canines	*Intrafollicular theory:* Dentigerous cyst is caused by fluid accumulation between reduced enamel epithelium and enamel surface which result in a cyst in which crown is located within the lumen. *Extrafollicular theory:* Dentigerous cyst may arise by proliferation and cystic transformation of islands by odontogenic epithelium in connective tissue wall of dental follicle or even outside dental follicle and this transformed epithelium then unite with lining follicular epithelium forming cystic cavity around tooth crown	Small cyst by intraoral approach. Larger cyst involves surgical drainage and marsupialization
Eruption cyst	Erupting deciduous or permanent teeth	It develops as a result of separation of dental follicle from around the crown of an erupting tooth which is within the soft tissues overlying bone	In some cases, cyst rupture spontaneously which lead to tooth eruption. If cyst does not rupture excision of roof of cyst is done

Contd…

Contd…

Cyst	Etiology	Pathogenesis	Management
Odontogenic keratocyst	–	• Cyst arises from dental lamina which poses the growth potential • It also arises from proliferation from basal cells as a residue/remanent oral epithelium	• Commonly OKCs are treated by enucleation with curettage • Most of surgeons recommend peripheral osteotomy of bone cavity • Other group of surgeons undergo chemical cauterization by Carnoy's solution
Adenomatoid odontogenic cyst	Impacted tooth	Cystic hamartoma arising from odontogenic epithelium	• Enucleation with curettage • In some lesions marsupialization is done.
Lateral periodontal cyst	Inflammation by pocket content near alveolar crest at lateral root surface of tooth Developing tooth germ	• From proliferation of cell rest of malassez in PDL • From proliferation and cystic transformation of rest of dental lamina • From reduced enamel epithelium	Conservative enucleation is done
Gingival cyst of adult	Traumatic injury	• Cystic transformation of dental lamina • Traumatic implantation of surface epithelium • From postfunctional rest of dental lamina	Local surgical excision is done
Gingival cyst of newborn	–	Proliferation of remnants of dental lamina after tooth formation	No management
Palatal cyst of new born	–	• Due to entrapment of epithelium during formation of secondary palate • Epstein pearls occur along midpalatal raphae and presumably arise from epithelium entrapped along line of fusion • Bohn's nodules are scattered over hard palate near soft palate junction and are derived from minor salivary glands	No management is required. They are self-healing
Glandular odontogenic cyst	–	Arises from epithelial lining of dental lamina which has ability to induce formation of dental tissues	Enucleation or curettage is carried out
Calcifying odontogenic cyst	–	Arises from epithelial lining of dental lamina which has ability to induce formation of dental tissues	Enucleation and curettage should be done
Nasolabial cyst	Development	• From non-odontogenic fissural cyst • Develop from remnants of nasolacrimal duct or arising from epithelial lining of floor of mouth	It is removed intraorally through surgical approach
Nasopalatine cyst	• Trauma • Bacterial infection • Blocked duct of mucous gland	From epithelial remnants of nasopalatine duct which undergo proliferation and cystic transformation	Enucleation is done
Median palatal cyst	–	Develops from epithelium entrapped along embryonic line of fusion of lateral palatal shelves of maxilla	Surgical enucleation
Anterior median lingual cyst	–	Develops from epithelial entrapment between lateral tubercles of developing tongue	Incision and drainage
Periapical cyst	Carious tooth	• Arises from epithelial residues in periodontal ligament as a result of inflammation. • Pathogenesis occur in: - Phase of initiation - Phase of proliferation - Phase of cystification - Phase of enlargement	• Nonsurgical treatment followed by apicocectomy • Enucleation or marsupialization if lesion is large
Residual cyst	• Incompletely removed periapical granuloma. • If impacted tooth or carious tooth removed and cystic lesion is not recognized	Originates in residual epithelium of cell rests from PDL of lost tooth	Enucleation with primary closure
Traumatic cyst	Trauma	It results due to osteosclerosis resulting from a disturbed circulation caused by trauma creating an unequal balance of osteoclasts and repair of bone	Surgical exploration

Contd…

Contd...

Cyst	Etiology	Pathogenesis	Management
Aneurysmal bone cyst	History of trauma	It arises as an osseous arteriovenous fistula and thereby creates via its hemodynamic forces secondary reactive lesion of bone	Surgical curettage or excision
Mucocele	• Trauma to salivary duct • Obstruction to salivary duct	Obstruction or trauma results in extravasation of mucus in connective tissue. Due to continuous accumulation of mucus and pooling of saliva, a cavity develops which has no epithelial lining	Sharp and blunt dissection followed by excision of minor salivary gland
Ranula	Trauma to excretory ducts	It occurs when the extravasated mucus passes through mylohyoid muscle in submandibular region	Sublingual gland is removed by intraoral approach
Thyroglossal duct cyst		It may arises from the residues of the duct at any point of foramen cecum through neck of thyroid gland	Surgical excision along with cyst tract
Cystic hygroma	Developmental	Arises as the lymphatic spaces communicates with each other to form large thin walled cyst	Surgical excision along with cyst tract
Dermoid and epidermoid cyst	Trauma	It arises from epithelial rests persisting in midline after fusion of mandible and hyoid branchial arches	Intraoral lesions are removed by surgical excision through a midline incision in free edge of lingual frenum from behind the tip of tongue down to its attachment in mandible
Branchial cleft cyst		Arises from: • Epithelial remanent of branchial cleft • Residual cervical sinus epithelium • Cystic changes within cervical lymph nodes of epithelial inclusion	Complete surgical excision by cervical or intraoral approach

Q.11. Write short note on branchial cyst.

(Feb 2002, 10 Marks)

Ans. This is a cystic neck swelling in the lateral aspect of the neck, which is a result of a persisting cervical sinus formed by the second branchial cleft.

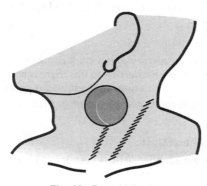

Fig. 18: Branchial cyst.

Pathogenesis

It arises from:

♦ Epithelial remnant of branchial cleft
♦ Residual cervical sinus epithelium
♦ Cystic changes within cervical lymph nodes of epithelial inclusion

Clinical Features

♦ Swelling is seen in the neck beneath anterior border of upper third of sternomastoid muscle.
♦ Swelling is smooth, soft, fluctuant and transilluminant with the sensation of half-filled double hot water bottle.

♦ It is seen commonly in late adolescent and during third decade of life.
♦ Swelling is painless unless it is infected.
♦ Mobility of swelling is restricted because of adherence to sternomastoid muscle.
♦ It contain cholesterol crystals which is from the lining of mucus membrane which consists of sebaceous gland. Cheesy toothpaste like material is typical.

Treatment

♦ Cyst should be excised under general anesthesia.
♦ Branchial cyst is in relation to carotid, hypoglossal nerve, glossopharyngeal nerve, spinal accessory nerve, posterior belly of digastrics and pharyngeal wall. Medially, it is close to posterior pillar of tonsils. During excision all the above structures should be taken care of.
♦ Sclerotherapy with OK–432 (Picibanil) is effective and is done under ultrasonography guidance.

Complications

♦ Since the wall is rich in lymphatic tissue, it can undergo secondary infection with pain and swelling.
♦ Recurrent infection.

Q.12. Write short note on plunging ranula.

(Oct 2007, 5 Marks)

Ans. When ranula extends in submandibular region through the deeper part of posterior margin of mylohyoid muscle, it is known as plunging ranula.

♦ It is an intraoral ranula with cervical extension.
♦ It is cross fluctuant across mylohyoid.
♦ It can arise from both submandibular and sublingual salivary gland as mucus retention cyst which reaches neck

by passing across the mylohyoid muscle presenting as soft, fluctuant, nontender, dumbbell-shaped swelling in the submandibular region.

♦ It is bidigitally palpable.

♦ Ultrasonography and/or MRI is diagnostic.

♦ It is treated by surgical excision through neck approach along with excision of submandibular and sublingual salivary glands.

♦ Small plunging ranula is often excised per orally along with excision of sublingual salivary gland.

Q.13. Write short note on cyst. *(Nov 2008, 5 Marks)*

Ans. Cyst is defined as "A pathological cavity having fluid, semifluid or gaseous contents and which is not created by accumulation of pus." **—Kramer (1974)**

♦ True cysts are lined by epithelium while false cysts are not lined by epithelium.

General Examination of Cyst

♦ *Location:* Most of the congenital cystic swellings have a typical location wherein diagnosis can be made with fair accuracy. A few examples are:
  • *Branchial cyst:* Anterior triangle partly covered by upper one-third of sternomastoid
  • *Dermoid cyst:* Midline, outer or inner canthus of the eye

♦ *Shape:* Majority of the cystic swellings are round or oval.
  • *For example subhyoid bursitis:* Transverse oval cystic swelling in the midline of the neck
  • *Thyroglossal cyst:* Vertically placed oval swelling in the midline of the neck
  • *Sebaceous cyst:* Hemispherical swelling

♦ *Surface:* Almost all the cystic swellings in the skin and subcutaneous tissue have smooth surface.

♦ *Consistency:* Fluctuation is positive in all cystic swellings. However, depending on the contents the fluctuation may be different, which an experienced surgeon can diagnose.
  • *Soft cystic:* Thyroglossal cyst, meningocele, lymph cyst.
  • *Tensely cystic:* Ganglion.
  • *Putty or tooth paste:* Sebaceous cyst

♦ *Transillumination test:* Cystic swelling which contains clear fluid show positive transillumination.

♦ *Mobility:* Almost all cystic swellings in skin, subcutaneous tissue or in deep plane are freely mobile. At times, this is not true due to various anatomical factors:
  • *Branchial cyst:* Restricted mobility is due to its adherence to sternomastoid muscle.
  • *Thyroglossal cyst:* Transverse mobility is absent because cyst is tethered by remnant of thyroglossal duct.

♦ *Sign of compressibility:* Swelling which have communication with cavity or with tissue spaces give positive sign of compressibility.

♦ *Pulsations:* Aneurysms are characterized by expansile pulsations and when the swelling pushes the vessel anteriorly transmission pulsation is obtained.

Complications of Cyst

♦ *Infection:* For example, sebaceous cyst

♦ *Calcification:* For example, hematoma, hydatid cyst

♦ *Pressure effects:* Ovarian cyst pressing iliac veins

♦ *Hemorrhage:* In thyroid cyst.

Q.14. Write short note on mucous cyst of lower lip.

(May/Jun 2009, 5 Marks)

Ans. It is also known as mucocele.

Etiology

♦ Due to obstruction of salivary duct

♦ Trauma to secretory acini.

Clinical Features

♦ They are common and occur on the inner aspect of lower lip. They may also occur on palate, cheek, tongue and floor of the mouth.

♦ They occur most frequently during third decade of life.

♦ The patient complains of painless swelling. The swelling may suddenly develops at meal time and may drain simultaneously at interval.

♦ The swelling is round, oval or smooth.

♦ The superficial cyst appears as bluish mass and if inflamed it is fluctuant, soft, nodular and dome-shaped elevation.

Treatment

Surgical removal is done by sharp and blunt dissection followed by excision of minor salivary gland.

Q.15. Write short note on mucous cysts.

(Dec 2009, 5 Marks)

Ans. Mucous cysts are of two types, i.e., mucous extravasation cyst and mucus retention cyst.

Mucous Extravasation Cyst

It is the swelling caused by pooling of saliva at injured minor salivary gland.

Etiology

Trauma to minor salivary gland duct causes extravasation of mucus in connective tissue, due to this there is accumulation of mucous in connective tissue with continuous pooling of saliva.

For clinical features and treatment, refer to Ans. 14 of same chapter.

Mucous Retention Cyst

It is also known as salivary duct cyst. It is a true cyst.

Etiology

Obstruction to the minor salivary gland leads to retention of saliva, continuous pressure due to retention leads to dilatation of duct and forms a cyst.

Clinical Features

♦ It more commonly occur in older individuals.

♦ Most common site is parotid gland. Intraorally, it is seen over buccal mucosa, lips and floor of mouth.

♦ It is a slow-growing lesion, soft, fluctuant swelling which appear bluish in color.

Treatment

Surgical excision is treatment of choice.

Q.16. Write short note on types of cysts of oral cavity. Describe ranula. *(Jun 2010, 5 Marks)*

Ans. *For types of cysts of oral cavity refer to classification of cysts given in Ans. 8 of same chapter. For ranula refer to Ans. 5 of same chapter.*

Q.17. Give classification, clinical features and complications of cysts. *(Aug 2011, 10 Marks)*

Ans. Cyst is defined as "A pathological cavity having fluid, semifluid or gaseous contents and which is not created by accumulation of pus." **—Kramer (1974)**

Classification of Cysts

♦ *Congenital cyst*
  • *Dermoids:* Sequestration dermoid cyst
  • *Tubulodermoids:* Thyroglossal cyst, postanal dermoid, ependymal cyst, urachal cyst
  • *Cyst of embryonic remnants:* cyst from paramesonephric duct and mesonephric duct, cyst of urachus and vitel-lointestinal duct cyst.
♦ *Acquired cyst*
  • *Retention cysts:* sebaceous cyst, bartholin's cyst, parotid cyst, breast cyst.
  • *Distention cyst:* lymph cyst, ovarian cyst, colloid goiter
  • *Exudation cyst:* Dursa, hydrocele, pancreatic pseudocyst
♦ *Cystic tumors:* Dermoid cyst of ovary, cystadenomas
♦ *Traumatic cyst:* Hematoma, implantation dermoid cyst
♦ *Degenerative cyst:* Tumor necrosis
♦ *Parasitic cyst:* Hydatid cyst, cysticercosis cellulosae, trichinosis.

Clinical Features of Cysts

♦ Hemispherical swelling which is smooth, fluctuant, nontender and well localized.
♦ Some cysts are transilluminant
♦ Presentation varies depending on anatomical location and pathology
♦ Cyst can be single or multiple.
♦ Cysts leads to the compression of adjacent structures

♦ This leads to infection, sinus formation, hemorrhage, calcification and cachexia.

Complications of Cysts

♦ *Infection:* For example, sebaceous cyst
♦ *Calcification:* For example, hematoma, hydatid cyst
♦ *Pressure effects:* Ovarian cyst pressing iliac veins
♦ *Hemorrhage:* In thyroid cyst
♦ *Torsion:* Ovarian dermoid
♦ Transformation into malignancy
♦ Ovarian cachexia.

Q.18. Define and describe differentiating features of dermoid cyst and sebaceous cyst. *(Jan 2012, 5 Marks)*

Ans.

Features	Dermoid cyst	Sebaceous cyst
Definition	It is a cyst which occurs due to inclusion of epithelium beneath the surface which later get sequestered	It is a retention cyst which occur due to blockage of duct of sebaceous gland causing cystic swelling
Etiology	It is congenital	It is acquired
Location	Midline of body, along the line of fusion	Occurs anywhere except palm and sole
Sign of indentation	Uncommon	Very common
Punctum	Absent	Present
Skin fixation	Absent	Skin is fixed at the site of punctum
Bony defect	Present	Absent
Mobility	It is restricted	Mobile
Intracranial communication	Rare	Absent
Treatment	Excision is done under general anesthesia	Excision is done under local anesthesia

Q.19. Name the treatment modalities and differentiating features of ranula and sublingual dermoid.

(Jan 2012, 5 Marks)

Or

Describe differentiating features sublingual dermoid and ranula.

(Jan 2017, 3 Marks)

Ans. Difference between ranula and sublingual dermoids.

Features	Ranula	Sublingual dermoid
Treatment modality	Sublingual gland is removed by intraoral approach.	Excision should be done
Definition	It is an extravasation cyst arising from sublingual glands or mucus glands of Nuhn or glands of Blandin in floor of mouth	Sublingual dermoids develop in relation to submandibular duct, lingual nerve and stylohyoid ligament
Features	Blue, smooth, soft, fluctuant brilliantly transilluminant swelling	It is smooth, soft, fluctuant, nontender and nontransilluminant swelling
Position	It is laterally placed	It can be laterally or medially placed

Q.20. Name the treatment modalities and differentiating features of dental cyst and dentigerous cyst.

(Jan 2012, 5 Marks)

Or

Write difference between dental cyst and dentigerous cyst.

(Mar 2016, 3 Marks)

Or

Write difference between periapical cyst and dentigerous cyst.

(Feb 2014, 3 Marks)

Ans.

Features	Dental cyst/periapical	Dentigerous cyst
Treatment modality	Nonsurgical treatment followed by apicoectomy Enucleation or marsupialization if lesion is large	• Small cyst by intraoral approach • Larger cyst involves surgical drainage and marsupialization
Origin	Originates due to fluid accumulation in reduced enamel epithelium	Originates due to periradicular inflammatory changes which leads to proliferation of epithelium
Association	Associated with and occurs in relation to apex of nonvital tooth	Associated with and occurs in relation to impacted tooth
Type of cyst	Inflammatory cyst	Odontogenic cyst
Site	Maxillary anterior teeth are commonly affected	Mandibular third molars and maxillary canines are affected
Radiology	Rounded radiolucency at apex of vital or nonvital tooth	Well-defined radiolucency along with hyperostotic borders and is visible around an unerupted tooth
Infection	Common	Not common
Complication	Osteomyelitis	Ameloblastoma

Q.21. Name the treatment modalities and differentiating features of thyroglossal cyst and subhyoid bursitis.

(Jan 2012, 5 Marks)

Ans.

Features	Thyroglossal cyst	Subhyoid bursitis
Treatment modality	Surgical excision along with cyst tract	Excision under general anesthesia
Definition	It is a swelling occurring in the neck in any part along the line of thyroglossal tract	In subhyoid bursitis due to constant friction inflammatory fluid collects in bursa leading to bursitis
Site	Present beneath the foramen cecum, in floor of mouth, suprahyoid, subhyoid and on thyroid cartilage	Horizontally placed midline swelling between lower part of hyoid bone and thyrohyoid membrane
Features	Swelling is smooth, soft, fluctuant, nontender, mobile and transilluminant	Swelling is smooth, soft, fluctuant, and non-transilluminant
Movement of swelling	Swelling move upward with deglutition but not while protruding the tongue out	Swelling move upward with deglutition as well as while protruding the tongue out

Q.22. Write short note on sequestration dermoid.

(Aug 2012, 5 Marks)

Ans. It occurs at the line of embryonic fusion, due to inclusion of epithelium beneath the surface which later gets sequestered forming a cystic swelling in the deeper plane.

♦ It is congenital type.
♦ Common sites are:
  • Forehead, neck, postauricular dermoid.
  • External angular dermoid.
  • Root of nose.
  • Sublingual dermoid.
  • Anywhere in midline or in the line of fusion.
♦ Dermoids occurring in the skull may extend into the cranial cavity.

♦ When it occurs as an external angular dermoid, it extends into the orbital cavity, or it can extend into any cavity in relation to its anatomical location (e.g., thorax, abdomen).

Types of Angular Dermoid

♦ *External angular dermoid:* It is a sequestration dermoid if situated over the external angular process of the frontal bone. Outer extremity of eyebrow extend over some part of swelling. This feature differentiate it from swelling arising from lacrimal gland. It can extend to orbital cavity also.

♦ *Internal angular dermoid:* It is a sequestration dermoid cyst in central position near the root of the nose. It occurs in frontonasal suture line. It mimics swelling from lacrimal sac or mucocele of frontal sinus. Mucocele of frontal sinus is due to blockage of frontonasal duct.

Clinical Features

- Painless swelling in the line of embryonic fusion.
- Seen in second or third decades of life.
- It is smooth, soft, nontender and fluctuant and nontransilluminating
- There is presence of resorption and indentation of bone beneath.
- Impulse on coughing may be present only if there is intracranial extension.

Complications

- Infection
- Hemorrhage
- Surface ulceration
- Calcification.

Investigations

- X-ray skull or part
- CT-scan head or part.

Treatment

Excision is done under general anesthesia. Often formal neurosurgical approach is required by raising cranial osteocutaneous flaps.

Q.23. Enumerate midline swelling of neck. Describe thyroglossal cyst in brief. *(Apr 2018, 5 Marks)*

Ans.

Midline Swelling of Neck

- Ludwig's angina
- Enlarged submental lymph node
- Sublingual dermoid cyst
- Thyroglossal cyst
- Subhyoid bursitis
- Goiter of thyroid, isthmus and pyramidal lobe
- Enlarged lymph node and lipoma in substernal space of burns
- Retrosternal goiter
- Thymic swelling
- Bony swelling arising from the manubrium sterni.
  For thyroglossal cyst in brief refer to Ans. 3 of same chapter.

Q.24. Write short answer on dermoid cyst.
(Sep 2018, 3 Marks) (Feb 2019, 3 Marks) (Oct 2019, 3 Marks)

Ans. Dermoid cyst is the cyst which is lined by squamous epithelium consisting of desquamated cells. Contents of the cyst are thick and sometimes toothpaste like which is a mixture of sweat, sebum and desquamated epithelial cells and sometimes even the hair are also seen.

Clinical Types of Dermoid Cyst

Congenital/Sequestration Dermoid

- It occurs along the line of embryonic fusion, due to the dermal cells being buried in deep plane.
- Cells which get sequestrated in subcutaneous plane proliferate and become liquefy to form cyst.
- At it grow, it indents mesoderm which explain the bony defects caused by dermoid cyst in skull and facial bone.

- As they are congenital, but they manifest as swelling at the time of childhood or later in life.
- They can occur anywhere in midline of body or face:
  - External and internal angular dermoid cyst: It occurs at fusion lines of frontonasal and maxillary process.
  - Median nasal dermoid cyst: At root of nose at fusion lines of frontal process.
  - In suprasternal space of burns
  - Sublingual dermoid cyst
  - Preauricular dermoid cyst: In front of auricle
  - Postauricular dermoid cyst: Behind the auricle.

Types of Angular Dermoid

- **External angular dermoid:** It is a sequestration dermoid situated over the external angular process of the frontal bone. Outer extremity of the eyebrow extends over some part of the swelling. This feature differentiates it from swelling arising from the lacrimal gland. It may extend in orbital cavity also.
- **Internal angular dermoid:** It is a sequestration dermoid cyst in central position near the root of nose. It occurs in frontonasal suture line. It is rare. It mimics the swelling from lacrimal sac or mucocele of frontal sinus.

Clinical Features of Congenital Cyst

- It manifest during childhood or adulthood. Few of the cases are also seen in 30–40 years of age group.
- Patient is present with the painless slow-growing swelling.
- Swelling is smooth soft, cystic, nontender and fluctuant.
- Paget's test is positive, i.e., swelling is fixed with two fingers and summit is indented to get yielding sensation due to fluid.
- Transillumination test is negative
- Rarely, it is putty like in consistency
- There will be resorption and indentation of the bone beneath.
- Impulse on coughing may be present only if there is intracranial extension.
- Its differential diagnosis consists of sebaceous cyst, lipoma, neurofibroma.

Complications of Congenital Dermoid Cyst

- Infection
- Hemorrhage
- Rupture
- Suppuration: Abscess
- Surface ulceration and calcification
- Ovarian dermoid: Torsion
- Pressure effects if there is intracavitary extension like into cranial cavity, thoracic cavity, etc.

Implantation Dermoid Cyst

- It is mainly seen in women, tailors and agriculturists who sustain repeated minor sharp injuries.
- After following a sharp injury, few of the epidermal cells get implanted into subcutaneous plane. Here, they develop in implantation dermoid cyst.
- This is seen in finger, palm and sole of the foot.
- As cyst develop in the areas where skin is thick and keratinized, it feel firm to hard in consistency, smooth,

tensely cystic, nontransilluminating and is often adherent to skin.

Teratomatous Dermoid Cyst

♦ Basically teratoma is the tumor which arises from totipotential cells. So, it has ectodermal, endodermal and mesodermal elements, such as hair, teeth, cartilage, bone, etc.

♦ Common sites associated are ovary, testis, retroperitoneum and mediastinum.

Tubuloembryonic Dermoid Cyst

It arises from ectodermal tubes. Few of the examples are thyroglossal cyst, postanal dermoid cyst and ependymal cyst of brain.

Treatment

Excision is under general anesthesia. Often formal neurosurgical approach is required by raising cranial osteocutaneous flaps.

15. ORAL CAVITY, LIP, AND PALATE

Q.1. Write note on leukoplakia. *(Dec 2010, 3 Marks)*

Or

Write briefly leukoplakia. *(Dec 2010, 5 Marks)*

Or

Answer briefly on leukoplakia. *(Mar 2016, 3 Marks)*

Or

Write in brief about leukoplakia. *(July 2016, 5 Marks)*

Or

Write short answer on leukoplakia.

(Apr 2019, 3 Marks)

Or

Describe etiology, pathology and treatment of leukoplakia. *(Oct 2019, 5 Marks)*

Ans. Leukoplakia is defined as a white patch or plaque that cannot be characterized clinically or pathologically as any other disease and is not associated with any physical or chemical causative agent except use of tobacco. First International Conference on Oral Leukoplakia Malmo, Sweden (1984) or modified WHO definition (1984).

Etiology

♦ **Tobacco:** Tobacco is widely used in two forms—
  • *Smokeless tobacco:* Chewable tobacco and snuff. When tobacco is chewed, various chemical constituents leach out, such as nitrosonornicotine, nicotine, pyridine and N picoline. Alkaline pH: 8.2–9.3 acts as local irritants and leads to alterations of mucosa.
  • *Smoked tobacco:* Cigar, cigarette, beedi and pipe. Smoking tobacco is harmful as this smoke contains polycyclic hydrocarbons, beta naphthylamine, nitrosoamines, carbon monoxide, nicotine, all of which acts as source of irritation. Heat also plays a major role. Heat induces

alterations in tissues increasing reddening and stippling of mucosal surface.

♦ **Alcohol:** Whether the use of alcohol itself is an independent etiological factor in the development of leukoplakia is still questionable. Its effect, at best may be synergistic to other well-known etiological factors (physical irritants). Alcohol leads to irritation and burning sensation of oral mucosa. Alcohol facilitates entry of carcinogen in exposed cells of oral mucosa and alters the oral epithelium as well as its metabolism.

♦ **Chronic irritation:** Continuous trauma or local irritation in the oral cavity leads to leukoplakia. Irritation or trauma can be caused by malocclusion, ill-fitting dentures, sharp tooth or broken tooth, hot spicy food and root piece.

♦ *Candida albicans:* As a possible etiological factor in leukoplakia and its possible role in malignant transformation is still unclear. About 10% of oral leukoplakias satisfy the clinical and histological criteria for chronic hyperplastic candidiasis.

♦ **Viruses:** The possible contributory role of viral agents, such as human papillomavirus 16 and 18 in the pathogenesis of oral leukoplakia particularly with regard to exophytic verrucous leukoplakia.

♦ **Vitamin deficiency:** Serum levels of vitamin A, B12, C, beta-carotene and folic acid were significantly decreased in patients with oral leukoplakia than compared to normal patients.

♦ **Genetic factor:** Relatively little is known yet with regard to possible genetic factors in the development of leukoplakia.

Clinical Features

♦ Usually, the lesion occurs in 4th, 5th, 6th and 7th decades of life.

♦ Buccal mucosa and commissural areas are most frequent affected sites followed by alveolar ridge, tongue, lip, hard and soft palate, etc.

♦ Oral leukoplakia often present solitary or multiple white patches.

♦ The size of lesion may vary from small well localized patch measuring few millimeters in diameter.

♦ The surface of lesion may be smooth or finely wrinkled or even rough on palpation and lesion cannot be removed by scrapping.

♦ The lesion is whitish or grayish or in some cases, it is brownish yellow in color due to heavy use of tobacco.

♦ In most of the cases, these lesion are asymptomatic, however in some cases, they may cause pain, feeling of thickness and burning sensation, etc.

Pathology

Leukoplakia occurs more often on buccal mucosa, tongue and floor of the mouth. Plaques may be solitary or multiple and vary from small lesions to large patches. Leukoplakia shows a spectrum of histopathologic changes, from increased surface keratinization without dysplasia to invasive keratinizing squamous cell carcinoma. Leukoplakic lesions are well defined with demarcated margins. The frequency of malignant transformation in leukoplakia is 10%.

Differential Diagnosis

♦ *Lichen planus:* Shows Wickham's straie
♦ *Syphilis:* Split papule or condyloma latum is seen
♦ *Leukoedema:* Shows faint milky appearance with folded and wrinkled pattern. Most commonly seen on buccal mucosa.

Treatment/Management

Removal of etiological factors may lead to the reversal or elimination of disease.

Conservative Treatment

♦ Vitamin therapy is given to patient. Vitamin A should be given to apply topically.
♦ Along with vitamin A, vitamin E should be given this leads to inhibit metabolic degeneration.
♦ Nystatin therapy is given to eliminate candidal infection.
♦ Vitamin B complex can be given as supplemental therapy.

Surgical Treatment

Conventional Surgery

♦ Incision is made around the lesion including the safe margins.
♦ Incision is deep and wide.
♦ Affected area is undermined and is dissected from underlying tissue.
♦ Sliding mucosal flap should be prepared for covering the wound.
♦ Fine iris scissors and skin hook is used for decreasing trauma.
♦ Extensive undermining of mucosal flap should be carried out so that when flap is advanced into its position, amount of tension will be minimum.
♦ As mobilization of mucosal flap is completed, it is advanced and free edges are approximated by multiple interrupted silk sutures.

Fulguration

It is a technique in which there is destruction of tissues by high voltage electric current and the action is controlled by movable electrode. This is done by electrocautery and electrosurgery.

Laser

Laser peel: It is used to remove the lesion which involves relatively large surface area.

Procedure

♦ Beam of laser is highly defocussed and should be kept at distant from the tissue.
♦ Initially, not any effect is seen on the tissue plane.
♦ Beam of laser should be gradually brought closer in focus, but remains in defocussed mode until tissue have white appearance and it begins to blister.
♦ Blistering usually occur at the basement membrane.
♦ The technique is extended over the rest of the lesion to be peeled.
♦ White area is then grafted with tissue forcep or hemostat.

Q.2. Describe clinical feature and treatment of submucous fibrosis. *(Apr 2008, 5 Marks) (Oct 2007, 5 Marks)*

Ans. OSMF is defined as "An insidious chronic disease affecting any part of oral cavity and sometime pharynx. Although occasionally preceded by and/or associated with vesicle formation, it is always associated with juxta-epithelial inflammatory reaction followed by fibroelastic changes in lamina propria, with epithelial atrophy leading to stiffness of oral mucosa and causing trismus and inability to eat."

—**Pindborg (1966)**

Clinical Features

♦ It occurs during 20–40 years of age.
♦ Most commonly involved sites are buccal mucosa, retromolar area, uvula, soft palate, palatal fauces, tongue, lips, pharynx and esophagus.
♦ Onset of disease is insidious or develop over the period of 2–4 years.
♦ Initially, the patient complains of burning sensation in the mouth, particularly during taking hot and spicy foods.
♦ It is often accompanied or followed by the formation of multiple vesicles over the palate or ulcers or inflammatory reactions in other parts of oral mucosa.
♦ There can be either excessive salivation or decreased salivation (xerostomia) along with recurrent stomatitis.
♦ Patients also develop defective gustatory sensation.
♦ In the initial phases of the disease, palpation of the mucosa elicits a "wet-leathery" feeling.
♦ Petechial spots may also be seen in the early stages of the disease over the mucosal surfaces of tongue, lips and cheek, etc.
♦ Oral mucous membrane is very painful upon palpation at this stage.
♦ One of the most important characteristic features of oral submucous fibrosis is the gradual stiffening of the oral mucosa with progressive reduction in the mouth opening.
♦ Stiffness of the oral mucosa and the subsequent trismus develops gradually within a few years after the development of the initial symptoms.
♦ In the advanced stage of OSF, the oral mucosa losses its resiliency to a great extent and it becomes blanched and stiff. Severe trismus develops at this stage.
♦ Because of stiffness of the lips and the tongue patients are unable to blow whistles or even blow out a candle.
♦ Oral mucosa is symmetrically affected on both sides of the mouth and it shows extreme pallor.
♦ Oral submucous fibrosis often causes a blanched opaque (white marble-like) appearance of the mucosa, on which, there may be occasional presence of leukoplakic or erythroplakic patches.
♦ Palpation of the mucosa often reveals many vertical white fibrous bands on the inner aspect of the cheek.
♦ Patients of OSMF often develops difficulty in deglutition, referred pain in the ear or deafness and nasal intonation of voice.
♦ Depapillation of the tongue with recurrent or sometimes persistent glossitis occurs. Later on the tongue becomes stiff and shows restricted movements.
♦ Uvula become 'bud-like' or hockey stick shaped or become shrunken.

Treatment

Supportive Treatment

♦ Diet rich with the vitamins along with iron preparation should be given to the patient.
♦ IM injection of iodine B complex is given to the patient. During early phase low doses are given and later on high doses are effective.
♦ Local injection of hydrocortisone in the lesional area is of value.
♦ Intralesional injection of hyaluronidase can be given.
♦ Systemically 100 mg/day of hydrocortisone is effective in reducing the burning sensation.
♦ About 2 mL injection of placentrex intralesional is effective.
♦ Lycopene as an antioxidant should be given to the patient.
♦ Vitamin E along with hyalurodinase and dexamethasone is effective.
♦ Intralesional injection of interferon gamma helps in increment in mouth opening.

Surgical Treatment

♦ *Conventional surgery:*
  • *Tongue mucosa as a graft:* The fibrous bands are excisioned and tongue mucosa as a flap is used.
  • Implantation of fresh human placenta can be done following the surgical excision of fibrous bands.
  • Fibrotic bands are excisioned and nasolabial flap is taken for reconstruction.
  • Bilateral palatal flap is taken for generally covering of exposed area.
♦ *Laser:*
  • Patient should be incorporated with general anesthesia. CO_2 LASER incise the buccal mucosa and vaporizes mucosal connective tissue.
♦ *Cryosurgery:* It helps in providing the relief from the local lesions.

Q.3. Describe about etiology, clinical features and treatment of epulis. *(Sep 2001, 15 Marks)*

Ans.
♦ Epulis means upon gum.
♦ It refers to solid swelling situated on the gum.
♦ Localized enlargement of gingiva is mainly known as epulis.
♦ It arises from alveolar margin of jaw.
♦ Epulis can originate from the bone, periosteum or the mucous membrane.

Types of Epulis

Granulomatous Epulis/Pyogenic Granuloma

♦ It is also called false epulis or pyogenic epulis.
♦ Precipitating factors are: carious tooth, dentures, poor oral hygiene.

Clinical Features

♦ The important point is that it does not contain pus while its name is pyogenic epulis.
♦ Pregnancy epulis refer to this variety.
♦ It is a mass of granulation tissue around the carious tooth on the gum.
♦ It is a soft to firm fleshy mass and bleed on touch.

Treatment

♦ Extraction of associated carious tooth.
♦ Removal of local irritation as ill-fitting denture.
♦ Excision of granulation tissue.
♦ Pregnancy epulis regress spontaneously after delivery.

Fibrous Epulis

It is the most common type of epulis.

Clinical Features

♦ Arises from periosteum at the neck of teeth.
♦ It is localized inflammatory hyperplasia of gum.
♦ It occurs in response to local irritation.
♦ It is composed of fibrous tissue and blood vessels.
♦ It is a firm polypoidal mass, slowly growing and nontender.

Treatment

Excision of growth and removal of local irritants.

Giant Cell Epulis/Myeloid Epulis

This is the osteoclastoma causing ulceration and hemorrhage of gingiva.

Clinical Features

♦ It is less common, purple and pedunculated tumor.
♦ It is an "osteoclastoma" arising in the jaw.
♦ It present as hyperemic vascular edematous, soft to firm gums with indurated underlying mass due to expansion of the bone.
♦ It may ulcerate and result in hemorrhage.
♦ Multinucleated giant cells are found in histology.
♦ It is more rapidly growing tumor than any other epulis.

Treatment

♦ Small tumors are treated by curettage.
♦ Large tumors are treated by radical excision.

Carcinomatous Epulis

Squamous cell carcinoma of alveolus and gingiva, present localized, hard, indurated, swelling with ulceration.

Clinical Features

♦ This is an "epithelioma" arising from mucous membrane of alveolar margin.
♦ It presents as a nonhealing, painless ulcer.
♦ It slowly infiltrates the bone.
♦ Hard regional lymph nodes are due to metastasis.

Treatment

Treated by wide excision, which include removal of segment of the bone.

Congenital Epulis

♦ This is a benign condition seen in a newborn arising from the gum pads.
♦ This is the variant of granular cell myeloblastoma originating from the gums.
♦ This is common in girls and more common in upper jaw mainly in canine or premolar area.

♦ Congetinal epulis is a well localized swelling from the gum which bleeds on touch.

♦ Excision of congenital epulis should be done.

Myelomatous Epulis

♦ This occurs mainly in leukemic patients.

♦ Treatment of leukemia resolves this condition.

Fibrosarcomatous Epulis

It is the fibrosarcoma arising from the fibrous tissue of gums.

Q.4. Write short note on epulis.
(Dec 2012, 5 Marks) (Aug 2012, 5 Marks)
(Apr 2008, 5 Marks) (Feb 2015, 5 Marks)
(Dec 2009, 5 Marks) (Apr 2017, 4 Marks)

Ans. *Refer to Ans. 3 of same chapter.*

Q.5. Classify tumors of jaw. How will you treat a case of epulis? *(Mar 2000, 15 Marks)*

Ans.

Classification of Tumors of Jaw

♦ **Swelling arising from the gums (epulis)**
  • Congenital epulis
  • Fibrous epulis
  • Pregnancy epulis
  • Giant cell epulis
  • Myelomatous epulis
  • Sarcomatous epulis
  • Carcinomatous epulis

♦ **Swelling arising from the dental epithelium (odontomes):**
  • Ameloblastoma
  • Compound odontome
  • Enameloma
  • Cementoma
  • Dentinoma
  • Odontogenic fibroma and myxoma
  • Radicular odontome
  • Composite odontome

♦ **Cysts arising in relation to dental epithelium:**
  • Dental cyst
  • Dentigerous cyst

♦ **Swelling arising from the mandible or maxilla:**
  • Osteoma and osteoblastoma
  • Torus palatinus and mandibularis
  • Fibrous dysplasia
  • Osteoclastoma
  • Osteosarcoma
  • Secondaries
  • Giant cell reparative granuloma

♦ **Surface tumors:**
Tumors from the surface which extend into the jaw.
  • Ossifying fibroma
  • Osteofibrosis of maxilla
  • Ivory osteoma of jaw
  • Leontiasis ossea (diffuse osteitis)
  • Carcinoma extending into the jaw
Also refer to Ans. 3 of same chapter for epulis.

Q.6. Write in short adamantinoma. *(Dec 2010, 3 Marks)*

Or

Write short answer on adamantinoma.
(Apr 2018, 3 Marks) (Feb 2019, 3 Marks)

Ans. In 1885, Malassez coined the term adamantinoma. In 1934, Churchill replaced the term adamantinoma with ameloblastoma.

Ameloblastoma is defined as "usually unicentric, non-functional, intermittent growth, anatomically benign and clinically persistent"   **—Robinson**

Pathogenesis

Ameloblastoma originates from:
♦ Epithelial rest of Malassez.
♦ Epithelium of odontogenic cysts
♦ Disturbances in developing enamel organ
♦ Basal cells of surface epithelium
♦ Heterotrophic epithelium.

Clinical Features

♦ It occurs during 2nd, 3rd and 4th decades of life.
♦ Predilection for males is seen.
♦ It is seen in molar ramus area in mandible and in third molar area including maxillary sinus and floor of nose in maxilla.
♦ Tumor start as a lesion of bone and later on expands the bone.
♦ Patient complains of asymmetry of face.
♦ Teeth in the lesional area are displaced.
♦ Pain and paresthesia is present if lesion involves any of the nerve.
♦ As the tumor enlarges palpation leads to crepitus also known as egg shell crackling.

Investigations

♦ *Clinically:* Presence of swelling in posterior mandible with expansion as well as egg shell crackling.
♦ *Radiographically:* Honey comb or soap bubble appearance in posterior region of mandible. Labial and lingual plate expansion is also seen.
♦ *Biopsy:* Biopsy of the lesion is needed for the confirmation of diagnosis so that histological type of ameloblastoma is diagnosed.

Treatment/Management

♦ Ameloblastomas are generally slow-growing but locally invasive tumors and have a high recurrence rate after treatment.
♦ Curettage of ameloblastomas, which was favored in the past, is now not advocated because of the high recurrence rate associated with it.
♦ Ameloblastomas are best treated by resection of the lesion with a marginal clearance of 1.5–2 cm of normal bone to prevent recurrence.
♦ The lesion may be resected as block resection with or without continuity defect based on the integrity of inferior cortex.

- Radiologically, a minimum of 1 cm residual mandible inferior cortex is required postoperatively to prevent pathologic fracture.
- Inferior alveolar nerve should be sacrificed if it lies within the lesion.
- Maxillary ameloblastomas are particularly dangerous, partly because the bones are considerably thinner than those of the mandible and present less effective barriers to spread. Therefore, radical excision is essential, preferably maxillectomy.
- Peripheral ameloblastomas are treated by excision, as usually there is no alveolar bone involvement. If prior biopsy indicates involvement of bone, block resection with continuity defect is the choice of treatment.

Q.7. Discuss the differential diagnosis of jaw swellings. Describe investigation, clinical features and treatment of adamantinoma. *(Mar 1997, 15 Marks)*

Or

Write differential diagnosis of different types of swellings of jaw. *(Feb 2019, 5 Marks)*

Ans.

Differential Diagnosis of Jaw Swellings

- *Swelling arising from the mucoperiosteum, i.e., epulis. It has five varieties:*
  1. Fibrous
  2. Granulomatous
  3. Myeloid
  4. Sarcomatous
  5. Carcinomatous.
- *Swellings arising from tooth germs, i.e., odontomes. The different varieties are:*
  - Epithelial odontomes
    – Dental cyst
    – Dentigerous cyst
    – Adamantioma.
  The following are the rare varieties:
  - *Connective tissue odontomes*
    – Fibrous
    – Cementous
    – Sarcomatous.
  - *Composite odontomes (i.e. arising from both epithelial and connective tissue elements):*
    – Radicular
    – Compound follicular
    – Composite complex.
- *Osseous tumors: Any bone tumor can affect jaw*
  - *Benign:*
    – Fibro-osseous group
    – Paget's disease
    – Osteoclastoma.
  - *Malignant tumors:*
    – Osteosarcoma
    – Squamous cell carcinoma

    – Burkitt's tumor
    – Columnar cell carcinoma of maxillary antrum.
- *Inflammatory group:*
  - Alveolar abscess
  - Osteomyelitis
  - Actinomycosis.

For investigation, clinical features and treatment of adamantinoma refer to Ans. 6 of same chapter.

Q.8. Write short note on Vincent's angina.
(Sep 2005, 5 Marks) (Jan 2012, 5 Marks)

Ans. It is an acute ulceromembranous stomatitis or acute ulcerative gingivitis.

This disease is caused by Vincent's organism—*Borrelia vincentii* an anaerobic spirochete and fusiformis.

Precipitating Factors

- Malnutrition, diabetes mellitus, carious tooth, war seasons, winter, etc.
- The disease starts in the intergingival defects as a deep penetrating ulcer, which results in a spontaneous gingival hemorrhage.
- Once infections spread to tonsillar region, it is called as Vincent's angina. Very severe painful condition.

Clinical Features

- Common in children and young adults between 20 and 40 years of age.
- It is a gangrenous devastating stomatitis which begins in mucus membrane of corner of mouth or cheek which progress rapidly to involve entire thickness of lips or cheek or both with necrosis and sloughing of entire tissue which is observed in poorly nourished children and debilitated adults.
- It start from lips extend to gums, spread to cheeks, bone, soft tissues and skin leading to extensive tissue loss with severe toxemia.
- There is presence of excessive salivation, fetid odor with destruction, discharge and toxic features.

Investigations

- Culture of *Borrelia vincentii*
- X-ray of involved part shows bony destruction.

Treatment

- Systemic antibiotics, i.e., higher doses of penicillin and metronidazole should be given.
- High protein and vitamin rich diet should be given through nasogastric intubation.
- Wound irrigation is done and liberal excision of dead tissue should be carried out.
- Blood transfusion is given.
- Later on patient require flaps to cover the defect.

Q.9. Write short note on tumors of jaw.

(Sep 2006, 10 Marks)

Or

Write short note on swelling of jaw.

(Feb 2015, 5 Marks)

Or

Discuss etiology, clinical features and treatment of tumor of jaw.

(Sep 2007, 10 Marks)

Or

Describe swelling of the jaw and its management.

(Apr 2007, 15 Marks)

Ans. *For classification refer to Ans. 5 of same chapter.*

Tumor of jaw	Etiology	Clinical features	Treatment/management
Epulis	• Carious tooth • Dentures • Poor oral hygiene	• In congenital epulis a well localized swelling is seen over the gum which is firm and bleeds on touch • In fibrous epulis swelling is red in color, firm/hard, sessile or pedunculated. It is painless	Excision should be done
Ameloblastoma	• Irritation in posterior region of mandible • Infection • Trauma • Dietary deficiency • Virus	• It occurs during 2nd, 3rd and 4th decades of life • Predilection for males is seen • It is seen in molar ramus area in mandible and in third molar area including maxillary sinus and floor of nose in maxilla • The tumor start as a lesion of bone and later on expands the bone • Patient complains of asymmetry of face • Teeth in the lesional area are displaced • Pain and paresthesia is present if lesion involves any of the nerve • As the tumor enlarges palpation leads to crepitus also known as egg shell crackling	• Ameloblastomas are generally slow-growing but locally invasive tumors and have a high recurrence rate after treatment • Curettage of ameloblastomas, which was favored in the past, is now not advocated because of the high recurrence rate associated with it • Ameloblastomas are best treated by resection of the lesion with a marginal clearance of 1.5–2 cm of normal bone to prevent recurrence. • Lesion may be resected as block resection with or without continuity defect based on the integrity of inferior cortex • Radiologically, a minimum of 1 cm residual mandible inferior cortex is required post-operatively to prevent pathologic fracture • Inferior alveolar nerve should be sacrificed if it lies within the lesion • Maxillary ameloblastomas are particularly dangerous, partly because the bones are considerably thinner than those of the mandible and present less effective barriers to spread. Therefore, radical excision is essential, preferably maxillectomy • Peripheral ameloblastomas are treated by excision, as usually there is no alveolar bone involvement. If prior biopsy indicates involvement of bone, block resection with continuity defect is the choice of treatment
Compound odontome	• Genetic transmission • Local trauma • Infection	• Slow growing, nonfiltrating lesion • Occur commonly in maxilla in incisor-canine region • Seen in 2nd and 3rd decades • Permanent teeth fail to erupt due to interference from compound odontome	Enucleation
Enameloma	Trauma	• Commonly seen in bifurcation or trifurcation of roots • Common site is maxillary molar • Appears as tiny globule of enamel adhering to the root	It should be removed if leading to periodontal diseases
Cementoma	–	• Painless boney expansion of jaw is present. • Occur during 15–30 years • Mandible is more commonly affected and the affected teeth are mandibular first molar, second and third molars • Slow-growing lesion which expand and resorb medial and lateral cortical plates	Extraction of associated tooth and complete enucleation of mass

Contd...

Contd...

Tumor of jaw	Etiology	Clinical features	Treatment/management
Dentinoma	–	• Seen in 2nd and 3rd decades • Seen in mandibular molar region and is associated with impacted tooth • Patient complains of swelling with pain	Surgical excision with curettage
Odontogenic fibroma	Irritation associated with overextended margins of faulty restoration and due to deposition of calculus	**Central** • Occurs during 2nd and 3rd decades • Female predilection is seen • Maxilla is more commonly affected • Appear as asymptomatic, progressive enlargement of jaw • Mobility of associated teeth is seen **Peripheral** • Lesion appear as pink, firm, sessile or pedunculated mass on attached gingiva • Mandible is commonly affected	**Central** Enucleation and curettage **Peripheral** Excision is done
Osteoma	–	• Seen in age group <30 years • Patient complaints of pain which worsen in night • Local soft tissue swelling is present	Excision or curettage

Fibrous dysplasia	• Genetic
	• Developmental
	• Endocrine
		• Monostotic fibrous dysplasia
		  - It involves only one bone and pigmented skin lesions are present
		  - The sites which affected are maxilla, mandible, ribs and femur
		  - It occurs in children younger than 10 years and both the sexes are equally affected
		  - Maxilla is more commonly affected than the mandible and most of the changes occur in posterior region. The most common area involved is premolar area
		  - There is presence of unilateral facial swelling which is slow-growing with intact overlying mucosa
		  - Swelling is painless but patient may feel discomfort
		  - There is presence of enlarging deformities of alveolar process mainly buccal and labial cortical plates
		  - In mandible, there is protrusion of inferior border of mandible
		• Polystotic fibrous dysplasia
		  - It is seen during first and second decades of life
		  - Female predilection is seen with male to female ratio of 1:3
		  - Most common sites to be involved are skull, facial bones, clavicle, thighs, shoulder, chest and neck
		
		  - Café-au-lait spots are seen over the skin which are irregular in shape and are light brown melanotic spots
		  - Patient complains of recurrent bone pain
		  - There is expansion of jaws and asymmetry of facial bones which leads to enlargement and deformity
			• Surgical removal of the lesion should be done.
			• Osseous contouring is done to correct the deformities so that aesthetics of patient should be improved.

Contd...

Contd...

Tumor of jaw	Etiology	Clinical features	Treatment/management
Ossifying fibroma	–	• Slow-growing painless expansile lesion which replaces normal bone as it enlarges • Patient complains of facial asymmetry • Seen between 2nd and 4th decades • Female predilection is seen	• The lesions have capsule and are enucleated by intraoral approach • Large lesions which distort the jaws requires local resection with grafting of bone

Q.10. Name the treatment modalities and differentiating features of adamantinoma and osteoblastoma.

(Jan 2012, 5 Marks)

Ans.

Features	Admantinoma	Osteoclastoma
Age	Childhood or early adult life	25–30 years
Rate of growth	Slow-growing tumor	Rapidly growing tumor
Expansion	Mostly the outer table of jaw bone	Both inner and outer table are expanded
Pain	It rarely causes pain	It is painless
Fungation	Some fungates in very late case to the exterior	Usually not fungate
X-ray appearance	Fine honey-comb appearance	Soap-bubble appearance with large cysts and fine or ill-defined trabeculae
Histology	Peripheral columnar cells with central core of star cells with large vacuoles in the cytoplasm	Multinucleated giant cells are many in number
Radiosensitive	No radiosensitive	Radiosensitive
Malignancy	It is locally malignant tumor	May turn into malignancy
Treatment modalities	Ameloblastomas are best treated by resection of the lesion with a marginal clearance of 1.5–2 cm of normal bone to prevent recurrence	Curettage and conservative surgical excision is done

Q.11. Classify oral mucosal lesions. Describe the clinical features and histopathological features of submucosal fibrosis. *(Sep 2004, 20 Marks)*

Ans.

Classification of Oral Mucosal Lesions

♦ **Genodermatous:**
  • White sponge nevus
  • Hereditary benign intraepithelial dyskeratosis
  • Pachyonychia congenita
  • Porokeratosis
  • Darier's disease
  • Pseudoxanthoma elasticum.

♦ **Noninfective disease**
  • *Vesicular:*
    – Erythema multiforme
    – Pemphigus
    – Bullous lichen planus.
  • *Nonvesicular:* Lichen planus.
  • *Collagen disorders:*
    – Lupus erythematous
    – Scleroderma.
  • *Degenerative:* Oral submucous fibrosis.
  • *Pigmentation:*
    – Anemia
    – Addison's disease
    – Racial pigmentation

OSMF is defined as "An insidious chronic disease affecting any part of oral cavity and sometime pharynx. Although occasionally preceded by and/or associated with vesicle formation, it is always associated with juxtaepithelial inflammatory reaction followed by fibroelastic changes in lamina propria, with epithelial atrophy leading to stiffness of oral mucosa and causing trismus and inability to eat."

—Pindborg (1966)

Clinical Features

♦ It is caused during 20–40 years of age.
♦ Females are affected more than males.
♦ In OSMF fibrotic changes are frequently seen in buccal mucosa, retromolar area, vulva, tongue, etc.
♦ Initially patient complains of burning sensation in the mouth, particularly during taking hot and spicy foods.
♦ There can be excessive salivation, decreased salivation and defective gustatory sensation.
♦ In initial phase of disease palpation of mucosa elicits a "wet leathery" feeling.
♦ In advanced stage, the oral mucosa losses its resilience and become blanched and stiff and thereby causing trismus.
♦ Palpation of mucosa often reveals vertical fibrous bands.

Histopathology

Microscopically, OSMF reveals following features:
♦ Overlying hyperkeratinized, atrophic epithelium often shows flattening and shortening of rete pegs.
♦ There can be variable degree of cellular atypia or epithelial dysplasia.

- In OSMF dysplastic changes are found in epithelium which include nuclear pleomorphism, severe intercellular edema, etc.
- Stromal blood vessels are dilated and congested and there can be areas of hemorrhage.
- Underlying connective tissue stroma in advanced stage of disease shows homogenization and hyalinization of collagen fibers.
- Decreased number of fibroblastic cells and narrowing of blood vessels due to perivascular fibrosis are present.
- There can be presence of signet cells in some cases.

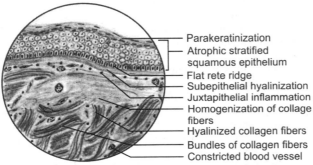

Parakeratinization
Atrophic stratified squamous epithelium
Flat rete ridge
Subepithelial hyalinization
Juxtapithelial inflammation
Homogenization of collage fibers
Hyalinized collagen fibers
Bundles of collagen fibers
Constricted blood vessel

Fig. 19: Oral submucous fibrosis
(For color version see Plate 3).

Q.12. Write the oral manifestations of systemic disease.
(Apr 2010, 5 Marks) (Sep 2004, 5 Marks)

Ans.

Oral Manifestations of Systemic Disease

Syphilis

The oral manifestations of syphilis are given in the following Table.

Tuberculosis

Oral manifestations of tuberculosis

- Tuberculous infection in oral cavity may produce nodules, vesicles, fissures, plaque, granulomas or verrucal papillary lesions.
- The tuberculous lesions of oral cavity are tuberculous ulcers, tuberculous gingivitis and tuberculosis of salivary gland.
- Tongue is most common location for the occurrence, besides this palate, gingiva, lips, buccal mucosa, alveolar ridge and vestibules may also be affected.

- *Tongue leison:* Tuberculous lesion of tongue develops on the lateral borders and appears as single or multiple ulcers which are well defined, painful, firm and yellowish gray in color.
- *Lip lesions:* The lesions produce small, nontender, granulating ulcer at mucocutaneous junction.
- *Gingival lesions:* These lesions produce small granulating ulcers with concomitant gingival hyperplasia.
- *Tuberculous lesion of jaw bone:* Chronic osteomyelitis of maxilla and mandible may occur and infection reaches to bone via blood or root canal or extraction socket. Tuberculous osteomyelitis of jaw bone produces pain, swelling, sinus or fistula formation.

Leprosy

Oral manifestations of leprosy

- In oral cavity, the disease produces tumor like lesions called as "lepromas" which are found on lips, gingiva, tongue and hard palate.
- Oral lesion appears as yellowish soft or hard sessile growth which have tendency to breakdown and ulcerate.
- Ulceration, necrosis and perforation of palate.
- Fixation of palate with loss of uvula.
- Difficulty in swallowing and regurgitation.
- Cobblestone appearance of tongue with loss of taste sensation.
- Chronic gingivitis, periodontitis and candidiasis are present.
- The enamel hypoplasia of teeth, pinkish discoloration of teeth and tapering of teeth is present.

Herpes Zoster

Oral Manifestations of Herpes Zoster

- Herpes zoster may involve the face by infection of trigeminal nerve, mainly first branch.
- There is usually involvement of skin and oral mucosa supplied by trigeminal nerve.
- Lesions of the oral mucosa are extremely painful vesicles which may be found on the buccal mucosa, tongue, pharynx and larynx and uvula.
- This vesicle generally ruptures and leaves the area of erosion.
- The erosive ulcers heal up in a few days without scar formation.
- In herpes zoster, neuralgic pain in oral cavity stimulates tooth ache.
- The pain may persist long after the lesion heals up and the condition is known as postherpetic neuralgia.

Characteristic	Primary syphilis	Secondary syphilis	Tertiary syphilis
Site	Chancre occurs at the site on entry of *Treponema*. It occurs on lip, oral mucosa, and lateral surface of tongue, soft palate and gingiva	Mucus patches are present on tongue, buccal mucosa, pharyngeal region and lips. • Split papules develop at commissure of lips	Gumma can occur anywhere in jaw but more frequent site is palate, mandible and tongue
Appearance	It has narrow copper colored slightly raised borders with reddish brown base in centers.	Mucus patches appears as slightly raised grayish white lesions surrounded by erythematous base. Split papules are cracked in middle giving "Split pea appearance"	Gumma manifests as solitary, deep punched out mucosal ulcer

Contd...

Contd...

Characteristic	Primary syphilis	Secondary syphilis	Tertiary syphilis
Symptom	Intraoral chancres are slightly painful due to secondary infection and are covered with grayish white film.	Mucus patches are painless mild-to-moderately painful	In gumma the breathing and swallowing difficulty may be encountered by the patients
Signs	White sloughy material is present	Snail tract ulcers and raw bleeding surfaces are present	Perforation of palatal vault is present.
Tongue	Tongue lesion may be commonly seen on lateral surface of anterior two-thirds or on dorsal surface and often there is enlargement of foliate papilla	Tongue gets fissured.	Numerous small healed gumma in tongue results in series of nodules or sparse in deeper area of organ giving tongue an upholstered or tufted appearance

Q.13. Write short note on lipoma.

(Aug 2012, 5 Marks) (Sep 2008, 5 Marks)
(Nov 2008, 5 Marks) (Sep 2007, 5 Marks)

Or

Write short answer on lipoma. *(Oct 2019, 3 Marks)*

Ans. Lipoma is a benign neoplasm arising from yellow fat. Often it can be hyperplasia or combination of neoplasm and hyperplasia.

♦ It is the most common benign tumor
♦ It is also called as universal tumor (ubiquitous tumor) as it can occur anywhere in the body except brain.

Types of Lipoma

♦ *Localized (encapsulated):* Localized lipoma is encapsulated with yellowish orange color.
♦ *Diffuse (nonencapsulated):* Diffuse lipomas are not encapsulated and not localized. It is common in palm, sole, head, neck. It is seen in subcutaneous and intermuscular tissues.
♦ *Superficial lipomas:* They are more common; common in subcutaneous plane. It is common in back, neck, proximal extremities and abdomen. It is commonly <5 cm, but can attain large size.
♦ *Deep lipomas:* They are commonly intramuscular, but often may be intermuscular; often both intra- and intermuscular (infiltrating lipoma). They are common in lower limbs (45%), trunk (17%), shoulder and upper limb. They attain large size compared to superficial lipomas.
♦ *Single lipoma:* It is common. It is usually superficial in subcutaneous plane but can be deep also.
♦ *Multiple lipomas:* They are 15% common; common in males (6:1). Common in back, shoulder and upper arm; can be symmetrical. It can be associated with many syndromes like multiple endocrine neoplasia (MEN), Cowden's, Frohlich syndromes, etc.
♦ *Hibernoma:* Benign tumor arising from brown fat is called as hibernoma (reddish brown), which has got serpentine vascular elements.
♦ *Fibrolipoma:* Lipoma with fibrous component is called as fibrolipoma.
♦ *Naevolipoma:* Lipoma with telangiectasis is called as naevolipoma.

♦ *Neurolipoma:* (with nerve tissue and is painful), angiolipoma (with vascular element), myolipoma, chondroid lipoma, spindle cell lipoma, pleomorphic lipoma-are different types
♦ Depending on the type of nonadipose component associated.

Clinical Features

♦ Localized swelling, which is lobular (surface), nontender.
♦ Often fluctuant like feel but actually not (because fat in body temperature remains soft). It is usually nontransilluminant.
♦ Mobile, with edges slipping between the palpating finger (slip sign).
♦ Skin is free.
♦ Lipomas may be pedunculated at times.
♦ It is rare in children.
♦ Pain in lipoma may be due to neural element or compression to nerves or adjacent structures. Angiolipoma was being highly vascular is commonly tender.
♦ Trunk is the most common site; nape of neck and limbs are next common.
♦ Clinically lipoma can be single, multiple or diffuse.

Differential Diagnosis

♦ *Neurofibroma:* It moves horizontally but not longitudinally along the line of nerve. Neurofibroma is firmer.
♦ Cystic swellings like dermoid, sebaceous cyst.
♦ *Liposarcoma:* All lipomas are benign. Large lipoma should be differentiated from liposarcoma.

Investigations

♦ Ultrasound or CT or MR imaging is done in deep or large or intracavitary lipomas.
♦ FNAC or incision biopsy is needed in large or deep or intracavitary lipomas to confirm it as benign.

Complications

♦ Myxomatous changes—occurs in retroperitoneal lipoma.
♦ Saponification
♦ Calcification—11% mineralization.
♦ Submucosal lipoma can cause intussusception and so intestinal obstruction.

Treatment

♦ Excision should be done if lipomas are painful. Small lipoma is excised under local anesthesia and larger one under general anesthesia.

♦ Percutaneous liposuction is relatively new treatment option

Q.14. Discuss differential diagnosis of submandibular swelling. *(Dec 2010, 8 Marks)*

Ans. Differential diagnosis of submandibular swellings. Submandibular swellings are of three types, i.e.:

♦ **Acute**
  • **Stones:** *Refer to Ans. 6 of chapter SALIVARY GLAND*
  • **Stenosis:** Most commonly occur as complication of Ludwig's angina
  • **Sialectasia:** It is an aseptic dilatation of salivary ductules causing grape like dilatation.
      It present as a smooth, soft, fluctuant, non-transilluminating swelling which increases in size during mastication. It is tender initially. It last for many days being asymptomatic.
  • **Acute lymphadenitis:** Very often, poor oral hygiene or a caries tooth produces painful, tender, soft enlargement of these lymph nodes. Extraction of tooth or with improvement of oral hygiene, lymph nodes regress.

♦ **Recurrent acute**
  • Stones
  • Stenosis
  • Sialectasis.

♦ **Chronic**
  • Sialosis
  • Autoimmune diseases
  • Neoplasms.

Chronic tuberculous lymphadenitis: Can affect these nodes along with upper deep cervical lymph nodes. These nodes are firm and matted.

Secondaries in the submandibular lymph node arises from carcinoma of cheek, tongue, palate. The nodes are hard with or without fixity.

Non-Hodgkin's lymphoma: It can involve submandibular lymph nodes along with horizontal group of lymph nodes in neck. The nodes are firm and rubbery in consistency.

Q.15. Describe different types of odontomes and their management. *(Oct 2003, 15 Marks)*

Ans. Odontome is defined as "tumor formed by an overgrowth of complete dental tissue". **—Broca**

In WHO classification of odontogenic tumors (2017) odontomes are classified as benign mixed epithelial and mesenchymal odontogenic tumor. Under this heading two types of odontomas are there:

♦ Complex odontoma
♦ Compound odontoma.

Compound Odontome

It is defined as "A tumor like malformation (hamartoma) with varying numbers of tooth like elements (odontoids)".

—WHO

Pathogenesis

It is produced by repeated divisions of tooth germ or by multiple budding off from dental lamina with formation of many tooth germs.

Clinical Features

♦ It is a painless slow growing lesion.
♦ It occurs commonly in maxilla in incisor-canine region.
♦ Male and females are equally affected.
♦ It is seen during 2nd and 3rd decades of life.
♦ At times permanent teeth fails to erupt.

Radiographic Features

Compound odontoma appears as collection of tooth-like structures surrounded by radiolucent zone.

Management

♦ Surgical removal by enucleation is the treatment of choice.
♦ Odontomas can be approached by intraoral mucosal incision and removal of adequate overlying bone to expose lesion.
♦ Removal of entire soft tissue portion is recommended to prevent recurrence.

Complex Odontome

It is defined as "a tumor like malformation (hamartoma) in which enamel and dentin and sometimes cementum is present".

—WHO

Pathogenesis

It develops from dental lamina or enamel organ in place of normal tooth.

Clinical Features

♦ Painless slowly growing lesions.
♦ They form hard masses.
♦ Mandible is more frequently affected.
♦ When the lesion becomes large it leads to expansion of bone and facial symmetry.
♦ Adjacent teeth may be displaced.

Radiographic Features

It appear as irregular dense radiopaque mass surrounded by thin radiolucent area overlying displaced unerupted tooth.

Management

♦ Enucleation or curettage is done if odontoma is source of obstruction to erupting teeth.
♦ Large complex odontomas should be cut in segments for removal in order to conserve normal bone and prevent jaw fracture.

Q.16. Write brief on odontomes. *(Dec 2010, 5 Marks) (Dec 2009, 5 Marks)*

Ans. *Refer to Ans. 15 of same chapter.*

Q.17. Write in brief tumors of tongue. *(Dec 2009, 5 Marks)*

Ans. Following are the tumors of tongue:

Benign

♦ Fibroma
♦ Granular cell myoblastoma
♦ Glomus tumor
♦ Leiomyoma
♦ Rhabdomyoma
♦ Neurofibroma
♦ Keratoacanthoma
♦ Traumatic neuroma
♦ Papilloma
♦ Pyogenic granuloma
♦ Adenoma
♦ Hemangioma
♦ Lymphangioma

Malignant

♦ Squamous cell carcinoma
♦ Adenocarcinoma
♦ Transitional cell carcinoma
♦ Verrucous carcinoma
♦ Mucoepidermoid carcinoma
♦ Reticular cell carcinoma
♦ Lymphosarcoma
♦ Angiosarcoma
♦ Kaposi's sarcoma
♦ Melanoma
♦ Rhabdomyosarcoma.

Benign Tumors

♦ **Fibroma:** It is a painless, sessile, dome-shaped or pedunculated lesion with smooth contour. On tongue it is present as circumscribed nodule. Color of tumor is pink and its surface is smooth consistency ranges from soft to firm and elastic.
♦ **Granular cell myoblastoma:** It occur over the dorsum of tongue. It is single, firm, submucosal nodule which is present within the substance of tongue.
♦ **Glomus tumor:** It is present over dorsum of tongue. Lesion is small usually <1 cm. Color of lesion ranges from red to purple. It is tender.
♦ **Leiomyoma:** It is present in circumvallate papillae of tongue. It is a slow-growing painless lesion which is mostly pedunculated.
♦ **Rhabdomyoma:** It is a well circumscribed tumor mass, painless and growth is slow.
♦ **Neurofibroma:** It has diffuse involvement over tongue. Sessile or pedunculated elevated small nodules of various sizes are present. Due to its diffuse involvement it leads to macroglossia.
♦ **Keratoacanthoma:** Lesion is tender, present as an elevated umblicated or crateriform with depressed central core which represent plug of keratin.
♦ **Neuroma:** It presents as small swelling or nodule over the tongue.

♦ **Papilloma:** It is an exophytic lesion with cauliflower-like surface. Projections are pointed or blunt. Appearance is due to presence of deep clefts.
♦ **Hemangioma:** Part of tongue or entire tongue is involved. Loss of mobility of tongue. Color of tumor is bluish.
♦ **Lymphangioma:** It involves dorsal and ventral surfaces of tongue. Presence of irregular nodularity over surface of tongue with grape-like projections which are gray and pink in color.

Malignant Tumors

♦ **Squamous cell carcinoma:** Nonhealing ulcer present over the tongue. Edges of ulcer are everted and base is indurated. Ulcer bleeds on touch.
♦ **Transitional cell carcinoma:** Lesion arises from the base of tongue. Lesion is ulcerated with granular eroded appearance.
♦ **Malignant melanoma:** A deep pigmented area is seen over the tongue which is ulcerated and hemorrhagic.
♦ **Verrucous carcinoma:** Pebbly surface is present which is keratinized. Have rugae like folds with cleft in between.

Q.18. Write short note on cavernous lymphangioma.

(Dec 2010, 5 Marks)

Ans. It is a congenital localized cluster of dilated lymph sacs in the skin and subcutaneous tissue that has failed to join the normal lymph system during development period.

Clinical Features

♦ It is present at birth.
♦ It is common on face, mouth, lips and tongue.
♦ Disfigurement is present over the child which is noticed by his/her parents.
♦ Lesion is soft, lobulated and is fluctuant.
♦ It is a brilliant transilluminant larger lymphatic swelling with multiple communicating lymphatic cysts.
♦ It often extends in deeper plane like muscle. It is common on face, mouth, lips and tongue.

Differential Diagnosis

♦ *Hemangioma:* It occurs at posterior triangle of neck. Hemangioma is soft, cystic and fluctuant. Its transillumination is negative and sign of compressibility is positive.
♦ *Lipoma:* It is a soft lobular swelling with fluctuation. While palpating edge of lipoma slips between palpating fingers. Both transillumination and compressibility tests are negative.
♦ *Cold abscess:* It is a soft, cystic, fluctuant swelling with negative transillumination. It is located at the carotid triangle.

Management

♦ Surgical excision of lesion is done for removing complete bulk of lesion. All the loculi or cysts should be removed.

♦ As lymphangioma extends to the muscle plane, to avoid recurrence careful examination should be done.

Complications

♦ As the size of lymphangioma is large, it can lead to difficulty in breathing in both neonates and infants.
♦ Secondary infection can occur in lymphangioma
♦ In mediastinum it can lead to dyspnea, dysphagia because of compression of trachea.

Q.19. Write short note on oral submucous fibrosis.

(Aug 2011, 5 Marks)

Or

Write in brief on submucous fibrosis.

(Feb 2013, 5 Marks)

Ans. *Refer to Ans. 2 of same chapter.*

Q.20. Write short note on acute laryngitis.

(Aug 2011, 5 Marks)

Ans. Acute laryngitis may occur as an isolated infection or as a part of a generalized bacterial or viral upper respiratory tract infection.

Etiology

♦ Infection, i.e., viral
♦ Excessive use of voice, i.e., in teaching, public speaking, singing
♦ Leisure activities, such as cheering at sport event
♦ Inhalation of smoke or fumes
♦ Aspiration of caustic chemicals.

Clinical Features

♦ It begins with hoarseness of voice.
♦ Pain is present while speaking or swallowing.
♦ Presence of dry cough
♦ Fever, malaise, restlessness and dyspnea
♦ Shortness of breadth
♦ Throat clearing
♦ Laryngeal edema.

Treatment

♦ Primary treatment involves resting of voice.
♦ For viral infection symptomatic care includes an analgesic and throat lozenges for pain relief.
♦ Bacterial infections require antibiotic therapy, i.e., 250 mg of cefuroxime twice daily.
♦ Severe acute laryngitis requires hospitalization.
♦ When laryngeal edema results in airway obstruction tracheostomy should be done.

Q.21. Discuss briefly stridor. *(May/Jun 2009, 5 Marks)*

Or

Write briefly on stridor. *(Aug 2011, 5 Marks)*

Ans. Stridor is an abnormal, high-pitched sound produced by turbulent airflow through a partially obstructed airway at the level of the supraglottis, glottis, subglottis, and/or trachea.

♦ Stridor is a symptom, not a diagnosis or disease, and the underlying cause must be determined.

♦ Stridor may be inspiratory, expiratory, or biphasic depending on its timing in the respiratory cycle.
♦ Inspiratory stridor suggests a laryngeal obstruction, while expiratory stridor implies tracheobronchial obstruction.
♦ Biphasic stridor suggests a subglottic or glottic anomaly.
♦ In addition to a complete history and physical, as well as other possible additional studies, most cases require flexible and/or rigid endoscopy to adequately evaluate the etiology of stridor.

Pathophysiology

Gases produce pressure equally in all directions; however, when a gas moves in a linear direction, it produces pressure in the forward vector and decreases the lateral pressure. When air passes through a narrowed flexible airway in a child, the lateral pressure that holds the airway open can drop precipitously (the Bernoulli principle) and cause the tube to close. This process obstructs airflow and produces stridor. Stridor may result from lesions involving the CNS, the cardiovascular system, the GI system, and the respiratory tract.

Etiology

Stridor may occur as a result of:

♦ Foreign bodies (e.g., aspirated foreign body, aspirated food bolus)
♦ Tumor (e.g., laryngeal papillomatosis, squamous cell carcinoma of larynx, trachea or esophagus)
♦ Acute lymphatic leukemia (ALL) (T-cell ALL can present with mediastinal mass that compresses the trachea and causes inspiratory stridor)
♦ Infections (e.g., epiglottitis, retropharyngeal abscess, croup)
♦ Subglottic stenosis (e.g., following prolonged intubation or congenital)
♦ Airway edema (e.g., following instrumentation of the airway, tracheal intubation, drug side effect, allergic reaction)
♦ Subglottic hemangioma (rare)
♦ Vascular rings compressing the trachea
♦ Many thyroiditis, such as Riedel's thyroiditis
♦ Vocal cord palsy
♦ Tracheomalacia or tracheobronchomalacia (e.g., collapsed trachea)
♦ Congenital anomalies of the airway are present in 87% of all cases of stridor in infants and children.
♦ Vasculitis.

Treatment

Medical Care

♦ Immediate tracheal intubation should be done.
♦ Expectant management with full monitoring, oxygen by facemask, and positioning the head on the bed for optimum conditions (e.g., 45–90°).
♦ Use of nebulized racemic adrenaline epinephrine (0.5–0.75 mL of 2.25% racemic epinephrine added to 2.5–3 mL of normal saline) in cases where airway edema may be the cause of the stridor.

- Use of dexamethasone (Decadron) 4–8 mg IV, 8–12 hourly in cases where airway edema may be the cause of the stridor; note that some time (in the range of hours) may be needed for dexamethasone to work fully.
- Use of inhaled Heliox (70% helium, 30% oxygen); the effect is almost instantaneous. Helium, being a less dense gas than nitrogen, reduces turbulent flow through the airways. Always ensure an open airway.
- In obese patients elevation of the panniculus has shown to relieve symptoms by 80%.

Surgical Care

- Certain conditions, such as severe laryngomalacia, laryngeal stenosis, critical tracheal stenosis, laryngeal and tracheal tumors and lesions (e.g., laryngeal papillomas, hemangiomas, others), and foreign body aspiration, require surgical correction.
- Occasionally, tracheotomy is done to protect the airway to bypass laryngeal abnormalities and stent or bypass tracheal abnormalities.
- Other conditions, such as retropharyngeal and peritonsillar abscess, may have to be dealt with on an emergent basis.

Q.22. Write briefly on lesions of lips. *(Dec 2009, 5 Marks)*

Ans. Following are the lesions of lips:

Developmental Lesions

- Congenital lip pits
- Commissural lip pits
- Double lip
- Cleft lip

Inflammatory Lesions

- Glandular cheilitis
- Angular cheilitis
- Granulomatous cheilitis
- Contact cheilitis
- Actinic cheilitis
- Eczematous cheilitis
- Exfoliative cheilitis
- Plasma cell cheilitis
- Cheilitis due to drugs

Lip Carcinoma

Miscellaneous

- Actinic elastosis
- Lip ulcers

Developmental Lesions of Lip

Congenital Lip Pits

- It is also known as congenital fistula.
- *Pathogenesis:* It occur due to failure of union of embryonic sulcus of lip which leads to persistent lateral sulci on embryonic mandibular arch.
- *Features:* It more commonly occurs in females; vermilion border of lip is commonly involved. Lower lip is involved;

lesion is present in form of depression; on palpation mucous secretion is seen from the base of lip pit.
- *Treatment:* Surgical excision is done.

Commissural Lip Pits

- They are mucosal invagination which arises at vermilion border of lip.
- *Pathogenesis:* Its occurrence is due to failure of normal fusion of embryonic maxillary and mandibular processes.
- *Features:* Males are commonly affected; it present as unilateral or bilateral pit at corners of mouth on vermilion border. Its size ranges from a shallow depression to an open tract measuring 4 mm; On palpation less amount of saliva ooze out.
- *Treatment:* Surgical excision is done.

Double Lip

- It is a fold of excessive tissue over inner mucosa of lip.
- *Pathogenesis:* It arises during second week of gestation because of persistence of sulcus between pars glabrosa and pars villosa of lip.
- *Features:* Inner aspect of lip is involved; at times when the upper lip become tensed, double lip give appearance of cupid bow.
- *Treatment:* Surgical excision is done.

Cleft Lip

- Cleft lip results from abnormal development of the median nasal and maxillary process.
- *Pathogenesis:* This is due to imperfect fusion of maxillary process with median nasal process which produce lateral cleft lip and due to failure of fusion of two median nasal processes which produce central cleft lip.
- *Features:* Patient has difficulty in sucking; defective speech is present, i.e., patient is unable to speak word, such as B, F, M, P and V.
- *Treatment:* Millard's criteria is use to undertake surgery for cleft lip, i.e., Rule of ten, i.e., 10 pound in weight; 10 weeks old; 10 g% hemoglobin; Millard cleft repair by rotating local nasolabial flaps; proper postoperative management, such as control of infection, training for sucking, swallowing and speech.

Inflammatory Lesions of Lip

- *Glandular cheilitis:* Lower lip is mostly affected and the lip become enlarged, become firm and get everted. It mainly occurs due to sun exposure.
- *Angular cheilitis:* In it cracking of lips is seen from the corners. Main cause is nutritional deficiency.
- *Actinic cheilitis:* It is a premalignant lesion. Occurs due to sun exposure. Lower lip is mostly affected. Lip become dry and scaly. If scales are removed bleeding points are seen.

Lip Carcinoma

Vermilion border of lip and mucosa is the main site of carcinoma of lip. It is common in the western elderly, white people, especially those people exposed to sunlight.

Clinical Features

♦ Elderly males are affected in 90% of cases.
♦ Nonhealing ulcer or growth is a common presentation.
♦ Lesion appears in the form of white plaque of nonhealing ulcers.
♦ Edges are everted and indurated, this is characteristic of carcinoma.
♦ Ulcer contain slough in floor.
♦ Bleeding may occur from ulcer.
♦ Pain and paresthesia may occur.
♦ Lesion may get fixed to the subcutaneous structure of lip.
♦ Ulcer spreads and destroys the tissue of lip and chin.
♦ Submental and submandibular lymph nodes are involved, lymph node becomes hard and may be fixed.

Treatment

♦ If lesion is <2 cm, then curative radiotherapy, either brachytherapy or external beam radiotherapy. It gives a good cure.
♦ If tumor is >2 cm, wide excision is done. Excision of lower lip up to one-third can be sutured primarily, in layers keeping vermilion border in proper apposition without causing any microstomia.
♦ Excision of more than one-third of the lip requires reconstruction using different flaps.

Q.23. Write short note on stridor and its emergency treatment. *(Aug 2012, 5 Marks)*

Ans. *Refer to Ans. 21 of same chapter.*

Q.24. Write short note on tongue tie. *(Aug 2012, 5 Marks)*

Ans. It is also known as ankyloglossia.

Ankyloglossia is the condition which arises when the inferior frenulum attaches to the bottom of tongue and subsequently restricts free movements of the tongue.

Clinical Features

♦ Males are affected more commonly than females
♦ It can cause feeding problems in infants
♦ Tongue movements become restricted.
♦ It causes speech defects especially articulation of the sounds l,r,t,d,n,th,sh and z
♦ It leads to persistent gap between the mandibular incisors.
♦ When attempt is made for sticking the tongue out a V shaped notch is seen at the tip of tongue.
♦ As high frenal attachment is present and patient has periodontal problems.
♦ During protrusion, lateral margin and tip of tongue is everted with dorsal mid part heaping.

Management

Tongue tie should be treated surgically under the local anesthesia.

Procedure

♦ Local anesthesia should be given to the patient.
♦ Retract the tongue and held the tongue by traction suture. This makes frenum taut and easily visible for surgical release.

♦ Take a sharp scissor and made a cut of 1–2 cm midway between the tip of tongue and lingual surface of mandible. Cut should be given in such a way that blade of scissor should be parallel to floor of mouth.
♦ Place a hemostat across frenal attachment at base of tongue and keep it clamped for 3 minutes. This provide bloodless field for surgery.
♦ As hemostat is removed, place an incision through area of previously closed hemostat.
♦ Care should be taken not to injure submandibular duct, papilla and blood vessels under floor of mouth.
♦ Wound margins are carefully undermined should be approximated and closed without tension, i.e., in linear fashion.

Q.25. Describe diagnostic features and treatment of aphthous ulcers of tongue. *(Jan 2012, 5 Marks)*

Ans.

Diagnostic Features

Diagnosis of aphthous ulcers is made on basis of clinical examination:

♦ **Minor aphthous ulcers:** Painful round ulcer with yellow base and red margins. Size of the lesion is 0.4–1 cm.
♦ **Major aphthous ulcers:** Large and deep ulcers. Size may reach to 5 cm. They restrict the mobility of tongue and uvula.
♦ **Herpetiform aphthous ulcers:** These ulcer are numerous and very painful. They are small 1–2 mm in diameter. They occur in crops.

Treatment

♦ **Minor aphthous ulcers:** Topical corticosteroid ointment is applied over ulcer 4–5 times a day. Nutritional supplements should be given. Oral hygiene should be maintained.
♦ **Major aphthous ulcer:** Chlorhexidine gluconate should be given. Triamcinolone acetate is locally applied, choline salicylate gel is given.
♦ **Herpetiform aphthous ulcer:** Nutritional supplements should be given. Oral hygiene should be maintained. Chlorhexidine or tetracycline mouthwash will lead to rapid heading.

Q.26. Write short note on myeloid epulis. *(Apr 2015, 3 Marks)*

Ans. It is also known as giant cell epulis.

Origin

Two views are given over the origin of myeloid epulis:

1. It is an osteoclastoma arising from the peripheral part of jaw and so present under the gums.
2. It is an inflammatory hyperplasia. Granuloma extends in the body of bone where it produces cyst-like structure and is surrounded by shell of bone giving the pseudo appearance of osteoclastoma.

Clinical Features

♦ Myeloid epulis is found on gingival margin between teeth anterior to permanent molars.

- Swelling is round, soft and is maroon or purplish in color.
- Tumor is painless.
- Its consistency is firm and surface is smooth.

Investigations

- After doing biopsy on microscopical examination there is presence of fibrous tissue with rich vascularity and giant cells of foreign body type.
- X-ray examination shows typical soap bubble appearance of osteoclastoma.

Complications

- Ulceration
- Serious hemorrhage

Treatment

- If swelling is small the treatment is curettage along with filling the cavity with cancellous bone chips.
- If tumor is large radical excision of bone is done along with the grafting.

Q.27. Define, describe clinical features and principles of treatment of leukoplakia. *(Jan 2017, 5 Marks)*

Ans. Leukoplakia is defined as a white patch or plaque that cannot be characterized clinically or pathologically as any other disease and is not associated with any physical or chemical causative agent except use of tobacco. First International Conference on oral leukoplakia Malmo, Sweden (1984) or Modified WHO Definition (1984).

Clinical Features

- Usually the lesion occurs in 4th, 5th, 6th and 7th decades of life.
- Buccal mucosa and commissural areas are most frequent affected sites followed by alveolar ridge, tongue, lip, hard and soft palate, etc.
- Oral leukoplakia often present solitary or multiple white patches.
- The size of lesion may vary from small well localized patch measuring few millimeters in diameter.
- The surface of lesion may be smooth or finely wrinkled or even rough on palpation and lesion cannot be removed by scrapping.
- The lesion is whitish or grayish or in some cases it is brownish yellow in color due to heavy use of tobacco.
- In most of the cases these lesion are asymptomatic, however in some cases they may cause pain, feeling of thickness and burning sensation, etc.

Principles of Treatment

- Take thorough history and do proper clinical examination.
- Remove the causative factor
- Excisional or incisional biopsy should be done.
- Manage the lesion by oral medication or by eliminating the lesion
- Long-term follow up should be done at every 3 months interval.
- At each review submandibular and cervical lymph nodes should be checked for signs of metastasis.

Q.28. Name cysts and tumors of "lower jaw" with diagnostic features and method to treat them. *(Jan 2017, 20 Marks)*

Ans. Cysts of lower jaw (see below Table).

Name of cyst in lower jaw	Diagnostic features	Methods to treat
Dentigerous cyst	• *Clinical diagnosis:* Expansion of swelling in posterior area of mandible • *Radiological:* Presence of well defined radiolucency associated with impacted teeth with hyperostotic border • *Laboratory diagnosis:* It is usually composed of thin connective tissue wall with a thin layer of stratified squamous epithelium lining the lumen. Rete peg formation is absent except in case of secondarily infected cyst. Connective tissue wall is frequently quite thickened and composed of very loose fibrous connective tissue. Inflammatory cells commonly infiltrate connective tissue. It also shows Rushton bodies within the lining epithelium which are peculiar linear and often curved hyaline bodies	• *Surgical removal:* Small lesions are enucleated. Larger lesions undergo surgical drainage along with marsupialization. • *Decompression:* Short section of rubber is placed in preformed surgical opening in cyst which remains open and allows the drainage.
Odontogenic keratocyst	• *Radiological diagnosis:* Extension of radiolucency in anteroposterior direction along with the undulating border • *Laboratory diagnosis:* Presence of corrugated or wrinkled parakeratin surface. Presence of prominent palisaded basal cell layer having picket fence or tombstone appearance. Connective tissue shows satellite or daughter cysts	• *Enucleation:* Enucleation is done with vigorous curettage • *Peripheral osteotomy:* It is done in bony cavity to reduce the chances of recurrence • *Chemical cauterization:* Chemical cauterization of bony cavity along with intraluminal injection of carnoy's solution is done which leads to the freezing of cyst from bony wall which allow easier removal of cyst • *Decompression:* This is done by polyethylene drainage tube which is kept inside the bony cavity

Contd...

Contd...

Name of cyst in lower jaw	Diagnostic features	Methods to treat
Paradental cyst	• *Radiological features:* Radiolucency is present which is distal to the third molar with intact PDL space • *Laboratory diagnosis:* Proliferating, nonkeratinized squamous epithelium lines the cyst. Fibrous capsule consists of mixed or chronic inflammation	Surgical enucleation is done
Solitary bone cyst	• *Radiological diagnosis:* Presence of well-defined radiolucency with vital tooth and there is history of trauma. • *Laboratory diagnosis:* Fragments of fibrin with enmeshed RBCs are seen. Hemorrhage and hemosiderin pigments are seen	• Enucleation or curettage should be done. • Intralesional steroid injection proved to be successful
Mandibular buccal infected cyst	• *Clinical diagnosis:* Patient is young, site is mandibular molar, buccal periostitis, vital pulp is present • *Radiological diagnosis:* Lamina dura is intact with expansion of buccal cortical plates	Enucleation of cyst is done without removing the associated tooth
Lateral periodontal cyst	• *Clinical diagnosis:* Normal color swelling visible at canine or premolar region • *Radiological:* Oval-shaped radiolucency present between roots of teeth along with hyperostotic borders • *Laboratory diagnosis:* Cyst is lined by the stratified squamous epithelium with connective tissue wall. Lumen of cyst shows focal thickened plaque of proliferating lining cell	Surgical excision is done along with removal of the offending tooth
Gingival cyst of adult	• *Clinical diagnosis:* Presence of blue color swelling of gingiva. It is dome shaped. • *Radiological:* Bony erosion is evident • *Laboratory diagnosis:* Cyst is lined by the stratified squamous epithelium with connective tissue wall. Lumen of cyst shows focal thickened plaque of proliferating lining cell	Surgical excision of the lesion is done
Dental lamina cyst	• *Clinical diagnosis:* Soft tissue elevation is present on alveolar ridge in infant which is white in color • *Laboratory diagnosis:* Presence of thin epithelial lining, shows lumen filled with desquamated keratin	No treatment is needed
Glandular odontogenic cyst	• *Radiological features:* Presence of multilocular appearance with scalloped margin • *Laboratory diagnosis:* Histologically, a cystic space is present lined by nonkeratinized epithelium. Mucus as well as cylindrical cells form part of epithelial component with mucinous material in cystic space	Enucleation or curettage should be done

Tumors of Lower Jaw

Name of tumor in lower jaw	Diagnostic features	Methods to treat
Ameloblastic fibroma	• *Radiological diagnosis:* CT scan can be helpful • *Laboratory diagnosis:* Presence of scattered islands of epithelial cell in a rosette form. Cells are present which resemble like ameloblasts. Mesenchymal component is of primitive connective tissue	Aggressive surgical excision should be carried out
Calcifying epithelial odontogenic tumor	• *Radiological diagnosis:* Typical snow driven appearance is present • *Laboratory diagnosis:* Presence of polyhedral epithelial cells present in large sheets. Calcification is present in form of Liesegang rings	Conservative surgical excision is done or simple enucleation can also be done
Dentinoma	• *Radiological diagnosis:* Presence of radiopaque mass along with crown of tooth • *Laboratory diagnosis:* Presence of irregular dentin in biopsy which is known as dentinoid	Surgical excision is done along with thorough curettage
Complex odontomea	• *Radiological diagnosis:* It shows disorganized mass of tooth structure. • *Laboratory diagnosis:* Mature tubular dentin is seen in biopsy	Local surgical excision is done
Ameloblastoma	• *Clinical diagnosis:* Presence of swelling in the posterior mandible along with bony expansion and egg shell crackling • *Radiological diagnosis:* Presence of characteristic honeycomb appearance, soap bubble appearance in posterior mandible along with bony expansion	Ameloblastomas are best treated by resection of the lesion with a marginal clearance of 1.5–2 cm of normal bone to prevent recurrence.

Contd...

Contd...

Name of tumor in lower jaw	Diagnostic features	Methods to treat
	• *Laboratory diagnosis:* Histopathologically various types of ameloblastomas are identified, i.e., follicular (islands of tumor cells with peripheral layer of cuboidal and columnar ameloblast like cells), plexiform (presence of network of interconnecting strands of cells, bounded by layer of columnar cells and between these layers stellate reticulum like cells are present), acanthomatous type, granular type, basal type and unicystic.	The lesion may be resected as block resection with or without continuity defect based on the integrity of inferior cortex. Radiologically, a minimum of 1 cm residual mandible inferior cortex is required postoperatively to prevent pathologic fracture. Inferior alveolar nerve should be sacrificed if it lies within the lesion.
Squamous odontogenic tumor	• *Radiological diagnosis:* Presence of semicircular radiolucency between the roots • *Laboratory diagnosis:* Histopathology shows presence of islands of squamous epithelium without peripheral palisaded polarized columnar cells	Conservative enucleation along with curettage is done
Odontogenic myxoma	• *Clinical diagnosis:* Presence of missing tooth along with hard swelling is suggestive of this disease • *Radiological diagnosis:* Tennis racquet pattern is characteristic. • *Laboratory diagnosis:* Presence of loosely arranged spindle shaped as well as stellate cells majority of which have long fibrillar process that tend to intermesh	Surgical excision is done along with resection of proper amount of bone
Peripheral odontogenic fibroma	• *Clinical diagnosis:* Attachment of sessile mass to gingiva • *Laboratory diagnosis:* Histopathology shows cellular fibrous connective tissue parenchyma along with the nonneoplastic islands, strands and cords of columnar or cuboidal cells	Surgical excision is done
Granular cell odontogenic tumor	• *Radiological diagnosis:* Inside the unilocular radiolucency calcification is seen. • *Laboratory diagnosis:* Histopathology show large eosinophilic granular cells. Small islands of odontogenic epithelium are scattered in area of granular cells.	Simple curettage is done
Periapical cemental dysplasia	• *Radiological diagnosis:* In early stage there is presence of radiolucency at apex of vital teeth with no loss of lamina dura. In mature stage radiopaque lesion is visible • *Laboratory diagnosis:* Histopathology shows periapical bone is replaced by the mass of fibrous tissue, various small round to oval calcifications are seen in fibrous tissue	Surgical excision of large lesions should be carried out
Benign cementoblastoma	• *Radiological diagnosis:* Surrounding of radiopaque lesion by radiolucent capsule attached to root surface. • *Laboratory diagnosis:* In histopathology there is presence of cementum like tissue which is deposited in globular pattern	Surgical excision of tumor along with the involved tooth Surgical excision of tumor mass along with root amputation and endodontic treatment is done

Q.29. Write long answer on types and causes of oral ulcer and their treatment. *(Apr 2018, 5 Marks)*

Ans. Aphthous ulcer is the most common type of nontraumatic, ulcerative condition of the oral mucosa.

Types of Oral Ulcer

Clinically, aphthous ulcers present three recognizable forms, namely:

1. Minor aphthous ulcers
2. Major aphthous ulcers
3. Herpetiform ulcers.

Minor Apthous Ulcer

♦ It is the most common type of aphthous ulcer of the oral cavity and it appears episodically either as single lesion or in clusters of 1–5 lesions.

♦ The ulcers are very painful, shallow, round or elliptical in shape and they measure about 0.5 cm in diameter with a crateriform margin.

♦ The lesion is usually surrounded by an erythematous "halo" and is covered by a yellowish, fibrinous membrane.

♦ Minor aphthous ulcers mostly develop over the nonkeratinized mucosa, e.g., lips, soft palate, anterior fauces, floor of the mouth and ventral surface of the tongue (gland bearing mucosa), etc.

♦ The ulcer lasts for about 7–10 days and then heals up without scarring but recurrence is common.

♦ New lesions may continue to appear during an attack for about 3–4 weeks period.

♦ Few lesions may be present in the mouth almost continuously.

Major Apthous Ulcers

♦ Major aphthous ulcers are less common than the minor form of the disease.

- These are larger, 0.5 cm in diameter and can be as big as several centimeters in diameter.
- Major aphthous ulcers are more painful lesions than the minor variety; and they persist in the mouth for longer durations as they take more time to heal.
- These lesions are considered to be the most severe among all types of aphthous and they often make the patients ill.
- Only one or two lesions develop at a time and are mostly seen over the lips, soft palate and fauces, etc. Besides involving the non-keratinzed mucosa, major aphthous ulcers can involve the masticatory mucosa as well, such as the dorsum of the tongue and gingiva, etc.
- The ulcer appears crateriform (owing to its increased depth), and it heals with scar formation in about 6 weeks time.
- Few lesions may look like malignant ulcers, moreover sometimes these lesions occur in association with HIV infections.
- Major aphthous ulcers often become secondarily infected and in such cases, the healing process is further delayed.

Herpetiform Ulcers

- Herpetiform type of aphthous ulcers produce recurrent crops of extremely painful, small ulcers in the oral mucosa, which resemble herpetic ulcers. However, these ulcers do not develop following vesiculations and exhibit no virus infected cells.
- Their numbers vary from few dozens to several hundreds and each ulcer is surrounded by a wide zone of erythema.
- Size of these ulcers ranges between 1–2 mm in diameter only. However on few occasions, small ulcers coalesce together to form large irregular ulcers.
- The ulcers last for several weeks or months.
- Children in their late teens often suffer from this disease and the lesions occur in both gland bearing mucosa as well as over keratinized mucosa.
- The lesions usually heal up within 1–2 week time.

Causes of Oral Ulcer

The exact etiology is not known and only the probable factors have been identified which are as follows:

- *Genetic predisposition:* The disease often affects several members of the same family and moreover identical twins are most frequently affected.
- *Exaggerated response to trauma:* The ulcer develops in those mucosal sites which are subjected to trauma in the past., e.g., tooth prick injury.
- *Immunological factors:* The disease may occur due to some autoimmune reactions, or in patients with immunosuppression, e.g., AIDS. Some investigators believe, then it is an immune complex-mediated type III or cell mediated type IV reaction.
- *Microbiologic factors:* The disease may be caused by herpes simplex virus type I or *S. sanguinis*.
- *Nutritional factors:* Deficiency of vitamin B12, folate and iron, etc., often reported in patients with aphthous ulcer; moreover supplementation of these elements may cause rapid recovery.

- *Systemic conditions:* Behcet's syndrome, Crohn's disease and celiac disease are associated with increased incidences of aphthous ulcer.
- *Hormonal imbalance:* Hormonal change during menstrual cycle may be associated with higher incidence of aphthous ulcer.
- *Non-smoking:* The disease almost exclusively occurs in nonsmokers or the people those who have given up smoke recently.
- *Allergy and chronic asthma:* Allergic manifestations to any medicines or foods (e.g., nuts and chocolates, etc.) may lead to the development of aphthous ulcer.
- *Miscellaneous factors:* Stress and anxiety.

Treatment

Medicinal Treatment

- Topical corticosteroid, i.e., 0.1% triamcinolone acetonide QDS is effective on daily use.
- Topical anesthetics, i.e., 2% viscous lidocaine, benzocaine and benzydamine hydrochloride can reduce pain. Topical protective emollient base can be given.
- Topical application of sucralfate 4 times a day has soothing effect on an ulcer.
- Topical tetracycline mouthwash QDS for 5–7 days provides good response.
- Beclomethasone spray is given in severe cases.
- In resistant cases systemic steroids can be given. Most commonly beclomethasone or prednisolone syrup in swish and swallow method is advised. In some cases prednisolone tablet 20–30 mg/day and beclomethasone 2–3 mg per day for 4–8 days can be given.

Surgical Treatment

Laser Surgery

Surgical removal of apthous ulcer should also be used. Laser ablation shortens the duration and decreases the associated symptoms. CO_2 or Nd:YAG lasers are used. Laser treatment requires frequent visits.

Local Cauterization

Application of 0.5% hydrogen peroxide, 1–2% of silver nitrate or silver nitrate caustic stick represents several older therapeutic methods which reduce duration of solitary oral ulcer.

Q.30. Write short answer on premalignant conditions of oral cavity. *(Apr 2018, 3 Marks)*

Ans. The premalignant condition is defined as "A generalized state of body, which is associated with significantly increased risk of cancer development".

Following are the premalignant conditions of oral cavity:

- *Leukoplakia:* Its incidence in those who smoke or chew pan is 20% while its incidence in nonsmokers is 1%. Its incidence in turning malignancy is 4–10% which increases with age, duration of pan chewing and smoking.
  For details refer to Ans. 1 of same chapter.

♦ *Erythroplakia:* It is a red velvety lesion which has incidence of malignancy till around 15%. It is 17–20 times more potentially malignant than leukoplakia.

♦ *Oral submucus fibrosis:* 4.5–7.6% of oral submucus fibrosis cases turn into malignancy. *For details refer to Ans. 2 of same chapter.*

♦ *Syphilitic glossitis:* Tertiary syphilis leads to chronic superficial glossitis which leads to carcinoma of tongue. This is rare nowadays.

♦ *Dyskeratosis congenita:* Reticular atrophy, nail dystrophy and leukoplakia in oral cavity.

♦ *Sideropenic dysphagia:* It is common in Scandinavian females. It leads to atrophy of epithelium and become potentially malignant. Proper iron therapy controls the disease and reduces the risk.

♦ *Chronic hyperplastic candidiasis:* It is common in commissures of mouth and tongue. Dense plaque of leukoplakia is common with curdy white patches due to *Candida albicans* infection. It is treated by systemic anti-fungals or surgical excision or laser therapy.

♦ *Papilloma of tongue or cheek*

♦ *Discoid lupus erythematosus*

♦ *Oral lichen planus*

Q.31. Define precancerous lesions of oral cavity and its management. *(Feb 2019, 5 Marks)*

Ans. Precancerous lesion is defined as "morphologically altered tissue in which cancer is most likely to occur than in its apparently normal counterpart". **—WHO (1972)**

Precancerous Leisons

♦ Leukoplakia.
♦ Erythroplakia.
♦ Mucosal changes associated with smoking habits.
♦ Carcinoma in situ
♦ Bowen disease.
♦ Actinic keratosis, cheilitis and elastosis.

Name of precancerous lesion	Management
Leukoplakia	*For details refer to Ans. 1 of same chapter*
Erythroplakia	• *Removal of cause:* First of all elimination of the suspected irritant should be done. • *Surgical stripping:* Definitive treatment for erythroplakia is controversial. So conservative surgical approach, such as surgical stripping is done with minimal damage to the deep tissues. • *Destructive techniques:* Laser ablation, electrocoagulation and cryotherapy is effective. • Proper clinical follow up is done for every 3 months for first postoperative year and every 6 months for additional 4 years. After this an annual evaluation with thorough head and neck examination is done.

Contd...

Contd...

Name of precancerous lesion	Management
Carcinoma in situ	Lesion can be surgically excised, cauterized and even exposed to solid carbon dioxide.
Actinic keratosis	• Cryotherapy should be done with liquid nitrogen. • Other therapies, such as topical application of 5-fluorouracil, curettage, electrodessication or surgical excision is done.

Q.32. Enumerate causes of jaw swelling. Describe clinical features and management of admantinoma of mandible. *(Oct 2019, 5 Marks)*

Ans. *For cause of jaw swelling refer to Ans. 9 of same chapter.*

For clinical features and management of admantinoma of mandible refer to Ans. 6 of same chapter.

16. CLEFT LIP AND PALATE

Q.1. Write short note on cleft lip. *(June 2015, 5 Marks) (Jan 2012, 5 Marks) (May/June 2009, 5 Marks) (Dec 2007, 3 Marks) (Apr 2007, 5 Marks) (Mar 2016, 5 Marks)*

Or

Describe briefly cleft lip. *(Apr 2017, 5 Marks)*

Or

Write in short about cleft lip. *(July 2016, 5 Marks)*

Or

Write short answer on cleft lip. *(Apr 2017, 3 Marks)*

Or

Write short note on principle of management of cleft lip. *(Feb 2019, 5 Marks)*

Ans. Cleft lip results from abnormal development of the median nasal and maxillary process.

Causes

♦ Increase parenteral age.
♦ Infection during pregnancy.
♦ Smoking and steroid therapy during pregnancy.
♦ Trauma and psychological stress during pregnancy.

Types of Cleft Lip

♦ *Central:* It is very rare and occurs due to failure of fusion of two median nasal processes (hare lip).

♦ *Lateral:* It is the most common variety, there is a cleft between the frenum and the lateral part of the upper lip. This is due to imperfect fusion of maxillary process with median nasal process. Lateral variety can be unilateral or bilateral.

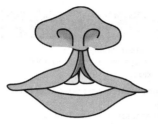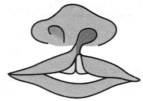

Fig. 20: Cleft lip.

- *Complete or incomplete:* In case of complete variety, cleft lip extend to the nose. In case of incomplete variety the cleft does not extend up to the nostrils.
- *Simple or compound:* Simple cleft lip is only cleft in the lip while compound refers to cleft lip associated with a cleft in the alveolus.

Clinical Features

- Patient has difficulty in sucking.
- Defective speech is present, i.e., patient is unable to speak word, such as B, F, M, P and V
- Presence of soft tissue mass in between the ends of bone which unite tongue to lip.
- In hare lip cleft lies in middle of lip.
- In incomplete cleft lip extension is from nostril to some distance forward
- In complete cleft lip extension is from nostril to palate.

Treatment

- Millard's criteria is use to undertake surgery for cleft lip, i.e., rule of ten, i.e., 10 pound in weight; 10 weeks old; 10 g% hemoglobin.
- If cleft lip is bilateral and is extensive two surgeries should be done to close the cleft. Surgery of one side should be done first and later on after few week surgery of second side is done.
- Millard's rotation advancement flap technique is commonly used. In this correction of both lip and nasal deformity is done. Realigning of muscles and of lip and their correct anatomical position is an important part of this repair. In this method a tilted cupid bow is rotated downwards following curved incision extending to columella. This allows rotation of misplace cupid's bow and philtral dimple in normal position. High rotation gap created is filled with triangular flap which consists of skin muscle and mucosa from upper part of lateral side of cleft. The resultant scar is hidden inside the nose or follows natural line of philtrum.
- *Hagedorn–LeMesurier repair:* In this method, medial lip element should be lengthened by introducing the quadrilateral flap which is developed from lateral lip element.
- *Tennison–Randall repair:* In this a cut is given on lower one-third of lip to correct upward tilt of cupid's bow by placing a Z-shape wire. Gap is filled with triangle of skin, muscle and mucosal flap from lower end of lateral lip element. In this resultant scar is Zigzag scar.

- Proper postoperative management, such as control of infection, training for sucking, swallowing and speech therapy should be done.

Principles of Cleft Lip Repair/Principles of Management of Cleft Lip

- Rule of 10 should be fulfilled.
- Before six months it should be operated.
- Infection should not be present.
- Millard advancement flap is used for unilateral cleft lip repair.
- Bilateral cleft lip repair can be done either in single or two stages.
- One stage bilateral cleft lip repair is done using Veau III method.
- Proper markings are made prior to surgery and incision should be over full thickness flap.
- Often 1:2,00,000 adrenalin injection is used to achieve hemostasis.
- Three layer lip repair should be done, i.e., mucosa, muscle and skin.
- Cupid's bow should be horizontal.
- Continuity of white line is maintained.
- Vermilion notching should not be present.

Q.2. Write short note on cleft palate. *(Feb 2015, 5 Marks)* *(2012, 5 Marks) (June 2010, 5 Marks)*

Ans. The palate is formed from the Y-shaped fusion of premaxilla and two palatine processes.

Imperfect fusion of these processes or developmental anomalies results in cleft palate.

Types

- **Complete cleft palate:**
  - Failure of fusion of palatine process and premaxilla result in complete cleft palate.
  - The nasal cavity and the mouth are interconnected.
  - This may be unilateral or bilateral.
- **Incomplete cleft palate:**
  - When the fusion of three component of palate takes place.
  - It starts from uvula and then backwards.
- **Various types:**
  - Bifid uvula
  - The whole length of soft palate is bifid.
  - The whole length of soft palate and posterior part of hard palate are involved.

Effects of Cleft Palate

- Interferers with swallowing and speech.
- Unable to make the constant sound, such as B, P, D, K and T.
- *Teeth:* Upper incisors may be small maxilla tends to be smaller. Teeth are crowded.
- *Nose:* Oral organisms contaminate the upper respiratory mucous membrane.
- *Hearing:* Even with repair, acute and chronic hearing problem can occur.

Management of Cleft Palate

♦ Cleft palate is usually repaired in 12–18 months. Early repair causes retarded maxillary growth. Late repair causes speech defect.
♦ Both soft and hard palates are repaired.
♦ Abnormal insertion of tensor palati is released. Mucoperiosteal flaps are raised in the palate which is sewed together.
♦ If maxillary hypoplasia is present, then osteotomy of the maxilla is done. With orthodontic teeth extraction and alignment of dentition is done.
♦ Regular examination of ear, nose and throat during follow-up period, i.e., postoperative speech therapy.
♦ Whenever complicated problems are present, staged surgical procedure is done.
♦ Wardill–Kilner push back operation or V–Y pushback palatoplasty by raising mucoperiosteum flaps based on greater palatine vessels.

V–Y Pushback Palatoplasty or Wardill–Kilner Pushback Palatoplasty

♦ In this palate is infiltrated by 1:2 adrenaline saline solution.
♦ Both mucoperiosteal flaps are raised, one from either side of palatal shelves and then nasal layers should be mobilized.
♦ Closure of palate is done in three layers, i.e., nasal layer, muscle layer and oral layer.
♦ In this procedure palatal lengthening is achieved by V–Y plasty. Hook of hamulus can be fractured to relieve tension on suture line by relaxing tensor palate muscle.

Secondary Management

♦ Hearing support is given using hearing aids if defect is present; control of otitis media.
♦ Speech problems occur due to velopharyngeal incompetence; articulation problems also can occur. Speech therapy is given. It is corrected by pharyngoplasty, veloplasty, speech devices.
♦ Dental problems, such as uneruption, unalignment are common. They should be corrected by proper dentist opinion, and reconstructive surgery.
♦ Orthodontic management with alveolar bone graft, maxillary osteotomy is done in 8–11 years.
♦ Veloplasty, dental implants, rhinoplasty, orthognathic surgeries, etc.

Q.3. Write short note on orthodontic treatment of cleft lip and palate. *(Sep 2004, 5 Marks)*

Ans. One of the clinical features common to cleft lip and palate is constricted and distorted maxillary arch. The severe the cleft, more severe the arch deformity due to collapse. Orthodontic treatment is necessary to correct the deformity.

Orthodontic treatment should be started during mixed dentition, and continued through the permanent dentition. Permanent teeth especially, those adjacent to cleft are malposed, often severely rotated, and poorly calcified. They certainly need to be orthodontia. If extracted, especially the supernumerary one.

Even with complete orthodontic treatment, there is maxillomandibular *discrepancy, which may need surgical correction in the form of maxillary advancement with or without mandibular pushback, with or without *genioplasty.

Q.4. Discuss about treatment of cleft palate. *(Mar 2008, 5 Marks)*

Ans. *Refer to Ans. 2 of same chapter.*

Q.5. Write about pathogenesis, classification, structural and functional problems of cleft lip and palate. Write note on principles of management. *(Feb 2013, 10 Marks)*

Ans.

Pathogenesis of Cleft Lip and Cleft Palate

♦ Cleft lip results from abnormal development of medial nasal process and maxillary process.
♦ Cleft palate occurs due to fusion of two palatine process.
♦ Defect in fusion of lines between premaxilla and palatine processes of maxilla one on each side.
♦ When premaxilla and both palatine processes do not fuse, it leads to complete cleft palate.
♦ Incomplete fusion of all three components lead to incomplete cleft palate.

Classification of Cleft Lip and Cleft Palate

Refer to Ans. 6 same chapter.

Functional and Structural Problems of Cleft Lip and Cleft Palate

♦ Difficulty in sucking and swallowing
♦ Speech is defective especially in cleft palate, mainly to phonate B,D,K,P,T and G
♦ Altered dentition or supernumerary teeth
♦ Recurrent upper respiratory tract infection
♦ Respiratory obstruction
♦ Hypoplasia of maxilla
♦ Cosmetic problem
♦ Chronic otitis media and middle ear problems.

Management of Cleft Lip and Cleft Palate

For management of cleft lip refer to Ans. 1 and for management of cleft palate refer to Ans. 2 of same chapter.

Q.6. Write briefly on classification of cleft lip and palate defects. *(Dec 2009, 5 Marks)*

Ans. Following are the classifications:

Davis and Ritchie (1922)

Group I: Prealveolar cleft
Group II: Postalveolar cleft
Group III: Alveolar cleft

Q3. *Discrepancy = An illogical or surprising lack of compatibility or similarity between two or more facts.
   *Genioplasty = Cosmetic surgery done on chin.

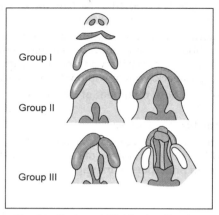

Fig. 21: Davis and Ritchie classification.

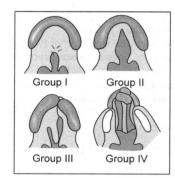

Fig. 22: Veau classification.

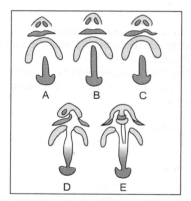

Fig. 23: Kernahan and Stark classification.

Veau (1931)

- *Group I:* Cleft of soft palate only
- *Group II:* Cleft of the hard and soft palate extending no further than the incisive foramen, thus involving the secondary palate alone.
- *Group III:* Complete unilateral cleft, extending from uvula to the incisive foramen, thus the uvula to the incisive foramen in the midline, then deviating to one side and usually extending through the alveolus at the position of the future lateral incisor tooth.

- *Group IV:* Complete bilateral cleft, resembling Group III with two clefts extending from the incisive foramen through the alveolus.

Kernahan and Stark (1958)

- Incomplete cleft of secondary palate
- Complete cleft of secondary palate
- Incomplete cleft of primary and secondary palate
- Unilateral complete cleft of primary and secondary palate.
- Bilateral complete cleft of the primary and secondary palate.

Harkins and Associates (1962)

- *Cleft or primary palate:*
  - Cleft lip
    - *Unilateral:* Right, left (extent; one-third, two-thirds, complete)
    - *Bilateral:* Right, left (extent: one-third, two-thirds, complete)
    - *Median* (extent: one-third, two-thirds, complete)
    - *Prolabium:* Small, medium, large
    - *Congenital scar:* Right, left, median (one-third, two-thirds, complete)
  - Cleft of alveolar process
    - *Unilateral:* Right, left (extent: one-third, two-thirds, complete)
    - *Bilateral:* Right, left (extent: one-third, two-thirds, complete)
    - *Median* (extent: one-third, two-thirds, complete)
    - *Submucous:* Right, left, median
    - Absent incisor tooth
- *Cleft of palate:*
  - Soft palate
    - *Posteroanterior:* One-third, two-thirds, complete
    - *Width:* Maximum
    - *Palatal shortness:* None, slight, moderate, marked
    - *Submucous cleft* (extent: one-third, two-thirds, complete)
  - Hard palate
    - *Posteroanterior* (extent: one-third, two-thirds, complete)
    - *Width:* Maximum (mm)
    - *Vomer attachment:* Right, left, absent
    - *Submucous cleft* (extent: one-third, two-thirds, complete)
- *Mandibular process clefts:*
  - *Lip extent:* One-third, two-thirds, complete
  - *Mandible* (extent: one-third, two-thirds, complete)
  Lip pits: Congenital lip sinuses
- *Naso-ocular:* Extending from the nasal region towards the medial canthus
- *Oro-ocular:* Extending from angle of the mouth towards the palpebral fissure
- *Oro-aural:* Extending from the angle of the mouth towards the tragus of ear.

Q.7. Describe the development of face and various congenital abnormalities of lip and palate.

(Dec 2010, 10 Marks)

Or

Write briefly on development of face.

(Feb 2013, 5 Marks)

Ans.

Development of Face

♦ Face is derived from the following structures that lie around the stomatodeum, i.e.:
  • Frontonasal process
  • The first pharyngeal (or mandibular) arch of each side.
♦ At this stage each mandibular arch forms the lateral wall of the stomatodeum.
♦ This arch gives off a bud from its dorsal end. This bud is called the maxillary process. It grows ventro-medially cranial to the main part of the arch which is now called the mandibular process.
♦ The ectoderm overlying the frontonasal process soon shows bilateral localized thickenings, that are situated a little above the stomatodeum. These are called the nasal placodes. The formation of these placodes is induced by the underlying forebrain. The placodes soon sink below the surface to form nasal pits.
♦ The pits are continuous with the stomatodeum below. The edges of each pit are raised above the surface. The medial raised edge is called the medial nasal process and the lateral edge is called the lateral nasal process.

Lower Lip

Mandibular processes of the two sides grow towards each other and fuse in the midline. They now form the lower margin of the stomatodeum. If it is remembered that the mouth develops from the stomatodeum, it will be readily understood that the fused mandibular processes give rise to the lower lip and to the lower jaw.

Upper Lip

Each maxillary process now grows medially and fuses, first with the lateral nasal process and then with the medial nasal process. The median and lateral nasal processes also fuse with each other. In this way the nasal pits are cut-off from stomatodeum. The maxillary processes undergo considerable growth. At the same time the frontonasal process becomes much narrower from side to side, with the result that the two external nares come close together.

The stomatodeum is now bounded above by the upper lip which is derived as follows:
♦ The mesodermal basis of the lateral part of the lip is formed from the maxillary process. The overlying skin is derived from ectoderm covering this process.
♦ The mesodermal basis of the median part of the lip (called philtrum) is formed from the frontonasal process. The ectoderm of the maxillary process however, overgrows this mesoderm to meet that of the opposite maxillary process in the midline. As a result, the skin of the entire upper lip is innervated by maxillary nerves.

The muscles of the face are derived from mesoderm of second branchial arch and are therefore supplied by the facial nerve.

Nose

Nose receives contributions from the frontonasal process, and from the medial and lateral nasal processes of the right and left sides. External nares are formed when the nasal pits are cut-off from the stomatodeum by the fusion of the maxillary process with the medial nasal process. External nares gradually approach each other. Mesoderm becomes heaped up in the median plane to form the prominence of the nose. Simultaneously, groove appears between the regions of the nose and the bulging forebrain. As the nose becomes prominent the external nares come to open downwards. The external form of the nose is thus established.

Cheeks

After the formation of the upper and lower lips, the stomatodeum (which can now be called the mouth) is very broad. In its lateral part, it is bounded above by the maxillary process and below by the mandibular process. These processes undergo progressive fusion with each other to form the cheeks.

Eye

The region of the eye is first seen as an ectodermal thickening, the lens placode, which appears on the ventrolateral side of the developing forebrain, lateral and cranial to the nasal placode.

The lens placode sinks below the surface and is eventually cut-off from the surface ectoderm. The developing eyeball produces a bulging in this situation. The bulging of the eyes are at first directed laterally and lie in the angles between the maxillary processes and the lateral nasal processes. With the narrowing of the frontonasal process they come to face forwards. The eyelids are derived from folds of ectoderm formed above and below the eyes, and by mesoderm enclosed within the folds.

External Ear

External ear is formed around the dorsal part of the first ectodermal cleft. A series of mesodermal thickenings (often called tubercles or hillocks) appear on the mandibular and hyoid arches where they adjoin this cleft. The pinna (or auricle) is formed by fusion of these thickenings.

Nasal Cavities

Nasal cavities are formed by extension of the nasal pits. These pits are at first in open communication with the stomatodeum. Soon the medial and lateral nasal processes fuse and form a partition between the pit and the stomatodeum. This is called the primitive palate and is derived from the frontonasal process.

The nasal pits now deepen to form the nasal sacs which expand both dorsally and caudally.

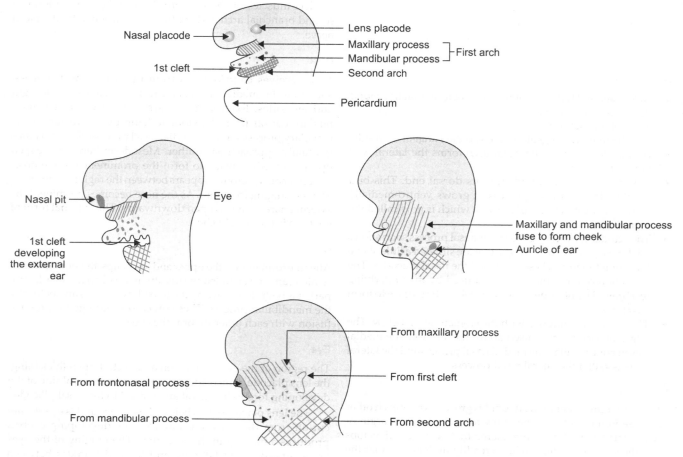

Fig. 24: Development of face.

The dorsal part of this sac is, at first, separated from the stomatodeum by a thin membrane called the bucconasal membrane (or nasal fin). This soon breaks down.

The nasal sac now has a ventral orifice that opens on the face (anterior or external nares) and a dorsal orifice that opens into the stomatodeum (primitive posterior nasal aperture).

The two nasal sacs are at first widely separated from one another by the frontonasal process. However, the frontonasal process becomes progressively narrower. This narrowing of the frontonasal process, and the enlargement of the nasal cavities themselves, bring them closer together.

This intervening tissue becomes much thinned to form the nasal septum.

The ventral part of the nasal septum is attached below to the primitive palate. More posteriorly the septum is at first attached to the bucconasal membrane, but on disappearance of this membrane it has a free lower edge. The nasal cavities are separated from the mouth by the development of the palate.

The lateral wall of the nose is derived, on each side, from the lateral nasal process. The nasal conchae appear as elevations on the lateral wall of each nasal cavity.

The original olfactory placodes form the olfactory epithelium that lies in the roof, and adjoining parts of thin walls, of the nasal cavity.

Congenital Abnormalities of Lip and Palate

Following are the congenital abnormalities of lip and palate:
♦ Congenital lip pits
♦ Commissural lip pits
♦ Double lip
♦ Cleft lip and cleft palate

Congenital Lip Pits

It is also known as congenital fistula.

Pathogenesis

It occurs due to failure of union of embryonic sulcus of lip which leads to persistent lateral sulci on embryonic mandibular arch.

Clinical Features

♦ It more commonly occurs in females.
♦ Vermilion border of lip is commonly involved. Lower lip is involved.
♦ Lips appear swollen

* Lesion is present in form of depression.
* On palpation mucous secretion is seen from the base of lip pit.

Treatment

Surgical excision is done.

Commissural Lip Pits

They are mucosal invagination which arises at vermilion border of lip.

Pathogenesis

Its occurrence is due to failure of normal fusion of embryonic maxillary and mandibular processes.

Clinical Features

* Males are commonly affected
* It present as unilateral or bilateral pit at corners of mouth on vermilion border
* Its size ranges from a shallow depression to an open tract measuring 4 mm
* On palpation less amount of saliva ooze out.

Treatment

Surgical excision is done.

Double Lip

It is a fold of excessive tissue over inner mucosa of lip.

Pathogenesis

It arises during second week of gestation because of persistence of sulcus between pars glabrosa and pars villosa of lip.

Clinical Features

* Inner aspect of lip is involved.
* At times when the upper lip become tensed, double lip give appearance of cupid bow.

Treatment

Surgical excision is done.

Cleft Lip and Cleft Palate

For cleft lip refer to Ans. 1 and for cleft palate refer to Ans. 2 of same chapter.

Q.8. Write short note on management of a case of unilateral cleft lip and palate repair. *(Apr 2015, 3 Marks)*

Ans.

Management of a Case of Unilateral Cleft Lip Repair

* For unilateral cleft lip repair most commonly used methods are Millard's rotation advancement flap and Tennison–Randall triangular flap method.
* Millard's cleft lip repair is done by rotating local nasolabial flaps.
* Majority of surgeons follow Millard criteria or "Rule of 10", i.e., at the time of repair hemoglobin should be >10 g%, age

is 10 weeks, weight is >10 pound and total leukocyte count is <10,000/cu mm.

Millard Rotation Advancement Flap

In this a tilted cupid bow is rotated downwards following curved incision extending to columella. This allows rotation of misplace cupid's bow and philtral dimple in normal position. High rotation gap created is filled with triangular flap which consists of skin muscle and mucosa from upper part of lateral side of cleft. The resultant scar is hidden inside the nose or follows natural line of philtrum.

Tennison–Randall Triangular Flap Repair

In this a cut is given on lower one third of lip to correct upward tilt of cupid's bow by placing a Z-shape wire. Gap is filled with triangle of skin, muscle and mucosal flap from lower end of lateral lip element. In this resultant scar is zigzag scar.

Management of Cleft Palate Repair

For details refer to Ans. 2 of same chapter.

Q.9. Write brief notes on treatment of cleft lip.

(Apr 2017, 2 Marks)

Ans.

Treatment of Cleft Lip

* Millard's criterion is used to undertake surgery for cleft lip, i.e., rule of ten, 10 pound in weight; 10 weeks old; 10 g% hemoglobin.
* If cleft lip is bilateral and is extensive two surgeries should be done to close the cleft. Surgery of one side should be done first and later on after few week surgery of second side is done.
* Millard's rotation advancement flap technique is commonly used. In this correction of both lip and nasal deformity is done. Realigning of muscles and of lip and their correct anatomical position is an important part of this repair. In this technique, medial lip element is rotated inferiorly and the lateral lip element is advanced into resulting upper lip defect. The columellar flap is then used to create nasal sill.
* *Hagedorn–LeMesurier repair:* In this method medial lip element should be lengthened by introducing the quadrilateral flap which is developed from lateral lip element.
* *Tennison–Randall repair:* In this method, medial lip element is lengthened by introducing a triangular flap from inferior portion of lateral lip element.
* Proper postoperative management, such as control of infection, training for sucking, swallowing and speech therapy should be done.

Q.10. Write classification of cleft lip and palate and its treatment. *(Apr 2018, 5 Marks)*

Ans. *For classification of cleft lip and palate refer to Ans. 6 of same chapter.*

* *For treatment of cleft lip refer to Ans. 9 of same chapter.*
* *For treatment of cleft palate refer to Ans. 2 of same chapter.*

17. ORAL CANCER

Q.1. Describe the etiology, pathology, clinical features and treatment of oral cancer. *(Apr 2008, 15 Marks)*

Ans.

Etiology

Etiological Factors of Oral Cancer

♦ *Tobacco smoking:*
  • Cigarettes
  • Bidis
  • Pipes
  • Cigars
  • Reverse smoking.
♦ *Use of smoking tobacco:*
  • Snuff dipping
  • Tobacco sachets
  • Tobacco chewing:
    – Betal chewing
    – Chewing of areca nut
    – Consumption of alcohol
    – *Diet and nutrition:* Vitamin A, B complex and C deficiency.
♦ *Dental factors:*
  • Chronic irritation from broken teeth.
  • Ill-fitting or broken prosthesis.
♦ *Ultraviolet radiation:* Actinic radiation
♦ *Viruses:*
  • Herpes simplex virus
  • Human papilloma virus
  • Human immunodeficiency virus (HIV)
  • Epstein–Barr virus
♦ *Immunosuppression:*
  • AIDS
  • Organ transplantation
♦ *Chronic infection:*
  • Candidiasis
  • Syphilis.
♦ *Occupational hazards:* Woollen textile workers.
♦ *Genetic factors:*
  • Oncogenes
  • Tumor suppressor genes
♦ *Pre-existing oral disease:*
  • Oral lichen planus
  • Oral submucous fibrosis
  • Leukoplakia.

Clinical Features

♦ Male predilection is seen.
♦ Carcinoma mostly occurs in the older age.
♦ *Site:* Most commonly involved are the posterior and lateral borders of tongue and lower lip and less frequently the floor of mouth, palate and buccal mucosa.
♦ Small lesion is asymptomatic.
♦ Large lesion may cause some pain or paresthesia and swelling.
♦ Patients complain of persistent ulcer in the oral cavity.

♦ Function of organ is impaired.
♦ *Appearance:* The clinical appearance of a carcinomatous ulcer is that one of irregular shape induration and raised everted edges.
♦ *Base:* Usually have broad base and are dome like or nodular.
♦ *Surface:* May range from granular to pebbly to deeply creviced.
♦ Surface may be entirely necrotic and have ragged whitish gray appearance.
♦ *Color:* It may be completely red or red surface may be sprinkled with white necrotic or keratin area.
♦ *Lymph nodes:* Superficial and deep cervical nodes are commonly affected.

Pathology

♦ Allelic imbalance [loss of heterozygosity (LOH)] has been identified in tumor suppressor gene.
  Damage to tumor suppressor gene may also involve damage to other genes involved in growth control, mainly those involve in cell signaling (oncogenes, especially some on chromosome 11 and chromosome 16)
♦ Changes in oncogenes can disrupt cell growth control, leading ultimately to uncontrolled growth of cancer.

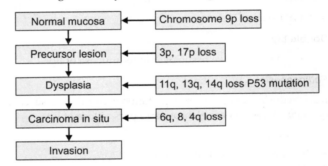

Management of Oral Cancer

Management should be curative or palliative:
♦ *Early growth without bone involvement*
  • Curative radiotherapy using cesium needles or iridium wires, i.e., brachytherapy.
  • Other option is wide excision wire 1–2 cm clearance. Often, the approach to the tumor is by raising the cheek flap (outside). After the wide excision, the flap is placed back (Patterson operation).
  • Presently advanced technology in radiotherapy, facilitates the use of external radiotherapy also. The incidence of dreaded complication like osteoradionecrosis mandible has been reduced due to better radiotherapy methods.
♦ *Growth with mandible involvement:* Here along with wide excision of the primary tumor hemimandibulectomy or segmental resection of the mandible or marginal mandibulectomy (using rotary electric saw) is done.
♦ *Operable growth with mandible involvement and mobile lymph nodes on the same side (confirmed by FNAC):* Along with wide excision of the primary, hemimandibulectomy and radical neck lymph node dissection is done (commando operation).

Wide excision of primary lesion, hemimandibulectomy with radical neck node dissection is called as composite resection.

♦ *Operable growth with mandible involvement; mobile lymph node on same side and opposite side:* Along with wide excision of the tumor, hemimandibulectomy, radical neck lymph node dissection on same side and functional block dissection on opposite side are done, retaining the internal jugular vein, sternomastoid and spinal accessory nerve.

♦ *Operable primary tumor with mobile lymph nodes on same side but without mandibular involvement:* Wide excision of primary tumor and radical neck lymph node dissection on same side are done. Mandible is not removed.

♦ *Fixed primary tumor or advanced neck lymph node secondaries:* Only palliative external radiotherapy is given to palliate pain fungation and to prevent anticipated torrential hemorrhage.

♦ Preoperative radiotherapy is often used in fixed lymph node to downstage the disease to make it operative.

♦ *Postoperative radiotherapy is given in T3 and T4 tumors:* N2 and N3 nodal status to reduce the recurrence and to improve the prognosis.

♦ Prophylactic block dissection has become popular in N0 diseases.

♦ *If growth is extending to upper alveolus:* Partial maxillectomy or total maxillectomy is done.

Reconstruction after Surgery

Flaps used for reconstruction after oral surgery:
♦ Forehead flap based on superficial temporal artery.
♦ Deltopectoral flap based on 1, 2 and 3 perforating vessels from internal mammary vessels.
♦ Pectoralis major myocutaneous flap (PMMF) based on thoracoacromial artery.
♦ Free microvascular flaps may be from radial artery forearm flap.
♦ For small defects—tongue flap, buccal flap, palatal mucoperiosteal flap.

Chemotherapy

♦ Drugs used are methotrexate, cisplatin, vincristine, bleomycin, adriamycin. Often it is given intra-arterially through external carotid artery using arterial pump or by increasing the height of the drip more than 13 feet, so as to attain a pressure more than systolic pressure. Chemotherapy can also be given IV or orally postoperatively.

♦ Initial chemotherapy to downstage the tumor followed by surgery and later again end with chemotherapy.

♦ Chemoradiotherapy is used in unresectable tumors as consecutive therapies.

Radiotherapy

♦ Early lesions are managed by radiotherapy.
♦ Radiotherapy is of two types, i.e., external radiotherapy and interstitial radiotherapy.
♦ In external radiotherapy large dose of 6,000 to 8,000 cGy units are given, i.e., 200 cGy units/day

♦ Interstitial radiotherapy is indicated in infiltrative small lesions. Cesium[137] or iridium wires are placed within the tumor. Minimal tissue resection is the basic advantage of this procedure.

Q.2. Briefly discuss the etiology, epidemiology, classification and principles of treatment of oral cancer.

(Feb 1999, 15 Marks)

Ans. Etiology: *For details refers to Ans. 1 of same chapter.*

Epidemiology

♦ Squamous cell carcinoma representing about 90% of all oral cancer, for this reason, oral squamous cell carcinoma is often designated as "oral cancer."

♦ On an average, oral squamous cell carcinoma represent about 3% of all cancer in males and about 2% of all cancer in females.

♦ The incidence of oral squamous cell carcinoma increases with age and most of the causes occur usually after the age of 40 years.

Classification

♦ *Oral cancer of epithelial tissue origin:*
  • Basal cell carcinoma
  • Squamous cell carcinoma
  • Verrucous carcinoma
  • Adenoid squamous cell carcinoma
  • Malignant melanoma

♦ *Oral cancer of mesenchymal tissue origin:*
  • Oral cancer of fibrous tissue
    – Fibrosarcoma
    – Malignant fibrous histiocystoma.
  • Oral cancer of adipose tissue
    – Liposarcoma.
  • Oral cancer of vascular tissue
    – Hemangiopericytoma
    – Hemangioendothelioma
    – Angiosarcoma.
  • Oral cancer of lymphoid tissue
    – Hodgkin's lymphoma
    – Non-Hodgkin's lymphoma
    – Burkitt's lymphoma
    – Leukemia.
  • Oral cancer of bone
    – Osteosarcoma
    – Ewing's sarcoma.
  • Oral cancer of neural tissue
    – Neurosarcoma
    – Neurofibrosarcoma
    – Neuroblastoma.
  • Oral cancer of muscle
    – Leiomyosarcoma
    – Malignant granular cell myoblastoma
  • Tumor of salivary gland
    – Mucoepidermoid carcinoma
    – Adenocarcinoma
    – Acinic cell carcinoma.

Principle of Treatment

Following are the principles of treatment of oral cancer:

♦ If only primary is present which is mucosal with size <2 cm without nodal spread, then wide local excision with supraomohyoid block dissection of same side is done (N0); primary may also be treated with curative brachytherapy or external beam teletherapy. If nodes are histologically positive then radical neck dissection is done.

♦ Larger mucosal primary with similar features are also treated similarly, but postoperative radiotherapy or/and chemotherapy is added depending on grading of the tumor.

♦ In all these types of lesions, if there are positive mobile neck nodes which is confirmed by FNAC, then radical neck dissection should be done.

♦ If primary lesion extends into adjacent soft tissue with mandibular involvement then mandibular resection is needed. Part is reconstructed using plates or bone graft taken from iliac crest or opposite 11th rib. 2.4 mm reconstruction plate with pectoralis major myocutaneous flap (PMMF) or nonvascularized bone graft (iliac crest cancellous chips) or vascularized bone graft from fibula/iliac crest/scapula are the present recommendations. Skin covering is done by split skin graft inside to mucosa or by appropriate flaps depending on the need and feasibility of donor area (PMMF/DP flap/forehead flap). Neck is addressed similarly. Postoperative EBRT and chemotherapy is needed either concurrent or sequential.

♦ If primary is advanced then chemotherapy with EBRT is used. If lesion reduces in size and becomes operable it is then operated accordingly.

♦ In fixed primary or secondary, radiotherapy with chemotherapy is used for palliation to relieve pain, fungation, sepsis.

♦ In advanced stage terminal events may be severe malnutrition, bleeding, sepsis, and bronchopneumonia.

♦ Posterior lesions has got poor prognosis than anterior lesions. Lip carries best prognosis depends on anatomical location, grading, lymph node status, soft tissue involvement and response of therapy.

Q.3. Write short note on *modalities of treatment of oral cancer.** *(Sep 2004, 10 Marks)*

Ans. Oral cancer is treated by surgery, radiotherapy and chemotherapy or by combination of these. The other developing techniques in the treatment of oral cancer are laser therapy, hormonal therapy, hyperthermia, etc.

Surgery

♦ The surgical treatment of oral cancer as a primary modality is excisional in nature.

♦ All clinical detectable tumor must be excised with adequate margins of adjacent normal tissue, to ensure that the residual element of the microscopic disease do not remain within the surgical field.

♦ The surgical treatment of oral carcinoma includes three important steps:

1. Wide excision of primary tumor
2. Neck dissection, i.e., surgical removal of involved lymph nodes present in the neck
3. Reconstruction of the resected region in the oral cavity

Lesion in Mandible

Surgical procedures that can be done for the resection of tumors in the mandible include:

♦ **Alveolectomy:** This is an intraoral procedure in which alveolus is removed alone. This is done for small alveolar lesions in the mandible.

♦ **Marginal mandibulectomy:** It is the surgical procedure which involves the removal of body of the mandible in the involved area leaving lower border of the mandible intact. This procedure is done in cases where the tumor involves body of the mandible but does not involve the lower border of the mandible.

♦ **Segmental resection:** It is the surgical procedure in which a segment of mandible including the lower border should be excised. Depending on the location of the tumor, this procedure is divided into two parts, i.e., anterior segmental or posterior segmental resection. Since the lower border of the mandible is also resected, it causes discontinuity of the mandible.

♦ **Hemimandibulectomy:** In this procedure excision of one half of the mandible is done. This is carried out in extensive tumors which involve the mandible. This could be for a tumor of the buccal mucosa or floor of the mouth infiltrating into the mandible. The soft tissues involved in the tumor are resected along with the mandible. The condyle is usually spared in these cases.

♦ **Disarticulating hemimandibulectomy:** In this surgical procedure, one half of the mandible including the condyle is excised.

Lesion in Maxilla

The different surgical options in the maxilla depending upon the size and extent of the tumor include:

♦ **Alveolectomy:** This is an intraoral procedure which involves removal of the involved part of the maxillary alveolus.

♦ **Subtotal maxillectomy:** In this removal of maxilla excluding the floor of the orbit and infraorbital rim.

♦ **Total maxillectomy:** Removal of maxilla including orbital floor as well as rim.

♦ **Radical maxillectomy:** It involves removal of orbital contents along with the maxilla.

♦ T1, T2 lesions involving only the maxillary alveolus should be incised with an adequate margin of normal tissue intraorally. Alveolectomy is done for these lesions. T3, T4 lesions with invasion into the maxillary antrum or nasal cavity require subtotal maxillectomy.

♦ Larger lesions eroding the floor of the orbit require total maxillectomy. Invasion of the tumor into the orbit requires removal of orbital contents and is called a radical maxillectomy. Alveolectomy can be done intraorally.

For all other procedures, a wide exposure of the maxilla is required. This can be achieved by the Weber Ferguson incision. This incision may have a subciliary or a brow extension for a better exposure of the maxilla.

Reconstruction

♦ Although cure rates have not changed much over the years, better function and appearance of the patient have been made possible by reconstructive techniques.

♦ Various surgical advances have provided means for soft tissue and hard tissue reconstruction of the excised region.

♦ Soft tissues used for reconstruction include:
  - Deltopectoral flap
  - Sternocleidomastoid flap
  - Pectoralis major flap

♦ These and various other flaps have revolutionized the reconstructive procedures.

Radiotherapy

♦ Radiotherapy is the treatment of the disease with ionizing or nonionizing radiation.

♦ Following methods are to be followed for radiotherapy:
  - *X-ray therapy:*
    - Superficial X-ray therapy 45–100 kV
    - Kilovoltage X-ray therapy 300 kV
  - Electron therapy
  - Surface applicator.
    - Interstitial implantation
      » Radiation is given externally by the use of X-ray generators.
      » Uninvolved areas of patient should be prevented by doing shielding.
      » Host tissues of patient should be protected from radiation by two methods, i.e., fractionation and multiple ports.
      » In fractionation instead of giving maximum radiation patient is given radiation in small increments for several weeks which provides time for normal tissues for recovery between dosages.
      » In multiple ports multiple beams are used which provide radiation to tumor from different angles. In this radiation delivery is on every 5th day a week.

Chemotherapy

♦ It is used in the treatment of malignant tumor. It selectively kill's tumor cells by virtue of cell kinetic proliferation character and cell biology.

♦ Chemicals which interferes with rapid growth of tumor cells are used for treating oral cancer.

♦ Vincristine, bleomycin and methotrexate in various combinations are used.

♦ Chemotherapy should be given intravenously but nowadays its intra-arterial injections can be given

♦ It produces only partial or temporary tumor regression.

♦ It may be used in combination with radiotherapy or surgery or as palliative treatment.

♦ Chemotherapy is most effective in the lesions which are confined to the soft tissues.

Q.4. Describe the causes, clinical features and management of carcinoma of tongue.

(Apr 2007, 15 Marks)

Or

Write a short note on carcinoma of tongue.

(June 2014, 5 Marks)

Ans. Carcinoma of tongue is mostly epidermoid carcinoma.

Responsible Features or Causes

♦ Poor oral hygiene
♦ Pipe smokers
♦ Chronic alcoholic
♦ Chewing of betel nut, tobacco and slaked lime
♦ Chronic irritation by sharp tooth
♦ Syphilis
♦ Leukoplakia
♦ Erythroplakia
♦ Sepsis
♦ Superficial glossitis
♦ Spices
♦ Susceptibility, vitamin deficiency
♦ Chronic hyperplastic candidiasis
♦ Human papillomavirus a possible cause

Pathological Types

♦ Nonhealing ulcer
♦ Proliferative growth
♦ Frozen tongue or indurated plaque
♦ Fissure variety

Clinical Features

♦ A bleeding ulcer is seen over the tongue.
♦ Pain in the tongue is due to involvement of lingual nerve. Pain can refer to the ear and lower temporal region.
♦ Disarticulation—difficulty in talking is due to disability of the tongue to move freely.
♦ Dysphagia is a common presentation from the carcinoma of posterior one-third.
♦ Fetor oris is due to infected necrotic growth.
♦ Ankyloglossia restricted mobility of the tongue. It is due to infiltration of the mouth or mandible.
♦ Bilateral massive enlargement of lower deep cervical nodes in an elderly patient is suggestive of carcinoma of posterior one-third.
♦ Painless ulcer or swelling is present on the tongue which later becomes painful.
♦ Excessive salivation is present and saliva is blood tinged.
♦ Visible ulcer can be seen on anterior two-thirds of tongue. Ulcer can bleed on touch; edge, base and surrounding areas are indurated. Often indurated area is more extensive than primary tumor. Edges are everted. Ulcer may cross the midline and extend to the floor or mouth/alveolus/mandible.
♦ Features of bronchopneumonia due to aspiration during lying down sleeping mainly to lower segment of lung.

Investigations

- Wedge biopsy
- FNAC of lymph nodes
- Indirect and direct laryngoscopy to see posterior third growth
- CT scan to see the extension of posterior third growth or to see status of lymph node secondaries.
- MRI to assess extent of primary tumor
- Chest X-ray to see bronchopneumonia
- Orthopantomogram

Management

Following is the management of the carcinoma of tongue:

- Wide excision with l cm clearance in margin and depth is done in tumor <l cm in size or in carcinoma in situ. Laser (CO_2/diode) can be used.
- Tumor between 1–2 cm in size, partial glossectomy is done with 2 cm clearance from the margin with removal of one-third of anterior two-thirds of the tongue.
- Tumor larger than 2 cm, hemiglossectomy is done with removal of anterior two-thirds of tongue on one side up to sulcus terminalis.
- Raw area in these procedures can be left alone when area is wide allowing it to granulate and heal by epithelialization. If area is small like in wide excision it can be closed by primary suturing. Wide raw area can also be covered with PMMF or quilted split-skin graft.
- Larger primary tumor can be given preoperative radiotherapy then later hemiglossectomy is done.
- Same side palpable mobile lymph nodes are removed by radical neck block dissection.
- Bilateral mobile lymph nodes are dealt with one side radical block and other side junctional block dissection with essentially retaining internal jugular vein (on opposite side) to maintain the cerebral venous blood flow. Other option is doing same side radical neck dissection and on opposite side supraomohyoid block dissection.
- Wide excision is done when growth is in the tip of the tongue.
- Posterior third growth can be approached by lip split and mandible resection, so as to have total glossectomy—Kochers approach. It is not done commonly as it carries significant morbidity and mortality due to difficulty in speech, swallowing, aspiration, sepsis.
- When mandible is involved hemimandibulectomy is done.
- The procedure that involves wide excision or hemiglossectomy, hemimandibulectomy and radical neck dissection together is called as commando operation.
- Reconstruction of tongue and other area after surgery: By deltopectoral flap, forehead flap, pectoralis major muscle flap, skin grafting.
- Prophylactic block dissection is becoming popular at present.

Radiotherapy

- In small primary tumor—brachytherapy using cesium or iridium needles.
- In large primary tumor initial radiotherapy is given to reduce the tumor size so that resection will be better later.

- Advanced primary as well as secondaries in neck are controlled by palliative external radiotherapy.
- Postoperative radiotherapy is given in large tumors to reduce the chances of relapse.
- In case of growth in posterior one-third of tongue radiotherapy is of curative as well as palliative mode.

Chemotherapy

- It is given in postoperative period and also for palliation.
- Price–Hill regimen is commonly used. Drugs are methotrexate, vincristine, adriamycin, bleomycin and mercaptopurine.
- It is either given intra-arterially, as regional chemotherapy through external carotid artery using arterial pump or through IV. It can be given orally also.

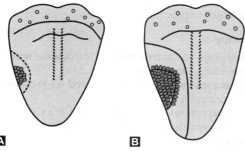

Figs. 25A and B: Glossectomy: (A) Partial glossectomy; (B) Hemiglossectomy.

Q.5. Discuss management of anterior two-thirds tongue carcinoma. *(Feb/Mar 2004, 10 Marks)*

Ans. Carcinoma of the tongue is a common lesion.

Carcinoma of the tongue occurs on the anterior 2/3, 50% of carcinoma is seen in this region.

Management

Following is the management of the carcinoma of anterior two-thirds of tongue:

Investigations

- Wedge biopsy
- FNAC of lymph nodes
- CT scan to see the status of lymph node secondaries
- MRI to assess extent of primary tumor
- Chest X-ray to see bronchopneumonia
- Orthopantomogram

Treatment

Surgery

- Wide excision with l cm clearance in margin and depth is done in tumor <l cm in size or in carcinoma in situ. Laser (CO_2/diode) can be used.
- Tumor between 1–2 cm in size, partial glossectomy is done with 2 cm clearance from the margin with removal of one-third of anterior two-thirds of the tongue.

- Tumor larger than 2 cm, hemiglossectomy is done with removal of anterior two-thirds of tongue on one side up to sulcus terminalis.
- Raw area in these procedures can be left alone when area is wide allowing it to granulate and heal by epithelialization. If area is small like in wide excision it can be closed by primary suturing. Wide raw area can also be covered with PMMF or quilted split-skin graft.
- Larger primary tumor can be given preoperative radiotherapy then later hemiglossectomy is done.
- Same side palpable mobile lymph nodes are removed by radical neck block dissection.
- Bilateral mobile lymph nodes are dealt with one side radical block and other side junctional block dissection with essentially retaining internal jugular vein (on opposite side) to maintain the cerebral venous blood flow. Other option is doing same side radical neck dissection and on opposite side supraomohyoid block dissection.
- Wide excision is done when growth is in the tip of the tongue.
- Reconstruction of tongue and other area after surgery: By deltopectoral flap, forehead flap, pectoralis major muscle flap, skin grafting.
- Prophylactic block dissection is becoming popular at present.

Radiotherapy

- In small primary tumor—brachytherapy using cesium or iridium needles.
- In large primary tumor initial radiotherapy is given to reduce the tumor size so that resection will be better later.
- Advanced primary as well as secondaries in neck are controlled by palliative external radiotherapy.
- Postoperative radiotherapy is given in large tumors to reduce the chances of relapse.

Chemotherapy

- It is given in postoperative period and for palliation.
- Price–Hill regimen is commonly used. Drugs are methotrexate, vincristine, adriamycin, bleomycin and mercaptopurine.
- It is either given intra-arterially as regional chemotherapy through external carotid artery using arterial pump or through IV. It can be given orally also.

Q.6. Write short note on Ca lip. *(Mar 2001, 10 Marks)*

Ans. Ca lip: Carcinoma of lip.

Vermilion border of lip and mucosa is the main site of carcinoma of lip.

It is common in the western elderly, white people, especially those people exposed to sunlight.

The lesions known as countryman's lip because it occurs commonly in agriculturists.

Etiology

- Excessive use of tobacco
- Leukoplakia and syphilis
- Placing *khaini* between lower lip and gum
- Heavy consumption of alcohol
- Radiation to the lip

Clinical Features

- Elderly males are affected in 90% of cases.
- Nonhealing ulcer or growth is a common presentation.
- Lesion appears in the form of white plaque of nonhealing ulcers.
- Edges are everted and indurated, this is characteristic of carcinoma.
- Ulcer contain slough in floor.
- Bleeding may occur from ulcer.
- Pain and paresthesia may occur.
- Lesion may get fixed to the subcutaneous structure of lip.
- Ulcer spreads and destroys the tissue of lip and chin.
- Submental and submandibular lymph nodes are involved, lymph node becomes hard and may be fixed.

Differential Diagnosis

- Leukoplakia
- Syphilitic chancre
- Keratocanthoma
- Ectopic salivary gland tumor
- Pyogenic granuloma

Treatment

- If lesion is <2 cm, then curative radiotherapy, either brachytherapy or external beam radiotherapy. It gives a good cure.
- If tumor is >2 cm, wide excision is done. Excision of lower lip up to one-third can be sutured primarily, in layers keeping vermilion border in proper apposition without causing any microstomia.
- Excision of more than one-third of the lip requires reconstruction using different flaps.

Methods

- Abbe–Estlander's rotation flap used for either upper or lower lip lesions located at the angle based on labial artery. Here base at a later stage need not be disconnected unlike in Abbe lip.
- *Fries modified Bernard facial flap:* Reconstruction using lateral facial flaps. It is used when defect is more than half of lip and midline.
- *Gillies fan flap:* It is a cheek flap usually bilateral but can be unilateral. Incision is full thickness around commissure extending into nasolabial fold and upper lip up to upper lip vermilion border. Flap which is based on labial vessels advanced towards the defect. Vermilion is reconstructed with tongue mucosal flap which is divided in 3 weeks.
- *Karapandzic flap:* It is the modified version of Gillie's flap used for lower lip defect with less angulations towards upper lip. Reverse Karapandzic flap is used for upper lip.
- Microvascular flaps.
- *Nasolabial flap:* It is used when defect is more than half of lip laterally or defect is in the floor of mouth.
- Cheek flap.
- Free radial artery flap
- *Abbe flap:* It is used for upper or lower lip lesions at the middle or the site other than angle based on labial artery.

Here at the later second stage base of the flap should be released once as flaps takes up.

- *'W' flap plasty:* It is done for lower lip middle tumor which is less than one-third of the lip.
- Johansen stepladder procedure is used for extensive carcinoma of lower lip.
- Other regular flaps, such as forehead flap, deltopectoral flap can also be used.
- Lymph nodes are dealt with by radical neck dissection on one side and functional block or supraomohyoid block dissection on other side. For central tumor N0 disease, bilateral elective (prophylactic) supraomohyoid dissection is done. For lateral tumor N0 disease, elective ipsilateral supraomohyoid dissection is done.
- Postoperative radiotherapy is given if tumor is large or if lymph nodes are involved.
- When mandible is involved, segmental resection is done.

Q.7. Write short note on etiology and treatment of carcinoma of cheek. *(Feb 2004, 6 Marks)*

Or

Describe clinical presentation and management of carcinoma buccal mucosa. *(Apr 2019, 15 Marks)*

Ans. The common carcinoma of cheek is squamous cell carcinoma.

This is also called verrucous carcinoma or tobacco chewers carcinoma of cheek.

Etiology

- All the 'S', i.e., smoking, spirit, syphilis, sharp tooth and spices.
- Premalignant lesions and conditions, i.e., leukoplakia, erythroplakia, OSMF, candidiasis, etc.
- Placing the quid of betel nut and tobacco in cheek mucosa.

Pathological Types

- A nonhealing ulcer
- An exophytic growth or verrucous carcinoma
- An infiltrative lesion, which involves adjacent structures, such as tongue, mandible, floor of mouth.

Clinical Features/Clinical Presentation

- Ulcer (painless to begin with) in the cheek which gradually increases in size in a patient with history of chewing pan and smoking is the most common presentation and initially it is painless.
- Pain occurs when it involves the skin, bone or if secondarily infected. Referred pain to the ear signifies involvement of lingual nerve.
- Halitosis which is bad odor breath is common.
- Involvement of retromolar trigone indicates that it is an advanced disease, as the lymphatics here communicate freely with the pharyngeal lymphatics.
- Everted edge, induration are the typical features of the ulcer.
- Mandible is examined bidigitally, for thickening, tenderness, irregularity and sites of fracture. Mandible may get involved by direct extension, through mandibular canal or through periodontal membrane. Loss of central part of mandible due

to destruction by tumor will cause pouting of lower lip with drooling of saliva, i.e., Andy Gump deformity.

- Mandibular canal is close to occlusive alveolar surface in elderly and edentulous patients to cause early mandibular spread in carcinoma.
- Trismus and dysphagia signify involvement of pterygoids or posterior extension.
- Occasionally, it may extend into the upper alveolus and to the maxilla causing swelling, pain and tenderness.
- Once involvement of soft tissue occurs, it may come out through skin as fungating lesion often with orocutaneous fistulas with saliva dribbling through fistula.
- Submandibular lymph nodes and upper deep cervical nodes are involved which are hard and nodular; initially mobile and later get fixed to each other and then to deeper structure.

Features of Advanced Carcinoma Cheek

- Involvement of retromolar trigone.
- Extension into the base of skull and pharynx
- Fixed neck lymph nodes
- Extension to the opposite side

Spread

- *Local spread:* Result in orosubcutaneous fistula and mandibular sinus.
- *Lymphatic spread:* Enlargement of submandibular lymph nodes.
- *Hematogenous spread:* Very rare.

Investigation

- Wedge biopsy, usually taken from two sites. Biopsy has to be taken from the edge as it contains active cells; not from the center as it is the area of necrosis. Malignant squamous cells with epithelial pearls (keratin pearls) are the histological features.
- FNAC from lymph nodes.
- CT scan is used to assess the extent of tumor into mandible, pterygoid region, in patient with trismus, with neck lymph nodes, with carotid involvement by lymph nodes.
- MRI is very useful in assessing the soft tissues, base of skull and perineural spread.
- Orthopantomogram to look for the involvement of mandible—destruction and fracture sites. Symphysis menti and lingual plate are not clearly appreciated. So often OPG may be supported with dental occlusion and intraoral X-rays.

Treatment/Management

Treatment should be curative or palliative.

- *Early growth without bone involvement:*
  - Curative radiotherapy using cesium needles or iridium wires, i.e., brachytherapy.
  - Other option is wide excision wire 1–2 cm clearance. Often, the approach to the tumor is by raising the cheek flap (outside). After the wide excision, the flap is placed back (Patterson operation).
  - Presently advanced technology in radiotherapy, facilitates the use of external radiotherapy also.

The incidence of dreaded complication like osteoradionecrosis mandible has been reduced due to better radiotherapy methods.

♦ *Growth with mandible involvement:* Here along with wide excision of the primary tumor hemimandibulectomy or segmental resection of the mandible or marginal mandibulectomy (using rotary electric saw) is done.

♦ *Operable growth with mandible involvement and mobile lymph nodes on the same side (confirmed by FNAC):* Along with wide excision of the primary, hemimandibulectomy and radical neck lymph node dissection is done (commando operation).

Wide excision of primary lesion, hemimandibulectomy with radical neck node dissection is called as composite resection.

♦ *Operable growth with mandible involvement; mobile lymph node on same side and opposite side:* Along with wide excision of the tumor, hemimandibulectomy, radical neck lymph node dissection on same side and functional block dissection on opposite side are done, retaining the internal jugular vein, sternomastoid and spinal accessory nerve.

♦ *Operable primary tumor with mobile lymph nodes on same side but without mandibular involvement:* Wide excision of primary tumor and radical neck lymph node dissection on same side are done. Mandible is not removed.

♦ *Fixed primary tumor or advanced neck lymph node secondaries:* Only palliative external radiotherapy is given to palliate pain fungation and to prevent anticipated torrential hemorrhage.

♦ Preoperative radiotherapy is often used in fixed lymph node to downstage the disease to make it operative.

♦ Postoperative radiotherapy is given in T3 and T4 tumors: N2 and N3 nodal status to reduce the recurrence and to improve the prognosis.

♦ Prophylactic block dissection has become popular in N0 diseases

♦ *If growth is extending to upper alveolus:* Partial maxillectomy or total maxillectomy is done.

Reconstruction after Surgery

Flaps used for reconstruction after oral surgery:
♦ Forehead flap based on superficial temporal artery.
♦ Deltopectoral flap based on 1, 2 and 3 perforating vessels from internal mammary vessels.
♦ Pectoralis major myocutaneous flap (PMMF) based on thoracoacromial artery.
♦ Free microvascular flaps may be from radial artery forearm flap.
♦ For small defects—tongue flap, buccal flap, palatal mucoperiosteal flap.

Chemotherapy

♦ Drugs used are methotrexate, cisplatin, vincristine, bleomycin, adriamycin. Often it is given intra-arterially through external carotid artery using arterial pump or by increasing the height of the drip >13 feet, so as to attain a pressure more than systolic pressure. Chemotherapy can also be given IV or orally postoperatively.

♦ Initial chemotherapy to downstage the tumor followed by surgery and later again end with chemotherapy.
♦ Chemoradiotherapy is used in unresectable tumors as consecutive therapies.

Radiotherapy

♦ Early lesions are managed by radiotherapy.
♦ Radiotherapy is of two types, i.e., external radiotherapy and interstitial radiotherapy.
♦ In external radiotherapy large dose of 6,000 to 8,000 cGy units are given, i.e., 200 cGy units/day
♦ Interstitial radiotherapy is indicated in infiltrative small lesions. Cesium 137 or iridium wires are placed within the tumor. Minimal tissue resection is the basic advantage of this procedure.

Q.8. Describe the pathology, clinical features and principles of treatment of head and neck cancer.
(Feb 2002, 20 Marks)

Ans. *For pathology, refer to Ans. 1 of same chapter.*

For clinical features, refer to Ans. 1 of same chapter.

For principles of treatment, refer to Ans. 2 of same chapter.

Q.9. Write short note on TNM classification of malignant tumors. *(Sep 1999, 10 Marks)*

Ans. TNM classification was given by **American Joint Committee on Cancer (AJCC):**

T is suggestive of primary tumor

N is suggestive of regional lymph nodes

M is suggestive of distant metastasis

T: Primary tumor

TX: Primary tumor cannot be assessed

T0: No evidence of primary tumor

Tis: Carcinoma in situ

T1: Tumor 2 cm of less in greatest dimension

T2: Tumor >2 cm but not more than 4 cm in greatest dimension

T3: Tumor more than 4 cm in greatest dimension

T4a (lip): Tumor invades through cortical bone, inferior alveolar nerve, floor of mouth or skin (chin or nose)

T4a (oral cavity): Tumor invades through cortical bone, into deep/extrinsic muscle of tongue (genioglossus, hyoglossus, palatoglossus and styloglossus), maxillary sinus or skin of face.

T4b (lip and oral cavity): Tumor invades masticatory space, pterygoid plates or skull base or encases internal carotid artery

N: Regional lymph nodes

NX: Regional lymph nodes cannot be assessed

N0: No regional lymph node metastasis

N1: Metastasis in a single ipsilateral lymph node, 3 cm or less in greatest dimension

N2a: Metastasis in a single ipsilateral lymph node, more than 3 cm but not more than 6 cm in greatest dimension

N2b: Metastasis in multiple ipsilateral lymph nodes, not more than 6 cm in greatest dimension

N2c: Metastasis in bilateral or contralateral lymph nodes, not more than 6 cm in greatest dimension

N3: Metastasis in a lymph node more than 6 cm in greatest dimension

M: Distant metastasis

MX: Distant metastasis cannot be assessed

M0: No distant metastasis

M1: Distant metastasis.

Stage Grouping of Oral Cancer

Stage 0	Tis	N0	M0
Stage I	T1	N0	M0
Stage II	T2	N0	M0
Stage III	T1	N1	M0
	T2	N1	M0
	T3	N0, N1	M0
Stage IVa	T1,T2,T3	N2	M0
	T4a	N0, N1, N2	M0
Stage IVb	Any T	N3	M0
	T4b	Any N	M0
Stage IVc	Any T	Any N	M1

Q.10. Difference between benign and malignant tumors.

(Aug 2018, 10 Marks)

Or

Enumerate difference between benign and malignant neoplasia.

(June 2014, 2 Marks)

Or

Describe differentiating features of benign and malignant tumors.

(Jan 2017, 3 Marks)

Ans.

Characters	Benign tumor	Malignant tumor
Age	May occur at any age	Usually after 40 years
Size	Usually small	Usually large
Growth	i. Slow growing	i. Rapidly growing
	ii. Expansive type of growth	ii. Invasive type of growth
Local infiltration	The surrounding structures are not involved	Involvement of surrounding structure is a characteristic feature
Fixity	Usually not fixed to the surrounding structures	Fix to the surrounding structure due to local invasion
Histological features	• Well differentiated • Well formed stromal cells • Few mitosis	• Less differentiated • Stroma is poorly formed • Mitosis numerous
Hemorrhage and ulceration tendency	Usually does not occur	More tendency towards hemorrhage and ulceration
Metastasis	Never occur	Metastasis frequent
Fetal to life	Usually not fatal to life, if death occur it is due to mechanical pressure and obstructive effects	Almost fatal, if untreated. Cause of death is mechanical and destructive effect

Q.11. Describe the clinical features and treatment of anterior 2/3 of tongue. *(Sep 2008, 10 Marks)*

Ans.

Clinical Features

- Painless ulcer or swelling on the tongue which later on may become painful. Pain is present in the tongue due to infection or ulceration or due to involvement of lingual nerve.
- Salivation is excessive and is often blood stained.
- Visible ulcer can be seen on anterior two-thirds of tongue. Ulcer can bleed on touch; edge, base and surrounding areas are indurated. Often indurated area is more extensive than primary tumor. Edges are everted. Ulcer may cross the midline and extend to the floor or mouth/alveolus/mandible.
- Fetor oris is due to infected necrotic growth.
- Ankyloglossia restricted mobility of the tongue. It is due to infiltration of the mouth or mandible.
- Disarticulation—difficulty in talking is due to disability of the tongue to move freely.
- Presence of palpable lymph nodes in the neck which are hard, nodular and get fixed to underlying tissues in advanced stages.

For treatment of anterior two-thirds of tongue, refer to Ans. 5 of same chapter.

Q.12. Discuss the etiology, clinical features and management of carcinoma of alveolus. *(Jan 2011, 10 Marks)*

Ans. *For etiology refer to Ans. 1 of same chapter.*

Clinical Features

- Early invasion of bone takes place mostly via the PDL and this causes extensive mobility and premature loss of the regional teeth.
- Extraction of tooth often leads to early bone invasion, which causes nonhealing or delayed healing of the extraction socket.
- Mandibular lesions often extend to the adjoining structures, e. g. labial mucosa, tongue, bone, floor of the mouth and the retromolar areas.
- Metastasis occurs often to the submandibular and deep cervical lymph nodes.
- Involvement of inferior alveolar nerve can lead to paresthesia.

Management

For management, refer to Ans. 3 of same chapter.

Q.13. Enlist premalignant lesions of oral cavity. Discuss clinical features, investigations and management of carcinoma of anterior two-thirds of tongue.

(Feb 2013, 10 Marks)

Ans.

Premalignant Lesions of Oral Cavity

- Leukoplakia
- Erythroplakia
- Mucosal changes associated with smoking habits
- Carcinoma in situ
- Bowen disease
- Actinic keratosis, actinic chelitis and actinic elastosis.

Clinical Features

♦ Painless ulcer or swelling on the tongue which later on may become painful. Pain is present in the tongue due to infection or ulceration or due to involvement of lingual nerve.

♦ Salivation is excessive and is often blood stained.

♦ Visible ulcer can be seen on anterior two-thirds of tongue. Ulcer can bleed on touch; edge, base and surrounding areas are indurated. Often indurated area is more extensive than primary tumor. Edges are everted. Ulcer may cross the midline and extend to the floor or mouth/alveolus/mandible.

♦ Fetor oris is due to infected necrotic growth.

♦ Ankyloglossia restricted mobility of the tongue. It is due to infiltration of the mouth or mandible.

♦ Disarticulation—difficulty in talking is due to disability of the tongue to move freely.

♦ Presence of palpable lymph nodes in the neck which are hard, nodular and get fixed to underlying tissues in advanced stages.

Investigations

♦ Wedge biopsy
♦ FNAC of lymph nodes
♦ CT scan to see the status of lymph node secondaries
♦ MRI to assess extent of primary tumor
♦ Chest X-ray to see bronchopneumonia
♦ Orthopantomogram

Management

Refer to Ans. 5 of same chapter.

Q.14. Write short note on incisional and excisional biopsy.
(Jan 2012, 5 Marks)

Or

Write short answer on incisional biopsy.
(Apr 2018, 3 Marks)

Or

Write short answer on incisional and excisional biopsy.   *(June 2018, 3 Marks)*

Ans.

Incisional Biopsy

♦ This is the excision of a portion of lesion for microscopic examination.

♦ This method is employed on large, diffuse lesions which has the size of 2 cm in its greatest dimension.

♦ This method can also be done on lesions suspected for malignancy.

♦ Aim of this method is to remove a portion of lesional tissue in question along with the sample of normal adjacent tissue for comparison.

Types

♦ *Punch biopsy:* This is done by using a surgical punch of diameter 4, 8 or 10 mm. This incisional biopsy is done in mass screening programs.

♦ *Wedge biopsy:* It is done by making the wedge shaped incision which begins 2–3 mm from normal tissue and penetrates in the region surrounding abnormal tissue. Tissue should always be incised narrow and deep.

Exisional Biopsy

♦ This procedure should be done for the small lesions which are clinically benign.

♦ In this complete lesion should be removed for examination and diagnosis. So it is both diagnostic and curative.

Application

♦ This procedure is performed on the lesions which need complete removal for diagnostic and therapeutic purposes.

♦ It is indicated in lesions which are diagnosed as benign and need complete removal

Advantages

♦ It allows histopathological examination of an entire lesion.

♦ Amount of tissue which is removed from one biopsy site, ensure adequate sample for various studies, such as culture, histopathology, immunofluorescence and electron microscopy.

Disadvantages

♦ If the tumor is highly infiltrative margin of excision cannot be exactly elicited, further surgery should be needed.

♦ Cancerous cells actively multiply at tumor margins, debulking of the mass results in residual cancer cells left behind.

♦ Excision needs greater precision and skill of surgeon.

Procedure of Incisional or Excisional biopsy

♦ **Anesthesia:** Give a block to anesthetize the region where specimen is to be obtained. Local infiltration and injections into the tissue which should be biopsied is avoided as it leads to the artifacts in the specimen. If a block is not effective give local infiltration atleast 1 cm away from the lesion.

♦ **Stabilization of tissue:** Soft tissue biopsies are done over the movable tissues of oral cavity, i.e., tongue, lips, etc. Dental assistant stabilizes the tissue by stretching it.

♦ **Hemostasis:** Gauze pieces are the best means for compressing the tissue and achieving hemostasis. Gauze piece can also be placed to cover the mouth of suction tip and is used to prevent the specimen from being sucked inside.

♦ **Incisions:** Use a sharp scalpel. Provide two incisions which form an elliptical incision and converge to form a V at the base, this provides a good specimen and a wound which is easy to close. Alternatively, a triangular-shaped incision can be made which converges in the form of a tip of a pyramid at the base. Incisions should be given parallel to the nerves and vessels in that region to avoid damage.

♦ **Handling of tissues:** Tissue which has to be removed should be handled carefully so that histopathological examination can be performed. A non-toothed tissue holding forceps is used and care is taken not to crush the tissues.

♦ **Care of specimen:** After removal of the tissues, the specimen is transferred to a bottle containing 10% formalin which should be at least 20 times the volume of the specimen obtained.

♦ **Surgical closure of wound:** Primary closure is possible in most cases. Where it is not possible, the tissues are undermined to facilitate closure.

Q.15. Write short note on hemimandibulectomy.
(Feb 2013, 5 Marks)

Ans. Hemimandibulectomy means half of the mandible is removed to excise the lesion which is involving that region.

Types of Hemimandibulectomy

♦ *Condyle sparing hemimandibulectomy:* This method is done for extensive lesions which involve both inferior and posterior borders of the mandible. The condyle can be spared if it is not involved. Sparing of the condyle allows the reconstruction procedure to be simpler. This is because there will be a segment for attachment of the reconstruction plate or bone graft.

♦ *Disarticulating hemimandibulectomy:* This procedure is done for extensive lesions which involve inferior border, posterior border and condyle. Condyle removal makes reconstruction a little more difficult as the condylar prosthesis has to be placed very carefully in condylar fossa without applying pressure inside the fossa. Reconstruction plates are available with the condylar prosthesis for reconstruction of hemimandibulectomy defects.

Basic Procedure for Hemimandibulectomy

♦ Depending on the extent of involvement a partial or hemimandibulectomy is done.

♦ Once the inferior border of the mandible is exposed masseter and medial pterygoid are reflected of from the buccal ramus of the mandible.

♦ Similarly temporalis muscle is reflected off the coronoid process and the mylohyoid muscle from the lingual surface of the mandible.

♦ A bone cut is made anterior to the lesion extending till the inferior border of the mandible using either a Gigli saw or bur.

♦ Once the cut is made the segment is rotated laterally, the inferior alveolar bundle entering the lingula is identified and ligated.

♦ The condyle is then freed from the lateral pterygoid muscle and the mandible is disarticulated.

♦ Hemostasis is achieved and closure is accomplished by approximating the buccal and lingual mucoperiosteal flaps.

♦ Similarly the lip and submandibular incisions are approximated and closed in layers.

♦ A drain may be inserted to avoid collection of fluid in dead space.

♦ Pressure dressing should be applied.

Q.16. Discuss etiology, pathology and treatment of carcinoma alveolar margin. *(Oct 2003, 15 Marks)*

Ans. *For etiology and pathology and treatment refer to Ans. 1 of same chapter.*

Q.17. Discuss briefly squamous cell carcinoma.
(Nov 2008, 5 Marks)

Ans. Squamous cell carcinoma is histological terminology for cancer arising from stratified squamous epithelium.

Squamous cell carcinoma of oral cavity, i.e., oral squamous cell carcinoma is the most common malignant tumor of oral cavity.

Etiology

Following are the etiological factors which lead to oral squamous cell carcinoma:

Tobacco smoking: Cigarettes, bidis, pipes, and cigars.

Reverse Smoking

♦ *Use of smokeless tobacco:* Snuff dipping, *gutka*, tobacco chewing, tobacco as a toothpaste.

♦ *Alcohol:* Drinking spirits, drinking wines, drinking beers

♦ *Diet anal nutrition:* Vitamin A, B-complex and C deficiency,

♦ Nutritional deficiency with alcoholism.

♦ *Dental factors:* Chronic irritation from broken teeth, Ill-fitting or broken prosthesis.

♦ *Radiations:* Actinic radiation, X-ray radiation

♦ *Viral infections:* Herpes simplex virus (HSV), human papillomavirus (HPV), human immunodeficiency virus (HIV), Epstein–Barr virus (EBV)

♦ *Chronic infections:* Candidiasis, syphilis

♦ *Genetic factors:* Oncogenes, tumor suppressor genes

♦ *Pre-existing Oral diseases:* Lichen planus, Plummer–Vinson Syndrome, DLE, OSMF

Clinical Features

♦ Carcinomas mostly occur in the 4th to 7th decades of life.

♦ Males are more commonly affected

♦ Lower lip is the most common site, the second most common site is the lateral border of the tongue. Among all intraoral sites, dorsum of the tongue and hard palate are the least common sites for oral squamous cell carcinoma.

♦ The initial lesion may be asymptomatic or can be presented as white or red nodule or fissure over the oral mucosa.

♦ Initially the lesion is usually painless.

♦ More advanced lesions present either as a fast enlarging, exophytic or invasive ulcer or sometimes as a large tumor mass or a verrucous growth.

♦ Ulcerated lesion often shows persistent induration around the periphery with an elevated and everted margin.

♦ The lesion can be painful either due to secondary infection or due to involvement of the peripheral nerves by the tumor cells. The lesion can also bleed easily.

♦ Floor of the mouth lesions often cause fixation of the tongue to the underlying structures with difficulty in speech and inability to open the mouth.

♦ When malignant tumor cells invade into the alveolar bone of either maxilla or mandible, they usually cause mobility or exfoliation of regional teeth.

♦ Involvement of inferior alveolar nerve often causes paresthesia of the lower teeth and the lower lip.

♦ Regional lymph nodes are often enlarged, tendered and fixed; some of these nodes can be stony hard in consistency.

♦ Untreated lesions may sometimes destroy the oral tissues and extend into the skin on the outer surface of the face to produce a nodular or lobulated growth on the facial skin, which appears as an extraoral discharging sinus.

♦ Pathological fracture of the jaw bone may sometimes occur in untreated cases due to extensive destruction of the bone by the tumor.

Histological Grading

Squamous cell carcinoma is divided in following categories by Broader also known as Broader's classification:
♦ Well-differentiated
♦ Moderately differentiated
♦ Poorly differentiated

Well-differentiated Squamous Cell Carcinoma

Most of the squamous cell carcinomas histologically belong to the well-differentiated category.
♦ In this lesion, the tumor epithelial cells to a large extent resemble the cells of the squamous epithelium both structurally and functionally.
♦ Tumor cells produce large amount of keratin in the form of "keratin pearls".
♦ Tumor cells invade into the underlying connective tissue, where the cells proliferate further and give rise to the formation of many epithelial islands within the connective tissue stroma.
♦ Tumor cells often exhibit dysplastic features, such as cellular pleomorphism, nuclear hyperchromatism, individual cell keratinization and altered nuclear-cytoplasmic ratio, loss of cohesion, etc.
♦ Prognosis is better.

Moderately Differentiated Squamous Cell Carcinoma

♦ The tumor cells are usually more severely dysplastic than that of the well-differentiated type.
♦ Tumor cells produce little or no keratin and these cells exhibit greater number of mitotic cell divisions.
♦ There is formation of epithelial islands or cell nests, etc., are diminished since these tumor cells do not differentiate or mature as much as the well-differentiated type of cells do.
♦ This tumor also carries a reasonably good prognosis.

Poorly Differentiated Squamous Cell Carcinoma

♦ In poorly differentiated squamous cell carcinoma, the malignant tumor cells produce no keratin.
♦ The tumor exhibits extensive cellular abnormalities with lack of normal architectural pattern and loss of intercellular bridges between the tumor cells.
♦ Mitotic cell division is extremely high and because of this, the neoplastic cells are often very immature and primitive looking and it is often very difficult even to recognize them as squamous epithelial cells.
♦ Prognosis is poor.

Treatment

Surgical excision is the treatment of choice.
For more details refer to Ans. 1 of same chapter.

Q.18. **What are the causes of secondaries in neck? Describe carcinoma of tongue in detail.**

(May/Jun 2009, 15 Marks)

Ans. Following are the causes of secondaries in neck:
♦ Submental lymph nodes: Infections and metastasis
♦ Submandibular lymph nodes: Infections and carcinoma
♦ Parotid: Eyelid tumors, parotid tumors and tuberculosis
♦ Prelaryngeal: Laryngeal carcinoma
♦ Pretracheal and paratracheal: Papillary carcinoma of thyroid and tuberculosis
♦ Upper anterior deep (jugulodigastric): Tonsillitis, carcinoma of posterior one-third of tongue, oropharyngeal carcinoma and tuberculosis
♦ Upper posterior deep: Tuberculosis, nasopharyngeal carcinoma
♦ Middle group: Papillary carcinoma of thyroid
♦ Lower anterior (jugulo-omohyoid): Carcinoma of tongue and carcinoma of thyroid
♦ Lower posterior (supraclavicular): Bronchogenic carcinoma, intra-abdominal malignancy and lymphoma
For carcinoma of tongue in detail refer to Ans. 4 of same chapter.

Q.19. **Describe incidence, spread, differential diagnosis and treatment of carcinoma of lips.**

(Dec 2009, 15 Marks)

Ans.

Incidence

Incidence of carcinoma of lip is 15% of head and neck cancers and 1% of all cancers.

Spread

Carcinoma of lip spreads to submental and submandibular lymph nodes (level I) and later to other neck nodes bilaterally.

Differential Diagnosis

♦ *Basal cell carcinoma:* It occurs only in upper lip
♦ *Pyogenic granuloma:* On palpation it is soft and bleeds easily.
♦ *Verrucous carcinoma:* Surface is papillomatous and white.
♦ *Necrotizing sialometaplasia:* Ulcers in this are painful with no raised borders, no hardening and characteristic histology.
♦ Keratoacanthoma
♦ Malignant melanoma.

Treatment

Refer to Ans. 6 of same chapter in detail.

Q.20. **Describe features to benign swelling turning malignant.** *(Jan 2012, 5 Marks)*

Ans.

Features of Benign Swelling Turning Malignant

♦ In benign swelling boundaries are encapsulated or well circumscribed but when it become malignant boundaries are poorly circumscribed and irregular.
♦ In benign swelling surrounding tissue is often compressed but when it turns malignant surrounding tissue is invaded.
♦ In benign swelling size is small but when it turns malignant size is large.
♦ In benign swelling secondary changes occur less often but when it turns malignant secondary changes occur more often.

- In benign swelling growth rate is slow but when it turns malignant growth rate is rapid.
- Benign swelling often compresses the surrounding tissues without invading or infiltrating them but when it turns malignant it infiltrate and invades adjacent tissues.
- In benign swelling metastasis is absent but when it turns malignant metastasis is frequently present.

Q.21. Describe the pathology, diagnosis and management of carcinoma of tongue. *(Aug 2012, 15 Marks)*

Ans.

Pathology

For pathology refer to Ans. 1 of same chapter.

Diagnosis

- Wedge biopsy is the golden rule for confirmation of diagnosis
- FNAC of lymph nodes is done to rule out invasion of cancer in lymph nodes.
- Indirect and direct laryngoscopy is done to see posterior one-third growth.
- CT scan is done to see extension of posterior one-third growth or to see status of advanced secondaries.
- MRI can also be done to assess the extent of primary tumor.
- Chest X-ray is done to see bronchopneumonia
- Orthopantomogram (OPG) is done to assess the bony involvement.
- Staging should be done by TNM classification

For management refer to Ans. 4 of same chapter.

Q.22. a. Enlist predisposing factors, premalignant lesions of oral cavity.

b. Discuss clinical features, investigations and management of carcinoma of tongue (anterior two- third) stage II. *(Aug 2012, 10 Marks)*

Ans.

a. Premalignant lesions are defined as "A morphologically altered tissue in which cancer is more likely to occur than its apparently normal counter part".

Following are the premalignant lesions:
- Leukoplakia
- Erythroplakia
- Mucosal changes associated with smoking habits
- Carcinoma in situ
- Bowen disease
- Actinic keratosis, chelitis and elastosis.
  Refer to Ans. 1 etiology part for predisposing features of premalignant lesions of oral cavity.

b. **Carcinoma of Tongue (anterior two-thirds) Stage II.**

Clinical Features

- Painless ulcer or swelling on the tongue which later on may become painful. Pain is present in the tongue due to infection or ulceration or due to involvement of lingual nerve.
- Salivation is excessive and is often blood stained.
- Visible ulcer can be seen on anterior two-thirds of tongue. Ulcer can bleed on touch; edge, base and surrounding areas are indurated. Often indurated area is more extensive than

primary tumor. Edges are everted. Ulcer may cross the midline and extend to the floor or mouth/alveolus/mandible.
- Fetor oris is due to infected necrotic growth.
- Ankyloglossia restricted mobility of the tongue. It is due to infiltration of the mouth or mandible.
- Disarticulation—difficulty in talking is due to disability of the tongue to move freely.
- Presence of palpable lymph nodes in the neck which are hard, nodular and get fixed to underlying tissues in advanced stages.

Investigations

- Biopsy is the golden standard to identify the carcinoma of tongue. Biopsy of the lesional margin is done and histopathological evaluation is done. Broader classification histologically divides oral cancer in various stages which are:
  - Well-differentiated squamous cell carcinoma
  - Moderately differentiated squamous cell carcinoma
  - Poorly differentiated squamous cell carcinoma
- FNAC of lymph nodes
- CT scan to see the status of lymph node secondaries.
- MRI to assess extent of primary tumor
- Chest X-ray to see bronchopneumonia
- Orthopantomogram

Treatment

Stage II tumor means T2N0M0, i.e., Tumor more than 2 cm but not more than 4 cm in its greatest dimensions. There is no regional lymph node metastasis and no distant metastasis. So following treatment can be done.

Surgery

- Wide excision with 1 cm clearance in margin and depth is done in tumor <1 cm in size or in carcinoma in situ. Laser (CO_2/diode) can be used.
- Tumor between 1–2 cm in size, partial glossectomy is done with 2 cm clearance from the margin with removal of 1/3rd of anterior two-thirds of the tongue.
- Tumor larger than 2 cm, hemiglossectomy is done with removal of anterior 2/3rd of tongue on one side up to sulcus terminalis.
- Raw area in these procedures can be left alone when area is wide allowing it to granulate and heal by epithelialization. If area is small like in wide excision it can be closed by primary suturing. Wide raw area can also be covered with PMMF or quilted split-skin graft.
- Larger primary tumor can be given preoperative radiotherapy then later hemiglossectomy is done.
- Same side palpable mobile lymph nodes are removed by radical neck block dissection.
- Bilateral mobile lymph nodes are dealt with one side radical block and other side junctional block dissection with essentially retaining internal jugular vein (on opposite side) to maintain the cerebral venous blood flow. Other option is doing same side radical neck dissection and on opposite side supraomohyoid block dissection.
- Wide excision is done when growth is in the tip of the tongue.

♦ Reconstruction of tongue and other area after surgery: By deltopectoral flap, forehead flap, pectoralis major muscle flap, skin grafting.

♦ Prophylactic block dissection is becoming popular at present.

Radiotherapy

♦ In small primary tumor—brachytherapy using cesium or iridium needles.

♦ In large primary tumor initial radiotherapy is given to reduce the tumor size so that resection will be better later.

♦ Advanced primary as well as secondaries in neck are controlled by palliative external radiotherapy.

♦ Postoperative radiotherapy is given in large tumors to reduce the chances of relapse.

Chemotherapy

♦ It is given in postoperative period and for palliation.

♦ Price–Hill regimen is commonly used. Drugs are methotrexate, vincristine, adriamycin, bleomycin and mercaptopurine.

♦ It is either given intra-arterially as regional chemotherapy through external carotid artery using arterial pump or through IV. It can be given orally also.

Q.23. Write short note on management of lower lip carcinoma. *(Mar 2006, 5 Marks)*

Ans.

Management of Lower Lip Carcinoma

♦ If lesion is <2 cm, then curative radiotherapy, either brachytherapy or external beam radiotherapy. It gives a good cure.

♦ Tumor is >2 cm, wide excision is done. Excision of lower lip up to one-third can be sutured primarily, in layers keeping vermilion border in proper apposition without causing any microstomia.

♦ Excision of more than one-third of the lip requires reconstruction using different flaps.

Methods

♦ *Abbe–Estlander's rotation flap:* It is done in lower lip lesions which located at the angle based on labial artery.

♦ *Abbe flap:* Done in lower lip lesions at the middle or at the site other than angle based on labial artery. In the later second stage base of the flap should be released once the flap takes up.

♦ *W flap plasty:* It is done for the lower lip middle tumor which is less than one-third of the lip.

♦ *Karapandzic flap:* It is done in lower lip defect with less angulation towards upper lip.

Q.24. Enumerate benign tumors around oral cavity. *(June 2015, 5 Marks)*

Ans.

Benign Tumors Around Oral Cavity

♦ Epithelial tissue
  • Papilloma
  • Keratoacanthoma

  • Squamous acanthoma
  • Nevus.

♦ Fibrous connective tissue
  • Fibroma
  • Fibrous hyperplasia
  • Fibrous epulis
  • Giant cell fibroma
  • Fibrous histiocytoma
  • Desmoplastic fibroma
  • Myxoma
  • Myxofibroma.

♦ Cartilage tissue
  • Chondroma
  • Chondroblastoma
  • Chondromyxoid fibroma.

♦ Adipose tissue
  • Lipoma
  • Angiolipoma.

♦ Bone
  • Osteoma
  • Osteoid osteoma
  • Osteoblastoma
  • Torus palatines or torus mandibularis
  • Osteomatosis.

♦ Vascular tissue
  • Hemangioma
  • Lymphangioma
  • Arteriovenous fistula
  • Glomus tumor.

♦ Neural tissue
  • Neurofibroma
  • Neurilemmoma
  • Ganglioneuroma
  • Traumatic neuroma
  • Melanotic neuroectodermal tumor of infancy.

♦ Muscles
  • Leiomyoma
  • Rhabdomyoma
  • Granular cell myoblastoma.

♦ Giant cell tumor
  • Central giant cell tumor
  • Peripheral giant cell tumor
  • Giant cell granuloma
  • Giant cell tumor of hyperthyroidism.

♦ Teratoma.

Q.25. Describe etiopathology, clinical feature and management of Ca of tongue. *(Apr 2017, 10 Marks)*

Ans.

Etiopathology of Carcinoma of Tongue

Benzopyrenes and nitrosamines in cigarette smoke and tobacco products, arecoline in areca nut are the carcinogenic agents; alterations in activity of genes on 3p, 9p and 17; E6 and E7 proteins of human papillomavirus inactivate p53 and retinoblastoma tumor suppressor gene later leading to overexpression of p16 presence of which is correlated with HPV associated carcinoma.

For clinical feature and management of carcinoma of tongue, refer to Ans. 4 of same chapter.

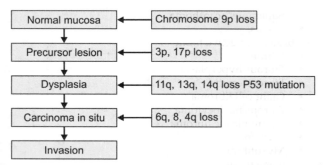

Q.26. Discuss etiology, clinical features and management of carcinoma alveolar margin. *(Jan 2018, 20 Marks)*

Ans. *For etiology, refer to Ans. 1 of same chapter*

For clinical features, refer to Ans. 12 of same chapter

For management, refer to Ans. 3 of same chapter

Q.27. Write on etiology, clinical features, staging and management of anterior two-thirds of carcinoma of tongue. *(Feb 2019, 10 Marks)*

Ans. *For etiology refer to Ans. 4 of same chapter.*

For staging refer to Ans. 9 of same chapter.

For clinical features refer to Ans. 11 of same chapter.

For management refer to Ans. 5 of same chapter.

Q.28. Write short answer on wedge biopsy.

(Oct 2019, 3 Marks)

Ans. Wedge biopsy is the type of incisional biopsy.

Wedge is an area at two meeting parts. For, e.g., thick to thin etc.

A wedge biopsy is made by a wedge shaped incision which begins 2–3 mm from the normal tissue and penetrates into the region surrounding the abnormal tissue. It is always better to incise the tissue narrow and deep than broad and shallow.

Procedure

♦ **Anesthesia:** A block is given to anesthetize the region where specimen is to be obtained. Local infiltration and injections into the tissue to be biopsied is avoided as it causes artifacts in the specimen. When a block is not effective, local infiltration is given at least l cm away from the lesion.

♦ **Stabilization of the tissue:** Soft tissue biopsies are usually done on movable tissues of the oral cavity, such as tongue, lips, etc. The assistant stabilizes the tissue by stretching it.

♦ **Hemostasis:** Use of high volume suction may cause aspiration of the specimen into the suction device. Gauze pieces can be used for compressing the tissue and achieving hemostasis. Also gauze piece can be placed to cover the mouth of the suction tip and used to prevent the specimen from being sucked in.

♦ **Incision:** A sharp scalpel is used. Here two incisions forming an elliptical incision and converging to form a V at the base provides a good specimen and a wound which is easy to close. Incisions are kept parallel to the nerves and vessels in that region to avoid damage.

♦ **Handling of tissues:** The tissue to be removed is to be handled carefully so that histopathological examination can be performed. A nontoothed tissue holding forceps is used and care is taken not to crush the tissues.

♦ **Specimen care:** After removal of the tissues, the specimen is transferred to a bottle containing 10% formalin that is atleast 20 times the volume of the specimen obtained.

♦ **Surgical closure of wound:** Primary closure is possible in most cases. Where it is not possible, tissues are undermined to facilitate closure.

Indications

♦ In diagnosis of vesicular or bullous lesions
♦ In diagnosis of ulcerative lesions
♦ For evaluating the lesions of uncertain origin.
♦ For diagnosing atypical appearing lesions, such as atypical mycobacterial infections.
♦ It is used to confirm or exclude the malignancy.

Advantages

♦ It is a simple procedure.
♦ It can be expertise by the physician.
♦ It is time conserving.
♦ There is low incidence of infection, bleeding or non-healing.
♦ Scaring is insignificant, so it is cosmetic.

Q.29. Write differences between incisional biopsy and excisional biopsy. *(Feb 2019, 5 Marks)*

Ans. Differences between incisional and excisional biopsy:

Incisional biopsy	Excisional biopsy
It is the biopsy which examines only the representative part of the lesion and normal adjacent tissue in order to make a definitive diagnosis before treatment.	This procedure removes the lesion completely at the time when the diagnostic procedure is being performed.
Lesions more than 1 cm in size or where there is greater suspicion of malignancy, in them this type of biopsy method is used	Lesions <1 cm in diameter can be excised by this method.
This technique can only be used as diagnostic method.	This technique at times is for both diagnosis and treatment of disease.
It is used to confirm or exclude the malignancy	If tumor is highly infiltrative thee margin of excision cannot be exactly elicited, further surgery will be needed. Furthermore cancerous cells actively multiply at tumor margins, debulking of mass may result in residual cancer cells left behind.

18. NECK

Q.1. Describe clinical features and treatment of carotid body tumor. *(Sep 1999, 4 Marks)*

Ans. It is also called as chemodectoma or potato tumor.

Definition: It is a non-chromaffin paraganglioma.

It most commonly arises near the bifurcation of common carotid artery.

It is a benign tumor.

Clinical Features

♦ It is usually unilateral.
♦ More common in middle age.
♦ Swelling (75%) in the carotid region of the neck which is smooth, firm, pulsatile and moves only side to side but not in vertical direction.
♦ It can often compress over esophagus and larynx.
♦ Headache, neck pain, dysphagia, syncope are other presentations.
♦ It can present with unilateral vocal cord palsy; can cause Horner's syndrome.
♦ Features of transient ischemic attacks due to compression over the carotids, "carotid body syncope."
♦ Thrill may be felt and bruit may be heard.
♦ It is located at the level of hyoid bone deep to anterior edge of the sternomastoid muscle in anterior triangle, vertically placed, round, firm 'potato' like swelling.
♦ Often tumor may extend into the cranial cavity along with internal carotid artery as dumbbell tumor.

Treatment

♦ If it is small, it can be excised easily as the tumor is situated in adventitia.
♦ When it is large, as commonly observed, complete excision has to be done followed by placing a vascular graft.
♦ During resection a temporary shunt is placed between common carotid below and internal carotid above to safeguard cerebral perfusion; external carotid artery is ligated. Venous or prosthetic graft is placed between common carotid and internal carotid arteries.

Q.2. Write in short torticollis. *(Sep 2002, 5 Marks)*

Ans. Torticollis or wry neck is a deformity in which the head is bent to one side with the chin point to the outer side.

In long standing cases there may be atrophy of the face on the affected side.

The different varieties of wry neck are:

♦ *Congenital:*
  • The diagnosis is made by a history of difficult labor, followed by the appearance of a sternomastoid tumor.
  • The affected muscle feels firm and rigid.
♦ *Traumatic:* Fracture dislocation of the cervical spine.
♦ *Rheumatic:* Sudden appearance of wry neck after an exposure to cold or draught is suggestive.
♦ *Inflammatory:* For example, from inflammed cervical lymph node.
♦ *Spasmodic:* When the sternomastoid of the affected side and the posterior cervical muscle of the opposite side are found in a state of spasm.
♦ *Compensatory:* For example, from scoliosis, defect in sight (ocular torticollis)
♦ From Pott's disease of the cervical spine.
♦ *From contracture:* For example, after burns, ulcer, etc.

Features

♦ Restricted neck movements
♦ Chin pointing towards opposite side
♦ Presence of squint

Treatment

Botulinus toxins have been used to inhibit the spastic contraction of affected muscle.

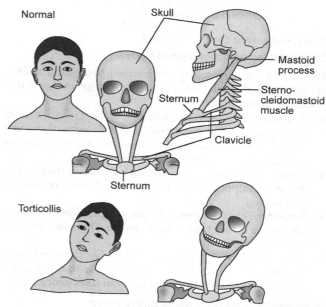

Fig. 26: Torticollis.

Q.3. Discuss the differential diagnosis of swelling in the lateral aspect of neck. *(Sep 2001, 15 Marks)*

Ans. It is classified according to their location in three triangles of the neck:

1. Submandibular or digastric triangle
   • Enlarged lymph node
   • Enlarged submandibular salivary gland
     – Calculus
     – Chronic sialadenitis
     – Cancer
     – Chronic diseases—autoimmune.
2. Carotid triangle
   • Aneurysm of carotid artery
   • Carotid body tumor
   • Branchial cyst
   • Neurofibroma vagus
   • Enlargement of thyroid gland
   • Lymph node swelling (cold abscess)
   • Laryngocele
   • Sternomastoid tumor.
3. In posterior triangle
   • *Solid swellings:*
     – Metastasis in lymph node
     – Tuberculosis
     – Lymphoma
     – Lipoma
     – Cervical rib
     – Pancoast tumor.
   • *Cystic swellings:*
     – Lymphangioma

- Hemangioma
- Cold abscess.
- *Pulsatile swellings:*
  - Subclavian artery aneurysm
  - Vertebral artery aneurysm.

Submandibular or Digastric Triangle

Enlarged Submandibular Lymph Node

They form a nodular swelling which is deep to deep fascia. They are palpable only in the neck. The nodes can get enlarged due to following conditions:

- *Acute lymphadenitis:* Very often, poor oral hygiene or a caries tooth produces painful, tender, soft enlargement of these lymph nodes. Extraction of the tooth or with improvement of oral hygiene, lymph nodes regress.
- Chronic tuberculous lymphadenitis can affect these nodes along with upper deep cervical nodes. The nodes are firm and matted.
- Secondaries in the submandibular lymph nodes arise from carcinoma of the cheek, tongue, palate. The nodes are hard with or without fixity.
- Non-Hodgkin's lymphoma can involve submandibular lymph nodes along with horizontal group of nodes in the neck. The nodes are firm or rubbery in consistency.

Submandibular Salivary Gland Enlargement

The common causes are chronic sialadenitis with or without a stone, tumors of the salivary gland or enlargement due to autoimmune diseases. They form irregular or nodular swelling. The diagnosis is confirmed by bidigital palpation of the gland. Enlarged submandibular gland is bidigitally palpable because the deep lobe is deep to mylohyoid muscle.

Carotid Triangle

- **Branchial cyst:** It is located in anterior triangle of neck. It is soft, cystic, fluctuant and transillumination negative.
- **Lymph node swelling (cold abscess):** Patient present with history of tuberculosis. Lymph nodes are firm and matted. Signs of inflammation are absent.
- **Aneurysm of carotid artery:** It is firm, fluctuant and transillumination negative swelling with presence of expansile pulsations. Bruit/thrill can be heard.
- **Carotid body tumor:** It is has a typical location, i.e., located at level of hyoid bone in upper part of anterior triangle of neck beneath anterior edge of sternomastoid muscle. On palpation it moves in transverse direction. Surface is smooth or lobulated, borders are round, oval in shape, vertically placed swelling.
- **Sternomastoid tumor:** Swelling is present in infants or children. It is tender, mobile sideways, medial and lateral borders are distinct. Both superior and inferior borders are continuous with the swelling.
- **Laryngocele:** It is a smooth, oval, boggy swelling which moves upwards on swallowing. Expansile cough impulse is present.
- **Neurofibroma of vagus nerve:** It produces swelling in carotid triangle in region of thyroid swelling. It is a vertically

placed oval swelling. On pressure over the swelling dry cough occurs and in some cases bradycardia can occur.

Posterior Triangle

Solid Swellings

- **Metastasis in lymph nodes:** Lymph nodes become enlarged and become fixed to the underlying structures. They become immobile and are stoney hard in consistency.
- **Tuberculosis:** Lymph nodes become enlarged mainly cervical. The nodes are firm and matted.
- **Lymphoma:** It can involve submandibular lymph nodes along with horizontal group of nodes in the neck. The nodes are firm or rubbery in consistency.
- **Lipoma:** It is a localized swelling with lobular surface, nontender. It is semifluctuant and nontransilluminant. It is mobile with edges slipping between palpating fingers.
- **Cervical rib:** It is an extra, rib present in the neck. A hard mass is visible or palpated in root of neck.
- **Pancoast tumor:** It is a tumor felt in the lower part of posterior triangle. It is hard in consistency, fixed, irregular and sometimes tender. Lower border of mass cannot be appreciated.

Cystic Swellings

- **Lymphangioma:** Skin vesicles contain watery or yellow fluid. Bleeding in vesicle turn into brown or black. Area is soft, spongy, often fluctuant with fluid thrill and translucency. It is noncompressible. Vesicles will not fade on pressure.
- **Hemangioma:** Swelling is warm and bluish in color, nonpulsatile, soft, fluctuant, transillumination negative. Compressibility is present. When the swelling is compressed between fingers blood diffuses under vascular spaces and when pressure is released it slowly fills up.
- **Cold abscess:** Patient present with history of tuberculosis. Lymph nodes are firm and matted. Signs of inflammation are absent.

Q.4. Write short note on swelling midline of neck.

(Sep 2006, 10 Marks)

Or

Write briefly on midline swellings of neck.

(Dec 2009, 5 Marks)

Ans. The midline swellings of neck are:

- Ludwig's angina
- Enlarged submental lymph node
- Sublingual dermoid cyst
- Thyroglossal cyst
- Subhyoid bursitis
- Goiter of thyroid, isthmus and pyramidal lobe
- Enlarged lymph node and lipoma in substernal space of burns
- Retrosternal goiter
- Thymic swelling
- Bony swelling arising from the manubrium sterni.

Ludwig's Angina

- This is an inflammatory edema of the floor of the mouth. It spreads to the submandibular region and submental region.

♦ Tense, tender, browny edematous swelling in the submental region with putrid halitosis is characteristic of this condition.

Enlarged Submental Lymph Nodes

The three important causes of enlargement:

1. *Tuberculosis:* Matted submental nodes, firm in consistency, with enlarged upper deep cervical lymph nodes, with or without evening rise of temperature are suggestive of tuberculosis.
2. Non-Hodgkin's lymphoma can present with submental nodes along with other lymph nodes in the horizontal group of nodes, such as submandibular, upper deep cervical, preauricular, postauricular and occipital lymph nodes (external Waldeyer's ring). Nodes are firm or rubbery, discrete without matting.
3. Secondaries in the submental lymph nodes can arise from carcinoma of the tip of the tongue, floor of the mouth, central portion of the lower lip. The nodes are hard in consistency and sometimes, fixed.

Sublingual Dermoid Cyst

♦ It is a type of sequestration dermoid cyst which occurs due to sequestration of the surface ectoderm at the site of fusion of the two mandibular arches. Hence, such a cyst occurs in the midline, in the floor of the mouth.
♦ When they arise from 2nd branchial cleft, they are found lateral to the midline. Hence, lateral variety.

Subhyoid Bursitis

♦ Accumulation of inflammatory fluid in the subhyoid bursa results in a swelling and is described as subhyoid bursitis.
♦ Bursa is located below hyoid bone and in front of thyrohyoid membrane.
♦ It is the swelling in front of neck in midline below hyoid bone.
♦ Swelling moves up with deglutition and is tender.

Thyroglossal Cyst

♦ It arises from thyroglossal tract or duct which extends from foramen cecum at base of tongue to isthmus of thyroid.
♦ It is common in females and is painless midline swelling. Swelling is deviated to left side.
♦ Thyroglossal cyst exhibits three types of mobilities, i.e.
  1. It moves upwards with deglutition
  2. Cyst moves with protrusion of tongue
  3. Swelling move sideways but not vertically as it is tethered by the thyroglossal duct.

Enlarged Isthmus of Thyroid Gland

Almost all the diseases of the thyroid gland result in enlargement of the isthmus. However, a solitary nodule and cysts can occur in relation to isthmus. The swelling moves with deglutition. However, it does not move on protrusion of the tongue.

Pretracheal and Prelaryngeal Lymph Nodes

These lymph nodes produce nodular swelling in the midline. One or two discrete nodes are palpable. They can enlarge due to following conditions:

♦ *Acute laryngitis:* The nodes are tender, soft.
♦ *Papillary carcinoma of thyroid:* The nodes are firm without matting, with or without evidence of thyroid nodule.
♦ *Carcinoma of the larynx:* The nodes are hard in consistency.

Thymic Swelling

♦ It is caused by an aneurysm of innominate or subclavian artery.
♦ It is a pulsatile swelling.

Lipoma in Suprasternal Space of Burns

♦ It is soft and lobular.
♦ Edge of lipoma slips under the palpating finger.

Q.5. Write short note on pulsatile swellings in neck.

(Dec 2009, 5 Marks)

Ans.

Pulsatile Swellings in Neck

♦ Carotid body tumor: *Refer to Ans. 1 of same chapter in detail*
♦ Aneurysm
  • Arterial hemangioma:
    – An abnormal communication between artery and vein results in AV fistula.
    – It is a soft, cystic, fluctuant, transillumination negative, pulsatile swelling.
    – A continuous bruit/murmur is characteristic.
    – On compressing the feeding artery, venous return to heart diminishes which leads to fall in pulse rate and pulse pressure.
  • Cirsoid aneurysms:
    – It is a rare variant of capillary hemangioma occurring in skin beneath which abnormal artery communicates with the distended veins.
    – Variant of capillary hemangioma
    – Pulsatile swelling
    – Involves bone
    – Treatment is ligation of feeding artery and excision of lesion.

Q.6. Describe various triangles of neck and their boundaries. Discuss the differential diagnosis of neck swelling. *(Jun 2010, 15 Marks)*

Ans. Each side of neck is the quadrilateral space which is subdivided by sternocleidomastoid into anterior triangle and posterior triangle. These triangles are further subdivided into:

♦ Anterior triangle
♦ Posterior triangle

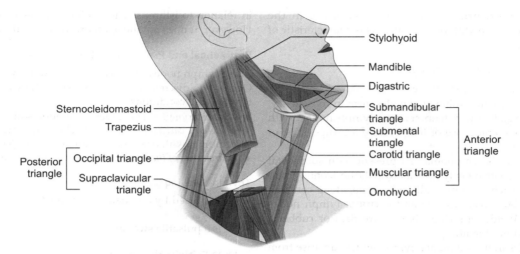

Fig. 27: Triangles of neck *(For color version see Plate 1).*

Anterior Triangle

Boundaries

- *Anterior:* Anterior midline of the neck extending from symphysis menti above to the middle of suprasternal notch below.
- *Posterior:* Anterior border of sternocleidomastoid
- *Base:* Lower border of the body of mandible and line joining the angle of mandible with the mastoid process
- *Apex:* Suprasternal notch, at the meeting point between anterior border of sternocleidomastoid and anterior midline.

Subdivisions of Anterior Triangle

The anterior triangle in subdivided by the diagastric muscle and superior belly of omohyoid into following:

- Submental triangle
- Digastric triangle
- Carotid triangle
- Muscular triangle.

Submental Triangle

This triangle is complete only when the neck is seen from the front. Each half of the triangle is visible when viewed from side.

Boundaries

- *On each side:* Anterior belly of diagastric
- *Base:* Body of hyoid bone
- *Apex:* Chin or symphysis menti
- *Floor:* Oral diaphragm formed by the mylohyoid muscles.

Digastric Triangle

Boundaries

- *Anteroinferior:* Anterior belly of digastric
- *Posteroinferior:* Posterior belly of digastric
- *Base:* Base of the mandible and an imaginary line joining the angle of mandible to the mastoid process

- *Apex:* Intermediate tendon of diagastric muscle bound down to hyoid bone by a facial sling.
- *Floor:* Is formed by mylohyoid muscle (anteriorly), hyoglossus muscle and small part of middle constrictor (posteriorly).
- *Roof:* Is formed by the investing layer of deep cervical fascia which splits to enclose the submandibular salivary gland.

Carotid Triangle

Boundaries

- *Superior:* Posterior belly of digastric and stylohyoid
- *Anteroinferior:* Superior belly of omohyoid
- *Posterior:* Anterior border of sternocleidomastoid
- *Roof:* Is formed by investing layer of deep cervical fascia
- *Floor:* Is formed by four muscles:
  1. Thyrohyoid
  2. Hyoglossus
  3. Middle constrictor of pharynx
  4. Inferior constrictor of pharynx.

Muscular Triangle

Boundaries

- *Anterior:* Anterior midline of the neck
- *Anterosuperior:* Superior belly of the omohyoid
- *Posteroinferior:* Anterior border of sternocleidomastoid.

Posterior Triangle

Boundaries

- *Anterior:* Posterior border of sternocleidomastoid
- *Posterior:* Anterior border of trapezius
- *Base:* Middle third of the clavicle
- *Apex:* Meeting point of sternocleidomastoid and trapezius on the superior nuchal line.
- *Roof:* Is formed by investing layer of deep cervical fascia stretching between sternomastoid and trapezius muscles
- *Floor:* Is muscular and is formed by following muscles

From Above Downwards

- Semispinalis capitis
- Splenius capitis
- Levator scapulae
- Scalenus posterior
- Scalenus medius
- Outer border of 1st rib.

Sub-divisions of Posterior Triangle

- Occipital triangle
- Supraclavicular triangle

Occipital Triangle (From Above Downwards)

- Occipital artery at apex
- Spinal part of accessory nerve
- Four cutaneous branches of cervical plexus of nerves
  1. Lesser occipital
  2. Great auricular
  3. Transverse cervical
  4. Supraclavicular
- Muscular branches of C3 and C4 nerves
- Dorsal scapular nerve.

Supraclavicular Triangle

- Trunks of brachial plexus of nerves with their branches
  - Dorsal scapular
  - Long thoracic
  - Nerve to subclavius.
- Subclavian artery—3rd part
- Subclavian vein
- External jugular vein
- Supraclavicular lymph nodes.

For differential diagnosis of neck swellings refer to Ans. 3 and Ans. 4 of same chapter.

Q.7. Enumerate different triangles of neck, its boundary, contents and its surgical importance.

(Feb 2019, 5 Marks)

Ans.

Enumeration of Different Triangles of Neck

- Anterior triangle
  - Submental triangle
  - Digastric triangle
  - Carotid triangle
  - Muscular triangle
- Posterior triangle
  - Occipital triangle
  - Supraclavicular triangle

Boundaries of Different Triangles of Neck

For details refer to Ans. 6 of same chapter.

Contents of Different Triangles of Neck

Contents of Submental Triangle

- Two to four small submental lymph nodes are situated in superficial fascia between anterior bellies of digastric muscles. They drain:

- Superficial tissues below the chin
- Central part of lower lip
- The adjoining gums
- Anterior part off floor of mouth
- Tip of tongue
- Small submental veins join to form the anterior jugular veins.

Contents of Digastric Triangle

Anterior Part of Triangle

Structures superficial to myelohyoid are:
- Superficial part of submandibular gland
- Facial vein and submandibular lymph node are superficial to it and facial artery deep to it.
- Submental artery
- Myelohyoid nerve and vessels
- The hypoglossal nerve.

Posterior Part of Triangle

- Superficial structures are:
  - Lower part of parotid gland
  - External carotid artery before it enter parotid gland
- Deep structures passing between the internal and external carotid arteries:
  - The styloglossus
  - The stylopharyngeus
  - The glossopharyngeal nerve
  - Pharyngeal branch of vagus nerve
  - The styloid process
  - A part of parotid gland
- Deepest structures include:
  a. Internal carotid artery
  b. Internal jugular vein
  c. The vagus nerve

Contents of Carotid Triangle

- **Arteries:**
  - Common carotid artery with carotid sinus and carotid body at its termination
  - Internal carotid artery
  - External carotid artery with its superior thyroid, lingual, facial, ascending pharyngeal and occipital branches.
- **Veins:**
  - Internal jugular vein
  - Common facial vein draining into internal jugular vein.
  - Pharyngeal vein which end in internal jugular vein.
  - Lingual vein which terminates in internal jugular vein.
- **Nerves:**
  - Vagus running vertically downwards
  - Superior laryngeal branch of vagus, dividing in external and internal laryngeal nerves.
  - Spinal accessory nerve running backward over internal jugular vein
  - Hypoglossal nerve running forward over external and internal carotid arteries
  - Sympathetic chain run vertically downward posterior to carotid sheath. Carotid sheath with its contents.
- **Lymph nodes:** Deep cervical lymph nodes are situated along internal jugular vein, and include jugulodiagastric node

below the posterior belly of digastric and jugulo-omohyoid node above the inferior belly of omohyoid.

Contents of Muscular Triangle

Infrahyoid muscles are the chief contents of the triangle.

These muscles may also be regarded arbitrarily as forming the floor of triangle. The infrahyoid muscles are:

a. Sternohyoid
b. Sternothyroid
c. Thyrohyoid
d. Omohyoid

Posterior Triangle

It is subdivided into occipital triangle and subclavian triangle.

Contents	Occipital triangle	Subclavian triangle

A. Nerves	• Spinal accessory nerve
	• Four cutaneous branches of cervical plexus
	  - Lesser occipital
	  - Greater auricular
	  - Anterior cutaneous nerve of neck
	  - Supraclavicular nerve
	• Muscular branches
	  - Two small branches to levator scapulae
	  - Two small branches to trapezius
	  - Nerve to rhomboids
	• C5, C6 roots of brachial plexus
		• Three trunks of brachial plexus
		• Nerve to serratus anterior
		• Nerve to subclavius
		• Suprascapular nerve

B. Vessels	• Transverse cervical • Occipital artery	• Third part of subclavian artery and vein • Suprascapular artery and vein • Commencement of transverse cervical artery and termination of corresponding vein • Lower part of external jugular vein
C. Lymph nodes	Supraclavicular and occipital lymph nodes	Few members of supraclavicular chain

Surgical Importance of Triangles of Neck

Anatomical landmarks can be useful during surgery of the neck. There are many triangles in the neck containing arteries, veins, nerves, lymph vessels and nodes, and other important structures. A better understanding of the anatomy of these triangles of the neck could help to minimize surgical injuries and make surgical dissections more efficient.

Q.8.   Write short note on Waldeyer's ring.
(Aug 2018, 10 Marks)

Ans. It is also known as Waldeyer's lymphatic ring.

It is of two type, i.e., inner and outer Waldeyer's ring.

1. Inner Waldeyer's lymphatic ring has adenoids above, lingual tonsil below and two palatine tonsils and tubal tonsils laterally one on each side.
2. Outer circular chain of nodes (outer Waldeyer's ring) has occipital, postauricular, preauricular, parotid, facial, submandibular, submental, superficial cervical and anterior cervical lymph nodes.

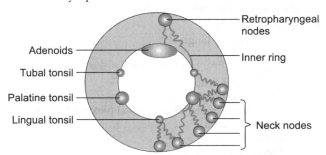

Fig. 28: Inner and outer Waldeyer ring anatomy
(For color version see Plate 1).

• **Facial nodes are:**
  – Superficial groups
    » Upper: Infraorbital
    » Middle: Buccinator
    » Lower: Supramandibular
  – Deep groups—in relation to pterygoids.
• **Submandibular lymph nodes:** Drain side of the nose; cheek; angle of the mouth; entire upper lip; outer part of the lower lip; the gums; side of the tongue.
• **Submental lymph nodes:** Drain from the central part of the lower lip, floor of the mouth and apex of the tongue.
• **Superficial cervical nodes:** They lie on outer surface of the sternomastoid around the external jugular vein. They drain the parotid region and lower part of the ear.
• **Deep cervical lymph nodes:** Upper deep cervical lymph nodes—jugulodigastric nodes below the digastric and infront of internal jugular vein.
• **Lower deep cervical lymph nodes:** Jugulo-omohyoid nodes—above the omohyoid and behind the internal jugular vein. They drain the ipsilateral half of head and neck, finally form a jugular lymph trunk from lower deep cervical nodes to join thoracic duct on the left side, and the junction of right subclavian and right jugular vein on right side.

Q.9.   Enumerate the indications of radical neck dissection and its types.
(Sep 2018, 5 Marks)

Ans.

Indications of Radical Neck Dissection

♦ In carcinoma of tongue and carcinoma of floor of mouth.
♦ In malignant melanoma
♦ In metastatic lymph nodes from both pharynx and upper esophagus

Types of Radical Neck Dissection

1. Classical radical neck dissection
2. Modified radical neck dissection
   - Type I (XI preserved)
   - Type II (XI nerve and internal jugular vein preserved)
   - Type III (XI nerve, internal jugular vein and sternocleidomastoid muscle preserved)
3. Selective neck dissection
   - Supraomohyoid type
   - Lateral type
   - Posterolateral type
   - Anterior compartment type
4. Extended radical neck dissection

Classic Radical Neck Dissection

It is resection of lymph nodes (level I to V), fat, fascia, sternocleidomastoid muscle, omohyoid muscle, internal jugular vein, external jugular vein, accessory nerve, submandibular salivary gland, lower part of parotid, prevertebral fascia - "en—block"(Criles' operation). Incision which is commonly made are Fischel T or modified Criles or MacFee incisions which are two parallel incisions, one at submandibular region, and another at supraclavicular region. Blood supply of the flap remains intact and so healing will be better without flap necrosis.

Modified Radical Neck Dissection

It is done only in selected cases where tumor is very well differentiated and less aggressive. Here one or more non-lymphatic structures are preserved. Medina classification is used for modified radical neck dissection types:

- Type I (XI preserved). N—preserved
- Type II (XI nerve and Internal jugular vein preserved). NV are preserved
- Type III (XI nerve, internal jugular vein and sternocleido-mastoid muscle preserved). NMV—preserved. It is called as functional neck dissection.

Selective Neck Node Dissection

Here one or more nodal levels in the neck are retained unlike radical neck dissection. It can be supraomohyoid, lateral neck (anterolateral), anterior (central) or posterolateral neck dissections.

- **Supraomohyoid neck dissection:** Removal of only fat, fascia, lymph nodes, muscles, submandibular salivary gland, with dissection above the omohyoid muscle is done. Done only in selected individuals with well-differentiated tumor and involvement of few submandibular lymph nodes (levels I, II, III are removed). It is also done in N0 lesions. Here ideally (done in N0 cases) alter dissection, frozen section biopsy should be done; if nodes are positive, modified radical neck dissection/radical neck dissection should be done depending on grading of the primary.
- **Lateral neck dissection:** It is done in laryngeal and pharyngeal primaries with clinically negative nodes. Levels II, III, IV are removed bilaterally.
- **Anterior dissection:** Level VI (pre, paratracheal) nodes are removed. It is done in carcinoma of thyroid.

- **Posterolateral dissection:** Levels II, III, IV, with suboccipital and postauricular or with level V are removed for cutaneous malignancies.

Extended Radical Dissection

Removal of one or more additional groups of lymphatics or removal of nonlymphatic structures with radical neck dissection is called as extended radical neck dissection. Additional nodes in the mediastinum are cleared (level VII). Nodes like level VI or parapharyngeal, retropharyngeal, external carotid artery, hypoglossal nerve, vagus nerve, parotid gland, mastoid tip—are addressed.

Other Types of Neck Dissections

- **Bilateral neck dissection:** Here internal jugular vein is preserved on one side. Always the side where the vein is preserved, is operated first. Ligating one internal jugular vein increases the intracranial pressure by three fold; both internal jugular veins ligations increase intracranial pressure by five fold. Intracranial pressure gradually falls over 8–10 days. For this reason pressure dressing should be avoided over the wound of neck dissection after surgery.
- **Commando operation (combined mandibular dissection and neck dissection operation):** It is en-block removal, which includes wide excision of primary tumor with hemimandibulectomy and neck block dissection, Examples: It is done usually in carcinoma of tongue or floor of the mouth; it is a composite resection of primary tumor, mandible and radical neck dissection.
- **Comprehensive neck dissection (Medina):** It means either radical neck dissection or modified radical neck dissection types of neck node dissections.

---

19. SALIVARY GLAND

Q.1. Describe surgical anatomy of parotid gland. Describe signs, symptoms and management of pleomorphic adenoma of parotid gland.

(Sep 2008, 5 Marks) (Sep 2005, 15 Marks)

Ans. Parotid gland is a major salivary gland.

Surgical Anatomy of Parotid Gland

- Parotid gland lies beneath the skin, in front and below the ear.
- Parotid gland is contained in the investing layer of the deep fascia of the neck which is known as parotid fascia.
- Parotid gland is separated from submandibular gland by a fascial thickening known as stylomandibular ligament.
- Parotid space is occupied by the parotid gland.
- From anterolateral edge of the gland, parotid duct or Stensen's duct passes lateral to the masseter muscle. Parotid duct turns medial at the anterior margin of the muscle, where it is related to the buccal fat pad or "boule de Bichat".
- Location of buccal pad is medial to the parotid duct, between the masseter and buccinator muscles.
- Stensen's duct pierces the buccinator muscle and enters the oral cavity at the level of the upper second molar tooth.

- At times accessory parotid tissue may extend along the Stensen's duct. A short accessory duct may enter the main duct.

Parotid Fascia

- Parotid fascia is mainly the splitting of general investing layer which envelops both parotid and submandibular glands forming the superficial and deep layers.
- Superficial layer is dense and tough while the deep layer is thin and weak.
- Stylomandibular ligament which lies between the styloid process and the angle of the mandible is derived from the deep layer. The ligament is tough, and separates the parotid from the submandibular gland.
- Communication of parotid space is medial with the lateral pharyngeal space and with the posterior area of the masticator space.
- Posterior area of the masticator space consists of masseter muscle, pterygoid muscles, the small pterygomandibular space and the space of the body of the mandible.
- As many intraparotid anatomic structures radiate from parotid gland, surgeon should be familiar with all those structures, especially those which should not be sacrificed.

Bed of the Parotid Gland

Complete removal of the parotid gland reveals the following structures:

- Internal jugular vein, i.e., one vein
- External carotid artery and internal carotid artery, i.e., two arteries
- IX, X, XI, and XII cranial nerves, i.e., four nerves

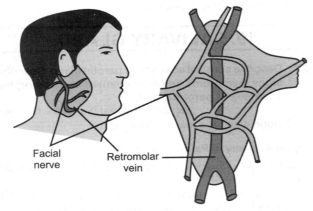

Facial nerve   Retromolar vein

Fig. 29: Surgical anatomy of parotid gland.

Signs and Symptoms (Clinical Features)

- Middle aged women around 40 years are commonly affected.
- Swelling is painless.
- Parotid swelling has following classical features:
  - It present as a swelling in front, below and behind the ear.
  - Raises ear lobule.
  - Retromandibular groove is obliterated.

- It is rubbery or firm
- Soft area indicates necrosis
- In long standing cases it can be hard
- Surface can be nodular
- Skin is stretched and becomes shiny
- Being a benign tumor it is neither adherent to the skin nor to masseter.
- After few years pleomorphic adenoma shows features of transformation into malignancy.

Management

- Surgery is the first line management.
- If only superficial lobe is involved, then superficial parotidectomy is done wherein parotid superficial to facial nerve is removed.
- Various steps in superficial parotidectomy:
  - Give incision, incision should start in front of tragus, vertically descend downwards, curve round the ear lobule till mastoid process and is carried till the neck.
  - Facial nerve should be recognized which lies 1 cm inferomedial to pointed end of tragal cartilage of external ear. Trace posterior belly of digastric till mastoid process. Facial nerve lies between muscle and tympanic plate.
  - Both facial nerve and retromandibular vein divides the parotid gland into deep and superficial lobes. Benign tumors do not invade faciovenous plane of Patey.
  - Gentle handling, good suction and nice hemostasis provide visibility to nerve.
  - Tumor along with lobe should be removed In Toto to avoid spillage.
- If both the lobes are involved then total conservative parotidectomy is done. In this, tumor along with the normal lobe is removed by retaining facial nerve. Avoid rupture of gland.

Q.2. Write short note on mixed parotid tumor.

(June 2014, 5 Marks) (Aug 2012, 5 Marks)
(Dec 2010, 3 Marks) (Nov 2014, 5 Marks)
(Dec 2015, 5 Marks)

Or

Write in short about mixed parotid tumor.

(July 2016, 5 Marks)

Or

Discuss about pleomorphic adenoma.

(Sep 2008, 5 Marks)

Or

Write short note on pleomorphic adenoma.

(Jan 2012, 5 Marks) (June 2010, 5 Marks)

Or

Write short answer on pleomorphic adenoma.
(June 2018, 5 Marks) (Feb 2019, 3 Marks)
(Oct 2019, 3 Marks)

Ans. Pleomorphic adenoma is also known as mixed parotid tumor or mixed salivary tumor.

- This is the most common tumor of the major salivary gland.
- Pleomorphic adenoma is benign epithelial tumor.
- Epithelial cells proliferate in strands or may be arranged in form of acini or cords.

Pleomorphic adenoma is mixed tumor because of the presence of epithelial cells, myoepithelial cells, mucoid material, pseudo-cartilage and lymphoid tissue.

Etiology

- **Dardick's theory:** A neoplastically altered epithelial cell with potential for multidirectional differentiation can be responsible for pleomorphic adenoma.
- **Differentiation of the ductal reserve cells:** Intercalated ductal reserve cells may be differentiated into ductal and myoepithelial cells and later on these cells undergo Mesenchymal metaplasia as they inherently consist of smooth muscle like properties.

Clinical Features

- It occurs in middle aged women around 40 years are commonly affected.
- It is usually unilateral, present as single painless, smooth, firm, lobulated mobile swelling in front of parotid with positive curtain sign, i.e., as the deep fascia is attached above to zygomatic bone, it acts as curtain, not allowing parotid swelling to move above the level of zygomatic bone. This is curtain sign.
- Obliteration of retromandibular groove is common.
- Ear lobule is raised or lifted.
- Swelling is rubbery or firm. Soft area indicates necrosis. In long standing cases it can be hard, surface can be nodular. Skin is stretched and becomes shiny.
- When deep lobe is involved, swelling is located in lateral wall of pharynx, posterior pillar and over soft palate. Deep lobe tumor passes through Patey's submandibular tunnel pushing tonsils, pharynx, soft palate often without any visible swelling or only small swelling when only deep lobe tumor is present.
- Being a benign tumor it is neither adherent to the skin nor to masseter.
- After few years pleomorphic adenoma shows features of transformation into malignancy.

Investigations

- *Fine needle aspiration cytology:* It is done to confirm diagnosis and rule out the malignancy.
- *CT scan:* This is to be done when tumor arises from deep lobe. It defines the extraglandular spread and extent of parapharyngeal disease as well as cervical lymph nodes.
- *FNAC of lymph nodes:* Palpable lymph nodes in neck are to be examined for malignancy.
- *X-ray of bones:* For seeing the bony resorption.
- MRI is the better method compared to CT scan. MRI provides better soft tissue delineation, i.e., superior perineural invasion.

Complications

- Recurrence in 5–50% of cases.
- Malignancy is seen in 3–5% of tumors
- Malignancy is seen in 10% of tumors in long duration.

Treatment

- Surgery is the first line treatment.
- If only superficial lobe is involved, then superficial parotidectomy is done wherein parotid superficial to facial nerve is removed.
- Various steps in superficial parotidectomy:
  - Give incision, incision should start in front of tragus, vertically descend downwards, curve round the ear lobule till mastoid process and is carried till the neck.
  - Facial nerve should be recognized which lies 1 cm inferomedial to pointed end of tragal cartilage of external ear. Trace posterior belly of digastric till mastoid process. Facial nerve lies between muscle and tympanic plate.
  - Both facial nerve and retromandibular vein divides the parotid gland into deep and superficial lobes. Benign tumors do not invade faciovenous plane of Patey.
  - Gentle handling, good suction and nice hemostasis provide visibility to nerve.
  - Tumor along with lobe should be removed In Toto to avoid spillage.
- If both the lobes are involved then total conservative parotidectomy is done. In this, tumor along with the normal lobe is removed by retaining facial nerve. Avoid rupture of gland.

Q.3. Write short note on acute parotitis.

(Aug 2012, 5 Marks)

Ans. Acute inflammation of parotid can occur due to bacterial or nonbacterial causes. This may be unilateral and bilateral.

Acute Nonsuppurative Parotitis (Mumps Parotitis)

It is an acute generalized viral disease with painful enlargement of salivary gland chiefly parotid.

Clinical Features

Fever, headache, muscular pain are usually found, both parotids are enlarged with pain and temperature.

Treatment

Only symptomatic treatment as analgesic and anti-inflammatory drugs.

Acute Suppurative Parotitis

- It is an acute inflammation of parotid gland caused by *Staphylococcus aureus*.
- *Streptococcus viridans* and pneumococci may be involved.
- *Pathogenesis:* The bacterium reaches to the salivary gland through the Stensen's duct. This is called as retrograde infection.

Clinical Features

♦ Pain and swelling on one side of face
♦ Browny edematous swelling over the parotid region with all signs of inflammation.
♦ Cellulitis of overlying skin
♦ Pus comes out on pressing the parotid gland.

Investigations

♦ Ultrasonography of parotid region should be done.
♦ Pus collected from duct orifice should be sent for culture and sensitivity
♦ Needle aspiration from the abscess is done to confirm formation of pus.

Treatment

♦ **Conservative line of management:**
  • It is indicative in stage of cellulitis with no evidence of abscess.
  • Maintain good oral hygiene.
  • Proper antibiotic mainly cloxacillin 500 mg 6 hourly along with metronidazole 400 mg 8 hourly.
♦ **Surgical treatment:**
  • Incision and drainage should be done under general anesthesia.
  • Incise the skin in front of tragus vertically and then parotid sheath is opened horizontally. Pus is drained by using the sinus forcep. This is known as Blair's incision. Antibiotics should be continued.
  • Proper hydration, mouthwash using povidone iodine or potassium permanganate solutions.

Q.4. Describe etiology, clinical features, investigations and management of submandibular gland stone.
(Feb 2013, 10 Marks)

Ans. This is a pathological condition characterized by formation of calcified mass (sialolith) within the salivary gland or its duct.

Etiology

The exact cause for sialolith or calculus formation is not clear but factors which contribute to its formation are:
♦ Stagnation of saliva
♦ Focus for sialolith formation resulting from ductal epithelial inflammation and injury.
♦ Poorly understood biological factors favoring precipitation of calcium salts.

Hilus is the most common site for the formation of sialolith but it can arise anywhere throughout the ductal system. 80% of all salivary duct stones develop in the submandibular or Warthin's duct. Predisposition of sialolith formation for the submandibular gland can be due to:
♦ Composition of secretion of submandibular salivary gland is more alkaline and viscous.
♦ Submandibular gland consists of higher concentration of calcium and phosphorus ions as compared to other major salivary glands.
♦ Both submandibular gland and duct are placed in such an anatomically dependent position that the flow of saliva is against gravity which gives more chances for stasis of saliva inside the ducts.
♦ Stagnation of secretions in Warthin's duct can also due to angulation of duct as it courses around the mylohyoid muscle and the vertical orientation of the distal duct segment.

Clinical Features

♦ Patient complains of periodic painful swelling when eating, interspersed with periods of remission.
♦ Occasionally patients report spontaneous extrusion of small calculi from the ducts.
♦ Most common finding on examination is point tenderness in the region of the hilum or, near Wharton's duct of the submandibular gland.
♦ Salivary secretion may be affected slightly.
♦ A gelatinous, cloudy, mucopurulent material is seen in basically clear and adequate saliva. This mucopurulent material is derived from the inflammatory ductal changes caused by calculus blockage and salivary stagnation.
♦ If treatment is not instituted early pronounced exacerbations are seen, characterized by an acute suppurative process with attendant systemic manifestations.
♦ Pus may exude from the duct orifice.
♦ Mucosa around the duct is inflamed, particularly in the floor of the mouth where swelling, redness and tenderness are present along the course of Wharton's duct.
♦ Glands are enlarged, tender and tense. Palpation of the gland and the duct causes pain and a flow of pus.

Investigations

♦ Occlusal radiograph
♦ *Intraoral periapical radiograph:* Submandibular stones are mostly radioopaque.
♦ Ultrasound (excellent non-invasive method)
♦ *Sialography:* A retrograde injection of a radiopaque dye as neohydriole into the duct of salivary gland. (Occluded submandibular salivary duct can be best observed by simple palpitation).

Treatment

♦ **Stone in the submandibular duct:**
  • Small stone in the distal part of the duct is removed manually.
  • Stone in deeper parts require operation. This can be removed by incising the mucosa over the floor of the mouth, after stabilizing the stone.
♦ **If the stone is present inside the gland:**
  This requires excision of submandibular salivary gland. Three steps of dissection of gland includes incision, mobilization and excision
  1. *Incision:* It should be a skin crease incision over the lower pole of the gland.
  2. *Mobilization of the gland:* Division of the facial artery twice, once in deeper plane on the posterolateral aspect and another at the superolateral aspect close to the lower border of the mandible which gives mobilization of the gland.

3. *Excision of the gland:* It is done by ligating and dividing the submandibular duct.

Q.5. Describe the etiology, clinical features and treatment of submandibular sialolithiasis. *(Feb 1999, 8 Marks)*

Ans. Sialolithiasis is the formation of hardened intraluminal deposits in ductal system of salivary gland which obstructs the normal flow of saliva.

For etiology refer Ans. 4 of same chapter.

Clinical Features

♦ It is usually seen in patients in the 5th to 8th decade of life.
♦ Recurrent swelling of the gland region is seen at the meal time.
♦ Recurrent episodes of acute, subacute or suppurative sialadenitis are present.
♦ Swelling is sometimes seen as hard lump present in the floor of the mouth or cheek.
♦ Submandibular salivary gland becomes tense and tender.
♦ Swelling and tenderness subside only to recur again during meal time.
♦ Large submandibular calculi can be seen as a swelling in the floor of the mouth.
♦ Stone may be palpable during bimanual palpation and may be movable up and down the duct.
♦ As in chronic infection and obstruction, the gland undergoes atrophy rarely, becomes indurated and when operated it is seen to be adherent to adjacent structures.

Treatment

Treatment is surgical.

Removal of Submandibular Calculi (Transoral Sialolithotomy)

♦ Place the patient in sitting position and give local anesthesia.
♦ Locate the stone accurately by using radiographs and palpation.
♦ Pass a suture behind the stone as well as below the duct to prevent stone from sliding backwards during removal.
♦ Retract the tongue for proper visualization.
♦ Palpate submandibular gland extraorally in submandibular region and is pushed upwards toward floor of mouth to fix intraoral tissues under tension. During this take care of lingual nerve and sublingual gland.
♦ If the sialolith is present posteriorly, incision should be placed slightly medially to avoid injury to the lingual nerve.
♦ Place a superficial incision through mucosa alone and give blunt dissection to reach the duct for preventing injury to the lingual nerve.
♦ If stone is more anteriorly placed, incision is given medial to plica sublingualis or else there are chances of injury to sublingual gland.
♦ Duct should be located at place where stone is lodged. As duct is located, a longitudinal incision is given directly over the duct where stone is located.
♦ Transverse incision should not be given as it retracts and gets divided completely and a salivary fistula may be formed.

♦ Incision given should reveal the stone and is of sufficient length to be removed easily. Stone can usually be removed easily with a forceps or a larger stone may need to be crushed into smaller pieces and removed.
♦ A probe is then passed from the caruncle to the region of stone to ensure patency of the duct in the anterior region.
♦ Incision on the duct need not be sutured. Incision in the floor of the mouth should be sutured with interrupted sutures.

Q.6. Write short note on sialolithiasis.

(May/June 2009, 5 Marks) (Sep 2007, 5 Marks)

Ans. Sialolithiasis is the formation of hardened intraluminal deposits in ductal system of salivary gland which obstructs the normal flow of saliva.

For etiology refer Ans. 4 and for clinical features and management, refer to Ans. 5 of same chapter.

Sialolith Composition

Sialolith is made up of:

♦ *Inorganic materials:* Calcium phosphate, calcium carbonate, combined with other salts, such as Mg, Zn, etc.
♦ Organic materials, i.e., glycoproteins, mucopolysaccharides and cellular debris.
♦ Aggregations of bacteria, clumps of epithelial cells, mucus, blood clots following trauma, are all suggested to form foci.

Q.7. Write short note on Warthin's tumor.

(Oct 2007, 5 Marks)

Ans.

♦ Warthin's tumor is also called adenolymphoma.
♦ It is a benign parotid tumor, it constitute about 10% of parotid tumors.
♦ Origin of adenolymphoma during development some parotid tissue gets included within lymph nodes which are present within the parotid sheath.
♦ It involves only superficial lobe of parotid gland.

Etiology

Smoking and radiation exposure can be the cause.

Clinical Features

♦ Middle aged or elderly males are commonly affected usually they are smokers.
♦ Can be bilateral, in some cases.
♦ It has smooth surface, round border with soft, cystic fluctuant swelling in lower pole often bilateral and is nontender.
♦ Classically, situated at the lower pole of parotid elevating the ear lobule.
♦ May be multicentric.
♦ This tumor affects only parotid gland.

Investigations

♦ Adenolymphoma produces "hot spot" in 99Technetium pertechnetate scan which is diagnostic.
♦ FNAC can be done
♦ Biopsy is done and histology reveals:

- Cyst is lined by a bilayered oncocytic epithelium, the inner cells of which are tall columnar with fine granular and eosinophilic cytoplasm and slightly hyperchromatic nuclei. The outer layer consists of basaloid cells.
- An eosinophilic coagulum is present within the cystic spaces.
- The numerous lymphocytic components may represent normal lymphoid tissue within which tumor is developed.

Treatment

It is best treated by superficial parotidectomy which spares the facial nerve.

Q.8. Write short note on parotid fistula.

(Jan 2011, 5 Marks)

Ans. It is an uncommon condition, which occurs after the surgery on the parotid gland.

It may arise from parotid duct or gland.

Types

- Duct fistula forms after superficial parotidectomy. It is profuse and often persisting. So duct should be ligated using nonabsorbable suture as far as possible, anteriorly to allow normal saliva drainage from deep lobe. If common duct is ligated deep lobe atrophies without causing any fistula.
- Gland fistula occurs from the raw surface after superficial parotidectomy. It is mild and symptom subsides in a month with anticholinergic drugs. Jacobsen tympanic neurectomy completely stops the secretion from the fistula in this type.

Etiology

- Rupture or bursting of parotid abscess.
- Inadvertent incision for drainage of parotid gland
- Penetrating injury to parotid gland
- As a complication after the superficial parotidectomy.

Clinical Features

- The chief complaint is an opening on the cheek, which discharges during meal.
- Excoriation of adjacent structure takes place.
- Tenderness and induration
- Trismus.

Diagnosis

- Sialography is done to find out origin of fistula whether from parotid gland or duct or ductules.
- Fistulogram or CT fistulogram should be done.
- Discharge study
- MRI

Treatment

- Anticholinergics: Hyoscine bromide (probanthine).
- Radiotherapy.
- Often exploration of fistula is required.
- Repair or reinsertion of the duct into the mucosa.

- Newman Seabrook operation: A probe is passed into the parotid duct through the opening in mouth. Another probe is passed through the fistula. Duct and fistula are dissected over the probe. After removal of the fistula tract severed duct ends are identified; and ends are trimmed. Probes are removed. A tantalum wire is passed into the duct across the severed ends and duct is sutured over it using 4 zero Vicryl. Tantalum stent is removed after 3 weeks.
- If still persists, auriculotemporal nerve which supplies secretomotor component of parotid is cut.
- If there is stenosis at the orifice of the Stenson's duct, papillotomy at the orifice may help.
- Total conservative parotidectomy is done in failed cases.

Q.9. Write short note on acute parotid abscess.

(Sep 1997, 6 Marks)

Ans. It is a result of an acute bacterial sialadenitis of the parotid gland.

- It is an ascending bacterial parotitis, due to reduced salivary flow, dehydration, starvation, sepsis, after major surgery, radiotherapy for oral malignancies and poor oral hygiene.
- Parotid fascia is densely thick and tough and so parotid abscess does not show any fluctuation until very late stage.
- Causative organism are *Staphylococcus aureus* (most common) *Streptococcus viridans* and often others like gram-negative and anaerobic organisms.

Clinical Features

- Pyrexia. malaise, pain and trismus.
- Red, tender, warm, well-localized, firm swelling is seen in the parotid region (brawny induration).
- Tender lymph nodes are palpable in the neck.
- Features of bacteremia are present in severe cases.
- Pus or cloudy turbid saliva may be expressed from the parotid duct opening.

Investigations

- Ultrasonography of parotid region should be done.
- Pus collected from duct orifice should be sent for culture and sensitivity
- Needle aspiration from the abscess is done to confirm formation of pus.

Treatment

- Antibiotics are started depending on culture report.
- When it is severely tender and localized, incision and drainage is done under general anesthesia. Skin is incised in front of tragus vertically and then parotid sheath is opened horizontally. Pus is drained using sinus forceps and is sent for culture. Antibiotics should be continued.
- Proper hydration, mouth wash using povidone iodine; potassium permanganate solutions, nutrition. Often patient with parotid infection needs admission and treatment.

Q.10. Write short note on sialadenitis. *(Mar 2008, 3 Marks)*

Ans. Sialadenitis is defined as the inflammation of the salivary gland.

Types

♦ Acute bacterial sialadenitis
♦ Chronic bacterial sialadenitis
♦ Chronic sclerosing sialadenitis/Kuttner's disease
♦ Allergic sialadenitis.

Etiology

♦ Microorganisms, i.e., *S. aureus, S. viridans*
♦ Predisposing factor, i.e., dehydration, malnutrition, cancer and surgical infections
♦ Poor oral hygiene
♦ *Drugs:* Anti-Parkinson, diuretics and antihistaminics.

Symptoms

♦ Fever
♦ Sudden onset of pain at the angle of jaw.

Sign

♦ Unilateral involvement of parotid gland is common

♦ Parotid gland is tender, enlarged and the overlying skin is warm and red
♦ Swelling causes elevation of the ear lobule.
♦ Intraorally, parotid papilla may be inflamed
♦ Cervical lymphadenopathy

Management

♦ Meticulous oral hygiene should be practiced
♦ Soft diet should be given
♦ High dose of parenteral antibiotic
♦ IV saline is given.

Surgical Treatment

If improvement does not occur surgical drainage of the affected gland should be performed.

Q.11. **Name the treatment modalities and differentiating features of parotid abscess and periodontal abscess.**

(Jan 2012, 5 Marks)

Ans. See Table below:

Features	Parotid abscess	Periodontal abscess
Treatment modality	Antibiotics should be started and if it is tender localized incision and drainage is done under general anesthesia	• Antibiotics should be started. Incision and drainage is given. • Debridement of root surface is done • If roots are denuded beyond apical third extraction of tooth is done
Pathogenesis	It is an ascending bacterial parotitis due to reduced salivary flow, dehydration, starvation, sepsis, major surgery, radiotherapy for malignancies and poor oral hygiene	It occurs in pre-existing periodontal pocket. Bacteria inside the pocket multiply and cause sufficient irritation
Location	Parotid gland	Gingiva
Features	Red, tender, warm, well localized firm swelling in parotid region	• Presence of swelling of soft tissues over the surface of involved root • Tooth becomes mobile and tender and pus drains from gingival crevice

Q.12. **Write in brief on Sjögren's syndrome.**

(Feb 2013, 5 Marks)

Or

Write short note on Sjögren's syndrome.

(Sep 2007, 3 Marks) (Mar 2008, 3 Marks)

Ans. It is a chronic inflammatory autoimmune disorder that affects salivary, lacrimal and other exocrine gland.

Types

♦ *Primary Sjögren's syndrome:* It is also known as Sicca syndrome. It consists of dry eyes, i.e., xerophthalmia and dry mouth, i.e., xerostomia.
♦ *Secondary Sjögren's syndrome:* It consists of dry eyes, i.e., xerophthalmia, dry mouth, i.e., xerostomia and collagen disorders, i.e., rheumatoid arthritis or systemic lupus erythematosus.

Clinical Features

♦ Xerostomia is present with unpleasant taste, soreness and difficulty in eating dry fruits.

♦ Patient also complains of xerophthalmia and arthralgia
♦ Severe tiredness is present.
♦ There is cobblestone appearance of tongue.
♦ There is often secondary acute bacterial sialadenitis and rapid progressive dental caries.
♦ Burning sensation present in the eyes.
♦ Parotid gland is predominantly affected, sometimes submandibular and minor glands can also be affected.

Investigations

♦ *Sialography:* Presence of snowstorm and branchless fruit laden tree appearance.
♦ *Rose bengal staining test:* Keratoconjunctivitis sicca is characterized by corneal keratotic lesion which stain pink when 'rose bengal' dye is used.
♦ *Schirmer test:* Lacrimal flow rate is measured by this test. In this test a strip of filter paper is placed in between eye and eyelid for determining degree of tears which is measured in millimeter. When flow is reduced to 5 mm in 5 minute sample, patient is considered positive for Sjögren's syndrome.

♦ *Sialometry:* In this salivary flow rate estimation is carried out. Stimulated flow rate in symptomatic primary and secondary Sjögren's syndrome is below 0.5–1 mL/min.

♦ *Sialochemistry:* In Sjögren's syndrome saliva of parotid gland is has twice total lipid content and high phospholipids and glycolipids.

♦ Blood investigations should be done.

Treatment

♦ Ocular lubricants, i.e., artificial tears should be used and provide relief.

♦ Xerostomia is managed by saliva substitutes.

♦ Frequent drinking of water is mandatory.

♦ Maintenance of oral hygiene is mandatory.

♦ Fluoride application should be done.

♦ Various saliva stimulants, i.e., pilocarpine, bromhexine and cevimeline are used.

♦ If salivary gland is enlarged to the extent that it is giving discomfort to the patient, then surgery is carried out.

Q.13. Classify tumors of parotid gland. Discuss clinical features and management of malignant parotid tumor. *(Jan 2018, 20 Marks)*

Ans.

Classification of Tumors of Parotid Gland

International Classification of Parotid Tumors

Epithelial

♦ Adenomas
  • Pleomorphic adenoma
  • Monomorphic adenoma
    – Adenolymphoma
    – Oxiphilic
    – Other type

♦ Mucoepidermoid—low grade malignancy

♦ Acinic cell tumor

♦ Carcinoma
  • Adenoid cystic carcinoma
  • Adenocarcinoma
  • Epidermoid carcinoma
  • Undifferentiated carcinoma
  • Carcinoma Ex pleomorphic adenoma

Nonepithelial

♦ Hemangioma

♦ Lymphangioma

♦ Neurofibroma

Metastatic

♦ Epidermoid carcinoma

♦ Malignant melanoma

Malignant Parotid Tumor

It is also known as carcinoma ex pleomorphic adenoma.

Clinical Features of Malignant Parotid Tumor

♦ It occurs from 2nd to 9th decade of life. But is common between 5th to 6th decades.

♦ Pain is very commonly present.

♦ Size of the tumor is very large and tumor can be associated with ulceration.

♦ These tumors can also lead to facial nerve palsy.

♦ Tumor gets fixed to underlying structures as well as to overlying mucosa or skin.

Management of Malignant Parotid Tumor

Radical Parotidectomy

♦ It is the removal of both the lobes of parotid, facial nerve, parotid duct, fiber of masseter, buccinators, pterygoids and radical block dissection of the neck.

♦ If there is no involvement of the facial nerve, it should be preserved. But, if facial nerve is removed it should be reconstructed by the greater auricular nerve or sural nerve

♦ Advanced tumor with the fixed nodes in neck may require radiotherapy but the response rate is poor.

Postoperative Radiotherapy

♦ This is useful to reduce the chances of relapse.

♦ Mainly external radiotherapy should be given.

Chemotherapy

♦ It is also given.

♦ Drugs given here depend on the tumor type.

♦ Intra-arterial chemotherapy is beneficial

♦ Overall efficacy of chemotherapy is less as compared to radiotherapy.

♦ 5FU, cisplatin, doxorubicin, epirubicin, cetuximab are used.

Q.14. Write short answer on Frey's syndrome. *(Sep 2018, 3 Marks)*

Ans. Frey's syndrome is also known as auriculotemporal syndrome or gustatory sweating.

It is due to injury to the auriculotemporal nerve, wherein postganglionic parasympathetic fibers from the otic ganglion become united to sympathetic nerves from the superior cervical ganglion (pseudosynapsis). There is inappropriate regeneration of the damaged parasympathetic autonomic nerve fibers to the overlying skin.

Auriculotemporal nerve has got two branches. Auricular branch supplies external acoustic meatus, surface of tympanic membrane, skin of auricle above external acoustic meatus. Temporal branch supplies hairy skin of the temple. Sweating and hyperesthesia occurs in this area of skin.

So, due to injury to auriculotemporal nerve whenever the act of mastication or chewing get started, there is increased sweating and hyperesthesia in region supplied by auriculotemporal nerve. So, it is known as auriculotemporal syndrome.

Causes

♦ Surgeries or accidental injuries to the parotid

♦ Surgeries or accidental injuries to temporomandibular joint

Features

♦ Flushing, sweating, erythema, pain and hyperesthesia in the skin over face innervated by the auriculotemporal nerve, whenever salivation is stimulated (i.e., during mastication).

♦ Condition causes real inconvenience to the patient.

♦ Involved skin is painted with iodine and dried. Dry starch applied over this area will become blue due to more sweat in the area in Frey's syndrome—minor's starch iodine test.

Treatment

♦ Initially conservative and reassurance. Most often they recover without any active treatment in 6 months. Antiperspirants, anticholinergics like scopolamine 3%, glycopyrrolate 1%, methyl sulfate, radiation 50 Gy are used.
♦ Occasionally (10%) they require surgical division of the tympanic branch of glossopharyngeal nerve below the round window of middle ear [i.e., intratympanic parasympathetic (Jacobsen nerve) neurectomy.]
♦ Dermal/fat graft; avulsion of auriculotemporal nerve; interposition of temporal fascia, fascia lata, sternomastoid muscle, acellular human dermal collagen; alcohol injection—are all tried.
♦ Latest treatment consists of injection of botulinum toxin in the affected skin.

Q.15. Write short answer on parotid abscess.

(Apr 2019, 3 Marks)

Ans. It is a result of an acute bacterial sialadenitis of the parotid gland.

♦ It is an ascending bacterial parotitis, due to reduced salivary flow, dehydration, starvation, sepsis, after major surgery, radiotherapy for oral malignancies and poor oral hygiene.
♦ Parotid fascia is densely thick and tough and so parotid abscess does not show any fluctuation until very late stage.
♦ Its causative organism are *Staphylococcus aureus* (most common), *Streptococcus viridans* and often others like gram-negative and anaerobic organisms.

Clinical Features

♦ Pyrexia, malaise, pain and trismus.
♦ Red, tender, warm, well-localized, firm swelling is seen in the parotid region (brawny induration).
♦ Tender lymph nodes are palpable in the neck.
♦ Features of bacteremia are present in severe cases.
♦ Pus or cloudy turbid saliva may be expressed from the parotid duct opening.

Investigations

♦ Ultrasonography of the parotid region.
♦ Pus collected from duct orifice is sent for culture and sensitivity.
♦ Needle aspiration from the abscess is done to confirm the formation of pus.

Treatment

Conservative Line of Management

♦ Maintain good hydration of patient in the postoperative period.
♦ Improvement in the oral hygiene by giving mouth washes with potassium permanganate ($KMnO_4$) solution or povidone iodine.

♦ Appropriate antibiotics against staphylococci, such as cloxacillin, are administered in the dose of 500 mg, 6th hourly along with metronidazole 400 mg, 8th hourly to treat anaerobic infections.
♦ It usually takes about 3–5 days for inflammation to subside.

Surgical Treatment when there is Pus

It is done under general anesthesia, give an adequate vertical incision in front of tragus of the ear till deep fascia. Open the deep fascia in two or three places and drain with blunt hemostat so as to avoid damage to facial nerve. It is known as Blair's method of drainage of parotid abscess. A drain tube has to be kept which can be removed after 3–4 days.

20. THYROID AND PARATHYROID GLAND

Q.1. Write short note on thyroid crisis. *(Sep 2009, 6 Marks)*

Or

Write short note on thyroid storm/crisis.

(Dec 2012, 5 Marks)

Ans. It is also known as thyroid crisis or thyroid storm.

♦ It occurs in a thyrotoxic patient inadequately prepared for thyroidectomy.
♦ Other causes are infection, trauma, pre-eclampsia, diabetic ketosis, emergency surgery and stress.
♦ It is an acute life-threatening metabolic state which is induced by excess release of thyroid hormones in individuals with thyrotoxicosis.

Etiology

♦ Previously thyroid storm was a common complication of toxic goiter surgery during intraoperative and postoperative stages.
♦ In modern era thyroid storm is seen in a thyrotoxic patient with intercurrent illness or surgical emergency.
♦ Most common cause of thyroid storm is intercurrent illness or infection.
♦ Various other causes which rapidly increase the thyroid hormone levels are radioiodine therapy, withdrawal of antithyroid drug therapy, vigorous thyroid palpation, iodinated contrast dye, ingestion of thyroid hormone and sepsis or infection.

Clinical Features

♦ Thyroid crisis is present in 12–24 hours after surgery; with severe dehydration, circulatory collapse, hypotension, hyperpyrexia, tachypnea, hyperventilation, palpitation, restlessness, tremor, delirium, diarrhea, vomiting and cardiac failure; later coma.
♦ Bayley's symptom complex of thyroid storm are insomnia, anorexia, diarrhea, vomiting, sweating, emotional instability, fever, tachycardia, aggravated toxic features, multiorgan dysfunction.

Treatment

- Patient should be sedated immediately with morphine or pethidine.
- Hyper pyrexia should be controlled by ice bag, rapid sponging, hypothermic blanket, and rectal ice irrigation.
- Oxygen is administered and IV glucose saline solution should be combat dehydration.
- Potassium may be added to control tachycardia.
- Hydrocortisone is often highly effective.
- Lugol's iodine should be given IV
- Propranolol should be used 20–40 mg 6 hourly.
- For atrial fibrillation, digitalis may be cautiously administered.
- Large dose of propylthiouracil orally, rectally or through Ryle's tube.
- Saturated solution of potassium iodide.

Q.2. Write short note on solitary thyroid nodule.

(Mar 2006, 5 Marks)

Or

Write long answer on clinical features and management of solitary thyroid nodule.   *(Sep 2018, 5 Marks)*

Ans.

- It is the end stage result of diffuse goiter.
- Almost all the thyroid swellings initially present as solitary nodule.
- Solitary thyroid nodule is a discrete lesion/nodule within the thyroid gland and or radiologically distinct from surrounding thyroid parenchyma.

Types

- Toxic solitary nodule—3% to 5% of solitary nodules of thyroid
- Nontoxic solitary nodule.

Based on Radioisotope Study

- **Hot:** Means autonomous toxic nodule. Normal surrounding thyroid tissue is inactive and so will not take up isotope. Nodule is overactive. It is 5% common of which only 5% can be malignant.
- **Warm:** Normally functioning nodule. Nodule and surrounding normal thyroid will take up the isotope (active). It is 10% common of which 10% can be malignant.
- **Cold:** Nonfunctioning nodule; may be malignant (need not be always). Nodule will not take up isotope (underactive). It is 80% common of which 20% are malignant.

Etiopathogenesis

- Puberty or pregnancy nodule
- Iodine deficiency nodule
- Adenoma
- Carcinoma
- Cyst.

Clinical Features

- Common in female, seen in age group 20–40 year.
- Long duration of swelling in front of neck, dyspnea, dysphagia.
- Various obstructive signs are present, i.e., stridor, tracheal deviation, neck vein engorgement.
- Single nodule is present.
- Hard area may suggest calcification and soft area necrosis.
- Sudden increase in size may occur due to hemorrhage.
- Solitary nodule has more tendencies to change in malignancy then multinodular goiter (MNG).

Complication

- Calcification in long standing.
- It may change into MNG.
- Sudden hemorrhage causes sudden enlargement of gland and even causes dyspnea.
- Patient may develop secondary thyrotoxicosis.

Investigations

- *Thyroid scan:* This is basically a radioactive scan which makes out a hot or cold nodule. Hot nodules are not malignant and are toxic while cold nodules are malignant but they can be a simple cyst.
- *Thyroid function tests:* T3, T4 and TSH are not of use as most of the nodules are euthyroid.
- *Ultrasound:* It shows either cystic or solid nodule. Solid swellings can be edema or carcinoma.
- *FNAC:* It shows benign or indeterminate or malignant and at times it is undiagnostic also.
- Power Doppler can be done to know vascularity of the gland. Vascularity is described in resistive index.
- Serum calcitonin estimation is done if FNAC confirms medullary carcinoma.
- CT scan or MRI can only be done in selective cases.
- X-ray of neck is done to see tracheal deviation.

Management

- Nontoxic benign nodule is treated with observation without any therapy. There is no role of any hormone therapy (L-thyroxine). Annual clinical examination and ultrasound neck is needed during essential follow-up: any nodule of 20% increase in size or more than 2 mm increase in diameter warrants a repeat FNAC and hemithyroidectomy may be considered. Compressive symptoms and cosmesis are the indications for surgery, i.e., hemithyroidectomy.
- Solitary toxic nodule needs initial antithyroid drugs and then radioactive iodine therapy (5 m curie); occasionally surgery is done, i.e., hemithyroidectomy.
- During thyroid surgery complete thyroid gland should be explored properly. Care to be taken not to miss any similar nodule in any other part of gland. If there are no nodules and only solitary nodule is found it is resected with normal surrounding thyroid tissue, i.e., resection enucleation.
- If nodule is situated at junction of isthmus and the lobe, hemithyroidectomy is done. Histopathology of excised

nodule is done. In histopathology report if there is presence of any evidence of malignancy immediate total thyroidectomy is done.

Q.3. Discuss difference in physiological, colloidal and nodular goiter. *(Sep 1999, 3 Marks)*

Ans.

Physiological Goiter

♦ It is called sporadic goiter
♦ Goiter is soft and diffuse
♦ Puberty, pregnancy goiter.

Colloidal Goiter

♦ It is the late stage of diffuse hyperplasia. TSH level have gone down and many follicles are inactive and full of colloid
♦ May be due to iodine deficiency.

Nodular Goiter

♦ The formation of nodules takes place due to fluctuating TSH stimulation and its level in circulation
♦ The nodule may be solid or cellular
♦ It may occur due to adenoma or carcinoma.

Q.4. Write short note on tetany. *(Feb 2013, 5 Marks)*

Ans. Tetany is a condition where is hyperexcitability of peripheral nerves.

Etiology

♦ It occur due the decrease in calcium level in blood.
♦ After thyroidectomy there is decreased level of parathormone in the blood which leads to hypocalcemia. It is temporary and lasts for 4–6 weeks.
♦ Other causes are neck dissection, hemochromatosis, Wilson's disease, DiGeorge syndrome.
♦ Severe vomiting, hyperventilation associated with respiratory alkalosis.
♦ Metabolic alkalosis
♦ Rickets, osteomalacia
♦ Chronic renal failure
♦ Acute pancreatitis

Clinical Features

♦ The first symptoms of tetany are tingling and numbness in the face, fingers, and toes.
♦ Cramps are present in hand and feet.
♦ Stridor is the dangerous complication of severe tetany due to spasm of muscles of respiration.
♦ Spasm of intraocular muscles lead to blurring of vision.
♦ *Carpopedal spasm or Trousseau's sign:*
  • It occurs in extreme cases and latent tetany.
  • Arm is flexed at elbow, wrist, and metacarpophalangeal joints but the interphalangeal joints are extended.
  • Thumb means towards the palm.

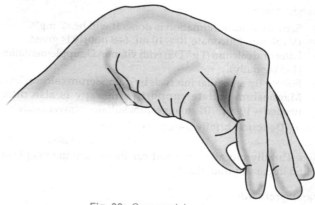

Fig. 30: Carpopedal spasm.

♦ *Chvostek's sign:*
  • It also occurs in latent tetany.
  • It indicates facial hyperexcitability.
  • If a tap is given to facial nerve infront of ear, twitching of eyelids, corners of mouth takes place.

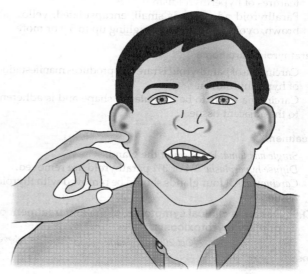

Fig. 31: Chvostek's sign.

♦ *Laryngeal spasm:*
  • Increased excitability of the laryngeal muscles produces laryngeal spasm.
  • This leads to blockage of respiratory passage and death may occur.
♦ Convulsions can occur in infants.

Diagnosis

It is confirmed by estimating serum calcium level which is <7 mg%.

Management

◆ Serum calcium estimation is done. It will be <7 mg%.
◆ IV calcium gluconate 10% 10 mL 6–8 hourly is given.
◆ Later oral calcium (1 g TDS) with vitamin D supplementation (1–3 µg daily).
◆ Follow-up at regular intervals by doing serum calcium level
◆ Magnesium sulfate supportive therapy is also often needed—10 mL 10% magnesium sulfate intravenously.

Q.5. Describe briefly parathyroid tumor.

(Sep 2002, 5 Marks)

Ans. Parathyroid adenoma and carcinoma are the neoplasm found in parathyroid gland.

Parathyroid Adenoma

◆ The most common tumor of the parathyroid gland is an adenoma.
◆ It may occur at any age and in either sex but is found more frequently in adult life.
◆ Most adenomas are first brought to attention because of excessive secretion of parathyroid hormones causing features of hyperthyroidism.
◆ Parathyroid adenoma is small, encapsulated, yellowish brown, ovoid nodular and weighing up to 5 g or more.

Parathyroid Carcinoma

◆ Carcinoma of parathyroid is rare and produces manifestation of hyperthyroidism
◆ Carcinoma tends to be irregular in shape and is adherent to the adjacent tissue.

Treatment

◆ *Single adenoma:* Excision of the gland.
◆ *Diffuse hyperplasia:* 3½ or 3¾ parathyroid are removed.
◆ *Carcinoma:* All four glands should be removed with thyroid tissue.

Q.6. Describe clinical symptoms, signs and treatment of primary thyrotoxicosis.

(Oct 2007, 15 Marks) (Sep 2006, 15 Marks)

Ans.

Symptoms

◆ Hyperactivity, excitability irritability and dysphoria
◆ Heat intolerance and swelling
◆ Palpitations
◆ Hyperreflexia, muscle wasting proximal myopothy without fasciculations
◆ Fatigue and weakness
◆ Weight loss with increased appetite
◆ Diarrhea and polyuria
◆ Oligomenorrhea and loss of libido
◆ Profuse sweating
◆ Goiter or enlarged thyroid gland

Signs

◆ Tachycardia is main sign which is present due to activation of thyrocardiac component

◆ Systolic hypertension is present
◆ Palms are hot and moist.

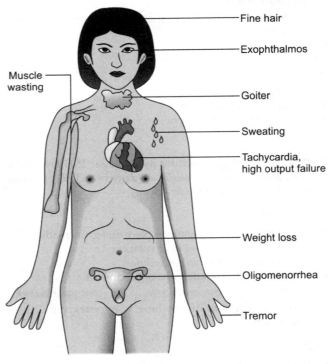

Fig. 32: Thyrotoxicosis.

◆ Presence of tremors, i.e., involuntary movement of body parts is present.
◆ Cardiac arrhythmias, i.e., atrial fibrillation and atrial tachycardia develops.
◆ Diaphoresis is present, i.e., excessive sweating is present.
◆ There is presence of powerful wide pulse pressure and good bounding pulse is present.
◆ Exaggerated deep tendon reflexes are seen.
◆ There is protrusion of eyes, i.e., exophthalmos with staring look.
◆ *Pretibial myxedema:* Thickening of skin due to mucin deposition over tibia.

Treatment

◆ *General:*
  • Allow the patient to take mental and physical rest.
  • Maintain nutrition of patient by giving nutritious diet.
  • If patient is anxious alprazolam 0.25–0.5 mg BD is given.
  • Most of the patients of thyrotoxicosis are fearful because of increased sympathetic activity. In such type of patient, propranolol 40–80 mg BD is given.
◆ *Drug therapy:*
  • Carbimazole is commonly used drug. It is started with 30 mg/day, adjustment of doses is made when patient come under control and maintenance dose is given, i.e., 10–20 mg/day.

- Potassium per chlorate 800 mg/day in divided doses is given and the dose is reduced with improvement in patient's condition.
- Iodides are given, i.e., sodium or potassium iodide 6–10 mg/day.
◆ *Surgery:* The commonly performed surgery is subtotal thyroidectomy, prior surgery antithyroids are given to make patient euthyroid. Potassium iodide 50–100 mg/day is given for 10–14 days.
◆ *Radioiodine treatment:* I^{131} is used and average effective dose is 8–10 millicuries.

Q.7. Write short note on hypothyroidism.
(Dec 2012, 5 Marks) (Apr 2007, 10 Marks)
Or
Write short answer on management of hypothyroidism. *(Apr 2018, 3 Marks)*
Ans. Inadequate release of thyroid hormone and its defective synthesis give rise to clinical synthesis of hypothyroidism.

Etiology

◆ After doing thyroidectomy
◆ Agenesis or dysgenesis
◆ Enzyme deficiency
◆ Iodine deficiency
◆ Hashimoto's thyroiditis
◆ Antithyroid drugs
◆ Radioiodine
◆ *Drugs:* Lithium, amiodarone

Forms of Hypothyroidism

◆ Cretinism
◆ Myxedema

Cretinism

Congenital absence of thyroid hormone leads to condition called as cretinism.
◆ A cretin has retarded physical and mental growth.
◆ Child is obese with pads of fat in supraclavicular region, coarse features, limbs which are stumpy, thick lips and tongue, protuberant abdomen, small eyes, coarse hairs and dry skin.
◆ TSH will be raised; T3 and T4 will be low.
◆ Cretinism will be treated by L-thyroxine once in a day in morning orally.

Myxedema

Myxedema is a clinical condition resulting from decreased circulating levels of T3 and T4. It is characterized by deposition of mucinous material causing swelling of skin and subcutaneous tissue.

Clinical Features

◆ *General:* There is tiredness, somnolence (prolong drowsiness or sleepiness), weight gain, cold intolerance and goiter.
◆ *Skin and subcutaneous tissue:* Coarse dry skin, puffiness of face with malar flush, baggy eyelids with swollen edematous appearance of supraclavicular regions, neck and lacks of hand and feet.
◆ *Cardiovascular and respiratory features:* Bradycardia, angina, cardiac failure, pericardial effusion and pleural effusion.
◆ *Neuromuscular features:* Aches and pains, cerebellar syndrome with slurred speech and ataxia, muscle cramps and stiffness.
◆ *Gastrointestinal features:* Constipation and ascites
◆ *Developmental:* Growth and mental retardation
◆ *Reproductive system:* Infertility, menorrhagia, hyperprolactinemia and galactorrhea.

Management

◆ In patient of myxedema adequate ventilation is maintained along with electrolyte balance and slow warming.
◆ Principle of therapy is replacement of deficient thyroid hormones.
◆ Replacement with L-thyroxine 100–150 µg/day. In old patients with ischemic heart disease initial therapy is with 25–50 µg/day and then gradually increased till the required dose. Drug may take at least a week to act. It is better to give the drug in morning hours to obviate sleeplessness.
◆ Initial rapid response is achieved by giving L-iodothyronine 20 µg TID.

Q.8. Etiology, clinical picture and treatment of Grave's disease. *(Sep 2008, 8 Marks) (Mar 2008, 8 Marks)*
Ans.

Etiology

Grave's disease is an autoimmune disease caused by production of autoantibodies that stimulate thyroid-stimulating hormone receptor.

Clinical Features

◆ There is presence of diffused goiter which is with or without bruit.
◆ Fever, anxiety and restlessness are present.
◆ There is weight loss, fatigue, sweating and heat intolerance.
◆ *Cardiovascular features:*
  • Tachycardia is present which persists during sleep.
  • Large pulse pressure is present with raised systolic blood pressure.
  • Cardiac arrhythmias are present.
  • Capillary pulsations may be seen.
◆ *Ocular manifestations:*
  • *Primary manifestations:* Proptosis, exophthalmos and ophthalmoplegia.
  • *Secondary manifestations:* Optic nerve compression, impaired convergence and exposure keratitis.
◆ *Gastrointestinal:* Weight loss, diarrhea and vomiting.
◆ *Reproductive system:* Oligomenorrhea and infertility.

Management

◆ *General:*
  • Allow the patient to take mental and physical rest.
  • Maintain nutrition of patient by giving nutritious diet.

- If patient is anxious alprazolam 0.25–0.5 mg BD is given.
- Most of the patients of thyrotoxicosis are fearful because of increased sympathetic activity. In such type of patient propranolol 40–80 mg BD is given.

- *Drug therapy:*
  - Carbimazole is commonly used drug. It is started with 30 mg/day, adjustment of doses is made when patient come under control and maintenance dose is given, i.e., 10–20 mg/day.
  - Potassium per chlorate 800 mg/day in divided doses is given and the dose is reduced with improvement in patient's condition.
  - Iodides are given, i.e., sodium or potassium iodide 6–10 mg/day.

- *Surgery:* The commonly performed surgery is subtotal thyroidectomy, prior surgery antithyroids are given to make patient euthyroid. Potassium iodide 50–100 mg/day is given for 10–14 days.

- *Radioiodine treatment:* I^{131} is used and average effective dose is 8–10 millicuries.

Q.9. Write short note on Hashimoto disease of thyroid.

(Dec 2007, 3 Marks)

Ans. It is an autoimmune disease.

It is also called as Hashimoto's thyroiditis or diffuse non-goitrous thyroiditis or struma lymphomatosa.

Clinical Features

- It is very common in women. Most common in perimeno-pausal females.
- There is painful, diffuse enlargement of both the lobes of thyroid gland which is firm, rubbery, tender and smooth.
- Initially both lobes of thyroid are present with toxic features but later they manifest with the features of hypothyroidism.
- Hepatosplenomegaly can be present.
- The condition can predispose to papillary carcinoma of thyroid.

Histology

- Histology is characterized by extensive lymphocytic infiltration resulting in destruction of thyroid follicles with variable degree of fibrosis.
- The thyroid follicles are destroyed by significant fibrosis.
- The deep eosinophilic staining thyroid follicular cell Askanazy cell, is characteristic.

Investigations

- FNAC can be done
- Assessment of T3, T4 and TSH levels
- *Thyroid antibodies assay:* Significant rise is observed in 85% of cases.
- ESR is very high, i.e., over 90 mm/hour.

Treatment

- L-thyroxine 0.2 mg/day is given as a supplementary dose.
- If there is compression on the trachea, isthmusectomy is done to relieve compression.

- If the goiter is big and causing discomfort, subtotal thyroidectomy can also be done.
- Steroid therapy often is helpful.

Complications of Hashimoto's Thyroiditis

- Permanent hypothyroidism
- Papillary carcinoma of the thyroid
- Malignant lymphoma.

Q.10. Discuss briefly myxedema. *(May/Jun 2009, 5 Marks)*

Ans. Myxedema is a clinical condition resulting from decreased circulating levels of T3 and T4. It is characterized by deposition of mucinous material causing swelling of skin and subcutaneous tissue.

Clinical Features

- *General:* There is tiredness, somnolence, weight gain, cold intolerance and goiter.
- *Skin and subcutaneous tissue:* Coarse dry skin, puffiness of face with malar flush, baggy eyelids with swollen edematous appearance of supraclavicular regions, neck and lacks of hand and feet.
- *Cardiovascular and respiratory features:* Bradycardia, angina, cardiac failure, pericardial effusion and pleural effusion.
- *Neuromuscular features:* Aches and pains, cerebellar syndrome with slurred speech and ataxia, muscle camps and stiffness.
- *Gastrointestinal features:* Constipation and ascites
- *Developmental:* Growth and mental retardation
- *Reproductive system:* Infertility, menorrhagia, hyperprol-actinemia and galactorrhea.

Investigation

- *Thyroid function test:* There is reduction in T3 and T4 levels and rise in serum thyroid stimulating hormone which indicates primary hypothyroidism. Reduction in T3 and T4 levels with TSH level below normal range is secondary hypothyroidism.
- *Serum cholesterol:* It is raised in primary thyroid failure.
- The fall in serum level is more than 50 mg/100 mL.
- Tendon reflex duration is prolonged.
- In ECG bradycardia, low voltage complexes and flattened or inverted T waves are present.

Management

- In patient of myxedema adequate ventilation is maintained along with electrolyte balance and slow warming.
- Principle of therapy is replacement of deficient thyroid hormones.
- Replacement with L – thyroxine 100 to 150 µg/day. In old patients with ischemic heart disease initial therapy is with 25–50 µg/day and then gradually increased till the required dose. Drug may take at least a week to act. It is better to give the drug in morning hours to obviate sleeplessness.
- Initial rapid response is achieved by giving L iodothyronine 20 µg TID.

Q.11. Write classification of thyroid swelling. Discuss treatment of simple goiter. *(Sep 2009, 10 Marks)*

Ans.

Classification of Thyroid Swelling

- **Simple nontoxic**
  - Diffuse hyperplastic:
    - Physiological
      » Puberty
      » Pregnancy.
    - Primary iodine deficiency
    - Secondary iodine deficiency:
      » Goitrogens of Brassica family, e.g., cabbage, soyabean
      » Excess dietary fluoride.
      » *Drugs:* PAS, lithium, phenylbutazone, thiocyanates, potassium perchlorate, antithyroid drugs, radioactive iodine.
      » Dyshormonogenetic goiter.
  - Colloid goiter.
  - Nodular goiter (multinodular).
  - Solitary nontoxic nodule.
  - Recurrent nontoxic nodule.
- **Toxic:**
  - Diffuse (primary)—Grave's disease.
  - Multinodular (secondary)—Plummer's disease.
  - Toxic nodule (solitary) (tertiary).
  - Recurrent toxicosis.
- **Neoplastic:**
  - Benign adenomas: Follicular, Hurthle cell.
  - Malignant:
    - Carcinomas: Papillary, follicular, medullary, anaplastic.
    - Lymphomas.
- **Thyroiditis**
  - Hashimoto's autoimmune thyroiditis.
  - De-Quervain's autoimmune thyroiditis.
  - Riedel's thyroiditis.
- **Rare causes:** Bacterial (suppurative), amyloid.

Treatment of Simple Goiter

- When entire gland is diseased total thyroidectomy is done.
- Subtotal thyroidectomy is done depending on the amount of gland involved, amount of normal gland existing and location of nodules. It is a commonly done procedure in multinodular goiter. Eight grams of thyroid tissue is retained in each lateral lobe.
- Often partial thyroidectomy or Hartley Dunhill operation (isthmus + one entire lateral lobe and opposite side subtotal or partial) is also done depending on the amount of diseased gland and normal tissues behind. Partial thyroidectomy is not well approved now.
- Postoperative L-thyroxine is often given to prevent any fluctuation in TSH level which may cause recurrent nodule formation.

Q.12. Write differential diagnosis between follicular carcinoma and medullary carcinoma of thyroid regarding etiopathology, clinical picture, metastasis and management.

(Jan 2011, 8 Marks)

Ans. See Table below:

Features of differential diagnosis	Follicular carcinoma	Medullary carcinoma
Etiopathology	It arises in a multinodular goiter mainly in cases of endemic goiter. Tumor cells line the blood vessels and get dislodged into systemic circulation producing secondaries in bones	It is sporadic or familial. It arises from parafollicular C cells which are derived from ultimobranchial body. It contains amyloid stroma in which malignant cells are dispersed. Spreads mainly to lymph nodes
Clinical picture	• Occurs during 30–50 years of age. • Presence of swelling in neck which is firm or hard and nodular. • If lung secondaries are present dyspnea, chest pain and hemoptysis are present. • Pulsatile secondaries in skull and bones.	• Occurs in middle age. • Thyroid swelling with enlargement of neck lymph nodes. • Presence of diarrhea and flushing • Associated with MEN syndrome. • Paraneoplastic syndrome like Cushing's and carcinoids
Metastasis	It spreads mainly through blood in bone, lungs and liver	It spreads both by lymphatics and blood
Management	• Total thyroidectomy is done along with central lymph node compartment dissection (Level VI) • Functional neck node dissection is done with preservation of sternocleidomastoid, spinal accessory nerve and internal juglar vein if nodes are present.	Total thyroidectomy is done along with central lymph node dissection (Level VI) even if there are no nodes in neck. Neck lymph nodes block dissection if lymph nodes are involved. External beam radiotherapy for residual tumor tissue

Q.13. Write short note on hyperthyroidism.

(Aug 2011, 5 Marks)

Or

Define hyperthyroidism, its signs and symptoms and its management. *(Feb 2019, 5 Marks)*

Ans. Hyperthyroidism is the condition resulting from the effect of excessive amounts of thyroid hormones on body. In hyperthyroidism pathology is in thyroid gland itself.

Etiology

♦ Exophthalmic goiter leads to hyperthyroidism. The condition is characterized by hyperplasia of thyroid gland and eye involvement.
♦ Pituitary diseases which occurs in or involves anterior lobe of pituitary gland.
♦ Toxic adenoma
♦ Multinodular goiter
♦ Ectopic thyroid tissue.

Clinical Features

Symptoms of Hyperthyroidism

♦ *Gastrointestinal system:* Weight loss in spite of increased appetite; diarrhea (due to increased activity at ganglionic level).
♦ *Cardiovascular system:* Palpitations; shortness of breath at rest or on minimal exertion; angina; irregularity in heart rate; cardiac failure in the elderly (CCF).
♦ *Neuromuscular system:* Undue fatigue and muscle weakness; tremor.
♦ *Skeletal system:* Increase in linear growth in children.
♦ *Genitourinary system:* Oligo or amenorrhea; occasional urinary frequency.
♦ *Integumentry system:* Hair loss, gynecomastia; pruritus; palmar erythema.
♦ *Psychiatry:* Irritability; nervousness; insomnia.
♦ *Sympathetic overactivity:* It causes dyspnea, palpitation, tiredness, heat intolerance, sweating, hyperactivity, irritability, nervousness, increased appetite and decrease in weight.
♦ Because of the increased catabolism, they have increased appetite, decreased weight and so also increased creatinine level which signify myopathy (due to more muscle catabolism).
♦ Fine tremor is due to diffuse irritability of gray matter.

Signs

Eye Signs in Toxic Goiter

♦ *Lid retraction:* Here upper eyelid is higher than normal; lower eyelid is in normal position. It is due to sympathetic overactivity causing spasm of involuntary smooth muscle part of the levator palpebrae superioris.
♦ *Von Graefe's sign (Lid Lag's sign):* It is inability of the upper eyelid to keep pace with the eyeball when it looks downwards to follow the examiner's finger. It is contraction/overactivity of the involuntary part of the levator palpebrae superioris muscle.
♦ *Dalrymple's sign:* Upper eyelid retraction, so visibility of upper sclera.
♦ *Stellwag's sign:* Absence of normal blinking—so staring look. First sign to appear. It is due to widening of palpebral fissure due to lid retraction and also due to contraction of voluntary part of levator palpebrae superioris muscle.
♦ *Jaffroy's sign:* Absence of wrinkling on forehead when patient looks up (frowns) with head in bent down/flexed position.
♦ *Moebius sign:* It is lack of convergence of eyeball. Defective convergence is dug to lymphocytic infiltration of inferior oblique and rectus muscle in case of primary thyrotoxicosis. There will be diplopia. It may be an early sign of eventual ophthalmoplegia.
♦ *Naffziger's sign:* With patient in sitting position and neck fully extended, protruded eyeball can be visualized when observed from behind.
♦ *Jellinek's sign:* increased pigmentation of eyelid margins.
♦ *Enroth sign:* Edema of eyelids and conjunctiva.
♦ *Rosenbach's sign:* Tremor of closed eyelids.
♦ *Gifford's sign:* Difficulty in everting upper eyelid in primary toxic thyroid. Differentiate from exophthalmos of other cause.
♦ *Loewi's sign:* Dilatation of pupil with weak adrenaline solution.
♦ *Knie's sign:* Unequal pupillary dilatation.
♦ *Cowen's sign:* Jerky pupillary contraction to consensual light.
♦ *Kocher's sign:* When clinician places his hands on patient's eyes and lifts it higher, patient's upper lid springs up more quickly than eyebrows.

Exophthalmos: It is proptosis of the eye. Exophthalmos is visible sclera first below the lower edge of iris and later eventually part of sclera will be visible.

♦ *Cardiac manifestations:* Tachycardia is commonly present. Others are pulsus paradoxus; wide pulse pressure; multiple extrasystoles; paroxysmal atrial tachycardia; paroxysmal atrial fibrillation; persistent atrial fibrillation.
♦ *Myopathy:* Weakness of proximal muscle occurs, i.e., arm muscles and front thigh muscles.
♦ *Pretibial myxoedema:* It is bilateral, symmetrical, shiny, red thickened dry skin with coarse hair in feet and the ankles.
♦ *Thyroid acropachy:* It is the clubbing of fingers and toes. Hypertrophic pulmonary osteoarthropathy can develop.
♦ *Other:* Thrill is felt in the upper pole of thyroid and also bruit on auscultation. Hepatosplenomegaly is also seen.

Treatment

Antithyroid Drugs

Drugs, such as carbimazole 5–10 mg 8 hourly is given for 12–16 months; Methimazole can also be given; Propylthiouracil is given 200 mg 8 hourly.

Surgery

♦ Before doing thyroid surgeries patient should become euthyroid.

♦ *Subtotal thyroidectomy:* Both lobes with isthmus are removed and a tissue equivalent to pulp of finger is retained at lower pole of gland bilaterally.

Radioiodine Therapy

♦ It destroys the cells and causes the complete ablation of thyroid gland. It should be given after the age of 45 years.

♦ Dosage is 5–10 millicurie.

Q.14. Define and classify goiters. Describe differentiating features between primary and secondary thyrotoxicosis along with medical treatment to make patient euthyroid. *(Jan 2012, 15 Marks)*

Ans. Diffuse enlargement of thyroid gland is described as goiter.

Classification of Goiter

♦ *Simple goiter:*
  • Puberty goiter
  • Colloid goiter
  • Iodine-deficiency goiter
  • Multinodular goiter.

♦ *Toxic goiter:*
  • Graves disease
  • Secondary thyrotoxicosis in multinodular goiter
  • Solitary nodule
  • Other causes.

♦ *Neoplastic goiter:*
  • Benign adenoma (follicular adenoma)
  • Malignant tumors are further classified into:
    – Primary
      » Well-differentiated carcinoma
        ▪ Papillary carcinoma
        ▪ Follicular carcinoma.
      » Poorly differentiated carcinoma
        ▪ Anaplastic carcinoma
      » Arising from parafollicular cells
        ▪ Medullary carcinoma.
      » Arising from lymphatic tissue
        ▪ Malignant lymphoma.
    – Secondary (metastasis): Malignant melanoma, renal cell carcinoma, breast carcinoma produce secondaries in the thyroid, due to blood spread.

♦ *Thyroiditis:*
  • Granulomatous thyroiditis
  • Autoimmune thyroiditis
  • Riedel's thyroiditis.

♦ *Other rare causes of goiter:*
  • Acute bacterial thyroiditis
  • Thyroid cyst
  • Thyroid abscess
  • Amyloid goiters.

Differentiating Features between Primary and Secondary Thyrotoxicosis

Features	Primary thyrotoxicosis	Secondary thyrotoxicosis
Age	Occur in 15–25 years	Occur in 25–40 years
Symptoms and signs	It appear simultaneously	Duration is long
Skin over the swelling	It is warm	Not warm
Consistency	Soft and firm	Firm and hard
Surface	Smooth	Nodular
Auscultation	Bruit is commonly heared	Bruit is uncommon
Eye signs	Found commonly	Found rarely
Predominant symptoms	Of central nervous system	Of cardiovascular system
Pretibial myxedema	Can be found	Never found

Medical Treatment to Make Patient Euthyroid

♦ Carbimazole 10 mg 6–8 hourly intervals daily, till the patient is euthyroid, after 8–12 weeks dosage may be reduced to 5 mg 8 hourly. Last dose is given in the evening before surgery.

♦ Propylthiouracil is given as 200 mg 8 hourly.

♦ Lugol's iodine, i.e., 5% iodine in 10% potassium iodide solution: 10 drops TDS for 2 weeks before operation to reduce vascularity.

♦ Thyroxine 0.1 mg daily to prevent TSH stimulation which may increase size and vascularity of the gland.

Q.15. Enlist midline neck swellings. Describe surgical anatomy of thyroid gland with reference to embryology, blood supply relationship and nerves related to thyroid gland. *(Aug 2012, 10 Marks)*

Ans.

Enlisting of Midline Swellings of Neck

The midline swellings of neck are:

♦ Ludwig's angina
♦ Enlarged submental lymph node
♦ Sublingual dermoid cyst
♦ Thyroglossal cyst
♦ Subhyoid bursitis
♦ Goiter of thyroid, isthmus and pyramidal lobe
♦ Enlarged lymph node and lipoma in substernal space of burns
♦ Retrosternal goiter
♦ Thymic swelling
♦ Bony swelling arising from the manubrium sterni.

Surgical Anatomy of Thyroid Gland

With Reference to Embryology

♦ It develops from median down growth (midline diverticulum) of a column of cells from the pharyngeal floor between first and second pharyngeal pouches.

- By 6 weeks of time the central column, which becomes thyroglossal duct, gets reabsorbed.
- The duct bifurcates to form thyroid lobes.
- Pyramidal lobe is formed by a portion of the duct.

With Reference to Blood Supply

Artery Supply

- Superior thyroid artery is a branch of external carotid artery, enters the upper pole of the gland, divides into anterior and posterior branches and anastomoses with ascending branch of inferior thyroid artery. Upper pole is narrow, hence ligation is easy.
- Inferior thyroid artery is a branch of thyrocervical trunk and enters the posterior aspect of the gland. It supplies the gland by dividing into 4–5 branches which enter the gland at various levels (not truly lower pole).
- Thyroidea ima artery is a branch of either brachiocephalic trunk or direct branch of arch of aorta and enters the lower part of the isthmus in about 2–3% of the cases.

Venous Drainage

- Superior thyroid vein drains the upper pole and enters the internal jugular vein. The vein follows the artery.
- Middle thyroid vein is single, short and wide and drains into internal jugular vein.
- Inferior thyroid veins form a plexus which drain into innominate vein. They do not accompany the artery.
- Kocher's vein is rarely found (vein in between middle and inferior thyroid vein).

With Reference to Nerve Supply

- *External laryngeal nerve:* Vagus gives rise to superior laryngeal nerve, which separates from vagus at skull base and divides into two branches. The large, internal laryngeal nerve is sensory to the larynx. The small external laryngeal nerve runs close to the superior thyroid vessels and supplies cricothyroid muscle (tensor of the vocal cord) and is sensory to upper half of the larynx. This nerve is away from the vessels near the upper pole. Hence, in thyroidectomy, the upper pedicle should be ligated as close to the thyroid as possible.
- *Recurrent laryngeal nerve:* It is a branch of vagus, hooks around ligamentum arteriosum on the left and subclavian artery on the right, runs in tracheoesophageal groove near the posteromedial surface. Close to the gland, the nerve lies in between (anterior or posterior) the branches of inferior thyroid artery. Hence, inferior thyroid artery should be ligated away from the gland, to avoid damage to recurrent laryngeal nerve. On right side it is 1 cm within the tracheoesophageal groove. The nerve traverses through the gland in about 5–8% of cases. The nerve may be very closely adherent to the posteromedial aspect of the gland. Nerve not seen may be far away in the tracheoesophageal groove.
- *Non-recurrent laryngeal nerve* is found in about 1 in 1,000 cases. Nerve has a horizontal course. In 25% of the cases it is within the ligament of Berry.

Q.16. Write the differential diagnosis of malignant tumors of thyroid with special reference to their management. *(Feb 2014, 8 Marks)*

Ans.

Features	Papillary	Follicular	Anaplastic	Medullary
Etiology	Irradiation	Endemic	Unknown	Sporadic or familial
Age	20–40	30–50	50 and above	Middle age
Diagnosis	Thyroid swelling with lymph node	Thyroid swelling, metastasis-bone	Thyroid swelling, local fixity, stridor	Difficult to diagnose clinically
Histology	Orphan Annie-eyed nuclei, psammoma bodies	Angioinvasion, capsular invasion	Poorly differentiated cells	Amyloid stroma like carcinoid
Spread	Lymphatic	Blood	Local infiltration	Lymphatic, blood
Investigation	FNAC	Frozen section	FNAC, biopsy	FNAC, calcitonin
Management	• Total or near thyroidectomy with central node compartment dissection (level IV) • Suppressive dose of L-thyroxine 0.3 mg OD life long • Modified radical neck dissection type III is required if lymph nodes are involved • If small lymph nodes are present 'Berry pickling may be done	• Total thyroidectomy is done along with central lymph node compartment dissection (level VI) • Functional neck node dissection is done with preservation of sternocleidomastoid, spinal accessory nerve and internal jugular vein if nodes are present	• External radiotherapy is done • Tracheostomy and isthemectomy relieve respiratory obstruction temporarily • Adriamycin as chemotherapy	• Total thyroidectomy is done along with central lymph node dissection (level VI) even if there are no nodes in neck • Neck lymph nodes block dissection if lymph nodes are involved • External beam radiotherapy for residual tumor tissue
TSH dependence	Yes	Yes	No	No
Hormone production	Very rare	Very rare	No	Calcitonin, 5HT, ACTH
Prognosis	Excellent	Good	Worst	Bad

Q.17. Write on classification of thyroiditis with clinical picture, etiology and management.

(Nov 2014, 10 Marks)

Ans.

Classification

Revised American Thyroid Association Classification

♦ Acute thyroiditis

♦ Subacute thyroiditis (De Quervain's)
♦ Chronic autoimmune thyroiditis or Hashimoto's disease
♦ Postpartum and silent thyroiditis
♦ Riedel's thyroiditis.

Classification of Thyroiditis in Relation to Inflammation Response and Clinical Course

Predominant inflammatory cell	Name of thyroiditis	Synonyms	Subcategories	Clinical course
Neutrophil	Acute thyroiditis	• Acute suppurative thyroiditis • Infectious thyroiditis	• Bacterial thyroiditis • Mycobacterial thyroiditis • Fungal thyroiditis • Parasitic thyroiditis	Acute
Macrophage/ histiocyte	Subacute granulomatous	• De Quervain thyroiditis • Subacute thyroiditis		Subacute
	Thyroiditis	• Painful subacute thyroiditis • Post-viral thyroiditis • Giant cell thyroiditis • Subacute nonsuppurative thyroiditis • Pseudotuberculous thyroiditis • Struma granulomatosa		
	Infectious granulomatous thyroiditis	• Infectious thyroiditis	• Tuberculosis • Fungal thyroiditis	Subacute to chronic
	• Sarcoidosis • Granulomatous vasculitis			Subacute to chronic to subclinical
	Other granulomatous reactions	Multifocal granulomatous folliculitis	• Reaction to hemorrhage • Reaction to surgery • Foreign body reaction	Subclinical
	Palpation thyroiditis			
Lymphocyte	Chronic lymphocytic thyroiditis	• Hashimoto's thyroiditis • Autoimmune thyroiditis • Struma lymphomatosa	• Classic • Fibrous variant • Atrophic or fibrous atrophy variant	Chronic
	Silent thyroiditis	• Sporadic thyroiditis • Painless thyroiditis • Painless sporadic thyroiditis • Painless thyroiditis with hyper-thyroidism • Silent thyrotoxic thyroiditis • Subacute lymphocytic thyroiditis • Atypical subacute thyroiditis • Spontaneously resolving thyroiditis • Lymphocytic thyroiditis with spontaneously resolving hyperthyroidism	• Juvenile variant • Hashitoxicosis variant	Subacute
	Postpartum thyroiditis • Focal lymphocytic thyroiditis • Invasive fibrous thyroiditis	Painless postpartum thyroiditis • Nonspecific thyroiditis • Focal autoimmune thyroiditis • Riedel thyroiditis • Fibrosing thyroiditis • Sclerosing thyroiditis		Subclinical Chronic

Etiology, Clinical Picture and Management of Thyroiditis

Type of thyroiditis	Etiology	Clinical picture	Management	
			Investigation	Treatment
Granulomatous or subacute or de Quervain's Thyroiditis	Virus, i.e., either mumps or coxsackie virus	• Occur in young individuals • Patient complaints of fever, bodyache and painful enlargement of thyroid gland • Gland is enlarged, tender, soft to firm with few symptoms of hyperthyroidism occur initially	• T3 and T4 levels are high • FNAC is useful	Conservative treatment is given in form of analgesics and short course of prednisolone
Autoimmune or Hashimoto's thyroiditis or struma lymphomatosa	Autoimmune	• It commonly occur in women at perimenopause. • Initially symptoms of mild hyperthyroidism, i.e., hashitoxicosis can be present • Later on there is presence of permanent hypothyroidism • Thyroid gland is firm to hard and at times rubbery in consistency, smooth or irregular and can involve a lobe or entire gland	• ESR is very high, i.e., about 90 mm/hour. • Thyroid antibody assay is done • If goiter is big and lead to discomfort, subtotal thyroidectomy can be done	• Thyroxine 0.2 mg/day is given • If there is presence of compression over trachea, isthmusectomy is done
Riedel's thyroiditis	Collagen disorder	• It is common in males • There is presence of swelling with irregular surface • Involvement of trachea, esophagus, internal jugular vein, etc., causes dysphagia and dyspnea • Consistency is stony hard • There is presence of stridor • Berry's sign is positive • Goiter is small	• FNAC is mandatory to rule out carcinoma • T3 and T4 can be low • Radioisotope will not show any uptake	• Treatment with thyroxine is given to treat hypothyroidism • Isthmectomy is done to relieve compression on airway

Q.18. Describe classification, clinical features and management of thyroid neoplasia. *(Feb 2015, 10 Marks)*

Or

Write about clinical features of papillary and follicular carcinoma of thyroid and management.

(Jan 2018, 15 Marks)

Ans.

Classification of Thyroid Neoplasia

♦ Benign
  • Follicular adenoma—colloid, embryonal, fetal
  • Hurthle cell adenoma
  • Colloid adenoma
  • Papillary adenoma.

♦ Malignant (Dunhill classification)
  • *Differentiated:*
    – Papillary carcinoma
    – Follicular carcinoma
    – Papillofollicular carcinoma behaves like papillary carcinoma of thyroid
    – Hurthle cell carcinoma behaves like follicular carcinoma.
  • *Undifferentiated:*
    – Anaplastic carcinoma
  • Medullary carcinoma
  • Malignant lymphoma
  • Secondaries in thyroid from colon, kidney, melanoma and breast.

Clinical Features and Management of Thyroid Neoplasias

Name of thyroid neoplasia	Clinical features	Management	
		Investigation	Treatment
Papillary carcinoma	• It occurs commonly in young females • It presents as soft or hard or firm, solid or cystic, solitary or multinodular thyroid swelling • Often discrete lymph nodes are palpable in lower deep cervical region and thyroid may or may not be palpable. If thyroid is not palpable it is known as occult	• FNAC of thyroid nodule demonstrate colloid filled follicles with papillary process • Radioisotope shows cold nodule • TSH level in blood is high	• Total or near total thyroidectomy, with central node compartment dissection (level IV) • Suppressive dose of L-thyroxine is 0.3 mg OD life long • Modified radical neck dissection type III is required if lymph nodes are involved

Contd...

Contd...

Name of thyroid neoplasia	Clinical features	Management	
		Investigation	Treatment
	• Some of the patients who reported late have fixed nodes in neck and fixed thyroid to trachea with or without recurrent laryngeal nerve paralysis	• Plain X ray of neck shows fine calcification • CT scan in neck to identify nonpalpable nodes in neck	• Radioactive iodine therapy (I131) is indicated if tumor is more than 4 cm or if there is extra thyroid involvement or lymph node involvement or multicentric
Follicular carcinoma	• It occurs commonly in females and peak age group is around 40 years • There is presence of swelling in the neck which is firm or hard and nodular • There is presence of tracheal compression and stridor • If lung secondaries are present there is presence of dyspnea, hemoptysis and chest pain • Involvement of recurrent laryngeal nerve leads to hoarsness of voice • Pulsatile secondaries in skull and long bones	• Frozen section biopsy is done • Thyroid scan demonstrate cold nodule • Alkaline phosphatase level is checked if high, scanning of bone is done • Plain X-ray of bone shows osteolytic lesion	• Total thyroidectomy, with central node compartment dissection (level IV) • Functional neck node dissection is done with preservation of sternocleidomastoid, spinal accessory nerve and internal jugular vein if nodes are present clinically or by imaging • L-thyroxine 0.1 mg OD is given life long • If secondaries are detected therapeutic dose radiation I¹³¹ is given. L-thyroxine should be stopped 7 days before radiation therapy • Secondaries in bone are treated by external radiotherapy • Internal fixation should be done whenever there is presence of pathological fracture
Anaplastic carcinoma	• It is common in elderly women which are of 60–70 years of age • Patients are present with the rapidly growing thyroid swelling of short duration • Surface of swelling is irregular and consistency is hard • There is presence of stridor and hoarseness of voice due to tracheal obstruction • Dysphagia is also present • Tumor is fixed to the skin • Positive Berry's sign, i.e., involvement of carotid sheath leads to absence of carotid pulsation • Isthmus is also involved along with lateral lobes	• FNAC is diagnostic	• Tracheostomy and isthmectomy provide temporary relieve in obstruction • External radiotherapy is done • Adriamycin is used in chemotherapy
Medullary carcinoma	• There is presence of thyroid swelling with neck lymphadenopathy • Presence of diarrhea and flushing • There is presence of hypertension, pheochromocytoma and mucosal neuromas when associated with MEN II syndrome • Sporadic and familial type of cases are seen in adults while cases with MEN II syndrome occur in young age group	• FNAC shows amyloid deposition with dispersed malignant cells and C cell hyperplasia • Level of calcitonin will be high. Unstimulated calcium serum more than 100 pg/mL is suggestive of medullary carcinoma of thyroid • CT of neck and chest is done to identify nodes • 111 indium octreotide scanning is useful for detection of medullary carcinoma	• Total thyroidectomy with central node dissection in all patients along with maintenance dose of L-thyroxine • Neck lymph node block dissection when lymph nodes are involved • External beam radiotherapy is given for residual tumor disease • Adriamycin is used in chemotherapy • All the members of patient's family are evaluated for serum calcitonin and if the levels are high, they should undergo prophylactic total thyroidectomy

Q.19. Etiopathology, clinical picture and management of a case of secondary thyrotoxicosis. Write indication, contraindication and complication of methods applied for the treatment. *(Apr 2015, 8 Marks)*

Ans. Secondary hyperthyroidism is the result of abnormal, excessive thyroid-stimulating hormone (TSH) release and stimulation of the thyroid resulting in excessive T4 release.

Etiopathology of Secondary Thyrotoxicosis

♦ **Autoimmune:** Here the thyroid IgG antibodies stimulate thyroid to produce more hormone. This mechanism causes diffuse enlargement of thyroid along with the hyperfunction. The antibodies which are directed specifically against TSH receptors are known as thyroid receptor antibodies. There is presence of circulating antibodies and lymphocytic infiltration of thyroid tissue.

♦ **Genetics:** Association of HLA B8 DR3 and DR4 indicates the genetic susceptibility to environmental factors, such as viruses and bacteria which may produce antibodies which cross react with TSH receptors and causes thyrotoxicosis.

Clinical Picture of Secondary Thyrotoxicosis

♦ It occurs during 25–40 years of age.
♦ Swelling is present for the long time while symptoms remain for shorter duration.
♦ Skin over the swelling is not warm.
♦ Consistency of the swelling is firm to hard and surface is nodular.
♦ On auscultation bruit is commonly heard.
♦ Cardiovascular symptoms are predominant, i.e., Tachycardia—may be atrial fibrillation, presence of wide pulse pressure, extrasystole and/or heart failure.
♦ CNS and GIT manifestations are less predominant.
♦ Internodular tissues of gland are overactive.

Management

Antithyroid Drugs

Carbimazole and propylthiouracil should be given. Treatment should be started 48 hours later and should be continued till radioiodine has had its effect till 6 weeks. Carbimazole should be given in dose of 40–60 mg, treatment should be continued for 12–18 months.

Indication

♦ In all patients preoperatively.
♦ In patients not willing for surgery.
♦ In recurrence after surgery.

Contraindication

♦ In cases with hypersensitivity
♦ Anemia or leukemia
♦ Kidney or liver disease.

Complications

♦ Agranulocytosis
♦ Arthralgia
♦ Skin rashes
♦ Fever.

Radioactive iodine

I^{131} should be given 150 microcuries per gram orally.

Indication

♦ In patients over the age of 40 years.
♦ Toxicity recurring after previous subtotal thyroidectomy.

♦ In very nervous patients who have fear of surgery.
♦ In patients with severe thyrotoxic heart disease.

Contraindications

♦ In patients under 45 years of age because of high incidence of hypothyroidism.
♦ During pregnancy and lactation.

Complication

♦ Hypothyroidism
♦ Worsening ophthalmopathy
♦ Risk for cancer and birth defects in long standing cases.

Subtotal Thyroidectomy

♦ If cardiac symptoms are controlled well and risk of anesthesia is acceptable, subtotal thyroidectomy is done.
♦ Before surgery, it should be remembered that patient should be euthyroid. Antithyroid drugs should be stopped two weeks before surgery and is replaced by potassium iodate 170 mg daily orally.
♦ In the surgery, both lobes with isthmus are removed and a tissue equivalent to the pulp of finger is retained at lower pole of gland on both sides.

Indications

♦ In recurrent thyrotoxicosis after 12–18 month course of antithyroid drugs under the age of 40 years.
♦ In cases with sensitivity reactions to antithyroid compounds.
♦ In severe thyrotoxicosis not responding to medical treatment.
♦ In tracheal compression.

Contraindications

In patients showing evidence of marked exophthalmos.

Complications

♦ Hemorrhage
♦ Hematoma formation
♦ Edema of glottis
♦ Injury to recurrent laryngeal nerve
♦ Tetany.

Q.20. Write short note on parathormone.

(Feb 2015, 5 Marks)

Ans.

♦ Parathormone is secreted by chief cells whenever serum calcium falls.
♦ Parathormone stimulate osteoclast cells for bone resorption, kidney for promoting calcium reabsorption and production of 1, 25 dihydroxy vitamin D and gastrointestinal tract to promote absorption of calcium and phosphorus.
♦ Half-life of parathormone is 4 minutes.
♦ In normal persons, the parathormone is balanced by calcitonin.

Actions of Parathormone

♦ It increases absorption of calcium from gut.
♦ It mobilizes calcium from the bone.

♦ It increases calcium reabsorption from renal tubules and promote excretion of phosphate.

Q.21. Classify thyroid swellings. Describe pathogenesis, clinical features and management of multinodular goiter. *(Dec 2015, 10 Marks)*

Or

Write on pathogenesis clinical features and management of multinodular goiter.

(Feb 2019, 10 Marks)

Ans. *For classification of thyroid swelling refer to Ans. 11 of same chapter.*

Multinodular Goiter

Multinodular growth is a discordant growth with structurally and functionally altered thyroid follicles which present multiple nodules in thyroid.

Pathogenesis

Flowchart 13: Pathogenesis of multinodular goiter.

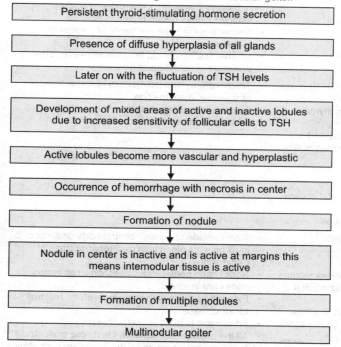

Clinical Features

♦ Multinodular goiter is more common in females. Female to male ratio is 10:1
♦ It occurs during the age of 20–40 years.
♦ It is a slowly progressive disease.
♦ There is presence of multiple nodules of various sizes which are present in both lobes and in isthmus which are firm, nodular, nontender and does not move with deglutition.
♦ Swelling remain in front of neck, dyspnea is present due to tracheomalacia.

♦ Dysphagia is also present.
♦ Hard areas suggest calcification and soft areas are suggestive of necrosis.

Management

Management part consists of both investigations and treatment:

Investigations

♦ T3, T4, TSH and ultrasound neck and FNAC. FNAC should be done from the most dominant and suspected nodule. Ultrasound-guided FNAC is more reliable. This method identifies impalpable nodules, their number, nature of nodule and vascularity of nodule.
♦ *X-ray neck:* It shows rim of calcification which shows displacement and compression of trachea.
♦ *Indirect laryngoscopy:* It shows the mobility of vocal cords.
♦ *Radioisotope iodine scan:* It should be done in selected patients only.
♦ Complete blood picture, routine urine examination, fasting and postprandial blood sugar, serum calcium estimation should be done.

Treatment

Treatment for multinodular goiter is surgical.
♦ When complete gland is affected total thyroidectomy should be done.
♦ Subtotal thyroidectomy is carried out depending on amount of gland involved and amount of normal gland left along with location of nodules. In this 8 g of thyroid tissue is retained in each lateral lobe.
♦ Postoperatively L-thyroxine is given to prevent any fluctuation in TSH which can lead to recurrent nodule formation.

Prevention

♦ When patient develop goiter in puberty he/she should be supplemented with 0.1–0.2 mg of L-thyroxine.
♦ Patient should be given iodine rich diet.
♦ Goitrogenic diet, i.e., cabbage and goitrogenic drugs should be avoided.

Q.22. Describe classification, clinical features, treatment and complications of thyroid malignancy.

(Jan 2016, 10 Marks)

Ans.

Classification of Thyroid Malignancy Or Dunhill Classification

♦ Differentiated (80%)
  • Papillary carcinoma (60%)
  • Follicular carcinoma (17%)
  • Papillofollicular carcinoma
  • Hurthle cell carcinoma.
♦ Undifferentiated (20%)
  • Anaplastic carcinoma (13%)
♦ Medullary carcinoma (6%)
♦ Malignant lymphoma (4%)
♦ Secondaries in thyroid—from colon, kidney, melanoma, breast.

Clinical Features and Treatment of Thyroid Malignancy

Name of thyroid malignancy	Clinical features	Treatment
Papillary carcinoma	• It occurs commonly in young females • It presents as soft or hard or firm, solid or cystic, solitary or multinodular thyroid swelling • Often discrete lymph nodes are palpable in lower deep cervical region and thyroid may or may not be palpable. If thyroid is not palpable it is known as occult • Some of the patients who reported late have fixed nodes in neck and fixed thyroid to trachea with or without recurrent laryngeal nerve paralysis	• Total or near total thyroidectomy, with central node compartment dissection (level IV) • Suppressive dose of L-thyroxine is 0.3 mg OD life long • Modified radical neck dissection type III is required if lymph nodes are involved • Radioactive iodine therapy (I^{131}) is indicated if tumor is more than 4 cm or if there is extrathyroid involvement or lymph node involvement or multicentric
Follicular carcinoma	• It occurs commonly in females and peak age group is around 40 years • There is presence of swelling in the neck which is firm or hard and nodular • There is presence of tracheal compression and stridor • If lung secondaries are present there is presence of dyspnea, hemoptysis and chest pain • Involvement of recurrent laryngeal nerve leads to hoarseness of voice • Pulsatile secondaries in skull and long bones	• Total thyroidectomy, with central node compartment dissection (level IV) • Functional neck node dissection is done with preservation of sternocleidomastoid, spinal accessory nerve and internal jugular vein if nodes are present clinically. Or by imaging • L-thyroxine 0.1 mg OD is given life long • If secondaries are detected therapeutic dose radiation I^{131} is given. L-thyroxine should be stopped 7 days before radiation therapy • Secondaries in bone are treated by external radiotherapy • Internal fixation should be done whenever there is presence of pathological fracture
Anaplastic carcinoma	• It is common in elderly women which are of 60–70 years of age • Patients are present with the rapidly growing thyroid swelling of short duration • Surface of swelling is irregular and consistency is hard • There is presence of stridor and hoarsness of voice due to tracheal obstruction • Dysphagia is also present • Tumor is fixed to the skin. • Positive Berry's sign, i.e., involvement of carotid sheath leads to absence of carotid pulsation • Isthmus is also involved along with lateral lobes	• Tracheostomy and isthmectomy provide temporary relieve in obstruction • External radiotherapy is done • Adriamycin is used in chemotherapy
Medullary carcinoma	• There is presence of thyroid swelling with neck lymphadenopathy • Presence of diarrhea and flushing • There is presence of hypertension, pheochromocytoma and mucosal neuromas when associated with MEN II syndrome • Sporadic and familial type of cases are seen in adults while cases with MEN II syndrome occur in young age group	• Total thyroidectomy with central node dissection in all patients along with maintenance dose of L-thyroxine • Neck lymph node block dissection when lymph nodes are involved • External beam radiotherapy is given for residual tumor disease • Adriamycin is used in chemotherapy • All the members of patient's family are evaluated for serum calcitonin and if the levels are high, they should undergo prophylactic total thyroidectomy

Complications of Thyroid Malignancy

Complications of thyroid malignancy are associated with the thyroidectomy procedure followed as surgical treatment in most of thyroid malignancies. So following are the complications:

Hemorrhage

♦ Chances of reactionary hemorrhage are present which is more dangerous and occurs within 6–8 hours after surgery. It occurs due to slipping of ligature, coughing, etc.

♦ Tension hematoma develop deep-to-deep fascia it compresses the larynx.

Respiratory Obstruction

It occur due to hematoma or laryngeal edema, due to tracheomalacia or bilateral recurrent laryngeal nerve palsy.

Recurrent Laryngeal Nerve Palsy

It can be transient or permanent. Transient recover in 3 weeks to 3 months. It presents with hoarseness of voice, aphonia, aspiration and ineffective cough.

Hypoparathyroidism

It is temporary and due to vascular spasm of parathyroid glands. It occurs on 2nd and 5th postoperative day. It presents with weakness, positive Chvostek's sign, carpopedal spasm and convulsion.

Thyrotoxic Crisis

It occurs in thyrotoxic patient which is inadequately prepared for thyroidectomy.

Injury to External Laryngeal Nerve

It leads to weakening of cricothyroid muscle which causes alteration in pitch of voice, voice fatigue, breathy voice and frequent throat clearing.

Hypothyroidism

It reveal clinically after 6 months.

Stitch Granuloma

It can occur with or without sinus formation and is seen after the use of nonabsorbable suture material.

Q.23. Describe differentiating features of primary and secondary thyrotoxicosis. *(Jan 2017, 3 Marks)*

Ans. Following are the differences between primary and secondary thyrotoxicosis:

Features	Primary thyrotoxicosis	Secondary thyrotoxicosis
Age	Occur in 15–25 years	Occur in 25–40 years
Symptoms and signs	It appear simultaneously	Duration is long
Skin over the swelling	It is warm	Not warm
Consistency	Soft and firm	Firm and hard
Surface	Smooth	Nodular
Auscultation	Bruit is commonly heard	Bruit is uncommon
Eye signs	Found commonly	Found rarely
Predominant symptoms	Of central nervous system	Of cardiovascular system
Pretibial myxedema	Can be found	Never found

Q.24. Write short note on complication of thyroid surgery.
(Jan 2017, 5 Marks)

Ans. Complications of thyroid surgery can be divided into three parts, i.e., minor, rare, or major.

♦ **Minor complications:** Postoperative surgical site seromas, poor scar formation.
♦ **Rare complications:** Damage to the sympathetic trunk.
♦ **Major complications:**
  • *Bleeding:* Present with neck swelling, neck pain, and/ or signs and symptoms of airway obstruction (e.g., dyspnea, stridor, hypoxia).
  • *Injury to recurrent laryngeal nerve:* Present with postoperative hoarseness or breathlessness.
  • *Hypoparathyroidism:* Signs of hypocalcemia, i.e., circumoral paresthesias, mental status changes,

tetany, carpopedal spasm, laryngospasm, seizures, QT prolongation on ECG, and cardiac arrest.
  • Thyrotoxic storm
  • *Injury to superior laryngeal nerve:* Mild hoarseness or decreased vocal stamina.
  • *Infection:* Manifests as superficial cellulitis or as an abscess.

Q.25. Classify goiter. Discuss clinical features, investigations and management of multinodular goiter.
(Apr 2017, 15 Marks)

Ans. *For classification of goiter refer to Ans. 14 of same chapter.*

For clinical features, investigations and management of multinodular goiter refer to Ans. 21 of same chapter.

Q.26. Enumerate the midline swelling in neck. How to diagnose a case of thyroid swelling?
(Aug 2018, 10 Marks)

Ans.

Enumeration of Midline Swelling of Neck

♦ Ludwig's angina
♦ Enlarged submental lymph node
♦ Sublingual dermoid cyst
♦ Thyroglossal cyst
♦ Subhyoid bursitis
♦ Goiter of thyroid, isthmus and pyramidal lobe
♦ Enlarged lymph node and lipoma in substernal space of burns
♦ Retrosternal goiter
♦ Thymic swelling
♦ Bony swelling arising from the manubrium sterni.

Diagnosis of a Case of Thyroid Swelling

Following is the diagnosis of the case of thyroid swelling:

Based on the Complaints and History Taking

♦ **Duration of swelling:** Long duration of thyroid swelling is indicative of the benign condition., e.g., multinodular goiter and colloid goiter. Short duration with rapid growth is indicative of malignancy, such as anaplastic carcinoma. Majority of thyroid swellings does not cause pain.
♦ **Rate of growth:**
  • In benign disease, swelling is slow growing.
  • If growth is rapid, it can be 'de novo' malignancy or malignancy which is developing in benign lesion., e.g., follicular carcinoma in multinodular goiter.
  • Sudden increase in the size of swelling with pain is indicative of hemorrhage in multinodular goiter.
♦ **Dyspnea:** It is the difficulty in breathing of patient with goiter due to:
  • Tracheal infiltration
  • Anaplastic carcinoma
  • Lower border not seen
  • Retrosternal goiter
  • Tracheomalacia
  • Long standing multinodular goiter
  • Cardiac failure
  • Secondary thyrotoxicosis

- Small goiter, rapid growth is indicative of anaplastic carcinoma infiltrating the trachea.
- When lower border is not visible, it means there is retrosternal goiter.
- Hyperthyroidism producing arryhthmias causes congestive cardiac failure which produces dyspnea and orthopnea.
- Long standing multinodular goiter compresses on tracheal cartilage and produces pressure atrophy of tracheal cartilages. This is known as tracheomalacia.
- Hoarsens of voice: This is indicative of malignancy. This always occurs in carcinoma of thyroid which infiltrates recurrent laryngeal nerve.

Based on Examination

Inspection

- Swelling should be located in front of the neck, it extend from one sternomastoid to another sternomastoid, vertically from suprasternal notch to thyroid cartilage.
- Surfaces of various thyroid swellings are:
  - Smooth surface: Adenoma, puberty goiter and Grave's disease
  - Irregular surface: Carcinoma of thyroid
  - Nodular: Multinodular thyroid
- Thyroid swelling moves up with deglutition, but restriction of movement can be due to:
  - Malignancy with fixity to trachea
  - Restrosternal goiter
  - Large goiter due to its size
  - Due to previous surgery.
- Movement on tongue protrusion is suggestive of thyroglossal cyst. This test is performed when there is a nodule or a cyst in the region of isthmus of thyroid gland. This test has no relevance in cases of multinodular goiter and other thyroid swellings.

Palpation

- Confirm the size, shape, surface and border. Local rise in temperature is the feature of toxic goiter. Very large nodular surface is bosselated surface.
- *Consistency:*
  - Soft: In grave's disease and colloid goiter
  - Firm: In adenoma and multinodular goiter
  - Hard: It is suggestive of carcinoma and calcification in multinodular goiter.
- Confirm the movement with deglutition by holding the thyroid gland.
- Intrinsic mobility of thyroid gland is restricted in carcinoma due to infiltration inside the trachea.
- When only one lobe is enlarged sternomastoid contraction test is done. Here examiner keeps hand on the side of chin, opposite to side of the lesion and ask patient to push his/her hand against the resistance provided. If gland is less prominent, this is indicative that swelling is deep to sternomastoid muscle.
- *Chin test:* It is done in multinodular goiter where both of the lobes are enlarged. Ask the patient to bend the chin downward against the resistance given. This produces contraction of both sternomastoid and strap muscle and gland become less prominent.

- *Special test:*
  - Crile's method: It is indicated when doubtful nodule is present. Thumb should be kept over the suspected area of nodule and ask the patient to swallow.
  - Lahey's method: This can be done from both front and behind. In order to palpate right lobe, push gland to right side and feel nodule in posteromedial aspect of gland. Lobe becomes more prominent and so nodules are appreciated better.
  - Pizzillo's method: This is done in obese patients especially short neck individuals. Ask the patient to clasp his/her hands and press against the occiput with head extended. Thyroid gland becomes more prominent and palpation becomes better.
  - Kocher's test: If a gentle compression is given on lateral lobe, it produces stridor, now the test is positive. It is due to scabbard trachea. Long standing multinodular goiter leading to tracheomalacia and carcinoma with infiltration in trachea can give rise to stridor.
- *Position of trachea:* In solitary nodule cases which are confined to single lobe, trachea is deviated to opposite side. In multinodular goiter, trachea needs not to be deviated due to symmetrical enlargement off both the lobes.
- *Palpation of lymph nodes:* In neck, if the lymph nodes are significant, it is indicative of papillary carcinoma of thyroid.
- *Palpation of common carotid artery:* In large multinodular goiter, common carotid artery may be pushed laterally. So pulsations are felt in posterior triangle. Carcinoma of thyroid engulfs the carotid sheath. Consequently pulsations can be absent. Absent carotid artery pulsation is known as Berry sign positive.

Q.27. Write short note on goiter and its management.

(Sep 2018, 5 Marks)

Ans. *For definition and classification refer to Ans. 14 of same chapter.*

- Most common cause for the goiter is iodine deficiency.
- Main symptom of the goiter is swelling of the thyroid gland which eventually becomes noticeable lump inside the throat. Following symptoms occur when goiter enlarges significantly in size, i.e.:
- Hoarseness of voice
- Coughing
- Feeling of tightness in throat
- Dysphagia
- Dyspnea

Management

For details refer to Ans. 11 of same chapter.

Q.28. Enumerate different types of thyroid swelling and management of colloid goiter. *(Apr 2019, 5 Marks)*

Ans. *For enumeration of thyroid swellings refer to Ans. 11 of same chapter.*

Management of Colloid Goiter

Investigations

- **Complete blood picture:** Routine urine examination and fasting and postparandial blood sugar is done to rule out the diabetes mellitus.
- **X-ray of neck:** Anteroposterior and lateral view.

- Look for compression of trachea: To check the feasibility of intubation during anesthesia.
- To rule out the retrosternal extension: Soft tissue shadow is to be seen.
- **Flexible laryngoscopy:** This is done to see the vocal cord mobility.
- **Ultrasonography:** This is most useful investigation mainly in solitary nodule. It can also detect clinically impalpable lymph nodes in neck.
- **CT scan:** It is done when clinician suspect retrosternal extension, doubtful resectability or large lymph nodes in neck.

Treatment

- Thyroid hormone replacement therapy is prescribed for iodine deficiency. Hormone replacement inhibits thyroid stimulating hormone (TSH) and allows the thyroid to recover.
- A large goiter that is unresponsive to medical management or restricts swallowing and breathing may require partial or complete removal of the thyroid gland.
  - *Total thyroidectomy:* It is the choice in recent times but complications, such as recurrent laryngeal nerve paralysis and hypocalcemia due to removal of parathyroid glands can be avoided. So it is desirable to do total thyroidectomy. It gives permanent quick cure to patient.
  - *Subtotal thyroidectomy:* In this surgery, parts of right and left lobes and complete isthmus is removed in flush with tracheal surface leaving behind little tissue in tracheoesophageal groove to protect recurrent laryngeal nerve and parathyroid gland.
- If the goiter is producing too much thyroid hormone, treatment with radioactive iodine, antithyroid medication, or surgery may be necessary.

Q.29. Write short note on recurrent laryngeal nerve.

(Aug 2018, 10 Marks)

Ans. Recurrent laryngeal nerve is a branch of vagus which hooks around ligamentum arteriosum on the left and subclavian artery on right and runs in tracheoesophageal groove near posteromedial surface. Close to the gland, nerve lies in between anterior or posterior branches of inferior thyroid artery.

Recurrent Laryngeal Nerve at Surgery

Recurrent laryngeal nerve is identified with careful dissection through its entire course.

- Lack of color: It is whitish.
- It shows lack of elasticity.
- It shows lack of pulsation.
- It has longitudinal course and is longitudinal vein on surface.
- It is located at riddle's triangle, i.e., between the inferior thyroid artery superiorly, carotid artery laterally and trachea medially. From here recurrent laryngeal nerve run upward to enter larynx at greater cornue of thyroid cartilage. Many branches of nerve and variations should be remembered while dissecting here.

Anomalies of Recurrent Laryngeal Nerve

- Nerve traverses via the gland in 5–8% of cases.
- Nerve may be very closely adherent to posteromedial aspect of gland.
- If nerve is not seen—it can be far away in tracheoesophageal groove.
- Nonrecurrent, recurrent laryngeal nerve is seen in 1 in 1,000 cases. It has horizontal course.
- In 25% of cases, it is within the ligament of Berry.

---

21. TONSILS

Q.1. Write short note on peritonsillar abscess.

(Sep 2000, 10 Marks)

Ans. Peritonsillar abscess is also called as "Quinsy".

Collection of pus in peritonsillar space, i.e., between capsule of tonsil and superior constrictor muscle is known as peritonsillar abscess or quinsy.

Etiology

- As a sequelae of acute tonsillitis.
- De novo.

Causative Organisms

- *Streptococcus pyogenes*
- *Staphylococcus aureus*
- Anaerobic organisms

Mechanism

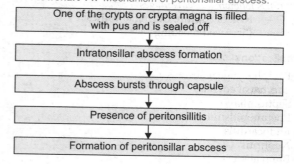

Flowchart 14: Mechanism of peritonsillar abscess.

One of the crypts or crypta magna is filled with pus and is sealed off
Intratonsillar abscess formation
Abscess bursts through capsule
Presence of peritonsillitis
Formation of peritonsillar abscess

Clinical Features

General Features

- Presence of high-grade fever with chills and rigors.
- Malaise, bodyache and headache.
- Nausea and constipation.

Local Features

- Severe unilateral throat pain
- Odynophagia leading to dehydration
- Hot potato speech
- Foul breath
- Poor orodental hygiene
- Ipsilateral earache
- Trismus.

Examination

- *Tonsils, pillars, soft palate:* Congestion of the involved side.
- *Uvula:* Swollen and pushed to the opposite side.
- Region of soft palate and anterior pillar above the tonsil appears bulged.
- Mucous covering the tonsil.
- Cervical lymph nodes are enlarged and tender.
- *Torticollis:* Head tilted to the involved side.

Treatment

Conservative Treatment

- Hospitalization is done and IV fluids should be given.
- IV antibiotics for aerobic and anaerobic organisms should be given
- Analgesics should be started
- *Oral hygiene:* Hydrogen peroxide and warm saline mouth gargles should be started.

Surgical treatment

- *Incision and drainage:*
  - If no response to conservative management and frank pus is present, incision and drainage is done.
  - Incision site: Point of maximum bulge above the upper pole of tonsil, just lateral to the meeting point of lines drawn at the base of uvula and along the anterior pillar. Once the incision is made, sinus forceps is inserted into the incision to open up the abscess.
- *Interval tonsillectomy:*
  - Interval tonsillectomy is done 4–6 weeks following quinsy.
  - *Abscess or hot tonsillectomy done in the presence of abscess has following disadvantages:*
    - Risk of rupture during anesthesia
    - Increased bleeding.

Complications

- Parapharyngeal abscess
- Laryngeal edema
- Septicemia
- Pneumonitis/lung abscess
- Endocarditis
- Nephritis
- Brain abscess
- Jugular vein thrombosis.

Q.2. Write short note on quinsy.   *(Sep 2005, 5 Marks)*

Ans. *Refer to Ans. 1 of same chapter.*

Q.3. Write short answer on Singer's nodule.

(Apr 2018, 3 Marks)

Ans. Vocal nodules are fibrous thickenings of vocal folds at the junction of middle and anterior third and are the result of vocal abuse. They are known as Singer's nodule in adults and screamer's nodule in children.

- In these speech therapy is the preferred treatment.
- Some of the lesions will resolve spontaneously in most of the cases.
- Occasionally nodules will need to be surgically removed using modern microlaryngoscopic dissection or laser

techniques, but speech therapy will be required for post-operative voice rehabilitation.

---

22. STOMACH

Q.1. How we differentiate between malignant and benign ulcer and management?   *(Jan 2018, 10 Marks)*

Or

Write differences between benign and malignant ulcers.   *(Sep 2018, 5 Marks)*

Ans. Benign ulcer and malignant ulcer are the types of gastric ulcer.

Features	Malignant ulcer	Benign ulcer
Mucosal folds	Effacing mucosal folds	Converging mucosal folds till margin
Site	Greater curvature	95% less curvature
Margin	Irregular margin	Regular margin
Floor	Necrotic slough on floor	Granulation tissue on floor
Edge	Everted edge	Punching or sloping edge
Surrounding area	Surrounding areas show nodules, ulcer and irregularities	Surrounding area and rugae are normal
Size and extent	Large and deep	Small, deep up to part of muscle
Bleeding	Present	Absent
Luminal	Endoluminal	Exoluminal

Management of Benign Ulcer

Drugs like H_2 blockers, proton-pump inhibitors, carbenoxolone (biogastrone, sucralfate, prostaglandins which coats the ulcer and so creates a mucosal barrier) helps in reducing or eliminating the symptoms of benign ulcer.

Management of Malignant Ulcer

- But asymptomatic ulcer may exist silently and may turn into malignancy. So surgery is the preferred line of treatment. Partial gastrectomy and Billroth I gastroduodenal anastamosis is done.
- Type IV proximal gastric ulcer is difficult to manage. It is treated by subtotal gastrectomy. Often distal gastrectomy with selective sleeve like extension cut along the lesser curve to remove the ulcer is done—Pauchet's procedure.
- *Other surgical procedures:*
  - **de Miguel's antrectomy:** Distal antrectomy, pylorectomy with excision of ulcer along with gastroduodenal anastomosis is done. It preserves gastric reservoir function, shows less recurrence rate and less operative morbidity.
  - **Maki's pylorus preserving gastrectomy:** Hemigastrectomy with excision of pyloric ulcer but retaining 2 cm prepyloric stomach. It is only used in type l gastric ulcer.

Even though it has got fewer incidences of postoperative diarrhea and dumping, it has got high recurrence rate.

♦ HSV with excision of ulcer
♦ *Kelling Madlener procedure:* It is antrectomy and excision of proximal gastric ulcer type IV.
♦ *Csendes procedure:* It is subtotal gastrectomy with sleeve extended resection along the lesser curve for type IV proximal gastric ulcer.

Q.2. Write short answer on Virchow's node.
(Feb 2019, 3 Marks)

Ans. Rudolf Ludwig Karl Virchow, in 1849, noted the involvement of left supraclavicular node in relation to the junction of the thoracic duct, adjacent to medial to internal jugular vein; this end node drains through few lymphatics into the left jugular trunk and to thoracic duct. Reflux from thoracic duct into this node occurs easily in abdominal malignancy.

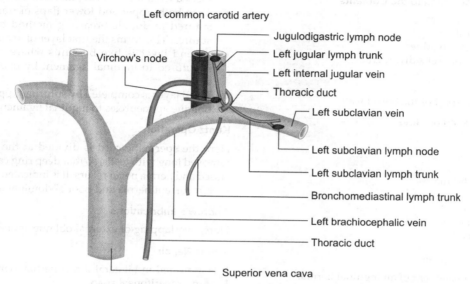

Fig. 33: Virchow's node *(For color version see Plate 2).*

♦ 40 years later, Troisier reported many abdominal cancers presenting with left supraclavicular lymph node involvement as external indicator and so coined the term Virchow's node and sign is called as Troisier sign.
♦ At the level of left C7 transverse process, thoracic duct arches behind the carotid sheath and internal jugular vein and joins the junction of internal jugular vein and left subclavian vein; this Virchow's (end node along the thoracic duct) is located medial to this junction behind the muscular lateral head of the left sternocleidomastoid muscle or in between the two heads.
♦ Virchow's node is also called as 'signal node' or seat of the devil' node.
♦ Virchow's node is actually part of the lower deep cervical node (level IV).
♦ Its surface marking almost corresponds to end of the thoracic duct, i.e., just above the sternal angle of the clavicle 1.5 cm left of the midline. Node is just medial to this point.

23. HERNIA

Q.1. Enumerate the different hernia of the body. Write the management and complication of inguinal hernia.
(Aug 2018, 10 Marks)

Ans. Hernia is defined as an area of weakness or disruption of the fibromuscular tissues of the body wall.

Enumeration of Different Hernia of the Body

Classification I (Clinical)

♦ *Reducible hernia:* Hernia gets reduced on its own or by the patient or by the surgeon. Intestine reduces with gurgling sound and it is difficult to reduce the first portion. Omentum is doughy and it is difficult to reduce the last portion. Expansile impulse on coughing is present.
♦ *Irreducible hernia:* Here contents cannot be returned to the abdomen due to narrow neck, adhesions, overcrowding. Irreducibility predisposes to strangulation.
♦ *Obstructed hernia:* It is an irreducible hernia with obstruction, but blood supply to the bowel is not interfered. It eventually leads to strangulation.
♦ *Inflamed hernia:* It is due to inflammation of the contents of sac., e.g., appendicitis, salpingitis. Here hernia is tender but not tense; overlying skin is red and edematous.
♦ *Strangulated hernia:* It is an irreducible hernia with obstruction to blood flow. The swelling is tense, tender, with no impulse on coughing and with features of intestinal obstruction. Features of intestinal obstruction may be absent in case of omentocele, Richter's hernia, Littre's hernia.

♦ *Occult (inguinal) hernia:* Hernia swelling is clinically not detectable but presents with groin pain; there may not be any expansile impulse on coughing.

Classification II

Congenital—common: It occur in a preformed sac/defect, clinically may present at a later period due to any of the precipitating causes like in direct inguinal hernia.

Classification III: According to the Contents

♦ Omentocele—omentum
♦ Enterocele—intestine
♦ Cystocele—urinary bladder
♦ Littre's hernia—Meckel's diverticulum
♦ Maydi's hernia
♦ Sliding hernia
♦ Richter's hernia—part of the bowel wall

Classification IV: Based on Sites

♦ Inguinal hernia
♦ Femoral hernia
♦ Obturator hernia
♦ Diaphragmatic hernia
♦ Lumbar hernia
♦ Spigelian hernia
♦ Umbilical hernia
♦ Epigastric hernia

Management of Inguinal Hernia

Following is the management of an inguinal hernia:
♦ **Herniotomy:** Excision of hernia sac is done. Repair is not required. This is carried out in children.
♦ **Hernioplasty:** Here, strengthening of posterior wall is done mostly by prolene mesh which is also known as Lichtenstein repair. This can be done by open or laparoscopic method. Hernioplasties are of two types:
  1. *Lichtenstein repair:* Strengthening of posterior wall of inguinal canal is done by prolene mesh. Mesh is of polypropylene. In preparation of mesh corners can be cut to provide round shape. Slit is provided on lateral border of mesh at junction of lower one-third and upper two-thirds to allow spermatic cord to pass through. Two of the slit ends should be overlapped. Fibroblasts and capillaries grow over mesh, converting it in thick fibrous sheath and strengthening the posterior wall. Mesh is fixed inferiorly to lacunar and inguinal ligaments, medially to overlap rectus sheath and fixed to fascia over pubic bone. Medially, the mesh overlaps the pubic tubercle and is sutured over the tissue of symphysis. Laterally, two of the tails are placed beyond deep ring and get sutured. Inferiorly, it is sutured to inguinal and lacunar ligament and superiorly to conjoined tendon. Few interrupted sutures put to fix it to transversalis fascia. Laterally, an artificial deep ring is created by crossing of both upper and lower leaves of the mesh. For attaining this, slit is given on the one side of mesh.
  2. *Prolene nylon dressing:* Suturing of conjoined tendon to inguinal ligament without tension in criss-cross manner

by using prolene suture material. It is preferred in both direct and indirect hernias.

Other Surgeries for Inguinal Hernia

Shouldice Repair

This is the tensionless method where only local tissues are used.
♦ As inguinal canal is opened, herniotomy is done.
♦ Transversalis fascia, which form the posterior wall get incised from internal ring till pubic tubercle.
♦ Then both upper and lower flaps of transverse fascia get sutured in double breasting method by nonabsorbable sutures. This forms the first layer of shouldice repair.
♦ Second layer is like Bassini's where conjoined tendon is sutured to inguinal ligament by using nonabsorbable sutures.
♦ Third layer is completed by suturing upper flap of external oblique aponeurosis to inguinal ligament.

Kuntz Operation

Here the spermatic cord is divided at the deep ring and is removed long with testis, so that deep ring can be permanently closed and hernia never recurs. It is indicated in elderly patients with recurrent hernia and poor abdominal muscle tone.

Andrew's Imbrications

Here, overlapping of external oblique aponeurosis is done.

Nyhus Repair

It is indicated in bilateral direct hernia, here a broad mesh is kept in preperitoneal space.

Stoppa Repair

It is a tension free type of hernia repair. This is performed by wrapping lower part of the parietal peritoneum with prosthetic mesh and placing it at preperitoneal level over Fruchaud's myopectineal orifice.

Marcy Repair

Here simple high ligation of the sac combined with tightening of internal ring is done.

Complications of Hernia

♦ **Irreducibility:** It occurs because of adhesion formed between omentum, sac and the contents. Irreducibility leads to dull aching pain.
♦ **Obstructed hernia:** Irreducible hernia along with obstruction to lumen of gut gives rise to obstructed hernia. Clinically it produces severe colicky abdominal pain, abdominal distention, vomiting and step ladder peristalsis.
♦ **Strangulated hernia:** It is irreducibility along with obstruction and impairment of blood supply to intestine.

24. OPERATIVE SURGERY

Q.1. Describe briefly tracheostomy.

(Jan 2011, 5 Marks) (Sep 2010, 10 Marks)

Or
Write short note on tracheostomy.
(Nov 2015, 5 Marks) (Dec 2009, 5 Marks)
(Apr 2008, 5 Marks) (Oct 2007, 5 Marks)
Or
Write briefly on tracheostomy. *(Jan 2016, 5 Marks)*
Or
Write in briefly about tracheostomy.
(July 2016, 5 Marks)
Or
Discuss indication, operative procedure and complication of tracheostomy. *(Sep 2005, 18 Marks)*
Or
Describe indication, procedure and complication of tracheostomy. *(Feb 2015, 10 Marks)*

Ans. Tracheostomy refers to a surgical entry into trachea through anterior wall to secure airway for oxygenation.

Classification/Types

♦ *Depending on the method of initial insertion:*
  • Surgical
  • Percutaneous (needle).
♦ *Depending on the intended duration:*
  • Temporary tracheostomy
  • Permanent tracheostomy.
♦ *Depending on situation demanding the procedure:*
  • Emergent tracheostomy
  • Urgent tracheostomy
  • Elective tracheostomy.

Indications

♦ To secure and clear the airway in upper respiratory tract obstruction (actual or potential).
♦ To secure and maintain a safe airway in patients with injuries to the face, head or neck and following certain types of surgery to the head and neck in unstable cervical spine fracture.
♦ To facilitate the removal of bronchial secretions where there is poor cough effort with sputum retention.
♦ To protect the airway of patients who are at high risk of aspiration, that is patients with incompetent laryngeal and tongue movement on swallowing, e.g., neuromuscular disorders, unconsciousness, head injuries, stroke, etc.
♦ To enable long-term mechanical ventilation of patients, either in an acute ICU setting or sometimes chronically in hospitals.
♦ To facilitate weaning from artificial ventilation in acute respiratory failure and prolonged ventilation.

Contraindications

♦ Children under 5 years of age.
♦ Pre-existing pathology of larynx, e.g., carcinoma
♦ Lack of experience and knowledge of cricothyroidotomy.
♦ Cervical trauma.

Procedure

♦ *Step I:* Skin from the chin to below the clavicles is sterilely prepared.
♦ *Step II:* Local anesthesia with vasoconstrictor is infiltrated in skin and deeper tissues.
♦ *Step III:* Skin of the neck over second tracheal ring is identified and an incision is placed horizontally along natural cervical skin crease.
♦ *Step IV:* Sharp dissection following the skin incision is done to cut across platysma muscle.
♦ *Step V:* Blunt dissection is given parallel to long axis of trachea for separating submuscular tissues until isthmus is identified.
♦ *Step VI:* A cricoids hook engages the space between cricoids and first tracheal ring pull trachea upward. Blunt dissection is continued longitudinally through pretracheal fascia.
♦ *Step VII:* Entrance in trachea
  • A linear incision is made through interspace between second and third tracheal rings.
  • Midportion of third or fourth tracheal ring is removed for creating tracheal window.
  • An inferiorly placed U-shaped flap also known as Bjork flap incorporates the ring below the tracheal incision is raised and sutured to the skin at inferior margin.
♦ *Step VIII:* Tube is placed and is secured to neck. Tube is inserted vertically downward into the trachea avoiding damage to the tracheal mucosa of posterior wall. The tube is secured by suturing the flanges to the neck skin. This is followed by tying the flanges of tube with thread encircling the neck taking care to avoid strangulation.

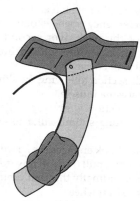

Fig. 34: Tracheostomy tube.

Complications

Complications are as follows:
♦ **Immediate complications (perioperative period)**
  • Hemorrhage
  • Misplacement of tube
  • Pneumothorax
  • Tube occlusion
  • Surgical emphysema
  • Loss of the upper airway

- **Delayed complications (postoperative period; <7 days)**
  - Tube blockage with secretions or blood.
  - Partial or complete tube displacement.
  - Infection of the stoma site.
  - Infection of the bronchial tree (pneumonia).
  - Ulceration and/or necrosis of trachea.
  - Mucosal ulceration by tube migration
  - Risk of occlusion of the tracheostomy tube in obese or fatigued patients who have difficulty extending their neck.
  - Tracheoesophageal fistula formation.
  - Hemorrhage.
- **Late complications (late postoperative period; >7 days)**
  - Granulomata of the trachea may cause respiratory difficulty when the tracheostomy tube is removed.
  - Tracheal dilation, stenosis, persistent sinus or collapse (tracheomalacia)
  - Scar formation requiring revision.
  - Blocked tubes may occur at any time, especially if secretions become thick, the secretions are not managed appropriately (suction) and humidification is not used.
  - Hemorrhage.

Q.2. Discuss emergency tracheostomy.

(Feb/Mar 2004, 10 Marks)

Ans. Emergency tracheostomy is performed within 2–3 minutes in an emergency situation when patient is anoxic and requires immediate oxygenation and verification to avoid cerebral hypoxia.

Procedure

- *Step I and II:* Preparation of skin and local anesthesia is not performed in emergency tracheostomy.
- *Step III:* Skin of the neck over second tracheal ring is identified and an incision is placed horizontally along natural cervical skin crease.
- *Step IV:* Sharp dissection following the skin incision is done to cut across platysma muscle.
- *Step V:* Blunt dissection is given parallel to long axis of trachea for separating submuscular tissues until isthmus is identified.
- *Step VI:* A cricoids hook engages the space between cricoids and first tracheal ring pull trachea upward. Blunt dissection is continued longitudinally through pretracheal fascia.
- *Step VII:* Entrance in trachea
  - A linear incision is made through inter-space between second and third tracheal rings.
  - Midportion of third or fourth tracheal ring is removed for creating tracheal window.
  - An inferiorly placed U-shaped flap also known as Bjork flap incorporates the ring below the tracheal incision is raised and sutured to the skin at inferior margin.
- *Step VIII:* Tube is placed and is secured to neck. Tube is inserted vertically downward into the trachea avoiding damage to the tracheal mucosa of posterior wall. The tube is secured by suturing the flanges to the neck skin. This is followed by tying the flanges of tube with thread encircling the neck taking care to avoid strangulation.

Q.3. Write short note on diathermy.

(Jan 2011, 3 Marks) (Nov 2014, 5 Marks)

Ans. It is also known as electrocautery.

It is the method to control bleeding or to cut the tissues during surgery.

Types

- **Based on type of current used:**
  - Unipolar cautery
  - Bipolar cautery.
- **Based on type of action:**
  - Coagulation cautery
  - Cutting cautery
  - *Blended current:* Combination both coagulation and cutting cautery.

Uses

- For coagulation of bleeding during surgery to achieve hemostasis.
- For cutting muscles, fascia, etc.
- For laparoscopic surgical procedures.
- To remove small cutaneous lesions.

Disadvantages

- It leads to infection.
- For the cauterization of normal tissues.
- It has problem of explosion.
- It can cause diathermy burn to the patient at the site where diathermy plate is used.
- It can cause burn injury or electrical shock to surgeon and assisting personnel.

Q.4. Classify suture material. Add a small note on catgut.

(Feb 2013, 5 Marks)

Or

Enumerate absorbable and nonabsorbable suture material.

(Feb 2019, 5 Marks)

Ans.

Classification of Suture Material

Classification I

- *Absorbable suture material:*
  - Plain catgut
  - Chromic catgut
  - Vicryl
  - Dexon
  - Maxon
  - Polydioxanone suture material
  - Monocryl
  - Biosyn.
- Nonabsorbable suture material
  - Silk
  - Polypropylene

- Polyethylene
- Cotton
- Linen
- Steel, polyester, polyamide, nylon.

Classification II

- *Natural:*
  - Catgut
  - Silk
  - Cotton
  - Linen.
- *Synthetic:*
  - Vicryl, dexon, PDS, maxon
  - Polypropylene, polyethylene, polyester, polyamide.

Classification III

- *Braided:* Polyester, polyamide, Vicryl, Dexon, silk
- *Twisted:* Cotton, linen.

Classification IV

- *Monofilament:* Polypropylene, polyethylene, PDS, catgut, steel
- *Multifilament:* Polyester, polyamide, Vicryl, Dexon, silk, cotton.

Classification V

- Coated
- Uncoated.

Catgut

Catgut was the first absorbable suture material available.

- Original word was kitgut, i.e., Kit means fiddle and present form arise thorough confusion with kit = cat.
- Another explanation of origin of cat in catgut is it is an abbreviation of cattle which originally denoted not only the cows but all types of livestock.
- Catgut is derived from natural source which is purified collagen tissue derived from serous layer of cow's intestine or submucous fibrous layer of sheep intestine.
- Catgut is pseudofilamentous in nature, i.e., microscopically it is made up of multiple filaments which are processed in such a way that they are twisted in ground together and polished to produce the appearance of monofilament suture material.
- As it is composed of collagen fibers, chances of degradation are present, i.e., the material should be kept moist.
- Commercial supply of this material is as the package soaked in isopropyl alcohol which act as preservative.
- Resorption of catgut is via enzymatic digestion through proteolytic enzymes and phagocytosis.
- When catgut is placed inside the tissues, it looses its tensile strength under 10–15 days, this is resorbed under 2–3 months.

Types of Catgut

It is of three types, i.e.

- Plane gut

- Chromic gut
- Fast absorbing surgical gut

Plane Gut

- At the time of suturing, it should be dry or else it become stiff and difficult to handle.
- It breaks easily as it consists of weak areas along its length due to manufacturing process.
- It is easily degraded by enzymatic action and inflammatory reaction is present during this procedure.
- Bacterial adhesion is more as compared to nylon and polypropylene.
- Tensile strength of this material is poor. Tensile strength lost in 7–10 days
- This is used to suture subcutaneous tissue, muscle and suturing circumcision in children.

Chromic Gut

- It is the plain surgical gut which is tanned with the chromic salts.
- This is done to decrease reactivity of tissue and increase in tensile strength.
- Chromic gut has better knot security as compared to plane gut.
- Coating by chromic salts increases its resistance to resorption. As plain gut looses its strength by 10–15 days, chromic gut takes the double of this time, i.e., 3–4 weeks.
- Resorption gets completed after 90 days.
- Chromic gut produces tissue reaction which is less as compared to plain gut.
- It is used for suturing muscle. Fascia, ligating pedicles, etc.

Fast Absorbing Gut

- When plain surgical gut is treated by heat to allow rapid resorption it is known as fast absorbing gut.
- This is designed for use on skin.
- Its tensile strength lost from 5–7 days and get resorbed by 2–4 weeks.

Q.5. Enlist indications, types of tracheostomy. Add a note on steps of tracheostomy and enlist its postoperative complications. *(Feb 2013, 10 Marks)*

Ans. *For indications, types, steps of tracheostomy and postoperative complications refer to Ans. 1 of same chapter.*

Q.6. Write short note on indications of tracheostomy.
(June 2010, 5 Marks) (May/Jun 2009, 5 Marks)

Or

Write briefly on indications of tracheostomy.
(Dec 2010, 5 Marks)

Or

Write short answer on indications of tracheostomy.
(June 2018, 3 Marks)

Ans. *For indications refer to Ans. 1 of same chapter.*

Q.7. Describe briefly suture materials. *(Apr 2017, 5 Marks)*

Ans. Suture materials are used to hold the several tissues in close approximation.

Properties of an Ideal Suturing Material

- It should produce less tissue reaction.
- There should be adequate strength of suture material to withstand stress.
- It should be easily sterilized.
- It is easy to handle within the tissues.
- It should have good knot tying properties.
- It should have less capillary action.

Classification of Suture Materials

- *Based on the degradation of material within the tissues:*
  - Absorbable
  - Nonabsorbable
- *Based on the source of materials:*
  - Natural, e.g., silk
  - Synthetic, e.g., polyglycolic acid
  - Metallic, e.g., stainless steel
- *Based on the number of filaments in the suture material:*
  - Monofilament
  - Multifilament
  - Pseudomonofilament
- *Based on the diameter of the thread in cross section:*
  - 1 – 0 to 10 – 0. With an increase in number of zeros, diameter of material reduces
- *Based on the coating applied on the material:*
  - Teflon coated
  - Chromic coated, etc.

Description of Suturing Materials

Absorbable Materials

- They loose their strength into the tissues and degrades under 60 days, e.g., catgut, polyglycolic acid, polyglactin 910 (Vicryl), polydiaxanone, polyglecaprone, polytrimethylene carbonate, Polyglytone 6211, etc.
- These sutures undergo enzymatic degradation by natural enzymes present in the body.
- They are used in deep layer suturing and suturing of wounds in patient who do not come for removal of sutures.

Nonabsorbable Suture Materials

- They are not degraded by the body.
- Suture removal has to be done after end of healing phase.
- Examples are silk, nylon and polyester.

Monofilament Suture Material

- It is known as monofilament as they are made up of single strand.
- They produce the advantage of least capillary effect.
- They decrease the chances of infection.
- *Examples:* In monofilament absorbable is monocryl and nonabsorbable is polyamide, polyester, etc.
- They have major disadvantage of memory effect due to which material come to its original position and this leads to loosening of knot.

Multifilament Suture Material

- It is known as multifilament as it is made up of multiple thin strands of suture material which are either rolled, twisted or braided together to form uniform strand of thread.

- They are easy to handle and have good knot tying properties.
- Knot placed cannot get slipped.
- They are used at places where good strength is needed to hold the wound edges together.
- It has more capillary action and can act as source of infection.
- Example is black braided silk.

Pseudomonofilament

- This suture material is made up of numerous strands of fiber which are processed by twisting, grinding and polishing to produce a monofilamentous appearance.
- Example is catgut.

Based on Diameter of Thread in Cross-section

- Suture materials are labeled from 1 – 0 to 10 – 0.
- With an increase in number of zeros, diameter of material reduces.
  - 10 – 0: Used for microsurgery repair
  - 5 – 0, 6 – 0: Suturing for skin on face
  - 4 – 0, 5 – 0: Used for suturing in extremities
  - 3 – 0: For scalp sutures
  - 3 – 0, 4 – 0: Commonly used in most of the oral surgical procedures.

Q.8. Write brief answer on types of sutures.

(Apr 2017, 5 Marks)

Ans.

Types of Sutures

Interrupted Sutures

Interrupted sutures are most common type of suture and are universally used.

Used to close oral mucosal incisions and skin wounds.

Technique

- Needle should be held two-thirds the distance from tip of needle with needle holder.
- Needle is passed via one side of the flap perpendicular to the tissues and brought out along the curvature of needle.
- Needle is now passed via other flap at same distance from edge of the flap and also at the same depth.
- It is brought out of the flap along with suture material till 3–4 cm of free end of suture material is left.
- Now needle should be held in the left hand and wound around the needle holder once or twice depending on the type of knot.
- Free end of suture material is grasped with beaks of needle holder.
- Material which is wound around the needle holder is made to slip over the beaks by slow pulling on needle end of suture material. Free end of suture material should be pulled minimally.
- Knot is stabilized in the manner that it comes to one side of the flap. It should not rest along edges of wound.
- For completion of knot, hold needle in left hand and roll suture material around the beaks of needle holder in opposite direction. Now again grasp free end of suture material and slide suture material over free end to stabilize the knot.
- Hold both the free ends and needle end of suture material taut for assistant to trim them with scissors leaving 3–4 mm.

Mattress Sutures

Horizontal Mattress Sutures

They are used in areas where there is underlying bony defect.

Technique

♦ Needle is first passed via one flap and at same vertical level through other flap similar to placing of an interrupted suture but the knot is not placed.
♦ Needle is now passed at the distance 3–4 mm parallel horizontally where the needle was passed through the second flap.
♦ Now it is passed via the first flap at same vertical level as last bite.
♦ In this way, the needle comes back via the same flap where it is started at a distance of 3–4 mm from entry point.
♦ Now the knot is placed and is stabilized over that side.

Vertical Mattress Suture

They are used to close skin wounds mainly in areas where edges of skin tend to invert.

Technique

♦ In this needle is first passed far away from wound edges and then nearer or at a more superficial level.
♦ Needle is passed via one wound edge taking a deep bite of tissue almost 4–8 mm from wound edge.
♦ It is now passed through other edge at same depth and brought out. Knot is still not placed.
♦ Needle is now turned around and passes backward through second flap at a level closer to wound edges.
♦ Needle is now passed via one flap at same superficial level and is brought out. In this way, both edges suture material are on the same side.
♦ Knot is now placed and stabilized on side where the suture first began.

Continuous Sutures without Locking

They are used to suture large wounds. Intraorally, they are used when full quadrant alveoloplasty is done.

Technique

♦ At first time place the interrupted suture.
♦ While cutting the suture ends, cut the free ends leaving the suture material with needle behind.
♦ Needle is now passed via flaps of wound alternately to get continuous oblique sutures all along the length of wound.
♦ At the end of wound, knot is placed by loop of the suture and the needle end of suture material.

Continuous Sutures with Locking

Technique

♦ First of all an interrupted suture is placed.
♦ Now the needle is passed through the loop made by suture material.
♦ Assistant should be made to follow the suture by holding suture material close to the tissues where needle was last passed via the loop.

♦ Each time needle pass through the flap and under the suture loop, assistant should hold suture material tightly close to the tissue to prevent suture material slipping and becoming loose.
♦ At end of suture line the knot is made with suture loop and the needle end of suture material.

Subcuticular Sutures

They are used for closing the cosmetic wounds.

Technique

♦ For this type of suturing technique nonabsorbable monofilament suture is used.
♦ First the suture is passed via skin at one end of the wound such that the needle is brought in the wound.
♦ Needle is now passed alternately through opposite wound edges completely in subcuticular layer without piercing the skin and without placing the knot anywhere in the wound.
♦ At the end, needle should be brought again through edge of the wound through skin.
♦ Pull the suture material tightly to get good approximation of wound edges without any bunching.
♦ Trim the suture materials to leave long ends and taped on both ends to secure from slipping.

Q.9. Write brief answer on endotracheal intubation.

(Apr 2017, 5 Marks)

Ans. Endotracheal intubation is the most basic skill which is acquired by an anesthesiologist. Endotracheal intubation consists of introduction of a tube inside trachea for maintaining the patency and protecting the airway as well as to ensure proper oxygenation and ventilation.

Endotracheal intubation is the definitive way of maintaining the airway in patients who need muscle paralysis as well as intermittent positive pressure ventilation.

Whenever general anesthesia is given and needs to be maintained for long periods, endotracheal intubation is done.

Indications

♦ For inducing general anesthesia for long time, i.e., >1–2 hours.
♦ To maintain patency of the airway in unconscious patients.
♦ For protecting lungs from aspiration of regurgitated gastric contents.
♦ For ensuring proper delivery of adequate tidal volumes to the lungs.
♦ For clearing excessive as well as retained secretions from the lungs.

Contraindications

♦ *In cases where upper airway integrity is lost, i.e.:*
  • In extensive maxillofacial injury with bilateral fractures of mandible and maxillae.
  • Injuries to the neck along with laryngeal rupture
  • Large tumors of upper airway.

In above conditions, endotracheal intubation may be extremely difficult and even dangerous. In above situations, tracheostomy may be a better choice.

Technique

- A pillow of 7–10 cm should be positioned under patient's head which enables mild flexion at the cervical spine.
- Head is then extended at the atlanto-occipital joint. This is known as intubating position or "sniffing position".

Procedure

- Endotracheal intubation can be done in multiple ways, i.e., can be done either orally or nasally; can be done either under direct vision or indirectly by fiberoptic scope. It can be done blindly when visualization of the glottis by direct means is not possible and fibreoptic scope is not available. In such cases, if the regular antegrade technique, i.e., mouth or nose to larynx or a retrograde intubation, i.e., larynx to mouth can be tried.
- In the retrograde technique, pass a guide wire from the cricothyroid membrane upward inside the mouth or nose and an endotracheal tube is guided over it into the larynx.
- Procedure of endotracheal intubation is done with the patient anesthetized but can also be carried out with the patient awake after administering local anesthesia to upper airway when a difficult intubation is anticipated.
- Many of the airway adjuncts are available for use when a difficult airway is encountered, especially when it is unanticipated. These include oropharyngeal airway, nasopharyngeal airway, laryngeal mask airway and Combitube®.

Complications

Immediate

- Trauma to the teeth, lips, tongue, pharynx or larynx.
- Hemodynamic changes, such as tachycardia, hypertension, myocardial ischemia.
- Misplaced tube, i.e., accidental extubation and esophageal intubation

Delayed

Laryngeal granuloma, laryngeal or subglottic stenosis.

Q.10. Write brief notes on incision and drainage.

(Apr 2017, 2 Marks)

Ans. Incision and drainage is the surgical procedure carried out to relieve the pus.

- Mainly incision and drainage is done in pyogenic abscess.
- Incision and drainage is contraindicated in cold abscess.
- During incision and drainage position of the patient should be supine, prone or lateral depending upon site of abscess.

Procedure

- For this procedure, preferred anesthesia is general anesthesia because abscess is multiloculated and infiltration of lignocaine into the abscess cavity does not act because of the acidic pH of the pus. However, a superficial abscess which is pointing can be managed without general anesthesia.

- Provide a stab incision over the most prominent part of the swelling, i.e., part which is red, skin is thinned out over it and is pointed.
- As incision is given and pus comes out of the swelling, it should be sent for culture and sensitivity.
- A sinus forceps or finger is introduced now inside the abscess cavity and all the loculi present inside the cavity should be broken. As fresh blood oozes out, this indicates the completion of procedure.
- Cavity should be irrigated with hydrogen peroxide solution or iodine solution.
- If size of the cavity is large, it should be packed by roller gauze which is soaked in iodine and it is removed after 24–48 hours. Packing helps in controlling the bleeding and due to the pack the opening of abscess cavity does not close. By 7–10 days, the cavity collapses spontaneously and granulation tissue fills up the cavity and healing takes place.
- An abscess should not be closed, as it contains bacteria, etc. It should be drained out.

Postoperative Management

- Proper antibiotics should be given to the patient.
- Control of diabetes should be done, if patient is diabetic.
- Regular dressing of wound is done by antiseptic solution.

Q.11. Write short note on laparoscopic surgery or minimal access surgery.   *(Jan 2017, 10 Marks)*

Ans.

Advantages of Laparoscopic Surgery

- Relatively less painful compared to open surgery. Trauma of access is very less.
- Shorter hospital stay and early return to work.
- Faster postoperative recovery.
- Better visualization of the anatomy, i.e., better approach for dissection and visualization of other parts of abdomen for any other pathology.
- Instrumental access to different abdominal locations is many times better compared to open method.
- Minimal scar on the abdomen.

Instruments Used

- Zero degree laparoscope is commonly used. Side viewing scopes are also used to have better visualization 30°.
- Cold light source either halogen lamp or xenon lamp is used. Halogen lamp is used commonly and is cheaper. Xenon lamp gives high visualization.
- *Camera:* 3 chip camera is commonly used with high resolution
- Video—monitor to display images.
- CO_2 insufflator.
- Long fine dissectors like in open surgical techniques.
- Hooks and spatulas are used along with cautery for dissection.
- Clip applicators
- Needle holders
- Endostaplers
- Veress needle

- Suction—irrigation apparatus.
- Trocars of different sizes—10 mm, 5 mm.
- Reducers to negotiate smaller instruments through larger ports.

Preparation

Always general anesthesia. Other preparations are same as for open method.

Technique

- Pressure bandages are applied to both legs to improve the venous return and to decrease the stasis.
- Head end of the table is lowered to have easier insertion of veress needle and scope.
- Ryle's tube and Foley's catheter are essential before insertion of the trocars.
- Pneumoperitoneum is created using veress needle through umbilical incision. Access can be achieved by open method through an umbilical incision. Carbon dioxide is commonly used to create pneumoperitoneum.
- Pneumoperitoneum is created up to a pressure of 15 mm Hg which distends the abdominal cavity adequately to have proper visualization of the abdominal contents.
- Laparoscope is inserted through the umbilical port (10 mm).
- Abdomen is evaluated for any pathology. Liver, gallbladder, pelvic organs are visualized.
- Additional ports (3–4) through trocars are placed depending on the procedure to be done. It may be either 5 mm port or 10 mm port. These ports are placed in such a way to have a proper triangulation of instruments for dissection.
- To use clip applicator 10 mm port is required.

Physiologic Changes due to Pneumoperitoneum

- Carbon dioxide causes hypercapnia, acidosis and hypoxia.
- Pneumoperitoneum exerts pressure on the IVC, decreases the venous return and so the cardiac output.
- It increases the arterial pressure also.
- It compromises the respiratory function by compressing over the diaphragm impairing the pulmonary compliance.

Complications

- Carbon dioxide narcosis and hypoxia.
- Sepsis—subphrenic abscess, pelvic abscess, septicemia.
- IVC compression
- Bleeding
- Leak from the site, e.g., bile leak.
- Organ injury during insertion of ports, e.g., major vessels, bowel, mesentery, liver.
- Subcutaneous emphysema and pneumomediastinum.
- Gas emboli, though is rare but fatal.
- Postoperative shoulder pain due to irritation of diaphragm.
- Cardiac dysfunction due to decreased venous return.
- Injury to the abdominal wall vessels and nerves.
- Cautery burn to abdominal structures.
- Abdominal wall hernias.
- Wound infection.
- Mortality—0.5%.

Relative Contraindications

- Patients with compromised cardiac status
- Peritonitis
- Previous abdominal surgeries
- Bleeding disorders
- Morbid obesity
- Third trimester of pregnancy
- Portal hypertension.

Basic Laparoscopic Surgeries

- *Laparoscopic cholecystectomy:* This is indicated in gallstones, cholecystitis, biliary colic
- *Laparoscopic appendicectomy:* This is indicated in acute appendicitis.

Q.12. Write short note on robotic surgery.

(Jan 2018, 10 Marks)

Ans. Robotic surgery is a type of minimally invasive surgery. "Minimally invasive" means that instead of operating on patients through large incisions, we use miniaturized surgical instruments that fit through a series of quarter-inch incisions.

- When performing surgery with the da Vinci Si—the world's most advanced surgical robot—these miniaturized instruments are mounted on three separate robotic arms, allowing the surgeon maximum range of motion and precision. The da Vinci's fourth arm contains a magnified high-definition 3-D camera that guides the surgeon during the procedure.
- The surgeon controls these instruments and the camera from a console located in the operating room. Placing his fingers into the master controls, he is able to operate all four arms of the da Vinci simultaneously while looking through a stereoscopic high-definition monitor that literally places him inside the patient, giving him a better, more detailed 3-D view of the operating site than the human eye can provide.
- Every movement he makes with the master controls is replicated precisely by the robot.
- When necessary, the surgeon can even change the scale of the robot's movements: If he selects a three-to-one scale, the tip of the robot's arm will move just one inch for every three inches the surgeon's hand moves. And because of the console's design, the surgeon's eyes and hands are always perfectly aligned with his view of the surgical site, minimizing surgeon fatigue.
- The ultimate effect is to give the surgeon unprecedented control in a minimally invasive environment. Utilizing this advanced technology, surgeons are able to perform a growing number of complex urological, gynecological, cardiothoracic and general surgical procedures. Since these procedures can now be performed through very small incisions, patients experience a number of benefits compared to open surgery, including:
  - Less trauma on the body
  - Minimal scarring, and
  - Faster recovery time.

Q.13. Write short note on benefits of robotic surgery.

(Sep 2018, 5 Marks)

Ans. Benefits of robotic surgery are:

- **Enhanced visualization:** The high power camera and in-built optic system ensures amplified—visual picture ensuring perception of high quality images in real clinical situation.
- **Elimination of physiologic tremors and scale motion:** The unit eliminates hand tremors, fulcrum effect of instruments especially when insertion of endoscopes is involved. The torque, force and scale motion are greatly reduced leading to better surgery lower iatrogenic injury ensuring safer surgery.
- **Multiarticulated instruments:** Simultaneous, coordinated handling of multiple instruments, such as drill, suction and electrocautery units in controlled environment.
- **Fatigue reduction:** The unit instills a confidence, reduces time of surgery owing to clear field, precision and accurate manipulation. All of these lead to a reduced surgical time as well as fatigue reduction to the surgical team.
- **Restore proper hand-eye coordination:** High resolution robotic handling ensures proper hand-eye coordination.
- **Telesurgery:** The modality ensures distance remote surgery as surgeons console can be kept away and the remaining unit can be connected through high speed internet.

25. NEUROLOGICAL INJURIES

Q.1. Write short note on trigeminal neuralgia.

(Feb 2013, 5 Marks) (June 2015, 5 Marks)
(Mar 2006, 5 Marks) (Jan 2016, 5 Marks)
(Jan 2012, 5 Marks) (Aug 2011, 5 Marks)
(June 2010, 5 Marks) (Sep 2009, 5 Marks)
(Apr 2008, 5 Marks) (Oct 2007, 5 Marks)

Or

Answer briefly on trigeminal neuralgia.

(Mar 2016, 3 Marks)

Or

Write in short about trigeminal neuralgia.

(July 2016, 5 Marks)

Or

Discuss the treatment of trigeminal neuralgia.

(Sep 2010, 10 Marks)

Or

Write short answer on trigeminal neuralgia.

(Apr 2018, 3 Marks)

Or

Write short note on management of trigeminal neuralgia. *(Feb 2019, 5 Marks)*

Ans. It is also called as Tic Douloureux, trifacial neuralgia or Fothergill's disease.

Trigeminal neuralgia is an extremely painful condition along the distribution of any branches of trigeminal nerve.

Etiology

- Dental pathosis at times leads to trigeminal neuralgia.
- Due to excessive traction divisions of trigeminal nerve are affected which leads to trigeminal neuralgia.
- Allergic and hypersensitivity reaction may lead to trigeminal neuralgia.
- Mechanical factors, such as pressure caused by aneurysms of internal carotid artery.
- Secondary lesions, such as carcinomas of maxillary antrum, carcinoma of nasopharynx leads to trigeminal neuralgia.

Clinical Features

- It occurs in middle age and older people.
- Female predilection is seen.
- Pain is paroxysmal in nature, last for few minutes and is of extreme intensity.
- Pain is usually limited to the distribution of trigeminal nerve and is unilateral. At times pain is bilateral too.
- Pain is provoked by obvious stimuli to the face. A touch, a draft of air, any movement of face as in talking, chewing, yawning or swallowing.
- Pain attacks are precipitated by touching some "trigger zone" on the face, i.e., vermilion border of lip, the ala of nose, the cheek and around the eyes. Patient usually avoid touching of skin over these areas. Patient has unshaven face, avoid brushing, undergo dental extraction.
- Objective signs or sensory loss are demonstrated on examination.
- Onset of pain is sudden and tends to persist for weeks or months before remitting spontaneously.

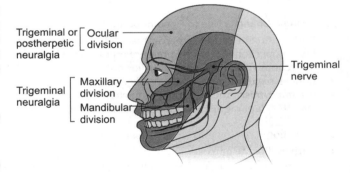

Fig. 35: Trigeminal neuralgia.

Treatment

Medical Treatment

- Carbamazepine (tegretol) has a special effect on the paroxysmal pain. This is considered to be the best conservative treatment for trigeminal neuralgia. As an initial dose, 100 mg twice daily till relief is established.
- *Dilantin:* Diphenylhydantoin, an anticonvulsant drug has been recommended, effective when given orally, 300–400 mg/day.
- Recently, baclofen an antispastic drug is also being used.
- A combination of dilantin and carbamazepine may also be given.

- Clonazepam an antiepileptic found to be useful.
- Anti-inflammatory agents, such as indomethacin and short course of steroids have been found to be useful.

Surgical Treatment

- *Infection of the nerve with anesthetic solution:* Local anesthetics of various types injected near the peripheral branches of the trigeminal nerve to serve to provide temporary relief from pain.
- *Injection of the nerve with alcohol:*
  - The most popular material, alcohol, can be placed directly into the area where a nerve exits from the skull or more peripherally.
  - When alcohol contracts the nerve, neurolysis occurs distal to the injection site.
  - Generally, 95% alcohol is used or procaine or monocaine 2%, chloroform 5%, absolute alcohol 70%, Ringer's solution 23% can also be used.
- *Nerve sectioning and nerve evolution (peripheral neurectomy):* This procedure is more lasting and effective than an injection with alcohol. Peripheral neurectomy results in high degree of success in elimination of pain.
- *Electrocoagulation of gasserian ganglion:* Diathermy apparatus is placed in the gasserian ganglion to coagulate and destroy it.
- *Percutaneous radiofrequency trigeminal neurolysis:* It is performed by insertion of temperature monitoring electrode through foramen ovale into trigeminal ganglion. Advantages include decreased mortality and morbidity and permanent cure.
- *Rhizotomy:* Actual cutting of trigeminal sensory root results in permanent anesthesia in most patients.
- *Bulbar trigeminal tractotomy:* The descending tract of the trigeminal nerve may be cut in the area of medulla oblongata to induce loss of pain and temperature sensation.

Q.2. Write short note on Bell's palsy.
(Nov 2014, 3 Marks) (Dec 2015, 5 Marks)
(Feb 2013, 5 Marks) (Aug 2012, 5 Marks)

Ans. It is also called as 7th nerve paraplegia or facial palsy.

Etiology

- *Cold:* It occurs after exposure to cold.
- *Trauma:* Extraction of teeth or injection of local anesthetic may damage the nerve and causes subsequent paralysis.
- *Surgical procedure:*, such as removal of parotid gland tumor in which the facial nerve is sectioned can also cause facial paralysis.
- *Tumors:* Tumors of the cranial base, parapharyngeal space and infratemporal fossa cause facial nerve palsy.
- *Familial:* Familial and hereditary occurrence is also reported in case of Bell's palsy.
- Facial canal and middle ear neoplasms may lead to Bell's palsy.

Clinical Features

- It occur in older age group.
- Female predilection is most common.

- There is presence of paralysis over one side of the face.
- Drooping of angle of mouth is present over the affected side and saliva is drooling from the affected side.
- Patient is unable to raise the eyebrow of the affected side.
- Patient is unable to close the eye over affected side and tears continuously roll down.
- Eyeball roll upward when attempted to close the eye, this is known as Bell's phenomenon.
- Over the affected side, patient has lost the taste sensation.
- Patient complaints of pain in or behind the ear.
- Presence of numbness over the affected side of face.
- Patient has mask like appearance when he/she tries to smile.
- There is difficulty in blowing or clenching.
- Obliteration of nasolabial fold
- Presence of wide palpebral fissure
- Presence of epiphora.

Treatment

Medicinal Treatment

- Patients with Bell's palsy have excellent prognosis. Treatment of Bell's palsy is controversial as spontaneous recovery is present.
- Treatment is given to the patients who have onset of paralysis under 1–4 days of an initial visit.
- Corticosteroids, i.e., prednisolone 1 mg/kg or 60 mg per day for 6 days followed by the taper of 10 days.
- Antiviral drugs can be given in the patients in which bell's palsy is associated with herpes infection.
- In Bell's palsy eye of the patient is at risk for drying which cause corneal abrasion and corneal ulcer. Eye care consists of inducing the artificial tears in daytime along with eyeglasses. At night eye lubricant can be used.

Surgical treatment

- Surgical treatment for Bell's palsy is surgical decompression and anastomosis of the nerve. In this facial and hypoglossal nerve get anastomosed which helps in restoring the partial function.
- Nerve grafting using greater auricular nerve, sural nerve, lateral cutaneous nerve of thigh or hypoglossal nerve.
- Suspension of angle of mouth to zygomatic bone using temporal fascia sling.
- *Lateral tarsorrhaphy:* This prevent corneal ulceration
- *Medial canthus reconstruction:* To decrease epiphora
- Cross facial nerve transplantation from opposite side using its insignificant branches.
- Dynamic neurovascular muscle graft
- Upper lid gold weights to protect cornea.

Q.3. Discuss etiology and management of injury of facial nerve. *(Feb/Mar 2004, 10 Marks)*

Ans. Injuries of facial nerve causes facial palsy or Bell's palsy.

Etiology of Facial Paralysis

- *Congenital:* Mobius syndrome (uncommon and poorly understood)

- *Traumatic:*
  - Birth injury
  - Iatrogenic injury at the time of surgeries, e.g., surgery for parotid gland surgery etc.
  - Blunt or penetrating trauma to nerve.
  - Fracture of the temporal bone can lead to facial nerve injury.
- *Infections:*
  - Virally mediated diseases, i.e., herpes zoster, mumps, coxsackie virus and mononucleosis.
  - Bacterial infections, i.e., sequelae to otitis media, Lyme disease, mastoiditis.
- *Inflammatory conditions:* Sarcoidosis
- *Neoplastic:* Tumors of the parotid gland (typically malignant tumors)
  - Facial nerve schwannomas
  - Acoustic neuromas
  - Neoplasms of the brain, such as brainstem tumors.
- *Idiopathic:*
  - Bell`s palsy is most common type of facial paralysis. It occurs due to virally induced inflammation of the nerve resulting in compromise of the function of nerve, swelling and vascular supply to the nerve.
  - Melkersson–Rosenthal syndrome
  - Myasthenia gravis.

Management

Facial nerve repair can be done by following surgical methods, i.e.:

- Direct repair
- Cable nerve grafting
- Nerve substitution techniques.

Direct Repair

Preoperative Details

- Direct repair of the facial nerve is the best method to rehabilitate the paralyzed face. By this method, there are chances of restoring spontaneous, emotional expression to the face.
- Direct repair is indicated in cases where the length of nerve is adequate and reapproximation of the nerve is possible without tension along the nerve.
- It involves restoring the continuity of the both ends of the nerve directly by using sutures.
- For the successful repair of nerve, it is mandatory that functional motor unit be available to receive the innervations, i.e., facial musculature should not have undergone excessive atrophy and there should be no fibrosis at the motor end plate which prevent reinnervation.

Technique of Direct Repair

- Parotidectomy incision is given and the nerve is exposed. Identify the nerve and its branches. If the intratemporal portion of the nerve is injured, this area is exposed with the help of a mastoidectomy.

- As identification is over, the nerve is followed distally as required.
- Handle the nerve as atraumatically as possible. Surgery should be performed by using a surgical microscope. This allows precise alignment of the nerve ends.
- 2–3 sutures should be placed by using 8–0 to 10–0 fine monofilament sutures. Sutures are usually placed through the epineurium.
- Perineurial, endoneurial and interfascicular suturing should also be done.
- Most important relationship is the size match of endoneurial surfaces. This must be inspected with magnification, and if a mismatch is seen, then one end may be trimmed in a beveled fashion to obtain a better surface area.

Cable Nerve Grafting

- If sufficient length is not present to approximate the nerve primarily, cable grafting is done.
- Patient must be informed about the operation of the donor site.
- Commonly used nerves are greater auricular nerve, sural nerve, lateral femoral cutaneous nerve, etc.

Technique

- Great auricular nerve is located by drawing a line between angle of jaw and mastoid tip. Bisect this line at a right angle by great auricular nerve as it passes around the posterior border of the sternocleidomastoid muscle just behind the external jugular vein.
- Sural nerve may be located between lateral malleolus and Achilles tendon. It lies deep or posterior to the saphenous vein. Sural nerve then runs superiorly up to back of lower leg in a subcutaneous plane until it descends between the two heads of the gastrocnemius toward the popliteal fossa and its origin off the tibial nerve. Sural nerve can be harvested either by giving a single long incision from the ankle to popliteal fossa (depending on the length of nerve required) or a series of shorter transverse incisions. The nerve may be dissected under direct vision with the single incision, or by employing a fascia stripper and making the stepwise incisions. Nerve grafting should be done same as for primary repair. In cable grafting, it may be helpful to obtain enough nerve graft length to allow the graft to have some redundancy between the ends of facial nerve. This provides a C or S shape and ensures tension-free coaptation.
- Graft should lie in healthy and vascularized recipient site which is free of scar tissue.
- Epineurium should be intact and 10–0 sutures may be used to repair the nerve without tension.
- A soft silicone tube can be used which surround the anastomotic site to prevent in growth of scar tissue inside the surgical site and also to keep cut axons approximated.

Nerve Substitution Techniques

There are two types of nerve substitution techniques:

1. Hypoglossal facial anastomosis
2. Cross face grafting

Hypoglossal Facial Nerve Anastomosis

It is the most standard procedure to reanimate the face when proximal end of the facial nerve is not present or undergone degeneration and the peripheral aspect of nerve is still viable.

This procedure can be done as a primary procedure, i.e., it can be done along with the surgical procedure that lead to the sacrifice of the facial nerve or as a secondary procedure, i.e., when facial nerve paralysis is noticed postoperatively.

Technique

♦ Parotidectomy incision is given and facial nerve is exposed. Identify the nerve as it exits the stylomastoid foramen. It is sharply transected here in this region.

♦ Identify the hypoglossal nerve in the neck by following the posterior belly of the digastric muscle to the hyoid bone. Nerve is followed distally to gain length for the anastomosis.

♦ Transect descendens hypoglossi to gain length and mobilization for the anastomosis.

♦ Transect hypoglossal nerve distally and approximate it to the facial nerve passing medial or lateral to the digastrics muscle. The nerve ends are then grafted together.

Cross Face Grafting

♦ This procedure attempts to connect the branches of paralyzed facial nerve to the corresponding branches on the normal side.

♦ It is done in cases where the proximal end of the nerve is not available for repair but the mofor end plates on the paralyzed side should be functional for the success of this procedure.

♦ This procedure is not possible in cases in which the nerve has been paralyzed for over a year.

Technique

♦ Very commonly sural nerve is used to carry nerve to opposite side as it consists of adequate length to thread across from one end of the face to another. It is indicated in cases where multiple branches are to be anastomosed. Great auricular nerve may be used in cases when a single nerve is grafted.

♦ Dissect affected side first and identify all the branches. If multiple branches should be grafted they are identified and exposed a little beyond the parotid gland.

♦ Expose the normal facial nerve and the donors should be taken from distal border of the parotid gland.

♦ Now identify sural nerve and the branches should be tunneled across the face. First suture the nerve graft to the normal side and then to the chosen branch on the paralyzed side.

♦ For good healing meticulous hemostasis and the use of drains to prevent the formation of hematoma is essential.

♦ Some iatrogenic weakness is expected on the donor side after this procedure and the patient must be warned of this before going for procedure.

Postoperative Care of the Patient

♦ As return of function takes few months with each of these procedures, attention to patient care should be given, such as eye protection.

♦ Various adjunctive procedures, i.e., gold weight eyelid implants or brow lift may be considered.

♦ Re-exploration and revision should be done if improvement is not seen in one year following grafting.

Q.4. Discuss the management of head injury.

(Mar 2003, 15 Marks)

Ans. Initial assessment of head injuries must follow advanced trauma and life support (ATLS) guidelines with an initial primary survey, then resuscitation followed by secondary survey then definite management, such as airway, breathing, circulation, disability and exposure.

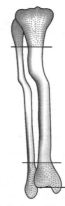

Fig. 36: Malunion of fracture of bone.

Important Histories of Head Injury

♦ Period of loss of unconsciousness
♦ Period of post-traumatic amnesia
♦ Cause and circumstances of injury
♦ Presence of headache and vomiting.

Physical Examination Includes

♦ Thorough general examination.
♦ Local examination for evidence of injury, skull fractures.
♦ Determination of conscious level by Glasgow coma scale.

Investigations

♦ *X-ray skull:* To look for fracture, relative position of calcified pineal gland, presence of intracranial air.
♦ Serum electrolyte measurement is done
♦ Blood grouping and cross matching of blood is done.
♦ *CT scan:* Plain (not contrast) to look for cerebral edema, hematoma, midline shift, fractures, ventricles, brainstem injury.
♦ Carotid arteriography
♦ Investigations for other injuries, such as ultrasound of abdomen.
♦ Monitoring of intracranial pressure.

Glasgow Coma Scale

I. Eye Opening

- Spontaneous: 4
- To speech: 3
- To pain: 2
- Nil: 1

II. Best Motor Response

- Obeys command: 6
- Localizes pain: 5
- Withdrawal to pain: 4
- Flexion to pain: 3
- Extension to pain: 2
- Nil: 1

III. Verbal Response

- Oriented: 5
- Confused: 4
- Inappropriate words: 3
- Incomprehensible: 2
- Nil: 1

Coma Score = E + M + V

Total score is 15

Mild head injury score 13–15

Moderate head injury score 9–12

Severe head injury score less than 8 (3–8)

Any patient who has a coma score of 7 or less than 7 is said to be in coma.

Pupillary response should be elicited to determine whether there is incipient transtentorial habitat, with oculomotor palsy and responses recorded.

General Management

- Management of head injuries includes ventilation, surgery, ICU management of intracranial pressure, cerebral perfusion pressure and oxygenation.
- Management of patients having head injury is based on Glasgow coma scale following the resuscitation.
- Patients with mild injury, i.e., having Glasgow comma scale of 14–15 should be admitted to the ward where thorough neurological examinations are performed.
- If patient with mild head injury subsequently deteriorate neurologically, CT scan of patient's head should be done and local neurosurgical unit should be contacted.
- Mild head injury patients should remain under observation until complete neurological recovery occur. Such patients are discharged to the responsible adult which can take good care of such patient at home for few days.
- Patients with Glasgow comma scale of 13 or less should undergo for CT scan of their head. If there is presence of acute lesion on CT scan or there is presence of diffuse cerebral edema should referred to local neurosurgical unit. CT scan should also be sent to the unit. A provisional radiography report should also be sent to referring hospital.
- If there is presence of compound depressed skull fracture, severely depressed fracture, CSF otorrhea and rhinorrhea patient should be referred to neurosurgical unit.

- Airways are protected by using mouth gag, endotracheal intubation or tracheostomy whenever required.
- Throat suction, bladder and bowel care as well as good nursing is essential.
- After evacuation of hematoma patient should be admitted to ICU and ventilated to a PCO_2 of 4 to 4.5 Kpa.
- A central line, arterial line and urinary catheter should be inserted.
- Head of bed should be positioned 40 degrees up and patient is given analgesia (fentanyl)
- IV fluids are administered should be isotonic. It is administered till nasogastric tube is inserted for feeding.
- ICP monitor should be inserted intraparenchymally to measure ICP and CPP (ideally should be <25 mm Hg and CPP should be about 70 mm Hg) If CPP is low, ionotropic agent should be used.
- Mannitol or frusemide could lower the ICP if it is not controlled by these agents then EEG burst suppression therapy with a barbiturates, ventriculator or lumber CSF drainage to be considered.
- Antibiotics, such as penicillin, ampicillin are given to prevent risk of meningitis.

Surgical Management

- Burr hole is made and hematoma is evacuated.
- *Surgery is done in case when:*
  - Consciousness is decreasing continuously.
  - Pupil becomes fixed or dilated.
  - Pulse rate becomes <60/minute.

Surgical Management

Craniotomy is done and cranial flap is raised. Clot is evacuated applying hitch stitches between dural layer and scalp.

Q.5. Write short note on danger area of face.

(Sep 2005, 5 Marks)

Ans. Dangerous area of face extends from corner of mouth to bridge of nose. It is basically the area of upper lip and lower part of nose.

- Infection from this area spreads through deep facial vein to pterygoid plexus and from pterygoid plexus to communicating vein and from communicating vein to cavernous sinus which can lead to life-threatening cavernous sinus thrombosis.
- Mainly due to the special nature of blood supply to human nose and the surrounding area there is possibility for retrograde infections from nose to spread to brain.
- One of the misconception is present that veins of head does not have one way valves as it is present in other veins of circulatory system. Reality is venous valves are not absent but there is communication between facial vein and cavernous sinus and the direction of blood flow which leads to spread of infection from face.
- Boils and pimples present in the area of upper lip and lower part of nose should never be squeezed and pricked by a needle, by doing so the infection spreads to cavernous sinus causing cavernous sinus thrombosis.

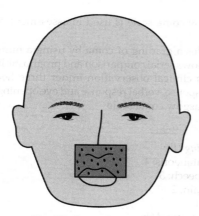

Fig. 37: Danger area of face.

Q.6. Write short note on facial palsy.
(May/June 2009, 5 Marks) (Mar 2007, 5 Marks)

Or

Write brief note on facial palsy. *(Apr 2017, 2 Marks)*

Ans. Facial palsy refers to the paralysis of facial muscles.
It is of two types:
  i. Upper motor neuron palsy
  ii. Lower motor neuron palsy or Bell's palsy

Upper Motor Neuron Palsy

♦ It affects mainly muscles of lower part of face and is never complete.
♦ It is seldom isolated palsy.
♦ The emotional movements are preserved.
♦ There is no muscle contracture.
♦ There is no reaction of degeneration.
♦ Electromyography and nerve conduction is normal.

Lower Motor Neuron Palsy or Bell's Palsy

It is also called as 7th nerve paraplegia or facial palsy.

Etiology

♦ *Cold:* It occurs after exposure to cold.
♦ *Trauma:* Extraction of teeth or injection of local anesthetic may damage the nerve and causes subsequent paralysis.
♦ *Surgical procedure:*, such as removal of parotid gland tumor in which the facial nerve is sectioned can also cause facial paralysis.
♦ *Tumors:* Tumors of the cranial base, parapharyngeal space and infratemporal fossa cause facial nerve palsy.
♦ *Familial:* Familial and hereditary occurrence is also reported in case of Bell's palsy.
  Facial canal and middle ear neoplasms may lead to Bell's palsy.

Clinical Features

♦ It is in older age group.
♦ Female predilection is most common.
♦ There is presence of paralysis over one side of the face.
♦ Drooping of angle of mouth is present over the affected side and saliva is drooling from the affected side.

♦ Patient is unable to raise the eyebrow of the affected side.
♦ Patient is unable to close the eye over affected side and tears continuously roll down.
♦ Eyeball rolls upward when attempted to close the eye, this is known as Bell's phenomenon.
♦ Over the affected side, patient has lost the taste sensation.
♦ Patient complaints of pain in or behind the ear.
♦ Presence of numbness over the affected side of face.
♦ Patient has mask-like appearance when he/she tries to smile.
♦ There is difficulty in blowing or clenching
♦ Obliteration of nasolabial fold
♦ Presence of wide palpebral fissure
♦ Presence of epiphora.

Treatment

Medicinal Treatment

♦ Patients with Bell's palsy have excellent prognosis. Treatment of Bell's palsy is controversial as spontaneous recovery is present.
♦ Treatment is given to the patients who have onset of paralysis under 1–4 days of an initial visit.
♦ Corticosteroids, i.e., prednisolone 1 mg/kg or 60 mg per day for 6 days followed by the taper of 10 days.
♦ Antiviral drugs can be given in the patients in which bell's palsy is associated with herpes infection.
♦ In Bell's palsy eye of the patient is at risk for drying which cause corneal abrasion and corneal ulcer. Eye care consists of inducing the artificial tears in day-time along with eyeglasses. At night, eye lubricant can be used.

Surgical Treatment

♦ Surgical treatment for Bell's palsy is surgical decompression and anastomosis of the nerve. In this facial and hypoglossal nerve get anastomosed which helps in restoring the partial function.
♦ Nerve grafting using greater auricular nerve, sural nerve, lateral cutaneous nerve of thigh or hypoglossal nerve.
♦ Suspension of angle of mouth to zygomatic bone using temporal fascia sling.
♦ *Lateral tarsorrhaphy:* This prevents corneal ulceration
♦ *Medial canthus reconstruction:* To decrease epiphora
♦ Cross facial nerve transplantation from opposite side using its insignificant branches
♦ Dynamic neurovascular muscle graft
♦ Upper lid gold weights to protect cornea

Q.7. Classification of peripheral nerve injuries with methods of treatment of cut injured nerve.
(Jan 2011, 8 Marks)

Ans.

Classification of Peripheral Nerve Injuries

♦ **Seddon's Classification**
  • **Neurapraxia:** It is a temporary physiological paralysis of nerve conduction. Here recovery is complete.
  • **Axonotmesis:** Division of nerve fibers or axons with intact nerve sheath. Reaction of degeneration is distally with near complete recovery.
  • **Neurotmesis:** Here complete division of nerve fibers with sheath occurs. Degeneration occurs proximally up

to the first node of Ranvier as well as distal to the injury. Recovery is incomplete even after nerve suturing. There is complete loss of motor and sensory functions with loss of reflexes. If the nerve is mixed type other than pure motor or sensory recovery is still poorer.

- **Neuromas:**
  - True neuroma or false neuroma
  - End neuroma or side neuroma.

♦ **Sunderland's classification**
  - *Conduction block:* Temporary neuronal block
  - Axonotmesis but endoneurium is preserved.
  - Axonotmesis with disruption of endoneurium, but perineurium is preserved
  - Here disruption of endo and perineurium has occurred but endoneurium is intact.
  - Neurotmesis with disruption of endoneurium, perineurium and epineurium has occurred.

Treatment of Cut Injured Nerve

Usually, microscope or loup is used for nerve suturing.

♦ *Epineurorrhaphy:* Only epineurium is sutured using interrupted sutures.

♦ *Epi-perineurorrhaphy:* Initially, perineural sheath and then epineurium is sutured.
  - If nerve is lacerated marker stitches are placed at cut end site to identify the nerve for suturing at later period.
  - If nerve suturing fails or it cannot be done, tendon transfer is done at later period after 4–6 months.

Nerve suturing can be:

♦ *Primary repair:*
  - It is done immediately after injury.
  - Nerve ends are minimally trimmed very close using a blade.
  - Fascicles of the nerve are oriented correctly.
  - Two stay sutures are placed to keep the orientation properly.
  - Usually, epineural suturing is done using 8 zero polypropylene interrupted sutures.
  - 6–8 sutures are placed for large peripheral nerve like median or ulnar nerve.
  - For or small nerve like digital nerve, only 2–3 sutures are placed.

♦ *Secondary repair:*
  - It is done at a later period.
  - It is in a pre-existing scar tissue.
  - Here first nerve ends, but proximal and distal are identified, carefully dissects; adequately.
  - Proximal neuroma and distal glioma trimmed for l cm to expose the normal fascicles of nerve ends.
  - Often guide sutures of silk may be present which were placed earlier during exploration of trauma.
  - Once nerve ends are clean, it is sutured alike primary suturing with stay sutures, with proper alignment of fascicles, followed by epineural suturing.
  - Here as epineurium is thicker, suturing is easier.

Q.8. Describe briefly Glasgow coma scale.
(Jun 2010, 5 Marks) (Dec 2010, 5 Marks)

Ans. Glasgow coma scale is used in assessment of conscious level.

- It provides a grading of coma by using a numerical scale which allows serial comparison and prognostic information.
- It relates clinical observation under three headings, i.e., motor response, verbal response and eye opening. Following is the Glasgow coma scale

Glasgow Coma Scale

♦ *Eye opening (E):*
  - Spontaneous: 4
  - To speech: 3
  - To pain: 2
  - Nil: 1

♦ *Motor response (M):*
  - Obeys command: 6
  - Localizes pain: 5
  - Withdrawal to pain: 4
  - Flexion to pain: 3
  - Extension to pain: 2
  - Nil: 1

♦ *Verbal response (V):*
  - Oriented: 5
  - Confused: 4
  - Inappropriate words: 3
  - Incomprehensible: 2
  - Nil: 1

Coma Score = E + M + V

Total score is 15

Mild head injury score 13 to 15

Moderate head injury score 9 to 12

Severe head injury less than 8 (3 to 8).

Q.9. Write short note on peripheral nerve injuries.
(Jan 2016, 5 Marks) (Dec 2010, 5 Marks)
(Mar 2016, 5 Marks)

Ans. *For classification, refer to Ans. 7 of same chapter.*

Etiology

♦ *Traumatic:* Either closed or open injury
♦ *Inflammatory:* Leprosy, diphtheria, herpes zoster
♦ Lead and arsenical poisoning
♦ Alcoholism
♦ Diabetes mellitus
♦ Vitamin B_1 deficiency
♦ Porphyria
♦ Neurofibroma and other neural tumors
♦ Idiopathic.

Clinical Features

♦ Loss of sensory, motor, autonomous and reflex functions.
♦ Secondary changes in the skin and joint.

Management

♦ **Medicinal**
  - *Steroids:* They reduce the edema around nerve and is useful in neurapraxia. Prednisolone 5–10 mg is effective.

- *Nerve tonics:* Vitamin B$_1$, B$_6$, B$_{12}$, they are supposed to facilitate nerve fiber regeneration and are useful in cases of neuropraxia and axonotmesis.
- In the cases with acute neuralgic pain, drugs, such as carbamazepine or gabapentin can be prescribed. It is purely symptomatic treatment.
- *Physiotherapy:* In the form of electrical nerve stimulation (TENS) and in cases of motor nerve exercises and massage therapy can be given.
- **Surgical**
  - *Decompression:* It is used, if nerve compression occurs resulting into neuropraxia. It is usually done when nerve due to bone deposition in the nerve canal; there is pressure on the nerve leading to neuropraxia. Here, enlargement of the canal boundaries is done to relieve the pressure on the nerve.
  - *Anastomosis:* It is microsurgical repair of the severed ends of the nerve. It is useful, when there is no loss of nerve tissue as in accidental clean surgical by transection of the nerve.
  - *Cross innervation:* It is useful when there is motor nerve deficit due to a lesion in the course of the nerve. In this repair, a nerve is grafted to connect the affected nerve to the normal functional nerve on the other side of the body using microsurgical repair.
  - *Nerve grafts:* It is use of a nerve segment from one part of the body to reconstruct and repair an affected nerve in some other part using microsurgical technique.
  - Glasgow coma scale gives clear idea about neuronal injury.
  - Autonomic disturbances with bradycardia, systolic hypertension, deep and slow respiration, Cheyne-Stokes ventilation.
  - Cushing's triad of raised intracranial pressure is obvious, i.e., bradycardia, hypertension and respiratory irregularity.
  - Features, such as restlessness, irritability, headache, vomiting and progressive deterioration are common.

Q.10. Write briefly on clinical features of head injury.

(Aug 2011, 5 Marks)

Ans.

Clinical Features of Head Injury

- Unequal pupil size is potentially a sign of a serious brain injury.
- Symptoms are dependent on the type of traumatic brain injury (diffuse or focal) and the part of the brain that is affected.
- Unconsciousness tends to last longer for people with injuries on the left side of the brain than for those with injuries on the right.
- With mild traumatic brain injury, the patient may remain conscious or may lose consciousness for a few seconds or minutes.
- Other symptoms of mild traumatic brain injury include headache, vomiting, nausea, lack of motor coordination, dizziness, difficulty in balancing, lightheadedness, blurred

vision or tired eyes, ringing in the ears, bad taste in the mouth, fatigue or lethargy, and changes in sleep patterns.
- Cognitive and emotional symptoms include behavioral or mood changes, confusion, and trouble with memory, concentration, attention, or thinking.
- A person with a moderate or severe traumatic brain injury may have a headache that does not go away, repeated vomiting or nausea, convulsions, an inability to awaken, dilation of one or both pupils, slurred speech, aphasia (word-finding difficulties), dysarthria (muscle weakness that causes disordered speech), weakness or numbness in the limbs, loss of coordination, confusion, restlessness, or agitation.
- Common long-term symptoms of moderate-to-severe traumatic brain injury are changes in appropriate social behavior, deficits in social judgment, and cognitive changes, especially problems with sustained attention, processing speed, and executive functioning.
- Alexithymia, a deficiency in identifying, understanding, processing, and describing emotions occurs in 60.9% of individuals with traumatic brain injury.
- Cognitive and social deficits have long-term consequences for the daily lives of people with moderate-to-severe traumatic brain injury, but can be improved with appropriate rehabilitation.
- When the pressure within the skull (intracranial pressure) rises too high, it can be deadly. Signs of increased intracranial pressure include decreasing level of consciousness, paralysis or weakness on one side of the body, and a blown pupil, one that fails to constrict in response to light or is slow to do so.
- Cushing's triad, a slow heart rate with high blood pressure and respiratory depression is a classic manifestation of significantly raised intracranial pressure.
- Anisocoria, unequal pupil size, is another sign of serious traumatic bone injury.
- Abnormal posturing, a characteristic positioning of the limbs caused by severe diffuse injury or high intracranial pressure, is an ominous sign.

Q.11. Describe features to extradural hematoma.

(Jan 2012, 5 Marks)

Ans.

Features to Extradural Hematoma

- Patient soon regain consciousness and again after 6–12 hour start deteriorating (Lucid interval).
- Later the patient presents with confusion, irritability, drowsiness, hemiparesis on same side of the injury. Initially pupillary constriction and later pupillary dilatation occurs on the same side, finally becomes totally unconscious—Hutchinson pupils.
- Death can occur, if immediate surgical intervention is not done.
- Features of raised intracranial pressure, such as high blood pressure, bradycardia, vomiting is also seen. Occasionally, convulsions may be present.
- Wound and hematoma in the temporal region of scalp may be seen.

♦ Glasgow coma scale gives clear idea about neuronal injury.

♦ Autonomic disturbances with bradycardia, systolic hypertension, deep and slow respiration, Cheyne–Stokes ventilation.

♦ Cushing's triad of raised intracranial pressure is obvious, i.e., bradycardia, hypertension and respiratory irregularity.

♦ Features, such as restlessness, irritability, headache, vomiting and progressive deterioration are common.

Q.12. **Describe the types, pathology, clinical features and management of peripheral nerve injuries.**

(June 2014, 10 Marks)

Ans. *For types, refer to classification part of Ans. 7 of same chapter.*

For clinical features and management, refer to Ans. 9 of same chapter.

Pathology

Guillain–Barré Syndrome

♦ Guillain–Barré syndrome is one of the most common life-threatening diseases of the peripheral nervous system.

♦ It is a rapidly progressive acute demyelinating disorder affecting motor axons that results in ascending weakness that may lead to death from failure of respiratory muscles over a period of only several days.

♦ It appears to be triggered by an infection or a vaccine that breaks down self-tolerance, thereby leading to an autoimmune response.

♦ Associated infectious agents include *Campylobacter jejuni*, Epstein–Barr virus, cytomegalovirus, and human immunodeficiency virus.

♦ The injury is most extensive in the nerve roots and proximal nerve segments and is associated with mononuclear cell infiltrates rich in macrophages.

♦ Both humoral and cellular immune responses are believed to play a role in the disease process.

Chronic Inflammatory Demyelinating Polyneuropathy

♦ Chronic inflammatory demyelinating polyneuropathy (CIDP) typically manifests as a symmetric demyelinating disease.

♦ Both motor and sensory abnormalities are common, such as difficulty in walking, weakness, numbness, and pain or tingling sensations.

♦ CIDP is immune-mediated and occurs at increased frequency in patients with other immune disorders, such as systemic lupus erythematosus and HIV infection.

♦ CIDP follows a chronic, relapsing-remitting or progressive course.

♦ The peripheral nerves show segments of demyelination and remyelination.

♦ In long-standing cases, chronically regenerating Schwann cells may concentrically wrap around axons in multiple layers in an onion-skin pattern.

Toxic and Vasculitic Forms of Peripheral Neuropathy

♦ Drugs and environmental toxins that interfere with axonal transport or cytoskeletal function often produce peripheral neuropathies. The longest axons are most susceptible, so the resulting clinical presentation is often most pronounced in the distal extremities.

♦ Peripheral nerves are often damaged in many different forms of systemic vasculitis including polyarteritis nodosa, Churg–Strauss syndrome, and Wegener granulomatosis. Overall, peripheral nerve damage is seen in about a third of all patients with vasculitis at the time of presentation. The most common clinical picture is that of mononeuritis multiplex with a painful asymmetric mixed sensory and motor peripheral neuropathy. Patchy involvement also is apparent at the microscopic level, as single nerves may show considerable interfascicular variation in the degree of axonal damage.

Leprosy

♦ There is peripheral nerve involvement in both lepromatous and tuberculoid leprosy.

♦ In lepromatous leprosy, Schwann cells are often invaded by *Mycobacterium leprae*, which proliferate and eventually infect other cells. There is evidence of segmental demyelination and remyelination and loss of both myelinated and unmyelinated axons. As the infection advances, endoneurial fibrosis and multilayered thickening of the perineurial sheaths occur. Clinically, these patients develop a symmetric polyneuropathy that prominently involves pain fibers; the loss of sensation that results contributes to the tissue injury of the disease.

♦ Tuberculoid leprosy shows evidence of active cell-mediated immune response to *M. leprae*, with nodular granulomatous inflammation situated in the dermis.

♦ The inflammation injures cutaneous nerves in the vicinity; axons, Schwann cells, and myelin are lost, and there is fibrosis of the perineurium and endoneurium. With this form of leprosy, patients have much more localized nerve involvement but do develop areas of abnormal sensation from the injury.

Diphtheria

♦ Peripheral nerve involvement results from the effects of the diphtheria exotoxin and begins with paresthesias and weakness; early loss of proprioception and vibratory sensation is common.

♦ The earliest changes are seen in the sensory ganglia, where the incomplete blood-nerve barrier allows entry of the toxin.

♦ There is selective demyelination of axons that extends into adjacent anterior and posterior roots as well as into the mixed sensorimotor nerve.

Varicella–Zoster Virus

♦ This virus is one of the few that produce lesions in the peripheral nervous system.

♦ Latent infection of neurons in the sensory ganglia of the spinal cord and brain stem follows chickenpox, and reactivation leads to a painful, vesicular skin eruption in the distribution of sensory dermatomes (shingles), most frequently thoracic or trigeminal.

♦ The virus may be transported along the sensory nerves to the skin, where it establishes an active infection of epidermal cells. In a small proportion of patients, weakness is also apparent in the same distribution. Although the factors giving rise to reactivation are not fully understood, decreased cell-mediated immunity is of major importance in many cases.

♦ Affected ganglia show neuronal destruction and loss, usually accompanied by abundant mononuclear inflammatory infiltrates. Regional necrosis with hemorrhage may also be found.

♦ Peripheral nerve shows axonal degeneration after the death of the sensory neurons. Focal destruction of the large motor neurons of the anterior horns or cranial nerve motor nuclei may be seen at the corresponding levels. Intranuclear inclusions generally are not found in the peripheral nervous system.

Q.13. Write on type of nerve injuries with methods of repair of cut nerves. *(Apr 2015, 7 Marks)*

Ans. *For types of nerve injuries refer to Ans. 7 of same chapter and for methods of repair of cut nerves, refer to Ans. 9 of same chapter.*

Q.14. Enumerate the cranial nerves. *(Jan 2017, 5 Marks)*

Ans. Following are the cranial nerves:

♦ Cranial nerve I: Olfactory (smell)
♦ Cranial nerve II: Optic (sight)
♦ Cranial nerve III: Oculomotor (moves eyelid and eyeball and adjusts the pupil and lens of the eye)
♦ Cranial nerve IV: Trochlear (moves eyeballs)
♦ Cranial nerve V: Trigeminal (facial muscles including chewing; facial sensations)
♦ Cranial nerve VI: Abducens (moves eyeballs)
♦ Cranial nerve VII: Facial (taste, tears, saliva, facial expressions)
♦ Cranial nerve VIII: Vestibulocochlear (auditory)
♦ Cranial nerve IX: Glossopharyngeal (swallowing, saliva, taste)
♦ Cranial nerve X: Vagus (control of PNS, e.g., smooth muscles of GI tract)
♦ Cranial nerve XI: Accessory (moving head and shoulders, swallowing)
♦ Cranial nerve XII: Hypoglossal (tongue muscles—speech and swallowing)

Q.15. Describe differentiating features of Bell's palsy and trigeminal neuralgia. *(Jan 2017, 3 Marks)*

Ans.

Bell's palsy	Trigeminal neuralgia
It is also known as idiopathic facial paralysis	It is also known as Tic douloureux, trifacial neuralgia or Fothergill's disease
It affects facial nerve	It affects trigeminal nerve
It is caused due to cold, trauma, during surgical procedures, ischemia, familial, tumors and due to facial canal and middle ear neoplasms	It is caused due to various factors, such as dental pathosis, excessive traction, allergies, mechanical factors, anomalies of superior cerebellar artery and due to secondary lesions
It begins abruptly as paralysis of facial musculature, unilaterally.	It occurs more commonly over the right side and lower portion of face is more commonly affected.

Contd...

Contd...

Bell's palsy	Trigeminal neuralgia
Pain is present over side of face which is involved. Intensity of pain is low.	Pain is present which is paroxysmal and last for few seconds to few minutes and is of extreme intensity.
Pain is particularly present within the ear, temple, mastoid area and angle of jaw.	Pain is confined to trigeminal zone.
Trigger zones are absent.	Trigger zones are present which precipitate an attack when touched. Trigger zones are at vermilion border of lip, ala of nose, cheeks, around eyes
Eye of the affected side cannot be closed and wrinkles are absent on that side. Watering of eye is present as patient is unable to close his/her eye.	Eye of the affected side can be closed easily and wrinkles are present on that side
Due to muscular paralysis, there is dropping of corner of mouth, from which saliva may dribble.	No drooling of saliva present.
Patient save his face easily, brush easily.	Patient avoid shaping, avoid brushing of teeth and undergo indiscriminate dental extraction

Q.16. Enumerate branches of facial nerve.
(June 2018, 3 Marks)

Ans.

Branches of Facial Nerve

♦ Within the facial canal
  • Greater petrosal nerve
  • Nerve to stapedius
  • Chorda tympani nerve
♦ At exit from stylomastoid foramen
  • Posterior auricular
  • Digastric
  • Stylohyoid
♦ Terminal branches within the parotid gland
  • Temporal
  • Zygomatic
  • Buccal
  • Marginal mandibular
  • Cervical
♦ Communicating branches with adjacent cranial and spinal nerves

26. FRACTURES OF BONE

Q.1. Describe different types of mandibular fractures, their clinical presentation and treatment.
(Jan 2012, 10 Marks)

Or

Describe various types of mandibular fractures, their clinical presentation and treatment.
(Mar 2016, 7 Marks)

Or

Classify fractured mandible and discuss clinical features and management of fracture mandible.
(July 2016, 10 Marks)

Or

Write short answer on types of fractures mandible with diagram. *(June 2018, 3 Marks)*

Or

Write short answer on fracture mandible.
(Apr 2019, 3 Marks)

Ans.

Types of Mandibular Fracture

Dingman and Natvig Anatomic Classification

♦ *Midline:* Fractures between central incisors.
♦ *Symphysis:* Fractures occurring within the area of symphysis.
♦ *Parasymphysis:* Bounded by vertical lines distal to canine teeth.
♦ *Body:* From distal symphysis to a line coinciding with the alveolar border of the masseter muscle usually including third molar.
♦ *Angle:* Triangular region bounded by the anterior border of masseter muscle to posterosuperior attachment of the masseter muscle.
♦ *Ramus:* Bounded by superior aspect of the angle to two lines forming an apex at the sigmoid notch.
♦ *Condylar process:* Area of condylar process superior to the ramus region.
♦ *Coronoid process:* Includes coronoid process of the mandible superior to ramus region.
♦ *Dentoalveolar process:* Region that would normally contain the teeth

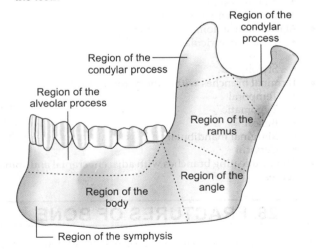

Fig. 38: Different types of mandibular fractures.

Clinical Presentation/Clinical Features

Fracture at Angle

♦ Swelling at the angle externally and there may be obvious deformity.

♦ Laceration of skin or mucosa.
♦ Step deformity behind the last molar tooth may be visible which is more apparent, if no teeth are present in the molar region.
♦ Undisplaced fractures are usually revealed by the presence of a small hematoma adjacent to the angle on either the lingual or buccal side, or both.
♦ Anesthesia or paresthesia of the lower lip may present on the side of the fracture.
♦ Inability to close the jaw causing premature dental contact.
♦ Occlusion is often deranged. Movements of the mandible are painful and range of movements are reduced.
♦ Trismus to some degree is usually present.
♦ Anterior open bite is seen in bilateral angle fracture.
♦ Ipsilateral open bite is seen in unilateral angle fracture.

Fracture of Body

♦ Physical signs and symptoms, such as swelling and bone tenderness similar to that as seen in fracture of angle of mandible.
♦ Even slight displacement of the fracture causes derangement of the occlusion.
♦ Premature contact occurs on the distal fragment because of the displacing action of muscles attached to the ramus.
♦ Fractures between adjacent teeth tend to cause gingival tears.
♦ When there is gross displacement, inferior dental artery may be torn and this can give rise to severe intraoral hemorrhage.
♦ Sublingual hematoma or ecchymosis in floor of mouth.
♦ Flattened appearance of lateral aspect of face.
♦ Inability to open or close the jaw.
♦ Crepitation on palpation.

Fracture of Symphysis and Parasymphysis

♦ These fractures are commonly associated with fractures of one or both the condyles.
♦ This fracture may be missed, if occlusion is undisturbed locally.
♦ Presence of bone tenderness and a small lingual hematoma may be the only physical signs.
♦ Sublingual hematoma or ecchymosis in floor of mouth.
♦ Posterior open bite or unilateral open bite is seen in parasymphysis fracture. Posterior crossbite can result from midline symphysis fractures.
♦ Crepitation on palpation is noted in symphyseal fracture.
♦ An inability to close the jaw causing premature dental contact.
♦ A retruded chin can be caused by bilateral parasymphyseal fracture.
♦ Fracture line is often oblique which allows over-riding of the fragments with lingual inversion of the occlusion on each side.

Fracture of Ramus

♦ They are uncommon.
♦ Flattened appearance of the lateral aspect of face.
♦ Inability to open or close the jaw.
♦ Swelling and ecchymosis usually noted both extraorally and intraorally.

Tenderness over the ramus and movements produce pain over the same area.

Severe trismus is present.

Fracture of Coronoid Process

The fracture can be caused by direct trauma to the ramus but is rarely in isolation. It is usually considered to result from reflex contracture of the powerful anterior fibers of the temporalis muscle.

This fracture is difficult to diagnose clinically.

Tenderness over anterior part of the ramus.

Painful limitation of movement, especially during protrusion of the mandible may be found.

Treatment

Refer to Ans. 3 of same chapter.

It depends upon the line of fracture.

Oblique fracture shows bad prognosis.

Spiral fracture shows good prognosis due to increased surface area.

Q.2. Write short note on fracture mandible.
(Feb 2015, 5 Marks) (Sep 2005, 8 Marks)
Or
Write short note on fracture of mandible.
(Mar 2006, 5 Marks)
Or
Write briefly on fracture of mandible.
(Aug 2011, 5 Marks)
Or
Write short note on types of mandibular fractures with diagrams *(June 2010, 5 Marks)*
Ans. *Refer to Ans. 1 of same chapter.*

Q.3. Discuss in brief management of a case of fracture of mandible. *(Sep 2009, 5 Marks)*
Or
Discuss management of fracture of mandible.
(Jan 2011, 10 Marks) (Feb/Mar 2004, 10 Marks)
Or
Write brief answer on management of fractured mandible. *(Apr 2017, 7, 5 Marks)*
Ans.

Management of Mandibular Fracture

Reduction
  • Open reduction
  • Closed reduction.

Fixation.

Immobilization.

Prevention of infection and rehabilitation.

Reduction of Mandibular Fracture

Reduction of fracture is the process to bring the fractured fragments into alignment.

Reduction is of two types, i.e., closed and open reduction.

Closed Reduction

In closed reduction method, the fractured fragments are brought into an alignment without actually exposing the fractured bone ends, occlusion is the key to reduction.

Reduction by manipulation

It is done in fresh cases of fracture where displacement of the fractured fragments is due to muscle spasm:

Carried out under local anesthesia.

After anesthesia is given, the dislocated fragments of the mandible are held between the finger and thumbs on each side of the fractured line.

The fragments are shaken up and down to disengage them or to break the fibrous union.

When normal occlusion is achieved the fragments are fixed in position.

Various methods used for close reduction of mandibular fracture are:
  • Arch bar fixation
  • Bridle wire
  • Figure of 8 wiring
  • Gilmer's direct wiring
  • Eyelet wiring
  • Essig's wiring
  • Stout's continuous loop wiring
  • Risdon's wiring.

Reduction by traction

Traction is a procedure by which the fractured dislocated fragments are subjected to a continuous gradual pull by elastic bands.

Open Reduction

It is a procedure by which we expose the fractured bone ends and bring them into alignment under direct vision.

The fractured bone can exposed by intraoral or extraoral approach.

The extraoral approach is preferred to avoid contamination.

As depending on the areas to accessed various surgical approaches are used in open reduction.

Symphysis, parasymphysis and body of the mandible can be approached via intraoral incisions given in labial mucosa. Extraoral incision can be used to approach these regions. Symphysis can be approached via an incision placed in submental region in skin crease. Body of mandible can be approached by submandibular approach.

Angle of mandible should be approached via intraoral incision placed on third molar region which extends to anterior border of ramus. Extraorally the angle of mandible can be approached via Risdon's incision.

Ramus of mandible can be approached via retromandibular incision.

Coronoid process can be approached via intraoral incision placed high on anterior border of ramus of mandible.

Condyle of the mandible can be approached via various incisions, i.e., preauricular, retromandibular and submandibular, etc.

♦ Aligned bone is held in position with the help of wire, screws or bone plates as per requirement.

Fixation of Mandibular Fracture

♦ In this phase, the fractured fragments are fixed, in their normal anatomical relationship to prevent displacement and achieve proper approximate fixation.

♦ If a closed reduction is done, the fractured fragments are fixed and immobilized in anatomically reduced position by means of wire which are placed around teeth, i.e., interdental wiring. Various wiring techniques are used and each of them are used in various types of mandibular fractures. Wiring techniques used are Bridle wire, Figure-of-8 wiring, Gilmer's direct wiring, eyelet wiring, Essig's wiring, stout's continuous loop wiring and Risdon's wiring.

♦ If an open reduction is done the fixation can be:
  • *Non-rigid fixation:* By use of transosseous wires or wire osteosynthesis
  • *Semi-rigid fixation:* By use of monocortical miniplates or lag screws
  • *Rigid fixation:* By use of dynamic compression plates

Immobilization

♦ In this phase, the reduced and fixed fragments of bone are immobilized for certain period for healing to occur.

♦ A fixation device is given to stabilize the reduced fragments into their normal anatomical position till clinical bony union takes place.

♦ For mandibular fracture, period of immobilization should be 4–6 weeks.

♦ If mandibular condyle is fractured, then period of immobilization is for 2–3 weeks.

Prevention of Infection and Rehabilitation

♦ Proper antibiotic regimen should be given to the patient to prevent intraoperative and postoperative complications.

♦ If there is presence of gap between the bony ends, proper bone graft should be given.

♦ After 4–6 weeks as fracture is healed, jaw regain some of its strength, patient should be encouraged to be on a normal diet and use the jaw as before he/she use it prior to the trauma.

Q.4. Describe briefly cause of malunion of fracture of bone. *(Mar 1998, 5 Marks)*

Ans. The malunion means union of fragments in a defective position.

The most common deformity is angulations, beside this there may be overlapping with shortening and malrotation.

The causes of malunion are:

♦ Fracture was not reduced properly.

♦ After reduction replacement occurs within the plaster for this a check X-ray after a week is advisable in certain fractures anticipating redisplacement, e.g., fracture of both bones of the forearm.

♦ Growth disturbance due to injury to the epiphyseal cartilage may lead to malunion; fracture separation of an epiphysis does not lead to growth disturbance as the fracture occurs through the metaphyseal plate keeping the epiphyseal cartilage intact.

Site of malunion are those where the bone is cancellous so union occurs as a rule, but malunion complicates due to imperfect position of the bone ends. These sites are fracture neck and the supracondylar fracture of humerus, collar fracture, fracture through the condyles of the tibia, etc.

Q.5. Describe briefly general treatment of fracture of bone. *(Dec 2010, 7 Marks)*

Ans. **General management of fracture of bone:**

♦ Early treatment (neurovascular problems)

♦ The principle of management of fracture is to deal with life-saving problems first

♦ This means paying attention to ABC (airway, breathing and circulation) and to the neurovascular status

For reduction, immobilization and rehabilitation, refer to Ans. 8 of same chapter.

Q.6. Describe briefly causes of delayed union of fracture of bone. *(Sep 2002, 5 Marks)*

Ans. When the procedure of healing a fracture is slower than the normal speed, then it is called delayed union.

Causes

♦ *Severe initial injury:* This is most probably due to associated soft tissue damage which allows diffusion of hematoma and also due to the blood supply to the bone fragments.

♦ *Infection of fracture hematoma:* Healing fails because of the cellular element which is required for the production of bone at the production of pus.

♦ Soft tissue interposition between the fracture fragments may so separate them that it is physically impossible for them to unite.

♦ A poor blood supply at the fracture site.

♦ *Inadequate immobilization:* Excessive movement at the fracture site during the healing phase may produce delayed union because the fracture site is constantly 'refractured' by the movement.

♦ Compound fracture (when more than two segments) or open fracture.

Q.7. Describe different types of fracture of mandible and their management. *(Mar 2007, 10 Marks)*

Ans. *For different types of fracture of mandible refer to Ans. 1 and for management, refer to Ans. 3 of same chapter.*

Q.8. Discuss the classification, general principles of treatment and healing of fracture.
(Feb/Mar 2004, 15 Marks)

Or

Define and classify fractures. Discuss general principles of management of fractures.
(Sep 2008, 8 Marks)

Or

Describe fracture and give principles of fracture management and healing. *(May/Jun 2009, 15 Marks)*

Or

Describe fracture. Give principles of fracture management and healing. *(June 2018, 5 Marks)*

Ans. Fracture is defined as break in the continuity of lamellar pattern of bone.

Classification of Fracture of Bone

♦ *Closed or simple fracture:* When the outer skin is not injured due to fracture. Fracture side dose not communicate to the outer surface.

♦ *Open or compound fracture:* In this type, outer tissue also broken down and fracture site communicate with outer surface.

♦ *Comminuted fracture:* When the bone is broken down into more than two segments. It show bad prognosis.

♦ *Impacted fracture:* When one fragment enters into another segment.

♦ *Green stick fracture:* Only the bone is bent-like a green stick. Fracture is incomplete and occurs in children.

♦ Transverse, oblique and spiral fracture.

  • It depends upon the line of fracture.
  • Oblique fracture shows bad prognosis.
  • Spiral fracture shows good prognosis due to increased surface area.

General Principles of Treatment of Fracture

The three fundamental principles of fracture treatment—reduction, immobilization and preservation of function, i.e., rehabilitation.

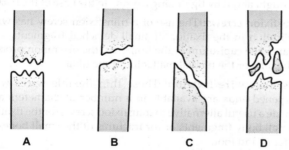

Figs. 39A to D: Types of fracture; (A) Transverse fracture; (B) Oblique fracture; (C) Spiral fracture; (D) Comminuted fracture.

Reduction

This first principle must be qualified by the words 'if necessary'. In many fractures reduction is unnecessary, either because there is no displacement or because the displacement is immaterial to the final result.

If it is judged that perfect function can be restored without undue loss of time, despite some uncorrected displacement of the fragments, there is clearly no object in striving for perfect anatomical reduction. Indeed, meddlesome intervention may sometimes be detrimental, especially if it entails open operation.

Methods of Reduction

When reduction is decided upon it may be carried out in three ways:

1. By closed manipulation
2. By mechanical traction with or without manipulation
3. By open operation.

Manipulative reduction

Closed manipulation is the standard initial method of reducing most common fractures. It is usually carried out under general anesthesia, but local or regional anesthesia is sometimes appropriate. The technique is simply to grasp the fragments through the soft tissues, to disimpact them if necessary, and then to adjust them as nearly as possible to their correct position.

Reduction by mechanical traction

When the contraction of large muscles exerts a strong displacing force, some mechanical aid may be necessary to draw the fragments out to the normal length of the bone. This particularly applies to fractures of the shaft of the femur, and to certain types of fracture or displacement of the cervical spine. Traction may be applied either by weights or by a screw device, and the aim may be to gain full reduction rapidly at one sitting with anesthesia, or to rely upon gradual reduction by prolonged traction without anesthesia.

Operative reduction

When an acceptable reduction cannot be obtained, or maintained, by these conservative methods, the fragments are reduced under direct vision at open operation. Open reduction may also be required for some fractures involving articular surfaces, or when the fracture is complicated by damage to a nerve or artery. When operative reduction is resorted to, the opportunity should always be taken to fix the fragments internally to ensure that the position is maintained.

Immobilization

Like reduction, this second great principle of fracture treatment must be qualified by the words 'if necessary'. Whereas some fractures must be splinted rigidly, many do not require immobilization to ensure union, and excessive immobilization is actually harmful in some.

Indications for Immobilization

There are only three reasons for immobilizing a fracture:
1. To prevent displacement or angulation of the fragments
2. To prevent movement that might interfere with union
3. To relieve pain.

If in a given fracture, none of these indications applies, then there is no need for immobilization.

Methods of Immobilization

When immobilization is seemed necessary, there are four methods by which it may be effected:

♦ By a plaster of Paris cast or other external splint
♦ By continuous traction
♦ By external fixation
♦ By internal fixation.

Immobilization by plaster, splint or brace.

For most fractures, the standard method of immobilization is by a plaster of Paris cast.

Plaster technique

The plaster bandages are applied in two forms: round-and-round bandages and longitudinal strips or 'slabs' to reinforce a particular area. Round-and-round bandages must be applied smoothly without tension, the material being drawn out to its full width at each turn. Slabs are prepared by unrolling a bandage to and fro upon a table: an average slab consists of about 12 thickness.

The slabs are placed at points of weakness or stress and are held in place by further turns of plaster bandage. A plaster is best dried simply by exposure to the air: artificial heating is unnecessary.

Other external splints: Apart from plaster of Paris, splints that are in general use are mostly those for the thigh and leg and for the fingers. Individual splints may also be made from malleable strips of aluminum, from wire, or from heat-moldable plastic materials, such as polyethylene foam. Rarely, a halo-thoracic splint is used for an unstable fracture of the cervical spine. This consists of a metal 'halo' or ring that is screwed to the skull and joined by bars to a plaster or plastic splint enclosing the chest.

Cast bracing (functional bracing): A brace has come to be understood as a supportive device that allows continued function of the part. Cast bracing, or functional fracture bracing (to use a better term), is a technique in which a fractured long bone is supported externally by plaster of Paris or by a mouldable plastic material in such a way that function of the adjacent joints is preserved and use of the limb for its normal purposes can be resumed. Functional bracing is used mainly for fractures of the shaft of femur or tibia.

Immobilization by Sustained Traction

In some fractures—notably, those of the shaft of the femur and certain fractures of the shaft of the tibia or of the distal shaft of the humerus—it may be difficult or impossible to hold the fragments in proper position by a plaster or external splint alone. This is particularly so when the plane of the fracture is oblique or spiral, because the elastic pull of the muscles, then tends to draw the distal fragment proximally so that it overlaps the proximal fragment. In such a case, the pull of the muscles must be balanced by sustained traction upon the distal fragment, either by a weight or by some other mechanical device.

Immobilization by External Fixation

Strictly, immobilization in plaster or in a splint might be regarded as external fixation. By convention, however, the term external fixation is used to imply anchorage of the bone fragments to an external device, such as a metal bar through the medium of pins inserted into the proximal and distal fragments of a long bone fracture. In its simplest form, external fixation may be provided by transfixing each fragment with a Steinmann pin and incorporating the protruding ends of the pins in a plaster of Paris splint. This simple method is now seldom used, and fixation is now by means of rigid bars or a frame.

Methods of internal fixation: The following methods are currently in general use:

♦ Metal plate held by screws or locking plate (with screws fixed to the plate by threaded holes)
♦ Intramedullary nail, with or without cross-screw fixation for locking
♦ Dynamic compression screw-plate
♦ Condylar screw-plate
♦ Tension band wiring
♦ Transfixion screws.

The choice of method depends upon the site and pattern of the fracture.

Plate and screws: This method is applicable to long bones. Usually, a single six-hole plate suffices, but an eight-hole plate may be preferred for larger bones.

Locking plate: A newer concept is the 'locking plate', that uses screws with heads that are threaded and when tightened lock into matching threads in the holes of the plate. This produces a more rigid fixation in terms of length and angle, which is particularly valuable in comminuted fractures in osteoporotic bone. It can also be inserted with less stripping of soft tissue that preserves bone vascularity, particularly in the metaphyseal region.

Intramedullary nail: This technique is excellent for many fractures of the long bones, especially when the fracture is near the middle of the shaft. It is used regularly for fractures of the femur and tibia, and less commonly in the humerus.

Compression screw-plate: The compression screw-plate (dynamic hip screw) is a standard method of fixation for fractures of the neck of the femur and for trochanteric fractures. The screw component, which grips the femoral head, slides telescopically in the barrel to allow the bone fragments to be compressed together across the fracture. This compression effect is brought about by tightening a screw in the base of the barrel.

Transfixion screws: The use of a transfixion screw has wide application in the fixation of small detached fragments—for instance the capitulum of the humerus, the olecranon process of the ulna or the medial malleolus of the tibia.

Kirschner wire fixation: These thin flexible wires with sharpened ends are available in a number of diameters and provide a useful alternative to transfixion screws for the fixation of small bony fragments or for fractures of the small bones in the hand and foot.

Tension band wiring: This technique of fixation is most commonly used in the patella and olecranon, but can be applied to other small metaphyseal fragments, such as the medial malleolus. It uses the mechanical principle of converting the tensile stresses of the muscles acting on the bone fragment, into a compressive force at the fracture site.

Rehabilitation

Improved results in the treatment of fractures owe much to rehabilitation, perhaps the most important of the three great principles of fracture treatment. Reduction is often unnecessary; immobilization is often unnecessary; rehabilitation is always essential. Rehabilitation should begin as soon as the fracture comes under definitive treatment. Its purpose is twofold: first, to preserve function so far as possible while the fracture is uniting and second, to restore function to normal when the fracture is united. This purpose is achieved not so much by any passive treatment as by encouraging patients to help themselves. The two essential methods of rehabilitation are active use and active exercises.

Active Use

This implies that the patient must continue to use the injured part as naturally as possible within the limitations imposed by necessary treatment. The degree of function that can be retained depends upon the nature of the fracture, the risk of redisplacement of the fragments, and the extent of any necessary splintage. Although in some injuries rest may be necessary in the early days or weeks, there should be a graduated return to activity as soon as it can be allowed without risk.

Active Exercises

These comprise exercises for the muscles and joints. They should be encouraged from an early stage. While a limb is immobilized in a plaster or splint, exercises must be directed mainly to the preservation of muscle function by static contractions. The ability to contract a muscle without moving a joint is soon acquired under proper supervision. When restrictive splints are no longer required, exercises should be directed to mobilizing the joints and building up the power of the muscles. Finally, when the fracture is soundly united, treatment may be intensified, movements being carried out against gradually increased resistance until normal power is regained.

Healing of Fracture

Healing of fracture takes place in three steps:
1. **Hematoma and granulation tissue formation**
    - After fracture a hematoma is formed due to rupture of blood vessels
    - Inflammatory changes start at the site of fracture
    - Hematoma is gradually resorbed
    - The necrotic debris is removed by neutrophils and macrophages
    - Collagen fibers are laid down at the site of union of fracture
    - Capillaries and collagen fiber form granulation tissue which covers the fracture site, it takes about 15 days
    - Bone ends are now united at fracture site, by weak fibrous band.
2. **Callous formation**
    - Calcification of newly formed fibrous tissue takes place after 3 weeks
    - Matrix becomes ossified and is called 'Callous'
    - Callous is distributed along the fractured site
    - Callous provides a firm and rigid bridge at the fracture segments.
3. **Mature bone formation**
    - Callus is now replaced by a lamellar bone. The bone undergoes remodeling and comes in normal morphology
    - Haversian system develops in bone
    - Bony union takes place in about 2–3 months.

Q.9. How will you manage a case of ankylosis of TMJ?

(Sep 2000, 15 Marks)

Ans. Ankylosis is a Greek term means "stiff joint".
- TMJ ankylosis: There is immobility of joint, the jaw function get affected. Hypomobility to immobility of the joint can lead to inability to open the mouth from partial to complete
- Two main factors predisposing to the ankylosis are trauma and infection, in or around the joint region.

Management of TMJ Ankylosis

The treatment of TMJ ankylosis is always surgical.

The internationally accepted protocol for the management of TMJ ankylosis
- Early surface intervention
- *Aggressive resection:* A gap of at least 1–1.5 cm should be created.
- Ipsilateral coronoidectomy and temporalis myotomy.
- Contralateral coronoidectomy and temporalis myotomy.
- Lining of the glenoid fossa region with temporalis fascia.
- Reconstruction of the ramus with costochondral graft.
- Early mobilization and aggression physiotherapy for at least 6 month postoperatively.
- Regular long-term follow-up.
- To carry out cosmetic surgery at the later date when the growth of the patient is complete.

Principles of Management
- Removal of the ankylosed mass of bone to mobile the jaw.
- Reconstruction of joint and maintenance of vertical height of ramus.
- Prevention of recurrence.
- Restoration of occlusion and maintain function.
- Correction of secondary facial deformity.

Step-by-Step Treatment of Ankylosis
- *Use of brisement force:* Forced opening of the jaw by mouth gag under general anesthesia. It is used in case of fibrous ankylosis.
- *Surgical lysis:* Opening of joint by preauricular approach and destroy union of condyle and glenoid fossa.

Condylectomy
- This procedure is done in cases of fibrous or partial ankylosis where the anatomical features of joint are not completely changed.
- Condylectomy procedure should be started by giving the preauricular incision.
- Now a horizontal osteotomy cut is given by the help of bur at the level of condylar neck.
- Section the head of the condyle till the level of neck and separate it from superior attachment.
- Stump of the condyle at neck is smoothened and wound is closed in layers.
- As unilateral condyle leads to deviation of mandible at operated side on mouth opening and in cases of bilateral ankylosis open bite is present due to loss of vertical rami. So when condylectomy is done, after recontouring an alloplastic material is used for maintain space, provide proper occlusion as well as joint movements.

Gap Arthroplasty

♦ Gap arthroplasty is the procedure which involves the creation of an anatomical gap in an ankylosed segment to form artificial joint space.

♦ In patients with complete bony ankylosis anatomical features of joint are very difficult to appreciate as they get covered by the bone. So in complete bony ankylosis cases a gap in the bone is made for separating ramus of mandible from ankylosed mass in glenoid fossa.

♦ Now two horizontal bony cuts are given in superior aspect of ramus and the wedge of bone between the two cuts is removed. Take care while removing the bone from medial aspect as it is close to maxillary artery and carotid canal. Remove the bone by using large round bur till medial bone gets thinned out completely to remove by osteotome.

♦ There is recommendation of leaving gap of about 1–1.5 cm laterally and medially for preventing the reankylosis.

Interpositional Arthroplasty

♦ In cases of gap arthroplasty chances of reankylosis are present, if bony cuts come in contact.

♦ So to avoid this an interpositional material is inserted in between the two cut ends which avoid contact between them and decreases the chances of reankylosis.

♦ Various materials are used which can be autogenous or alloplastic.

♦ Autogenous materials used for interpositioning are cartilaginous graft, temporal muscle, temporal fascia, fascia, dermis while alloplastic materials used are metallic and nonmetallic. In metallic ones, there are tantalum plate, stainless steel, titanium, gold and in nonmetallic ones there are Teflon, acrylic, ceramic and elastic.

Q.10. Write on management of maxillofacial injuries.
(Dec 2009, 15 Marks)

Ans. Management of maxillofacial injuries

Prehospital Care

♦ *General airway:* Administer oxygen and maintain a patent airway. Maintain an immobilized cervical spine at all times. Clear the mouth of any foreign body or debris, and suction any blood present.

♦ *Intubation:* Intubate, if indicated. Have the cricothyroidotomy and tracheotomy tray set up prior to an initial attempt at intubation. Consider conscious sedation intubation, if distortions of the mandible and maxilla exist because a tight seal with the mask may not be possible when bagging. Consider nasotracheal intubation, if massive oropharyngeal edema is present. Consider orotracheal intubation, if midface or upper face trauma is present. If unable to intubate the patient nasotracheally or endotracheally, cricothyroidotomy is the next procedure of choice

♦ *Breathing:* Assess breath sounds. Check tube placement.

♦ *Circulation:* Do not remove impaled foreign bodies that can result in worsening of damage and bleeding. Control hemorrhage with direct pressure. Obtain large-bore intravenous access bilaterally.

♦ *Disability:* Assess the patient using the Glasgow coma scale. Perform a brief neurologic examination. Note any change in mental status.

♦ *Exposure:* Expose patients, but keep them warm. Remove all clothing and accessories. Recover all avulsed hard and soft tissue, and transport them in damp gauze with no ice and very little manual manipulation.

Medical and Surgical Therapy

♦ *General medical therapy:* Administer oxygen and, isotonic crystalloid fluids. Administer packed red blood cells if the patient is bleeding excessively. Tetanus prophylaxis is indicated.

♦ *Antibiotics:* For facial lacerations, use cefazolin (Ancef, Kefzol). For oral cavity lacerations, use clindamycin or penicillin. For fractures communicating with the sinus, use amoxicillin. For fractures with dural tears or CSF leaks, use vancomycin and a third-generation cephalosporin.

♦ *Pain management:* Use oral medications for minor injuries and parenteral medications if the patient cannot take oral medications [i.e., nothing by mouth (NPO)]. For anti-inflammatory control, use ibuprofen, naproxen, or ketorolac (toradol). For central control, use narcotics (e.g., codeine, oxycodone, hydrocodone, meperidine, morphine).

Frontal Bone Fractures

♦ Of great concern is the patency of the nasofrontal duct. If this duct is blocked, surgery is indicated.

♦ Blockage may result in mucopyocele or abscess.

♦ Nondisplaced anterior sinus wall fractures are treated by observation.

♦ Displaced anterior sinus wall fractures with severe comminution and mucosal injury require neurosurgery, oral and maxillofacial surgery, otolaryngology, or plastic surgery for bone grafting and frontal sinus obliteration.

♦ Treatment of posterior sinus wall fractures is controversial and variable.

♦ Posterior sinus wall fractures are examined for displacement, dural tears, and cerebrospinal fluid leakage.

♦ Non-displaced fractures with a cerebrospinal fluid leak may be observed for 5–7 days while undergoing treatment with intravenous antibiotics. Frontal sinus obliteration is indicated, if a cerebrospinal fluid leak persists.

♦ Surgical treatment of displaced fractures with no cerebrospinal fluid leak is based on the severity of comminution.

♦ Mild comminution requires an osteoblastic flap and sinus obliteration.

♦ Comminution of greater than 30% of the posterior sinus wall require the neurosurgeon to remove the posterior table allowing the brain to expand into the frontal sinus, this is known as cranialization.

♦ Displaced sinus wall fractures with a cerebrospinal fluid leak and minimal-to-mild comminution requires sinus obliteration.

♦ Moderate-to-severe comminution requires sinus cranialization.

Orbital Floor Fractures

♦ Blow-out fractures of the orbital floor require consultation with an ophthalmologist and maxillofacial trauma specialist (e.g., oral and maxillofacial surgeon, otolaryngologist or plastic surgeon).

♦ Several approaches are available including subciliary, subtarsal, transconjunctival, and transconjunctival with lateral canthotomy. The subciliary approach has most complications (e.g., ectropion) and the transconjunctival approach the least complications.

♦ However, when major surgical exposure is necessary, a transconjunctival approach with or without a lateral canthotomy incision is recommended.

♦ Orbital floor repair via subtarsal approach.

Nasal Fractures

♦ Nasal fractures should be managed between days 2–10. This allows time for resolution of the edema and therefore assists in obtaining the best reduction possible.

♦ After 10 days, achieving good closed reduction results may be difficult and it may be necessary to wait for as long as 6 months to obtain satisfactory good results via an open reduction technique.

Nasoethmoidal (NOE) Fractures

♦ Fractures with suspected or detected dural tears require consultation with a neurosurgeon, and the patients should be admitted for observation and intravenous antibiotics.

♦ An ophthalmologist should be consulted for repair of the lacrimal apparatus, if disrupted.

♦ An oral and maxillofacial surgeon, plastic surgeon, or otolaryngologist should be consulted for repair of nasal bones, medial canthus, and the nasofrontal duct.

Zygomatic Arch Fractures

♦ Patients with isolated minimally displaced fractures to the zygomatic arch usually do not require treatment, unless it caused a facial asymmetry.

♦ Marked displacement and/or impingement of the coronoid process of the mandible, preventing the patient from opening their mouth, requires admission and an open reduction via transoral (Keen) or temporal (Gillies) approach.

♦ In cases of a severe comminuted fracture, an open reduction with internal fixation (ORIF) may be required.

Zygomaticomaxillary Complex Fractures

♦ When the impact is sufficient to sustain a fracture of the zygomaticomaxillary (ZMC) consultation with an ophthalmologist is warranted to rule out ocular injury. Like the zygomatic arch fracture, surgical treatment of a ZMC fracture is indicated when a cosmetic deformity or functional loss is noted.

♦ Waiting 4–5 days for the edema to be reduced is helpful to properly assess the situation.

♦ The standard of care is open reduction and internal fixation with miniplates and screws. The orbital floor is frequently explored and repaired, if necessary.

Maxillary Fractures

♦ When the impact is severe enough to cause mobility of the maxilla or to a part of it, the patient should be placed in intermaxillary fixation and open reduction with internal fixation should be performed at the piriform rim and zygomaticomaxillary buttress.

♦ Patients with a maxillary fracture should be placed on sinus precautions, and if they have subcutaneous emphysema, they should be placed on antibiotics because some of the bacterial flora could have been forced by the air into the subcutaneous planes.

Mandibular Fractures

♦ Management is provided by an oral and maxillofacial surgeon, otolaryngologist or plastic surgeon.

♦ Temporary stabilization in the emergency department can be addressed with the application of a Barton bandage.

♦ Bring the teeth into occlusion and wrap the bandage around the crown of the head and jaw. This stabilizes the jaw and greatly reduces pain and hemorrhage.

♦ A symphysis or body fracture can be reduced temporarily with a bridal wire (a 24-gauge wire wrapped around 2 teeth on either side of the fracture). This greatly reduces hemorrhage, pain and infection.

♦ Nondisplaced mandibular fractures may be treated by closed reduction and intermaxillary fixation for 5–6 weeks. However many patients do not want to be closed down for that length of time and prefer open reduction.

♦ Initially, the fracture is stabilized with intermaxillary fixation followed by open reduction and rigid fixation using titanium miniplates, mandibular plates, or reconstruction plates, depending on where the fracture is located.

♦ Nondisplaced fractures of the condyle require intermaxillary fixation for 10 days, followed by physiotherapy to help restore improved function.

♦ Ankylosis of the joint is extremely rare and is believed to be caused by an untreated intracapsular injury or fracture.

Panfacial Fractures

♦ At the time of surgery, tracheostomy or submandibular intubation is required.

♦ A submandibular intubation, which avoids a tracheostomy, is performed by first intubating orally, and then surgically bringing the tube out through the submandibular space.

♦ Nasoendotracheal intubation is definitely contraindicated.

♦ Facial bones are repositioned beginning at the cranium. After the occlusion is established by intermaxillary fixation, the remaining facial bones are repaired with open reduction and internal fixation.

Q.11. **Write short note on types of mandibular fracture with diagrams.** *(Jun 2010, 5 Marks)*

Ans. *For types of mandibular fractures, refer to Ans. 1 of same chapter.*

Q.12. **Write short note on maxillofacial injuries.** *(Dec 2010, 5 Marks)*

Ans. Maxillofacial injuries are due to road-traffic accidents, assaults, bullet injuries or sport injuries.

Classification

- Fracture of lower third which comprises of mandible
- Fracture of middle third which comprises of maxilla, zygoma and nose
- Fracture of upper third of face involving part of orbit and frontal bones.

Soft Tissue Injuries

- Lacerations, contusion, cut wounds, etc.
- Eyelid injuries with black eyes
- *Facial nerve injury:* Primary repair is required
- *Parotid duct injury:* Primary Anastomosis of injured duct is done, with fine polyethylene cannula kept as stent inside the duct which is removed in 14 days.
- *Lacrimal apparatus injuries:* Here the duct is sutured with fine nylon thread in canaliculus which is kept for three months.

Injuries to Facial Bones

- *Fracture nose:* Nasal bones are most commonly injured bones in face. Patient presents with pain and swelling in the nose with deviation and displacement. Here reduction of the fractured nasal bones and nasal septum under general anesthesia is done. Later position is maintained by nasal packs from inside (which is removed in 7 days) and by a nasal plaster from outside (which will be kept for 14 days). Procedure is done using Walsham and Asch forceps.
- Injuries to the maxilla
- Zygomatic bone injuries.
- Mandibular bone fracture and mandibular dislocation.
- *Orbital bone fracture:* Presents with diplopia, enophthalmous, sensory loss in the area of infraorbital nerve.
- Infraorbital ecchymosis of the orbit is called Panda sign.

Clinical Features

- Localized swelling due to hematoma
- Facial edema
- Bleeding with open wounds
- Asymmetry which is clinically confirmed by observing supraorbital ridges, nasal bridge
- Localized tenderness
- Step deformity
- Trismus
- Diplopia
- Features of associated injuries, such as intracranial, abdominal or thoracic injuries.

Investigations

- X-ray face
- CT scan of head and jaw

Management

- As the initial assessment, evaluation and management of life-threatening injury get completed compound fracture should be treated in following manner, i.e.:
  - Hemostasis should be achieved.

- For type I and type II compound fractures cephazolin or clindamycin are the choice of drugs while for type III compound fractures aminoglycoside is given.
- Tetanus vaccination should be given.
- Irrigation as well as debridement of the wound should be carried out immediately.
- In cases with type II and type III compound fractures serial irrigation and debridement is recommended for every 24–48 hours till clean surgical wound is confirmed. Close the wound when it get clean fully.
- Management of open fracture depends on its type and its site. Later on wound is stabilized temporarily or definitively.
- If coverage of soft tissue after injury is not proper soft tissue transfer or free flap is given to the patient when fracture is treated.

Q.13. Describe diagnostic features and treatment of temporomandibular joint dislocation.

(Jan 2012, 5 Marks)

Ans. Temporomandibular joint dislocation occurs when condyle is displaced forcefully anteriorly out of the articular fossa but lie in the capsule of joint.

Diagnostic Features

- *Clinical diagnosis:* Patient complains of difficulty in swallowing. Saliva is seen drooling over chin. Severe pain is present in area over temporal fossa. The place where the condylar head is normally placed, at that area depression is seen. There is also presence of anterior open bite along with gagging of molar teeth.
- *Radiographical diagnosis:* Due to dislocation of the condyle articular fossa space appears to be empty.

Treatment

- **Nonsurgical treatment:**
  - *Acute dislocation:* It is done within 72 hours. Manual reduction can be done. It can be done with or without use of anesthesia. Patient should be sit upright on the chair. Clinician should wear the gloves. Thumbs of the clinician are positioned over lower molar teeth bilaterally. Index fingers are placed under inferior border of mandible. Posterior aspect of mandible is depressed inferiorly to depress the condyle, while the chin is elevated anteriorly and entire mandible is pushed backwards with palm. Mandible is moved downwards, backward and upward, manipulating the condyle back in position.
  - *Chronic dislocation:* Manual reduction is done under general anesthesia.
- **Surgical treatment:**
  - *Alteration of ligaments:*
    - By injecting the sclerosing agent in capsular space of TMJ.
    - Strengthening ligaments by surgically exposing temporal fascia and suturing flap of fascia on capsular ligament.

- *Alteration of musculature:*
  - By closed condylectomy: Gigli saw is used to intraorally bisect the condylar neck.
  - Ligation of coronoid process to zygomatic arch anterior to articular tubercle
- *Alteration of bony structure:*
  - By condylectomy
  - Eminectomy, i.e., reduction of height of eminences.

Q.14. Describe etiology, pathology and treatment of acute osteomyelitis. *(Aug 2012, 15 Marks)*

Ans. Osteomyelitis is the inflammation of medullary portion of bone.

Etiology

- Direct spread of infection from dental pulp into the mandible.
- Spread of infection in the mandible from presenting suppurative odontogenic infections.
- Spread of infection following removable of tooth without proper asepsis and antibiotic coverage.
- Compound fracture of mandible with exposure of bone outside the mucosa.
- Postradiation secondary infection.
- Infection to the pre-existing bony lesions, e.g., Paget's disease of bone and fibrous dysplasia.

Pathology

Flowchart 15: Pathology of acute osteomyelitis.

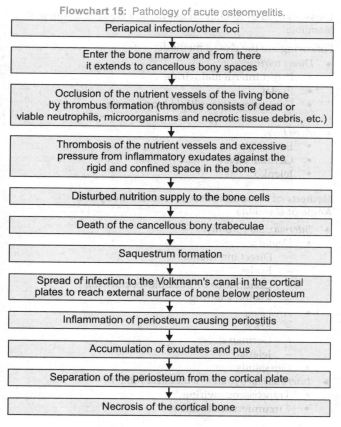

```
Periapical infection/other foci
        ↓
Enter the bone marrow and from there
it extends to cancellous bony spaces
        ↓
Occlusion of the nutrient vessels of the living bone
by thrombus formation (thrombus consists of dead or
viable neutrophils, microorganisms and necrotic tissue debris, etc.)
        ↓
Thrombosis of the nutrient vessels and excessive
pressure from inflammatory exudates against the
rigid and confined space in the bone
        ↓
Disturbed nutrition supply to the bone cells
        ↓
Death of the cancellous bony trabeculae
        ↓
Saquestrum formation
        ↓
Spread of infection to the Volkmann's canal in the cortical
plates to reach external surface of bone below periosteum
        ↓
Inflammation of periosteum causing periostitis
        ↓
Accumulation of exudates and pus
        ↓
Separation of the periosteum from the cortical plate
        ↓
Necrosis of the cortical bone
```

Treatment

The treatment include:
- Conservative treatment.
- Surgical treatment.
  - The goal of management is:
    - Attenuate and eradicate proliferating pathological organism.
    - Promote healing.
    - Re-establish vascular permeability.

Successful Treatment Based on

- Early diagnosis.
- Bacterial culture and sensitivity test.
- Adequate and prompt antibiotic therapy.
- Adequate pain control.
- Proper surgical intervention.
- Reconstruction (if indicated).

Conservative Treatment

- Complete bed rest.
- *Supportive therapy:* It includes nutritional support in form of high protein and high caloric diet and adequate multivitamins.
- *Dehydration control:* Hydration orally or through IV fluid.
- *Blood transfusion:* When RBC and Hb is low.
- *Control of pain:* Analgesic and sedation.
- *Intravenous antimicrobial agents:* Penicillin.

Surgical Treatment

Surgical intervention is done under antibiotic cover, started at least 1–2 days prior to the procedure.

Incision and Drainage

- Done as soon as possible.
- It relives pain and pressure caused by pus accumulation.
- Extraction of loose or offending teeth.
- *Debridement:* Followed by incision and drainage thorough debridement of affected area should be carried out.
- The area may be irrigated with hydrogen peroxide and saline thrice a day.
- Any foreign body, necrotic tissue or small sequestrum should be removed.
- Drainage for the body and angle of the mandible area is established through extraoral submandibular skin incision.
- Intraoral drainage can be established for the body of mandible.
- Sequestrum formed should be removed, if it can be gently picked up (sequestrectomy).

Q.15. Write short note on osteomyelitis. *(Apr 2015, 3 Marks)*

Or

Write short note on osteomyelitis of jaw.

(Dec 2009, 5 Marks)

Ans. Osteomyelitis may be defined as an inflammatory condition of bone that begin as an infection of medullary cavity and Haversian system of the cortex and extends to involve the periosteum of the affected side.

Osteomyelitis more frequently occurs in mandible than in maxilla.

Classification of Osteomyelitis

♦ **Acute osteomyelitis**
  • Acute suppurative osteomyelitis
  • Acute subperiosteal osteomyelitis
  • Acute periostitis.
♦ **Chronic osteomyelitis**
  • Nonspecific type:
    – Chronic intramedullary osteomyelitis
    – Chronic focal sclerosing osteomyelitis
    – Chronic diffuse sclerosing osteomyelitis
    – Chronic osteomyelitis with proliferative periostitis
    – Chronic subperiosteal osteomyelitis
    – Chronic periostitis.
  • Specific type:
    – Tuberculous osteomyelitis
    – Syphilitic osteomyelitis
    – Actinomycotic osteomyelitis.
♦ **Radiation-induced osteomyelitis.**
♦ **Idiopathic osteomyelitis.**

Pathogenesis

For details refer to Ans. 14 of same chapter.

Clinical Features

♦ Pain and tenderness is minimal.
♦ Nonhealing bony and overlying soft tissue wounds with indurations of soft tissues.
♦ Thickened or wooden character of bone.
♦ History of chronic discharge in oral cavity or on face through the sinus present.
♦ Pathological fracture may occur.
♦ Teeth in area tend to become loose and sensitive to palpation and percussion.
♦ Lymphadenopathy is present.

Treatment

Treatment of Acute Osteomyelitis

For details refer to Ans. 14 of same chapter.

Treatment of Chronic Osteomyelitis

Done by sequestrectomy and saucerization (removal of bony cavity).

Sequestrectomy

♦ Removal of sequestrum.
♦ It may be carried out under proper cover of antibiotics.
♦ Small sequestra are removed under local anesthesia.
♦ General anesthesia may be given for the removal of bigger sequestrum.
♦ Sequestra from lower border of mandible are best removed by extraoral approach using Risdon's incision.
♦ From ramus, it may be removed by retromandibular incision.
♦ From condyle by preauricular incision.

♦ Coronoid process is best approached by or intra oral incision given along the anterior border of ramus of the mandible.
♦ After removal of the sequestrum the residual granulation tissue is curetted till white shining bone appears.
♦ Bleeding is controlled by pressure pack.
♦ When complete infection has been eradicated the wound can be closed by primary closure.
♦ When the elimination of the infection is doubtful, a glove drain or a rubber drain is kept in place and is changed every 24 hours till no discharge from the bone, is seen.

Saucerization

♦ Removal of bony cavity.
♦ It consists of elimination for bony cavity in the jaw bone to avoid collection of blood and formation of large hematoma which is liable to get infected.
♦ It is simple procedure for eliminating the dead space in bone.
♦ Saucerization is carried out by existing the wall of the bony cavity by means of Rongeur bone-cutting forceps or burs.
♦ The bone is smoothen by file.
♦ The wound can be partially or completely closed depending upon the amount of suppuration.

Q.16. Write the close methods of reduction and immobilization of fracture of long bone and fracture body and angle of mandible. *(Dec 2012, 10 Marks)*

Ans. *For close methods of reduction and immobilization of fracture of long bone refer to Ans. 8 of same chapter.*

Close Method of Reduction of Fracture Body and Angle of Mandible

Following are the closed methods:
♦ *Direct wiring:*
  • Direct interdental wiring
  • Eyelet
  • Continuous or multiple loop wiring
  • Risdon's wiring.
♦ *Arch bars:*
  • Erich
  • German silver
  • Jelenko.

Methods of Immobilization of Fracture Body and Angle of Mandible

♦ *Intermaxillary fixation:*
  • *Dental wiring:*
    – Direct interdental
    – Eyelet
    – Continuous or multiple loop wiring
    – Risdon's wiring.
  • *Arch bars:*
    – Erich
    – German silver
    – Jelenko.
  • *Cap splints*
♦ *Intermaxillary fixation with osteosynthesis:*
  • Transosseous wiring
  • Circumferential wiring

- External pin fixation
- Bone clamps.
♦ *Osteosynthesis without intermaxillary fixation:*
  - Noncompression small plates
  - Compression plates
  - Mini plates.

Direct Interdental Wiring

In this a prestretched soft stainless steel wire of 0.35 mm thickness and 15 cm in length is taken. Middle portion of the wire should be twisted around the tooth. Free ends of the wire are twisted together and form a plaited tail which is 3 cm in length. In this way, all other teeth are attached by the wires and then twisted.

Risdon's Wiring

Risdon's wiring is a commonly utilized method of horizontal wire fixation.

♦ Use when all teeth are present.
♦ A 26 gauge, 25 cm long wire is passed around the neck of the 2nd molar on each side so that both ends of wire extend to buccal side. Than the ends of both wires twisted together for their entire length. So that the strong base wires is formed on either side, coming towards midline from each second molar.
♦ The excess wire is cut and the ends are checked in interdental space.
♦ The base wire is secured to individual tooth by using additional interdental wires.
♦ The one of small wire is passed from the distal surface of the tooth below the base wire and brought out towards the lingual side and then brought out on the buccal surface from mesial interdental space above the base wire.
♦ Both ends are again grasped together and twisted, cut and finished in interdental space.
♦ Each tooth is engaged in the same manner to the base wire, so that the base wire is fully secured to the dental arch.
♦ Two types of horizontal wiring after strong fixation and prevent supraeruption.

Arch Bars

Arch bar are used for immobilization of jaw during management of fractured jaw.

♦ There are many types of arch bars available.
♦ Rigid types are made by half round stainless steel wire of 18 and 21 gauge.
♦ The read-made arch bars are available (Erich arch bar) These are consider better as these are soft, easy to adapt and have hooks.
♦ The arch bars are indicated when there are not enough teeth in the arch for conventional Risdon's wiring or when all teeth in arch cannot be secured due to poor periodontal condition of teeth.
♦ The arch bar should be perfectly adapted to the teeth in the arch because if the bar is not fitted, it can cause orthodontic movement.

♦ The arch is adapted by starting from distal most point in the arch.
♦ A sharp bend is given at the edge of wire to be pushed into the interdental space between 2nd and 3rd molar to avoid slippage of arch bar.
♦ It is adapted progressing to midline and finishing on other end.
♦ Arch bar should not cross the fracture line.
♦ The bar should be cut and adapted to each fragment separating.
♦ The arch bar is secured in place by using ligature wire passed around each individual tooth.
♦ One end of the wire coming below the arch bar and above it in the buccal side and then finished.
♦ Care is taken that hooks on the arch bar are directed upward in the maxilla and downward in mandible.

Transosseous Wiring

The direct wiring of the fractured ends after exposing and reducing the fractured fragment.

♦ *There are two method of wiring:* The upper border wiring and lower border wiring, in case of angle and body of the mandible.
♦ The upper border wiring is done intraorally just below the alveolus and lower border wiring is done by extraoral approach.
♦ The edges of bony fragments are cleaned and reduced with the help of "Bone-holding" device.
♦ Holes are drilled in the bone using an electric or "hand drill".
♦ Drilling is done under constant jet of normal saline solution.
♦ The holes should be drilled at a distance of atleast 5 mm from the fractured site.
♦ A no 26-gauge wire is passed through the holes across the fracture line and tightened by trusting the two ends.

Miniplates

♦ In multiple mandibular fractures, accurate reduction and establishment of normal occlusion is tuf, so it is advisable to secure the normal occlusion through interdental wiring, before the miniplate osteosynthesis is performed.
♦ Following reduction, the osteosynthesis lines should be established. The adaptation of the bone plate is done by bending pliers.
♦ Adapted bone plate should lie passively over the contour of external cortex, and it is confirmed that there should not be any gap between the plate and the bone.
♦ The miniplate is fixed in its specific position with the screws.
♦ In fractures of the angle of the mandible, plate is located on the posterior fragment, medial to the external oblique line, this is done so that it can be bent over the surface and the posterior screws are placed in sagittal direction.
♦ In cases with simultaneous fractures of the alveolar process or if impacted third molar teeth are present, the plate may be fixed to the outer surface of the mandible which correspond to the position in the course of line of tension.
♦ When fracture is present between the canine and premolars, mental nerve may be damaged by applying the plate. In such

cases, it is recommended to place concave section of plate between screw holes precisely at the exit point of the nerve.

♦ In some of the very exceptional cases, transposition of nerve to lower level may be indicated. To reduce the effect of torsional forces in symphysis region between mental foramina, it is mandatory to use two parallel plates.

♦ In the cases of comminuted fractures or in cases where there are detached triangular pieces of bone, longer plates with six or more screws should be used.

Q.17. Write short note on methods of immobilization of fracture body of mandible. *(Feb 2014, 5 Marks)*

Ans. *For details of methods of immobilization of fracture body of mandible, refer to Ans. 16 of same chapter.*

Q.18. Write short note on compound fracture.
(Dec 2015, 5 Marks)

Or

Compound fracture. Definition and management.
(Aug 2018, 10 Marks)

Ans. Compound fracture is also known as open fracture.

If the bone breaks in such a way that bone fragments stick out through the skin or a wound penetrates down to the broken bone, the fracture is called as compound fracture. For example, when a pedestrian is struck by the bumper of a moving car, the broken shinbone may protrude through a tear in the skin and other soft tissues.

Since compound fractures often involve more damage to the surrounding muscles, tendons, and ligaments, they have a higher risk for complications and take a longer time to heal.

This type of fracture is particularly serious because once the skin is broken, infection in both the wound and the bone can occur.

Classification of Compound Fractures (Gustilo et al. and Anderson's)

♦ *Type I:* Wound is smaller than 1 cm, clean and generally caused by fractured fragment which pierces the skin. This is a low energy injury.

♦ *Type II:* Wound is longer than 1 cm, not contaminated and is without major soft tissue damage or defect. It is also a low energy injury.

♦ *Type III:* Wound is longer than 1 cm with significant soft tissue disruption. Mechanism involves high energy trauma, resulting in severe unstable fracture with varying degrees of fragmentation.

♦ *Type IIIA:* Wound has sufficient soft tissue to cover the bone without need for local or distant flap coverage.

♦ *Type IIIB:* Disruption of soft tissue is extensive, such as local or distant flap coverage is necessary to cover the bone. Wound may be contaminated, serial irrigation and debridement procedures are necessary to ensure clean surgical wound.

♦ *Type III C:* Any open fracture associated with an arterial injury requires repair is considered as Type IIIC.

Etiology

♦ Compound fractures are caused by high-energy trauma, most commonly from a direct blow, such as from a fall or motor vehicle collision.

♦ These fractures can also occur indirectly, such as a high-energy twisting type of injury.

Management

Management of compound fracture is divided into two parts, i.e., investigations and treatment.

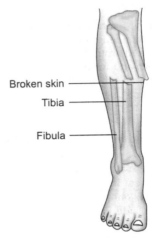

Fig. 40: Compound fracture.

Investigations

♦ X-rays will show how complex the fracture is.

♦ Routine blood and urine tests provide information about the general health.

Treatment

♦ Antibiotics are started as soon as possible in the emergency room. Severity of injury determines which antibiotics are given. Tetanus shot should be given. Cefazolin/clindamycin is given the type I and type II open fractures while for type III fractures aminoglycoside is given.

♦ Injury will be covered with a sterile dressing. Doctor will gently put the bones back into alignment to prevent the fragments from causing further damage to soft tissues. Then splint should be applied to injured limb to protect it and keep it from moving until patient is taken to surgery.

♦ **Débridement:** During this procedure, surgeon will remove all dirt and foreign bodes, as well as any contaminated and unhealthy skin, muscle, and other soft tissues. The bone is also cleaned of all dirt and other foreign material. Any unattached pieces of bone are removed. Severely contaminated bone fragments are also discarded. This bone loss can be corrected later with additional surgeries.

♦ **Irrigation.** After débridement, the wound is cleansed and irrigated with several liters of saline.

♦ It is important to stabilize the broken bones as soon as possible to prevent further soft tissue damage. The broken bones in an open fracture are typically held in place using external or internal fixation methods. These methods require surgery.

♦ For type II and type III compound fractures, serial irrigation and debridement is done till clean surgical wound is achieved.

Internal fixation: During the operation, the bone fragments are first repositioned (reduced) into their normal alignment, and then held together with special screws or by attaching metal plates to the outer surface of the bone. The fragments may also be held together by inserting rods down through the marrow space in the center of the bone. These methods of treatment can reposition the fracture fragments very exactly. Because open fractures may include tissue damage and be accompanied by additional injuries, it may take time before internal fixation surgery can be safely performed.

External fixation: Depending on the injury, surgeon may use external fixation to hold bones in general alignment. In external fixation, pins or screws are placed into the broken bone above and below the fracture site. Then the orthopedic surgeon repositions the bone fragments. The pins or screws are connected to a metal bar or bars outside the skin.

- As fixation gets completed the skin should be sutured.
- In complex wounds, flaps should be place to cover the injury.

Local flap. The muscle tissue from the involved limb is rotated to cover the fracture. A patch of skin taken from another area of the body (graft) is placed over this.

Free flap. Some wounds may require a complete transfer of tissue. This tissue is often taken from the back or abdomen. A free flap coverage procedure requires the assistance of a microvascular surgeon to ensure the blood vessels connect and circulation is established.

Complications

Compound fractures are serious injuries and, therefore, serious complications are associated with them:

- Infection is the most common complication of open fractures. Infection can occur early, during the healing phase of the fracture, or even later. In general, the greater the extent of soft tissue damage, the greater the risk for infection. If an infection becomes chronic (osteomyelitis), it may lead to further surgeries and amputation.
- Compound fractures may have difficulty healing. If your fracture is failing to heal, further surgery may be required. Surgery to promote healing usually includes placing a bone graft over the fracture, as well as new internal fixation components.
- Acute compartment syndrome may develop. This is a painful condition that occurs when pressure within the muscles builds to dangerous levels. Unless the pressure is relieved quickly, permanent disability and tissue death may result.

Q.19. Describe etiology, pathology, clinical features and treatment of acute osteomyelitis. What is the sequel of poorly treated osteomyelitis?

(Jan 2016, 10 Marks)

Ans. Acute osteomyelitis is a rapidly destructive, pus producing infection which is capable of destructing the bone.

For etiology, pathology and treatment of acute osteomyelitis refer to Ans. 14 of same chapter.

Clinical Features

- There is presence of deep intense pain.
- Patient complaints of intermittent fever.
- Signs of acute infection are present, i.e., bodyache, malaise, leukocytosis, raised ESR, etc.
- Presence of paresthesia or anesthesia of lower lip as inferior alveolar nerve is involved.
- Acute infection is present in the tooth and pus discharge is seen from gingival crevice.
- Presence of mobility of involved teeth.

Sequel of Poorly Treated Osteomyelitis

- If the infection is left untreated, an abscess may develop in the bone and surrounding tissue. In time, this may burst on to the skin and leave a tract, i.e., sinus between the infected bone and surface of the skin.
- Blood infection, i.e., septicemia develop which cause serious illness.
- If the infection follows a fracture, then there is a chance that the fracture will not heal, i.e., there is non-union of fracture.
- Compression of other structures occur next to the infection.
- Some bone infections are caused by methicillin-resistant *S. aureus* (MRSA) which is difficult to clear with antibiotics.
- Persistent infection of the bone, i.e., chronic osteomyelitis sometimes develops and can be difficult to clear.

Q.20. Classify fractures. Describe etiology, clinical features and management of compound fractures.

(Mar 2016, 10 Marks)

Ans.

Classification of Fractures

- *Based on plane of fracture surface:*
  - *Linear fractures:* Fracture which run parallel to long axis of bone.
  - *Transverse fracture:* Fracture in right angle with axis of bone
  - *Oblique fracture:* Fracture with oblique fracture line
  - *Spiral fracture:* Fracture with spiral fracture line
  - *Comminuted fracture:* Fracture with splintered or crushed bone with more than two fragments.
  - *Segmental fracture:* Fracture where a part of bone is completely separated from are not bone with same diameter.
- *Based on etiology of fracture:*
  - Traumatic fractures
  - Pathological fractures
  - Stress fractures
- *Based on condition of soft tissue:*
  - *Close or simple fracture:* This fracture lacks communication between site of fracture and exterior of body
  - *Open or compound fracture:* In this, fracture a wound is present through the adjacent or overlying soft tissue communicates outside the body.
- *Special fractures:*
  - *Depressed fracture:* It is common in skull bone
  - *Fracture-dislocation:* Anterior dislocation of shoulder along with fracture neck of humerus.

- Fracture involving a joint
- *Complex fracture:* These fractures involve major nerves and vessels.

Clinical Features of Compound Fracture

♦ Swelling or bruising over a bone.
♦ Deformity of an arm or leg.
♦ Pain in the injured area that gets worse when the area is moved or pressure is applied.
♦ Loss of function in the injured area.

♦ Bone appears protruding from the skin.
♦ Bleeding is present at the fracture site.
♦ Presence of contamination of fracture site by mud, dirt, etc.
♦ Victim heard a bone break or snap or heard a grating sensation.

For etiology and management of compound fractures, refer to Ans. 18 of same chapter.

Q.21. Describe differentiating features of Le Fort Type I, II and III fractures. *(Jan 2017, 3 Marks)*

Ans. See Table below:

Differentiating features of Le Fort type I, II, and III fractures.

Features	Le Fort type I	Le Fort type II	Le Fort type III
Synonyms	It is also known as Guerin's fracture or floating fracture or horizontal fracture of maxilla or low level fracture	It is also known as pyramidal fracture	It is also known as craniofacial disjunction or high level fracture or suprazygomatic fracture
Fracture line	Fracture line runs horizontally above the floor of nasal cavity involving lower third septum, palate, alveolar process of maxilla and lower third of pterygoid plates of maxilla	Fracture line run from nasal bone at top most, fracture run laterally towards lacrimal bones, medial wall of orbit, infraorbital margin, through medial to infraorbital foramen and backward below the zygomaticomaxillary area through lateral wall of maxillary sinus and pterygoid plates. Zygoma is intact with skull base.	Fracture line runs parallel to skull base. It passes through the nasal bone, lacrimal bone, ethmoid bone, optic foramen, inferior orbital fissure, pterygomaxillary fissure and lateral orbital wall with frontozygomatic suture. With zygomatic arch.
Etiology	Occur due to strong blow with sharp object at the level above tooth bearing region	Occur from strong force applied in central region at the level of nasal bones.	Occur due to strong blow to face at level of orbit either from lateral or frontal direction
Features	• Bleeding from nose • Posterior gagging of occlusion • Upper lip swelling • Palatal ecchymosis • Occlusion derangement • Floating maxilla	• Edema of middle third of face • Bilateral circumorbital and subconjunctival ecchymoses • Nasal bleeding/obstruction/deformity • Dish face deformity of face • Diplopia • Retroposition of maxilla with posterior gagging • Limitation of ocular movements • CSF rhinorrhea • Tenderness and separation of infraorbital margin	• Lengthening of face • Enophthalmos, ocular level depression • Hooding of eyes, occlusal plane tilting • Entire facial skeleton moves as a single block • Tenderness and separation of suture line • Trismus • Teeth malalignment • *Guerin sign:* Hematoma at greater palatine foramen is present.

27. ADVANCED METHODS OF SURGERY AND RADIOLOGY

Q.1. Write short note on CT scan. *(Apr 2008, 5 Marks)*

Or

Write briefly on CT scan. *(Dec 2010, 5 Marks)*

Ans. Computed tomography scan was invented by Godfrey Hounsfield in 1963.

Working of CT Scan

Narrow X-ray beams are passed from rotating X-ray generator through the gantry where patient is placed. When X-ray pass through the tissues, some of the X-rays get absorb and some pass through, depending on the tissue density, different grades of absorption in different tissues are detected through sensitive detectors which are translated to a Gray scale image by a computer. Density of tissues is numbered as Hounsfield Number (HN).

Contrast Agents

♦ *Ionic:* Water soluble iodide dyes, such as sodium diatrizoate, meglumine iothalamate. They are cheaper but often toxic and cause anaphylaxis.
♦ *Non-ionic* are safer but expensive, such as iohexol, iopamiro.

Indications

♦ Trauma-like head injury, chest injury. Abdomen trauma: in trauma only plain CT scan is taken.
♦ Neoplasms: To see the exact location, size, vascularity, extent and operability.
♦ *Inflammatory conditions:* In various sites, such as in pseudocyst of pancreas.

Contraindications

- In pregnancy.
- In restless patient.

Advantages

- 1–2 mm sized sections are possible.
- Amount of exposure to radiation is less
- More accurate, sensitive and specific.
- Small lesions are detected.

Disadvantages

- Interpretation by experienced radiologist is done
- Artifacts can be present
- Cost is high.

Q.2. Write short note on biopsy.   *(Feb 2013, 5 Marks)*

Or

Write short answer on biopsy and its types.

(Feb 2019, 3 Marks)

Ans. Biopsy is the removal of tissue from the living organism for the purpose of microscopic examination and diagnosis.

Types of Biopsy

- **Excisional biopsy:** If a lesion is totally excised for histological evaluation it is called as excisional biopsy.
- **Incisional biopsy:** When only a small section of tissue is removed from the lesion for the purpose of histological evaluation it is called as incisional biopsy.
- **Fine needle aspiration cytology (FNAC):** It is done by aspirating tissue material inside a lesion which is later on diagnosed microscopically after preparing a smear.
- **Frozen section biopsy:** It is performed in order to get an immediate histological report of a lesion. The tissue is obtained from the lesion and is kept in deep freeze and than frozen tissue is sectioned and stained to get a prompt diagnosis.

Procedure of Biopsy

- **Anesthesia:** Give a block to anesthetize the region where specimen is to be obtained. Local infiltration and injections into the tissue which should be biopsied is avoided as it leads to the artifacts in the specimen. If a block is not effective give local infiltration atleast 1 cm away from the lesion.
- **Stabilization of tissue:** Soft tissue biopsies are done over the movable tissues of oral cavity, i.e., tongue, lips, etc. Dental assistant stabilizes the tissue by stretching it.
- **Hemostasis:** Gauze pieces are the best means for compressing the tissue and achieving hemostasis. Gauze piece can also be placed to cover the mouth of suction tip and is used to prevent the specimen from being sucked inside.
- **Incisions:** Use a sharp scalpel. Provide two incisions which form an elliptical incision and converge to form a V at the base, this provides a good specimen and a wound which is easy to close. Alternatively, a triangular-shaped incision can be made which converges in the form of a tip of a pyramid at the base. Incisions should be given parallel to the nerves and vessels in that region to avoid damage.

- **Handling of tissues:** Tissue which has to be removed should be handled carefully so that histopathological examination can be performed. A non-toothed tissue holding forceps is used and care is taken not to crush the tissues.
- **Care of specimen:** After removal of the tissues, the specimen is transferred to a bottle containing 10% formalin which should be atleast 20 times the volume of the specimen obtained.
- **Surgical closure of wound:** Primary closure is possible in most cases. Where it is not possible, the tissues are undermined to facilitate closure.

Q.3. Write short note on FNAC.   *(Nov 2008, 5 Marks)*

Or

Write short note on fine needle aspiration cytology.

(Aug 2011, 5 Marks)

Or

Write short answer on FNAC.

(Sep 2018, 3 Marks) (Apr 2019, 3 Marks)

Ans. FNAC is also called as fine needle aspiration cytology.

- FNAC is the microscopic examination of aspirate which is obtained by penetrating a fine needle in the lesion.
- FNAC is a procedure for rapid diagnosis.

Procedure

- Position the needle over the target area in the lesion.
- As the needle is penetrated and is positioned a plunger is pulled to apply negative pressure.
- Negative pressure should be released as needle remains in target tissue.
- Needle is withdrawn and defumed air is withdrawn outside.
- Drop of aspirate is taken on the slide and is thoroughly spreaded.
- Fix the slide by keeping it in 95% of alcohol for one hour.
- Staining with PAP stain should be done.

Indications

- Help in diagnosis of swellings of head and neck region.
- Part of initial diagnostic work-up of lymphadenopathy, metastatic lesion or lymphomas.
- Helps in distinguishing benign from malignant and cystic lesions from inflammatory lesions.
- Aids in diagnosis for salivary gland pathologies.
- Helps to identify the cause for enlarged lymph nodes.

Advantages

- It is minimally invasive.
- It is safe, fast and cost effective method.
- It is less time consuming.
- It do not spread the tumors, disrupt the field for surgical dissection.

Q.4. Write briefly on Laser.   *(Dec 2010, 5 Marks)*

Or

Write short note on Laser in surgery.

(Dec 2015, 5 Marks) (June 2014, 5 Marks)

Ans. Molecules are placed in a compact area and power is passed through this so as to activate the molecules. Molecules get activated at different periods and move in different directions, which they hit to each other releasing energy. This energy is allowed to act through optical system to the area, wherever required. It is named depending on the molecules used as:

♦ Argon laser.
♦ Neodymium Yttrium Aluminum Garnet Laser (Nd: YAG Laser)
♦ CO_2 laser.
♦ Neon laser.
♦ Holmium laser.
♦ Erbium laser.

Uses of Laser

♦ In cranial surgery in children.
♦ In ENT it is used to treat vocal cord lesions, laryngeal lesions.
♦ In ophthalmology, it is very useful in retinal surgery
♦ In general surgery:
  • In bleeding duodenal ulcer.
  • For palliative decoding of tumors in carcinoma esophagus.
  • In carcinoma of rectum.
  • In treatment of hemorrhoids (lst and 2nd degree).
  • In resection of bladder tumor.
  • In cervical cancer.
  • To achieve bloodless field.
  • Often in making incisions in abdomen and other places.

Precautions

♦ All reflecting instruments should be avoided otherwise laser gets reflected and injure normal tissues or the working team in the OT
♦ All should wear protective spectacles to their eyes.

Advantages

♦ Provide bloodless field
♦ It is fast
♦ Small lesions can be removed easily and completely.

Disadvantage

Availability and cost factors.

Q.5. Write short note on cryosurgery or laser in surgery.
(Dec 2012, 5 Marks)

Or

Write short note on cryosurgery. *(Feb 2015, 5 Marks)*

Ans.

Cryosurgery

♦ It is the method of destruction of tissues by controlled cooling.
♦ It consists of an automatic defrosting device with cryoprobe.
♦ Commonly nitrous oxide is used as it is easily available, cheaper and have optimum temperature required for other procedures.
♦ Other gases used are CO_2, liquid nitrogen, Freon.

Mode of Action

♦ It produces intracellular crystallization, dehydration and denaturation of proteins and cell death.
♦ It causes the obliteration of microcirculation and so cell death.

Indications

♦ To remove warts and lesions in the skin.
♦ Cryotherapy for piles.
♦ For chronic cervicitis.

Advantages

♦ Relatively bloodless and painless.
♦ Adequate control of extent and depth in freezing
♦ Equally effective.

Disadvantages

♦ Can cause infection.
♦ Discharge from the site.

For Laser in surgery refer to Ans. 4 of same chapter.

Q.6. Write short note on brachytherapy.
(Aug 2012, 5 Marks)

Ans. It is radiation given with source close to the tumor.

♦ It is given using iridium 192 cesium 137.
♦ It is curative radiotherapy.
♦ It is used in carcinoma of oral cavity, penis, breast, cervix and bladder.
♦ Radiation material placed in the cavity is called intracavitary radiotherapy.
♦ Radiation material is inserted into the tissues—interstitial radiotherapy.
♦ Implants can be kept permanently or temporarily.
♦ Radioactive material is placed into the cavity/tissue through applicators under general anesthesia.
♦ Intraoperative radiotherapy is also becoming popular. It has only localized effect with adjacent tissue being spared.

Advantages

♦ High, localized, continuous dose of radiotherapy.
♦ Deeper and adjacent tissues get spared
♦ Dose rate is high in short time.
♦ Side effects are less.
♦ It is curative and effective in early cancers.
♦ Surgery is avoided and part is retained.

Disadvantages

♦ Technique is difficult.
♦ Availability of facility.
♦ Produces local complications, such as displacement/erosion.

Q.7. Describe briefly different types of biopsy.
(Apr 2017, 5 Marks)

Ans.

Types of Biopsies

♦ Incision biopsy—wedge biopsy
♦ Excision biopsy
♦ Trucut biopsy
♦ Pap smear

- FNAC
- Frozen section biopsy
- Punch biopsy
- Ultrasound-guided biopsy
- Brush biopsy
- Laparoscopic biopsy
- CT-guided biopsy
- Thoracoscopic biopsy
- Endoscopic biopsy (gastroscopic or colonoscopic or through ERCP or through cystoscopy)
- Proctoscopic biopsy
- Open biopsy either laparotomy or thoracotomy or craniotomy using Dancly's brain cannula

Incision Biopsy

- This is the excision of a portion of lesion for microscopic examination.
- This method is employed on large, diffuse lesions which has the size of 2 cm in its greatest dimension.
- This method can also be dome on lesions suspected for malignancy.
- Aim of this method is to remove a portion of lesional tissue in question along with the sample of normal adjacent tissue for comparison.

Types of Incision Biopsy

- *Punch biopsy:* This is done by using a surgical punch of diameter 4, 8 or 10 mm. This incisional biopsy is done in mass screening programs.
- *Wedge biopsy:* It is done by making the wedge-shaped incision which begins 2–3 mm from normal tissue and penetrates in the region surrounding abnormal tissue. Tissue should always be incised narrow and deep.

Excision Biopsy

- This procedure should be done for the small lesions which are clinically benign.
- In this, complete lesion should be removed for examination and diagnosis. So it is both diagnostic and curative.

Trucut Biopsy

It is done using a specialized device wherein gun with trucut tip is inserted into the surface tissue/organ and gun is fired to close the punching needle of to catch and cut the adequate tissue. It is done in prostrate, breast and surface tumors.

FNAC

- This is the cytological study of tumor cells to find out the disease and also confirm whether it is malignant or not.
- It is done by using 23 or 24 gauge needle fixed to specialized syringes which create negative pressure for aspiration and contents are smeared on slides.
- It is contraindicated in testicular tumor.

Frozen Section Biopsy

- It is done when biopsy report is needed at earliest.
- It is done in pathology set-up existing adjacent to operation theater.

- In this an unfixed fresh tissue is frozen (using carbon dioxide) in a metal and sections are made and stained.
- Advantage of this technique is that, it is quick and surgeon can decide further steps in surgery.

Ultrasound-guided or CT-guided

- This procedure is conducted with large needle with assisted CT scan equipment.
- Simultaneous CT scan allow identification and visualization of exact size of tumor on computer screen.
- It enables operator to guide the needle in tumor and obtain several samples of tissue.
- Tissues then later examined by histopathologist.

Brush Biopsy

- In this, a brush biopsy kit is supplied by the manufacturer which consists of brush biopsy instrument, bar-coded glass slide, alcohol-based fixative and protective plastic case for mailing and instruction sheet.
- In this, nylon brush is designed to collect cells from all layers of epithelium including basal cell layer of epithelium.
- Procedure includes application of firm pressure on lesion rotating brush 5–10 times. After this nylon brush is manipulated on glass slide so more cells are spread over the slide.
- Slide is analyzed by computer program designed for pathological review.
- Results are interpreted as negative, positive or typical.

28. STERILIZATION

Q.1. Write short note on sterilization in surgery.

(Feb 2013, 5 Marks) (Sep 2006, 5 Marks)

Or

Write short note on sterilization.

(Apr 2008, 5 Marks) (Mar 2016, 5 Marks)

Ans. Sterilization is the complete removal of all types of microbes. It can be attempted by one of the following methods of sterilization.

1. Heat method: Dry heat or moist heat
2. Ionizing radiation
3. Ethylene oxide gas.

Heat Method

- *Dry heat:* The most common apparatus, which works on the principles of dry heat, is hot air oven. The hot air oven, which has controlled cycles,160°C for one hour are suitable for killing bacteria on materials, which are not penetrated by steam. Dry heat oxidize the bacterial cytoplasm, e.g., glassware, oils, petroleum jelly.
- *Moist heat:* Steam kills bacteria by coagulating cytoplasm and is an extremely efficient sterilizer when used under increased pressure, when the temperature exceeds 100°. Autoclave is the apparatus used which causes sterilization by moist heat within 30 min. The autoclave work at

temperature of 121°C at 15 Ibs pressure per square inch for 15–20 minutes.

Ionizing Radiation

Gamma rays are lethal, non-charged, ultrashort, wavelength rays with great penetrating power from a radioactive isotope, such as cobalt-60, disposable plastic syringes, sutures and rubber glass are examples.

Ethylene Oxide Gas

It is a highly toxic inflammable gas, which kills all types of microbes including bacterial spores. CO_2 is mixed with ethylene oxide gas to reduce likelihood of explosion. The gas diffuses well through items, such as plastic materials, swab and paper.

Q.2. Discuss the asepsis and antiseptic measures in oro-dental surgery patient. *(Dec 2007, 8 Marks)*

Ans. Asepsis means precaution taken before any surgical procedure against development of infection.

♦ Antisepsis means all surgical procedures done after taking precautions.

♦ The concept of asepsis can be applied in any clinical setting.

♦ The element requiring careful attention is equipment or supplies. Medical and dental equipment can be sterilized by chemical treatment, radiation, gas, or heat. Personnel can take steps to ensure sterility by assessing that sterile packages are dry and intact and checking sterility indicators, such as dates or colored tape that changes color when sterile.

♦ Besides overall attention to the clinical environment and equipment, clinicians need to be attentive to their own practices and those of their peers in order to avoid inadvertent contamination.

♦ Aseptic technique is most strictly applied in the operating room because of the direct and often extensive disruption of skin and underlying tissue. Aseptic technique helps to prevent or minimize postoperative infection. The patient is prepared by shaving hair from the surgical site, cleansing with a disinfectant, such as iodine, and applying sterile drapes.

♦ In all clinical settings, handwashing is an important step in asepsis. In general settings, hands are to be washed when visibly soiled, before and after contact with the patient, after contact with other potential sources of microorganisms, before invasive procedures, and after removal of gloves. Patients and visitors should also be encouraged to wash their hands. Proper handwashing for most clinical settings involves removal of jewelry, avoidance of clothing contact with the sink, and a minimum of 10–15 seconds scrubbing hands with soap, warm water, and vigorous friction.

♦ A surgical scrub requires use of a long-acting, powerful, antimicrobial soap, careful scrubbing of the fingernails, and a longer period of time for scrubbing. Institutional policy usually designates an acceptable minimum length of time required. Thorough drying is essential, as moist surfaces invite the presence of pathogens. Contact after handwashing with the faucet or other potential contaminants should be avoided. The faucet can be turned off with a dry paper towel, or, in many cases, through use of foot pedals. Despite this careful scrub, bare hands are always considered potential sources of infection. An important principle of aseptic technique is that fluid (a potential mode of pathogen transmission) flows in the direction of gravity. With this in mind, hands are held below elbows during the surgical scrub and above elbows following the surgical scrub.

♦ Sterile surgical clothing or protective devices, such as gloves, facemasks, goggles, and transparent eye/face shields serve as a barrier against microorganisms and are donned to maintain asepsis in the operating room. This practice includes covering facial hair, tucking hair out of sight, and removing jewelry or other dangling objects that may harbor unwanted organisms. This garb must be done with deliberate care to avoid touching external, sterile surfaces with nonsterile objects including the skin. This ensures that potentially contaminated items, such as hands and clothing remain behind protective barriers, thus prohibiting inadvertent entry of microorganisms into sterile areas. Personnel assist the surgeon to wear gloves and garb and arrange equipment to minimize the risk of contamination.

♦ Donning sterile gloves requires specific technique so that the outer glove is not touched by the hand. A large cuff exposing the inner glove is created so that the glove may be grasped during donning. It is essential to avoid touching nonsterile items once sterile gloves are applied; the hands may be kept interlaced to avoid inadvertent contamination. Any break in the glove or touching the glove to a nonsterile surface requires immediate removal and application of new gloves.

♦ Asepsis in the operating room or for other invasive procedures is also maintained by creating sterile surgical fields with drapes. Sterile drapes are sterilized linens placed on the patient or around the field to delineate sterile areas. Drapes or wrapped kits of equipment are opened in such a way that the contents do not touch nonsterile items or surfaces. Aspects of this method include opening the furthest areas of a package first, avoiding leaning over the contents, and preventing opened flaps from falling back onto contents.

Other principles that are applied to maintain asepsis include:

♦ All items in a sterile field must be sterile.

♦ Sterile packages or fields are opened or created as close as possible to time of actual use.

♦ Moist areas are not considered sterile.

♦ Contaminated items must be removed immediately from the sterile field.

♦ Only areas that can be seen by the clinician are considered sterile, i.e., the back of the clinician is not sterile.

♦ Gowns are considered sterile only in the front, from chest to waist and from the hands to slightly above the elbow.

♦ Tables are considered sterile only at or above the level of the table.

♦ Nonsterile items should not cross above a sterile field.

♦ There should be no talking, laughing, coughing, or sneezing across a sterile field.

♦ Personnel with colds should avoid working while ill or apply a double mask.

♦ Edges of sterile areas or fields (generally the outer inch) are not considered sterile.

♦ When in doubt about sterility, discard the potentially contaminated item and begin again.

♦ A safe space or margin of safety is maintained between sterile and nonsterile objects and areas.

♦ When pouring fluids, only the lip and inner cap of the pouring container is considered sterile. The pouring container should not touch the receiving container, and splashing should be avoided.

♦ Tears in barriers are considered breaks in sterility.

Q.3. Write short note on autoclave.

(Aug 2012, 5 Marks) (Apr 2017, 4 Marks)

Or

Write short answer on sterilization by autoclave.

(Apr 2019, 3 Marks)

Ans. It is the means of moist heat sterilization.

♦ It is the method of choice for sterilization of instrument as it eliminates even resistant spore forming microorganisms, fungi, viruses along with vegetative microorganisms.

♦ It works on principle of steam under pressure.

♦ It has two pressure cycles:
  1. 15 psi pressure at 121°C for 30 minutes.
  2. 30 psi pressure at 134°C for 3–5 minutes also known as flash method.

Mechanism of Action

Steam is the mixture of heat and water vapor. As it comes in contact with any cool surface it get condensed and heat is released from water. This heat is taken by surface it comes in contact with. Heat goes on penetrating deeper layers of object. Steam and air move in vertical direction and the movement is quicker penetration of steam into the material, it is also better, if articles are placed vertically in autoclave.

Advantages

♦ It is economical.

♦ Penetration is good.

♦ Cycle time is short.

♦ It is monitored easily.

♦ No exhaust or special chemicals are to be required.

Disadvantages

♦ Carbon steel gets damaged.

♦ Moisture retention is present.

Q.4. Write short note on methods of sterilization of dental instrument. *(Aug 2012, 5 Marks)*

Ans.

Methods for Sterilization of a Dental Instrument

♦ Placing the instrument presoaking solutions, i.e., phenolic compounds prevents drying of debris and also helps in microbial killing.

♦ Autoclaving is the most accepted method of sterilization of surgical instruments as it eliminates bacteria, viruses, fungi and spores. It works on the principle of steam under pressure of 15 lb at 121°C for 20 minutes or 30 lb at 134°C for 3 minutes. It has excellent penetration, facilitating exposure of all instrument surfaces to the steam.

♦ Dry heat ovens or the unsaturated chemical vapor sterilizers are the other means of sterilization. Hot air ovens require 160°C and 2 hours for sterilization.

♦ Ultraviolet light may kill microorganisms that are directly exposed to the light; however, the light may not reach all the surface of an instrument. A temperature of 160°C–170°C maintained for l hour is capable of sterilization.

♦ Glass bead sterilizers are used to sterilize endodontic files and burs in beads. They require 10 seconds for sterilization.

Q.5. Write briefly on chemical sterilization.

(Jan 2016, 2 Marks)

Ans. Chemical sterilization is also known as cold sterilization.

Following are the various chemicals used in chemical sterilization:

Name of chemical	Target	Mechanism of action	Materials sterilized
Glutaraldehyde	Cell wall or outer membrane of bacteria	• In gram-positive bacteria and fungi crosslinking of protein occur • In gram-negative bacteria, there is removal of magnesium and there is release of some phospholipids • In virus, there is inhibition of DNA synthesis	Corrugated rubber, anesthetic tubes, plastic endotracheal tubes, metal instruments and polythene tubing
Formaldehyde	DNA of bacteria	It reacts with carboxyl and sulfhydryl groups. Hydroxyl group also reacts with nucleic acid and inhibit RNA and DNA synthesis by crosslinking proteins	Operation theaters
Chlorhexidine and quaternary ammonium compounds	Cytoplasmic membrane of bacteria	It causes membrane damage which involves phospholipid bilayers. Low concentration of this affect membrane integrity and high concentration leads to congealing of cytoplasm	For preparation of skin for surgery
Phenols	Cytoplasmic membrane of bacteria	It leads to leakage of potassium and other intercellular constituents. It also causes uncoupling of oxidative phosphorylation which leads to irreversible cell damage.	For disinfecting the surfaces
Halogens, i.e., chlorine and iodine	DNA of bacteria	It causes DNA synthesis	For preparation of skin for surgery

Q.6. Write difference between sterilization and disinfection. *(Apr 2017, 2 Marks)*

Ans.

Sterilization	Disinfection
Sterilization is a process by which articles are freed of all microorganisms both in vegetative and spore state.	It is the process of removal of pathogenic microorganisms to the level where it can no more cause disease.
Not applicable to living tissue	Applicable to inanimate objects
Agents used for sterilization are known as sterilants	Agents used for disinfection are known as disinfectants
Examples of methods of sterilization are sunlight, drying, heating, radiation and filtration	Examples of disinfectants are phenols, halogens, aldehydes, oxidizing agents, etc.
It is sporicidal	It is not sporicidal
It includes both physical and chemical methods	It includes mainly chemical methods and some of radiation methods
It is a well-defined process strictly done under proper quality control	It does not require any strict protocol
This method guarantee total control in preventing infection	It never assures complete prevention from acquiring the infection

29. UPPER LIMB ISCHEMIA

Q.1. Write short note on cervical rib. *(Sep 2009, 5 Marks)*

Ans. This is an extra rib present in the neck in about 1–2% of the population.

♦ Commonly, unilateral and in some cases, it is bilateral.
♦ It is more frequently encountered on the right side.
♦ It is the anterior tubercle of the transverse process of the 7th cervical vertebra which attains excessive development and results in cervical rib.

Types of Cervical Rib

♦ *Type I:* Free end of the cervical rib is expanded into a hard, bony mass which can be felt in the neck.
♦ *Type II:* Complete cervical rib extends from C7 vertebra posteriorly to the manubrium anteriorly.
♦ *Type III:* Incomplete cervical rib, which is partly bony, partly fibrous.
♦ *Type IV:* A complete fibrous band which gives rise to symptoms but cannot be diagnosed by X-ray.

Clinical Features

♦ It is common in young females.
♦ Dull aching pain in the neck is caused by expanded bony end of cervical rib.
♦ Upper limb ischemia is usually present.
♦ Ulnar nerve paralysis or weakness manifest as paralysis, of interosseous muscles.
♦ A hard mass may be movable or visible or palpable in neck.

♦ On palpation a thrill and on auscultation, a bruit can be heard in cases of poststenotic dilatation.

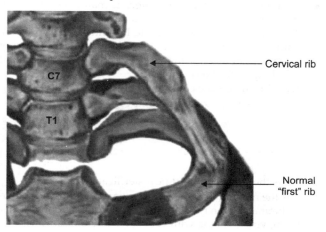

Fig. 41: Types of cervical rib.

Differential Diagnosis

♦ *Cervical spondylosis:* This should be considered as a possibility in patients above the age of 40 years.
♦ *Cervical disc protrusion and spinal cord tumors:* May mimic cervical rib with predominant neurological feature.
♦ Carpal tunnel syndrome can occur due to various causes, such as myxoedema, rheumatoid arthritis, etc. Predominant features of median nerve involvement, more so in menopausal women gives a clue to the diagnosis.
♦ Raynaud's phenomenon.

Treatment

♦ *Conservative:* Patients with mild neurological symptoms are managed by shoulder girdle exercises or correction of faulty posture.
♦ *Surgery:*
   • Excision of cervical rib including periosteum: This is called extraperiosteal excision of cervical rib. This is included with cervical sympathectomy, if vascular symptoms are predominant.
   • If there is a thrombus in the subclavian artery, it is explored and thrombus is removed and the artery is repaired.
   • At exploration, if cervical rib is not found, divide scalenus anterior muscle. This is called scalenotomy.
   • If hyperabduction syndrome is diagnosed, pectoralis minor is divided from its insertion into the coracoid process.

30. RECTUM AND ANAL CANAL

Q.1. Write short note on Goodsall's rule. *(Nov 2008, 5 Marks)*

Ans. It is also known as Goodsall's (1900) rule.

Goodsall's Rule

♦ Fistulas with an external opening in relation to the anterior half of the anus is of direct type.

♦ Fistulas with external openings in relation to posterior half of the anus, has a curved track may be of horseshoe type, opens in the midline posteriorly and may present with multiple external opening all connected to a single internal opening.

♦ Per rectal (P/R) examination shows indurated internal opening usually in the midline posteriorly.

♦ Most of the fistulas are on posterior half of anus.

♦ Probing in the ward and fistulogram in the ward before surgery using Lipiodol is not advisable as it may cause recrudescence of inflammation. It can be done with adequate precaution. Probing is done under general anesthesia gently with care without creating extensions.

31. MISCELLANEOUS

Q.1. Write short note on Sushruta. *(Feb 2015, 5 Marks)*

Ans. Sushruta, one of the earliest surgeons of the recorded history (600 BC) is believed to be the first individual to describe plastic surgery.

♦ Sushruta who lived nearly 150 years before Hippocrates vividly described the basic principles of plastic surgery in his famous ancient treatise Sushruta Samhita.

♦ He is dubbed as the "Founding Father of Surgery" and the Sushruta Samhita is identified as one of the best and outstanding commentary on Medical Sciences of Surgery.

♦ He is said to have been a physician originally of South India active in Varanasi.

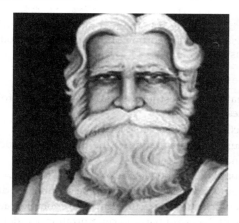

Fig. 42: Sushruta.

♦ His period is usually placed between the period of 1200–600 BC.

♦ One of the earliest known mention of the name is from the Bower Manuscript (4th or 5th century), where Sushruta is listed as one of the ten sages residing in the Himalayas.

♦ Sushruta has described surgery under eight heads Chedya (excision), Lekhya (scarification), Vedhya (puncturing), Esya (exploration), Ahrya (extraction), Vsraya (evacuation) and Sivya (suturing).

♦ The Sushruta Samhita, in its extent form, in 184 chapters contains descriptions of 1,120 illnesses, 700 medicinal plants, 64 preparations from mineral sources and 57 preparations based on animal sources.

♦ The text discusses surgical techniques of making incisions, probing, extraction of foreign bodies, alkali and thermal cauterization, tooth extraction, excisions, etc.

♦ The Sushruta's contribution in the field of Plastic Surgery can be enumerated as follows:

  • Rhinoplasty (cheek)

  • Classification of mutilated earlobe defects and techniques for repair of torn earlobes (15 different types of otoplasties)

  • Cheek flap for reconstruction of absent ear lobe.

  • Repair of accidental lip injuries and congenital cleft lip.

  • Piercing children's ear lobe with a needle or awl.

  • Use of suture materials of bark, tendon, hair and silk.

  • Needles of bronze or bone (circular, two finger-breadths wide and straight, triangular bodied, three finger - breadths wide)

  • Classification of burns into four degrees and explaining the effect of heat stroke, frostbite, and lightening injuries.

  • Fourteen types of bandaging capable of covering almost all the regions of the body and different methods of dressings with various medicaments.

  • Use of wine to dull the pain of surgical incisions.

  • Described 20 varieties of sharp instruments (sastra) and 101 types of blunt instruments (yantra) and their handling techniques.

  • Systematic dissection of cadavers.

  • Advocated the practice of mock operations on inanimate objects, such as watermelons, clay plots and reeds.

  • Use of leeches to keep wounds free of blood clots.

  • A code of ethics for teachers as well as students.

Q.2. Write short note on surveyor. *(Apr 2015, 3 Marks)*

Ans. Surveyor is the one of the member of trauma team. Surveyor are of two types, i.e., primary surveyor and secondary surveyor.

Primary Surveyor (Surgical Resident)

♦ Performs the primary survey, relaying all pertinent findings to the team.

♦ May perform the secondary survey, relaying all pertinent findings to the team.

♦ Performs or assists in the performance of any life-saving procedures at the direction of the team leader.

Secondary Surveyor (Surgical Resident or Intern)

♦ Assists with the "exposure" aspect of the primary survey and applies warm blankets.

♦ May perform the secondary survey, relaying all pertinent findings to the team.

♦ Performs or assists in the performance of any life-saving procedures at the direction of the team leader.

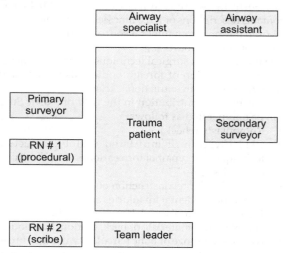

Fig. 43: Various members which comprises of trauma team and their position with respect to traumatically injured patient.

Surveying in Maxillofacial Injuries

Primary Survey

♦ Identify the airway compromise from fracture or hemorrhage.

♦ Bilateral anterior fractures of mandible have risk of falling back of tongue.

♦ Orotracheal intubation should be needed.

♦ By help of mouth props and epistaxis balloons hemorrhage should be controlled.

♦ Anterior and posterior nasal packing can be needed.

Secondary Survey

♦ Orbital rim, zygomatic arches and mandible should be palpated to identify fractures.

♦ Eyes should be examined: Restricted eye movement is suggestive of orbital fracture.

♦ Subconjunctival hemorrhage can be suggestive of fracture of skull.

♦ Proptosis and ophthalmoplegia can be suggestive of retrobulbar hemorrhage.

♦ Sensation should be assessed in maxillary branch of trigeminal nerve.

♦ Check intracanthal distance which should be 30–35 mm. If distance is more than mentioned range, it is suggestive of nasoethmoid fracture.

♦ Intraoral examination is necessary. Assess the occlusion and intraoral hematomas.

Q.3. Write briefly on Louis Pasteur. *(Jan 2016, 2 Marks)*

Ans. Louis Pasteur was a French chemist and microbiologist renowned for his discoveries of the principles of vaccination, microbial fermentation and pasteurization.

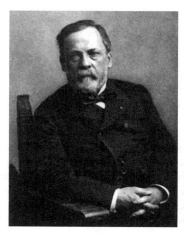

Fig. 44: Louis Pasteur.

♦ He is remembered for his remarkable breakthroughs in the causes and preventions of diseases, and his discoveries have saved countless lives ever since.

♦ He reduced mortality from puerperal fever, and created the first vaccines for rabies and anthrax. His medical discoveries provided direct support for the germ theory of disease and its application in clinical medicine.

♦ He is best known to the general public for his invention of the technique of treating milk and wine to stop bacterial contamination, a process now called pasteurization.

♦ He is regarded as one of the three main founders of bacteriology, together with Ferdinand Cohn and Robert Koch, and is popularly known as the "Father of Microbiology"

Q.4. Write short note on local anesthesia.

(June 2014, 5 Marks) (Sep 2018, 5 Marks)

Ans. Local anesthesia is defined as a condition of loss of pain sensation over a portion of the anatomy without loss of consciousness.

Properties of Local Anestheisa

The ideal local anesthetic should possess the following properties:

♦ Its action must be reversible.

♦ It must be non-irritating to the tissues and produces no secondary local reaction.

♦ It should have a low degree of systemic toxicity.

♦ It should have a rapid onset and be of sufficient duration.

♦ It should have potency sufficient to give complete anesthesia without the use of harmful concentration solution.

♦ It should have sufficient penetrating properties to be effective as a topical anesthetic.

♦ It should be relatively free from producing allergic reactions.

♦ It should be stable in solution and undergo biotransformation readily within the body.

♦ It should be either sterile or capable of being sterilized by heat without deterioration.

Techniques of Local Anesthesia

♦ **Surface anesthesia:** Local anesthetic spray is applied by spray, solution or cream to skin or the mucus membrane.

♦ **Infiltration anesthesia:** Local anesthetic is injected in tissue which is to be anesthetized. Both surface as well as infiltration anesthesia makes up topical anesthesia.

♦ **Field block:** Subcutaneous injection of local anesthetic agent is given in area which borders the field to be anesthetized.

♦ **Peripheral nerve block:** Local anesthesia is given in vicinity of peripheral nerve to anesthetize nerve's area, of innervations.

♦ **Plexus anesthesia:** Local anesthesia is given in vicinity of plexus of nerve, often inside the tissue compartment which limits diffusion of drug away from site of injection.

♦ **Epidural anesthesia:** In this local anesthetic solution is injected in the epidural space where it acts primarily on spinal nerve roots. Depending on site of anesthesia and volume injected, anesthetized area varies from limited areas of abdomen or chest to large regions of body.

♦ **Spinal anesthesia:** It is given at lumbar spine in CSF where it acts on spinal nerve root and at the part of spinal cord. Anesthesia occurs from legs to abdomen or chest.

♦ **Regional anesthesia:** In this method, circulation of blood over a limb is interrupted by tourniquet, than large volume of local anesthetic is injected into the peripheral vein. Now the drug fills the venous system of limb and diffuses in the tissues where peripheral nerves and nerve endings anesthetize. Effect of anesthesia is limited to the area which gets excluded from blood circulation and resolves as circulation is restored.

Uses of Local Anesthesia

♦ *In dentistry:* Surface or infiltration anesthesia is used during restorative procedures or extractions. Regional nerve blocks are used in oral surgical procedures.

♦ *Ophthalmic surgeries:* Surface anesthesia and topical anesthetics are used. In eyes, retrobulbar block can also be given.

♦ *In head and neck surgery:* Field block, peripheral nerve block and plexus anesthesia is used.

♦ *During heart and lung surgeries:* Epidural anesthesia is combined with the general anesthesia.

♦ *In abdominal surgery:* Epidural or spinal anesthesia is combined with the general anesthesia.

♦ *In gynecological and urological procedures:* Spinal or epidural anesthesia is given.

♦ *In skin and peripheral vascular surgery:* Topical anesthesia, field block, peripheral nerve block or epidural anesthesia can be given.

Complications of Local Anesthesia

♦ *Local complications*
  • Needle breakage
  • Paresthesia
  • Facial nerve paralysis
  • Trismus
  • Hematoma
  • Burning on giving injection
  • Infection
  • Edema
  • Soft tissue injury
  • Sloughing of tissues
  • Postanesthetic intraoral lesion

♦ *Systemic complications:*
  • Toxicity
  • Idiosyncrasy
  • Allergy
  • Anaphylactic reactions.

Q.5. Write short answer on sequelae of inflammation.

(Apr 2018, 3 Marks)

Ans. The inflammatory process can culminate into one of the following outcomes;

♦ *Resolution:* It means complete return to normal tissue following acute inflammation. This occurs when tissue changes are slight and the cellular changes are reversible e. g. resolution in lobar pneumonia.

♦ *Healing:* Healing by fibrosis takes place when the tissue destruction in acute inflammation is extensive so that there is no tissue regeneration. But when tissue loss is superficial, it is restored by regeneration.

♦ *Suppuration:* When the pyogenic bacteria causing acute inflammation result in severe tissue necrosis, the process progresses to suppuration. Initially, there is intense neutrophilic infiltration. Subsequently, mixture of neutrophils, bacteria, fragments of necrotic tissue, cell debris and fibrin comprise pus which is contained in a cavity to form an abscess. The abscess, if not drained, may get organized by dense fibrous tissue, and in time, get calcified.

♦ *Chronic inflammation:* Persisting or recurrent acute inflammation may progress to chronic inflammation in which the processes of inflammation and healing proceed side by side.

Q.6. What are the side effects of steroids?

(Sep 2018, 5 Marks)

Ans. Following are the side effects of steroids:

♦ **Cushing's habitus:** Abnormal fat distribution which leads to characteristic appearance with rounded face, narrow mouth, supraclavicular hump, obesity of trunk with relatively thin limbs.

♦ **Fragile skin and purple striae:** Present typically on thighs and lower abdomen, easy bruising, telangiectasis, hirsutism. Cutaneous atrophy localized to the site occurs with topical application as well.

♦ **Hyperglycemia:** It may be glycosuria, precipitation of diabetes.

♦ **Muscular weakness:** Proximal (shoulder, arm, pelvis, thigh) muscles are primarily affected. Myopathy occurs occasionally, warrants withdrawal of the corticoids.

♦ **Susceptibility to infection:** Long-term therapy with steroids leads to flare up of opportunistic infections, such as viral, fungal and bacterial.

- **Delayed healing:** There is delayed healing of wounds and surgical incisions.
- **Peptic ulceration:** Risk is doubled; bleeding and silent perforation of ulcers may occur. Dyspeptic symptoms are frequent with high dose therapy.
- **Osteoporosis:** Especially involving vertebrae and other flat spongy bones. Compression fractures of vertebrae and spontaneous fracture of long bones can occur, especially in the elderly.
- **Avascular necrosis:** Avascular necrosis of head of femur, humerus, or knee joint is an occasional abrupt onset complication of high dose corticosteroid therapy.
- **Eye:** Posterior subcapsular cataract may develop after several years of use, especially in children. Glaucoma may develop in susceptible individuals after prolonged topical therapy.
- **Growth retardation:** It occurs in children even with small doses if given for long periods. Large doses do inhibit growth hormone secretion, but growth retardation may, in addition, be a direct cellular effect of corticoids. Recombinant growth hormone given concurrently can prevent growth retardation, but risk/benefit of such use is not known.
- **Psychiatric disturbances:** Presence of mild euphoria frequently accompanies high dose steroid treatment. This may rarely progress to manic psychosis. Nervousness, decreased sleep and mood changes occur in some patients. Rarely, a depressive illness may be induced after long-term use.
- **Suppression of hypothalamo-pituitary-adrenal (HPA) axis:** This occurs depending both on dose and duration of therapy. In time, adrenal cortex atrophies and stoppage of exogenous steroid precipitates withdrawal syndrome consisting of malaise, fever, anorexia, nausea, postural hypotension, electrolyte imbalance, weakness, pain in muscles and joints and reactivation of the disease for which they were used. Subjected to stress, these patients may go into acute adrenal insufficiency leading to cardiovascular collapse.

Q.7. Enumerate the antitubercular drugs.

(Sep 2018, 5 Marks)

Ans.

- **First line:** These drugs have high antitubercular efficacy as well as low toxicity and are used routinely. The first line drugs are isoniazid, streptomycin, rifampin, pyrazinamide, ethambutol.
- **Second line:** These drugs have low antitubercular efficacy or high toxicity or both and are used in special circumstances. The second line drugs used are thiacetazone, para-amino salicylic acid, ethionamide, cycloserine, kanamycin, amekacin, capeomycin.
- **Newer drugs:** Ciprofloxacin, ofloxacin, clarithromycin, azithromycin, rifabutin.

Q.8. Write short note on role of thymus on our body.

(Sep 2018, 5 Marks)

Ans. T cell develops from pre-T cell. The thymus is the site for T cell development. The epithelial cells play an important role in the development of bone marrow-derived prethymic cells into mature T cells.

Role in Lymphopoiesis

The role of the thymus in lymphopoiesis is significant.

- Stem cells from bone marrow that reach the superficial part of the cortex divide repeatedly to form smaller lymphocytes.
- It has been proposed that during these mitoses, the DNA of the lymphocytes undergoes numerous random mutations, as a result of which different lymphocytes acquire the ability to recognize a very large number of different proteins and to react to them.
- As it is not desirable for lymphocytes to react against the body's own proteins, all lymphocytes that would react against them are destroyed. It is for this reason that 90% of lymphocytes formed in the thymus are destroyed within three to four days.
- The remaining lymphocytes that react only against proteins foreign to the body are thrown into the circulation as circulating, immunologically competent T lymphocytes. They lodge themselves in secondary lymph organs, such as lymph nodes, spleen, etc., where they multiply to form further T lymphocytes of their own type when exposed to the appropriate antigen.

Thymus as a Primary Lymphoid Organ

Thymus is regarded as a primary lymphoid organ along with bone marrow.

- It has been observed that, within the thymus, lymphocytes are not allowed to come into contact with foreign antigens, because of the presence of the blood-thymic barrier. It has also been stated that because of this thymocytes do not develop into large lymphocytes or into plasma cells, and do not form lymphatic nodules.
- Recently, it has been postulated that the medulla of the thymus (or part of it) is a separate "compartment". After thymocytes move into this compartment they probably come into contact with antigens presented to them through dendritic macrophages. Such contact may be necessary step in making T lymphocytes competent to distinguish between foreign antigens and proteins of the body itself.
- The proliferation of T lymphocytes and their conversion into cells capable of reacting to antigens, probably takes place under the influence of hormones produced by epithelial cells of the thymus. T lymphocytes are also influenced by direct cell contact with epitheliocytes. Hormones produced by the thymus may also influence lymphopoiesis in peripheral lymphoid organs. This influence appears to be especially important in early life, as lymphoid tissues do not develop normally if the thymus is removed.
- Thymectomy has much less influence after puberty as the lymphoid tissues have fully developed by then.

Endocrine Role of Thymus

A number of hormones produced by the thymus have now been identified as follows:

- *Thymulin:* Thymulin enhances the function of various types of T cell, especially that of suppressor cells.
- *Thymopoietin:* Thymopoietin stimulates the production of cytotoxic T cells. The combined action of thymulin and thymopoietin allows precise balance of the activity of cytotoxic and suppressor cells.
- *Thymosin:* Thymosin α-1 stimulates lymphocyte production and also the production of antibodies. Thymosin β-4 is produced by mononuclear phagocytes.
- Thymic humoral factor controls the multiplication of helper and suppressor T cells.

Q.9. Enumerate the branches of external carotid artery.

(Sep 2018, 5 Marks)

Ans. It gives off 8 branches which are:

Anteriorly

- Superior thyroid artery
- Lingual artery
- Facial artery

Posteriorly

- Occipital artery
- Posterior auricular artery

Medially

Ascending pharyngeal artery.

Terminally

- Maxillary artery.
- Superficial temporal artery.

MULTIPLE CHOICE QUESTIONS

As per DCI and Examination Papers of Various Universities

1 Mark Each

1. Adamantinoma or ameloblastoma may be seen in all, *except*:
   a. Odontogenic epithelium
   b. Femur bone
   c. Tibia bone
   d. Stalk of pituitary

2. The most common tumor in the minor salivary gland, which spreads through neural sheath is:
   a. Acinar cell carcinoma
   b. Adenoid cystic carcinoma
   c. Mucoepidermoid carcinoma
   d. Pleomorphic adenoma

3. In submandibular gland surgery, the nerve least likely to be injured is:
   a. Hypoglossal nerve
   b. Lingual nerve
   c. Inferior alveolar nerve
   d. Mandibular branch of facial nerve

4. Hyperparathyroidism is characterized by the following, *except*:
   a. Generalized osteoporosis
   b. Osteosclerosis
   c. Hypercalcemia
   d. Renal calculus

5. True about Warthin tumor of salivary gland is:
   a. Malignant neoplasm
   b. Rapidly growing tumor
   c. Gives a "Hot" pertechnetate scan
   d. Gives a "Cold" pertechnetate scan

6. In fracture, mandible osteosynthesis or rigid fixation is done by all, *except*:
   a. Bone grafting
   b. Miniplates
   c. Leg screws
   d. Arch bar

7. The cleft lip is best repaired at the age of:
   a. 5 months
   b. One year of age
   c. 6–8 years of age
   d. At puberty

8. Sjögren's syndrome is characterized by all, *except*:
   a. Xerostomia
   b. Keratoconjunctivitis
   c. Rheumatic arthritis
   d. Enlargement of salivary gland

9. The X-ray of jaw shows "Honeycomb" appeerence, the diagnosis is:
   a. Granulomatous epulis
   b. Osteoclastoma
   c. Ameloblastoma
   d. Dentigerous cyst

10. The most common cause of thyroiditis is:
    a. Riedle's thyroiditis
    b. Hashimoto's thyroiditis
    c. Subacute thyroiditis
    d. Cervicofacial actinomycosis

11. The skin grafting is not done in infection with:
    a. *Pseudomonas*
    b. *E. coli*
    c. β-hemolyticus streptococci
    d. Staphylococci

12. The most common presenting complaint of medullary carcinoma of thyroid is:
    a. Diarrhea
    b. Dysphagia
    c. Flushing
    d. Hoarseness of voice

13. What is the advantage of chromic catgut over plain catgut suture in deep wounds?
    a. Greater strength
    b. Greater ease to use
    c. Delayed resorption
    d. Less tissue reaction

14. An allograft is transfer of tissue between:
    a. Sister to brother
    b. Unrelated donor
    c. Same individual
    d. Monozygotic twins

15. Hyperparathyroidism is characterized by following, *except*:
    a. Generalized osteoporosis
    b. Hypercalcemia
    c. Osteosclerosis
    d. Renal stone formation

Answers:

1. b. Femur Bone	2. b. Adenoid cystic...	3. c. Inferior alveolar...	4. b. Osteosclerosis
5. c. Gives a "Hot"...	6. a. Bone grafting	7. a. 5 months	8. d. Enlargement of...
9. c. Ameloblastoma	10. b. Hashimoto's...	11. c. β-hemolyticus...	12. a. Diarrhea
13. d. Less tissue...	14. a. Sister to brother	15. c. Osteosclerosis	

16. Ameloblastoma may be seen in all, *except*:
    a. Jaws
    b. Pituitary stalk
    c. Tibia
    d. Hip bone

17. The papillary carcinoma of thyroid having all, *except*:
    a. Most common thyroid cancer
    b. Psammoma bodies seen
    c. Encapsulated
    d. Blood borne metastasis is common

18. In cleft lip operation, all the stitches are removed on:
    a. 2nd day
    b. 4th–5th day
    c. 10th day
    d. 14th day

19. A patient presents with neck swelling and respiratory distress few hours after thyroidectomy, the next management would be:
    a. Open immediately
    b. Tracheostomy
    c. Wait and watch
    d. Oxygen by mask

20. In facial injury with voluntary control lost over tongue, the best emergency treatment to prevent tongue from falling back is by:
    a. Definitive treatment
    b. Oropharyngeal airway
    c. Towel clipping of tongue
    d. Deep traction suture of tongue

21. Skin is best:
    a. Dressing
    b. Cosmetic
    c. Layer
    d. Cover

22. Tissue is best
    a. Antibiotic
    b. Antiseptic
    c. Meat
    d. Culture

23. Rh-incompatibility in pregnant woman causes:
    a. Neonatal jaundice
    b. Placenta previa
    c. Hydrops fetalis
    d. Acute renal failure

24. Hemophilia is due to congenital deficiency of:
    a. Factor III
    b. Factor VII
    c. Factor IX
    d. Factor VIII

25. Hepatitis B virus is:
    a. DNA virus
    b. RNA virus
    c. Flavi virus
    d. Incomplete RNA virus

26. Edge of a malignant ulcer is:
    a. Raised
    b. Undermined
    c. Sloping
    d. Everted

27. Most rapid diagnosis of tuberculosis can be done with:
    a. Polymerase chain reaction
    b. ZN staining
    c. Bacterial culture
    d. Tuberculin test

28. Most suitable antibiotic in gas gangrene is:
    a. Cloxacillin
    b. Penicillin
    c. Gentamicin
    d. 3rd generation cephalosporin

29. Most ancient plastic surgery was performed in:
    a. Greece
    b. Rome
    c. Egypt
    d. India

30. HIV-1 virus is considerably less infective than Hepatitis-B:
    a. True
    b. False

31. FNAC is useful in all thyroid carcinomas, *except*:
    a. Papillary
    b. Follicular
    c. Medullary
    d. Anaplastic

32. The open methods of reduction and immobilization of fracture body of mandible are all, *except*:
    a. Miniplates
    b. Transosseous wiring
    c. Lag screws
    d. Arch bar

33. Hormones produced by medullary carcinoma of thyroid are:
    a. Calcitonin
    b. Prostaglandins
    c. Serotonin
    d. All a, b and c
    e. None

Answers:
16. d. Hip bone	17. d. Blood borne	18. b. 4th–5th day	19. b. Tracheostomy
20. c. Towel clipping...	21. d. Cover	22. b. Antiseptic	23. c. Hydrops fetalis
24. c. Factor IX	25. a. DNA virus	26. d. Everted	27. b. ZN staining
28. b. Penicillin	29. d. India	30. a. True	31. b. Follicular
32. b. Transosseous...	33. a. Calcitonin		

34. A patient with a fistula and chronic pus discharge from lower face and mandible is most commonly suffering from:
    a. Dental cyst
    b. Vincent angina
    c. Ludwig angina
    d. Actinomycosis

35. Axonotmesis is:
    a. Rupture of nerve fibers in an intact sheath
    b. Rupture of nerve sheath only
    c. Rupture of nerve fibers and nerve sheath
    d. Physiological paralysis of nerve fibers

36. 'Tetany' is caused by all, *except*:
    a. Hypoparathyroidism
    b. Rickets
    c. Osteomalacia
    d. Hyperparathyroidism

37. The most common tumor of minor salivary gland is:
    a. Mucoepidermoid
    b. Acinic cell carcinoma
    c. Adenoid cystic carcinoma
    d. Pleomorphic adenocarcinoma

38. The most common site of thyroglossal cyst is:
    a. Suprahyoid
    b. Subhyoid
    c. Floor of mouth
    d. At the level of cricoid cartilage

39. Common type of cleft lip is:
    a. Mid line
    b. Unilateral
    c. Bilateral
    d. Cleft lip combined with cleft palate

40. Immediate management of a patient with multiple fracture and fluid loss includes the infusion:
    a. Blood
    b. Dextran
    c. Normal saline
    d. Ringer lactate

41. What is cognizable medicolegal situation?
    a. Fracture
    b. Abrasion
    c. Ecchymosis

42. Surgical incision heal by:
    a. First intension
    b. Second intension

43. Sulfur granules are seen in pus of:
    a. Carbuncle
    b. Abscess
    c. Actinomycosis
    d. Erysipelas

44. Tourniquet is the best treatment for bleeding venous ulcer in lower limb:
    a. True
    b. False

45. Normally, cyst is diagnosed by eliciting fluctuation test:
    a. True
    b. False

46. Hypertrophied scar usually is result of healing by:
    a. Second intension
    b. First intension

47. Hemophilia is transferred genetically by:
    a. Autosomes
    b. Sex chromosomes
    c. Mitochondria
    d. Golgi complex

48. Involvement of lymph nodes by secondaries from a cancer is:
    a. Stoney hard
    b. Soft
    c. Firm
    d. Fluctuant

49. The edge of tubercular ulcer is:
    a. Everted
    b. Raised
    c. Undermined
    d. Sloping

50. Universal blood donor belongs to blood group:
    a. A
    b. B
    c. AB
    d. O

51. Unilateral cleft lip is more common on:
    a. Right side
    b. Left side
    c. Median
    d. None of the above

52. Which type of thyroid cancer has the best prognosis?
    a. Papillary
    b. Follicular
    c. Medullary
    d. Anaplastic

Answers: 34. d. Actinomycosis   35. c. Rupture of nerve...   36. d. Hyperparathyroidism 37. a. Mucoepidermoid
38. b. Subhyoid   39. b. Unilateral   40. d. Ringer lactate   41. a. Fracture
42. a. First intension   43. c. Actinomycosis   44. b. False   45. a. True
46. a. Second intension   47. b. Sex chromosomes   48. a. Stoney hard   49. c. Undermined
50. d. O   51. b. Left side   52. a. Papillary

53. The most common form of actinomycosis is:
    a. Thoracic
    b. Fasciocervical
    c. Liver
    d. Right iliac fossa

54. Radiologically, the 'Honeycomb' appearance is seen in:
    a. *Myeloid epulis*
    b. *Granulomatous epulis*
    c. *Ameloblastoma*
    d. *Dentigerous cyst*

55. Skin grafting is absolutely contraindicated in which infection:
    a. *Staphyloccocus*
    b. *Pseudomonas*
    c. *Proteus*
    d. *Streptococcus hemolyticus*

56. The structure preserved in functional block dissection in papillary carcinoma thyroid are all, *except*:
    a. Sternomastoid muscle
    b. Internal jugular vein
    c. Spinal accessory nerve
    d. Enlarged lymph nodes

57. The swelling in neck moves with deglutition are all, *except*:
    a. Thyroglossal cyst
    b. Subhyoid bursitis
    c. Pretracheal lymph nodes
    d. Branchial cyst

58. Highly transilluminated, cystic and compressible swelling in posterior triangle of neck is:
    a. Cystic hygroma
    b. Branchial cyst
    c. Thyroglossal cyst
    d. Dermoid cyst

59. Recurrent laryngeal nerve is in close relation or associated with:
    a. Superior thyroid artery
    b. Inferior thyroid artery
    c. Superior thyroid vein
    d. Inferior thyroid vein

60. Advantages of Vicryl suture material over chromic catgut are all, *except*:
    a. Delayed resorption
    b. Less tissue reaction
    c. Greater strength
    d. Cheap then chromic

61. Open methods of treatment of fracture mandible are all, *except*:
    a. Miniplates
    b. Transosseous wiring
    c. Bone plating
    d. Arch bar

62. The cysts containing cholesterol crystals are all, *except*:
    a. Periapical cyst
    b. Dentigerous cyst
    c. Branchial cyst
    d. Dermoid cyst

63. A patient has lacerated untidy wound in leg and attended the casualty after two hours. The wound should be:
    a. Sutured immediately
    b. Debrided and sutured immediately
    c. Debrided and sutured secondarily
    d. Clean and dress only

64. A 80-year-old edentulous patient with midline tumor of lower jaw involving alveolar margin the treatment of choice is:
    a. Hemimandibulectomy
    b. Marginal mandibulectomy
    c. Commando's operation
    d. Segmental mandibulectomy

65. Not a feature of De Quervains disease:
    a. Autoimmune etiology
    b. Increased ESR
    c. Tends to regress spontaneously
    d. Painful and associated with enlargement of thyroid

66. Highest chances of malignancy in oral cavity is due to:
    a. Leukoplakia
    b. Lichen planus
    c. Erythroplakia
    d. Aphthous ulcers

67. Which of the following causes maximum bleeding?
    a. Partial arterial tear
    b. Complete arterial tear
    c. Artery caught between fractured ends of bone
    d. Intimal tear

68. All are the pulsating swellings, *except*:
    a. Plexiform hemangioma
    b. Carotid aneurysm
    c. Primary thyrotoxicosis
    d. Sternomastoid tumors

Answers: 53. b. Fasciocervical   54. c. Ameloblastoma   55. d. *Streptococcus*...   56. d. Enlarged lymph...
57. d. Branchial cyst   58. a. Cystic hygroma   59. b. Inferior thyroid artery 60. a. Delayed resorption
61. d. Arch bar   62. a. Periapical cyst   63. b. Debrided and...   64. d. Segmental...
65. a. Autoimmune...   66. c. Erythroplakia   67. a. Partial arterial tear   68. d. Sternomastoid...

69. Early multiple painful ulcers on tongue are seen in all, *except*:
    a. Aphthous ulcers
    b. Carcinomatous ulcer
    c. Tubercular
    d. Herpes

70. Incisional or open biopsy should not be taken from all, *except*:
    a. Malignant melanoma
    b. Parotid gland
    c. Tongue and cheek
    d. Thyroid gland

71. Admantinoma or ameloblastoma may be seen in all, *except*:
    a. Odontogenic epithelium
    b. Femur bone
    c. Tibia bone
    d. Stalk of pituitary

72. The X-ray of jaw shows 'honeycomb' appearance:
    a. Granulomatous epulis
    b. Osteoclastoma
    c. Ameloblastoma
    d. Dentigerous cyst

73. In fracture mandible osteosynthesis or rigid fixation is done by all, *except*:
    a. Bone grafting
    b. Miniplates
    c. Leg screw
    d. Arch bar

74. The most common site of thyroglossal cyst is:
    a. Suprahyoid
    b. Subhyoid
    c. Floor of the mouth
    d. At the level of cricoids cartilage

75. The papillary carcinoma thyroid is having all, *except*:
    a. Most common thyroid cancer
    b. Psammoma bodies are seen
    c. Encapsulated
    d. Blood-borne metastasis is common

76. In cleft lip operation all stitches after operation are removed on:
    a. 3rd day
    b. 4th–5th day
    c. 10th day
    d. 14th day

77. A 14-year-old child presented with progressive cervical lymph node enlargement since 3 month. The diagnosis can be achieved by:
    a. X-ray soft tissues of neck
    b. CBP ESR
    c. Lymph node biopsy
    d. CT scan of neck

78. Structure preserved in modified radical neck dissection in:
    a. Internal jugular vein
    b. Sternomastoid muscle
    c. XI nerve
    d. X nerve

79. Advantages of vicryl suture material over chromic catgut are all, *except*:
    a. Delayed resorption
    b. Less tissue reaction
    c. Greater strength
    d. Cheaper than chromic

80. The swelling in neck moves with deglutition are all, *except*:
    a. Thyroglossal cyst
    b. Subhyoid bursa
    c. Pretracheal lymph nodes
    d. Branchial cyst

81. Hand of surgeon can be rendered aseptic by washing:
    a. True
    b. False

82. Biopsy can be taken with as needle:
    a. True
    b. False

83. Abscess should always be sutured closed after drainage:
    a. True
    b. False

84. Skin should not be sutured by nonabsorbable sutures:
    a. True
    b. False

85. Heat sensitive surgical items can be best sterilized in a well-equipped OT by:
    a. Formalin chambers
    b. 2% glutaraldehyde
    c. Ethylene oxide
    d. Ionizing radiation

86. One of the following is an example of painless midline neck swelling:
    a. Branchial cyst
    b. Thyroglossal cyst
    c. Cystic hygroma
    d. Carotid body tumor

Answers: 69. b. Carcinomatous...   70. c. Tongue and cheek   71. d. Stalk of pituitary   72. c. Ameloblastoma
73. a. Bone grafting   74. b. Subhyoid   75. d. Blood-borne...   76. b. 4th to 5th day
77. c. Lymph node...   78. c. XI nerve   79. a. Delayed resorption   80. c. Pretracheal lymph...
81. b. False   82. a. True   83. a. True   84. b. False
85. c. Ethylene oxide   86. b. Thyroglossal cyst

87. Jaw tumors associated with unerupted tooth is:
    a. Dental cyst
    b. Dentigerous cyst
    c. Admantinoma
    d. Giant cell granuloma

88. Hyperparathyroidism is characterized by the following, *except*:
    a. Generalized osteoporosis
    b. Osteosclerosis
    c. Hypercalcemia
    d. Renal calculus

89. The cleft lip is repaired at the age of:
    a. 5 months
    b. 1 year ago
    c. 6–8 years
    d. At puberty

90. Most common cause of thyroiditis is:
    a. Riedel's thyroiditis
    b. Hashimoto's thyroiditis
    c. Subacute thyroiditis
    d. Viral thyroiditis

91. Immediate management of patient with multiple fracture and loss of blood with shock is the infusion of:
    a. Dextrosaline
    b. Dextran
    c. Blood
    d. Ringer's lactate

92. Bone metastasis is common in which type of thyroid cancer:
    a. Medullary
    b. Follicular
    c. Papillary
    d. Anaplastic

93. The most common type of cleft lip is:
    a. Unilateral
    b. Bilateral
    c. Midline
    d. None of the above

94. A patient has wide eyes, nervousness, raised systolic BP and weight loss. Most probable diagnosis is:
    a. Hypothyroidism
    b. Hyperthyroidism
    c. Hyperparathyroidism
    d. Hypoparathyroidism

95. Collar stud abscess occurs in:
    a. Cervical TB lymphadenitis
    b. Peritonsillar abscess

    c. Pyogenic lymphadenitis
    d. Retropharyngeal abscess

96. In long surgical procedure intubation method:
    a. Nasotracheal tube with cuff
    b. LMA
    c. Nasotracheal tube with cuff
    d. Endotracheal tube

97. Knife used for harvesting split thickness skin graft is:
    a. Husson's knife
    b. Bard Parker knife
    c. Humby's knife
    d. Foley's knife

98. Rapid infusion of blood causes:
    a. Acute left heart failure
    b. Pulmonary edema
    c. Ankle edema
    d. Respiratory distress

99. The best vein for total parenteral nutrition is:
    a. Subclavian vein
    b. Femoral
    c. Brachial vein
    d. Saphenous

100. In the blood bank platelets are stored at:
    a. 180°C for 1 year
    b. 2–40°C for 35 days
    c. 20–240°C for 3–5 days
    d. 20–250°C for 35 days

101. The best dressing for open wounds is:
    a. Skin
    b. Amnion
    c. Opsite
    d. Tulle grass

102. Reactionary hemorrhage occurs:
    a. Within 24 hours of surgery
    b. After 48 hours of surgery
    c. After 72 hours of surgery
    d. After 7–14 days of surgery

103. The treatment of choice for stage I cancer larynx:
    a. Radical surgery
    b. Chemotherapy
    c. Radiotherapy
    d. Surgery followed by radiotherapy

104. In an emergency tracheostomy incision is:
    a. Vertical
    b. Oblique
    c. Horizontal
    d. Paramedian

Answers:	87. b. Dentigerous cyst	88. b. Osteosclerosis	89. a. 5 months	90. b. Hashimoto's...
	91. d. Ringer's lactate	92. c. Papillary	93. a. Unilateral	94. b. Hyperthyroidism
	95. a. Cervical TB...	96. d. Endotracheal tube	97. c. Humby's knife	98. b. Pulmonary edema
	99. a. Subclavian vein	100. c. 20–240°C for 3–5...	101. a. Skin	102. a. Within 24 hours...
	103. c. Radiotherapy	104. c. Horizontal		

105. Punched out edge is characteristic of ulcer:
    a. Tuberculosis
    b. Rodent ulcer
    c. Syphilitic
    d. Nonspecific

106. Loss of differentiation of tumor cells is called as:
    a. Metaplasia
    b. Dysplasia
    c. Anaplasia
    d. Hyperplasia

107. The muscle which is resected in classical neck dissection is:
    a. Sternohyoid
    b. Sternomastoid
    c. Sternothyroid
    d. Sternocricoid

108. Painless ulcer of tongue is due to:
    a. Dysplasia
    b. Syphilis
    c. Tuberculosis
    d. None of the above

109. A patient having tumor of maxillary sinus manifest with excessive rolling tears from his eye, likely due to obstruction of:
    a. Nasolacrimal duct
    b. Conjunctival sac
    c. Lacrimal gland
    d. None of the above

110. Basal cell carcinomas:
    a. Usually metastasize to regional lymph nodes
    b. Common on the face and neck
    c. Common in females
    d. Radioresistant

111. All the following are congenital cysts, *except*:
    a. External angular dermoid cyst
    b. Sebaceous cyst
    c. Branchial cyst
    d. Thyroglossal cyst

112. Ranula is a condition which occurs in:
    a. Preauricular area
    b. Nasolabial angle
    c. Medial angle of orbit
    d. Floor of the mouth

113. Commonest premalignant lesion of oral cancer:
    a. Leukoplakia
    b. Syphilitic ulcer
    c. Apthous ulcer
    d. Erythroplakia

114. Undermined edge is the characteristic of:
    a. Rodent
    b. Syphilitic
    c. Tuberculosis
    d. Squamous cell carcinoma

115. Duct of parotid gland is known as:
    a. Stenson's duct
    b. Wharton's duct
    c. Nasolacrimal duct
    d. Bartholin's duct

116. Largest number of lymph nodes are present in which area:
    a. Axilla
    b. Groin
    c. Neck
    d. Abdomen

117. Marjolin's ulcer is:
    a. Wet gangrene
    b. Dry gangrene
    c. Premalignant
    d. Malignant

118. Which of the following is congenital?
    a. Sebaceous cyst
    b. Hypothyroidism
    c. Cystic hygroma
    d. Vincent's angina

119. Bell's palsy occurs due to injury to:
    a. Recurrent laryngeal nerve
    b. Facial nerve
    c. Trigeminal nerve
    d. Ulnar nerve

120. Most common cyst for thyroglossal cyst is:
    a. Suprahyoid
    b. Subhyoid
    c. Level of cricoids
    d. Floor of mouth

121. Which neck swelling moves with swallowing?
    a. Submandibular cyst
    b. Thyroid cyst
    c. Supraclavicular lymph node
    d. Sternomastoid tumor

122. All are true about cystic hygroma, *except*:
    a. Pulsatile
    b. May cause respiratory obstruction
    c. Common in neck
    d. Brilliant translucent

Answers: 105. c. Syphilitic   106. c. Anaplasia   107. b. Sternomastoid   108. a. Dysplasia
109. a. Nasolacrimal duct   110. b. Common on the...   111. b. Sebaceous cyst   112. d. Floor of the...
113. a. Leukoplakia   114. c. Tuberculosis   115. a. Stenson's duct   116. c. Neck
117. d. Malignant   118. c. Cystic hygroma   119. b. Facial nerve   120. b. Subhyoid
121. b. Thyroid cyst   122. a. Pulsatile

123. In management of thyroglossal cyst:
    a. Central portion of hyoid excised
    b. Sternothyroid muscle dissected
    c. Isthmusectomy
    d. Strap muscles excised

124. FNAC is useful in all the following tumors of thyroid, *except*:
    a. Papillary carcinoma
    b. Anaplastic carcinoma
    c. Thyroiditis
    d. Follicular carcinoma

125. Everted edge is characteristic of.............ulcer:
    a. TB
    b. Malignant
    c. Syphilitic
    d. Healing

126. Most common histological type of thyroid carcinoma is:
    a. Medullary type
    b. Follicular type
    c. Papillary type
    d. Anaplastic type

127. There was sudden increase in the size of thyroid swelling along with pain. Most likely cause is:
    a. Malignant change
    b. Nodular goiter
    c. Hemorrhage within the thyroid cyst
    d. Colloid goiter

128. Cystic compressible swelling in the posterior triangle of neck which is translucent is:
    a. Cystic hygroma
    b. Branchial cyst
    c. Thyroglossal cyst
    d. Dermoid cyst

129. Sistrunk's operation is done in:
    a. Parotid tumor
    b. Thyroglossal fistula
    c. Branchial cyst
    d. Cystic hygroma

130. Complications of total thyroidectomy include all, *except*:
    a. Airway obstruction
    b. Hoarsness
    c. Hemorrhage
    d. Hypercalcemia

131. Hyperparathyroidism is characterized by the following, *except*:
    a. Generalized osteoporosis
    b. Renal calculi
    c. Hypercalcemia
    d. Osteosclerosis

132. After thyroidectomy patient developed stridor within two hours. All are likely cause of stridor, *except*:
    a. Hypocalcemia
    b. Recurrent laryngeal nerve palsy
    c. Laryngomalacia
    d. Wound hematoma

133. Which of the following is not the component of Glasgow coma scale?
    a. Eye opening
    b. Motor response
    c. Verbal response
    d. Mini mental status

134. All of the following swellings move with deglutition, *except*:
    a. Subhyoid bursitis
    b. Thyroid nodule
    c. Thyroglossal cyst
    d. Dermoid cyst

135. Treatment of choice for gallbladder stone is:
    a. Lap cholecystectomy
    b. Open cholecystectomy
    c. Cholecystostomy
    d. Partial cholecystectomy

136. Rodent ulcer is a feature of:
    a. Squamous cell carcinoma
    b. Basal cell carcinoma
    c. Malignant melanoma
    d. Venous ulcer

137. Which of the following is not a premalignant condition?
    a. Erythroplakia
    b. Leukoplakia
    c. Lipoma
    d. Bowen's disease

138. A young lady of 19 years presented in ER with the complaint of pain in right iliac fossa associated with nausea and vomiting. On examination she is having tachycardia, raised body temperature, with localized tenderness and guarding in right iliac fossa. The most probable diagnosis is:
    a. Acute cholecystitis
    b. Renal colic
    c. Lymphadenitis
    d. Acute appendicitis

Answers: 123. a. Central portion of ... 124. d. Follicular carcinoma 125. b. Malignant　126. c. Papillary type
127. a. Malignant change　128. a. Cystic hygroma　129. b. Thyroglossal fistula 130. d. Hypercalcemia
131. d. Osteosclerosis　132. a. Hypocalcemia　133. d. Mini mental status　134. d. Dermoid cyst
135. b. Open cholecy...　136. b. Basal cell carcinoma 137. c. Lipoma　138. d. Acute appendicitis

139. With reference to patient in above mentioned question (A young lady of 19 years......). What is the investigation of choice?
    a. X ray abdomen
    b. USG abdomen
    c. CT abdomen
    d. MRI

140. Murphy's triad consists of all, *except*:
    a. Pain
    b. Fever
    c. Jaundice
    d. Vomiting

141. Most common donor site for split thickness skin graft is:
    a. Abdomen
    b. Scalp
    c. Thigh
    d. Shoulder

142. Lateral aberrant thyroid is:
    a. Follicular thyroid carcinoma
    b. Papillary thyroid carcinoma
    c. Metastatic cervical lymph node of papillary thyroid carcinoma
    d. Medullary thyroid carcinoma

143. Which nerve is most likely to be injured during superficial parotidectomy?
    a. Facial nerve
    b. Great auricular nerve
    c. Trigeminal nerve
    d. None of the above

144. All are true for malignant melanoma, *except*:
    a. Caused by UV rays
    b. Never metastasize to regional lymph nodes
    c. Xeroderma pigmentosa increases risk
    d. WLE is treatment of choice

145. Which of the following is not the risk factor for Ca tongue?
    a. Hepatitis B
    b. Smoking
    c. Tobacco
    d. Alcoholism

146. True for keloid is:
    a. Has zero recurrence rate after surgery
    b. Surgery gives better outcome
    c. Can be treated with intralesional corticosteroids
    d. None of the above

147. Post-thyroidectomy immediate life-threatening complication is:
    a. Compressing hematoma
    b. RLN injury
    c. Hypocalcemia
    d. None of the above

148. LeFort fracture is:
    a. Fracture of proximal end of femur
    b. Transfacial fracture of midface
    c. Fracture of distal end of femur
    d. None of the above

149. DVT is a risk factor for:
    a. Pulmonary embolism
    b. Excessive bleeding
    c. Shock
    d. TIA

150. Which of the following has feco-oral route of transmission?
    a. HBV
    b. HPV
    c. HEV
    d. HIV

151. Sterilization of surgical instruments is done by:
    a. Autoclaving
    b. Flaming
    c. Boiling
    d. None of the above

152. Most common cause of food poisoning is:
    a. *Clostridium tetani*
    b. *Clostridium perfringens*
    c. *Clostridium botulinum*
    d. *Clostridium difficile*

153. Cocks peculiar tumor is:
    a. Papilloma
    b. Infected sebaceous cyst
    c. Cylindroma
    d. Squamous cell carcinoma

154. Sistrunk operation is done for:
    a. Thyroglossal cyst
    b. Plunging ranula
    c. Thyroglossal fistula
    d. Branchial cyst

155. Commonest site for branchial cyst:
    a. Lower 1/3rd anterior border SCM muscle
    b. Upper 1/3rd anterior border SCM muscle
    c. Lower 1/3rd posterior border SCM muscle
    d. Upper 1/3rd posterior border SCM muscle

156. Common site of fracture of mandible:
    a. Neck
    b. Angle
    c. Mantle
    d. Canine fossa

Answers: 139. b. USG abdomen 140. c. Jaundice 141. c. Thigh 142. b. Papillary thyroid...
143. a. Facial nerve 144. b. Never metastasize... 145. a. Hepatitis B 146. c. Can be treated...
147. c. Hypocalcemia 148. b. Transfacial fracture...149. a. Pulmonary... 150. c. HEV
151. a. Autoclaving 152. b. *Clostridium*... 153. b. Infected sebaceous... 154. a. Thyroglossal cyst
155. b. Upper 1/3rd... 156. a. Neck

157. Sebaceous cyst does not occur at:
    a. Scalp
    b. Scrotum
    c. Sole
    d. Back

158. Hypovolemic shock manifest when the % of blood loss exceeds:
    a. 10%
    b. 15%
    c. 30%
    d. 40%

159. Commonest cause of hyperparathyroidism is:
    a. Single adenoma
    b. Multiple adenoma
    c. Single gland hyperplasia
    d. Multiple gland hyperplasia

160. Erysipelas is caused by:
    a. *Staphylococcus aureus*
    b. *Staphylococcus albus*
    c. *Streptococcus pyogens*
    d. *Haemophilus*

161. Plexiform neurofibromatosis commonly affects which cranial nerve:
    a. 7
    b. 5
    c. 6
    d. 8

162. Pitting edema indicates as excess of how much fluid in tissue space:
    a. 2.5 L
    b. 3.5 L
    c. 4.5 L
    d. 5.5 L

163. Most common site of carcinoma of tongue is:
    a. Dorsum aspect
    b. Ventral aspect
    c. Tip
    d. Anterior 2/3rd lateral aspect

164. Parotid tumor which spreads perineurally:
    a. Mucoepidermoid carcinoma
    b. Epidermoid carcinoma
    c. Pleomorphic adenoma
    d. Adenoid cystic carcinoma

165. Adenolymphoma refers to:
    a. Warthin's tumor
    b. Adenocarcinoma
    c. Pleomorphic adenoma
    d. Adenoid cystic carcinoma

166. What is ranula?
    a. Retention cyst of sublingual gland
    b. Retention cyst of submandibular gland
    c. Extravasation cyst of sublingual gland
    d. Extravasation cyst of submandibular gland

167. Potato tumor of neck is also called as:
    a. Ganglioneuroma
    b. Nuerofibroma
    c. Chemodectoma
    d. Angiomyolipoma

168. Which of the following does not move on deglutition?
    a. Sublingual dermoid
    b. Thyroid nodule
    c. Pretracheal lymph node
    d. Thyroglossal cyst

169. Cleft lip is due to nonfusion of:
    a. Maxillary process with lateral nasal process
    b. Maxillary process with medial nasal process
    c. Maxillary process with mandibular process
    d. All of above

170. Most common malignancy in maxillary antrum:
    a. Mucoepidermoid carcinoma
    b. Adenocystic carcinoma
    c. Adenocarcinoma
    d. Squamous cell carcinoma

171. Malignancy in multinodular goiter is most often:
    a. Anaplastic carcinoma
    b. Follicular carcinoma
    c. Medullary carcinoma
    d. Papillary carcinoma

172. In submandibular gland surgery the nerve least likely to be injured is:
    a. Inferior alveolar nerve
    b. Hypoglossal nerve
    c. Lingual nerve
    d. Mandibular branch or nerve

173. Serous salivary secretion is produced by:
    a. Parotid gland
    b. Submandibular gland
    c. Sublingual gland
    d. None of the above

174. About cleft upper lip all are correct, *except*:
    a. Median is the most common
    b. Lateral is most common on left side
    c. Best time for repair is earliest possible time (3 months)
    d. Repair is mainly for cosmetic purposes

Answers: 157. c. Sole   158. d. 40%   159. a. Single adenoma   160. c. *Streptococcus*...
161. b. 5   162. c. 4.5 L   163. d. Anterior 2/3rd...   164. d. Adenoid cystic...
165. a. Warthin's tumor   166. c. Extravasation cyst...   167. c. Chemodectoma   168. a. Sublingual dermoid
169. b. Maxillary process...   170. d. Squamous cell...   171. d. Papillary...   172. b. Hypoglossal nerve
173. a. Parotid gland   174. a. Median is the most...

175. All of the following are predisposing factors for cancer tongue, *except*:
    a. Cigarette smoking
    b. Spicy food
    c. Septic tooth
    d. Sjogren's syndrome

176. Correct statement about dentigerous cyst include following, *except* that it:
    a. Occurs in children and adolescents in relation to a missing tooth.
    b. Is more common in the upper than in the lower jaw.
    c. Presents as a globular swelling expanding the jaw.
    d. Is lined with squamous epithelium.

177. Which of the following is not a complication of submandibular gland excision?
    a. Frey's syndrome
    b. Anesthesia of the ipsilateral tongue
    c. Weakness of the cornerstone of mouth
    d. Anesthesia of submental skin

178. Which of the following is not a branch of the facial nerve?
    a. Temporal
    b. Orbital
    c. Zygomatic
    d. Buccal

179. About pleomorphic adenoma of the parotid gland, all the following statements are true, *except*:
    a. It has epithelial and mesenchymal components
    b. The tumor is painless
    c. It has an incomplete capsule
    d. The tumor is usually present deep to the facial nerve

180. About cold abscess of the neck, all the following statements are true, *except*:
    a. It is usually caused by caseation of tuberculous lymphadenitis
    b. The condition is mildly painful with low-grade fever
    c. Antituberculous treatment is an essential part of treatment
    d. Drainage is achieved by incision

181. Midline cystic swelling in the neck, moves up and down with deglutition and with protrusion of the tongue:
    a. Thyroid cancer
    b. Branchial cyst
    c. Thyroglossal cyst
    d. Ranula

182. Most common site of lymph node enlargement in Hodgkin's lymphoma is:
    a. Abdominal
    b. Cervical
    c. Axillary
    d. Mediastinal

183. Secondary hemorrhage is usually due to:
    a. Trauma
    b. Slipped ligature
    c. Infection
    d. All of the above

184. Sebaceous cyst is characterized by the following, *except* that it:
    a. Is due to obstruction of sebaceous gland
    b. Is lined by stratified squamous epithelium
    c. Contains a yellow plutaceous greasy material known as sebum
    d. May occur in palm and soles

185. The most serious complication of blood transfusion is:
    a. Pyrogenic reactions
    b. Thrombophlebitis of recipient vein
    c. Circulatory overloading
    d. Incompatibility reaction

186. Most common site of actinomycosis:
    a. GIT
    b. Head and neck
    c. Breast
    d. Lungs

187. Is a clinical defined swelling which is the first choice of investigation:
    a. USG
    b. CT Scan
    c. MRI
    d. PET Scan

188. Everted edge is characteristic of which ulcer:
    a. Healing
    b. Tubercular
    c. Malignant
    d. Venous

189. Marjolin ulcer is:
    a. Arterial
    b. Venous
    c. Malignant
    d. Healing

190. Common cancer of oral cavity is:
    a. Melanoma
    b. Lymphoma
    c. Sarcoma
    d. Squamous cell carcinoma

Answers: 175. b. Spicy food   176. b. Is more in the...   177. a. Frey's syndrome   178. b. Orbital
179. d. The tumor is...   180. b. The condition is...   181. c. Thyroglossal cyst   182. b. Cervical
183. d. All of the above   184. d. May occur in palm...   185. d. Incompatibility...   186. a. GIT
187. a. USG   188. c. Malignant   189. c. Malignant   190. d. Squamous cell...

191. Loss of differentiation (poorly) of tumor cell is called:
    a. Metaplasia
    b. Dysplasia
    c. Anaplasia
    d. Hyperplasia

192. The best routine management for multinodular goiter is by:
    a. Hemithyroidectomy
    b. Partial thyroidectomy
    c. Bilateral wedge resection
    d. Subtotal thyroidectomy

193. Nasopharyngeal carcinoma mostly arises from:
    a. Roof
    b. Posterior wall
    c. Anterior wall
    d. Fossa of Rosenmuller

194. After a swelling has been clinically defined the most commonly adviced investigation is:
    a. X-ray
    b. Ultrasound
    c. FNAC
    d. MRI

195. Branchial cyst is best differentiated from cold abscess by:
    a. Fluctuation
    b. Transillumination
    c. Contains cholesterol crystals
    d. Contain blood

196. Mask use in operation theater:
    a. Protects patient from getting infection
    b. Protects the doctor
    c. None is protected
    d. Should not be used

197. A punched out edge is characteristic of which ulcer:
    a. Tubercular ulcer
    b. Rodent ulcer
    c. Syphilitic ulcer
    d. Malignant

198. Cystic hygroma is:
    a. Lymphangiecatsia
    b. Sebaceous cyst
    c. Dermoid cyst
    d. Hemangioma

199. Following facial injury, nasal secretion can be differentiated from CSF, rhinorrhea on estimation of:
    a. Sodium
    b. Glucose
    c. Potassium
    d. Chloride

200. In a patient with pneumothorax and circulatory collapse first action should be:
    a. Immediate chest X-ray
    b. Oxygen inhalation
    c. Insertion of chest drain/needle
    d. Tracheostomy

201. The most common indication for removal of sublingual salivary gland is:
    a. Neoplasm
    b. Sialadenosis
    c. Ranula
    d. Lymphoma

202. Cleft palate repair is ideal at age of:
    a. 6 months
    b. 16–18 months
    c. 12–24 months
    d. >2 years

203. In tongue cancer the site least affected is:
    a. Lateral margin
    b. Ventral surface
    c. Dorsal surface
    d. Tip

204. Weakest part of mandible where fractures occur:
    a. Neck of condyle
    b. Angle of mandible
    c. Midline
    d. Canine fossa

205. The most common fracture of face is that of:
    a. Mandible
    b. Maxilla
    c. Zygoma
    d. Nasal bone

206. Sinus disease is best demonstrated by:
    a. CT scan
    b. Plain X-ray
    c. Tomography
    d. Ultrasound

207. Gillies approach is reduction of:
    a. Blow out fracture
    b. Nasal bone fracture
    c. Zygoma fracture
    d. Orbital bone

208. 80% of all salivary stones occur in:
    a. Parotid
    b. Submandibular
    c. Submaxillary
    d. Sublingual

Answers: 191. b. Dysplasia   192. d. Subtotal...   193. d. Fossa of Rosenmuller 194. b. Ultrasound
195. c. Contains...   196. b. Protects the...   197. c. Syphilitic ulcer   198. a. Lymphangiecatsia
199. b. Glucose   200. c. Insertion of...   201. c. Ranula   202. b. 16 to 18 months
203. c. Dorsal surface   204. a. Neck of condyle   205. d. Nasal bone   206. a. CT scan
207. c. Zygoma fracture   208. b. Submandibular

209. The carotid body is a:
    a. Pressure receptor
    b. pH receptor
    c. Osmo receptor
    d. Schwannoma

210. The suture that maintains strength for the longest time is:
    a. Vicryl
    b. PDS
    c. Chromic catgut
    d. Plain catgut

211. Neoplasm of laryngopharynx are most common in:
    a. Lateral wall
    b. Piriform fossa
    c. Medial wall
    d. Postcricoid region

212. Most common primary malignant thyroid tumor is:
    a. Papillary
    b. Follicular
    c. Anaplastic
    d. Medullary

Answers: 209. c. Osmo receptor   210. b. PDS   211. b. Piriform fossa   212. a. Papillary

FILL IN THE BLANKS

As per DCI and Examination Papers of Various Universities

1 Mark Each

1. Duct of parotid gland is known as ....
Ans. Stensen's duct

2. Duct of submandibular gland is known as ....
Ans. Wharton's duct

3. Branches of facial nerve are (any three) ...., ... and ....
Ans. Temporal, zygomatic and buccal

4. Two premalignant lesions are .... and ....
Ans. Leukoplakia and erythroplakia

5. The most common site of thyroglossal cyst is ....
Ans. Subhyoid

6. FNAC cannot distinguish between a benign .... and .... carcinoma of thyroid.
Ans. Follicular adenoma and follicular

7. The triad of thyroid swelling (goiter), thyrotoxicosis and exopthalmosis is seen in ....
Ans. Grave's disease

8. The swelling which moves on deglutition and also a protrusion of tongue is ....
Ans. Thyroglossal cyst

9. Infection in floor of mouth along with inflammatory swelling in the neck is called as ....
Ans. Ludwig's angina

10. The most commonly used local anesthetic agent is ....
Ans. Lignocaine

11. The term 'Ubiquitous tumor' is usually referred to ....
Ans. Fibrous tumor

12. The line of demarcation is usually seen between a living zone and dead zone is ....
Ans. Gangrene

13. Wash leather slough appearance of floor of ulcer is seen in .... ulcer.
Ans. Syphilitic

14. The abbreviation FNAC stands for ....
Ans. Fine Needle Aspiration Cytology

15. CSF rhinorrhea is seen in .... fossa fractures.
Ans. Anterior

16. A patient with multiple discharging sinuses along with faciocervical involvement is most probably suffering from ....
Ans. Cervicofacial actinomycosis

17. The organ most sensitive to hypovolemic shock is ....
Ans. Brain, heart and lung

18. Mandible is most commonly fractured at ....
Ans. Condyles

19. Undermined edge is seen in .... ulcer.
Ans. Tuberculous ulcer

20. Submandibular gland lies on .... muscle.
Ans. Hyoglossus

21. The most commonly used absorbable suture material for closure of intraoral wound is ....
Ans. Catgut

22. The most common site of enlargement of lymph nodes in Hodgkin's lymphoma is ....
Ans. Cervical region

23. The nerve most likely to get injured in parotid gland surgery is ....
Ans. Facial nerve

24. Father of Antiseptic surgery is ....
Ans. Joseph Lister

25. Commonest site for carcinoma tongue is ....
Ans. Anterior two-thirds part

26. The most common indication for doing tracheostomy is ....
Ans. In head, neck and facial injuries

27. Father of Plastic Surgery is ....
Ans. Sir Harold Gillies

28. True or False: Antisepsis is better than asepsis ....
Ans. False

29. Most common method of instrument sterilization is ....
Ans. Autoclave

30. True/False: Cancrum oris is often associated with malnutrition
Ans. True

31. Tissue is best antiseptic. Yes or No
Ans. Yes

32. Metabolism of Ca^{2+} and PO_4^- is regulated by...... .... hormone
Ans. Parathyroid

33. Biopsy and histopathological examination achieves final diagnosis of a lump. (True or false)
Ans. True

34. Medullary thyroid cancer can cause diarrhea. (True or false)
Ans. True

35. Cacinomatous masses are often hard. (True or false)

Ans. True

36. Most common salivary gland tumor is ....

Ans. Pleomorphic adenoma

37. Universal blood donor group is .... and universal blood recipient group is ....

Ans. O negative, AB positive

38. Most common bacteria involved in abscess formation is ....

Ans. *Staphylococcus aureus*

39. The difference between sinus and fistula is ....

Ans. Fistula a pathway that leads from an internal cavity or organ to the surface of the body. A sinus tract is an abnormal channel that originates or ends in one opening.

40. Consistency of a malignant tumor on palpation is ....

Ans. Hard

41. Catgut is manufactured from ....

Ans. Submucosa of jejunum of sheep

42. Most commonly employed method of sterilization in OT is ....

Ans. UV radiation or formaldehyde

43. Edges of malignant ulcer is ....

Ans. Everted

44. 'Slipping sign' is observed in ....

Ans. Lipoma

45. A line of demarcation is usually seen between living and dead zone in ....

Ans. Gangrene

46. .... discovered germ theory of diseases.

Ans. Louis Pasteur

47. .... performed first rhinoplasty.

Ans. Joseph Constantine Carpue

48. .... pioneered aseptic surgery.

Ans. Joseph Lister

49. Rodent ulcer edge is ....

Ans. Beaded

50. The first sign in hypovolemic shock is .... in pulse.

Ans. Increase

51. FNAC achieves better diagnosis than biopsy. (True or false)

Ans. False

52. Cancrum oris is generally associated with malnutrition. (True or false)

Ans. True

53. Tetanus has both tonic and clonic convulsions. (True or false)

Ans. True

54. Metastatic lymph nodes have .... consistency.

Ans. Stony hard

55. Aphthous ulcers are painful and multiple. (True or false)

Ans. True

56. Primary healing achieves better function than secondary healing. (True or false)

Ans. True

57. Skin grafting can spoil the cosmetic appearance. (True or false)

Ans. True

58. Carbuncles are seen commonly in nondiabetics. (True or false)

Ans. False

59. Mothers are carriers and fathers are sufferer in ....

Ans. Hemophilia

60. Universal tumor is the name given to ....

Ans. Lipoma

61. Neurotmesis involves rupture of both................... and ....

Ans. Neuron sheath and axons

62. Line of demarcation is the feature of .... gangrene.

Ans. Wet

63. Discoverer of system of human blood groups ....

Ans. Landsteiner

64. Edge of tubercular ulcers is...................

Ans. Undermined

65. Consistency of metastatic lymph nodes is ....

Ans. Hard

66. Plastic surgery was invented in ....(country).

Ans. India

67. Venous bleeding is .... in color and flows...................

Ans. Dark in color and flows continuously

68. In lymphoma lymph nodes are .... in consistency.

Ans. Rubbery

69. Sharp instruments should not be sterilize by ....

Ans. Boiling

70. .... suffer from hemophilia while .... transmit it.

Ans. Males suffer from hemophilia while females transmit it

71. Calcium and phosphate in blood and bones are regulated by ....

Ans. Calcitonin

72. .... is the most common site for keloid.

Ans. Nape of the neck

73. ....is known as hydrocele of neck.

Ans. Serous cyst

74. Branches of facial nerve are .... and .... (any two).
Ans. Temporal and mandibular

75. Hilton method is used for the treatment of ....
Ans. Abscess

76. Boil is also called as furuncle. (True or false)
Ans. True

77. Clean-incised surgical wound is healed by primary intension. (True or false)
Ans. True

78. Cold abscess is caused by tuberculosis. (True or false)
Ans. True

79. Abscess of peritonsillar space is called as ....
Ans. Quinsy

80. Cystic hygroma is a brilliantly transilluminant swelling. (True or false)
Ans. True

81. Edge of squamous cell carcinoma is....................
Ans. Everted

82. Repair of cleft lip should be done at the age of ....
Ans. 3–6 months

83. Cellulitis is commonly caused by the microorganism ....
Ans. *Streptococcus pyogenes*

84. Hemophilia is caused by deficiency of................
Ans. Factor VIII

85. Tuberculous ulcer has a punched out edge. (True or false)
Ans. False

86. Thyroglossal cyst moves on deglutition. (True or false)
Ans. True

87. Consistency of tuberculous lymph node is hard. (True or false)
Ans. False

88. Granulomatous epulis is...................in consistency.
Ans. Soft

89. 5 cardinal signs of inflammation................
Ans. Rubor, Calor, Tumor, Dolor, Functio laesa

90. Gas gangrene is caused by........................(Name of organism)
Ans. *Clostridium perfringens*

91. ....cranial nerves are affected in plexiform neurofibromatosis.
Ans. 5th, 9th and 10th

92. Punched out edges are seen in......................ulcer.
Ans. Syphilitic

93. Contusion is a type of closed wound. (True or false)
Ans. True

94. Keratocanthoma arising from.................
Ans. Pilosebaceous glands

95. Ranula is a mucus retention cyst.................(True or false)
Ans. True

96. In autologous transfusion, patient's own blood is used ....(True or false)
Ans. True

97. Crushed wounds are closed after debridement. (True or false)
Ans. False

98. PMMC flap is supplied by....................
Ans. Thoracoacromial artery and its venae comitantes

VIVA-VOCE QUESTIONS FOR PRACTICAL EXAMINATION

1. What is an abscess?

Ans. It is a cavity which is filled with pus and is lined by a pyogenic membrane.

2. What is pyemic abscess?

Ans. In this, multiple abscesses are formed from the infected emboli in pyemia.

3. What is pyemia?

Ans. It is the condition where there is formation of secondary foci of suppuration in various body parts.

4. What is bacteremia?

Ans. It is the condition where the bacteria circulate in blood stream.

5. What is septicemia?

Ans. It is the condition where multiple clinical manifestations arise as toxins are liberated by the bacteria in the bloodstream.

6. What is toxemia?

Ans. It is the condition where toxins either derived from bacteria or from chemical circulate in the bloodstream.

7. What is the another name of gas gangrene?

Ans. Clostridial myonecrosis

8. Gas gangrene comes under which type of gangrene?

Ans. Moist gangrene

9. What is the most characteristic feature of gas gangrene?

Ans. There is presence of profuse discharge of brown, foul smelling fluid in between sutures and crepitus is also present.

10. Name various organisms which leads to gas gangrene.

Ans. *Clostridium welchii, Clostridium septicum, Clostridium histolyticum, Clostridium oedematiens*

11. Name the exotoxins released by *Clostridium tetani*?

Ans. Tetanospasmin and Tetanolysin

12. How much is the incubation period of tetanus?

Ans. It is from 3 days to 3 weeks.

13. What is Tetanus neonatorum?

Ans. It is the contamination of the cut surface of umbilical cord of neonate which causes spasm of respiratory muscles.

14. What is latent tetanus?

Ans. At times when wound are ignored *Clostridium tetani* rest in them for months and years but when suitable conditions come the bacteria multiply and tetanus develops.

15. Which is the earliest symptom of tetanus?

Ans. Trismus

16. What do you mean by risus sardonicus?

Ans. It is the anxious expression of the patient suffering from the tetanus.

17. Which is the most common form of actinomycosis?

Ans. Cervicofacial actinomycosis

18. In which disease, Leonine facies are seen?

Ans. Lepromatous leprosy

19. Name the peripheral nerve which is commonly affected in leprosy.

Ans. Ulnar nerve

20. What is carbuncle?

Ans. Carbuncle is the infective gangrene of skin and subcutaneous tissue.

21. What is cellulitis?

Ans. It is the condition in which there is nonsuppurative spreading inflammation of subcutaneous and fascial planes.

22. Name the microorganism which leads to cellulitis.

Ans. *Streptococcus pyogenes*

23. What is erysipelas?

Ans. It is the spreading inflammation of the skin and subcutaneous tissues due to the infection caused by *Streptococcus pyogenes*.

24. Which is the characteristic sign of erysipelas?

Ans. Milian's ear sign.

25. Define cyst.

Ans. A pathological cavity having fluid, semifluid or gaseous contents and which is not created by accumulation of pus.

26. What is a fracture?

Ans. It is the loss of continuity of bone.

27. Name the fracture occurring in the children.

Ans. Greenstick fracture

28. What is callus?

Ans. It is the new bone formed at the site of fracture.

29. What is neuropraxia?

Ans. It is the temporary physiological paralysis of nerve conduction.

30. What is axonotmesis?

Ans. It is the division of nerve fibers or axons with intact nerve sheath.

31. What is neurotmesis?

Ans. In this, there is complete division of nerve fibers with sheath occurs.

32. What is an ulcer?

Ans. It is the break in continuity of the epithelium.

33. **Name the parts of an ulcer.**
Ans. Edge, margin, floor and base.

34. **Which disease shows rolled out ulcer?**
Ans. Squamous cell carcinoma and adenocarcinoma

35. **Name the disease which consists of undermined ulcer.**
Ans. Tuberculosis

36. **What is cleft palate?**
Ans. Cleft palate occur due to defect in fusion of lines between premaxilla and palatine processes of maxilla one on each side.

37. **What is cleft lip?**
Ans. Cleft lip occurs due to defect in fusion of median nasal process along with maxillary process.

38. **Name the surgical treatment which is used for unilateral cleft lip repair.**
Ans. Millard advancement flap

39. **At what age cleft lip repair is done?**
Ans. Between 3 to 6 months

40. **What is rule of ten?**
Ans. When baby is of 10 lbs weight, 10 week old and has 10 g% of hemoglobin cleft lip repair is done.

41. **Name the prosthetic device which covers palatal defects in patients having cleft palate.**
Ans. Obturator

42. **At what age cleft palate repair has to be done.**
Ans. Between 12 to 15 months of age.

43. **Name the classification which is represented symbolically as Y for cleft lip and cleft palate.**
Ans. Kernahan classification

44. **Which is the tumor known as universal tumor or ubiquitous tumor?**
Ans. Lipoma

45. **Which is the most common site of carcinoma of lip?**
Ans. Vermilion border of lip

46. **Name the carcinoma which does not metastatize.**
Ans. Basal cell carcinoma

47. **Which is the most common site for occurrence of carcinoma of tongue?**
Ans. Lateral border of tongue

48. **What is commando's operation?**
Ans. In this, there is hemiglossectomy with the block dissection of the lymph nodes.

49. **Bedsore represents which type of an ulcer.**
Ans. Trophic ulcer.

50. **Which condition is known as quinsy?**
Ans. Peritonsillar abscess

51. **How are the lymph nodes in oral carcinoma?**
Ans. Hard and fixed lymph nodes

52. **How are the lymph nodes in Hodgkin's lymphoma?**
Ans. Rubbery and elastic

53. **How is the edge of ulcer in syphilis and aphthous ulcer.**
Ans. Punched out

54. **Name type of ameloblastoma which has maximum chances of turning into malignancy.**
Ans. Granular cell ameloblastoma

55. **Name the disease in which tracheostomy is mandatory.**
Ans. Ludwig's angina

56. **While performing tracheostomy, which is the site of entrance inside the trachea.**
Ans. Second and third tracheal ring is the site of entrance

57. **Name the disease in which Trottler's triad is seen.**
Ans. Nasopharyngeal carcinoma

58. **Name the most common complication which arises after doing the tracheal intubation.**
Ans. Sore throat is the most common complication.

59. **Which is the major advantage of tracheostomy?**
Ans. The procedure increases the dead space up to 50%.

60. **What is the another name of Ringer's lactate solution?**
Ans. Hartmann's solution.

61. **At how much temperature does the blood is stored in the blood bank.**
Ans. 4°C ± 2°C

62. **How much is the shelf life of stored blood in blood banks?**
Ans. 3 weeks

63. **At how much temperature, does whole blood is stored in the blood bank?**
Ans. 4–8°C

64. **At what temperature does fresh frozen plasma is stored?**
Ans. –40–50°C

65. **Name the method which is commonly used to stop the bleeding?**
Ans. Applying the pressure over the injured area.

66. **In how much time after the surgery reactionary hemorrhage occur?**
Ans. In 24 hours of surgery.

67. **Name the derivatives of plasma.**
Ans. Plasma, platelet rich plasma, fibrinogen, albumin, cryoprecipitate.

68. **What are the synthetically prepared solutions?**
Ans. Fluorocarbons, gelatin, dextran.

69. **How much is the blood transfusion rate?**
Ans. It is 1 unit for 4–6 hours

70. **Name the solution which is given to the patient who get burn?**
Ans. Human albumin 4.5%

71. **Which is the most common cause of the death in burn patient?**

Ans. Oligemic shock

72. **Name some of the topical agents used in cases of burn.**

Ans. Silver nitrate, silver sulphadiazine, cerium nitrate

73. **What are plasma expanders?**

Ans. They are the high molecular weight substances which exert colloidal osmotic pressure and when they are infused intravenously, they retain fluid in the vascular compartment, e.g., dextran and human albumin.

74. **What is shock?**

Ans. Shock is a state of poor perfusion with impaired cellular metabolism manifesting with severe pathophysiological abnormalities. It is due to circulatory collapse and tissue hypoxia.

75. **Which type of graft is given in deep skin burns?**

Ans. Split thickness graft.

76. **What is an allograft?**

Ans. It is the graft which is given from individual of same species.

77. **What is a heterograft?**

Ans. It is the graft taken from one specie to another species.

78. **What is keloid?**

Ans. Keloid is the defect in maturation and stabilization of collage fibrils. In this normal collagen bundles are absent.

79. **What is Buerger's disease?**

Ans. Buerger's disease is the inflammation and thrombosis in small and medium-sized blood vessels, typically in the legs and leading to gangrene. It has been associated with smoking

80. **Name the most common ulcer which occur in the leg.**

Ans. Venous ulcer

81. **Name the most common cause which leads to hypothyroidism.**

Ans. Autoimmune thyroiditis

82. **Name the cyst which moves while protruding the tongue.**

Ans. Thyroglossal cyst

83. **Where is thyroglossal cyst located?**

Ans. Just near to the hyoid bone

84. **Name the thyroid malignancy which occur most commonly.**

Ans. Papillary carcinoma of thyroid.

85. **What is ranula?**

Ans. It is the cystic swelling which is present at the floor of mouth and is the retention cyst of sublingual gland.

86. **Name the salivary gland in which there is maximum chances of formation of stones.**

Ans. Submandibular salivary gland.

87. **What is the duct of parotid gland?**

Ans. Stensen's duct

88. **What is the duct of submandibular duct known as?**

Ans. Wharton's duct

89. **Name the most common parotid gland tumor.**

Ans. Pleomorphic adenoma

90. **What is an adenoma?**

Ans. All the benign tumors which arises from the glandular epithelium are known as adenomas.

91. **Where is pleomorphic adenoma located in parotid gland?**

Ans. At the tail of parotid gland

92. **Name the salivary gland tumor which gets spread surrounding the nerves.**

Ans. Adenoid cystic carcinoma

93. **What is the feature in diagnosis except biopsy which gives conformational diagnosis of Warthin's tumor in comparison to other salivary gland tumors.**

Ans. Warthin's tumor shows hot spot in Scintiscan while other salivary tumors show cold spot.

94. **Name the nerve which cannot get preserved, while doing the parotid surgery.**

Ans. Facial nerve

95. **Name the tumors which metastasize to the parotid gland.**

Ans. Malignant melanoma and epidermoid carcinoma of skin

96. **What is Sjögren's syndrome?**

Ans. It is the triad of xerostomia, keratoconjunctivitis sicca and rheumatoid arthritis.

97. **Name the route by which papillary carcinoma of thyroid spread and follicular carcinoma of thyroid spread.**

Ans. Papillary carcinoma spread via lymphatic route while follicular carcinoma spreads via hematogenous route.

98. **What is thyroid storm?**

Ans. It is the thyrotoxic reaction which occurs under 3–4 days after thyroid surgery. This occur, if the thyrotoxic patient has not been brought down to euthyroid state before the thyroid surgery.

99. **What is Patey's operation?**

Ans. It is the superficial parotidectomy.

100. **What is goiter?**

Ans. Goiter is the enlargement of the thyroid gland.

101. **Name the goiter which has maximum chances of undergoing malignancy?**

Ans. Nodular goiter

102. **Name some of the goitrogens.**

Ans. Cabbage, cauliflower, turnip, kale, sprouts. Antithyoid drugs, thiocyanate, etc.

103. **In bilateral recurrent laryngeal nerve paralysis, what is the life-saving measure?**

Ans. Immediate tracheostomy.

ADDITIONAL INFORMATION

Thyroid Swellings on Scintiscanning

Hot nodule	It is overactive and takes up isotope but surrounding gland does not. This also actively secrete excess thyroid hormone
Warm	This is active, both swelling as well as normal thyroid tissue takes up an isotope
Cold	This is underactive and it does not take an isotope

Various Surgical Procedures and Anatomical Structures Injured during the Procedures

Surgical procedure	Anatomical structure injured
Parotidectomy	Facial nerve
Brachial cyst excision	Hypoglossal nerve and accessory nerve
Ranula excision	Submandibular duct
Submandibular gland excision	Lingual nerve, hypoglossal nerve, marginal mandibular branch of facial nerve

Various Hemorrhage and Arteries Involved in them

Name of hemorrhage	Artery involved
Extradural	Middle meningeal artery
Intracerebral bleed	Lenticulostriate arteries
Subarachnoid	Rupture of berry aneurysm
Subdural	Communicating veins or cortical bridging veins

Various Thyroid Carcinomas and their Spread

Name of thyroid carcinoma	Spread
Papillary carcinoma	Lymphatic route
Follicular carcinoma	Hematogenous route
Anaplastic carcinoma	Direct route
Medullar carcinoma	Lymphatic route

Wayne's Clinical Diagnostic Index for Thyrotoxicosis

Symptoms	Present	Absent
Palpitations	+2	------
Excessive sweating	+3	------
Appetite increased	+3	------
Appetite decreased	------	-3
Weight increased	------	-3
Weight decreased	+3	---------
Preference for cold	+5	---------
Preference for hot	---------	-5

Signs	Present	Absent
Palpable thyroid	+3	-3
Exopthalmos	+2	---------
Lid retraction	+2	---------
Finger tremor	+1	---------
Bruit over thyroid	+2	-2
Atrial fibrillation	+4	---------
Pulse rate (>90/min)	+3	---------
Pulse rate (>80/min)	-------	-3

Various Signs of Thyrotoxicosis

Name of sign	Description
Dalrymple's sign	Upper sclera is seen because of retraction of upper eye lid
Joffroy's sign	As patient is asked to look upward with head fixed, there is absence of wrinkling on forehead
Moebius sign	Eye balls fail to converge
Stellwag's sign	There is absence of normal wrinkling
Von Graffe's sign	As patient is asked to look down, his upper eyelid fails to follow rotation of an eyeball and so lags behind

Types of Laryngeal Nerve Paralysis

Type of laryngeal nerve paralysis	Description
Unilateral	It produces whispering voice. No airway obstruction present
Bilateral	It leads to dyspnea. Tracheostomy should be done
Superior	It leads to paralysis of cricothyroid muscle. It leads to weak and husky voice

Various Staphylococcal Infections with their Description

Staphyloccocal skin infection	Description
Boil	Hair follicle infection which proceed to suppuration and central necrosis. It is common on face, neck and head
Carbuncle	It is the infective gangrene of subcutaneous tissue which occurs at nape of neck. There is presence of skin sloughing and discharge of pus
Impetigo	It is a bulla which soon ruptures, erodes and forms a crust. It is an intradermal infection
Stye	It is an infection of an eyelash follicle

Various Clostridium Species and Infections Produced by them

Name of clostridium species	Infection
C. tetani	Tetanus
C. perfringens	Gas gangrene
C. difficile	Pseudomembranous colitis
C. botulinum	Food poisoning

Various types of Tetanus

Type of tetanus	Description
Acute tetanus	Incubation period is <10 days
Chronic tetanus	Incubation period is till one month
Delayed or latent tetanus	Organism remain latent in wound for months or years
Local tetanus	Leads to local contracture of muscles
Cephalic tetanus	Irritation and paralysis of cranial nerves. More often facial nerve is affected
Bulbar tetanus	Extensive spasm of muscles of deglutition and respiration

Types of Gas Gangrene

Type of gas gangrene	Description
Clostridial cellulitis	Crepitant infection which involve necrotic tissue, but there is no involvement of healthy muscle. It is characterized by foul smelling and seropurulent infection of wound
Fulminating type	Spread is very fast. Associated with intense toxemia
Group type	This is limited to one group of muscles
Massive type	It involve whole muscle mass of one limb
Single muscle type	This is limited to one muscle only

Various Streptococcal Species and Infections Produced by them

Name of streptococcal species	Infection
S. pyogenes	Cellulitis, erysipelas, glomerulonephritis, necrotizing fasciitis, scarlet fever, rheumatic fever, tonsillitis
S. viridians	Septicemia and endocarditis
Anaerobic streptococci	Liver abscess

Elements of Primary Survey

♦ A refers to airway management
♦ B refers to breathing and ventilation
♦ C refers to circulation and hemorrhage control
♦ D refers to dysfunction of CNS
♦ E refers to exposure in controlled environment

Important Points about Cleft Lip and Cleft Palate

Negros have less incidence of cleft lip/palate
Mongolians have high incidence of cleft lip/palate
In males cleft lip is common
In females cleft palate is common
Most common are unilateral clefts to occur, i.e., 80%
Least common are bilateral clefts to occur, i.e., 20%
Unilateral clefts occur more commonly on left side

Name of Cleft Lip and Cleft Palate Repair Techniques

Unilateral cleft lip repair technique	• Millards rotation advancement technique • Mirault–Blair–Brown triangular flap technique • Le Mesurier triangular flap techniques • Tenninson–Randall Z shape incision technique
Bilateral cleft lip repair technique	• Millards rotation advancement technique • Mirault–Blair–Brown triangular flap technique • Le Mesurier triangular flap techniques • Tenninson–Randall Z shape incision technique • V-Y flap techniques
Cleft palate repair techniques	• Von Langen back technique • Furlow • The three flap or V-Y technique • Vomer flap technique

Bone Grafting in Cleft Palate at Recommended Ages

Type of bone grafting	Age recommended
Primary bone grafting	Less than two years
Early secondary bone grafting	2 to 4 years
Secondary bone grafting	6 to 15 years
Late secondary bone grafting	In adults

Various Tumors and their Location

Name of the tumor	Location
Carotid body tumor or potato tumor or chemodectoma	Beneath anterior edge of sternomastoid
Ulcerated sebaceous cyst or Cock's peculiar tumor	Scalp
Lipoma or ubiquitous tumor	Can occur anywhere
Strenomastoid tumor or congenital torticollis	Middle of sternomastoid muscle
Extradural abscess or Pott's puffy tumor	Skull

Parts of an Ulcer

♦ **Margin:** This is the junction between normal epithelium and an ulcer

- **Edge:** This is the area between margin and floor of an ulcer
- **Floor:** This is an exposed surface of an ulcer
- **Base:** This is an area on which ulcer rest. This is better felt than seen

Various Ulcers and their Description

Name of an ulcer	Description
Bazin's ulcer	It is seen in young adult females
Cryopathic ulcer	It occur because of cold injury and chilblain
Marjolins ulcer	This is the malignant ulcer occur due to scar or burn
Martorell ulcer	It is basically a hypertensive ulcer
Rodent ulcer	It is also known as basal cell carcinoma
Trophic ulcer	It is also known as bed sore ulcer
Tropical ulcer	It occur because of Vincent's infection

Various Types of Ulcers and their Edges

Name of an ulcer	Type of an edge
Apthous ulcer	Regular punched out
Healing ulcer	Sloping edge
Rodent ulcer	Rolled out edge
Squamous cell carcinoma	Edge is raised, everted and indurated
Syphilitic ulcer	Regular punched out ulcer
Traumatic ulcer	Irregular margins
Tuberculous ulcer	Undermined
Nonspecific ulcer	Shelving edge

Type of Lymph Nodes in Various Diseases

Type of a lymph node	Disease
Elastic and rubbery	Hodgkin's lymphoma
Fixed and hard	Carcinoma
Firm, discrete and shotty	Syphilis
Matted	Tuberculosis

Various Terminologies

Terminology	Meaning
Hypertrophy	Increase in size of cells and increase in size of an organ
Hyperplasia	Increase in number of cells
Metaplasia	Reversible change of one epithelial cell to another
Dysplasia	It refers to disordered cellular development
Anaplasia	This is the loss of differentiation of tumor cells from where they arise
Carcinoma in situ	It resemble like a cancer but without invasion across basement membrane

Levels of Axillary Lymph Nodes

Levels of axillary lymph node	Description
Level I or low axilla	Lymph nodes lateral to lateral border of pectoralis minor muscle
Level II or mid axilla	Lymph nodes deep or posterior to pectoralis minor muscle and interpectoral lymph nodes
Level III or high axilla	Apical lymph nodes and those medial to medial margin of pectoralis minor muscle, excluding those which are designated as subclavicular or infraclavicular

Trotter's Triad

- Ipsilateral temporoparietal neuralgia (due to trigeminal nerve)
- Palatal paralysis (due to vagus nerve)
- Conducive deafness (due to Eustachian tube blockade)

Various Parenteral Fluids with their Composition and indications

Name of the parenteral fluid	Composition	Indications
Plasma, albumin 4.5%	• Albumin • Sodium • Potassium • Chloride • Bicarbonate	In severe burns
5% dextrose	Low sodium and potassium concentration	In postoperative period when there is decrease in sodium excretion
0.9% Isotonic saline	High concentration of sodium and chloride	In vomiting During gastric or duodenal aspiration
Ringer's lactate Or Hartmann's solution	• Sodium • Potassium • Chloride in concentration similar to plasma	In hypovolemic shock

Various Blood Substitutes

Name of blood substitute	Contents
Plasma and its derivatives	• Albumin • Cryoprecipitate • Fibrinogen • Plasma • Platelet rich plasma
Various synthetically prepared solutions	• Dextran • Fluorocarbons • Gelatin • Hydroxyethyl starch

Various Replacements and their Conditions

Name of replacement	Condition
Cryoprecipitate	Hemophilia
Fibrinogen	Disseminated intravascular coagulation
4.5% human albumin	Burns
Packed red cells	Anemia, elders and small children
Platelet concentrate and Platelet rich plasma	Thrombocytopenia

Various Formulas used in Burn

Timing	Moore's formula	Evan's formula	Brooke's formula
1st 24 hours	• Ringer's lactate: 1,000–4,000 mL • Normal saline is 1,000 mL • 5% dextrose is 1,500–5,000 mL • Colloid containing fluid: 7.5% of body weight	• Normal saline is 1 mL/kg/%burn • 5% dextrose is 2,000 mL • Colloid containing fluid is 1 mL/kg/%burn	• Ringer's lactate is 1 mL/kg/%burn • Colloid containing fluid is 1 mL/kg/% burn • 5% dextrose is 2,000 mL
2nd 24 hours	• Ringer's lactate: 1,000–4,000 mL • Normal saline is 1,000 mL • 5% dextrose is 1,500–5,000 mL • Colloid containing fluid: 2.5% of body weight	• Normal saline is 0.5 mL/kg/%burn • 5% dextrose is 2,000 mL • Colloid containing fluid is 0.5 mL/kg/%burn	• Ringer's lactate and colloid containing fluid is ½ to ¾ of above mentioned amount • 5% dextrose is 2,000 mL

Types of Grafts

Type of graft	Description
Allograft or homograft	Transfer of graft from one individual to another of same species
Heterograft	Transfer of graft from one individual to another individual of different species
ISO or synergistic graft	This is the graft transplant between identical twins
Hetrotropic graft	Transplant which is positioned at different site
Orthotropic graft	Transplant which is positioned at its anatomical site
Autogenous graft	This is the graft taken and received by same individual

Various Blood Products and their Storages

Name of blood product	Method of storage
Autologous blood	It can be stored till three weeks
Fresh frozen plasma	At -30°C with 2 years of shelf life
Packed red cells	These are stored in saline adenine glucose-mannitol (SAG-M) solution to increase shelf life till 5 weeks at 2–6°C
Platelets	At 20–24°C with shelf life of 5 days

Various Types of Thyroplasty

- **Type I:** There is medial displacement of vocal cord
- **Type II:** There is lateral displacement of vocal cord to improve airway
- **Type III:** To shorten or relax the vocal cord
- **Type IV:** To lengthen or tighten the vocal cord.

Various Markers of Cancer

Name of the marker	Name of cancer
Oncofetal antigens • Alpha-fetoprotein (AFP) • Carcinoembryonic antigen (CEA)	• Hepatocellular carcinoma, Nonseminomatous germ cell tumor of testis • Breast cancer, bowel cancer, bladder cancer
Enzymes • Prostrate acid phosphatase (PAP) • Neuron specific enolase (NSE)	• Carcinoma of prostrate • Oat cell carcinoma of lung and Neuroblastoma
Secreted cancer antigens • CA-125 • CA-15-3	• Carcinoma of ovary • Carcinoma of breast
Hormones • Calcitonin • Catecholamines and vanillyl mandelic acid (VMA)	• Medullary carcinoma of thyroid • Pheochromocytoma and neuroblastoma
Cytoplasmic proteins • Immunoglobulins • Prostrate specific antigens	• Multiple myeloma and other gammopathies • Carcinoma of prostrate

American Society of Anesthesiologists (ASA) Classification of Physical Status

Type of ASA	Description
Type I	Normal healthy patient
Type II	Patient with mild to moderate systemic disease
Type III	Patient with severe systemic disease that limit activity but is non incapacitating
Type IV	Patient with severe systemic disease that limit activity and is a constant threat to life
Type V	Moribund patient not expected to survive 24 hours with or without operation
Type VI	Clinically dead patient being maintained for harvesting of organs

Swellings of Head and Neck

- **Swellings in midline**
  - Lipoma
  - Sublingual dermoid
  - Submental lymph nodes
  - Thyroid gland enlargement
  - Thyroglossal cyst
- **Lateral swellings in neck**
  - Branchial cyst
  - Lipoma
  - Lymph node swelling
  - Salivary gland enlargement
  - Thyroid enlargement
- **Acute swellings in neck**
  - Acute lymphadenitis
  - Boil
  - Carbuncle
  - Ludwig's angina
- **Cysts demonstrating cholesterol crystals**
  - Branchial cyst
  - Cystic hygroma
  - Dental cyst
  - Dentigerous cyst
  - Old hydrocele
  - Thyroglossal cyst
- **Swellings that move with deglutition**
  - Enlarged pretracheal lymph nodes which are fixed to trachea
  - Laryngocele
  - Subhyoid bursal cyst or subhyoid bursitis
  - Thyroid swelling
  - Thyroglossal cyst

Schedule and Timing Protocol for Cleft Repair

- Palatal obturator: 0–1 year
- Primary cleft lip surgery: 3rd month
- Palatal repair: 9–12 months
- Tympanic tube: 6–12 months
- Speech therapy/pharyngoplasty: 2–7 years
- Bone grafting of jaw: 9–11 years
- Orthodontics: 8–18 years
- Rhinoplasty/orthognathic surgery: 15–18 years

Advanced Trauma Life Support (ATLS) Guidelines

Injuries are diagnosed and treated according to the ABCDE (Airway, Breathing, Circulation, Disability, and Exposure) sequence. Only when the abnormalities belonging to the letter should be evaluated and are treated as efficacious as possible an one can continue with the next letter. If there is deterioration of the patient condition during assessment, one should return to 'A'.

A: Airway with Cervical Spine Protection

- The airway is the first priority in trauma care.
- All patients should be 100% oxygen through a non-rebreathing mask. Airway should not be compromised when the patient talks normally. A hoarse voice or audible breathing is suspicious. Facial fractures and the soft tissue injury of neck can compromise airway, while patients in a comma are not capable of keeping their airway patent. Endotracheal intubation is the most definite way to secure the airway.
- In 'A' the cervical spine needs to be immobilized. When 'A' is secure, one can continue with B.

B: Breathing and Ventilation

- Tension pneumothorax, massive hemothorax, flail thorax accompanied by pulmonary contusion compromise breathing.
- Most clinical problems in 'B' can be treated with relatively simple measures as endotracheal intubation, mechanical ventilation, needle thoracocentesis, or tube thoracostomy.

C: Circulation with Hemorrhage Control

- Circulation is the third priority in the primary survey. Circulatory problems in trauma patients are usually caused by hemorrhage. The first action should be to stop the bleeding.
- Blood pressure and heart rate are measured; two intravenous lines are started, and blood it obtained for laboratory investigation.

D: Disability-Neurologic Status

- Disability should be assessed as the fourth priority, and this includes assessment of the neurological status.
- The Glasgow coma score (GCS) is used to evaluate the severity of head injury. This score is arrived at by scoring eye opening, best motor response and best verbal response. Patients who open their eyes spontaneously, obey commands and are normally oriented score a total of 15 points. The worst score is 3 points.
- A decreased GCS can be caused by a focal brain injury, such as epidural hematoma, a subdural hematoma or a cerebral contusion.

E: Environment and Exposure

Environment and exposure represent hypothermia, burns and possible exposure to chemical and radioactive substances and should be evaluated and treated as the fifth priority in primary survey.

Degrees of Frostbite

- 1st degree frostbite: Here there is hyperemia and edema of skin
- 2nd degree frostbite: Here there is hyperemia, vesicle formation and partial thickness necrosis of skin
- 3rd degree frostbite: Here there is necrosis of entire skin thickness and variable thickness of underlying subcutaneous tissue.
- 4th degree frostbite: Here there is necrosis of entire skin thickness and all underlying structures leading to gangrene of affected part.

Severity of Burn

- 1st degree burn: There is simple hyperemia of skin with slight edema of epidermis. There is only microscopic destruction of superficial layers of epidermis. It heals rapidly and without scarring and is not considering while estimating the magnitude of burn.
- 2nd degree burn: Complete thickness of epidermis gets destroyed. Blebs and vesicles get formed between dermis and epidermis. This is the hallmark of second degree burn. It can be divided into mild and severe varities. In severe cases, there is not enough epithelium left, so the resurfacing of burnt area is not usually possible and so skin grafting is necessary.
- 3rd degree burn: There is complete destruction of dermis and epidermis with irreversible destruction of dermal appendages and epithelial elements including sensory nerves. Skin grafting is obligatory.

Another type of Classification for Severity of Burns

- **Partial thickness burn:** It involves the whole thickness of epidermis and sometimes the superficial part of dermis. Spontaneous regeneration of epithelium is expected and skin grafting is not necessary. Sensation of skin remains and pin prick test is positive.
- **Full thickness burn:** It involves whole thickness of epidermis and total depth of dermis. So spontaneous regeneration is not possible and skin grafting is necessary. As sensory nerves are also destroyed, sensation is lost and pin prick test is negative.

Complications of Head Injury

Early complications:
- Leakage of CSF
- Aerocele
- Meningitis
- Fat metabolism
- Brain stem injury
- Posterior fossa compression
- Pituitary failure

Late complications:
- Chronic subdural hematoma
- Post-traumatic epilepsy
- Headache
- Hydrocephalus

Common Cancers in Salivary Gland in Descending Order

- Mucoepidermoid carcinoma
- Adenoid cystic carcinoma
- Adenocarcinoma
- Epidermoid carcinoma
- Undifferentiated carcinoma
- Carcinoma arising in pleomorphic adenoma

Paraneoplastic Syndrome Endocrinopathies

Name of disorder	Ectopic hormone	Associated cancer
Cushing's syndrome	ACTH	• Small cell carcinoma of lung • Medullary carcinoma of thyroid
Gynecomastia	HCC	Choriocarcinoma
Hypercalcemia	PTH-related protein calcitriol	• Renal cell carcinoma • Primary squamous cell carcinoma of lung • Breast carcinoma • Malignant lymphomas
Hypocalcemia	Calcitonin	Medullary carcinoma of thyroid
Hypoglycemia	Insulin-like factor	Hepatocellular carcinoma
Hyponatremia	Antidiuretic hormone	Small cell carcinoma of lung
Secondary polycythemia	Erythropoietin	• Renal cell carcinoma • Hepatocellular carcinoma

Common Edges seen in Surgical Practice

Edge of an ulcer	Characteristic feature
Undermined edge	Tuberculosis
Punched out edge	Syphilitic ulcer
Sloping edge	Healing traumatic or venous ulcer
Raised and pearly white beaded edge	Rodent ulcer or basal cell carcinoma
Rolled out or everted edge	Squamous cell carcinoma or ulcerated adenocarcinoma
Shallow, irregular and often indistinct edges	Venous ulcers

1. DEVELOPMENTAL DISTURBANCES OF ORAL AND PARAORAL STRUCTURES

Q.1. Write notes on xerostomia.

(Sep 2011, 3 Marks) (Feb 2013, 5 Marks)

Write short notes on xerostomia.

(Apr 2017, 5 Marks)

Ans. Xerostomia or dryness of mouth is not a disease, but a symptom of different diseases.

Xerostomia produces serious negative effects on patient's life affecting the dietary habits, nutritional status, speech, taste and increase susceptibility to dental caries.

Etiology

The causes of xerostomia are classified into two categories:

1. Temporary causes
2. Permanent causes

Temporary Causes

♦ *Psychological:* Anxiety and depression are well recognized as causes of reduced salivary flow.
♦ *Duct calculi:* Blockages of a duct of major salivary gland mainly submandibular produces dryness of affected side.
♦ *Sialoadenitis:* Inflammation of salivary glands can cause reduced secretions.
♦ *Drug therapy:* A wide variety of drugs, i.e., anticholinergic, tricyclic antidepressants, bronchodilators and histamines may cause xerostomia.

Permanent Causes

♦ *Salivary gland aplasia:* The congenital absence of salivary glands leads to xerostomia.
♦ *Sjogrens syndrome:* This is the combination of dry mouth, dry eyes and often rheumatoid arthritis.
♦ *Radiotherapy:* The distressing cause of xerostomia is therapeutic radiography for head and neck tumors.

Clinical Features

♦ Unilateral dryness with pain or discomfort and swelling in affected gland.
♦ Drying and burning sensations are present, but mucosa appears normal.
♦ Due to lack of saliva mucosa will appear dry, atrophic and more often pale and translucent.
♦ Soreness, burning and pain of mucous membrane and tongue are common symptoms.

Treatment

It is advisable to promote salivary stimulation by using sugar free chewing gum which is affected and convenient.

Q.2. Write notes on microdontia. *(Mar 2000, 5 Marks)*

Ans. Microdontia is the term used to describe the teeth which are smaller than the normal.

There are three types of microdontia:

1. True generalized microdontia
2. Relative generalized microdontia
3. Microdontia involving the single tooth

1. **True generalized microdontia:** In true generalized microdontia, all the teeth are smaller than the normal. Its occurrence is reported in the cases of pituitary dwarfism. The teeth are well formed and are small.
2. **Relative generalized microdontia:** In relative generalized microdontia, the normal or slightly smaller than normal teeth are present in the jaws that are somewhat larger than the normal and there is an illusion of true microdontia.
3. **Microdontia involving the single tooth:** It is a common condition which more commonly affects maxillary lateral incisor and third molar. Lateral incisor becomes peg shaped.

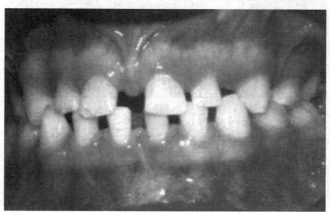

Fig. 1: Microdontia *(For color version, see Plate 2).*

Q.3. Write short note on benign migratory glossitis.

(Dec 2010, 3 Marks) (Aug 2011, 5 Marks)

Or

Write short note on geographic tongue.

(Jan 2018, 4 Marks)

Ans. Geographic tongue is a multifocal, patchy irregular area of depapillation of tongue characterized by frequent remissions and recurrences.

Clinical Features

♦ It is seen in children as well as in adults.
♦ Geographic tongue clinically presents multiple, irregular, well demarcated, patchy erythematous areas on dorsum of tongue with desquamation of filiform papilla.
♦ Although filiform papilla are absent in desquamated zone, the fungiform papillae remain present which appear as few red dots projecting on the surface.

♦ Geographic tongue is a painless, asymptomatic condition, however on few occasions it may produce soreness or burning sensations.

♦ Remissions of initial lesions always followed by fresh recurrent lesions which involves new areas of tongue surface.

Histopathology

♦ The condition show hyperparakeratinization of covering epithelium of the tongue with loss of filiform papillae.

♦ Intercellular edema and accumulation of neutral polymorphs is often seen in layers of epithelium.

♦ Mild inflammatory cell infiltration is present in underlying connective tissue.

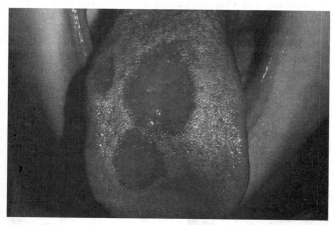

Fig. 2: Geographic tongue *(For color version, see Plate 2)*.

Q.4. Write short note on dilaceration. *(Jan 2012, 5 Marks)*

Ans. Dilaceration refers to an angulation or a sharp bend or a curve in the root and crown of the formed tooth.

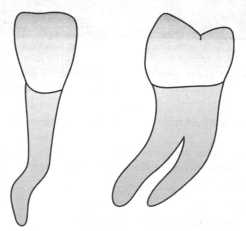

Dilaceration
Fig. 3: Dilaceration.

It occurs due to the mechanical trauma to calcified portion of partially formed teeth which lead to the displacement of calcified portion in different direction.

♦ The curve or the bend may occur anywhere along the length of the root, sometimes at the cervical portion, at other times midway along the root or even just at the apex of the root depending on the amount of root formed when injury occurs.

♦ Dilacerated teeth cause problems at the time of extraction, if operator is unaware of condition, so preoperative roentgenograms before any surgical procedure are carried out.

Q.5. Write short answer on Dens Invaginatus.
(Oct 2019, 3 Marks)

Or

Write short note on Dens in dente.
(July 2016, 5 Marks)

Ans. Oehlers describe dens invaginatus.

♦ Dens in dente or dens invaginatus is the deep surface invagination of crown or root which is lined by the enamel.

♦ Dens invaginatus is a developmental variation which is thought to arise as the result of invagination in the surface of tooth crown before calcification has occurred.

♦ The causes of the condition are increased localized external pressure, focal growth, retardation and focal growth stimulation in certain areas of tooth bud.

♦ The permanent maxillary lateral incisors are the teeth most commonly involved.

Types

♦ Coronal dens invaginatus
♦ Radicular dens invaginatus

Coronal Dens Invaginatus

♦ This is seen more frequently as compared to radicular dens invaginatus.

♦ In their decreasing order, teeth affected by this anomaly are permanent lateral incisors, central incisors, premolars, canines and molars.

♦ This is commonly seen in maxillary teeth.

♦ Variation in the depth of invagination is seen from slight enlargement of cingulum pit to deep infolding which extend to apex.

♦ Coronal dens invaginatus is of three types viz:
  • *Type I:* Exhibit invagination which is confined to the crown.
  • *Type II:* Extends below CEJ and ends in a blind sac that may/may not communicate with adjacent dental pulp.
  • *Type III:* It extends through the root and perforates in apical or lateral radicular area without any immediate communication with the pulp.

♦ Occasionally invagination can be rather large and resemble a tooth inside a tooth, i.e., it is known as dens in dente.

♦ In some of the other cases, invagination can be dilated and disturb the formation of tooth which lead to anomalous development of tooth known as dilated odontome.

♦ Roentgenographically, it is recognized as a pear-shaped invagination of enamel and dentin with a narrow constriction at the opening on the surface of the tooth and closely approximating the pulp in its depth.

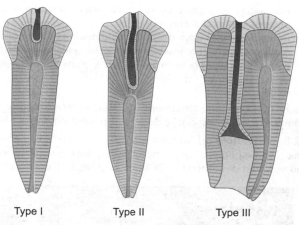

Type I   Type II   Type III

Fig. 4: Coronal dens invaginatus.

Radicular Dens Invaginatus

- This condition is rare.
- This condition arises secondary to proliferation of Hertwig's epithelial root sheath, with formation of strip of enamel that extends along surface of root.
- Roentgenographically, affected tooth shows enlargement of root. On close examination there is presence of dilated invagination which is lined by the enamel with opening of invagination situated along lateral aspect of root.

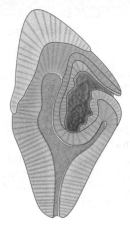

Fig. 5: Radicular dens invaginatus.

Treatment

- Type I invagination, opening should be restored after the eruption to prevent development of caries and pulpal inflammation.
- In large invagination content of lumen and carious dentine is removed and then calcium hydroxide base may be placed.
- Type III invaginations require endodontic therapy.

Q.6. Write a note on anodontia. *(Sep 2008, 3 Marks)*

Ans. Anodontia is defined as the condition in which there is congenital absence of teeth in oral cavity.

Etiology of Anodontia

The causes of anodontia are:

- Hereditary factor
- Environmental factor
- Familial factor
- Syndrome associated
- Radiation injury to the developing tooth germ.

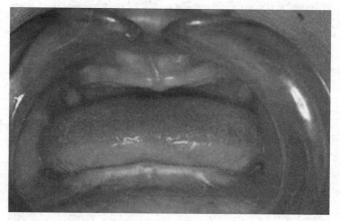

Fig. 6: Anodontia *(For color version, see Plate 2)*.

Anodontia is of two types:

1. *Complete anodontia:* There is congenital absence of all the teeth.
2. *Partial anodontia:* Congenital absence of one or few teeth.

Anodontia can also be divided into following types:

True anodontia: It occurs due to failure of development or formation of tooth in jaw bone.

Pseudoanodontia: It refers to the condition in which teeth are present within the jaw bone, but are not clinically visible in the mouth, as they have not erupted, e.g., impacted teeth.

False anodontia: It is the condition in which teeth are missing in the oral cavity because of their previous extraction.

Complete Anodontia

- It is the condition in which there is neither any deciduous tooth nor any permanent tooth present in the oral cavity.
- It is usually seen in association with hereditary ectodermal dysplasia. A complete anodontia is a common feature of hereditary ectodermal dysplasia however in many cases cuspids are present in this disease.
- Complete anodontia occurs among children those who have received high doses of radiation to the jaws as infants for therapeutic extraction.

Partial Anodontia

- It is a common phenomenon and is characterized by congenital absence of one or few teeth.
- In partial anodontia any tooth can be congenitally missing.
- Third molars are most frequently observed congenitally missing teeth.

♦ Mandibular first molar and the mandibular lateral incisor are least likely to be missing.

Q.7. Write note on amelogenesis imperfecta.

(Dec 2010, 8 Marks)

Ans. Amelogenesis imperfecta is also known as hereditary enamel dysplasia or hereditary brown enamel.

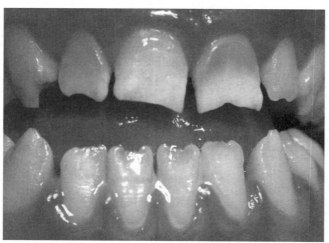

Fig. 7: Amelogenesis imperfecta *(For color version, see Plate 2).*

♦ Amelogenesis imperfecta is a heterogeneous group of hereditary disorders of enamel formation affecting both deciduous or permanent teeth.

♦ Disease involves only the ectodermal part of the tooth, i.e., enamel.

♦ It is of three types:
   1. Hypoplastic type
   2. Hypocalcified type
   3. Hypomature type

   1. *Hypoplastic type:* In this, the enamel thickness is usually far below the normal since disease affects the stage of matrix formation. In this stage, the teeth exhibit complete absence of enamel from crown surface or there may be a very thin layer of enamel in some focal areas.

   2. *Hypocalcification type:* This is due to disturbance in the process of early mineralization of enamel. In this stage, the enamel is soft and can easily be removed with blunt instrument.

   3. *Hypomaturation type:* This occurs due to interruption in the process of maturation of enamel. Here the enamel is of normal thickness, but it does not have normal hardness and is translucent. The enamel can be pierced with an explorer tip with firm pressure.

Clinical Features

♦ Color of teeth is mostly chalky white but sometimes it can be yellow or even dark brown.

♦ Contact points in proximal surfaces are mostly open while the occlusal surfaces and incisal edges are severely abraded.

♦ Enamel may have a cheesy consistency which is easily removable from tooth surface.

♦ Amelogenesis imperfecta does not increase the susceptibility of teeth to dental caries.

♦ In amelogenesis imperfecta, the enamel is of near normal hardness and has some white opaque flecks at incisal areas of teeth. These types of teeth are known as snow-capped teeth.

Treatment

There is no definite treatment of amelogenesis imperfecta. Composite veneering can be done to improve esthetics of teeth.

Q.8. Write note on mottled enamel. *(Feb 1999, 5 Marks)*

Ans. Mottled enamel is a type of hypoplasia due to fluoride and was first described by GV Black and Frederick S Mckay.

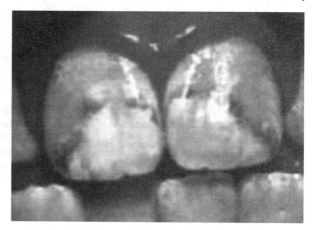

Fig. 8: Mottled enamel *(For color version, see Plate 2).*

Etiology

It is caused due to ingestion of fluoride containing water during the time of tooth formation which may result in mottled enamel.

Pathogenesis

Mottled enamel is due to the disturbance of ameloblasts during formative stage of tooth development.

There is histological evidence of cell development which is likely that the cell product, enamel matrix is defective or deficient. With higher level of fluoride, there is interference with calcification process of matrix.

Clinical Features

♦ There is white flecking or spotting of enamel.

♦ Mild changes are manifested by white opaque areas including tooth areas.

♦ Moderate and severe changes showing pitting and brownish staining of teeth.

♦ Corroded appearance of teeth.

♦ Those teeth which are moderately or severely affected may show a tendency of wear and even fracture of enamel.

Treatment

Mottled enamel frequently becomes stained an unsightly brown color. For cosmetic reasons it has become the practice to bleach the affected teeth with hydrogen peroxide.

Q.9. Enumerate various anomalies of teeth affecting number, size and shape. Describe one condition from each. *(Sep 1999, 15 Marks)*

Ans.

Enumeration of Anomalies Affecting Number of Teeth

♦ Anodontia
♦ Hypodontia
♦ Hyperdontia, i.e., natal teeth, neonatal teeth, premature eruption.

See anodontia in description. For anodontia, refer to Ans. 6 of same chapter.

Anomalies Affecting Shape of Teeth

♦ Gemination
♦ Twinning
♦ Fusion
♦ Concrescence
♦ Dilaceration
♦ Talon cusp
♦ Dens invaginatus
♦ Dens evaginatus
♦ Taurodontism
♦ Hypercementosis
♦ Enamel pearl
♦ Mulberry molar
♦ Globodontia
♦ Hutchinson's incisor

See dens invaginatus in description. For dens invaginatus, refer to Ans. 5 of same chapter.

Anomalies Affecting Size of Teeth

♦ Microdontia
♦ Macrodontia

See microdontia in description. For microdontia, refer to Ans. 2 of same chapter.

Q.10. Enumerate the developmental anomalies associated with the teeth. Describe factors associated with acquired enamel hypoplasia. *(Sep 1999, 15 Marks)*

Ans.

Anomalies Affecting Hard Tissues of Oral Cavity

The anomalies which affect the hard tissues of oral cavity are:

♦ Amelogenesis imperfecta or hereditary enamel dysplasia or hereditary brown enamel or hereditary opalescent teeth.
♦ Environmental enamel hypoplasia
♦ Dentinogenesis imperfecta
♦ Dentin dysplasia.
♦ Regional odontodysplasia or odontodysplasia or odontogenic dysplasia, odontogenesis imperfecta or ghost teeth
♦ Dentin hypocalcification

Factors Associated with Acquired Enamel Hypoplasia

There are two types of factors which are associated with acquired enamel hypoplasia:

1. Local factor
2. Environmental/systemic factor

1. *Local factors:* The local factors are infection, trauma, radiotherapy and idiopathic factors.
   • When local infection or trauma causes damage to ameloblasts cells during odontogenesis, it may result in defect in enamel formation in isolated permanent tooth and this is known as focal enamel hypoplasia.

   The focal enamel hypoplasia is caused due to periapical spread of infection from a carious deciduous tooth or trauma to the deciduous tooth, the tooth affected in this process is commonly known as turner's tooth.

2. *Environmental or systemic factors:* The systemic or environmental disturbances in the functioning of ameloblasts at specific period of time during odontogenesis often manifest as horizontal line of small pits or grooves or enamel surfaces. This line on tooth surface indicates zone of enamel hypoplasia and corresponds to time of development and duration of insult. The factors in following stages:
   • *Prenatal period:* The prenatal infections are rubella, syphilis.
     – There is presence of internal disease
     – There are excess fluoride ions
   • *Neonatal period:* During this period, enamel hypoplasia is caused due to:
     – Hemolytic disease of newborn
     – Birth injury
     – Premature delivery
     – Prolong labor
     – Low birth weight
   • *Postnatal period:* During this period, enamel hypoplasia is due to:
     – Sever childhood infection.
     – Prolong fever due to infectious disease in childhood
     – Nutritional deficiency
     – Hypocalcaemia
     – Rickets
     – Celiac disease.

For anomalies affecting number of teeth, affecting shape of teeth and affecting size of teeth, refer to Ans. 9 of same chapter.

Q.11. Write notes on gemination and fusion.
(Mar 2001, 5 Marks)

Or

Write short answer on fusion and gemination.
(Apr 2019, 3 Marks)

Ans.

Gemination

♦ Gemination is a developmental anomaly which refers to partial development of two teeth from single tooth bud following incomplete division.
♦ The structure is usually one with two completely or incompletely separated crowns that have a single root and a root canal.

♦ The condition is seen in both deciduous and permanent dentition.

♦ It appears to exhibit hereditary tendency.

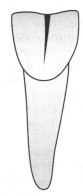

Fig. 9: Gemination.

Fusion

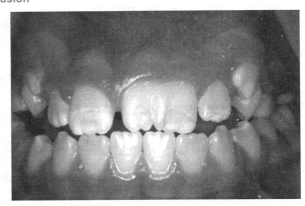

Fig. 10: Fusion *(For color version, see Plate 3).*

♦ Fusion is defined as union of two adjacent normal tooth germs at level of dentin during development.

♦ One of the most important criteria for fusion is that fused tooth must exhibit confluent dentin.

♦ Both permanent and deciduous dentition are affecting in case of fusion, although it is more common in deciduous teeth.

♦ Fusion can be complete or incomplete and its extent will depend on stage of odontogenesis at which fusion takes place.

♦ The incisor teeth are more frequently affected in both the dentitions during the condition.

Q.12. Write short note on taurodontism. *(Sep 2005, 5 Marks)* *(Jan 2017, 5 Marks) (Dec 2007, 3 Marks)*

Ans. Taurodontism is a dental anomaly in which the body of tooth is enlarged at the expense of the roots. Actually taurodontism means the bull shape appearance of the tooth.

Clinical Features

♦ Affected tooth in taurodontism has elongated pulp chamber with the rudimentary root formation.

♦ Tooth becomes rectangular in shape with minimum constriction at the cervical area.

♦ Taurodontism commonly affects multirooted permanent molar teeth and sometimes the premolar teeth.

♦ The bifurcation or trifurcation may be a few millimeter above the apices of the roots.

♦ Patient with hypodontia may have taurodontism.

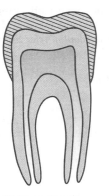 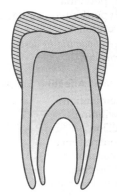

(A) Normal tooth   (B) Taurodontism

Figs. 11A and B: Taurodontism.

Treatment

No specific treatment is required.

Q.13. Write in brief on supernumerary teeth.

(Sep 2018, 5 Marks)

Ans. Presence of any extra tooth in dental arch in addition to normal series of teeth is known as supernumerary teeth.

Classification

♦ **According to the morphology**

• *Conical:* This small peg-shaped conical tooth is supernumerary tooth.

• *Tuberculate:* This type of supernumerary tooth possesses more than one cusp or tubercle. It is of barrel shaped and may be invaginated.

• *Supplemental:* It refers to the duplication of the teeth in normal series. The most common tooth is permanent maxillary lateral incisor.

• *Odontome:* This represents the hamartomatous malformation.

♦ **According to location**

• *Mesiodens:* They are located between two upper central incisor.

• *Distomolars:* They are located on the distal aspect of regular molar teeth in dental arch.

• *Paramolar:* They are located either in buccal or lingual aspect of normal molars.

• *Extra-lateral incisors:* They are more common in maxillary arch.

Clinical Features

♦ Supernumerary teeth cause crowding or malocclusion and give rise to cosmetic problem.

♦ These extra teeth are responsible for the increase caries incidence and periodontal problem.

♦ Multiple supernumerary teeth can occur in association with the conditions like Gardener's syndrome.

♦ Dentigerous cyst may sometimes develop from an impacted supernumerary tooth.

Treatment

♦ Supernumerary teeth should be extracted.

♦ Impacted supernumerary teeth should also be removed surgically since they can interfere with normal tooth alignment.

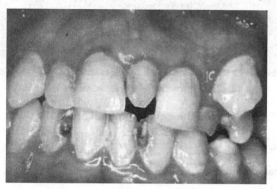

Fig. 12: Supernumerary teeth *(For color version, see Plate 3).*

Q.14. Write short note on dentinogenesis imperfecta.

(Mar 2006, 5 Marks)

Ans. Dentinogenesis imperfecta is an inherited disorder of dentin formation which affects deciduous and permanent dentition.

Classification

♦ **Sheild's Classification**
  • Dentinogenesis imperfecta Type I: Dentinogenesis imperfecta without osteogenesis imperfecta.
  • Dentinogenesis imperfecta Type II: Dentinogenesis imperfecta with osteogenesis imperfect
  • Dentinogenesis imperfecta Type III: It is a racial isolate in Maryland and is known as Brandywine type.

♦ **Extensive studies have shown that dentinogenesis imperfecta is clearly a disorder from osteogenesis imperfect, so the following revised classification is given:**
  • Dentinogenesis imperfecta 1: Dentinogenesis imperfecta without osteogenesis imperfecta (opalescent dentine). This corresponds to dentinogenesis imperfect Type II of Sheild's classification.
  • Dentinogenesis imperfecta 2: Brandywine type dentinogenesis imperfecta: This corresponds to dentinogenesis imperfect Type II of Sheild's classification.

There is no substitute in present classification for the category which is designated as Dentinogenesis imperfect Type I of Sheild's classification.

Etiology

Gene affected is present on chromosome 4 and it codes for DSPP (Dentine sialoprotein and phosphoprotein)

Clinical Features

♦ On eruption the teeth exhibit a normal contour and have opalescent amber like appearance.

♦ Few days after the eruption the teeth may achieve the normal color. Finally the teeth become gray or brownish in color with bluish reflection from enamel.

♦ In some cases, the affected teeth may exhibit hypomineralized areas on surface of enamel.

♦ Teeth are not particularly sensitive even when most of the surface enamel is lost.

♦ The dentin is soft and easily penetrable in dentinogenesis imperfecta, these teeth are not caries prone.

Histopathology

♦ Histopathologically the enamel appears normal in Dentinogenesis imperfecta. Mantle dentin is also nearly normal.

♦ Dentinal tubules are less in number per square unit area of dentin as compared to normal dentin. The tubules are often distorted, irregular in shape, widely spaced and larger in size.

♦ Pulp chamber and root canal are often obliterated by the abnormal dentin deposition.

♦ DEJ appears smooth or flattened instead of being scalloped.

♦ Large area of a tubular dentin is present.

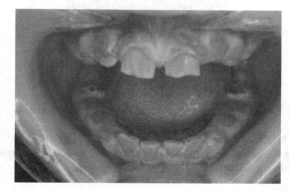

Fig. 13: Dentinogenesis imperfecta *(For color version, see Plate 3).*

Q.15. Write short note on median rhomboid glossitis.

(Dec 2009, 5 Marks) (Feb 2002, 5 Marks)
(Feb 2015, 5 Marks) (Jan 2016, 5 Marks)
Or
Write short answer on median rhomboid glossitis.
(May 2018, 3 Marks)

Ans. It is an asymptomatic, elongated, erythematous patch of atrophic mucosa on mid-dorsal surface of tongue.

Clinical Features

♦ Condition is seen mostly in the young adults.

♦ It is most common among the males.

♦ Lesion is located immediately anterior to the foramen cecum and circumvallate papillae in midline of dorsum of tongue.

♦ It starts as narrow, mildly erythematous area located along the median fissure of the tongue.

- Fully developed lesion of the median rhomboid glossitis appears diamond or lozenge-shaped area devoid of papilla.
- Color of lesion varies from pale pink to bright red.
- It is usually asymptomatic but occasionally causes slight soreness or burning sensation.

Histopathology

- Parakeratosis of surface epithelium
- Loss of papilla
- Thinning of supra papillary epithelium
- Presence of acanthosis with elongation of rete ridges.
- Superficial layer of epithelium shows neutrophilic infiltration and there is presence of candida hyphae.
- Underlying connective tissue is vascular and is infiltrated by chronic inflammatory cells.
- The epithelium may show features of dysplasia.

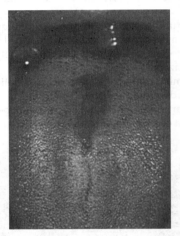

Fig. 14: Median rhomboid glossitis *(For color version, see Plate 3).*

Q.16. Write note on lingual thyroid. *(Aug/Sep 1998, 5 Marks)*

Ans. Accessory accumulation of functional thyroid gland tissue within the body of tongue is called lingual thyroid.

Clinical Features

- It is seen in females more commonly.
- In tongue, thyroid tissue appears as nodular exophytic mass measuring 2 to 3 cm in diameter and is located to foramen cecum.
- It can be present as smooth cystic swelling.
- Symptoms may vary which include change of voice, bleeding, pain, dysphagia, dyspnea and feeling of tightness in throat.

Histopathology

- Normal mature thyroid tissue, although embryonic or fetal thyroid gland tissue may also be seen.
- Thyroid nodules may exhibit colloid degeneration or goiter.
- Microscopic examination of human tongue removes at autopsy reveals remnant of thyroid tissue within tongue.

Treatment

Surgical excision should be done.

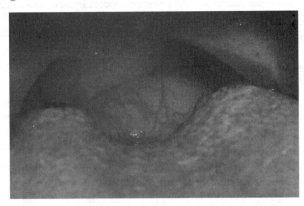

Fig. 15: Lingual thyroid *(For color version, see Plate 3).*

Q.17. Enumerate the developmental anomalies of tongue and describe any two. *(Mar 2007, 2.5 Marks)*

Ans.

Developmental Anomalies of Tongue

- Aglossia
- Microglossia
- Macroglossia
- Ankyloglossia or tongue tie
- Cleft tongue
- Fissured tongue
- Median rhomboid glossitis
- Geographic tongue
- Hairy tongue
- Lingual thyroid nodule
- Lingual varices

For detail, refer to median rhomboid glossitis (Ans. 15) and lingual thyroid (Ans. 16) of same chapter.

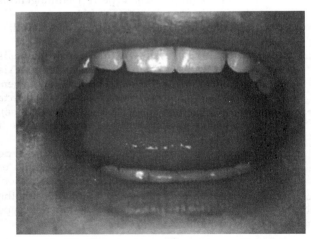

Fig. 16: Perleche *(For color version, see Plate 3).*

Q.18. Write short note on dentin dysplasia.

(Sep 2006, 5 Marks) (Jan 2012, 5 Marks)

Or

Write notes on dentin dysplasia. *(Feb 2013, 8 Marks)*

Ans. It is the autosomal dominant inherited disorder characterized by the defective dentin formation and abnormal pulp morphology.

♦ The condition is also known as "rootless teeth".
♦ It is classified into two types
  • *Type I:* Radicular dentin dysplasia
  • *Type II:* Coronal dentin dysplasia

Type I: Radicular Dentin Dysplasia

It represents a peculiar disturbance in the development of radicular dentin.

Clinical Features

♦ It affects both deciduous and permanent dentition.
♦ Root of teeth is defective and the crown portion of teeth is normal both structurally and morphologically.
♦ In some cases, the crown of teeth reveals slight bluish or brownish tendency.
♦ Because of presence of functionally unstable short roots, the affected teeth exhibit mobility.

Histopathology

♦ Enamel and mantle dentin are normal.
♦ Remaining coronal and radicular dentin appear fused nodular mass comprising of tubular dentin and osteo dentin.
♦ Histological appearance of such defective mass of dentinal tissue often reveals what is called as "series of sand dunes" or "lava flowing around boulders".
♦ Normal and abnormal dentin is well demarcated and later reveals an abnormal distribution and orientation of dentinal tubules with whorled appearance.

Treatment

No specific treatment.

Type II: Coronal Dentin Dysplasia

It is an inherited disorder of dentin, which affects the coronal dentin.

Clinical Features

♦ Both deciduous and permanent teeth are affected.
♦ Permanent teeth are of normal color whereas deciduous teeth are amber gray color.

Histopathology

♦ Pulp chambers in permanent teeth are abnormally large and have a flame shaped.
♦ Pulp chamber contains many denticles.
♦ Root canal may be partially obliterated in apical third region.

Q.19. Write short note on concrescence.

(Sep 2007, 2.5 Marks)

Ans. Concrescence is defined as union of roots of two or more adjoining teeth due to deposition of cementum.

It is the type of fusion which is limited only to the roots of teeth and it occurs after the root formation of involved teeth is completed.

Etiology

♦ Traumatic injury
♦ Crowding of teeth
♦ Hypercementosis

Important Features

♦ Concrescence represents an acquired defect and it can occur in both erupted or unerupted.
♦ In concrescence beside cementum union or fusion does not occur between the enamel, dentin or pulp of involved teeth.
♦ Permanent maxillary molar are usually affected by this anomaly.

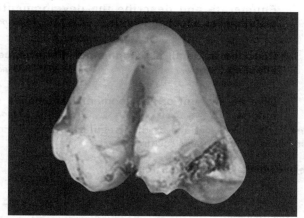

Fig. 17: Concrescence *(For color version, see Plate 4).*

♦ Concrescence can occur between normal molar and a supernumerary molar.
♦ Condition is seen in those areas of dental arch where roots of neighboring teeth lie close to one another.

Q.20. Write short note on Fordyce's granules.

(Jan 2016, 5 Marks) (Sep 2009, 3 Marks)

Ans. It is a developmental anomaly characterized by heterotrophic collection of sebaceous glands at various sites in oral cavity.

Pathogenesis

It is suggested that occurrence of sebaceous gland in the mouth may result from inclusion in the oral cavity of ectoderm having some of the potentialities of skin in the course of development of the maxillary and mandibular process during embryonic life.

Clinical Features

♦ They appear as yellow spots either separated from each other and remain in groups.

- They are seen bilaterally on the mucosa of cheeks opposite to molar tooth, on the inner surfaces of lips, retromolar area.
- They are also seen in the esophagus, female genitalia, male genitalia, nipples, palm and soles, parotid gland, larynx and orbit.

Histological Features

- They are unassociated with the hair follicles.
- Glands are superficial and may consist of only few or more tubules, all grouped around one or more ducts which open in the mucosa.
- Ducts may show keratin plugging.

Treatment

No treatment is required.

Q.21. Define anomaly. Describe in detail developmental anomalies of the tongue. *(Sep 2011, 8 Marks)*

Or

Enumerate and describe the developmental disturbances affecting tongue. *(Aug 2012, 15 Marks)*

Or

Describe in detail developmental disturbances affecting tongue. *(Apr 2015, 8 Marks)*

Or

Give an account of developmental anomalies of tongue. *(Mar 2016, 8 Marks)*

Ans. Anomaly is defined as the irregularity or deviation compared to the normal structure.

Developmental Anomalies of Tongue

- Aglossia
- Microglossia
- Macroglossia
- Ankyloglossia or tongue tie
- Cleft tongue
- Fissured tongue
- Median rhomboid glossitis
- Geographic tongue
- Hairy tongue
- Lingual thyroid nodule
- Lingual varices

For median rhomboid glossitis, refer to Ans. 15 of same chapter

For Lingual thyroid, refer to Ans. 16 of same chapter.

For Geographic tongue, refer to Ans. 3 of same chapter.

Aglossia

It is characterized by the complete absence of tongue

Microglossia

This is in reality a microglossia with extreme glossoptosis. In such cases, a rudimentary small tongue is observed. Due to the lack of muscular stimulus between alveolar arches they do not develop transversely and mandible does not grow in anterior direction.

Macroglossia

Macroglossia is an uncommon condition characterized by enlargement of tongue.

Type of Macroglossia

There are two broad categories under the heading of Macroglossia, i.e.:

- True macroglossia
- Pseudomacroglossia

Causes

- *Congenital and hereditary:*
  - Vascular malformations
  - Lymphangioma
  - Hemangioma
  - Hemihyperplasia
  - Cretinism
  - Beckwith-Wiedemann syndrome
  - Down syndrome
  - Mucopolysaccharidosis
  - Neurofibromatosis
- *Acquired:*
  - Edentulous patients
  - Amyloidosis
  - Myxedema
  - Acromegaly
  - Angioedema
  - Carcinoma and other tumors

Clinical features

- It most commonly occur in children.
- In infants, it is manifested by noisy breathing, drooling and difficulty in eating.
- Macroglossia result in lisping speech.
- Pressure of tongue against mandible and teeth produces lateral crenated border of tongue.
- Presence of open bite and mandibular prognathism is seen.
- Children with macroglossia often develop tongue thrusting habits, which may lead to malocclusion, open bite and diastema formation, etc.
- Macroglossia developing in adult people (as in acromegaly or in tumors, etc.) may produce spacing of teeth and distortion of the mandibular arch.
- Blockage of the pharyngeal airway due to macroglossia may result in a condition called obstruction sleep apnea.

Ankyloglossia

It is also known as tongue tie

Ankyloglossia is the condition which arises when the inferior frenulum attaches to the bottom of tongue and subsequently restricts free movements of the tongue.

Clinical Features

- Males are affected more commonly than females
- It can cause feeding problems in infants

♦ It causes speech defects especially articulation of the sounds l, r, t, d, n, th, sh and z

♦ It leads to persistent gap between the mandibular incisors.

Treatment

Frenulectomy is the treatment of choice.

Cleft Tongue

♦ It is a rare condition which arises due to lack of merging of lateral lingual swellings of this organ.

♦ A partial cleft tongue is more commonly seen.

♦ Partial cleft occurs because of incomplete merging and failure of groove obliteration by underlying mesenchymal proliferation.

Fissured Tongue

It is also known as scrotal tongue.

Clinical Features

♦ More common among males.

♦ No clinical symptom is seen in fissured tongue but collection of food debris and microorganisms in the fissures or grooves sometimes cause discomfort.

♦ Fissures or grooves often radiate freely in central groove on the dorsal surface in oblique direction.

♦ Large and deep fissures may be inter-connected and they separate the dorsum of the tongue into multiple lobules.

Histological Features

♦ There will be loss of filiform papillae from the surface mucosa.

♦ Neutrophilic microabscess formation within the epithelium.

♦ Hyperplasia of the rete pegs and increased thickness of the lamina propria.

♦ Mixed inflammatory cell infiltration in the connective tissue stroma.

Treatment

No treatment is required.

Hairy Tongue

♦ Hairy tongue is an unusual condition, which occurs due to hypertrophy of the filiform papilla of tongue along with loss of normal desquamation process.

♦ Abnormal hair-like growth of the papilla eventually leads to formation of a pigmented, thick, matted layer on the tongue surface often heavily coated with bacteria and fungi.

Etiology

♦ Poor oral hygiene

♦ Fungal infections

♦ Prolonged use of antibiotics

♦ Heavy smoking

♦ Excessive use of antiseptic mouth washes

♦ Chronic illness

♦ Lack of tooth brushing and consumption of soft foods with little or no roughage.

Pathogenesis

♦ Normally the keratinized surface layers of the tongue papillae are continuously desquamated through friction of the tongue with food, rough surface of the palate and the upper anterior teeth. Following desquamation, tongue papillae are replaced by newer epithelial cells from below.

♦ Lack of tongue movements due to local or systemic disease disturbs the regular desquamation process of the tongue papilla; especially the filiform papillae, which lengthens considerably and produces a hairy appearance on the tongue surface.

♦ Such hypertrophied papillae are often coated with microorganisms and become discolored.

Clinical Features

♦ Hairy tongue commonly affects the mid dorsum of the tongue.

♦ Hypertrophy of the filiform papillae produces a thick matted layer on the dorsal surface.

♦ Hypertrophied filiform papillae may grow up to half a centimeter long, which often brushes the soft palate and produces gagging sensations.

♦ There can be irritation to the tongue due to accumulation of food debris and microorganisms.

Treatment

♦ Removal of etiological factor.

♦ Proper cleaning of tongue.

Q.22. Describe environmental enamel hypoplasia.

(Mar 2011, 8 Marks)

Ans. Environmental enamel hypoplasia may be defined as an incomplete or defective formation of the organic enamel matrix of teeth.

Enamel hypoplasia (EH) is a quantitative defect associated with a reduced localized thickness of enamel, following disruption of the secretory phase of amelogenesis.

The enamel may be translucent or opaque, with single or multiple pits or grooves and partial or complete absence of enamel over significant areas of dentin. The enamel hypoplasia defects tend to occur in the incisal or cuspal one-third of the crown.

♦ Defect which is caused by environmental factors, either dentition may be involved and sometimes only a single tooth; both enamel and dentin are usually affected, at least to some degree.

♦ It is known that a number of different factors, each capable of producing injury to the ameloblasts, may give rise to the condition, including:

• Nutritional deficiency (vitamins A and D)

• Exanthematous diseases (e.g., measles, chickenpox, scarlet fever)

• Congenital syphilis

• Hypocalcemia

• Birth injury, prematurity and Rh hemolytic disease

• Local infection or trauma

• Ingestion of chemicals (chiefly fluoride)

• Idiopathic

- In mild environmental hypoplasia, there may be only a few small grooves, pits, or fissures on the enamel surface. If the condition is more severe, enamel may exhibit rows of deep pits arranged horizontally across the surface of the tooth. There may be only a single row of such pits or several rows indicating a series of injuries.
- In most severe cases, a considerable portion of enamel may be absent, suggesting a prolonged disturbance in the function of the ameloblasts.
- Hypoplasia results only if the injury occurs at the time teeth are developing, or more specifically during the formative stage of enamel development. Once the enamel has calcified, no such defect can be produced. Thus, knowing the chronologic development of the deciduous and permanent teeth, it is possible to determine from the location of the defect on the teeth the approximate time at which the injury occurred.

Enamel Hypoplasia Due to Vitamin A Deficiency

Although tissues of ectodermal origin, i.e., the epidermis is primarily affected in vitamin A deficiency, teeth also record this deficiency. Avitaminosis A is evidenced by marked metaplasia of the enamel organ, which results in defective enamel formation. This view originates from histological changes seen initially in the oral mucosa and extending to the degeneration of the epithelial-derived ameloblasts, which results in a hypoplastic enamel matrix. If vitamin A deficiency is severe, ameloblast cells will become completely atrophied, which results in an absence of enamel formation. In less severe cases, the columnar ameloblasts apparently shorten, and adjacent enamel exhibits hypoplasia. If vitamin A deficiency is relieved during subsequent tooth development, normal enamel is produced, although defective tissue is not repaired.

Enamel Hypoplasia Due to Vitamin D Deficiency

Vitamin D is essential for deposition of calcium and phosphorus in hard tissues. Its presence increases the absorption of dietary calcium and maintains proper levels of calcium and phosphorus in the blood. Primary deficiency of vitamin D results from insufficient exposure to the sun and insufficient dietary intake. Secondary deficiencies result from abnormal intestinal resorption. Secondary deficiencies may be overcome by alteration of dietary intake of calcium and phosphorus. A severe vitamin D deficiency in children results in rickets, a condition characterized by insufficient deposition of calcium salts in bony tissue. Dental features of rickets include enamel hypoplasia due to failure of tooth mineralization. Enamel hypoplasia is of pitted type.

Enamel Hypoplasia Due to Exanthematous Diseases

Some studies have indicated that exanthematous diseases, including measles, chickenpox and scarlet fever, are etiologic factors. In general, it might be stated that any serious nutritional deficiency or systemic disease is potentially capable of producing enamel hypoplasia, since ameloblasts are one of the most sensitive groups of cells in body in terms of metabolic function. The type of hypoplasia occurring from these deficiency or disease states is usually of the pitting variety. Since the pits tend to stain, the clinical appearance of the teeth may be very unsightly. Clinical studies indicate that most cases of enamel hypoplasia involve those teeth that form within the first year after birth, although teeth that form somewhat later may be affected. Thus the teeth most frequently involved are the central and lateral incisors, cuspids and first molars.

Enamel Hypoplasia Due to Congenital Syphilis

Congenital syphilis arises from transplacental fetal infection with *Treponema pallidum* acquired during pregnancy from an untreated mother. The disease is divided into an early stage that usually occur before 3 months, but may be seen up to 2 years, and late stage disease that occurs after 2 years. Late congenital syphilis affect the amelogenesis of the molars and incisors. Both Hutchinson teeth and mulberry molars are seen in about 65% of patients. These characteristic teeth present at around 6 years; they are centrally notched, widely spaced, peg-shaped upper permanent central incisors. Patients with congenital syphilis may also have mulberry molars, which are first molars dwarfed by a small occlusal surface, and are characterized by roughened lobulated hypoplastic enamel leading to caries. The surface has numerous poorly formed cusps which overcome to form a dome-shaped tooth, which is considerably narrower at the grinding surface than at its base.

Enamel Hypoplasia Due to Hypocalcemia

Tetany induced by a decreased level of calcium in the blood, may result from several conditions, the most common being vitamin D deficiency and parathyroid deficiency (parathyroprivic tetany). In tetany, the serum calcium level may fall as low as 6–8 mg per 100 mL, and at this level enamel hypoplasia is frequently produced in teeth developing concomitantly This type of enamel hypoplasia is usually of the pitting variety and thus does not differ from that resulting from a nutritional disturbance or exanthematous disease.

Enamel Hypoplasia Due to Birth Injuries

The neonatal line or ring, described by Schour in 1936 and present in deciduous teeth and first permanent molars, may be thought of as a type of hypoplasia because there is a disturbance produced in the enamel and dentin, which is indicative of trauma or change of environment at the time of birth.

Enamel Hypoplasia Due to Local Infection or Trauma

A type of hypoplasia occasionally seen is unusual in that only a single tooth is involved, most commonly one of the permanent maxillary incisors or a maxillary or mandibular premolar. There may be any degree of hypoplasia, ranging from a mild, brownish discoloration of the enamel to a severe pitting and irregularity of the tooth crown. Another frequent pattern of enamel defects seen in permanent teeth is caused by periapical inflammatory disease of the overlying deciduous tooth. The altered tooth is called Turner's tooth.

Q.23. Write short note on cleft lip. *(Jan 2012, 5 Marks)*

Ans. Cleft lip is a developmental anomaly characterized by wedge shaped defect in the lip which results from failure of two parts of the lip to fuse together at the time of development.

Etiology

◆ Nutritional factors, such as deficiency of or excess of vitamin A and deficiency of riboflavin.
◆ Maternal smoking (during pregnancy) is a very high-risk factor.
◆ Psychogenic, emotional or traumatic stress in pregnant mothers.
◆ Relative ischemia to the area due to defective vascular supply.
◆ Mechanical obstruction by enlarged tongue.
◆ High dose of steroid therapy during pregnancy.
◆ Localized mucopolysaccharide metabolism defect in the area.
◆ Infections.
◆ Substances, such as alcohol, drugs or toxins in the circulation.

Pathogenesis

◆ Cleft in lower lip usually occurs either due to failure of the copula to form the mandibular arch or due to persistence of the central groove of the mandibular process.
◆ Cleft of the upper lip and premaxilla occur due to failure of mesodermal penetration and subsequent obliteration of the ectodermal grooves between the median nasal process, lateral nasal process and the maxillary process, which occurs during the seventh week of intrauterine life.

Clinical Features

◆ Occur most commonly in males.
◆ Most common type of isolated cleft lip only is unilateral complete type.
◆ Breastfeeding is impossible to babies having cleft lip, as they cannot generate sufficient suction.
◆ There is difficulty in correct phonation and articulation of speech.
◆ Mental trauma to the child due to the unusual appearance.

Treatment

◆ Cosmetic repair of face and lips
◆ Proper development of speech
◆ Prevention of maxillary arch collapse

Q.24. Write short note on fluorosis. *(Feb 2013, 5 Marks)*

Ans. Fluorosis is a toxic manifestation of chronic fluoride intake.
◆ It can be described as a diffuse symmetric hypomineralization disorder of ameloblasts.
◆ Fluorosis is irreversible and only occurs with exposure to fluoride when enamel is developing.
◆ Instead of being a normal creamy-white translucent color, fluorosed enamel is porous and opaque.
◆ Teeth can resemble a ghostly white chalk colored (light refractivity is greatly reduced because the enamel's prism structure is defective).

◆ Cloudy striated (lines of demarcation) enamel, white specks or blotches, 'snow-capping', yellowish-brown spots, or brown pits on teeth are all characteristic of fluorosis.
◆ In its more severe form, fluorosed enamel is structurally weak (brittle) and prone to erosion and breakage, especially when drilled and filled.
◆ Even in the milder forms, there is increased enamel attrition.
◆ To prevent fluorosis from occurring in the most prominent and/or most susceptible teeth, the most critical time to avoid fluoride exposure is the first three to six years of a child's life.

Fejerskov et al. (1977) stated that the effect of fluoride on enamel formation can follow several possible pathogenic pathways:

◆ *Effect on ameloblasts:*
   • *Secretory phase:*
      – Diminished matrix production
      – Change of matrix composition
      – Change in ion transport mechanism
   • *Maturation phase:* Diminished withdrawal of protein and water
◆ Effect on nucleation and crystal growth in all stages of enamel formation
◆ Effect on calcium homeostasis generally with dental fluorosis as an indirect result
   • After the tooth erupts and calcification has been completed, ingested fluoride does not have adverse dental consequences.
   • Fluorosis is seen to affect mainly permanent dentition and very high fluoride levels (>10 ppm) are required in drinking water for it to cross placental barrier and affect primary dentition.

Also refer to Ans. 8 of same chapter.

Q.25. Enumerate the developmental disturbances affecting the structures of teeth and discuss in detail amelogenesis imperfecta. *(Feb 2013, 10 Marks)*

Or

Enumerate developmental disturbances affecting structures of teeth. Write in detail about amelogenesis imperfecta. *(July 2016, 10 Marks)*

Or

Enumerate developmental defects affecting tooth structure. Write in detail amelogenesis imperfecta.
(Feb 2019, 10 Marks)

Ans.

Developmental Disturbances Affecting Structure of Teeth

◆ Amelogenesis imperfecta
◆ Dentinogenesis imperfecta
◆ Enamel hypoplasia
◆ Dentin dysplasia
◆ Regional odontodysplasia
◆ Dentin hypocalcification

Amelogenesis Imperfecta

Amelogenesis imperfecta is a group of hereditary disorders characterized by alteration of the quantity and quality of enamel in humans and is frequently associated with a significant dental disease. —**Witkop and Sauk (1976)**

Classification of Amelogenesis Imperfecta

Witkop, 1988 Four major categories based primarily on phenotype (hypoplastic, hypomaturation, hypocalcified, hypomaturation-hypoplastic with taurodontism) subdivided into 15 subtypes by phenotype and secondarily by mode of inheritance.

- *Type I*–Hypoplastic
- *Type IA*–Hypoplastic, pitted autosomal dominant
- *Type IB*–Hypoplastic, local autosomal dominant
- *Type IC*–Hypoplastic, local autosomal recessive
- *Type ID*–Hypoplastic, smooth autosomal dominant
- *Type IE*–Hypoplastic, smooth X-linked dominant
- *Type IF*–Hypoplastic, rough autosomal dominant
- *Type IG*–Enamel agenesis, autosomal recessive
- *Type II*–Hypomaturation
- *Type IIA*–Hypomaturation, pigmented autosomal recessive
- *Type IIB*–Hypomaturation, X-linked recessive
- *Type IIC*–Hypomaturation, snow-capped teeth, X-linked
- *Type IID*–Hypomaturation, snow-capped teeth, autosomal dominant?
- *Type IIIA*–Autosomal dominant
- *Type IIIB*–Autosomal recessive
- *Type IV*–Hypomaturation-hypoplastic with taurodontism
- *Type IVA*–Hypomaturation-hypoplastic with taurodontism, autosomal dominant
- *Type IVB*–Hypoplastic-hypomaturation with taurodontism, autosomal dominant

For types and clinical features, refer to Ans. 7 of same chapter.

Histopathology

- There is a disturbance in the differentiation or viability of ameloblasts in the hypoplastic type, and this is reflected in defect in matrix formation up to and including total absence of matrix.
- In the hypocalcification type, there are defects of matrix structure and of mineral deposition.
- In the hypomaturation type, there are alterations in enamel rod and rod sheath structures.
- Ground section of the teeth involved showed very thin enamel, composed of laminations of irregularly arranged enamel prisms.

Radiographic Features

- The enamel may appear totally absent on the radiograph, or when present may appear as a very thin layer chiefly over the tips of cusps and on the inter-proximal surfaces.
- In other cases, the calcification of the enamel may be so affected that it appears to have the same approximate radiodensity as the dentin, making differentiation, between the two difficult.

Treatment

- There is no definite treatment of amelogenesis imperfecta.
- Composite veneering can be done to improve esthetics of teeth.

Q.26. Describe histologic features with diagram of ghost teeth. *(Nov 2008, 5 Marks)*

Ans. It is also known as regional odontodysplasia.

Following are the histologic features of ghost teeth:

- In ground section enamel thickness varies.
- Prism structure of enamel is irregular and it lacks laminated appearance.
- Dentin show clefts which are scattered through mixture of interglobular dentin and amorphous material.
- Reduction in amount of dentin is seen.
- Widening of predentin layer is present.
- Large areas of interglobular dentin are seen.
- Pulp contains free or attached pulp stones which exhibit tubules or have laminated calcification.
- Follicular tissue surrounding the crown is enlarged and exhibit collections of basophilic enamel like calcifications called as enameloid conglomerates.

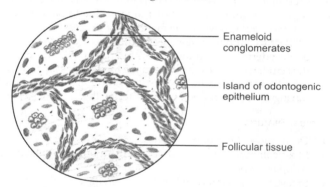

Fig. 18: Ghost teeth *(For color version, see Plate 4).*

Q.27. Write in detail enamel hypoplasia. *(May/Jun 2009, 10 Marks)*

Ans. *For enamel hypoplasia, refer to Ans. 22 of same chapter.*

Q.28. Classify enamel hypoplasia. Describe in detail about environmental factors causing enamel hypoplasia. *(Jan 2012, 15 Marks)*

Ans.

Classification of Enamel Hypoplasia

- *Mild:* Presence of few small grooves, pits and fissures on enamel
- *Moderate:* Presence of rows of deep pits arranged horizontally over surface.
- *Severe:* Portion of enamel may be absent

For environmental factors causing enamel hypoplasia, refer to Ans. 22 of same chapter.

Q.29. Write in brief on macroglossia. *(Jun 2010, 5 Marks)*

Or

Write short note on macroglossia. *(Jun 2017, 5 Marks)*

Ans. *Refer to Ans. 21 of same chapter.*

Q.30. Write short note on hypodontia. *(Aug 2012, 5 Marks)*

Ans. It is the developmental alteration in number of teeth.

♦ Hypodontia denotes the lack of development of one or more teeth.

♦ Oligodontia is a type of hypodontia which indicates lack of development of six or more teeth.

Etiology

♦ *Genetic:* Various syndromes are associated, such as hereditary ectodermal dysplasia, craniofacial dysostosis, etc.

♦ At present scenario evolution is there towards some teeth.

♦ X-ray radiation causing damage to developing tooth bud results in absence of teeth.

Clinical Features

♦ Hypodontia is very uncommon in deciduous dentition.

♦ When hypodontia is present it frequently involves lateral incisors.

♦ In permanent dentition, third molars are more commonly affected and after these second premolars and lateral incisors are absent.

♦ Hypodontia is also associated with microdontia.

Treatment

♦ Fixed prosthesis should be given to patient in form of bridges.

♦ Removable partial dentures can also be given.

Q.31. Discuss in detail about etiology, clinical features and treatment of cleft lip and palate. Add a note on syndromes associated. *(Aug 2012, 10 Marks)*

Ans. *For etiology, clinical features of cleft lip, refer to Ans. 23 of same chapter.*

Cleft Palate

Etiology of cleft lip and cleft palate is similar so for etiology, refer to Ans. 23 of same chapter.

Clinical Features

♦ It is seen more common in females as compared to males.

♦ Cleft is seen over the hard and soft palate and it can also be seen in cleft of soft palate alone.

♦ Extension of cleft palate varies, i.e., it involves uvula or soft palate, at times it extend over the complete palate, it also sometimes involve alveolar ridge unilaterally or bilaterally.

♦ Patient feels difficulty in drinking and eating since liquid and food regurgitates through the nose.

♦ Patient have problem in speaking.

♦ Upper lateral incisors of patient are short or may be absent.

♦ Crossbite is present.

Treatment of Cleft Lip and Cleft Palate

♦ Cleft palate is usually repaired in 12–18 months. Early repair causes retarded maxillary growth. Late repair causes speech defect.

♦ Both soft and hard palates are repaired.

♦ Abnormal insertion of tensor palati is released. Mucoperiosteal flaps are raised in the palate which is sewed together.

♦ If maxillary hypoplasia is present, then osteotomy of the maxilla is done. With orthodontic teeth extraction and alignment of dentition is done.

♦ Regular examination of ear, nose and throat during follow-up period, i.e., postoperative speech therapy.

♦ Whenever complicated problems are present, staged surgical procedure is done.

♦ Wardill-Kilner push back operation-by raising mucoperiosteum flaps based on greater palatine vessels.

♦ Hearing support is given using hearing aids if defect is present; control of otitis media.

♦ Speech problems occur due to velopharyngeal incompetence; articulation problems also can occur speech therapy is given. It is corrected by pharyngoplasty, veloplasty, speech devices.

♦ Dental problems, such as uneruption, unalignment are common. They should be corrected by proper dentist opinion, and reconstructive surgery.

♦ Orthodontic management with alveolar bone graft, maxillary osteotomy is done in 8–11 years.

Syndromes Associated with Cleft Lip and Cleft Palate

There are multiple syndromes associated but most common syndrome associated is Pierre-Robin syndrome. This syndrome is characterized by cleft palate, micrognathia and glossoptosis. Other syndromes associated are as follows:

♦ *Goldenhar syndrome:* Cleft palate, microstomia, hypoplastic zygomatic arch.

♦ *Marfan's syndrome:* Cleft palate, skeletal defects, ocular lens defect.

♦ *Down's syndrome:* Cleft palate, teeth anomalies, fissured tongue, malocclusion.

♦ *Patau syndrome:* Cleft lip and cleft palate, polydactyly and heart anomalies.

♦ *Orofacial digital syndrome:* Cleft lip, digital malformation, deformed facial features.

♦ *Treacher Collins syndrome:* Cleft lip and cleft palate, facial deformities.

♦ *Median cleft face syndrome:* Cleft palate, nasal cleft and frontonasal dysplasia.

♦ *Otopalatodigital syndrome:* Cleft palate, mandibular micrognathia, facial deformity.

♦ *Blepharocheilodontic syndrome:* Eye anomalies, cleft lip and palate, microdontia.

Q.32. Write short note on developmental disturbances in number of teeth. *(Dec 2012, 3 Marks)*

Or

Describe in detail developmental disturbances affecting number of teeth. *(Nov 2014, 8 Marks)*

Ans. Developmental disturbances in number of teeth

- Anodontia
- Hypodontia
- Hyperdontia

For anodontia in detail, refer to Ans. 6 of same chapter.

For hypodontia in detail, refer to Ans. 30 of same chapter.

Hyperdontia

- Hyperdontia is the development of an increased number of teeth.
- The additional teeth are known as supernumerary teeth.
- *For supernumerary teeth in detail, refer to Ans. 13 of same chapter.*
- Accessory teeth may be present at or shortly after birth.
- Teeth present in newborn baby are known as natal teeth while teeth arising in first 30 days of life are known as neonatal teeth.
- These teeth may represent predeciduous supernumerary teeth.

Q.33. Enumerate the different developmental disturbances of teeth on basis of size, number and shape. Describe in detail the developmental disturbances in structure of tooth. *(Mar 2013, 8 Marks)*

Ans. *For enumeration of developmental disturbances of teeth on basis of size, number and shape, refer to Ans. 9 of same chapter.*

Developmental Disturbances in Structure of Tooth

Following are the developmental disturbances in structure of tooth:

- Amelogenesis imperfecta or hereditary enamel dysplasia or hereditary brown enamel or hereditary opalescent teeth.
- Environmental enamel hypoplasia.
- Dentinogenesis imperfecta.
- Dentin dysplasia.
- Regional odontodysplasia or odontodysplasia or odontogenic dysplasia, odontogenesis imperfecta or ghost teeth.
- Dentin hypocalcification.

For amelogenesis imperfecta, refer to Ans. 7 and Ans. 25 of same chapter.

For environmental enamel hypoplasia, refer to Ans. 22 of same chapter.

For dentinogenesis imperfecta, refer to Ans. 14 of same chapter.

For dentin dysplasia, refer to Ans. 18 of same chapter.

Regional Odontodysplasia

It is also known as odontodysplasia or ghost teeth.

- In this both ectodermal and mesodermal, tooth components are affected.
- In this tooth is hypocalcified and hypoplastic.

Etiology

- Due to abnormal migration of neural crest cells
- Due to medication taken during pregnancy

- In local trauma or infection
- In cases of radiation therapy
- Due to somatic mutations
- Local circulatory deficiency

Clinical Features

- Both the dentitions, i.e., deciduous and permanent dentitions are affected.
- Slight female predilection is present.
- Maxillary teeth are more commonly involved as compared to mandibular teeth. More often involved are maxillary anterior teeth.
- Many of the affected teeth are failed to erupt.
- Erupted teeth have small irregular crowns that are yellow to brown with rough surface.
- Presence of caries and periapical inflammatory lesions are common.
- Gingival swelling is present adjacent to the affected tooth.

Histopathology

For histopathology, refer to Ans. 26 of same chapter.

Treatment

- Prosthetic replacement of teeth should be done.
- In some of teeth root canal should be done followed by capping of teeth.

Q.34. Enumerate the developmental disturbances affecting the structure of teeth and discuss in detail dentinogenesis imperfecta. *(June 2014, 10 Marks)*

Ans. *For enumeration of developmental disturbances affecting the structure of teeth, refer to Ans. 25 of same chapter.*

For dentinogenesis imperfecta in detail, refer to Ans. 14 of same chapter.

Q.35. Write short note on Turner's tooth. *(June 2014, 5 Marks)*

Ans. Turner's tooth is also known as Turner's hypoplasia.

It is a localized enamel hypoplasia caused due to local infection or trauma and tooth affected is known as Turner's tooth.

Pathogenesis

- If a deciduous tooth is affected by dental caries when crown of succeeding permanent tooth is formed, bacterial infection involving periapical tissues may occur and this disturbs the ameloblastic layer of permanent tooth bud which leads to hypoplastic crown.
- During trauma when deciduous tooth get lodged in alveolus and disturb the budding permanent tooth bud, this results in yellowish or brownish stain or pigmentation of enamel on labial surface, at times pitting of enamel and irregularity of tooth crown is also present.

Clinical Features

- The enamel defects vary from focal areas of white, yellow, or brown discoloration to extensive hypoplasia, which can involve the entire crown.

♦ Anterior teeth are involved less frequently because crown formation is usually complete before the development of any apical inflammatory disease in the relatively caries-resistant anterior deciduous dentition.

♦ Maxillary central incisors are affected in the majority of the cases; the maxillary lateral incisors are altered less frequently.

Q.36. Describe developmental disturbances affecting shape of tooth. *(Feb 2014, 8 Marks)*

Ans. Following are the developmental disturbances affecting shape of tooth:

♦ *Gemination: Refer to Ans. 11 of same chapter*
♦ Twinning
♦ *Fusion: Refer to Ans. 11 of same chapter*
♦ *Concrescence: Refer to Ans. 19 of same chapter*
♦ *Dilaceration: Refer to Ans. 4 of same chapter*
♦ Talon cusp
♦ *Dens invaginatus: Refer to Ans. 5 of same chapter*
♦ Dens evaginatus
♦ *Taurodontism: Refer to Ans. 12 of same chapter*
♦ *Hypercementosis: Refer to Ans. 6 of chapter regressive alterations of teeth*
♦ Enamel pearl
♦ Mulberry molar
♦ Globodontia
♦ Hutchinson's incisor.

Twinning

Cleavage of tooth germ leads to formation of supernumerary tooth which is duplicate image of tooth from which it is developed.

Talon Cusp

♦ It resembles as an eagle's talon which projects lingually from cingulum areas of a maxillary or mandibular permanent incisor.

♦ Talon's cusp is more prevalent in person's with Rubinstein-Taybi syndrome.

♦ It blends smoothly with the tooth except that there is deep developmental groove where cusp blends with sloping lingual tooth surface.

♦ Talons's cusp consists of normal enamel and dentin and consists of horn of pulp tissue.

♦ Major significance of talon's cusp is that there is occlusal interference and there is also high incidence of caries.

Dens Evaginatus

♦ It is also known as Leong's premolar, occlusal tuberculated premolar and occlusal enamel pearl.

♦ It is a developmental condition which appears clinically as an accessory cusp or a globule of enamel on occlusal surface between buccal and lingual cusps of premolar.

♦ Dens evaginatus occur due to proliferation and evagination of an area of the inner enamel epithelium and subjacent odontogenic mesenchyme into the dental organ during early development of tooth.

♦ Clinical significance is that the extra cusp may contribute to incomplete eruption, displacement of teeth and pulp exposure with subsequent infection following occlusal wear or fracture.

Enamel Pearl

♦ It is also known as enameloma or ectopic enamel.

♦ Enamel pearl is a nodule of enamel which is 1 to 2 mm in diameter which form on the root, at root bifurcation, at root trifurcation.

♦ Enamel pearl originates due to activity of remnants of Hertwig's epithelial before it get reduced to cell rest of Malassez.

♦ Clinical significance is that these pearls give rise to periodontal problems.

Mulberry Molar

♦ It occurs in syphilis.
♦ Posterior tooth is involved.
♦ In this hyperplastic enamel occur with the spherical aggregates or the globules over surface of dentin.

Globodontia

♦ Globodontia is the enlarged bulbous malformed posterior tooth with no discernable cusps or grooves. In this teeth have a clover leaf appearance.

♦ In globodontia relation between cusps and groove get eliminated.

♦ This condition occur both in deciduous or permanent dentition.

Hutchinson's Incisor

♦ It occurs in syphilis.
♦ In this incisal edge show notching.
♦ Tooth has shape of screw driver.

Q.37. Enumerate causes of enamel hypoplasia and describe amelogenesis imperfecta in detail. *(Feb 2013, 16 Marks)*

Ans.

Causes of Enamel Hypoplasia

♦ Nutritional deficiency (Vitamins A, C and D)
♦ Exanthematous diseases, i.e., measles, chickenpox and scarlet fever
♦ Congenital syphilis
♦ Hypocalcemia
♦ Birth injury, prematurity, Rh hemolytic disease
♦ Local infection or trauma
♦ Ingestion of chemicals, such as fluoride
♦ Idiopathic causes

For amelogenesis imperfecta in detail, refer to Ans. 25 of same chapter.

Q.38. Write short note on Melkersson–Rosenthal syndrome. *(Feb 2015, 5 Marks)*

Ans. This syndrome is the triad of cheilitis granulomatosa, fissured tongue, facial palsy.

- Melkersson–Rosenthal syndrome is occasionally a manifestation of Crohn disease or orofacial granulomatosis.
- A genetic predisposition may exist in Melkersson–Rosenthal syndrome.
- Histologically the swellings of syndrome consist of chronic inflammatory cell infiltration which shows peri and para vascular aggregation of lymphocytes, plasma cells and histiocytes. At places non-caseating granuloma formation is seen along with epithelioid cells and Langhans type giant cells.
- Six patterns of fissured tongue are associated with the Melkersson, Rosenthal syndrome, i.e., central longitudinal fissuring, transverse fissuring originating from central fissure, plication, lateral longitudinal fissuring, transverse fissuring with central fissure and lateral longitudinal fissuring.

Q.39. Write short note on talon's cusp. *(Feb 2015, 5 Marks)*

Ans. Talon's cusp is a well delineated accessory cusp which resembles as eagle's talon which project lingually from cingulum areas of maxillary or mandibular permanent incisor.

- Talon's cusp consists of normal enamel and dentin and has a horn of pulp tissue.
- Talon's cusp blends smoothly with the tooth except that there is deep developmental groove where the cusp blends with sloping lingual tooth surface.
- Due to presence of Talon's cusp patient's face the problem with esthetics. There is also presence of occlusal interference and high incidence of caries is also noticed.
- Talon's cusp is associated with Rubinstein-Taybi's syndrome as well as Sturge-Weber syndrome.

Q.40. Write short note on facial hemiatrophy.
(Dec 2015, 3 Marks)

Ans. It is also known as Parry-Romberg syndrome.

It is the slowly progressive atrophy of soft tissue mainly half of the face and is also characterized by wasting of subcutaneous fat which sometimes accompanied by atrophy of skin, cartilage, bone and muscle.

Clinical Features

- It occurs during first and second decades of life.
- Females are more commonly affected as compared to males.
- It occurs more commonly over the left side of face.
- Onset of facial hemiatrophy is marked by white line furrow.
- Earliest sign is the presence of painless cleft.
- Patients can show sharp line of demarcation which resemble as large scar in between normal and abnormal skin. This is known as Coup de sabre.
- Overlying the atrophic fat a bluish hue may appear on the skin.

Oral Manifestations

- Presence of severe facial hemiatrophy which leads to facial deformation and mastication.

- Presence of hemiatrophy of lips and tongue.
- Delayed eruption is present which leads to malocclusion.
- Presence of incomplete root formation.
- During opening the mouth jaw is deviated towards affected side.

Differential Diagnosis

- *Post-traumatic atrophy:* Brief history from patient is important.
- *Goldenhar syndrome:* It is non-progressive and is congenital.
- *Mandibulofacial dysostosis:* It is hereditary and cleft palate is present.

Treatment

- Surgical reconstruction is done.
- Malocclusion should be corrected by orthodontic treatment.

Q.41. Write short note on mesiodens. *(Apr 2017, 5 Marks)*

Ans. Mesiodens is a supernumerary tooth in maxillary anterior incisor region.

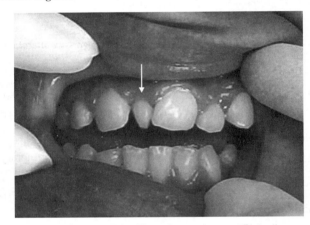

Fig. 19: Mesiodens *(For color version, see Plate 4).*

- Mesiodens represents one of the more common supernumerary teeth and can erupt spontaneously.
- Mesiodens supernumerary tooth was classified according to its location, i.e., it is located at or near to midline in incisal region of maxilla between the central incisors.
- According to the shape and size, two subclasses are considered in the classification of mesiodens; namely, eumorphic and dysmorphic. The eumorphic subclass is usually similar to a normal-sized central incisor, whereas the dysmorphic teeth have different shapes and sizes and are categorized into conical, tuberculate, supplemental and odontomes. Out of these conical form is most common type.
- Mesiodens may be seen as an isolated finding or as part of a syndrome, especially cleft lip and palate, cleidocranial dysostosis and Gardner's syndrome.
- Mesiodens can occur either as single tooth or it is paired. It can be impacted or inverted.
- Mesiodens is a small tooth consisting of cone-shaped crown and short root.
- Mesiodens can lead to retarded eruption, displacement or resorption of adjacent root.
- Mesiodens can frequently cause improper alignment.

♦ It usually results in oral problems, such as malocclusion, food impaction, poor esthetics, and cyst formation.

♦ Immediate removal of mesiodens is usually indicated in the following situations; inhibition or delay of eruption, displacement of the adjacent tooth, interference with orthodontic appliances, presence of pathologic condition, or spontaneous eruption of the supernumerary tooth.

Q.42. List developmental disturbances affecting the tooth. Discuss taurodontism and dilacerations.

(May 2018, 5 Marks)

Ans. Developmental disturbances affecting the tooth

Developmental Disturbances Affecting Structure of Tooth

♦ Amelogenesis imperfecta
♦ Dentinogenesis imperfecta
♦ Enamel hypoplasia
♦ Dentin dysplasia
♦ Regional odontodysplasia
♦ Dentin hypocalcification

Developmental Disturbances Affecting Number of Tooth

♦ Anodontia
♦ Hypodontia
♦ Hyperdontia

Developmental Disturbances Affecting Shape of Tooth

♦ Gemination
♦ Twinning
♦ Fusion
♦ Concrescence
♦ Dilaceration
♦ Talon cusp
♦ Dens invaginatus
♦ Dens evaginatus
♦ Taurodontism
♦ Hypercementosis
♦ Enamel pearl
♦ Mulberry molar
♦ Globodontia
♦ Hutchinson's incisor

Enumeration of Anomalies Affecting Size of Tooth

♦ Microdontia
♦ Macrodontia

For taurodontism in detail, refer to Ans. 12 of same chapter.

For dilacerations in detail, refer to Ans. 4 of same chapter.

Q.43. Write short note on Gardner's syndrome.

(Sep 2018, 5 Marks)

Ans. Gardner's syndrome is a rare disorder which is inherited as an autosomal dominant trait with near 100% penetrance.

Responsible gene has been mapped to the long arm of chromosome 5 and is identified as adenomatous polyposis coli (APC) tumor suppressor gene.

Gardner's syndrome is considered to be the part of spectrum of disease characterized by familial colorectal polyposis.

Gardner's syndrome consists of:

♦ Multiple polyposis of large intestine
♦ Osteomas of bones including long bones, skull and jaw
♦ Multiple epidermoid or sebaceous cysts of skin, mainly on scalp and back
♦ Occasional occurrence of desmoid tumors of soft tissue arise in 10% of affected patients
♦ Impacted supernumerary and permanent teeth

Histopathology

Osteomas are compact type. An individual lesion cannot be differentiated microscopically from solitary osteoma.

Treatment

♦ Major problem with patients of Gardner syndrome has high rate of malignant transformation of bowel polyps into invasive adenocarcinoma. Till age of 30 patients of Gardner syndrome will develop colorectal carcinoma. Prophylactic colectomy should be done.

♦ Removal of jaw osteomas and epidermoid cysts for cosmetic reasons can be indicated.

Q.44. Enumerate developmental anomalies of number and size of teeth and write in detail about anodontia.

(Feb 2019, 5 Marks)

Ans. *For enumeration of developmental anomalies of number and size of teeth, refer to Ans. 9 of same chapter.*

For anodontia in detail, refer to Ans. 6 of same chapter.

2. BENIGN AND MALIGNANT TUMORS OF ORAL CAVITY

Q.1. Enumerate white lesions of oral cavity. Describe leukoplakia in detail. *(June 2015, 10 Marks)*

Ans. The white lesions of oral cavity/orofacial region are as follows:

♦ **Hereditary condition:**
  • Leukoedema
  • White sponge nevus
  • Hereditary benign intraepithelial dyskeratosis
  • Keratosis follicularis
  • Tylosis syndrome.
♦ **Leukoplakia and malignancies:**
  • Chronic cheek biting
  • Friction or trauma associated leukoplakia
  • Tobacco associated leukoplakia
  • Carcinoma in situ
  • Squamous cell carcinoma
  • Verrucous carcinoma.
♦ **Dermatosis:**
  • Lichen planus
  • Lupus erythematous.
♦ **Inflammation:**
  • Mucous patches of syphilis
  • Candidiasis
  • Koplik spots of measles.

♦ **Miscellaneous conditions:**
- Oral submucous fibrosis
- Papilloma
- Lipoma
- Hairy tongue
- Geographic tongue
- Fordyce's granules.

Leukoplakia

Leukoplakia is defined as "a white patch or plaque that cannot be characterized, clinically or pathologically as any other disease and is not associated with any other physical or chemical causative agent except the use of tobacco". **—Axell et al, 1984**

Leukoplakia is defined as a predominantly white lesion of the oral mucosa that cannot be characterized as any other definable lesion. **—WHO (1997)**

Leukoplakia should be used to recognize white plaques of questionable risk having excluded (other) known diseases or disorders that carry no increased risk for cancer.

—Warnakulasuriya et al (2008).

Etiology of Leukoplakia

The common predisposing factors of leukoplakia are:

♦ *Tobacco:* It is used by large number of people in various forms, such as smoking of cigarette, cigar, biddies and pipes. All these types of tobacco habits are important for development of leukoplakia. It is believed that during smoking a large amount of tobacco end products are produced in oral cavity. The products in association with heat cause severe irritation to oral mucus membrane and finally result in development of leukoplakia.

♦ *Alcohol:* Alcohol leads to the entry of carcinogen into exposed cells and thus alters oral epithelium as well as its metabolism.

♦ *Candidiasis:* Chronic candidal infections are associated with leukoplakia.

♦ *Dietary deficiency:* Deficiency of vitamin A causes metaplasia and hyperkeratinization of epithelium which may result in development of leukoplakia.

♦ *Syphilis:* Syphilitic infections play minor role in causation of leukoplakia.

♦ *Hormonal imbalance:* Imbalance or dysfunction of both male and female sex hormones causes keratogenic changes in oral epithelium. These changes lead to the development of leukoplakia.

Modified Classification of Leukoplakia

L1	Size of leukoplakia <2 cm
L2	Size of leukoplakia 2 to 4 cm
L3	Size of leukoplakia >4 cm
Lx	Size not specified
P0	No epithelial dysplasia
P1	Distinct epithelial dysplasia
Px	Dysplasia not specified in pathology report

Oral Leukoplakia Staging System

Stage 1 – L1P0

Stage 2 – L2P0

Stage 3 – L3P0 Or L1L2P1

Stage 4 – L3P1

Histopathology

During leukoplakia variety of histologic changes are present which are related to:

♦ Keratinization pattern
♦ Changes in cellular layer
♦ Thickness of epithelium
♦ Alteration in underlying connective tissue stroma.

Keratinization Pattern

Leukoplakia generally presents hyperorthokeratinization or hyperparakeratinization or both with or without the presence of epithelial dysplasia.

♦ In case of leukoplakia an abnormal increase in the thickness of orthokeratin layer is seen in area of epithelium which is usually keratinized.

♦ An important histological criterion of leukoplakia is presence of hyperkeratinization of normally keratinized epithelium or some amount of parakeratin deposition in area of epithelium which are usually not keratinized.

♦ Epithelium dysplasia is more frequently associated with hyperkeratinized lesion.

Changes in Cellular Layer

Epithelial dysplasia is the hallmark of histologic changes seen in epithelium in case of leukoplakia. The criteria for epithelial dysplasia are:

Architecture and cytologic criteria for grading epithelial dysplasia given by who (2005)

Architecture criteria

♦ Irregular epithelial stratification
♦ Loss of polarity of basal cells
♦ Basal cell hyperplasia
♦ Drop shaped rete pegs
♦ Increased number of mitotic figures
♦ Abnormally superficial mitosis
♦ Dyskeratosis, i.e., premature keratinization in the cell
♦ Keratin pearls within rete ridges

Cytologic criteria

♦ *Anisonucleosis:* Abnormal variation in nuclear size
♦ *Nuclear pleomorphism:* Abnormal variation in nuclear shape
♦ Anisocytosis: Abnormal variation in cell size
♦ Cellular pleomorphism: Abnormal variation in cell shape
♦ Increased nuclear cytoplasmic ratio
♦ Increased nuclear size
♦ Atypical mitotic figures
♦ Increase in the number and size of nucleoli
♦ Hyperchromatism

Histopathology

♦ Classification of epithelial dysplasia is done on basis of its severity which is:
  • Mild epithelial dysplasia: It refers to the alteration which is limited to basal and parabasal cell layers.
  • Moderate epithelial dysplasia: It shows involvement from basal layer to midportion of spinous cell layer.
  • Severe epithelial dysplasia: It shows alterations from basal layer to the level above midportion of epithelium.
  • When complete thickness of epithelium, term carcinoma in situ is used.
♦ Histopathological report of leukoplakia should include a statement on absence or presence of epithelial dysplasia.

Thickness of the Epithelium

In leukoplakia, the thickness of epithelium is altered and it occurs in epithelial atrophy or acanthosis.

Alteration in Underlying Connective Tissue

In leukoplakia, there is often variable degree of destruction of collagen fibers and moreover chronic inflammatory cell infiltrate is also present in underlying connective tissue stroma.

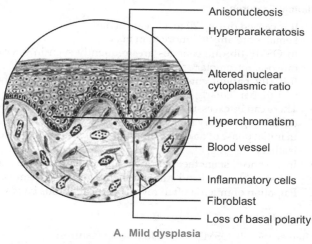

A. Mild dysplasia

— Anisonucleosis
— Hyperparakeratosis
— Altered nuclear cytoplasmic ratio
— Hyperchromatism
— Blood vessel
— Inflammatory cells
— Fibroblast
— Loss of basal polarity

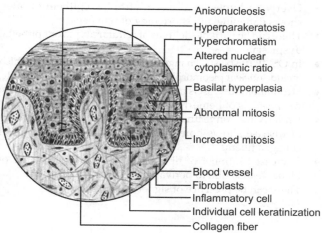

— Anisonucleosis
— Hyperparakeratosis
— Hyperchromatism
— Altered nuclear cytoplasmic ratio
— Basilar hyperplasia
— Abnormal mitosis
— Increased mitosis
— Blood vessel
— Fibroblasts
— Inflammatory cell
— Individual cell keratinization
— Collagen fiber

B. Moderate dysplasia

Figs. 20A and B: Leukoplakia *(For color version, see Plate 4).*

Clinical Features

♦ Usually the lesion occurs in 4th, 5th, 6th and 7th decades of life.
♦ Buccal mucosa and commissural areas are most frequent affected sites followed by alveolar ridge, tongue, hard and soft palate, etc.
♦ Oral leukoplakia often present solitary or multiple white patches.
♦ Size of lesion may vary from small well localized patch measuring few millimeters in diameter.
♦ The surface of lesion may be smooth or finely wrinkled or even rough on palpation and lesion cannot be removed by scrapping.
♦ Lesion is whitish or grayish or in some cases, it is brownish yellow in color due to heavy use of tobacco.
♦ In most of the cases, these lesion are asymptomatic, however in some cases they may cause pain, feeling of thickness and burning sensation, etc.

Q.2. Define and enumerate precancerous lesions. Describe in detail leukoplakia. *(Dep 2011, 8 Marks)*

Or

Define and enumerate precancerous lesions and conditions. Write in detail about histopathological features of leukoplakia. *(Aug 2011, 15 Marks)*

Or

Define precancerous lesions and conditions of oral cavity with examples. Describe leukoplakia in detail. *(Jan 2018, 10 Marks)*

Ans.

Premalignant Lesions or Precancerous Lesions

Premalignant lesions are defined as "A morphologically altered tissue in which cancer is more likely to occur then in its apparently normal counterpart".

The examples are:
♦ Leukoplakia
♦ Erythroplakia
♦ Mucosal changes associated with smoking habits
♦ Actinic cheilitis, actinic keratosis and actinic elastosis
♦ Bowen's disease
♦ Carcinoma in situ

Premalignant Condition or Precancerous Condition

The premalignant condition is defined as "A generalized state of body, which is associated with significantly increased risk of cancer development".

The examples are:
♦ Oral submucous fibrosis
♦ Syphilis
♦ Lichen planus
♦ Sideropenic dysphagia
♦ Lupus erythematosus
♦ Dyskeratosis congenita
♦ Xeroderma pigmentosum
♦ Epidermolysis bullosa.

For etiology, histopathology and clinical features of leukoplakia, refer to Ans. 1 of same chapter.

Q.3. Write notes on hairy leukoplakia. *(Mar 2003, 5 Marks)*

Ans. Hairy leukoplakia is HIV-associated mucosal disorder, which often involves lateral and ventral surfaces of tongue.

Homosexual man with HIV infection may develop white patchy lesion in oral cavity.

Clinical Features

♦ Clinically hairy leukoplakia occurs more frequently on the lateral border of the tongue however it can also occur on floor of the mouth, buccal mucosa, etc.

♦ The lesion often appears as white patch and is characterized by an irregular surface, exhibiting numerous linear vertical folds or projections, sometimes so marked to as resemble "Hairs".

♦ The lesions are always colonized by *Candida albicans*.

♦ Hairy leukoplakia probably occurs as an opportunistic infection caused by Epstein-Barr virus.

♦ Hairy leukoplakias are asymptomatic lesions and whenever they occur they occur on buccal mucosa, the lesions are smooth and homogeneous with straitened margin.

Histopathology

♦ A very characteristic finding in hairy leukoplakia is presence of subcorneal upper spinous layer zone made up of cytopathologically altered keratinocytes.

♦ Parakeratin layer is thick often colonized by candidal hyphae.

♦ The submucosa does not exhibit many inflammatory cell infiltrate.

Differential Diagnosis

♦ Lichen planus
♦ Verrucous leukoplakia
♦ Chronic tongue biting habits.

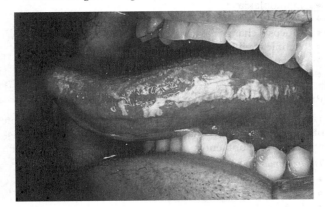

Fig. 21: Hairy leukoplakia *(For color version, see Plate 4).*

Q.4. Write notes on oral submucous fibrosis.

(Apr 2007, 10 Marks) (Dec 2007, 3 Marks)

Ans. OSMF is defined as "An insidious chronic disease affecting any part of oral cavity and sometime pharynx. Although occasionally preceded by and/or associated with vesicle formation, it is always associated with juxtaepithelial inflammatory reaction followed by fibroelastic changes in lamina propria, with epithelial atrophy leading to stiffness of oral mucosa and causing trismus and inability to eat." *Pindborg (1966)*

Etiology

The OSMF is caused due to:

♦ Excessive consumption of red chillies.
♦ Excessive "areca nut" chewing.
♦ Nutritive deficiency
♦ Immunological factors
♦ Genetic factors
♦ Protracted tobacco use
♦ Patient with deficiency of micronutrients.
♦ Use of lime with areca nut

Clinical Features

♦ It is caused during 20 to 40 years of age.
♦ Females are affected more than males.
♦ In OSMF fibrotic changes are frequently seen in buccal mucosa, retromolar area, uvula, tongue, etc.
♦ Initially patient complains of burning sensation in the mouth, particularly during taking hot and spicy foods.
♦ There can be excessive salivation, decreased salivation and defective gustatory sensation.
♦ In initial phase of disease palpation of mucosa elicits a "wet leathery" feeling.
♦ In advanced stage the oral mucosa loses its resilience and becomes blanched and stiff and thereby causing trismus.
♦ Palpation of mucosa often reveals vertical fibrous bands.

Histopathology

Microscopically OSMF reveals following features:

♦ Overlying hyper keratinized, atrophic epithelium often shows flattening and shortening of rete pegs.
♦ There can be variable degrees of cellular atypia or epithelial dysplasia.
♦ In OSMF dysplastic changes are found in epithelium which include nuclear pleomorphism, sever inter-cellular edema, etc.
♦ Stromal blood vessels are dilated and congested and there can be areas of hemorrhage.
♦ Underlying connective tissue stroma in advanced stage of disease shows homogenization and hyalinization of collagen fibers.
♦ Decreased number of fibroblastic cells and narrowing of blood vessels due to perivascular fibrosis are present.
♦ There can be presence of signet cells in some cases.

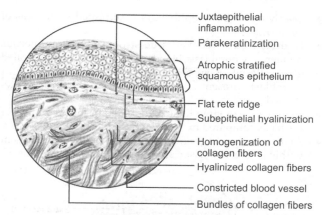

Fig. 22: Oral submucous fibrosis *(For color version, see Plate 5).*

Treatment

♦ Stoppage of all causing habits.
♦ Definitive treatment of OSMF includes intralesional injection of collagenase, corticosteroids and fibrinolysin, etc.
♦ Systemic administration of steroids in severe cases.

Q.5. Describe in brief histopathology of intraepithelial carcinoma. *(Mar 1994, 8 Marks)*

Ans. This is also called as carcinoma in situ

♦ Intraepithelial carcinoma is a condition which arises frequently on skin, but occurs also on mucous membrane including those of oral cavity.
♦ Metastasis is impossible in intra epithelial carcinoma.
♦ Bowen's disease is a special form of intraepithelial carcinoma occurring with some frequency on skin, particularly in patients who have had arsenic therapy and is often associated with development of internal or extra cutaneous cancer.

Histological Features

♦ Keratin may/may not be found on the surface of lesion but, if present, is more apt to be parakeratin rather than orthokeratin.

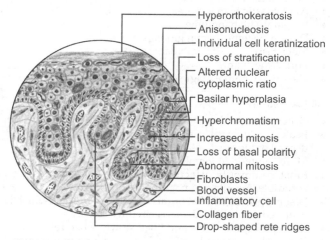

Fig. 23: Intraepithelial carcinoma *(For color version, see Plate 5).*

♦ In some instances, there appears to be hyperplasia of the altered epithelium while in others there is atrophy.
♦ An increased nuclear/cytoplasmic ratio and nuclear hyperchromatism is seen.
♦ Cellular pleomorphism is common
♦ There is loss of orientation of cells and loss of their normal polarity.
♦ Sometimes a sharp line of division between normal or altered epithelium extends from surface down to the connective tissue rather than a blending of epithelial changes.

Treatment

Treatment is done by surgery, radiotherapy or electrocautery.

Q.6. Describe etiology, histopathology and clinical features of carcinoma of tongue.

(Sep 2009, 6 Marks) (Dec 2009, 15 Marks)

Or

Describe in detail the etiology, clinical features and histopathology of squamous cell carcinoma of tongue. *(Dec 2015, 8 Marks)*

Ans.

Etiology

♦ Syphilis either an active case or past history of it coexistent with carcinoma of tongue. Syphilis is accepted as having strong association with development of dorsal tongue carcinoma. Arsenicals and heavy metals used to treat syphilis before advent of modern antibiotics have carcinogenic properties themselves and are responsible for some of earlier carcinoma development in this disease.
♦ Leukoplakia is the common lesion of tongue which leads to carcinoma of tongue.
♦ Carcinoma of tongue is due to poor oral hygiene, chronic trauma and use of alcohol and tobacco.
♦ Carcinoma of tongue is due to source of chronic irritation, such as carious or broken tooth or an ill-fitting denture.

Histopathology

♦ Cells are generally large and show distinct cell membrane.
♦ Nuclei of neoplastic cells are large.
♦ Carcinomas of tongue ranges from well differentiated keratinizing carcinoma to highly differentiated neoplasm.
♦ Changes of epithelial dysplasia are present.
♦ There is increased number of mitotic figure per field.
♦ *For histopathologic gradation, refer to Ans. 15 and Ans. 23 of same chapter.*

Clinical Features

♦ Most common presenting signs of carcinoma of tongue is painless mass or ulcer. The lesion becomes painful when it is secondarily affected.
♦ Tumor begins as superficially indurated ulcer with slightly raised borders and may proceed either to develop a fungating, exophytic mass or to infiltrate deep layers of tongue, producing fixation and induration without much surface change.

♦ If carcinoma is present on the dorsum of tongue, then patient has past or present history of syphilitic glossitis.
♦ Paresthesia of tongue frequently occurs due to invasion of lingual nerve by tumor cells.
♦ The common site where the lesion develops is lateral border of tongue and ventral surface of tongue.
♦ Initial lesions often appear as erythematous macules or nodules or fissured areas over the tongue.

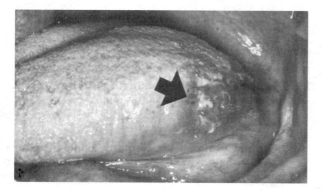

Fig. 24: Carcinoma of tongue (*For color version, see Plate 5*).

Q.7. Write short note on peripheral giant cell granuloma.
(Sep 2006, 5 Marks)

Or

Describe histologic features with diagram of peripheral giant cell granuloma. *(Nov 2008, 5 Marks)*

Or

Write short answer on peripheral giant cell granuloma.
(Oct 2019, 3 Marks)

Ans. Peripheral giant cell granuloma is the most common of giant cell lesions which arises from tooth bearing areas of jaw and appears as a purplish red nodule.

Clinical Features

♦ Lesion usually arises during mixed dentition or during third and fourth decade of life.
♦ It is most common in males.
♦ Its site in dentulous patient is interdental papilla. Mandible is more frequently affected than maxilla.
♦ Peripheral giant cell granuloma appears as a small, exophytic, well circumscribed, pedunculated lesion on gingival surface.
♦ Color of lesion varies from purplish red to darkish red.
♦ There can be bleeding from the surface either spontaneously or on provocation from instrument.
♦ Sometimes the peripheral cell granuloma can be aggressive in nature and such lesion may attain very large size and involves some teeth.
♦ In some cases, the lesion may develop with an 'hour-glass shape.'

Histopathology

♦ Peripheral giant cell granuloma present following histological features.

♦ Overlying covering epithelium is ulcerated with areas of hemorrhage.
♦ Underlying connective tissue stroma reveals numerous proliferating fibroblasts, blood capillaries and multinucleated giant cells, which are scattered throughout the lesion.
♦ Fibroblasts present in hypercellular stroma are spindle-shaped and have oval-shaped nuclei.
♦ Giant cells are large in size and contain more number of nuclei as compared to true giant cell tumor.
♦ Areas of hemorrhage and hemosiderin pigment are present within connective tissue stroma.

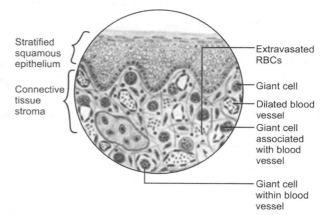

Fig. 25: Peripheral giant cell granuloma
(*For color version, see Plate 5*).

Treatment

Surgical excision with curettage.

Q.8. Write short note in hemangioma. *(Feb 2013, 5 Marks)*
Ans. Hemangiomas are lesions which are not present at birth, but they manifest within the first month of life, exhibit a rapid proliferative phase and slowly involute to non-existent.

Classification of Hemangiomas by Watson and McCarthy

♦ Capillary hemangioma
♦ Cavernous hemangioma
♦ Angioblastic hemangioma
♦ Racemose hemangioma
♦ Diffuse systemic hemangioma
♦ Metastasizing hemangioma
♦ Port-Wine stain
♦ Hereditary hemorrhagic telangiectasia

Clinical Features

♦ Occur most commonly in infants and children.
♦ Peak incidence of central hemangiomas is during 2nd decade of life.
♦ More common in females
♦ Most commonly affected bones are facial bones, i.e., mandible, maxilla and nasal bones.
♦ Lesion appears as a flat or raised lesion of mucosa which is deep red or bluish red and is circumscribed.
♦ Lesion is compressible and filled slowly when released.
♦ Intraorally commonly affected sites are lip, tongue, buccal mucosa and palate.

Histopathology

♦ There are several histopathologic types of hemangioma found in oral cavity, among them two very common types are:
  Capillary hemangioma
  Cavernous hemangioma.

Capillary Hemangioma

♦ They are histologically characterized by numerous, small, endothelial lined capillaries in lesion which are densely packed by erythrocytes.
♦ Cells of endothelial lining are single layered.
♦ Endothelial cells are spindle shaped.
♦ Capillaries are well formed and are present throughout the lesion.
♦ Fibrous connective tissue stroma is not well formed and is loosely arranged.

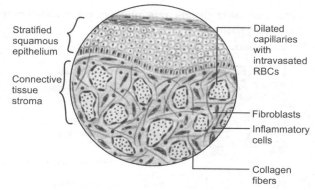

Fig. 26: Capillary hemangioma *(For color version, see Plate 5).*

Histopathology of Cavernous Hemangioma

♦ They are histologically characterized by large, irregularly shaped, dilated, endothelialized sinuses which contain large aggregates of erythrocytes.
♦ A single layer of flatted endothelial cell lines each sinus.
♦ Sinus lacks muscular coat on their walls.
♦ Large area of hemorrhage and hemosiderin pigments is often seen within cavernous hemangioma lesions.

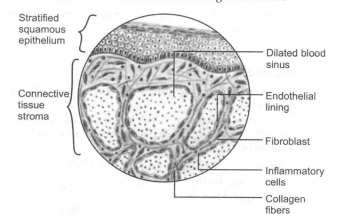

Fig. 27: Cavernous hemangioma *(For color version, see Plate 5).*

Treatment

Surgical excision is treatment of choice.

Q.9. Enumerate premalignant lesions and conditions describe in detail about leukoplakia.

(June 2010, 15 Marks)

Ans. *For enumeration of oral precancerous lesions and conditions, refer to Ans. 2 of same chapter and for leukoplakia in detail, refer to Ans. 1 of same chapter.*

Q.10. Describe precancerous lesion and condition. Describe in detail about oral submucous fibrosis.

(Sep 2004, 15 Marks)

Ans. *For description of precancerous lesion and condition, refer to Ans. 2 of same chapter in detail.*

For OSMF, refer to Ans. 4 of same chapter.

Q.11. Write notes on verrucous carcinoma.

(Dec 2007, 4 Marks) (Aug 2011, 10 Marks)
(Aug 2012, 5 Marks) (Feb 2015, 5 Marks)

Or

Discuss about verrucous carcinoma.

(Sep 2004, 8 Marks)

Or

Describe in detail clinical features, histopathology and treatment of verrucous carcinoma.

(Mar 2011, 8 Marks)

Or

Write short note on verrucous carcinoma.

(Jan 2016, 5 Marks)

Or

Write short answer on verrucous carcinoma.

(May 2018, 3 Marks)

Or

Write short answer on histopathology of verrucous carcinoma.

(Feb 2019, 3 Marks)

Ans. Verrucous carcinoma is a diffused papillary, non-metastasizing well differentiated malignant neoplasm of oral epithelium.

It is also known as Ackerman's tumor.

Clinical Features

♦ Tumor occurs during 60 years of life and males are more commonly affected.
♦ Common locations for verrucous carcinoma are gingiva, alveolar mucosa and buccal mucosa.
♦ Verrucous carcinoma presents as slow growing, exophytic, papillary growth having white pebbly surface.
♦ Carcinoma occurs either as single entity or there can be multiple lesions involving different parts of oral cavity.
♦ Lesions on buccal mucosa are sometimes very extensive and often cause pain, tenderness and difficulty in taking the food.
♦ Regional lymph nodes are often enlarged and tender.

Histopathology

♦ Hyperplastic epithelium often exhibits a papillary surface being covered by the thick layer of parakeratin.

♦ Massively enlarged bulb, such as acanthotic rete ridges are seen which invaginated into underlying connective tissue stroma.

♦ Many deep cleft like spaces lined by thick layer of parakeratin, these extend from the surface of epithelium and project deep into the center of bulbous rete ridges. This is known as parakeratin plugging.

♦ All bulbous rete ridges of the epithelium projects into the connective tissue and is known as pushing margin.

♦ The basement membrane is intact and underlying connective tissue shows inflammatory cell infiltration.

♦ Formation of epithelial pearls and microcytes are seen.

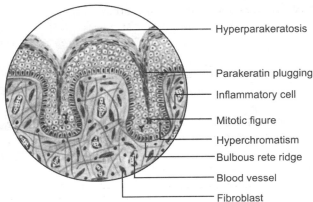

Fig. 28: Verrucous carcinoma *(For color version, see Plate 6).*

Labels:
- Hyperparakeratosis
- Parakeratin plugging
- Inflammatory cell
- Mitotic figure
- Hyperchromatism
- Bulbous rete ridge
- Blood vessel
- Fibroblast

Treatment

♦ Surgical excision or laser therapy is done.
♦ Prognosis should be good.

Q.12. Enumerate giant cell lesions and describe peripheral giant cell granuloma. *(Feb 2002, 15 Marks)*

Ans. *For enumeration of giant cell lesions, refer to Ans. 19 of same chapter. For peripheral giant cell granuloma, refer to Ans. 7 of same chapter.*

Q.13. Discuss about central giant cell granuloma.

(Sep 2005, 8 Marks)

Ans. Central giant cell granuloma is relatively a common benign intraosseous destructive giant cell lesion which affects anterior part of jaw bone.

Clinical Features

♦ Lesion occurs in young children and female predilection is present.

♦ Central giant cell granuloma affects the mandible more often than maxilla and occurs anterior to first molar.

♦ Central giant cell granuloma is a small, slow enlarging bony hard swelling of jaw which is painful on palpitation.

♦ Lesion causes expansion and distortion of cortical plates and there is presence of displacement or mobility of regional teeth.

♦ Central giant cell granuloma follow an aggressive course and in such cases, they produce fast enlarging, large, painful swelling in the jaw.

Histopathology

♦ Central giant cell granuloma exhibits fibrovascular connective tissue stroma, consisting of numerous stromal cell which are plum and spindle shaped and undergo frequent mitosis.

♦ Several areas of hemorrhage and hemosiderin pigmentations are also evident.

♦ Multiple multinucleated giant cells of varying size are dispersed throughout fibrous tissue stroma. Giant cells are found around the blood capillaries or near the area of hemorrhage and giant cells consist of 5 to 20 nuclei.

♦ Small foci of osteoids are often found near periphery of lesion.

♦ Little amount of chronic inflammatory cell infiltration in connective tissue stroma.

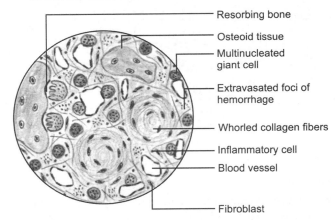

Fig. 29: Central giant cell granuloma *(For color version, see Plate 6).*

Labels:
- Resorbing bone
- Osteoid tissue
- Multinucleated giant cell
- Extravasated foci of hemorrhage
- Whorled collagen fibers
- Inflammatory cell
- Blood vessel
- Fibroblast

Radiological Features

♦ Radiographically the lesion produces multicellular radiolucent area in jaw with soap bubble appearance.

♦ Margin of lesion is scalloped and well demarcated.

♦ Resorption of roots of nearby teeth or divergence of roots is common feature.

Treatment

Surgical excision is done with curettage.

Q.14. Define epithelial dysplasia. Describe verrucous carcinoma. *(Mar 2007, 7.5 Marks)*

Ans. Epithelial dysplasia comprises a loss in the uniformity of individual cells or cytological atypia as well as a loss in their architectural orientation.

For verrucous carcinoma, refer to Ans. 11 of same chapter.

Q.15. Describe the histopathology of moderately differentiated squamous cell carcinoma.

(Sep 2006, 5 Marks)

Ans.

Histopathology

- In it the tumor cells are usually more severely dysplastic than of well differentiated type.
- Malignant epithelial cells produce little or no keratin and they exhibit greater number of mitotic division.
- Formation of epithelial islands is diminished since tumor cells do not mature properly.
- Malignant tumor cells are recognized as stratified squamous epithelial cells.

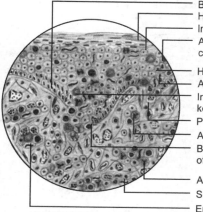

Basilar hyperplasia
Hyperparakeratosis
Increased mitosis
Altered nuclear cytoplasmic ratio
Hyperchromatism
Anisonucleosis
Individual cell keratinization
Prominent nucleoli
Abnormal mitosis
Break in the continuity of epithelium
Abnormal mitosis
Sheet of epithelial cells
Epithelial island

Fig. 30: Moderately differentiated squamous cell carcinoma (For color version, see Plate 6).

Q.16. Write notes on giant cell. *(Aug 2012, 5 Marks)*

Ans. Giant cells are multinucleated cells that commonly occur at sites of chronic inflammation mostly complicated by granuloma formation. Besides giant cells occurring in various lesions, there also exists physiological giant cells by virtue of the presence of multinucleated nature, present as a part of healthy tissues.

Multinucleated giant cells are highly stimulated cells of the monocyte-macrophage lineage at a terminal stage of maturation and studies have demonstrated that their multinucleated appearance is produced by cell–cell fusion rather than by nuclear division without cytokinesis.

Classification of Giant Cells

Giant cell can be classified based according to their occurrence in the body:

- Physiological giant cells:
  - Osteoclast
  - Striated muscle cells
  - Megakaryocytes
  - Syncytiotrophoblast
- Pathological giant cells:
  - Langhan's giant cells
  - Foreign body giant cells
  - Touton giant cells
  - Tumor giant cells
  - Warthin–finkeldey giant cells

Osteoclast

Osteoclasts are highly specialized for resorption of bone mineral and matrix through the coordinated secretion of hydrogen ions and proteolytic enzymes. Although most osteoclasts are large multinucleated cells, there are reports of mononuclear osteoclasts. Situated on the bone surface, it occupies a concavity surface of small bone spicules. An enlarged surface area created by plasma membrane infoldings, the ruffled border, characterizes the secretory or apical surface directed toward the bone. In routine histologic sections, the ruffled border appears striated and lightly stained. The presence of a ruffled border is an indication that the osteoclast is actively engaged in bone resorption. Each ruffled border is surrounded by a clear zone (or sealing zone), a cytoplasmic area rich in cytoplasmic actin filaments and devoid of major cytoplasmic organelles. Through close adaptation of the cell surface to the bone matrix, the clear zone establishes a seal between the bone resorption compartment and the interstitial fluid.

Striated Muscle

They are the muscles in which the cells exhibit cross striations at the light microscopic level.

It is further subclassified based on its location:

- Skeletal muscle
- Visceral striated muscle
- Cardiac muscle

Skeletal Muscle Cell

A skeletal muscle cell is a multinucleated syncytium. In skeletal muscle, each muscle fiber is a multinucleated syncytium. A muscle fiber is formed during development by the fusion of small, individual muscle cells called myoblasts. When viewed in cross section, the mature multinucleated muscle fibers reveal a polygonal shape with a diameter of 10 to 100 µm.

Visceral Striated Muscle

It is morphologically identical to skeletal muscle but is restricted to the soft tissues, namely the tongue, pharynx, lumbar part of diaphragm and upper part of esophagus. These play an essential role in speech, breathing and swallowing.

Cardiac Muscle

Cardiac muscle has the same type and arrangement of the contractile filament as skeletal muscle. In addition, cardiac muscle fibers exhibit densely staining cross bands called intercalated disks, that cross the fibers in a linear fashion or frequently in a way that resembles the rosters of a stairway. The intercalated disks represent a highly specialized attachment sites between adjacent cells. The linear cell—cell attachment of the cardiac muscle cells results in 'fibers' of variable length.

Megakaryocytes

Platelets are derived from large polypoid cells (cells whose nuclei contain multiple sets of chromosomes) in bone marrow are called megakaryocytes.

Syncytiotrophoblast

The syncytiotrophoblast is a continuous, normally uninterrupted layer that extends over the surfaces of all villous trees as well as over the inner surfaces chorionic and basal plates. The syncytiotrophoblast is a multinucleated protoplasmic mass without intercellular boundaries. From this mass emerge finger like projections, which penetrate through the endometrial epithelium into the endometrial stroma.

Langhans Giant Cell

They are characterized by location of the nuclei at the periphery of the cell in an acute configuration. They are seen in lesions, such as tuberculosis, sarcoidosis, leprosy and vasculitis. These are special, more highly organized forms than are 'foreign body' multinucleated giant cells. These giant cells may attain diameters of 40 to 50 μm. They have a large mass of cytoplasm containing 20 or more small nuclei arranged peripherally.

Foreign Body Giant Cell

Formation of foreign body giant cell is hallmark of the foreign body reaction and is harmful to implanted biomaterials because it contributes to the degradation of the bio-material and leads to stress cracking, tissue fibrosis and a chronic response. Foreign body giant cells are thought to be a source of chemokines that mediate the neutrophils and lymphocytes.

Touton Giant Cell

Touton giant cells are characterized by a ring of nuclei surrounding central eosinophilic zone and surrounded by a zone of pallor extending to the periphery of cell. These giant cells are seen in lesions with high lipid content, such as xanthoma, xanthogranuloma, fat necrosis. The characteristic appearance of 'Xanthelasmatic giant cell' of Touton is determined merely by the presence of demonstrable lipid in the cytoplasm.

Tumor Giant Cell

A feature of anaplasia is the formation of tumor giant cells, some possessing only a single huge polymorphic nucleus and others having two or more nuclei. These giant cells are not to be confused with inflammatory Langhans or foreign body giant cells, which are derived from macrophages and contain many small normal-appearing nuclei. In the cancer giant cell, the nuclei are hyperchromatic and large in relation to the cell.

Warthin-Finkeldey Giant Cell

The Warthin Finkeldey cells have up to 100 nuclei and contain spherical eosinophilic intracytoplasmic and intranuclear inclusions. They are present in viral infections like measles. Tompkins and Macaulay reported Warthin-Finkeldey giant cells in nasal secretions before the appearance of other clinical signs of measles, such as Koplik's spots and skin rash. These cells are found throughout the reticuloendothelial system and contain up to 100 nuclei.

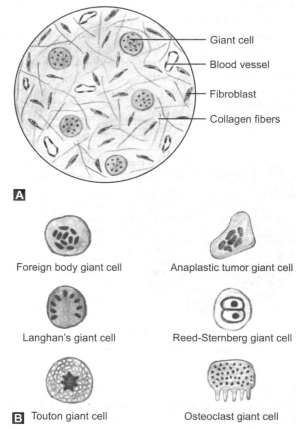

Figs. 31A and B: Giant cell *(For color version, see Plate 6).*

Q.17. Write notes on special stains. *(Mar 2000, 5 Marks)*

Ans. The special stains are:

van Gieson's Stain

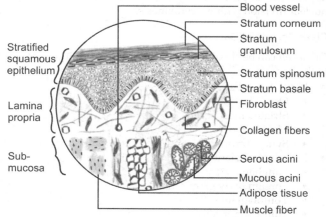

Fig. 32: van Gieson's stain *(For color version, see Plate 6).*

- It is a special stain which is used for connective tissue elements. It is used for differentiating between connective tissue fibers and muscle fibers.
- *Epithelium (cell and cytoplasm):* It takes greenish yellow stain.
- Collagen fibers are red
- Muscle fibers are yellow
- Nuclei of cells are blue black.

Mallory Stain

- It is a special stain for keratin that stains deep orange. It is used in hyperkeratotic lesions.
- The epithelium is royal blue.
- Collagen fibers are royal blue.
- Muscle fibers are royal blue.
- Keratin layers are orange.
- Nucleus is blue black.

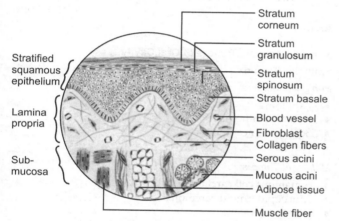

Fig. 33: Mallory stain *(For color version, see Plate 7).*

Periodic Acid Schiff's Stain or PAS Stain

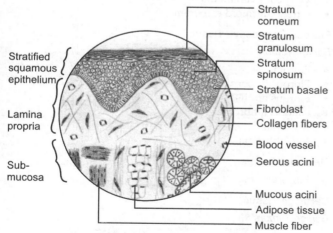

Fig. 34: PAS stain *(For color version, see Plate 7).*

- It is a special stain for mucopolysaccharide granules. These are prominently seen in basement membrane, intercellular spaces and keratin layer. It is used to detect continuity of basement membrane in intraepithelial carcinoma and squamous cell carcinoma.
- Epithelium and connective tissue is pink.
- Collagen fibers are pink.
- Muscle fibers are pink.
- Nucleus is blue black.
- Granules are of magenta color.

Masson's Trichrome Stain

It is a special stain used to differentiate between collagen fibers and muscle fibers. It demonstrates connective tissue disorders like leiomyosarcoma and rhabdomyosarcoma.

- Epithelium is red.
- Muscle fibers are bluish violet.
- Collagen fibers and blood vessels are blue.

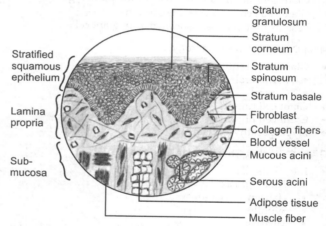

Fig. 35: Masson's trichrome stain *(For color version, see Plate 7).*

Q.18. Define premalignant lesion and condition. Describe etiology, clinical features and histopathology of oral submucous fibrosis. *(Sep 2007, 7.5 Marks)*

Or

Define precancerous condition and precancerous lesion. Discuss about etiology and histopathology of OSMF. *(Mar 2016, 8 Marks)*

Ans. The premalignant lesions are defined as morphologically altered tissue in which cancer is more likely to occur then in its apparently normal counterpart, e.g., leukoplakia, erythroplakia, nicotiana palati, stomatitis, dyskeratosis congenita, etc.

- The premalignant condition is defined as generalized state of body, which is associated with significantly increased risk of cancer, e.g., oral submucous fibrosis, syphilis, lichen planus, etc.
- *For etiology, clinical features and histopathology of OSMF, refer to Ans. 4 of same chapter.*

Q.19. Enumerate giant cell lesions. Describe in detail central giant cell granuloma.

(Sep 2007, 7.5 Marks)

Ans. Giant cell lesions of oral cavity are:

According to the Nature of Different Pathologic Conditions

♦ Infections
  • Bacterial
  • Viral
  • Fungal
  • Protozoal
  • Parasitic
♦ Fibro-osseous lesions and osteodystrophies
  • Immunologic
  • Idiopathic
  • Orofacial granulomatosis
  • Reaction to materials
  • Benign and malignant tumors

In this Classification, Giant Cells are Categorized into Three Categories

1. Giant cells are the main cause for the pathology
2. Giant cells characterize these lesions
3. Lesions that may be associated with giant cells

Main Cause for the Pathology

♦ Giant cell granuloma:
  • Peripheral
  • Central
♦ Giant cell tumors
♦ Giant cell fibroma
♦ Hyperparathyroidism

Giant Cells that Characterize Lesions

♦ Infections
  • Tuberculosis
  • Hansen's disease
  • Syphilis
  • Measles
♦ Granulomatous lesions
  • Wegener's granulomatosis
  • Orofacial granulomatosis
  • Pulse granuloma
  • Sarcoidosis
♦ Lesions in bone
  • Aneurysmal bone cyst
  • Cherubism
  • Paget's disease
♦ Foreign body lesions
  • Silicosis
  • Berylliosis
♦ Malignancies
  • Lymphoma—Hodgkin's disease
  • Bronchogenic carcinoma
  • Carcinoma of thyroid
♦ Miscellaneous
  • Xanthoma
  • Giant cell arteritis

Lesions that may be Associated with Giant Cell

♦ Malignancies
  • Multiple myeloma
  • Ewing's sarcoma
  • Fibrosarcoma
  • Chondrosarcoma

♦ Fibro-osseous lesions
  • Osteoblastoma
  • Fibrous dysplasia
  • Cemento-ossifying fibroma
  • Radicular cyst

Based on their Origin

♦ Epithelially derived, i.e., Warthin-finkeldey giant cells, tumor giant cells
♦ Stromally derived, i.e., Reed-sternberg giant cells.

For central giant cell granuloma, refer to Ans. 13 of same chapter.

Q.20. **Enumerate and classify non-odontogenic tumors of oral cavity. Write briefly about malignant melanoma.**

(Sep 2011, 8 Marks)

Or

Write short note on malignant melanoma.

(Feb 2019, 5 Marks)

Ans.

Non-odontogenic Tumors of Oral Cavity

Epithelial Tissue

Benign Tumors

♦ Papilloma
♦ Keratoacanthoma
♦ Squamous acanthoma
♦ Nevus

Malignant Tumors

♦ Squamous cell carcinoma
♦ Mucoepidermoid carcinoma
♦ Adenocarcinoma
♦ Basal cell carcinoma
♦ Transitional cell carcinoma
♦ Melanoma
♦ Verrucous carcinoma
♦ Intraepidermoid carcinoma

Fibrous Connective Tissue

Benign Tumors

♦ Fibroma
♦ Fibrous hyperplasia
♦ Fibrous epulis
♦ Giant cell fibroma
♦ Myxoma
♦ Myxofibroma.

Malignant Tumors

♦ Fibrosarcoma

Cartilage Tissue

Benign Tumors

♦ Chondroma
♦ Chondroblastoma
♦ Chondromyxoid fibroma.

Malignant Tumors

♦ Chondrosarcoma

Adipose Tissue

Benign Tumors

♦ Lipoma
♦ Angiolipoma.

Malignant Tumors

♦ Liposarcoma

Bone

Benign Tumors

♦ Osteoma
♦ Osteoid osteoma
♦ Osteoblastoma

Malignant Tumors

♦ Osteosarcoma
♦ Osteochondrosarcoma

Vascular Tissue

Benign Tumors

♦ Hemangioma
♦ Hereditary hemorrhagic telangiectasia
♦ Lymphangioma

Malignant Tumors

♦ Hemangioendothelioma

Neural Tissue

Benign Tumors

♦ Neurofibroma
♦ Neurilemmoma
♦ Schwannoma

Malignant Tumors

♦ Neurosarcoma
♦ Neurofibrosarcoma

Muscles

Benign Tumors

♦ Leiomyoma
♦ Rhabdomyoma

Malignant Tumors

♦ Leiomyosarcoma
♦ Rhabdomyosarcoma

Giant Cell Tumor

♦ Central and peripheral giant cell tumor
♦ Giant cell granuloma
♦ Giant cell tumor of hyperthyroidism.

Teratoma

Salivary Gland Tumor

Benign tumors

♦ Adenoma
♦ Warthin's tumor
♦ Pleomorphic adenoma.

Malignant tumors

♦ Mucoepidermoid carcinoma

♦ Adenocystic carcinoma
♦ Adenocarcinoma
♦ Acinic cell carcinoma
♦ Malignant change in pleomorphic adenoma

Lymphoid Tissue

Malignant tumors

♦ Hodgkin's and non-Hodgkin's lymphoma
♦ Lymphosarcoma
♦ Reticular cell sarcoma
♦ Ewing's sarcoma
♦ Burkitt's lymphoma
♦ Multiple myeloma
♦ Leukemia.

Malignant Melanoma

Malignant melanoma is a neoplasm of epidermal melanocytes. It is the third most common cancer of the skin.

Etiology

♦ *Sun exposure:* Persons who are exposed to the excess of sunlight develops malignant melanoma.
♦ *Artifical UV source:* PUVA therapy has been reportedly associated with risk of melanoma.
♦ *Socioeconomic status:* It is seen in high socioeconomic status since people of high socioeconomic status go for holidays.
♦ *Fare skin, freckles, red hair:* These characteristics increased the risk of melanoma.
♦ Melanotic nevi are the strong risk factors.
♦ *Genetic factors:* Familial melanoma and xeroderma pigmentosum are considered to be strong genetic factors for development of malignant melanoma.

Clinical Types of Malignant Melanoma

♦ **Superficial spreading melanoma:** Exists in a radial growth phase. Lesion present as tan, brown or black admixed lesion on sun exposed skin. Radial growth phase may last for several months to years.
♦ **Nodular melanoma:** It exists in a vertical growth phase. It present sharply delineated nodule with varying degrees of pigmentation. They may be pink or black.
♦ **Lentigo maligna melanoma:** Exists in a radial-growth phase. The lesion occur as macular lesion on malar skin of Caucasians.
♦ **Acral lentiginous melanoma:** Melanoma developing on the palms and soles as well as toe and fingers. It is characterized by macular lentiginous pigmented area around nodule.
♦ **Mucosal lentiginous melanoma:** Develops from mucosal epithelium that lines respiratory, gastrointestinal and genitourinary systems. It is more aggressive.
♦ **Amelanotic melanoma:** It is an erythematous or pink sometimes eroded nodule.

Clinical Features

♦ Oral melanomas initiate as macular pigmented focal lesions.
♦ Most of the lesions are pigmented excepting few non-pigmented lesions which referred to as "amelanotic melanomas", which appear as "slightly" inflamed looking areas.

◆ Pigmented lesions are often dark-brown, bluish-black or simply black in appearance.

◆ Initial macular lesions grow very rapidly and often result in a large, painful, diffuse mass.

◆ Surface ulceration is very common and beside; this, hemorrhage, paresthesia and superficial fungal infections are often present.

◆ As the tumor continues to grow, small satellite lesions can develop at the margin of the primary tumor.

◆ Like other epithelial malignant tumors, melanomas exhibit little or no induration at the periphery.

◆ Oral melanomas often cause rapid invasion and extensive destruction of bone. This often results in loosening and exfoliation of the regional teeth in the jaw.

◆ Widespread dissemination of the tumor cells occurs frequently in the lymph nodes as well as in the distant sites, e.g., the lung, liver, bone and brain, etc.

Histopathology

◆ Microscopically the malignant cells lie in nest or cluster of groups in an organoid fashion.

◆ Melanoma cells have large nuclei, often with prominent nucleoli and show nuclear pseudoinclusion.

◆ Cytoplasm of the cell is abundantly eosinophilic or optically clear.

◆ There is presence of large, epithelioid melanocytes distributed in pagetoid manner.

◆ When melanocytes penetrate the basement membrane a florid host cell response of lymphocytes develop.

◆ Macrophages or melanophages may be present.

◆ Vertical growth phase is characterized by the proliferation of malignant epithelioid melanocytes in the underlying connective tissues.

◆ These malignant melanocytes often exhibit extensive cellular pleomorphism and nuclear hyperchromatism.

◆ However, in some lesions melanin production by the tumor cells can be very little and on few occasions there can be virtually no melanin production.

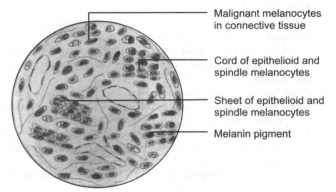

Malignant melanocytes in connective tissue

Cord of epithelioid and spindle melanocytes

Sheet of epithelioid and spindle melanocytes

Melanin pigment

Fig. 36: Malignant melanoma *(For color version, see Plate 7).*

Treatment

Radical surgery with prophylactic neck dissection is often advised.

Q.21. Describe in brief teratoma. *(Aug 2011, 5 Marks)*

Ans. A true teratoma is a developmental tumor composed of tissues from all three germ layers, i.e., ectoderm, mesoderm and endoderm:

◆ Such tumors are believed to derive from germ cells or entrapped totipotent blastomeres which can produce derivatives of all three germ layers.

◆ Teratomas are more common in ovaries and or testis and can be benign or malignant.

Clinical Features

◆ It is most commonly seen in infants.

◆ Orally, it involves soft palate and hard palate. Systemically, it involves testis, ovary, abdominal viscera and pineal region.

◆ It consist of teeth, sebaceous material and some hairs.

Histopathology

◆ H and E stained section show stratified squamous epithelium with epithelial appendages consisting of sebaceous glands, sweat glands, hairs, salivary glands, teeth.

◆ At times thyroid gland tissue and pancreatic tissue can be seen.

Treatment

Surgical excision of tumor should be done.

Q.22. Write in detail about Hodgkin's lymphoma.
(Aug 2011, 10 Marks)

Ans. It is also known as Hodgkin's disease.

◆ Epstein-Barr virus is considered to be the major cause.

◆ Patients with HIV infection have higher incidence of Hodgkin's disease.

Clinical Features

◆ It is most commonly seen in young adults and older individuals.

◆ More common in males as compared to females.

◆ Clinical signs and symptoms of the disease are protean

◆ There is painless enlargement of one or more cervical lymph nodes.

◆ Palpable painless cervical lymphadenopathy occurs in cervical area, axilla and less commonly in inguinal area and Waldeyer's ring and occipital nodes.

◆ Lymph nodes are firm and rubbery in consistency and overlying skin is normal.

◆ Symptoms are of unexplained weight loss, fever and night sweats.

Histopathology

◆ **Nodular sclerosis Hodgkin's disease**
  • Morphology show nodular pattern.
  • Broad bands of fibers divide node into nodules
  • Characteristic cell is lacunar type Reed-Sternberg Cell which has monolobated, multilobated nucleus and a small nucleolus with abundant and pale cytoplasm.

- ♦ **Mixed cellularity Hodgkin's disease**
  - Infiltrate is usually diffuse
  - Reed-Sternberg cells are of classic type, i.e., large with bilobate, double or multiple nuclei and a large eosinophilic inclusion like nucleolus.
- ♦ **Lymphocyte depleted Hodgkin's disease**
  - Infiltrate is diffuse and often appears hypocellular.
  - Large number of Reed-Sternberg cells and bizarre sarcomatous variants are present.
  - It is associated with older age and HIV positivity

- ♦ **Lymphocyte rich classic Hodgkin's disease**
  - Reed-Sternberg cells of the classic or lacunar type are observed with background infiltrate of lymphocytes.
- ♦ **Nodular lymphocyte-predominant Hodgkin's disease**
  - In this typical Reed-Sternberg Cell is not seen, instead a variant of Reed-Sternberg Cell, the lymphocytic and histiocytic cells or popcorn cells are seen within the background of inflammatory cells which are predominantly benign lymphocytes.

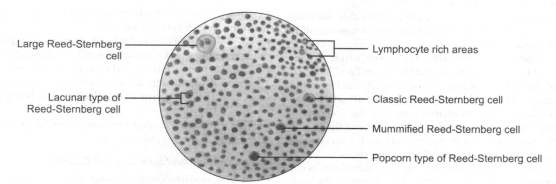

Fig. 37: Hodgkin's lymphoma *(For color version, see Plate 7).*

Treatment

Combination of radiotherapy and chemotherapy help in curing the disease.

Q.23. Write in detail on squamous cell carcinoma.
(May/June 2009, 10 Marks)

Enumerate all malignant epithelial neoplasms. Describe in detail histopathology of oral squamous cell carcinoma. *(Jan 2012, 10 Marks)*

Or

Enumerate malignant tumors of epithelial origin. Describe in detail about squamous cell carcinoma.
(Feb 2013, 10 Marks)

Ans. Malignant epithelial neoplasms/Tumors:
- ♦ Basal cell carcinoma
- ♦ Squamous cell carcinoma
- ♦ Verrucous carcinoma
- ♦ Adenoid squamous cell carcinoma
- ♦ Malignant melanoma
- ♦ Spindle cell carcinoma
- ♦ Primary intra-alveolar carcinoma
- ♦ Multicentric oral carcinoma.

Squamous Cell Carcinoma

- ♦ Squamous cell carcinoma is defined as a malignant epithelial neoplasm exhibit squamous differentiation as characterized by formation of keratin and/or presence of intercellular bridges. —**Pindborg et al, 1997**
- ♦ Squamous cell carcinoma is the commonest malignant epithelial tissue neoplasm of oral cavity. It is mostly derived from stratified squamous epithelium.

Etiology

Following are the etiological factors which lead to squamous cell carcinoma:
- ♦ *Tobacco smoking:* Cigarettes, bidis, pipes, cigars and reverse smoking.
- ♦ *Use of smokeless tobacco:* Snuff dipping, gutkha, tobacco chewing, tobacco as a toothpaste.
- ♦ *Alcohol:* Drinking spirits, Drinking wines, drinking beers
- ♦ *Diet anal nutrition:* Vitamin A, B-complex and C deficiency, Nutritional deficiency with alcoholism.
- ♦ *Dental factors:* Chronic irritation from broken teeth, Ill-fitting or broken prosthesis.
- ♦ *Radiations:* Actinic radiation, X-ray radiation
- ♦ *Viral infections:* Herpes simplex virus (HSV), Human papilloma virus (HPV), Human immunodeficiency virus (HIV), Epstein-Barr virus (EBV).
- ♦ *Chronic infections:* Candidiasis, syphilis
- ♦ *Genetic factors:* Oncogenes, Tumor suppressor genes
- ♦ *Pre-existing oral diseases:* Lichen planus, Plummer-Vinson Syndrome, discoid lupus erythematosus, OSMF.

Clinical Features

- ♦ Carcinomas mostly occur in the 4th to 7th decades of life.
- ♦ Males are more commonly affected
- ♦ Lower lip is the most common site, the second most common site is the lateral border of the tongue. Among all intraoral sites, dorsum of the tongue and hard palate are the least common sites for oral squamous cell carcinoma.
- ♦ Initial lesion may be asymptomatic or can be presented as white or red nodule or fissure over the oral mucosa.
- ♦ Initially the lesion is usually painless.

♦ More advanced lesions present either as a fast enlarging, exophytic or invasive ulcer or sometimes as a large tumor mass or a verrucous growth.

♦ Ulcerated lesion often shows persistent induration around the periphery with an elevated and everted margin.

♦ Lesion can be painful either due to secondary infection or due to involvement of the peripheral nerves by the tumor cells. Lesion can also bleed easily.

♦ Lesions of floor of mouth often cause fixation of the tongue to the underlying structures with difficulty in speech and inability to open the mouth.

♦ When malignant tumor cells invade into the alveolar bone of either maxilla or mandible, they usually cause mobility or exfoliation of regional teeth.

♦ Involvement of inferior alveolar nerve often causes paresthesia of the lower teeth and the lower lip.

♦ Regional lymph nodes are often enlarged, tendered and fixed; some of these nodes can be stony hard in consistency.

♦ Untreated lesions may sometimes destroy the oral tissues and extend into the skin on the outer surface of the face to produce a nodular or lobulated growth on the facial skin, which appears as an extraoral discharging sinus.

♦ Pathological fracture of the jaw bone may sometimes occur in untreated cases due to extensive destruction of the bone by the tumor.

Histological Features

Histological finding as given by **Broder's grading** for squamous cell carcinoma.

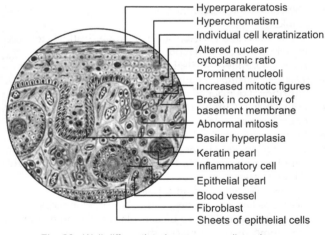

Fig. 38: Well-differentiated squamous cell carcinoma
(For color version, see Plate 8).

Well-differentiated Squamous Cell Carcinoma

♦ Most of the squamous cell carcinomas histologically belong to the well-differentiated category.

♦ In this lesion, the tumor epithelial cells to a large extent resemble the cells of the squamous epithelium both structurally and functionally.

♦ Tumor cells produce large amount of keratin in the form of "keratin pearls".

♦ Tumor cells invade into the underlying connective tissue, where the cells proliferate further and give rise to the formation of many epithelial islands within the connective tissue stroma.

♦ Tumor cells often exhibit dysplastic features like cellular pleomorphism, nuclear hyperchromatism, individual cell keratinization and altered nuclear-cytoplasmic ratio, loss of cohesion, etc.,

♦ Prognosis is better.

Moderately-differentiated Squamous Cell Carcinoma

♦ Tumor cells are usually more severely dysplastic than that of the well-differentiated type.

♦ Growth rate of individual cells is more rapid and this is reflected in greater number of mitotic figures.

♦ There is formation of epithelial islands or cell nests, etc., are diminished since these tumor cells do not differentiate or mature as much as the well differentiated type of cells do.

♦ This tumor also carries a reasonably good prognosis.

Also refer to Ans. 15 of same chapter.

Poorly-differentiated Squamous Cell Carcinoma

♦ In poorly-differentiated squamous cell carcinoma, the malignant tumor cells produce no keratin .

♦ The tumor exhibits extensive cellular abnormalities with lack of normal architectural pattern and loss of intercellular bridges between the tumor cells.

♦ Mitotic cell division is extremely high and because of this, the neoplastic cells are often very immature and primitive looking and it is often very difficult even to recognize them as squamous epithelial cells.

♦ Prognosis is poor.

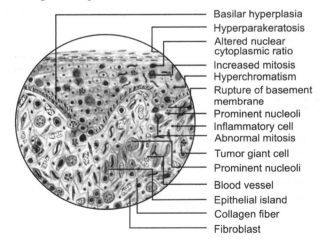

Fig. 39: Poorly-differentiated squamous cell carcinoma
(For color version, see Plate 8).

Investigations

♦ Biopsy of the involved area should be done for confirmation of diagnosis.

♦ Toluidine blue test should be done.

♦ Tumor markers, such as cytokeratins, epithelial membrane antigen, carcinoembryonic antigen (CEA) and alfa-fetoprotein should be used for detection of cancer.

Treatment

Surgical excision of the involved site is the treatment of choice.

Q.24. Write short note on leukoplakia. *(Feb 2013, 5 Marks)*

Or

Write short answer on leukoplakia.

(Sep 2018, 3 Marks)

Ans. *Refer to Ans. 1 of same chapter.*

Q.25. Define neoplasm. Describe in brief clinical features, X-ray details and histopathology of osteogenic sarcoma. *(Mar 2001, 15 Marks) (Sep 2008, 8 Marks)*

Or

Write short note answer on radiological features of osteosarcoma. *(Feb 2019, 3 Marks)*

Ans. "A neoplasm is an abnormal mass of tissue, the growth of which exceeds and is uncoordinated with that of the normal tissues and persists in the same excessive manner after cessation of the stimuli which evoked the change." —**Willis**

Osteogenic Sarcoma

It is a common malignant neoplasm arising from the bone and beside plasma and myeloma.

Clinical Features

♦ It occurs during 10–25 years of age in the jaw and males are more commonly affected.
♦ The tumor involves maxilla more often than mandible.
♦ A very fast enlarging, painful swelling of jaw, causes expansion and distortion of cortical plates.
♦ Severe facial deformity and difficulty in taking the food due to restricted jaw movement.
♦ Displacement and loosening of regional teeth.
♦ Ulceration, hemorrhage and pathological fracture of bone are commonly associated.

X-ray Details

The X-ray details of osteosarcoma are divided into following stages, i.e.:
♦ **Osteolytic stage**
  • It reveals moth eaten appearance.
  • Border of the lesion at this stage are ill-defined.
  • There is perforation and expansion of cortical plates.
  • Lamina dura is absent, i.e., it get destroyed.
  • Pathological fracture may be present.
  • Root resorption is present.
♦ **Mixed stage**
  • It is called as mixed because this stage show formation and destruction of bone.
  • It reveals honeycomb appearance.
  • Margins of lesion are ill defined.
♦ **Osteoblastic stage**
  • It reveals sun ray appearance.
  • At times subperiosteal bone laid down in layers which results in onion peel appearance.

• In osteosarcoma periosteum is elevated over the expanding tumor mass in a tent like fashion. At point on the bone where the periosteum begin to merge an acute angle between periosteum and bone is created which is known as Codman's Triangle.

Histopathology

♦ There will be presence of numerous, actively proliferating, spindle shaped, oval or angular, malignant osteoblast cells within cellular stroma.
♦ The malignant osteoblast cells exhibit cellular pleomorphism, abnormal increased mitosis and nuclear hyperchromatism
♦ Multiple areas of newly formed bone or osteoid tissue are often present within fibrous stroma.
♦ In chondroblastic variations the malignant tumor cells produce large amount of cartilaginous tissue within tumor.

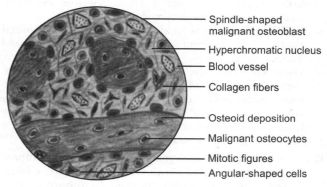

Spindle-shaped malignant osteoblast
Hyperchromatic nucleus
Blood vessel
Collagen fibers
Osteoid deposition
Malignant osteocytes
Mitotic figures
Angular-shaped cells

Fig. 40: Osteosarcoma *(For color version, see Plate 8).*

Q.26. Write short essay on osteosarcoma.

(Jan 2012, 5 Marks)

Or

Write short note on osteosarcoma.

(Aug 2012, 5 Marks) (Mar 2016, 3 Marks)

Ans. *Refer to Ans. 25 of same chapter.*

Q.27. Define oral submucous fibrosis. Describe in detail etiopathogenesis and histopathology of same.

(Apr 2008, 15 Marks)

Ans. OSMF is defined as "An insidious chronic disease affecting any part of oral cavity and sometime pharynx. Although occasionally preceded by and/or associated with vesicle formation, it is always associated with juxta-epithelial inflammatory reaction followed by fibroelastic changes in lamina propria, with epithelial atrophy leading to stiffness of oral mucosa and causing trismus and inability to eat."

—**Pindborg (1966)**

Etiopathogenesis

♦ **Betel nut:** Tannic acid and arecoline present in betel nut affect the vascular supply of oral mucosa leading to a neurotropic disorder. Nitrosation of arecoline causes formation of nitrosoguvacine and nitrosoguvacoline as well as 3 methylnitrosamino propionitrile which leads to alkylation of DNA. Metabolism of nitrosoguvacine and nitrosoguvacoline as well as 3 methylnitrosamino propionitrile causes formation of cyanoethyl. Cyanoethyl interacts with O-methyl guanine in DNA. Constant irritation by this leads to OSMF and exposure for long time leads to malignant transformation.

Recent concept: Arecoline in betel nut stimulates fibroblasts. Fibroblasts proliferates and produce collagen. Flavonoids, i.e., catechin and tannin in betel nut stabilizes collagen fibers which make them resistant to degradation by collagenase enzyme. Trismus is caused due to juxta-epithelial hyalinization as well as involvement of the secondary muscles. Increased muscle activity leads to glycogen depletion and reduced blood supply due to connective tissue changes leads to degeneration of muscle and also cause fibrosis.

♦ **Tobacco and lime:** Tobacco act as a local irritant which leads to OSMF. Lime causes local irritation as well as vesicle and ulcer formation in the oral mucosa.

♦ **Chillies:** Capsaicin is an active ingredient present in red chillies. It is the irritant in chillies which leads to oral submucous fibrosis.

♦ **Hereditary:** Presence of genetic susceptibility is present. Familial occurrence of OSMF is seen.

♦ **Immunological Studies:** It was found that human leukocyte antigen (HLA) A10, B7 and DR3 occur significantly more frequently in oral submucous fibrosis.

For histopathology, refer to Ans. 4 of same chapter.

Q.28. Enumerate premalignant lesions and conditions. Describe in detail about etiopathogenesis, clinical features, histopathology and treatment of oral submucous fibrosis. *(Jan 2012, 15 Marks)*

Or

Describe in detail about etiopathogenesis, clinical features, histopathology and treatment of oral submucous fibrosis. *(Aug 2012, 10 Marks)*

Or

Enumerate premalignant lesions and conditions in oral cavity. Describe in detail about oral submucous fibrosis (OSMF).

(Feb 2015 10 Marks) (Jun 2014, 10 Marks)

Or

List premalignant lesions and conditions. Discuss etiopathogenesis, clinical features and histopathology of oral submucous fibrosis.

(May 2018, 15 Marks)

Or

Discuss in detail oral submucous fibrosis.

(Oct 2019, 5 Marks)

Ans. *For enumeration of premalignant lesions and condition, refer to Ans. 2 of same chapter.*

For etiopathogenesis, refer to Ans. 27 of same chapter.

For clinical features, histopathology and treatment, refer to Ans. 4 of same chapter.

Q.29. Classify the non-odontogenic tumors of oral cavity and describe fibroma. *(Dec 2010, 16 Marks)*

Or

Write short answer on fibroma. *(May 2018, 3 Marks)*

Ans. *For classification of non-odontogenic tumors of oral cavity, refer to Ans. 20 of same chapter.*

Fibroma

It is a benign tumor of connective tissue origin.

Clinical Features

♦ It is a slow growing lesion and can be seen during 3rd, 4th and 5th decades of life.

♦ Female predilection is seen.

♦ It can occur anywhere in the oral cavity but most commonly it is seen on buccal mucosa along plane of occlusion. It also affects gingiva, tongue, buccal mucosa, lips and palate.

♦ Lesion appears as elevated nodule of normal color with smooth surface and a sessile or at times pedunculated base.

♦ Its size can ranges from several millimeters to centimeters.

♦ Lesion if traumatized it become painful.

♦ Color of the lesion is pink and texture is smooth.

♦ Consistency of lesion can be soft or firm or can be elastic.

♦ At times lesion is traumatized and become inflamed and show ulceration or hyperkeratosis.

Histopathology

♦ Lesion consists of stratified squamous epithelium which show shortening and flattening of rete pegs.

♦ Underlying connective tissue stroma show bundles of interlacing collagen fibers which are interspersed with numerous fibroblasts.

♦ There is presence of chronic inflammatory cell infiltrate consisting of lymphocytes and plasma cells.

♦ Areas of calcification and ossification can also be seen.

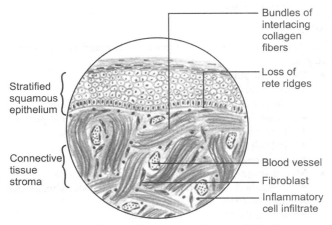

Fig. 41: Fibroma *(For color version, see Plate 8).*

Treatment

Excision of the lesion should be done.

Q.30. Write short note on fibroma H/P (histopathology).

(Mar 2013, 3 Marks)

Ans. *For H/P (histopathology) of fibroma, refer to Ans. 29 of same chapter.*

Q.31. Enumerate non-odontogenic connective tissue malignant tumors. Discuss in detail about clinical features, etiology and histopathology of fibrosarcoma. *(Mar 2013, 8 Marks)*

Ans.

Non-odontogenic Connective Tissue Malignant Tumors

♦ *Fibrous connective tissue:* Fibrosarcoma
♦ *Adipose Tissue:* Liposarcoma
♦ *Cartilage:* Chondrosarcoma
♦ *Bone*
  • Osteosarcoma
  • Osteochondrosarcoma
♦ *Vascular:*
  • Hemangioendothelioma
  • Angiosarcoma
  • Kaposi sarcoma
♦ *Neural tissue:* Neurosarcoma or Neurofibrosarcoma
♦ *Muscle:*
  • Leiomyosarcoma
  • Rhabdomyosarcoma
♦ *Lymphoid tissue:*
  • Hodgkin and non-Hodgkin lymphoma
  • Lymphosarcoma
  • Reticular cell sarcoma
  • Ewing's sarcoma
  • Burkitt's lymphoma
  • Multiple myeloma
  • Leukemia.

Fibrosarcoma

It is the malignant fibrous connective tissue tumor and is the malignant tumor of fibroblasts.

Clinical Features

♦ It arises at any age but mean age is 40 years.
♦ Male predilection is seen.
♦ It is most commonly seen in lower extremities, i.e., femur and tibia.
♦ In oral cavity tumor involves mandible, maxilla, maxillary sinus, lip and palate.
♦ Tumor is generally a large painless mass which lies deep to fascia and has ill-defined margin.
♦ Associated teeth become mobile.
♦ Tumors in starting show benign growth and later on they spread rapidly producing large tumor with ulceration and hemorrhage.
♦ They can also cause pathological fracture.

Etiology

♦ Most of the fibrosarcomas arise from preexisting lesions, such as Paget's disease, fibrous dysplasia chronic osteomyelitis, bone infarcts and in previously irradiated areas of bone.

♦ Congenital fibrosarcomas are thought to arise from genetic mutations.

Histopathology

Various histological grading of fibrosarcoma are:

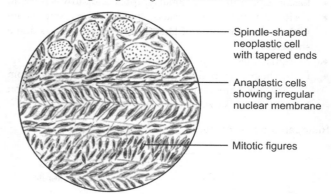

Spindle-shaped neoplastic cell with tapered ends

Anaplastic cells showing irregular nuclear membrane

Mitotic figures

Fig. 42: Fibrosarcoma *(For color version, see Plate 8).*

Well-differentiated

♦ In this multiple plump-shaped fibroblasts with pale eosinophilic cytoplasm, hyperchromatic spindle-shaped nuclei with tapered ends is seen.
♦ Malignant fibroblasts are dispersed in rich collagen area.
♦ Few mitotic figures are evident.

Intermediate Grade

♦ In this tumor show Herring bone pattern, i.e., parallel sheets of cells arranged in intertwining whorls.
♦ Cellularity is high.
♦ Cellular pleomorphism is evident.
♦ Areas of hyalinization can be appreciated.

High Grade

♦ Marked cellular atypia and mitotic activity is evident.
♦ This grade is highly anaplastic and pleomorphic with bizarre nuclei.

Q.32. Write short note on keratoacanthoma.

(June 2014, 5 Marks)

Or

Write short answer on keratoacanthoma.

(Oct 2019, 3 Marks)

Ans. It is also known as molluscum sebaceum, self-healing carcinoma or pseudocarcinoma.

It clinically and histologically resembles epidermoid carcinoma so it is mistaken as oral carcinoma.

Etiology

♦ Hereditary predisposition is present.
♦ Human papilloma virus (HPV) 26 or 37 can lead to keratoacanthoma.
♦ Sun exposure
♦ Chemical agents, such as coal tar and minerals

Clinical Features

♦ Its occurrence is at the age of 50 to 70 years. Male predilection is present.

♦ Intraorally, it is most commonly found on lips.

♦ Lesion is painful and regional lymphadenopathy is present.

♦ Lesion is elevated, umblicated with depressed central core with presence of plug of keratin. Lesion appears as dome shaped.

♦ Margins of lesion are sharply delineated.

♦ Lesion begins as small nodule which increases in size from 4 to 6 weeks. Later on it undergoes spontaneous regression from 6 to 8 weeks with scar formation.

Histopathological Features

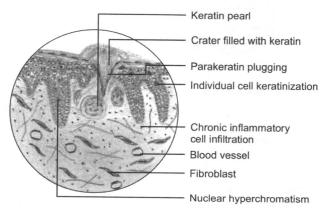

Keratin pearl
Crater filled with keratin
Parakeratin plugging
Individual cell keratinization
Chronic inflammatory cell infiltration
Blood vessel
Fibroblast
Nuclear hyperchromatism

Fig. 43: Keratoacanthoma *(For color version, see Plate 8).*

♦ Hyperplastic squamous epithelium growing into underlying connective tissue.

♦ Epithelial surface is covered by parakeratin or orthokeratin with parakeratin plugging.

♦ Pseudocarcinomatous infiltration typically present smooth, regular, well demarcated front which does not extend beyond the level of sweat gland.

♦ Connective tissue show chronic inflammatory cell infiltration.

♦ Most characteristic feature of lesion is seen at the margins where normal adjacent epithelium is elevated towards central portion of crater, later on an abrupt change in normal epithelium occurs as hyperplastic acanthotic epithelium is reached.

Treatment

Surgical excision.

Q.33. Write short note on Kaposi's sarcoma.

(Feb 2014, 3 Marks)

Ans. It is also known as multiple idiopathic hemorrhagic sarcoma of Kaposi.

♦ Kaposi's sarcoma is the multicentric proliferation of vascular or spindle cell components.

♦ Kaposi's sarcoma is currently associated with HIV/AIDS.

Clinical Features

Clinically, Kaposi's sarcoma is of four types, i.e.:

♦ Classic (Chronic)

♦ Endemic (Lymphadenopathic; African)

♦ Immunosuppression associated (Transplant)

♦ AIDS related.

Classic Type

♦ Development of cutaneous multifocal blue red nodules on the lower extremities.

♦ Lesion slowly increases in size and number with some of the lesions extinguishing and new ones forming on adjacent or distinct skin.

♦ Orally, soft bluish nodules occur on palatal mucosa or gingiva.

Lymphadenopathic

♦ Present in young African children.

♦ There is generalized or localized enlargement of lymph node chain which includes cervical lymph nodes.

♦ Disease follow fulminant course with visceral involvement and minimum skin or mucous membrane involvement.

Immunosuppression Associated

♦ It is usually seen in renal transplant patients.

♦ It occurs 1 to 2 years after transplantation

♦ Progression of disease is directly proportional to loss of cellular immunity of host.

AIDS Related

♦ Homosexual AIDS patients have maximum chances of developing Kaposi's sarcoma.

♦ Lesions occur on cutaneous lesions, i.e., along lines of cleavage and tip of nose.

♦ Oral lesions can occur anywhere in oral cavity, but predilection is for palatal mucosa and gingiva.

♦ Early oral mucosal lesions are flat and slight blue, red or purple plaques, either focal or diffuse and may be completely asymptomatic.

♦ Later on these lesions may be more deeply discolored and there is development of surface papules and nodules which may become exophytic and ulcerated. These lesions can also bleed.

♦ Cervical lymphadenopathy and salivary gland enlargement is seen.

Histopathology

Early lesion or Patch stage

♦ There is proliferation of small veins and capillaries around one or more preexisting dilated vessels.

♦ Slit like vessels are seen near periphery of preexisting blood vessel, skin adnexa and in between collagen fibers.

♦ Slit like vessels are lined by plump, mild atypical endothelial cells.

♦ There is presence of mononuclear inflammatory cell infiltrate consisting of mast cells, scattered erythrocytes and hemosiderin deposit.

Advance Lesion or Plaque Stage

♦ There is presence of increased numbers of increased capillaries and dilated vascular channels which are interspersed with proliferating sheets of sarcomatous cells with large number of extravasated erythrocytes.
♦ Slit like vessels without visible endothelial lining are interspersed with spindle cells.
♦ Lesional cells show enlarged, hyperchromatic nuclei with mild-to-moderate pleomorphism.

Nodular Stage

In all features are more prominent than plaque stage.

Q.34. Write short note on tori. *(Feb 2014, 3 Marks)*

Ans. Tori are of two types, i.e., torus palatinus and torus mandibularis

Torus Palatinus

It is a slow growing, flat based boney protuberance which occurs in midline of hard palate.

Clinical Features

♦ Women are affected more commonly.
♦ Torus palatinus can occur at any age. It reaches at its peak incidence at age of 30 years.
♦ It is an outgrowth in the midline of palate.
♦ It is spindle shaped, nodular or lobular.
♦ Mucosa overlying torus is intact and occasionally it appears blanched.
♦ It may become ulcerated if traumatized.
♦ Torus itself may be composed of dense compact bone or dense compact bone with center of cancellous bone.

Torus Mandibularis

It is an exostosis or outgrowth of mandible found on the lingual surface.

Clinical Features

♦ Growth on lingual surface of mandible occurs at mylohyoid line which is usually opposite to cuspid teeth.
♦ Mandibular tori are bilateral.
♦ Bilateral overgrowths are globular or they are multiple.

Treatment

For both tori treatment is surgical excision.

Q.35. Write short note on congenital epulis.

(Feb 2014, 3 Marks)

Ans. It is also known as congenital epulis of newborn or Neumann's tumor.

It is benign in nature and mostly occurs as single tumor.

Clinical Features

♦ Tumor is present at birth.
♦ It is located over maxillary or mandibular gingiva. But more common on maxillary.

♦ Lesion is pedunculated and is found on incisor region arising from crest of alveolar ridge or alveolar process.
♦ Lesion varies from few centimeters to millimeters.

Histology

♦ Presence of sheets of large closely packed cells showing fine, granular, eosinophilic cytoplasm which comprises the tumor mass.
♦ Numerous capillaries are present.

Treatment

Surgical Excision.

Q.36. Enumerate malignant epithelial tumors of oral cavity. Discuss about etiology, clinical features and histopathology of verrucous carcinoma.

(Feb 2014, 8 Marks)

Ans.

Enumeration of Malignant Epithelial Tumors of Oral Cavity

♦ Squamous cell carcinoma
♦ Intraepidermoid carcinoma
♦ Adenocarcinoma
♦ Metastatic carcinoma
♦ Basal cell carcinoma
♦ Transitional cell carcinoma
♦ Malignant melanoma
♦ Verrucous carcinoma
♦ Intraepidermoid carcinoma
♦ Spindle cell carcinoma
♦ Primary intra-alveolar carcinoma
♦ Adenoid squamous cell carcinoma.

For clinical features and histopathology of verrucous carcinoma, refer to Ans. 11 of same chapter.

Etiology

Tobacco: Verrucous carcinoma develops in tobacco chewers. It usually occurs in the buccal sulcus area where the person holds the tobacco most.

Q.37. Describe histopathology of well-differentiated squamous cell carcinoma. *(Mar 2006, 5 Marks)*

Ans. *For histopathology of well differentiated squamous cell carcinoma, refer to Ans. 23 of same chapter.*

Q.38. Write in brief lipoma. *(Feb 2013, 8 Marks)*

Or

Write short answer on oral lipoma.

(Apr 2019, 3 Marks)

Ans. Lipoma is a rare intraoral tumor.

It is a benign, slow growing tumor of mature fat cells.

Classification

On the basis of morphology

Superficial: It is a single, yellow, lobulated, painless lesion with sessile or pedunculated base.

Diffuse: It occurs in deeper tissues and produces a slight surface elevation.

Encapsulated: It is surrounded by a capsule.

Pathogenesis

♦ HMGI-C gene which is mapped to 12q15 is a member of high mobility group protein gene family, play a role in development of lipoma.

♦ Cells of lipoma are different metabolically as compared to normal fat cells. Precursors of fatty acid should be incorporated at faster rate in fat of lipoma as compared to normal fat and there is reduction in lipoprotein lipase activity.

Clinical Features

♦ It is mainly seen in adults with no gender predilection.

♦ Usually the size of lesion is 3 cm, but it can progress from 5 to 6 cm. It occurs in tongue, floor of the mouth, buccal mucosa, gingiva and mucobuccal or labial folds.

♦ Morphologically intraoral lipomas are classified as diffuse form, superficial and encapsulated form.

♦ Superficial form appear as single or lobulated, this is a painless lesion which is attached by either a pedunculated or sessile base.

♦ Oral lipoma is encapsulated have yellow surface discoloration and is freely mobile beneath the mucosa. It is soft to palpation.

♦ Lesion present in deeper part of tissue produces slight surface elevation which is more diffuse as compared to superficial type. On palpation diffuse form seem to be like cystic in consistency.

♦ Multiple head and neck lipomas are seen in neuro-fibromatosis, Gardner's syndrome, Proteus syndrome, multiple familial lipomatosis.

Histopathology

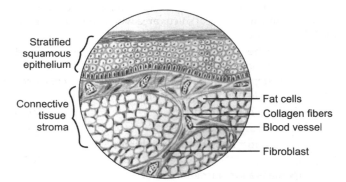

Fig. 44: Lipoma *(For color version, see Plate 9).*

♦ Lipoma consists predominantly of mature lymphocytes which are admixed with collagen streaks and is well demarcated from surrounding connective tissues.

♦ A thin fibrous capsule is present and distinct lobular pattern can be seen.

♦ Lesional fat cells are well appreciated infiltrating the surrounding tissues, perhaps producing long, thin extensions of fatty tissue which radiate from central tumor mass.

♦ When it is located inside striated muscle this variant is known as intramuscular lipoma, but extensive coverage of wide area of fibrovascular or stromal tissue is termed as lipomatosis.

♦ Occasionally lesions exhibiting excessive fibrosis between the fat cells is known as fibrolipoma, excess number of small vascular channels, i.e., angiolipoma, a myxoid background stroma, i.e., myxolipoma or areas with uniform spindle-shaped cells interspersed between normal adipocytes. It is also known as spindle cell lipoma.

♦ When the spindle cells appear somewhat dysplastic or mixed with pleomorphic giant cell with/without hyperchromatic, enlarged nuclei, it is called as pleomorphic lipoma.

♦ When the spindle cells are of smooth muscle origin, term myolipoma can be used or angiolipoma when smooth muscle appears to be derived from walls of arterioles.

♦ Rarely, chondroid or osseous metaplasia may be seen in lipoma.

♦ If bone marrow is present, term myelolipoma is given.

♦ On rare occasion isolated ductal or tubular adnexal structures are scattered throughout fat lobules, here term adenolipoma is applied.

♦ Perineural lipoma is also seen.

Treatment

Conservative surgical removal is treatment of choice for oral lipoma with occasional recurrences.

Q.39. Write short note on Ewing's sarcoma—histopathology.
(Nov 2014, 3 Marks)

Ans.

Histopathology of Ewing's Sarcoma

♦ The lesion consists of solid sheets of small round cells with very minimal stroma but at a few places connective tissue septae are present.

♦ Cells are round and small in shape along with scanty cytoplasm, nuclei of the cell is large round to oval in shape along with dispersed chromatin and hyperchromasia.

♦ Borders of cell are ill defined.

♦ Cells also show mitotic figures.

♦ Cells of the sarcoma are arranged in filigree pattern.

♦ Small vascular channels are also evident.

♦ Hemorrhage along with vascular lakes or sinuses are appreciated.

♦ Perivascular sparing and geographical necrosis is very common in Ewing's sarcoma.

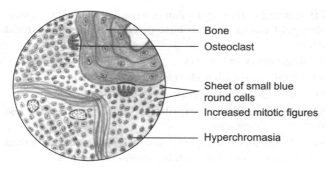

Labels: Bone, Osteoclast, Sheet of small blue round cells, Increased mitotic figures, Hyperchromasia

Fig. 45: Ewing's sarcoma *(For color version, see Plate 9).*

Q.40. Write short note on epithelial dysplasia.

(Nov 2014, 3 Marks)

Or

Write short answer on dysplasia. *(Sep 2018, 3 Marks)*

Ans. Epithelial dysplasia comprises a loss in the uniformity of individual cells or cytological atypia as well as a loss in their architectural orientation.

Dysplasia is a histopathological diagnosis which is made on the basis of presence of certain histological and cytological features in premalignant lesions and conditions.

Architecture and Cytologic Criteria for Grading Epithelial Dysplasia Given by WHO (2005)

Architecture Criteria

- Irregular epithelial stratification
- Loss of polarity of basal cells
- Basal cell hyperplasia
- Drop-shaped rete pegs
- Increased number of mitotic figures
- Abnormally superficial mitosis
- Dyskeratosis, i.e., premature keratinization in the cell
- Keratin pearls within rete ridges.

Cytologic Criteria

- *Anisonucleosis:* Abnormal variation in nuclear size
- *Nuclear pleomorphism:* Abnormal variation in nuclear shape
- *Anisocytosis:* Abnormal variation in cell size
- *Cellular pleomorphism:* Abnormal variation in cell shape
- Increased nuclear cytoplasmic ratio
- Increased nuclear size
- Atypical mitotic figures
- Increase in the number and size of nucleoli
- Hyperchromatism.

Grading of Epithelial Dysplasia

- Histopathological interpretation of potentially malignant disorders shows presence of epithelial dysplasia.
- There are numerous prognostic molecular markers but the epithelial dysplasia is considered to be the strongest predictor of future malignant transformation in potentially malignant disorders.

- Grading of epithelial dysplasia is divided into four categories:
  1. **Mild:** Cellular atypia and architectural disturbances limited to basal and parabasal layers.
  2. **Moderate:** Cellular atypia and architectural disturbances limited from basal to midportion of spinous cell layer.
  3. **Severe:** Cellular atypia and architectural disturbances from basal layer to a level above midpoint of epithelium.
  4. **Carcinoma in situ:** Theoretical concept of carcinoma in situ is that malignant transformation has occurred but invasion is absent. This is the most severe form of epithelial dysplasia and involves entire thickness of epithelium. This is cytologically similar to squamous cell carcinoma but architecturally the epithelial basement membrane remains intact and no invasion in connective tissue has occurred.

Q.41. Write short note on neurilemmoma.

(Feb 2014, 5 Marks)

Ans. It is also known as schwannoma.

It is a benign neural neoplasm of Schwann cell origin.

Clinical Features

- The lesion occurs most commonly in young and middle age adults.
- Neurilemmoma is a slow growing encapsulated tumor which arises in association with nerve trunk.
- Usually the tumor mass is asymptomatic, but tenderness or pain is present if tumor is causing pressure in associate nerves.
- Tumor may range from few millimeters to several centimeters in size.

Oral Manifestations

- It occurs commonly in oral cavity and the most common site of occurrence is tongue.
- The lesion is a single, circumscribed nodule of varying size which presents no pathognomonic features.
- Neurilemmoma also occur as central lesion in the mandible and arises from mandibular nerve.
- Centrally occurring lesion may lead to destruction of bone with expansion of cortical plates.
- Pain and paresthesia is common in centrally occurring lesions.

Histopathology

- Usually, the lesion presents two types of histologic patterns, i.e., Antoni A and Antoni B pattern.
- *Antoni A:* This pattern is made up of the cells which have spindle shape or elongated nuclei which are aligned to form a characteristic palisaded pattern and the intercellular fibers are arranged in parallel fashion between rows of nuclei. In some areas, these fibers show arrangement in shape of whorls or swirls. In the palisaded arrangement of cells around central acellular area eosinophilic areas are seen known as Verocay bodies.
- **Antoni B:** In this pattern, there is disordered arrangement of spindle cells and fibers in loose myxomatous stroma with areas of edema fluid and formation of microcysts.

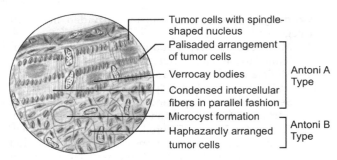

Fig. 46: Neurilemmoma *(For color version, see Plate 9).*

Treatment

Surgical excision is the treatment of choice.

Q.42. Enumerate the carcinomas of oral cavity. Describe staging and grading of squamous cell carcinoma.

(June 2015, 10 Marks)

Or

Write short note on TNM staging. *(Feb 2019, 5 Marks)*

Ans.

Carcinomas of Oral Cavity

- Squamous cell carcinoma
- Verrucous carcinoma
- Basaloid squamous cell carcinoma
- Adenoid squamous cell carcinoma
- Spindle cell carcinoma
- Adenosquamous carcinoma
- Undifferentiated carcinoma.

Staging of Squamous Cell Carcinoma

Staging is defined as extent of spread of tumor within the body.

Staging of squamous cell carcinoma is done by TNM classification which was given by **American Joint Committee on Cancer (AJCC)**

T is suggestive of primary tumor

N is suggestive of regional lymph nodes

M is suggestive of distant metastasis

T – primary Tumor

TX – Primary tumor cannot be assessed.

T0 – No evidence of primary tumor

Tis – Carcinoma in situ

T1 – Tumor 2 cm of less in greatest dimension

T2 – Tumor more than 2 cm but not more than 4 cm in greatest dimension

T3 – Tumor more than 4 cm in greatest dimension

T4a (Lip) – Tumor invades through cortical bone, inferior alveolar nerve, floor of mouth or skin (chin or nose).

T4a (Oral Cavity) – Tumor invades through cortical bone, into deep/extrinsic muscle of tongue (genioglossus, hyoglossus, palatoglossus and styloglossus), maxillary sinus or skin of face.

T4b (lip and oral cavity) – Tumor invades masticatory space, pterygoid plates or skull base or encases internal carotid artery

N – Regional lymph nodes

NX – Regional lymph nodes cannot be assessed

N0 – No regional lymph node metastasis

N1 – Metastasis in a single ipsilateral lymph node, 3 cm or less in greatest dimension.

N2a – Metastasis in a single ipsilateral lymph node, more than 3 cm, but not more than 6 cm in greatest dimension.

N2b – Metastasis in multiple ipsilateral lymph nodes, not more than 6 cm in greatest dimension.

N2c – Metastasis in bilateral or contralateral lymph nodes, not more than 6 cm in greatest dimension.

N3 – Metastasis in a lymph node more than 6 cm in greatest dimension.

M – Distant Metastasis

MX – Distant metastasis cannot be assessed

M0 – No distant metastasis

M1 – Distant metastasis.

Stage Grouping of Oral Cancer

Stage 0	Tis	N0	M0
Stage I	T1	N0	M0
Stage II	T2	N0	M0
Stage III	T1,	N1	M0
	T2,	N1	M0
	T3	N0, N1	M0
Stage IVa	T1,T2,T3,	N2	M0
	T4a	N0, N1, N2	M0
Stage IVb	Any T	N3	M0
	T4b	Any N	M0
Stage IVc	Any T	Any N	M1

Grading of Squamous Cell Carcinoma

Grading is defined as macroscopic and microscopic degree of differentiation of a tumor.

Squamous cell carcinoma is divided in following categories by Broder also known as Broder's classification:

Broader's Classification

- Grade I: Well differentiated—<25% undifferentiated cells
- Grade II: Moderately differentiated—<50% undifferentiated cells
- Grade III: Poorly differentiated—<75% undifferentiated cells
- Grade IV: Anaplastic/Pleomorphic—>75% undifferentiated cells

Q.43. Write short note on radiological features of osteosarcoma. *(Jan 2016, 5 Marks)*

Ans. The radiographic features of osteosarcoma are divided into following stages, i.e.:

- **Osteolytic Stage**
  - It reveals moth eaten appearance.
  - Border of the lesion at this stage are ill defined.
  - There is perforation and expansion of cortical plates.
  - Lamina dura is absent, i.e., it get destroyed.
  - Pathological fracture may be present.
  - Root resorption is present.
- **Mixed Stage**
  - It is called as mixed because this stage shows formation and destruction of bone.
  - It reveals honeycomb appearance.
  - Margins of lesion are ill defined.
- **Osteoblastic Stage**
  - It reveals sun ray appearance.
  - At times subperiosteal bone laid down in layers which results in onion peel appearance.
  - In osteosarcoma periosteum is elevated over the expanding tumor mass in a tent like fashion. At point on the bone where the periosteum begin to merge an acute angle between periosteum and bone is created which is known as Codman's Triangle.

Q.44. Write short note on papilloma. *(Mar 2016, 3 Marks)*

Or

Write short answer on squamous papilloma.

(Apr 2019, 3 Marks)

Ans. Papilloma is the benign proliferation of stratified squamous epithelium which result in papillary and verruciform mass.

Etiology

Papilloma is caused by human papilloma virus. Viral subtypes 6 and 11 are identified in 50% of oral papillomas.

Mode of Transmission

Exact mode of transmission is unknown but transmission is by sexual and non-sexual person to person contact, contaminated objects, saliva or breast milk.

Clinical Features

- Papilloma can be diagnosed at any stage but more commonly, it is seen in persons of 30 to 50 years of age.
- Papilloma occurs more commonly on tongue, lip and soft palate, but it can involve any of the surface.
- Papilloma is a soft, painless usually pedunculated, exophytic nodule with numerous finger like projections which impart cauliflower or wart like appearance.
- Lesion can be white, slightly red or normal in color depend on surface keratinization.
- Papilloma remains solitary and enlarges to the maximum size of 0.5 cm, but lesions of 3 cm are also reported.

Histopathology

- Papilloma is characterized by proliferation of keratinized stratified squamous epithelium which is arranged in finger like projections along with the fibrovascular cores.

- Its hallmark feature is proliferation of spinous cells in papillary pattern.
- Connective tissue core can show inflammatory changes. Presence of chronic inflammatory cells can be variably noted in connective tissue.
- Koilocytes, i.e., virus altered epithelial clear cells with small dark or pyknotic nuclei with perinuclear clear spaces are sometimes seen in prickle cell layer.

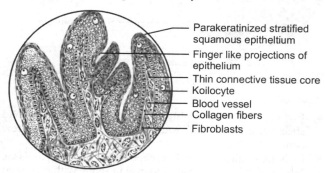

Parakeratinized stratified squamous epitheltium
Finger like projections of epithelium
Thin connective tissue core
Koilocyte
Blood vessel
Collagen fibers
Fibroblasts

Fig. 47: Papilloma (H and E Stain) *(For color version, see Plate 9).*

Treatment

Surgical excision should be done including the base of lesion.

Q.45. Write short note on Ewing's sarcoma.

(July 2016, 5 Marks)

Ans. Ewing's sarcoma is a small round cell tumor. It arises inside the bone.

Clinical Features

- It occurs predominantly in children and young adults between 5 to 25 years with median age of 13 years.
- It is more common in males as compared to females.
- Whites develop this tumor more commonly but in blacks not even single case is reported.
- Pain in Ewing's sarcoma is intermittent in nature.
- Swelling of the bone is earliest clinical sign.
- Long bones of extremities are more commonly affected besides these skull, clavicle, ribs, shoulder are also affected.
- Ewing's sarcoma in occur more commonly in mandible as compared to maxilla
- Paresthesia and loosening of teeth are common findings in Ewing's sarcoma of jaw.
- Appearance of jaw swelling is rapid and intraoral mass become ulcerated.
- Tumor commonly penetrates the cortex resulting in soft tissue mass which overlie affected area of bone.

Radiographic Features

- Most common finding is formation of layers of new subperiosteal bone which produces onion skin appearance of film.
- There is presence of irregular lytic bone destruction with ill-defined margins.

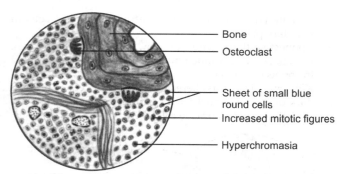

Bone
Osteoclast
Sheet of small blue round cells
Increased mitotic figures
Hyperchromasia

Fig. 48: Ewing's sarcoma (H and E stain)
(For color version, see Plate 9).

Histopathology

♦ Ewing's sarcoma is highly cellular which consists of solid sheets or mass of small round cells with little stroma, few connective tissue septa can also be seen.
♦ Cells are small and round in shape having scanty cytoplasm. Nuclei of cell is large round to oval in shape with dispersed chromatin and hyperchromasia. Borders of cell are indistinct.
♦ Cells are arranged in filigree pattern.
♦ Mitotic figures are commonly seen.
♦ Multiple small vascular channels are also present.
♦ Hemorrhage with vascular lakes or sinuses can be seen.
♦ There is also presence of geographic necrosis with perivascular sparing.
♦ Necrosis can be seen on the opposite side of fragment of bone.

Histological Differential Diagnosis

♦ Small cell osteosarcoma
♦ Peripheral neuroectodermal tumor of infancy
♦ Metastatic neuroblastoma
♦ Mesenchymal chondrosarcoma
♦ Malignant lymphoma
♦ Embryonal rhabdomyosarcoma.

Treatment

♦ Radical surgical excision should be done alone or coupled with X-ray radiation.
♦ Current treatment consists of combined surgery, radiotherapy and multidrug chemotherapy which led to 40 to 80% of survival rates.

Q.46. Write short note on features of epithelial dysplasia.

(July 2016, 5 Marks)

Ans. Following are the features of epithelial dysplasia:

Architecture and Cytologic Criteria for Grading Epithelial Dysplasia Given by WHO (2005)

Architecture Criteria

♦ Irregular epithelial stratification
♦ Loss of polarity of basal cells
♦ Basal cell hyperplasia
♦ Drop-shaped rete pegs
♦ Increased number of mitotic figures
♦ Abnormally superficial mitosis
♦ Dyskeratosis, i.e., premature keratinization in the cell
♦ Keratin pearls within rete ridges.

Cytologic Criteria

♦ *Anisonucleosis:* Abnormal variation in nuclear size
♦ *Nuclear pleomorphism:* Abnormal variation in nuclear shape
♦ *Anisocytosis:* Abnormal variation in cell size
♦ *Cellular pleomorphism:* Abnormal variation in cell shape
♦ Increased nuclear cytoplasmic ratio
♦ Increased nuclear size
♦ Atypical mitotic figures
♦ Increase in the number and size of nucleoli
♦ Hyperchromatism.

Q.47. Write short note on multiple myeloma.

(July 2016, 5 Marks)

Ans. Multiple myeloma is a relatively uncommon malignancy of plasma cell origin which often has multicentric origin within the bone.

Pathogenesis

Mutation of terminally differentiated B cells or early committed B cells lead to more differentiated plasma cells. Abnormal plasma cells probably arising from single malignant precursor which had undergone uncontrolled mitotic division and spreads throughout the body. Since the neoplasm develops from the single cell, all daughter cells which comprises of the lesional tissue have same genetic makeup and produce same proteins.

Clinical Features

♦ It occurs between 40 to 70 years of age.
♦ Male to female ratio is 4:1.
♦ Bone pain is present particularly in the lumbar spine.
♦ Pathological fractures are also present.
♦ Petechial hemorrhages of skin can be seen.
♦ Swelling over the areas of bony involvement can be seen.
♦ Metastatic calcification may involve the soft tissue and is due to hypercalcemia secondary to tumor related osteolysis.
♦ Amyloid deposits occur at periorbital region appearing waxy, firm, plaque like lesions.
♦ Death occurs due to renal failure as there is accumulation of abnormal proteins in renal tissue.

Oral Manifestations

♦ Mandible is commonly involved as compared to maxilla. Angle of mandible is commonly involved.
♦ Patient complaints of pain, numbness and swelling of jaw.
♦ Intraoral swelling is present which tends to be ulcerated, rounded and bluish red.
♦ Tongue may show diffuse enlargement and firmness or may have nodular appearance. Sometimes nodules are ulcerated.

Radiographic Features

Presence of multiple well defined, punched out radiolucency or ragged radiolucent lesions. This is evident on skull radiograph.

Laboratory Investigations

♦ *Urinary examination:* Light chain products found in urine of 30 to 50% of multiple myeloma patients are known as Bence Jones proteins.
♦ On serum protein electrophoresis most patients suffering from multiple myeloma have decreased quantity of

normal immunoglobulin and an abnormal monoclonal immunoglobulin protein peak, known as M spike. The immunoglobulin is usually of IgG or IgA class with monoclonal light chain component.

♦ Alkaline phosphatase levels are raised.

Histopathology

♦ There is presence of sheets of closely packed cells resembling plasma cells. Cells are round to oval in shape with eccentrically placed nucleus exhibiting chromatin clumping in cartwheel or checkerboard pattern.

♦ Perinuclear halo can also be seen.

♦ Russell bodies are seen in chronic inflammatory lesions with numerous typical plasma cells.

♦ Mitotic activity can be seen along with some frequency.

♦ If amyloid is present, it appears as homogenous, eosinophilic and relatively acellular.

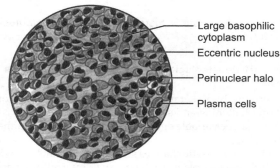

Fig. 49: Multiple myeloma *(For color version, see Plate 10).*

Treatment

♦ Multiple myeloma is treated by chemotherapeutic agents, such as melphalan and cyclophosphamide along with prednisolone.

♦ Oral bicarbonates, high fluid intake and corticosteroid decreases calcium levels.

♦ Local radiation therapy decreases painful bony lesions.

Q.48. Write short note on pathogenesis of oral submucous fibrosis. *(July 2016, 5 Marks)*

Ans. Basically pathogenesis of OSMF consists of disturbance in collagen metabolism via TGF–β. The whole procedure is described as:

Initial Event of Disease Process

According to **P. Rajalitha, S. Vali (2005)** initial event of the disease process is, oral mucosa which is indirect contact with betel quid (tobacco + areca nut + slaked lime + catechu and condominents) because of the habit which is the means of constant irritation. Major areca nut alkaloids are arecoline, arecaidine, arecolidine, guacoline and guacine. Out of all these arecoline is most abundant. These alkaloids undergo nitrosation and give rise to N–nitrosamines which have cytotoxic effects on cells. Important flavonoid components of areca nut are tannins and catechins. So all these alkaloids, flavonoids and microtrauma produced by friction of coarse fibers of areca nut leads to chronic inflammatory process which is characterized by presence of inflammatory cells, i.e.,

T cells and macrophages, these cells release and/or stimulate synthesis of various cytokines and growth factors. Increased susceptibility among individuals who are anemic due to iron or vitamin B12 deficiencies. It is because of increased fragility of mucosa by which there is more betel quid absorption.

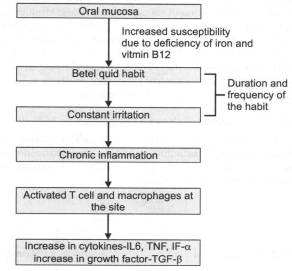

Fig. 50: Initial event of disease process.

Collagen Production Pathway as Regulated by TGF–β

Transforming growth factor-β (TGF–β) is a growth factor which regulate the collagen production pathway, it has autocrine activity. TGF–β activate procollagen genes which lead to production of more procollagen. TGF–β also increases secretion of procollagen–C–proteinase (PCP) and procollagen–N–proteinase (PNP) both of these are needed for conversion of procollagen to collagen fibrils.

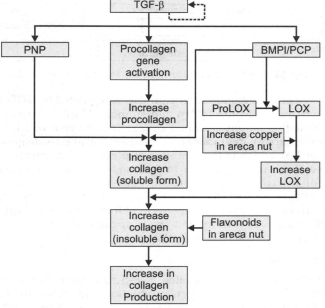

Fig. 51: Collagen production pathway as regulated by TGF-β.

In oral submucous fibrosis, there is increase in cross linking of collagen which results to increase in insoluble form. This is facilitated by increased activity and production of key enzyme Lysyl oxidase (LOX). PCP and bone morphogenetic protein 1 and increased copper in betel quid stimulate the activity of LOX which produces increase collagen which is insoluble. Flavonoids increases the cross linking of collagen fibers. These all steps lead to increase in collagen production. TGF–β strongly promote the expression of LOX both at mRNA and protein levels in various cell lines. LOX activity is important in formation of insoluble collagen due to cross linking. Process of cross linking provides tensile strength and mechanical properties to fibers as well as makes collagen fibers resistant to proteolysis.

Collagen Degradation Pathway as Regulated by TGF–β

There are also two main events modulated by TGF–β which also decreases collagen degradation, i.e., activation of tissue inhibitor of matrix metalloproteinase gene (TIMPs) and activation of plasminogen activator inhibitor (PAI) gene.

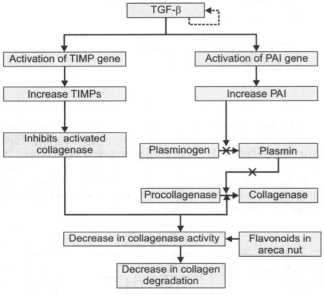

Fig. 52: Collagen degradation pathway as regulated by TGF-β.

Collagen degradation pathway as regulated by TGF-β activate genes for TIMPs and so more TIMP is formed. Now this inhibit activated collagenase enzyme which is necessary for degradation of collagen. It also activate gene for PAI which is the inhibitor of plasminogen activator, so there is no plasmin formation. Plasmin is needed for the conversion of procollagenase to active form of collagenase and absence of plasmin lead to absence of active collagenase. Flavonoids inhibit collagenase activity. Reduction in activity and levels of collagenase result in decrease in collagen degradation.

Overall Effect of TGF–β pathway

So, overall effect of activated TGF–β pathway is that there is an increase in collagen production and cross-linking (insoluble form) along with decrease in collagen degradation.

This produces an increased collagen deposition in subepithelial connective tissue layer of oral mucosa causing oral submucous fibrosis.

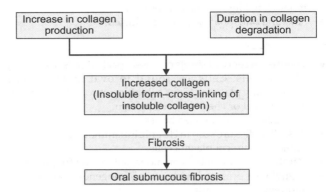

Fig. 53: Overall effect of TGF-β pathway.

Q.49. Write short note on histopathology of oral submucous fibrosis. *(Jan 2017, 5 Marks)*

Ans.

Common Histopathological Features of Oral Submucous Fibrosis

♦ Overlying hyperkeratinized or atrophic epithelium often shows flattening and shortening of rete pegs.
♦ There can be variable degrees of cellular atypia or epithelial dysplasia.
♦ In OSMF dysplastic changes are found in epithelium which include nuclear pleomorphism, sever intercellular edema, etc.
♦ Stromal blood vessels are dilated and congested and there can be areas of hemorrhage.
♦ Underlying connective tissue stroma in advanced stage of disease shows homogenization and hyalinization of collagen fibers.
♦ Decreased number of fibroblastic cells and narrowing of blood vessels due to perivascular fibrosis are present.
♦ There can be presence of signet cells in some cases.

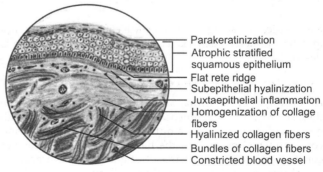

Fig. 54: Oral submucous fibrosis.

Histopathology Based on Various types of OSMF

Khanna JN and Andrade NN in 1995 given the group classification system for OSMF which consists of various groups of OSMF and their clinical and histological aspect. So following are the histological aspects as per the OSMF group:

Group of OSMF	Histological aspect
Group I or very early cases	• Presence of fine fibrillar collagen network interspersed with marked edema • Blood vessels are dilated and congested • Large aggregate of plump, young fibroblast present with abundant cytoplasm • Inflammatory cells mainly consist of polymorphonuclear leukocytes with few eosinophils • Epithelium is normal
Group II or early cases	• Juxtaepithelial hyalinization is present • Collagen present as thickened but separate bundles • Blood vessels are dilated and congested • Young fibroblast seen in moderate number • Inflammatory cells mainly consist of polymorphonuclear leukocytes with few eosinophils and occasional plasma cells • Flattening or shortening of epithelial rete pegs evident with degree of keratinization
Group III or moderately advanced cases	• Juxtaepithelial hyalinization present • Thickened collagen bundles faintly discernible, separated but very slight, residual edema • Blood vessels, mostly constricted • Mature fibroblasts with scanty cytoplasm and spindle-shaped nuclei • Inflammatory exudates consist mainly of lymphocytes and plasma cells • Epithelium markedly atrophic with loss of rete pegs • Muscle fibers seen interspersed with thickened and dense collagen fibers
Group IV A: Advanced cases	• Collagen hyalinized as smooth sheet • Extensive fibrosis obliterated the mucosal blood vessels and eliminated the melanocytes
Group IV B: Advanced cases with premalignant and malignant changes	• Fibroblasts were markedly absent within the hyalinized zones • Total loss of epithelial rete pegs • Mild-to-moderate atypia present • Extensive degeneration of muscle fibers evident

Q.50. Write short note on lymphangioma.

(Jan 2018, 5 Marks)

Ans. Lymphangioma is a benign hamartomatous tumor of lymphatic vessels.

Lymphangioma is thought to be developmental malformation of vessels which have poor communication with normal lymphatic system.

Types

Following are the types of lymphangiomas:
♦ *Lymphangioma simplex or capillary lymphangioma:* It consists of small thin walled capillaries.
♦ *Cavernous lymphangioma:* It consists of dilated lymphatic vessels with surrounding adventitia.
♦ *Cystic lymphangioma or cystic hygroma:* It consists of large, macroscopic cystic spaces with surrounding fibrovascular tissue and smooth muscle.

♦ *Benign lymphangioendothelioma:* In this lymphatic channels appear dissecting through dense collagen bundles.

Clinical Features

♦ Lymphangioma occur more commonly on head and neck.
♦ Cervical lymphangiomas are common in posterior triangle and are soft as well as fluctuant masses.

Oral Manifestations

♦ Most commonly lesion occurs on tongue and also seen on palate, buccal mucosa, gingiva and lips.
♦ Superficial lesions occur as papillary lesions which are of same color to surrounding mucosa or can be of red hue.
♦ Deep lesions appear as diffuse nodules or masses.
♦ Secondary hemorrhage in lymphatic spaces can cause some of vesicles to appear purple.
♦ Tongue involvement results in increase in size of tongue, i.e., macroglossia. Anterior dorsal part of tongue is commonly affected.
♦ Lip involvement can lead to macrocheilia.
♦ Small lymphangiomas are less than 1 cm in size and occur on alveolar ridge of black neonates.

Histopathology

♦ Lesion shows multiple, intertwining lymph vessels in loose fibrovascular stroma.
♦ Cavernous type show many dilated lymphatics with single layer of endothelial cells with flat nuclei and having lymph.
♦ Vessels which lie beneath surface epithelium replace connective tissue papillae and produce papillary surface change. This appears as translucent vesicle like clinical appearance.
♦ At times channels can be filled with blood which is known as hemangiolymphangioma.
♦ At times channels demonstrate proliferation of lymphatic channels with smooth muscle cells known as lymphangiomyoma.
♦ Cystic hygroma shows cyst like structures.

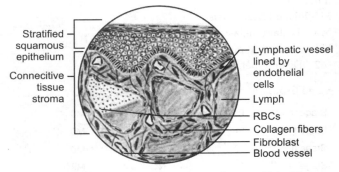

Fig. 55: Lymphangioma *(For color version, see Plate 10).*

Treatment

♦ Surgical removal should be done.
♦ Complete removal is impossible.
♦ Surgical debulking is the typical treatment provided.

Q.51. Write short note on TNM classification.

(Sep 2018, 5 Marks)

Ans. Staging of squamous cell carcinoma is done by TNM classification which was given by American Joint Committee on Carcinoma (AJCC)

T is suggestive of primary tumor

N is suggestive of regional lymph nodes

M is suggestive of distant metastasis

T - primary Tumor

TX - Primary tumor cannot be assessed.

T0 – No evidence of primary tumor

Tis – Carcinoma in Situ

T1 – Tumor 2 cm of less in greatest dimension

T2 – Tumor more than 2 cm, but not more than 4 cm in greatest dimension

T3 – Tumor more than 4 cm in greatest dimension

T4a (Lip) – Tumor invades through cortical bone, inferior alveolar nerve, floor of mouth or skin (chin or nose)

T4a (Oral Cavity) – Tumor invades through cortical bone, into deep/extrinsic muscle of tongue (genioglossus, hyoglossus, palatoglossus and styloglossus), maxillary sinus or skin of face.

T4b (lip and oral cavity) – Tumor invades masticatory space, pterygoid plates or skull base or encases internal carotid artery

N-Regional lymph nodes

NX - Regional lymph nodes cannot be assessed

N0 - No regional lymph node metastasis

N1- Metastasis in a single ipsilateral lymph node, 3 cm or less in greatest dimension

N2a - Metastasis in a single ipsilateral lymph node, more than 3 cm, but not more than 6 cm in greatest dimension

N2b - Metastasis in multiple ipsilateral lymph nodes, not more than 6 cm in greatest dimension

N2c - Metastasis in bilateral or contralateral lymph nodes, not more than 6 cm in greatest dimension

N3 - Metastasis in a lymph node more than 6 cm in greatest dimension

M – Distant Metastasis

MX – Distant metastasis cannot be assessed

M1 – No distant metastasis

M2 – Distant metastasis

Stage Grouping of Oral Cancer

Stage 0	Tis	N0	M0
Stage I	T1	N0	M0
Stage II	T2	N0	M0
Stage III	T1,	N1	M0
	T2,	N1	M0
	T3	N0, N1	M0
Stage IVa	T1,T2,T3,	N2	M0
	T4a	N0, N1, N2	M0
Stage IVb	Any T	N3	M0
	T4b	Any N	M0
Stage IVc	Any T	Any N	M1

Q.52. Define carcinoma and sarcoma. Give a detail account of verrucous carcinoma. *(Sep 2018, 5 Marks)*

Ans. Carcinoma: Malignant tumors of epithelial origin are known as carcinomas.

Sarcoma: Malignant mesenchymal tumors are known as sarcomas.

For verrucous carcinoma on detail, refer to Ans. 11 of same chapter.

Q.53. List benign and malignant lesions of vascular origin. Discuss hemangioma. *(Apr 2019, 5 Marks)*

Ans.

List of Benign and Malignant Lesions of Vascular Origin

Benign Lesions of Vascular Origin

♦ Hemangioma
♦ Sturge–Weber syndrome
♦ Hereditary hemorrhagic telangiectasia
♦ Arteriovenous fistula
♦ Glomus tumor
♦ Hemangiopericytoma
♦ Nasopharyngeal angiofibroma
♦ Lymphangioma
♦ Olfactory neuroblastoma

Malignant Lesions of Vascular Origin

♦ Malignant hemangioendothelioma
♦ Angiosarcoma

For hemangioma in detail, refer to Ans. 8 of same chapter.

3. TUMORS OF SALIVARY GLANDS

Q.1. Describe the clinical features, histology, pathogenesis and differential diagnosis of pleomorphic adenoma. *(Mar 2003, 15 Marks)*

Or

Classify salivary gland tumors. Describe in detail the clinical features, histolopathology and treatment of pleomorphic adenoma. *(Apr 2017, 10 Marks)*

Or

Write in detail about pleomorphic adenoma.

(Feb 2019, 5 Marks)

Or

Classify salivary gland tumors and write in detail about pleomorphic adenoma. *(Feb 2019, 10 Marks)*

Ans.

Salivary Gland Tumor Classification by WHO (2017)

♦ **Malignant tumors**
  • Mucoepidermoid carcinoma — 8430/3
  • Adenoid cystic carcinoma — 8200/3
  • Acinic cell carcinoma — 8550/3
  • Polymorphous adenocarcinoma — 8525/3
  • Clear cell carcinoma — 8310/3
  • Basal cell adenocarcinoma — 8147/3
  • Intraductal carcinoma — 8500/2
  • Adenocarcinoma, NOS — 8140/3

- Salivary duct carcinoma   8500/3
- Myoepithelial carcinoma   8982/3
- Epithelial-myoepithelial carcinoma   8562/3
- Carcinoma ex pleomorphic adenoma   8941/3
- Secretory carcinoma   8502/3*
- Sebaceous adenocarcinoma   8410/3
- Carcinosarcoma   8980/3
- Poorly differentiated carcinoma
  - Undifferentiated carcinoma   8020/3
  - Large cell neuroendocrine carcinoma   8013/3
  - Small cell neuroendocrine carcinoma   8041/3
- Lymphoepithelial carcinoma   8082/3
- Squamous cell carcinoma   8070/3
- Oncocytic carcinoma   8290/3

Uncertain malignant potential
- Sialoblastoma   8974/1

♦ **Benign tumors**
- Pleomorphic adenoma   8940/0
- Myoepithelioma   8982/0
- Basal cell adenoma   8147/0
- Warthin tumor   8561/0
- Oncocytoma   8290/0
- Lymphadenoma   8563/0*
- Cystadenoma   8440/0
- Sialadenoma papilliferum   8406/0
- Ductal papillomas   8503/0
- Sebaceous adenoma   8410/0
- Canalicular adenoma and other ductal adenomas   8149/0

♦ **Non-neoplastic epithelial lesions**
- Sclerosing polycystic adenosis
- Nodular oncocytic hyperplasia
- Lymphoepithelial sialadenitis
- Intercalated duct hyperplasia

♦ **Benign soft tissue lesions**
- Hemangioma   9120/0
- Lipoma/sialolipoma   8850/0
- Nodular fasciitis   8828/0

♦ **Hematolymphoid tumors**
- Extranodal marginal zone lymphoma of mucosa-associated lymphoid tissue (MALT lymphoma)   9699/3

These new codes were approved by the IARC/WHO Committee for ICD-0.

Pleomorphic adenoma or benign mixed tumor is most common neoplasm of salivary glands. The parotid gland is mostly affected by the tumor.

Clinical Features

- Pleomorphic adenoma develops in 5th and 6th decade of life.
- It produces slow growing, well delineated exophytic growth of salivary gland.
- Surface of lesion is smooth and lobulated and generally there is no pain.
- Neoplasm is usually soft or rubbery in consistency and is freely movable.
- Parotid gland lesion is usually superficial and often arises in superficial lobe as a small mass overlying angle of mandible or anterior to external ear.

- Sometimes, lesion can be multinodular and can assume an enormous size especially in long standing lesions.
- In buccal mucosa or lip pleomorphic adenoma presents small, painless, well defined, movable nodular lesion with intact overlying mucosa.

Histopathology

- Neoplasm often exhibits proliferation of glandular epithelial cells in form of diffuse sheet or clusters.
- Neoplastic cells are polygonal, spindle or stellate shape and have tendency to form duct like structures.
- Duct like structures are of varying size, shape, number and are widely distributed within lesion.
- Histologically, each duct like structure exhibits an inner row of cuboidal or columnar cells and outer row of spindle shape myoepithelial cells.
- Epithelial cells show "squamous metaplasia" and sometimes, there may be formation of keratin pearls by metaplastic epithelial cells.
- Connective tissue undergoes hyalinization to form structureless homogeneous material.
- Mucoid materials in myxochondroid are composed of glycosaminoglycans and consist mainly of chondroitin sulfate.
- Complete capsule is never present.

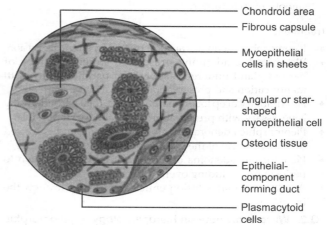

Fig. 56: Pleomorphic adenoma *(For color version, see Plate 10).*

Pathogenesis

- There is presence of myoepithelial cells and reserve cells arranged in intercalated duct.
- The intercalated duct reserve cells can differentiate into ductal and myoepithelial cells and the later can then undergo mesenchymal metaplasia.
- *Dardick's theory:* It is the most accepted theory. They state that a neoplastically altered epithelial cell with the potential for multidirectional differentiation may be histologically responsible for the pleomorphic adenoma.

Differential Diagnosis

- *Polymorphous low-grade adenocarcinoma:* It shows perineural growth and is infiltrative into periglandular tissue. It form small tubular structures or single cord of cells at periphery.

♦ *Carcinoma Ex pleomorphic adenoma:* Features of malignancy are seen in background of mixed tumor.

♦ *Epithelial myoepithelial carcinoma:* Two families of cells are seen, larger epithelial cells are arranged in tubular or acinar crystals and small myoepithelial cells seen mainly as "bipolar" spindly nuclei.

♦ *Warthin's tumor:* It consists of bilayered oncocytic epithelium, the inner cells of which are tall columnar with fine granular and eosinophilic cytoplasm and slightly hyperchromatic nuclei. The outer layer consists of basaloid cells.

♦ *Oncocytoma:* It consists of sheets of large polyhedral cells with abundant granular eosinophilic cytoplasm. These cells have centrally located nuclei which can vary from small and hyperchromatic to large and vesicular.

♦ *Mucoepidermoid carcinoma:* It consists of mixture of mucus producing cells ad squamous (epidermoid) cells. Mucus cells vary in shape and consist of foamy cytoplasm while epidermoid cells have squamoid features, polygonal shape, intercellular bridges and rarely keratinization. It is of three types, i.e., low grade, high grade and intermediate grade.

♦ *Adenoid cystic carcinoma:* It is a malignant tumor. It consists of mixture of myoepithelial cells and ductal cells which have varied arrangement. Three major patterns are cribriform, tubular and solid. It also shows increased nuclear atypia.

♦ Various mesenchymal tumors, such as nerve sheath tumor, smooth muscle tumor.

Treatment

♦ Pleomorphic adenomas are best treated by surgical excision.

♦ Pleomorphic adenoma present in superficial lobe of parotid gland undergoes superficial parotidectomy with identification and preservation of facial nerve.

♦ For tumors of deep lobe of parotid gland, total parotidectomy is necessary with preservation of facial nerve if possible.

♦ Pleomorphic adenoma in submandibular gland is treated by total removal of the gland along with tumor.

♦ Pleomorphic adenoma of hard palate is excised down to periosteum, including overlying mucosa.

♦ At other oral sites lesion enucleates easily through the incision site.

Q.2. Write short note on histopathology of pleomorphic adenoma. *(Mar 2013, 3 Marks)*

Or

Describe in brief histopathological features of pleomorphic adenoma. *(Aug 2011, 5 Marks)*

Or

Describe histopathology of pleomorphic adenoma. *(Mar 2006, 5 Marks)*

Ans. *Refer to Ans. 1 of same chapter.*

Q.3. Classify salivary gland diseases. Write about clinical features and histopathology of mucoepidermoid carcinoma. *(Sep 2007, 6 Marks)*

Or

Classify salivary gland neoplasm. Discuss in detail mucoepidermoid carcinoma. *(Sep 2005, 14 Marks)*

Or

Classify salivary gland disorders describe mucoepidermoid carcinoma. *(Aug 2012, 15 Marks)*

Or

Classify salivary gland tumors. Write in detail about mucoepidermoid carcinoma. *(July 2016, 10 Marks)*

Ans. Enumeration of salivary gland tumors.

Salivary Gland Tumor Classification by WHO (2017)

♦ **Malignant tumors**
- Mucoepidermoid carcinoma — 8430/3
- Adenoid cystic carcinoma — 8200/3
- Acinic cell carcinoma — 8550/3
- Polymorphous adenocarcinoma — 8525/3
- Clear cell carcinoma — 8310/3
- Basal cell adenocarcinoma — 8147/3
- Intraductal carcinoma — 8500/2
- Adenocarcinoma, NOS — 8140/3
- Salivary duct carcinoma — 8500/3
- Myoepithelial carcinoma — 8982/3
- Epithelial-myoepithelial carcinoma — 8562/3
- Carcinoma ex pleomorphic adenoma — 8941/3
- Secretory carcinoma — 8502/3*
- Sebaceous adenocarcinoma — 8410/3
- Carcinosarcoma — 8980/3
- Poorly differentiated carcinoma
  - Undifferentiated carcinoma — 8020/3
  - Large cell neuroendocrine carcinoma — 8013/3
  - Small cell neuroendocrine carcinoma — 8041/3
- Lymphoepithelial carcinoma — 8082/3
- Squamous cell carcinoma — 8070/3
- Oncocytic carcinoma — 8290/3

Uncertain malignant potential
- Sialoblastoma — 8974/1

♦ **Benign tumors**
- Pleomorphic adenoma — 8940/0
- Myoepithelioma — 8982/0
- Basal cell adenoma — 8147/0
- Warthin tumor — 8561/0
- Oncocytoma — 8290/0
- Lymphadenoma — 8563/0*
- Cystadenoma — 8440/0
- Sialadenoma papilliferum — 8406/0
- Ductal papillomas — 8503/0
- Sebaceous adenoma — 8410/0
- Canalicular adenoma and other ductal adenomas — 8149/0

♦ **Non-neoplastic epithelial lesions**
- Sclerosing polycystic adenosis
- Nodular oncocytic hyperplasia
- Lymphoepithelial sialadenitis
- Intercalated duct hyperplasia

♦ **Benign soft tissue lesions**
- Hemangioma — 9120/0
- Lipoma/sialolipoma — 8850/0
- Nodular fasciitis — 8828/0

♦ **Hematolymphoid tumors**
  • Extranodal marginal zone lymphoma of mucosa-associated lymphoid tissue (MALT lymphoma)   9699/3

These new codes were approved by the IARC/WHO Committee for ICD-0.

Mucoepidermal Tumor/Mucoepidermoid Carcinoma

Mucoepidermal tumor is an unusual type of malignant salivary gland neoplasm with varying degree of aggressiveness.

Pathogenesis

♦ It can occur due to entrapment of retromolar mucous glands in the mandible which undergo malignant transformation.
♦ Developmentally induced embryonic remnants of submaxillary gland within the mandible.
♦ Mucous secreting cells which are commonly found in pluripotential epithelial lining of dentigerous cyst associated with impacted third molars undergo neoplastic transformation.
♦ Neoplastic transformation as well as invasion from lining of maxillary sinus.

Clinical Features

♦ Tumor occurs at the age of 30 to 50 years.
♦ Tumor involves the parotid and minor salivary glands of palate, lips, buccal mucosa, tongue and retromolar areas.
♦ Tumor occurs as slowly enlarging painless mass which leads to the stimulation of pleomorphic adenoma.
♦ Facial nerve palsy and pain is present at times.
♦ Low-grade mucoepidermoid carcinomas is a slowly enlarging painless mass which rarely exceeds 5 cm in diameter.
♦ High-grade mucoepidermoid carcinomas grow rapidly and cause pain. It also infiltrates the surrounding tissues and metastatize to regional lymph nodes.

Histopathology

♦ Tumor is encapsulated and consists of three types of cells:
  1. Mucus secreting cells
  2. Epidermoid cells
  3. Intermediate type of cells.
♦ According to distribution of these cells the mucoepidermoid cells are divided into three grades:
  1. Well differentiated tumor or low-grade tumor
  2. Poorly differentiated tumor or high-grade tumor
  3. Intermediate-grade tumor
     – *Low-grade tumor:* They show well-formed glandular structures and prominent mucin filled with cystic space, minimal cellular atypia and high proportion of mucus cells.
     – *Intermediate grade tumor:* They have solid areas of epidermoid cells or squamous cells with intermediate basaloid cells. Cyst formation is seen but is less prominent than observed in low- grade tumor.

– *High-grade tumor:* They consist of cells present as solid nests and cords of intermediate basaloid cells and epidermoid cells, prominent nuclear pleomorphism and mitotic activity is noted. Necrosis and perineural invasion may be present.

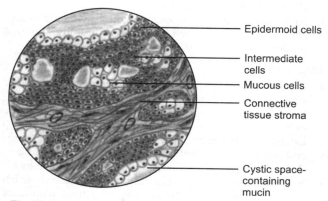

Fig. 57: Mucoepidermoid tumor *(For color version, see Plate 10).*

Differential Diagnosis

♦ Pleomorphic adenoma
♦ Squamous cell carcinoma
♦ Metastatic carcinoma
♦ Adenocarcinoma.

Treatment

Conservative excision with the preservation of facial nerve. The affected submandibular gland should be removed entirely. Treatment for minor gland is surgical.

Q.4. Enumerate the disease of salivary gland and describe in detail adenoid cystic carcinoma.
                    (Feb 2006, 6.5 Marks)

                    Or

Classify various diseases affecting salivary glands. Describe in detail adenoid cystic carcinoma.
                    (Apr 2008, 15 Marks)

                    Or

Classify salivary gland tumors. Describe in detail cylindroma.   *(Feb 2015, 10 Marks)*

Ans. *For enumeration of diseases, refer to Ans. 3 of same chapter.*

Adenoid Cystic Carcinoma/Cylindroma

♦ It is a malignant neoplasm arising from glandular epithelium of either major or minor glands.
♦ It is also known as cylindroma.

Clinical Features

♦ Tumor arises at the age of 50–70 years and is more common in females.
♦ It frequently affects parotid and other common sites are minor glands of palate, tongue, lacrimal glands, breast, prostrate, etc.

◆ Lesion produces, slow enlarging growth with frequent surface ulceration.

◆ Pain is common feature and neurological signs are anesthesia, paresthesia or palsy frequently develops.

◆ Often there is fixation of tumor to underlying structures along with the local invasion.

◆ It has marked tendency to spread through perineural spaces and usually invades well beyond the clinically apparent borders.

Histopathology

◆ It is characterized by the presence of numerous, small, darkly stained polygonal or cuboidal cells. Cells often resemble basal cells of oral epithelium and have hyperchromatic nuclei and minimum mitotic activity.

◆ Double layer of tumor cells are arranged in duct like pattern and contains eosinophilic coagulum at center, because of this lesion typically produces "Swiss Cheese appearance".

◆ Stroma of connective tissue tumor is hyalinized which surrounds tumor cells by forming structural pattern of many cylinders.

◆ Most striking feature of adenoid cystic carcinoma is spread of tumor cells via perineural or intraneural spaces. This is known as neurotrophism. This accounts for high rates in the recurrence of tumors.

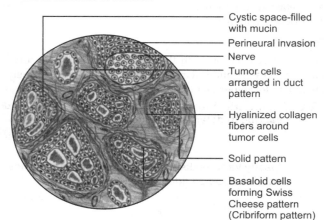

Cystic space-filled with mucin
Perineural invasion
Nerve
Tumor cells arranged in duct pattern
Hyalinized collagen fibers around tumor cells
Solid pattern
Basaloid cells forming Swiss Cheese pattern (Cribriform pattern)

Fig. 58: Adenoid cystic carcinoma *(For color version, see Plate 11).*

Treatment

By wide surgical excision.

Q.5. Write note on Sjogren's syndrome.
(Sep 2006, 5 Marks) (Dec 2007, 4 Marks)

Or

Write short note on Sjogren's syndrome.
(Mar 2006, 5 Marks) (Aug 2012, 5 Marks)

Or

Write in brief on Sjogren's syndrome.
(Jan 2012, 5 Marks)

Or

Write short answer on features of Sjogren's syndrome. *(Feb 2019, 3 Marks)*

Ans. It is a chronic inflammatory autoimmune disorder that affects salivary, lacrimal and other exocrine gland.

Types

◆ *Primary Sjögren's syndrome:* It is also known as Sicca syndrome. It consists of dry eyes, i.e., xerophthalmia and dry mouth, i.e., xerostomia.

◆ *Secondary Sjögren's syndrome:* It consists of dry eyes, i.e., xerophthalmia, dry mouth, i.e., xerostomia and collagen disorders, i.e., rheumatoid arthritis or systemic lupus erythematous.

Clinical Features

◆ Xerostomia is present with unpleasant taste, soreness and difficulty in eating dry fruits.

◆ Patient also complains of xerophthalmia and arthralgia

◆ Severe tiredness is present.

◆ There is cobble stone appearance of tongue.

◆ There is often secondary acute bacterial sialadenitis and rapid progressive dental caries.

◆ Burning sensation present in the eyes.

◆ Parotid gland is predominantly affected, sometimes submandibular and minor glands can also be affected.

Histopathology

◆ Initially infiltration of lymphocytes in intralobular ducts of involved salivary gland.

◆ There is atrophy of salivary gland acini and proliferation of ductal epithelial cells.

◆ Hyperplasia of ductal epithelium obliterates ductal lumen and there is formation of myoepithelial islands.

◆ In fully-developed lesions entire glandular tissue is replaced by myoepithelial islands which are surrounded by proliferating lymphoid tissue.

Treatment

◆ Use of systemic steroids

◆ Antibiotic eye drops

◆ Antifungal drugs

◆ Maintenance of oral hygiene.

Q.6. Write notes on mucoepidermoid carcinoma.
(Mar 2006, 2.5 Marks) (Mar 2007, 2.5 Marks)

Or

Write short note on mucoepidermoid carcinoma.
(June 2015 5 Marks)

Or

Describe the histopathology of mucoepidermoid carcinoma. *(Sep 2006, 5 Marks) (Jan 2010, 5 Marks)*

Ans. *Refer to Ans. 3 of same chapter.*

Q.7. Write short note on mucocele. *(Mar 2006, 5 Marks)*
(Apr 2007, 5 Marks) (Jan 2016, 5 Marks)

Ans. It is also called as mucus extravasation phenomenon or mucus escape reaction.

Mucocele is defined as swelling caused by pooling of saliva at the site of injured minor salivary gland.

Types

♦ **Mucus extravasation cyst:** In this mucus is extravasated into the connective tissue and is devoid of epithelial lining. It is also known as pseudocyst.

♦ **Mucus retention cyst:** In this mucin is retained in the dilated salivary excretory duct and is lined by epithelium. This is known as true cyst.

Clinical Features

♦ They are common and occur on the inner aspect of lower lip. They may also occur on palate, cheek, tongue and floor of the mouth.

♦ They occur most frequently during third decade of life.

♦ Patient complains of painless swelling. The swelling may suddenly develops at meal time and may drain simultaneously at interval.

♦ Swelling is round, oval or smooth.

♦ Superficial cyst appears as bluish mass and if inflamed it is fluctuant, soft, nodular and dome-shaped elevation.

Histopathological Features

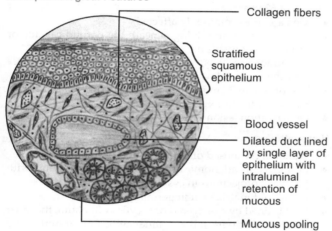

A. Mucous retention cyst

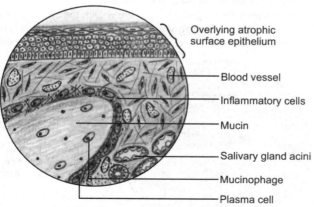

B. Mucous extravasation cyst

Figs. 59A and B: Mucocele *(For color version, see Plate 10)*

♦ In poorly defined cyst, it consists of irregularly shaped poorly defined pools which contain eosinophilic mucinous material, numerous vacuolated macrophages which are known as mucinophage.

♦ In well-defined cysts the periphery consists of granulation tissue or condensed fibrous tissue or both and is infiltrated by vacuolated macrophages, lymphocytes, polymorphonuclear leukocytes including eosinophils.

♦ Lumen of cyst like cavity is filled with eosinophilic coagulum.

Treatment

♦ Complete excision of cyst under local anesthesia should be done.

Q.8. Classify salivary gland neoplasms. Write about clinical features and histopathology of benign pleomorphic adenoma. *(Sep 2008, 6 Marks)*

Ans. *Refer to Ans. 3 for classification of salivary gland neoplasm and Ans. 1 for clinical features and histopathology of benign pleomorphic adenoma of same chapter.*

Q.9. Write short note on clinical features and histopatho-logy of cylindroma. *(Sep 2011, 3 Marks)*

Ans. Cylindroma is also known as adenoid cystic carcinoma.

For clinical features and histopathology refer to Ans. 4 of same chapter.

Q.10. Write short note on adenoid cystic carcinoma.
(Mar 2016, 3 Marks) (Jan 2012, 5 Marks)

Ans. *Refer to Ans. 4 of same chapter.*

Q.11. Classify salivary gland tumor. Write briefly about etiopathogenesis, clinical features, histopathology and radiographic findings of mucoepidermoid carcinoma. *(Sep 2011, 8 Marks)*

Or

Write about clinical features, etiopathogenesis and histopathology of mucoepidermoid carcinoma.
(Mar 2011, 5 Marks)

Ans. *For classification refer to Ans. 3 of same chapter.*

For clinical features and histopathology, refer to Ans. 3 of same chapter.

Etiopathogenesis

♦ As per the multicellular theory mucoepidermoid tumor arise from the excretory duct cells of salivary gland.

♦ During development, the retromolar mucous glands get entrapped in the mandible which undergo neoplastic transformation and leads to formation of intraosseous mucoepidermoid carcinoma.

For clinical features and histopathology, refer to Ans. 4 of same chapter.

Radiographic Findings

♦ Mucoepidermoid carcinoma appear as a unilocular or multilocular expanding mass.

♦ Margins are corticated, well defined.

- At times lesion show honeycomb or soap bubble appearance.
- Lamina dura of associated teeth is lost.
- Inferior border of mandible, buccal and cortical plates are displaced and thinned.

Q.12. Write short note on sialadenitis. *(Sep 2011, 3 Marks)*

Ans. Inflammation of salivary gland is known as sialadenitis.

Etiology

- *Viral Infections:* Mumps, CMV virus, Coxsackie virus and parainfluenza.
- Bacterial Infections
- Blockage of duct by sialolithiasis
- Congenital strictures
- Compression by adjacent tumor
- Recent surgeries of salivary glands.

Clinical Features

- It occurs most commonly in parotid gland.
- Affected gland is swollen and painful and overlying skin is warm and erythematous.
- Low-grade fever and trismus may be present.
- A purulent discharge is observed from the duct orifice.

Histopathology

- Accumulation of neutrophils is observed within the ductal system and acini.
- Chronic sialadenitis is characterized by scattered or patchy infiltration of parenchyma by lymphocytes and plasma cells.
- Atrophy of acini is common.

Sialographic Features

- It demonstrates ductal dilatation proximal to the area of obstruction.
- In acute sialadenitis sialography is contraindicated.
- In chronic sialadenitis stenson's duct may show a characteristic sialographic pattern known as sausaging which reflects a combination of dilatation plus ductal strictures from scar formation.

Treatment

- Antibiotics should be given to patient
- Proper hydration should be maintained
- If necessary go for surgical intervention.

Q.13. Classify salivary gland pathologies. Discuss in detail Warthin's tumor. *(Feb 2013, 10 Marks)*

Or

Write in detail on Warthin's tumor.

(Jan 2010, 10 Marks)

Or

Write short note on Warthin's tumor.

(Apr 2017, 5 Marks) (Feb 2013, 8 Marks)

Or

Write short answer on Warthin's tumor.

(Apr 2019, 3 Marks)

Or

Classify salivary gland tumors. Discuss Warthin's tumor.

(Oct 2019, 5 Marks)

Ans. *For classification of salivary gland pathologies, refer to Ans. 3 of same chapter.*

Warthin's Tumor

- It is also known as papillary cystadenoma lymphomatosum or adenolymphoma.
- It is the second most common tumor of salivary glands.

Pathogenesis

- According to the most accepted theory, the tumor arises in salivary gland tissue entrapped within periparotid or intraparotid lymph nodes during embryogenesis.
- According to Allegra, Warthin's tumor is a delayed hypersensitivity disease, the lymphocytes being an immune reaction to the salivary ducts which undergo oncocytic change.

Etiology

- Smoking
- Epstein Barr virus infection.

Clinical Features

- It occurs during 6th and 7th decades of life with average age of 62 years.
- Men are most commonly affected
- Tumor is superficial lying beneath the parotid capsule or protruding towards it.
- The tumor appear as a slow growing painless nodular mass over the angle of jaw. Lesion can be bilateral too.
- Tumor is 1 to 3 cm in diameter and is spherical in shape. Surface of the lesion is smooth
- On palpation lesion is firm and is nontender.

Histopathology

- Tumor is composed of epithelial and lymphoid tissue.
- Lesion is an adenoma undergoing cyst formation with papillary projections in cystic spaces.
- Lymphoid matrix exhibit germinal centers.
- Cyst is lined by a bilayered oncocytic epithelium, the inner cells of which are tall columnar with fine granular and eosinophilic cytoplasm and slightly hyperchromatic nuclei. The outer layer consist of basaloid cells.
- An eosinophilic coagulum is present within the cystic spaces.
- The numerous lymphocytic component may represent normal lymphoid tissue within which tumor is developed.

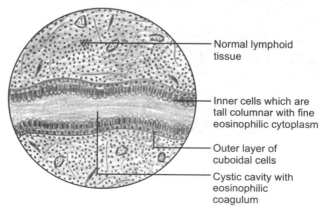

Fig. 60: Warthin's tumor *(For color version, see Plate 11).*

Treatment

Surgical excision is treatment of choice.

Q.14. Write short note on Warthin's tumor.
(Dec 2015, 3 Marks) (Nov 2008, 5 Marks)

Or

Describe in brief Warthin's tumor.
(May/Jun 2009, 5 Marks) (Feb 2014, 3 Marks)

Ans. *Refer to Ans. 13 of same chapter.*

Q.15. Classify salivary gland tumors and write in detail etiology, clinical features and histopathological features of adenoid cystic carcinoma. *(Dec 2012, 8 Marks)*

Ans. *For classification refer to Ans. 3 of same chapter.*

Etiology

♦ Some evidence supports an association with mutation on chromosome 6 and 12 and deletion of genetic material from chromosome 19.

♦ Adenoid cystic carcinoma is derived from neoplastic transformation of salivary acinar type cells and myoepithelial cells.

For clinical and histological features of adenoid cystic carcinoma, refer to Ans. 4 of same chapter.

Q.16. Enumerate benign and malignant tumors of salivary gland. Discuss in detail adenoid cystic carcinoma (ACC). *(June 2014, 10 Marks)*

Ans. *For benign and malignant tumors of salivary gland, refer to Ans. 3 of same chapter.*

For adenoid cystic carcinoma, refer to Ans. 4 and Ans. 15 of same chapter.

Q.17. Enumerate diseases of salivary gland. Write histopathology and etiology of mucoepidermoid carcinoma. *(Nov 2014, 8 Marks)*

Ans. *For enumeration of diseases of salivary gland and histopathology of mucoepidermoid carcinoma refer to Ans. 3 of same chapter.*

Etiology of Mucoepidermoid Carcinoma

Mucoepidermoid carcinoma is most commonly occurs due to radiation.

Q.18. Write short note on sialolithiasis. *(Apr 2015, 3 Marks)*

Ans. Sialolithiasis is also known as salivary duct calculi or salivary duct stone.

Sialolith are the calcified structures which develop within the salivary ductal system.

Pathogenesis

Salivary duct stone are formed by deposition of calcium salts around a central nidus which consists of altered salivary mucins, desquamated epithelial cells, bacteria, foreign bodies or products of bacterial decomposition.

Clinical Features

♦ Sialoliths occur during 2nd to 4th decades of life.

♦ Submandibular gland ductal system is the most common site for occurrence of sialolith.

♦ Sialoliths cause episodic pain or swelling of the affected gland during meal or thought of the meal.

♦ If it is not treated for longer time exacerbation of the lesion occur and systemic symptoms occur, such as malaise and fever.

♦ Pus can exude from the ductal orifice and surrounding soft tissues are inflamed.

♦ At times ulceration of the overlying mucosa is evident which allows calculus to extend in floor of oral cavity.

♦ Saliva can never be seen oozing out from the orifice of the affected duct.

Histopathology

♦ Calcified mass exhibit concentric lamellation which surrounds the nidus of amorphous deposits.

♦ Associated ductal epithelium shows squamous, oncocytic or mucus cell metaplasia.

♦ Periductal inflammation is also present.

♦ Ductal obstruction is frequently associated with acute or chronic sialadenitis of feeding gland.

Treatment

♦ Small calculi are removed by manipulation or increasing the salivation.

♦ Larger calculi require surgical exposure for removal.

Q.19. Classify salivary gland tumors. Describe in detail about pleomorphic adenoma. *(Jan 2016, 10 Marks)*

Ans. *For classification of salivary gland tumor, refer to Ans. 4 of same chapter.*

For pleomorphic adenoma in detail, refer to Ans. 1 of same chapter.

Q.20. List benign epithelial tumors of salivary gland. Discuss in detail pleomorphic adenoma.
(May 2018, 5 Marks)

Ans. Salivary Gland Tumor Classification by WHO (2017)

Benign tumors

♦ Pleomorphic adenoma 8940/0
♦ Myoepithelioma 8982/0
♦ Basal cell adenoma 8147/0
♦ Warthin tumor 8561/0
♦ Oncocytoma 8290/0
♦ Lymphadenoma 8563/0*
♦ Cystadenoma 8440/0
♦ Sialadenoma papilliferum 8406/0
♦ Ductal papillomas 8503/0
♦ Sebaceous adenoma 8410/0
♦ Canalicular adenoma and other ductal adenomas 8149/0
  • Non-neoplastic epithelial lesions
♦ Sclerosing polycystic adenosis
♦ Nodular oncocytic hyperplasia
♦ Lymphoepithelial sialadenitis
♦ Intercalated duct hyperplasia
  • Benign soft tissue lesions
♦ Hemangioma 9120/0
♦ Lipoma/sialolipoma 8850/0
♦ Nodular fasciitis 8828/0
  • Hematolymphoid tumors

- Extranodal marginal zone lymphoma of mucosa-associated lymphoid tissue (MALT lymphoma) 9699/3

These new codes were approved by the IARC/WHO Committee for ICD-0.

For pleomorphic adenoma in detail, refer to Ans. 1 of same chapter.

Q.21. Classify salivary gland tumors. Describe clinical features, histopathology and radiological features with treatment of adenoid cystic carcinoma.
(Sep 2018, 10 Marks)

Ans. *For classification, refer to Ans. 3 of same chapter.*

For clinical features, histopathology and treatment, refer to Ans. 4 of same chapter.

Radiographic Features

- Adenoid cystic carcinoma arising in palate or in maxillary sinus often show radiographic evidence of bone destruction.
- Its CT scan demonstrates the destructive lesion.

Q.22. List pseudocysts of oral cavity. Discuss in detail oral mucoceles.
(Oct 2019, 5 Marks)

Ans. Pseudocysts of oral cavity

- Solitary bone cyst
- Aneurysmal bone cyst

For oral mucocele in detail, refer to Ans. 7 of same chapter.

---

4. ODONTOGENIC TUMORS

Q.1. Classify odontogenic tumors describe in detail ameloblastoma of mandible.
(Nov 2008, 15 Marks)

Or

Describe in detail ameloblastoma.
(Jan 2010, 10 Marks)

Or

Describe in detail about clinical, radiographic, histopathological features of ameloblastoma.
(Jan 2012, 15 Marks)

Or

Classify odontogenic tumors and write in detail about ameloblastoma.
(Jan 2016, 10 Marks)
(Aug 2011, 15 Marks) (Dec 2012, 8 Marks)

Or

Classify odontogenic tumor and describe the clinical features, radiographic features and histological features of ameloblastoma.
(Feb 2013, 10 Marks)

Or

Classify odontogenic tumor. Describe in detail the clinical features, histopathology and treatment of ameloblastoma.
(Apr 2017, 10 Marks)

Or

Classify odontogenic tumors. Write in detail about histopathology of ameloblastoma.
(Feb 2019, 5 Marks)

Or

Define ameloblastoma. Write in detail clinical features, radiological features and histopathology of ameloblastoma.
(Feb 2019, 10 Marks)

Or

Draw a well-labeled histopathological diagram of plexiform ameloblastoma.
(Dec 2007, 3 Marks)

Ans.

Classification of Odontogenic Tumors by WHO (2017)

- Odontogenic carcinomas
  - Ameloblastic carcinoma
  - Primary intraosseous carcinoma, NOS
  - Sclerosing odontogenic carcinoma
  - Clear cell odontogenic carcinoma
  - Ghost cell odontogenic carcinoma
- Odontogenic carcinosarcoma
- Odontogenic sarcomas
- Benign epithelial odontogenic tumors
  - Ameloblastoma
    - Ameloblastoma, unicystic type
    - Ameloblastoma, extraosseous/peripheral type
    - Metastasizing ameloblastoma
  - Squamous odontogenic tumor
  - Calcifying epithelial odontogenic tumor
  - Adenomatoid odontogenic tumor
- Benign mixed epithelial and mesenchymal odontogenic tumors
  - Ameloblastic fibroma
  - Primordial odontogenic tumor
  - Odontoma
    - Odontoma, compound type
    - Odontoma, complex type
  - Dentinogenic ghost cell tumor
- Benign mesenchymal odontogenic tumors
  - Odontogenic fibroma
  - Odontogenic myxoma/myxofibroma
  - Cementoblastoma
  - Cemento-ossifying fibroma

Ameloblastoma

Ameloblastoma is defined as usually unicentric, non-functional, intermittent in growth, anatomically benign and clinically persistant.
—Robinson.

Pathogenesis of Ameloblastoma

The tumor may derive from the:

- Cell rest of enamel organ, either remnants of dental lamina or remnants of Hertwig's sheath, the epithelial rest cells of Malassez.
- Epithelium of odontogenic cyst.
- Disturbance of the developing enamel organ
- Basal cell of the surface epithelium of the jaw.

Histopathology

Histologically, the ameloblastoma shows neoplastic proliferation of odontogenic epithelial cells mostly in four distinct patterns:

- Follicular type
- Plexiform type
- Acanthomatous type
- Granular type

Follicular Type

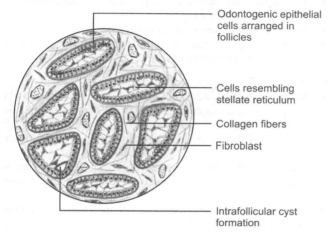

Fig. 61: Follicular ameloblastoma *(For color version, see Plate 11).*

- Neoplastic odontogenic epithelial cells proliferate in form of multiple discrete follicles and islands within fibrous connective tissue stroma.
- Each follicle like structure is bordered on the periphery by the single layer of tall columnar cells resembling ameloblasts like cells.
- Cells located at the center of follicle are loosely arranged and resemble stellate reticulum cells.
- Microcyst formation is often observed inside these follicles.

Plexiform Type

- Peripheral layer of cells are tall columnar in nature and often resemble ameloblast like cells.
- Cells situated at center portion of strands resemble stellate reticulum.
- Intervening connective tissue stroma is thin with minimum cellularity and shows multiple areas of cystification which may be either large or small in number.

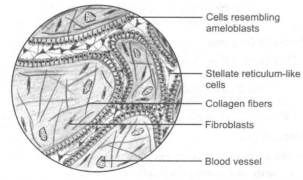

Fig. 62: Plexiform ameloblastoma *(For color version, see Plate 11).*

Acanthomatous Type

- Cells occupying the position of the stellate reticulum undergo squamous metaplasia, sometimes with keratin formation in the anterior portion of tumor islands.
- Occasionally, epithelial or keratin pearls may be observed.
- Areas of calcification may be found in the metaplastic squamous epithelium.
- It may be confused with squamous cell carcinoma.

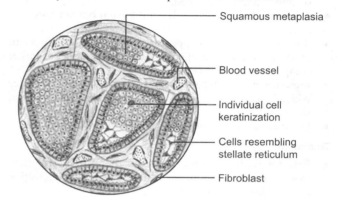

Fig. 63: Acanthomatous ameloblastoma *(For color version, see Plate 11).*

Granular Type

- There is marked transformation of the cytoplasm, usually of the stellate reticulum like cells that it takes a very coarse granular eosinophilic appearance.

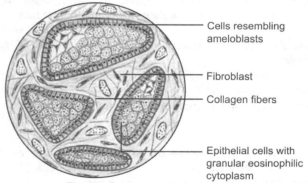

Fig. 64: Granular cell ameloblastoma *(For color version, see Plate 11).*

For more histopathology, refer to Ans. 9 of same chapter.

Clinical Features

- Ameloblastoma occurs in 2nd, 3rd, 4th and 5th decade of life.
- Mean age of occurrence is 32 years.
- Males are affected more commonly than females.
- Ameloblastoma in most of the cases involves mandible in molar ramus area.
- Clinically ameloblastoma presents slow enlarging, painless, ovoid and fusiform bony hard swelling of the jaw.

- Pain, paresthesia and mobility of regional teeth is present in some cases.
- Pathological fractures may occur in many affected bones.

Radiographical Appearance

- During the early stage, area of bone destruction is well defined and have hyperostotic borders.
- Outline of margins of lesion is smooth, well defined, scalloped and is corticated.
- Ameloblastomas are mostly multilocular but at times they are unilocular too.
- It reveals honeycomb appearance because of arrangement of septae. It also reveal soap bubble appearance if larger compartments are present.
- Presence of bony expansion and thinning of cortical plates which leaves thin egg shell of bone which is known as egg shell crackling.
- Extensive root resorption is seen in lesional area.

Treatment

- Patients with conventional solid or multicystic intra-osseous ameloblastoma are treated by simple enucleation to curettage to en bloc resection.
- Marginal resection is the most widely used treatment. But recurrence rate up to 15% are evident.
- Some surgeons adopt conservative approach by planning surgery after careful CT scan evaluation. Removal of tumor is done followed by peripheral ostectomy.
- Other surgeons advocate that margin of resection should be 1 to 1.5 cm past radiographic limits of tumor.

Q.2. Describe clinical features, histopathology and investigations associated with ameloblastoma.
(Mar 2003, 15 Marks)

Ans. *For clinical features and histopathology, refer to Ans. 1 of same chapter.*

For investigations, refer to radiographical features and histology of Ans. 1 of same chapter.

Q.3. Describe histopathology of ameloblastoma.
(Sep 2006, 5 Marks)

Or

Write short note on histological features of ameloblastoma. *(Sep 2005, 5 Marks)*

Ans. *Refer to Ans. 1 and Ans. 9 of same chapter.*

Q.4. Write short note on adenomatoid odontogenic tumor.
(Aug 2012, 5 Marks) (April 2007, 5 Marks)

Or

Write short note on histopathology of adenomatoid odontogenic tumor. *(Aug 2012, 5 Marks)*

Ans.

Adenomatoid Odontogenic Tumor

It is also called adenoameloblastoma or ameloblastic adenomatoid tumor.

Adenomatoid odontogenic tumor is uncommon, well circumscribed, odontogenic neoplasm characterized by the formation of multiple duct like structures by neoplastic epithelial cells.

Clinical Features

- Tumor usually occurs in younger age.
- Females are more commonly affected
- Lesion most typically appears in maxillary anterior region.
- Tumor presents a slow enlarging, small, bony hard swelling in maxillary anterior region.
- Sometimes, it occurs in premolar region
- There is displacement of regional teeth, mild pain and expansion of cortical bones.

Histopathology

- Microscopically, adenoid odontogenic tumor reveals neoplastic odontogenic epithelial cells, proliferating in multiple "duct like" patterns.
- Presence of these duct like structures often give glandular lesion.
- Each duct like structure is bordered on periphery by a single layer of tall columnar cells resembles ameloblastoma.
- Lumen of duct like structures are filled with the homogenous eosinophilic coagulum.
- Small foci of calcifications are often seen, which are scattered throughout the lesion.
- Droplets of amorphous (PAS positive) eosinophilic material are found between neoplastic cells.

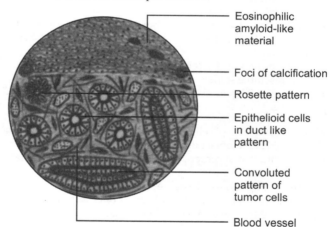

Fig. 65: Adenomatoid odontogenic tumor
(For color version, see Plate 12).

Differential Diagnosis

- Dentigerous cyst
- Odontomes
- Unicystic ameloblastoma
- CEOT
- CEOC.

Treatment

The treatment is surgical enucleation.

Q.5. Write short note on Pindborg tumor.
(Feb 2015, 5 Marks)

Or

Describe in brief Pindborg tumor.

(May/June 2009, 5 Marks)

Or

Write short note on CEOT.   *(Dec 2015, 3 Marks)*

Or

Write short answer on histopathology of Pindborg tumor.   *(Feb 2019, 3 Marks)*

Ans. Pindborg tumor is locally aggressive neoplasm, which is also known as calcifying epithelial odontogenic tumor.

Pathogenesis

♦ Some investigators suggest that the Pindborg tumor arises from remnant of cells in stratum intermedium layer of the enamel organ in tooth development. Some hypothesize that the Pindborg's tumor arises from the remnants of the primitive dental lamina.
♦ Definite etiology of neoplasm still remains enigmatic.

Clinical Features

♦ Tumor occur in middle age persons.
♦ Mandible is involved more often than maxilla.
♦ Molar region is more common site of occurrence followed by premolar region.
♦ Tumor presents a slow enlarging, painless swelling of jaw with expansion and distortion of cortical plates.
♦ Swelling is bony hard and clinically, it is well defined or diffused.
♦ Pain, paresthesia may develop on rare occasions and few lesions may be completely asymptomatic.

Histopathology

♦ Tumor reveals sheet of closely packed, polyhedral cells in noninflamed connective tissue stroma.
♦ Tumor cells contain oval-shaped nuclei and homogenous eosinophilic cytoplasm.
♦ Prominent intra cellular bridges and distinct cell boundaries are often found in the lesions.
♦ Some amount of homogenous, hyaline material is often deposited in between tumor cells called amyloid material.
♦ One of the most important histological characteristics of CEOT is the presence of several calcified masses in and around the tumor cells.
♦ Some Liesegang rings are also found.

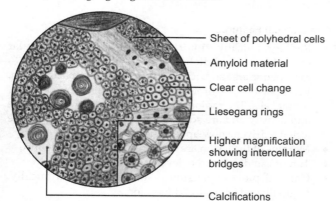

Fig. 66: Pindborg's tumor *(For color version, see Plate 12).*

Labels: Sheet of polyhedral cells; Amyloid material; Clear cell change; Liesegang rings; Higher magnification showing intercellular bridges; Calcifications

Treatment

Surgical enucleation is done.

Q.6. Write note on odontoma.

(Sep 2004, 5 Marks) (Feb 2002, 6 Marks)
(June 2015, 5 Marks) (Mar 2013, 3 Marks)

Or

Write short note on odontome.   *(Jun 2014, 5 Marks)*

Ans. Odontomas are hamartoma that contain both epithelial and mesenchymal dental tissue components.

Types of Odontoma

1. Complex odontoma
2. Compound odontoma.

Complex Odontoma

It is always benign and contains enamel, dentin and cementum which are not differentiated, so that structure of actual tooth is not identifiable.

Compound Odontoma

It is also benign. In compound odontomas, the enamel and dentin are laid down in such a fashion that the structure bears considerable anatomic resemblance to normal teeth, except that they are often smaller than typical teeth.

Clinical Features

♦ Lesion occurs among children or young adults.
♦ Both sexes are equally affected or slight male predominance is present.
♦ Maxilla is commonly affected. Odontomas are commonly seen in pericoronal area of permanent teeth.
♦ Odontoma produces large, bony, hard swellings of jaw, with expansion of cortical plates and displacement of regional teeth.
♦ If odontoma is located high in alveolus, they may tend to erupt in oral cavity by resorbing overlying bone and as a result there may be pain, inflammation, ulceration, etc.

Histopathology

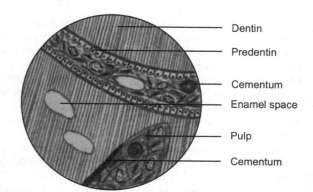

Fig. 67: Complex composite odontome *(For color version, see Plate 12).*

Labels: Dentin; Predentin; Cementum; Enamel space; Pulp; Cementum

♦ Fully developed compound odontoma reveals the presence of encapsulated mass of separate denticles, embedded in fibrous tissue stroma.

♦ The fully developed complex odontoma reveals an irregularly arranged but well-formed mass of enamel, dentin and cementum which is surrounded by fibrous tissue capsule.

♦ The dentinal tissues lie in the direct contact with connective tissue that resembles the dental pulp.

♦ Most of enamel tissues are fully calcified and appear as small empty space.

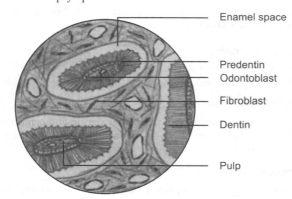

Fig. 68: Compound composite odontome
(For color version, see Plate 12).

Treatment

Surgical Enucleation.

Q.7. Write short note on histopathological variants of ameloblastoma. *(Sep 2011, 3 Marks)*

Or

Write in detail on histopathological types/variants of ameloblastoma. *(April 2008, 10 Marks)*

Ans. Following are the histopathological variants of ameloblastoma

♦ *Follicular type: Refer to Ans. 1 of same chapter*

♦ *Plexiform type: Refer to Ans. 1 of same chapter*

♦ *Acanthomatous Type: Refer to Ans. 1 of same chapter*

♦ *Granular cell type: Refer to Ans. 1 of same chapter*

♦ *Desmoplastic type:* There is presence of marked hyalinization of connective tissue stroma.

♦ *Basal cell type:* Tumor islands show basaloid pattern of cells.

♦ *Clear cell type:* Solid multicystic ameloblastoma may contain clear cells which are localized to the stellate reticulum like areas of follicular ameloblastoma.

♦ *Keratoameloblastoma and papilliferous keratoameloblastoma:* Ameloblastoma consisting partly of keratinizing cysts and partly of tumor islands with papilliferous arrangement

♦ *Mucous cell differentiation type:* Follicular ameloblastoma showing focal mucous cell differentiation.

♦ *Hemangiomatous ameloblastoma:* It is an ameloblastoma in which part of the tumor contain spaces filled with blood or large endothelial lined capillaries.

Q.8. Classify odontogenic tumors. Describe in detail etiopathogenesis, clinical features, radiology, histopathologic features and differential diagnosis of adenomatoid odontogenic tumor.

(Jan 2012, 10 Marks)

Or

Give classification of odontogenic tumors. Discuss about clinical features and histopathology of AOT.

(Nov 2014, 8 Marks)

Or

Classify odontogenic tumors. Write in detail about adenomatoid odontogenic tumor.

(July 2016, 10 Marks)

Or

Classify odontogenic tumors. Describe radiological and histopathological features of adenomatoid odontogenic tumor. *(Sep 2018, 5 Marks)*

Ans. *For classification, refer to Ans. 1 of same chapter.*

Etiopathogenesis

♦ Since adenomatoid odontogenic tumor occurs within tooth-bearing areas of jaw, it arises from reduced enamel epithelium during the presecretory phase of enamel organ development.

♦ Some category of authors also believes that it arises from dental lamina or from preexisting dentigerous cyst.

Radiology

♦ Radiographically tumor presents a well-circumscribed unilocular radiolucent area which consisted of impacted tooth or odontome and exhibits a smooth corticated border.

♦ Multilocular radiolucencies are also seen rarely with scalloped borders.

♦ At times radio-opaque foci is detectable within radiolucent lesion.

♦ As lesion progresses divergence of roots and displacement of teeth is seen.

For clinical features, histopathology and differential diagnosis, refer to Ans. 4 of same chapter.

Q.9. Classify odontogenic tumors. Write in detail about the clinical, radiological and histological features of calcifying epithelial odontogenic tumor.

(Mar 2006, 15 Marks)

Ans. *For classification of odontogenic tumor, refer to Ans. 1 of same chapter.*

For clinical and histological features of calcifying epithelial odontogenic tumor, refer to Ans. 5 of same chapter.

Radiological Features

♦ Radiographically tumor consists of either a unilocular or multilocular radiolucent defect with radiolucent to radiopaque area surrounding the crown of impacted tooth.

♦ Radiopacity is of proteinaceous material released by the tumor cells. The radiopaque structures are of varying size and density and are scattered all over which provides the lesion a driven snow appearance

♦ Margins of the lesion are scalloped and are well defined.

♦ Tumor can displace the developing tooth.

♦ Cortical plate expansion is also appreciated bucally, lingually and in vertical dimension.

Q.10. Classify odontogenic tumors and describe in detail Pindborg tumor. *(Feb 2013, 18 Marks)*

Ans. *For classification, refer to Ans. 1 of same chapter.*

For Pindborg tumor in detail, refer to Ans. 5 and Ans. 9 of same chapter.

Q.11. Classify and discuss ameloblastoma.

(May 2018, 5 Marks)

Ans. Ameloblastoma is classified, according to WHO and the International Agency for Research on Cancer, 2017, as a benign epithelial odontogenic tumor. It is further classified as:

Classification of ameloblastoma WHO 2017

♦ *Ameloblastoma:*
  • Ameloblastoma, unicystic type
  • Ameloblastoma, extraosseous/peripheral type
  • Metastasizing ameloblastoma

For ameloblastoma in detail, refer to Ans. 1 of same chapter in detail.

Q.12. Write short answer on histology of follicular ameloblastoma. *(Apr 2019, 3 Marks)*

Ans.

Histology of Follicular Ameloblastoma

♦ Neoplastic odontogenic epithelial cells proliferate in form of multiple discrete follicles and islands within fibrous connective tissue stroma.
♦ Each follicle like structure is bordered on the periphery by the single layer of tall columnar cells resembling ameloblasts like cells. Nuclei of these cells are located at opposite pole to basement membrane, i.e., reverse polarity.
♦ Cells located at the center of follicle are loosely arranged and resemble stellate reticulum cells of an enamel organ.
♦ Microcyst formation is often observed inside these follicles.

Q.13. Discuss unicystic ameloblastoma.

(Oct 2019, 3 Marks)

Ans. Unicystic ameloblastoma represents an ameloblastoma variant, presenting a cyst.

Pathogenesis

♦ Reduced enamel epithelium undergoing ameloblastic transformation along with subsequent development of cyst.
♦ Ameloblastoma arising in dentigerous cyst or the other type of cysts.
♦ Solid ameloblastoma mainly undergoing the cystic degeneration.
♦ Arising of the unicystic ameloblastoma is de novo (on its own).

Clinical Features

♦ It is mainly seen in younger patients during second decade of life.
♦ Mostly unicystic ameloblastomas are seen in the mandible mainly in posterior region.
♦ Lesion is mainly asymptomatic, although large lesions may lead to painless swelling of jaws.
♦ Numbness of lip is also present.
♦ In secondary infected lesions pain and discharge is present.

Radiographic Features

♦ It is a well circumscribed unilocular radiolucency along with sclerotic border.
♦ It is mainly associated with unerupted impacted mandibular third molar which resembles the dentigerous cyst.

Histopathology

Unicystic ameloblastoma is of three types, i.e.:

Luminal Unicystic Ameloblastoma

♦ Epithelial lining shows cuboidal or columnar basal cells which have hyperchromatic, palisading and polarized nucleus. There is also presence of cytoplasmic vacuolization, intercellular spacing and subepithelial hyalinization (Vicker's and Gorlin criteria)
♦ Overlying epithelial cells resemble stellate reticulum like cells.

Intraluminal Unicystic Ameloblastoma

♦ One or more nodules of epithelial lining project inside the cystic lumen. This is known as intraluminal unicystic ameloblastoma.
♦ These nodules can be relatively small or largely fill cystic lumen.
♦ In some of the cases, nodule of tumor projects inside the lumen demonstrates an edematous, plexiform pattern.

Intramural Unicystic Ameloblastoma

♦ Here, the fibrous wall of cyst is infiltrated by islands of follicular or plexiform ameloblastoma.
♦ Extent and depth of ameloblastic infiltration may vary considerably.

Treatment

♦ Unicystic ameloblastoma is treated by enucleation.
♦ As luminal variant does not infiltrate in surrounding bone, so no further treatment is done.
♦ Mural variant should be excised and further treatment depends on depth of epithelial invasion into the cystic wall.
  • In limited invasive lesions careful follow up is done.
  • In deep invasive lesions surgical intervention with long term follow up is done.

Q.14. Define hamartoma. List any four hamartomatous lesions. Discuss clinical features and histopathology of adenomatoid odontogenic tumor.

(Oct 2019, 5 Marks)

Ans. A benign tumor like nodule composed of an overgrowth of mature cells and tissues normally present in affected part, but often with one element predominating is known as hamartoma.

Four Hamartomatous Lesions

♦ Hemangioma
♦ Squamous odontogenic tumor
♦ Lymphangioma
♦ Hemangioma

For clinical features and histology of adenomatoid odontogenic tumor, refer to Ans. 5 of same chapter.

5. CYSTS OF ORAL CAVITY

Q.1. Define and classify cyst. Write in detail about dentigerous cyst.

(Mar 2006, 15 Marks) (Feb 2013, 18 Marks)

Or

Classify odontogenic cyst. Describe pathogenesis, clinical radiological and histopathologic features of dentigerous cyst. *(June 2015, 10 Marks)*

Or

Classify odontogenic cysts and describe clinical features, radiographic and histopathologic features of dentigerous cyst. *(Feb 2015, 10 Marks)*

Or

Classify odontogenic cyst. Describe pathogenesis, clinical, radiological features along with histopathology of dentigerous cyst.

(Jan 2018, 10 Marks)

Or

Write short answer on radiographic features and histopathology of dentigerous cyst.

(Oct 2019, 3 Marks)

Or

Classify odontogenic cyst. Discuss dentigerous cyst in detail. *(Apr 2019, 5 Marks)*

Ans. Cyst is defined as "A pathological cavity having fluid, semifluid or gaseous contents and which is not created by accumulation of pus." **—Kramer (1974)**

Classification of Cyst of Oral Cavity by Mervin Shear

I. Cysts of the Jaws

♦ *Epithelial:*
- *Developmental:*
  - *Odontogenic:*
    - » Gingival cyst of infants
    - » Odontogenic keratocyst (Neoplasm)
    - » Dentigerous cyst
    - » Eruption cyst
    - » Lateral periodontal cyst
    - » Gingival cyst of adults
    - » Botryoid odontogenic cyst
    - » Glandular odontogenic cyst
    - » Calcifying odontogenic cyst (neoplasm)
  - *Non-odontogenic:*
    - » Nasopalatine duct cyst
    - » Nasolabial cyst
    - » Midpalatal raphe cyst of infants
    - » Median palatine, median alveolar
    - » Median mandibular cyst
    - » Globulomaxillary cyst
- *Inflammatory:*
  - Radicular cyst, apical and lateral
  - Residual cyst
  - Paradental cyst and mandibular infected buccal cyst
  - Inflammatory collateral cyst
♦ *Nonepithelial (pseudocysts)*
- Solitary bone cyst
- Aneurysmal bone cyst

II. Cyst Associated With Maxillary Antrum

♦ Benign mucosal cyst of the maxillary antrum
♦ Postoperative maxillary cyst

III. Cyst of the Soft Tissues of Mouth, Face And Neck

♦ Dermoid and epidermoid cyst
♦ Lymphoepithelial cyst (branchial cyst)
♦ Thyroglossal duct cyst
♦ Anterior medial lingual cyst (intra lingual cyst of foregut origin)
♦ Oral cyst with gastric or intestinal epithelium
♦ Cystic hygroma
♦ Nasopharyngeal cyst
♦ Thymic cyst
♦ Cyst of salivary glands-mucous extravasation cyst
♦ Mucous retention cyst, ranula, polycystic disease of the parotid.
♦ Parasitic cyst-hydatid cyst, cysticercus cellulosae, trichinosis.

Classification of Odontogenic Cyst

WHO (2017) Classification of Odontogenic Cysts

♦ *Odontogenic cysts of inflammatory origin*
- Radicular cyst
- Inflammatory collateral cysts
♦ *Odontogenic developmental cysts*
- Dentigerous cyst
- Odontogenic keratocyst
- Lateral periodontal cyst and botryoid odontogenic cyst
- Gingival cysts
- Glandular odontogenic cyst
- Calcifying odontogenic cyst
- Orthokeratinized odontogenic cyst.

Dentigerous Cyst

♦ It is also called as follicular cyst or pericoronal cyst
♦ It is the odontogenic cyst that surrounds the crown of the impacted tooth.

Pathogenesis

♦ *Intrafollicular theory:* Dentigerous cyst is caused by fluid accumulation between reduced enamel epithelium and enamel surface which result in a cyst in which crown is located within the lumen.
♦ *Extrafollicular theory:* Dentigerous cyst may arise by proliferation and cystic transformation of islands by odontogenic epithelium in connective tissue wall of dental follicle or even outside dental follicle and this transformed epithelium then unite with lining follicular epithelium forming cystic cavity around tooth crown.

Clinical Features

♦ It is usually found in the children.

♦ Most lesions are present in the 2nd and 3rd decades with male predilection.

♦ Most common site of the cyst are the mandibular and maxillary third molar and maxillary cuspid areas, since these are most commonly impacted teeth.

♦ Generally, it is painless but may be painful if it is infected. Dentigerous cyst has potential to become an aggressive lesion with expansion of bone and subsequent facial asymmetry.

♦ There is extreme displacement of teeth, severe root resorption of adjacent teeth and pain.

Histopathological Features

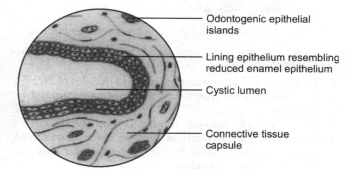

Odontogenic epithelial islands

Lining epithelium resembling reduced enamel epithelium

Cystic lumen

Connective tissue capsule

Fig. 69: Dentigerous cyst *(For color version, see Plate 12)*.

♦ The epithelial lining consists of two to four layers of flattened non-keratinizing cells and the epithelium and connective tissue interface is flat.

♦ It is usually composed of thin connective tissue wall with a thin layer of stratified squamous epithelium lining the lumen.

♦ Rete pegs formation is absent except in case of secondarily infected cyst.

♦ Connective tissue wall is frequently quite thickened and composed of very loose fibrous connective tissue.

♦ Inflammatory cells commonly infiltrate connective tissue

♦ It also shows Rushton bodies within the lining epithelium which are peculiar linear and often curved hyaline bodies.

♦ Content of cystic lumen is usually thin watery yellow fluid and is occasionally blood tinged.

Roentgenographic/Radiological Features

♦ There is presence of well-defined radiolucency having hyperostotic borders.

♦ An unerupted tooth is also seen around the radiolucency

♦ Cyst is unilocular but at times it appears multilocular.

♦ Bony margins of the cyst are well defined as well as sharp. If infection persists margins are ill defined.

♦ Cyst can envelop the crown symmetrically, but it can expand laterally from the crown of tooth. Tooth can also be displaced away in any direction.

♦ Resorption of roots of adjacent teeth can also be seen.

♦ Floor of maxillary sinus gets displaced with the expansion of cyst.

Q.2. Classify cysts of jaw. Describe pathogenesis, histopathology and clinical features and malignant potential of dentigerous cyst. *(Mar 2000, 15 Marks)*

Ans. *Refer to Ans. 1 of same chapter.*

Malignant Potential of Dentigerous Cyst

♦ Malignant potential of the epithelium of dentigerous cysts to ameloblastoma, epidermoid carcinoma and mucoepidermoid carcinoma.

♦ Development of an ameloblastoma is from rest of odontogenic epithelium or from lining epithelium of cyst is known as mural ameloblastoma.

♦ Mucoepidermoid carcinoma is the malignancy of salivary gland. The mucoepidermoid carcinoma is usually associated with lining epithelium of dentigerous cyst or dentigerous cyst which consist of mucous secreting cell.

♦ Epidermoid carcinoma can also develop from dentigerous cyst from rest of odontogenic epithelium or lining of epithelium of cyst.

Q.3. Write notes on dentigerous cyst. *(Feb 2006, 3 Marks)*

Or

Write short note on dentigerous cyst.
(Aug 2012, 5 Marks) (Apr 2008, 5 Marks)

Or

Write short essay on dentigerous cyst.
(Jan 2012, 5 Marks)

Ans. *Refer to Ans. 1 of same chapter.*

Q.4. Classify odontogenic cysts of oral cavity. Write about clinical features and histopathology of odontogenic keratocyst. *(Feb 2013, 10 Marks)*

Or

Write in detail on odontogenic keratocyst.
(June 2010, 10 Marks)

Or

Classify odontogenic cysts of oral cavity describe clinical features and histopathology of keratocyst.
(Dec 2010, 18 Marks)

Or

Classify odontogenic cysts and describe the clincial and histopathological features of odontogenic keratocyst (OKC) in detail. *(June 2014, 10 Marks)*

Or

Classify odontogenic cysts. Describe pathogenesis, clinical, radiological and histopathological features of odontogenic keratocyst. *(Jan 2016, 10 Marks)*

Or

Classify odontogenic cysts. Discuss clinical features, radiological features and histopathology of odontogenic keratocyst. *(Mar 2016, 8 Marks)*

Ans. *For classification, refer to Ans. 1 of same chapter.*

Odontogenic Keratocyst

Odontogenic keratocyst is a common cystic lesion of the jaw, which arises from the remnants of dental lamina.

- It is named as keratocyst because the cyst epithelium produces so much keratin that it fills the cyst lumen.
- Odontogenic cysts have more aggressive course than any other cystic lesion of jaw and for this reason these are sometimes known as benign cystic neoplasms.

Recent Concept of Odontogenic Keratocyst

- Keratocystic odontogenic tumor is now listed as 'odontogenic keratocyst (OKC)' in the 2017 classification of developmental odontogenic cysts.
- WHO 2005 classification reclassified this unique lesion as a neoplasm and renamed it as 'keratocystic odontogenic tumor' because of the high recurrence rate, aggressive clinical behavior, association with nevoid basal cell carcinoma syndrome, and mutations in the PTCH tumor suppressor gene. The WHO 2017 classification reverted back to the original and well accepted terminology of 'odontogenic keratocyst' because many papers showed that the PTCH gene mutation could be found in non-neoplastic lesions, including dentigerous cysts. It has also been reported that marsupialization is an effective treatment for the odontogenic keratocyst and may be associated with reversion of the epithelium to normal, and with lower recurrence rates, these features are not normally associated with neoplasia. So after considering all the available data, the WHO consensus group concluded that further research is needed, but at the present time, there was insufficient evidence to support a neoplastic origin of the odontogenic keratocyst. It was decided therefore that odontogenic keratocyst remains the most appropriate name for this lesion, and keratocystic odontogenic tumor was removed from the WHO 2017 classification of odontogenic cysts.

Pathogenesis

Odontogenic keratocyst mainly arises from the:
- Dental lamina or its remnants.
- Primordium of developing tooth germ or enamel organ.
- Sometimes from basal cell layer of oral epithelium.

Histopathological Features

- A parakeratin surface which is usually corrugated rippled or wrinkled.
- Uniformity of thickness of epithelium is generally between 6 to 10 cells in depth.
- Prominent palisaded, polarized basal cell layer often described as having a "picket fence" or "tombstone" appearance.
- Occasionally orthokeratin is found but if present, parakeratin is evident.
- Connective tissue shows "Daughter cells" or "Satellite cysts".
- Lumen of keratocyst may be filled with thin straw colored fluid or with thick creamy material.

- Sometimes a lumen contains a great deal of keratin while at other times it has little cholesterol as well as hyaline bodies at the site of inflammation.

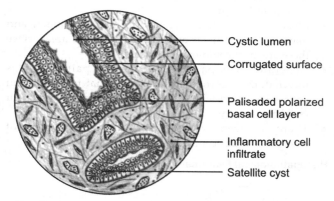

Fig. 70: Odontogenic keratocyst *(For color version, see Plate 12).*

Clinical Features

- Peak incidence is between 2nd and 3rd decades of life.
- It is found more frequently in males as compared to females.
- Mandible is affected more commonly than maxilla.
- In mandible, the majority of cysts occurs in ramus third molar area, followed by first and second molar area and then the anterior mandible.
- It is asymptomatic unless they become secondarily infected in which case patient complains of pain, soft tissue swelling and drainage.
- Occasionally, they experience paresthesia of lower lip and teeth.
- There is often one tooth missing from the dental arch.
- Expansion and thinning of bone may result in pathological fracture.
- Maxillary odontogenic keratocyst tends to be secondarily infected with greater frequency than the mandibular ones, due to its vicinity to maxillary sinus.

Radiological Features

- Odontogenic keratocyst is oval in shape and it extends to the body of mandible with mediolateral expansion.
- It is very small in size or it can exceed the diameter of 5 cm.
- Margins of the cyst are hyperostotic.
- Mostly odontogenic keratocyst is unilocular and have smooth borders while some of the cysts show irregular borders too.
- Radiolucency is seen in the cystic part which appears to be hazy if keratin is present in the cavity.
- Radiolucency is surrounded by thin sclerotic rim.
- In some of the cases perforation of lingual and buccal cortical plates is seen.
- Displacement of inferior alveolar canal is seen downwards.

Q.5. **Classify cysts of oral region. Discuss radicular cyst in detail.** *(Sep 2005, 16 Marks)*

Or

Write note on radicular cyst.
(Mar 2001, 5 Marks) (Feb 2013, 5 Marks)

Or

Write short note on radicular cyst.
(Aug 2012, 5 Marks) (Apr 2017, 5 Marks)

Or

Classify odontogenic cyst. Describe the pathogenesis, clinical, radiological and histopathogical features of radicular cyst. *(Jan 2017, 10 Marks)*

Or

Classify cyst of Jaws. Describe pathogenesis, clinical and radiological features with histopathology of radicular cyst. *(Sep 2018, 10 Marks)*

Ans. *For classification, refer to Ans. 1 of same chapter.*

Radicular Cyst

- It is also called as apical periodontal cyst or periapical cyst or dental root end cyst.
- It is an inflammatory odontogenic epithelial cyst.
- It is a common sequelae in progressive changes associated with bacterial invasion and death of the dental pulp.
- It most commonly occurs at the apices of the teeth.

Pathogenesis of Radicular Cyst

Radicular cyst develops due to the proliferation and subsequent cystic degeneration of the "epithelial cell rests of Malassez", in the periapical region of a nonvital tooth.

The process of development of this cyst occurs in various stages:
I. Phase of initiation
II. Phase of proliferation
III. Phase of cystification
IV. Phase of enlargement

I. **Phase of initiation:** During this phase, the bacterial infection of the dental pulp or direct inflammatory effect of necrotic pulpal tissue, in a nonvital tooth causes stimulation of the "cell rest of Malassez" which are present within the bone near the root apex of teeth.

II. **Phase of proliferation:** The stimulation to the cell rests of Malassez leads to excessive proliferation of these cells, which leads to the formation of a large mass or island of immature proliferating epithelial cells at the periapical region of the affected tooth.

III. **Phase of cystification:** Once a large bulk of the cell rest of Malassez is produced, its peripheral cells get adequate nutritional supply but its centrally located cells are often deprived of proper nutritional supply. As a result the central group of cells undergo ischemic liquefactive necrosis while the peripheral group of cells survive. This eventually gives rise to the formation of a cavity that contains a hollow space or lumen inside the mass of the proliferating cell rest of Malassez and a peripheral lining of epithelial cells around it.

IV. **Phase of enlargement:** Once a small cyst is formed, it enlarges gradually by the following mechanisms:
- Higher osmotic tension of the cystic fluid causes progressive increase in the amount of fluid inside its lumen and this causes increased internal hydrostatic tension within the cyst. The process results in cyst expansion due to resorption of the surrounding bone.
- The epithelial cells of the cystic lining release some bone resorbing factors, such as prostaglandins and collagenase, etc., which destroy the bone and facilitate expansion of the cyst.

Clinical Features

- It most commonly occurs on 3rd, 4th and 5th decades of the life.
- It is more common among the males.
- Maxillary anteriors are most commonly affected.
- Majority of cases are asymptomatic.
- It is associated with the nonvital tooth.
- Small cystic lesions are asymptomatic.
- Large lesions often produce a slow enlarging bony hard swelling of the jaw with expansion of cortical plates.
- Severe bone destruction produces "springiness" of jaw bone.
- If the cyst is secondarily infected it leads to the formation of the abscess, which is called "cyst abscess".

Histological Features

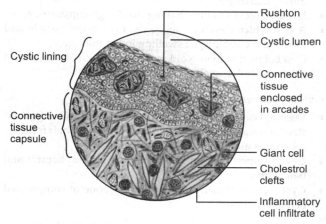

Fig. 71: Radicular cyst *(For color version, see Plate 13).*

- Radicular cyst is lined by the stratified squamous epithelium.
- It is lined by pseudostratified, columnar or respiratory type of epithelium.
- Hyaline bodies or Rushton bodies often found in the great numbers in the epithelium of apical periodontal cyst.
- Collagenous connective tissue makes the wall of radicular cyst.
- Abundant fibroblast can be identified within the cystic wall.
- Cystic wall presents inflammatory infiltrate which contains lymphocytes, plasma cells.
- Other histological findings within the cyst wall are erythrocytes, area of hemorrhage, occasional spicules of

dystrophic bone, multinucleated giant cells and cholesterol crystals.

Radiological Features

It is round or oval radiolucency of variable size which is generally well delineated and is most likely with marked radiopaque rim.

Treatment

- Root canal treatment
- Extraction of involved tooth
- Enucleation or marsupialization of large lesion is done.

Q.6. Write note on dermoid cyst.
(Oct/Nov 1992, 6 Marks)

Ans. It is also known as dermoid cystic tumor or cystic teratoma.

- It is a developmental cyst derived from the remnants of the embryonic skin.
- It is hamartomatous tumor containing multiple sebaceous glands and almost all skin adnexa, this may consist of substances, such as nails and dental cartilage like and bone like structures.

Clinical Features

- It occurs in young children.
- Dermoid cyst occurs most commonly on face, neck or scalp.
- In addition to skin dermoid cyst can be intracranial, intraspinal or perispinal.
- It is a painless swelling having the dough consistency.
- A cyst which develops above the mylohyoid muscle and presents the sublingual swelling in the midline.
- Cyst below the mylohyoid muscle presents submental and submandibular swelling in the midline.

Histological Features

- Dermoid cysts in the skin are lined by the orthokeratinized stratified squamous epithelium which exhibit hair follicles, sebaceous glands and erector pili muscles.
- Cavity lumen is often filled with the sebum, keratin and hair shafts.
- Cyst capsule is composed of narrow zone of compressed connective tissue.

Treatment

Surgical excision is done.

Q.7. Write note on epidermoid cyst. *(Sep 1999, 5 Marks)*

Ans. It is also called epidermoid inclusion cyst or epidermoid cyst or keratin cyst or sebaceous cyst.

- Epidermoid inclusion cysts are the result of implantation of epidermoid elements and its subsequent cystic transformation.

Clinical Features

- It is most common in 3rd and 4th decades of life.
- It is twice as common in men as in women.
- Common sites are face, trunk, neck extremities and scalp.

- Epidermoid cyst appears as firm, round, mobile, flesh colored to yellow or white subcutaneous nodules of variable size. In some patients, it contains melanin pigments.
- Discharge of foul smelling cheese like material is a common complaint.
- Sometimes cyst becomes inflamed and infected resulting in pain and tenderness.
- When located orally, it can cause difficulty in feeding, swallowing and even speaking.

Histological Features

- Cyst is lined by the stratified squamous epithelium with glandular differentiation.
- Cyst is filled with desquamated keratin disposed in a lamellar pattern.
- Dystrophic calcification and reactive foreign body reaction are seen associated with the cystic capsule.
- Pigmented epidermoid cyst may demonstrate melanin pigment in the wall and a keratin may present.
- A surrounding infiltrate of melanocytes and macrophages may be observed.

Treatment

Surgical excision is done.

Q.8. Write note on globulomaxillary cyst.
(Sep 1993, 6 Marks)

Ans. As per the older concept globulomaxillary cyst was a fissural cyst that arose from epithelium entrapped during fusion of the globular portion of the medial nasal process with the maxillary process.

- As per the recent concept globular portion of the medial nasal process is primarily united with the maxillary process and fusion does not occur. Therefore, epithelial entrapment should not occur during embryologic development of this area.
- All cysts in the globulomaxillary region, i.e., between the lateral incisor and canine teeth can be explained on an odontogenic basis.
- Many are lined by inflamed stratified squamous epithelium and are consistent with periapical cysts
- It was also theorized that some of these lesions may arise from inflammation of the reduced enamel epithelium at the time of eruption of the teeth.
- In some cases, cysts in the globulomaxillary area may be lined by pseudostratified, ciliated, columnar epithelium. Such cases provide credence to the fissural theory of origin.
- Since fissural cyst in this region probably does not exist, the term globulomaxillary cyst should no longer be used.
- When a radiolucency between the maxillary lateral incisor and canine is encountered, the clinician should first consider an odontogenic origin for the lesion.

Q.9. Write notes on benign cervical lymphoepithelial cyst.
(Mar 1994, 6 Marks)

Ans. Benign cervical lymphoepithelial cyst is also known as branchial cleft cyst.

Pathogenesis

It originates from cystic transformation of gland epithelium entrapped in the oral lymphoid aggregates during embryogenesis.

Clinical Features

♦ It is located superficially in the neck, close to the angle of mandible, anterior to sternocleidomastoid muscle.
♦ It occurs at all the ages with a fairly equal distribution from 1st to 6th decades.
♦ Neck lesions vary in size from small to very large.
♦ There is swelling, which may be progressive or intermittent and pain may also be a feature.
♦ Lymphoepithelial cyst generally present as an asymptomatic, circumscribed, movable swelling on lateral aspect of the neck.
♦ It may be unilateral or bilateral.

Histopathology

♦ Cystic cavity is lined by thin stratified squamous epithelium.
♦ Cyst is generally embedded in a circumscribed mass of lymphoid tissue.
♦ Capsule of the cyst also present variable amount of connective tissue, being infiltrated by lymphocytes, plasma cells, macrophages and some multinucleated giant cells.
♦ Cystic lumen is filled up with either a thin watery fluid or a thick gelatinous material.

Treatment

It is removed by local surgical incision.

Q.10. Write notes on odontogenic keratocyst.
(Mar 2007, 2.5 Marks) (Mar 2007, 2.5 Marks)
Ans. *Refer to Ans. 4 of same chapter.*

Q.11. Describe the histopathology of odontogenic keratocyst. *(Sep 2006, 5 Marks) (Sep 2011, 3 Marks)*
(Dec 2010, 3 Marks)

Or

Write in brief on histopathology of odontogenic keratocyst. *(Sep 2018, 5 Marks)*

Or

Write short note on histopathology of odontogenic cyst. *(Feb 2019, 5 Marks)*
Ans. *Refer to Ans. 4 of same chapter.*

Q.12. Define and classify cyst. Describe the clinical, radiological and histological features of radicular cyst. *(Sep 2006, 15 Marks)*
Ans. *For classification, refer to Ans. 1 of same chapter.*

For clinical, radiological and histological features of radicular cyst, refer to Ans. 5 of same chapter.

Q.13. Give the classification of oral cysts.
(Mar 2007, 4 Marks)
Ans. *Refer to Ans. 1 of same chapter.*

Q.14. Classify odontogenic cyst. Write in detail on radicular cyst. *(Apr 2007, 15 Marks)*
Ans.

Classification of Odontogenic Cyst

WHO (2017) Classification of Odontogenic Cysts

♦ Odontogenic cysts of inflammatory origin
  • Radicular cyst
  • Inflammatory collateral cysts
♦ Odontogenic developmental cysts
  • Dentigerous cyst
  • Odontogenic keratocyst
  • Lateral periodontal cyst and botryoid odontogenic cyst
  • Gingival cysts
  • Glandular odontogenic cyst
  • Calcifying odontogenic cyst
  • Orthokeratinized odontogenic cyst

Q.15. Enumerate nonodontogenic cysts of oral cavity. Write about histopathology of odontogenic keratocyst. *(Sep 2007, 5 Marks)*
Ans.

Nonodontogenic Cysts of Oral Cavity

According to Shear

♦ Nasopalatine duct cyst
♦ Median palatine, median alveolar and median mandibular cyst
♦ Globulomaxillary cyst
♦ Nasolabial cyst.

According to Gorlin

♦ Globulomaxillary cyst
♦ Nasoalveolar cyst
♦ Nasopalatine cyst
♦ Median mandibular cyst
♦ Anterior lingual cyst
♦ Dermoid and epidermoid cyst
♦ Palatal cyst of newborn infants.

According to WHO 2007

♦ Nasopalatine duct cyst.

For histopathology of odontogenic keratocyst, refer to Ans. 4 of same chapter.

Q.16. Write short note on pathogenesis of radicular cyst. *(Dec 2007, 3 Marks) (Sep 2011, 3 Marks)*
Ans. *Refer to Ans. 5 of same chapter.*

Q.17. Classify cysts of jaws. Describe in detail etiopathogenesis, clinical features, radiographic features and histopathologic features of periapical cyst. *(Jan 2012, 10 Marks)*
Ans. *For classification of cysts, refer to Ans. 1 of same chapter.*

For etiopathogenesis, clinical features, radiographic features and histologic features, refer to Ans. 5 of same chapter.

Q.18. Write note on eruption cyst. *(Mar 2011, 3 Marks)*

Ans. It is defined as odontogenic cyst with histologic features of a dentigerous cyst and that surrounds a tooth crown which has erupted through bone but not soft tissue and is clinically visible as a soft fluctuant mass on alveolar ridges.

Clinical Features

- Most commonly found in children.
- It arises most frequently anteriorly to first permanent molar.
- Lesion appears as circumscribed, fluctuant, often translucent swelling of alveolar ridge at site of erupting tooth.
- When the cystic cavity contains blood, swelling appears deep blue or purple so it is known as eruption hematoma.
- Swelling is painless since it is infected.

Histological Features

- On microscopic examination stratified squamous epithelium of overlying gingiva is seen.
- Epithelium is separated from cyst by a strip of dense connective tissue.
- There is presence of mild chronic inflammatory cell infiltrate.
- In non-inflamed areas epithelial lining of cyst is of reduced enamel epithelium.

Treatment

No treatment is necessary as cyst often ruptures spontaneously.

Q.19. Describe in brief reasons for recurrence of odontogenic keratocyst. *(May/Jun 2009, 5 Marks)*

Ans. Following are the reasons for recurrence of odontogenic keratocyst:

- Odontogenic keratocyst multiply in some patients including the occurrence of satellite cysts which may be retained during an enucleation procedure. If enucleation procedures are incomplete may be new cyst arise from retained satellite microcysts or retained mural cell islands.
- Linings of odontogenic keratocyst are thin and fragile and are difficult to enucleate. Portions of lining may remain left behind and lead to recurrence.
- When OKC is enucleated in a single piece chances of recurrence are low while when it is removed in multiple pieces chances of recurrence is high. This is because in multiple pieces at times remnants of cyst remain which lead to recurrence.
- OKCs may also arise from proliferation of basal cells of oral mucosa also known as basal cell hamartias in third molar region and ascending ramus of mandible. It was observed that there is perforation of overlying bone and firm adhesion of cyst to overlying mucosa. So when cysts were surgically removed overlying mucosa should be excised with them to prevent recurrence from residual basal cell proliferations. If overlying mucosa is not excised or it remains it leads to recurrence.

Q.20. Write short note on histopathology of COC. *(Dec 2012, 3 Marks)*

Ans. It is also known as calcifying odontogenic cyst or Calcifying epithelial odontogenic cyst.

Histopathology

- Epithelial lining of COC shows prominent basal cell layer consisting of palisaded columnar or cuboidal cells and hyperchromatic nuclei which are polarized away from basement membrane.
- Epithelium is 6–8 cell layer thick.
- Budding from the basal cell layer into adjacent connective tissue and epithelial proliferations into lumen are seen.

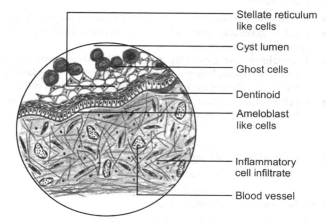

Fig. 72: Calcifying odontogenic cyst
(For color version, see Plate 13).

- *Ghost cells:* They are enlarged, ballooned shape, ovoid or elongated ellipsoid epithelial cells. They are eosinophilic. They are found in thick areas of epithelial lining. Cell outlines of these cells are well defined and at times they may be blurred. They are seen singly and also present in groups. Few ghost cells also show nuclear remnants. Ghost cells have abnormal type of keratinization and have affinity to calcify.
- Ghost cells also may remain in contact to connective tissue wall of cyst where they lead to foreign body reaction with formation of multinucleated giant cells.
- An atubular dentinoid is also seen in the wall close to epithelial lining and also in relation to epithelial proliferations.
- Dentinoid found particularly in contact with masses of ghost cells.

Q.21. Classify cysts of oral region. Give a detailed account of clinical, radiological and histopathological features of odontogenic keratocyst.

(Mar 2013, 8 Marks)

Or

Classify cyst of jaw. Write in detail clinical radiological and histopathological features of odontogenic keratocyst. *(Apr 2015, 8 Marks)*

Ans. *For classification, refer to Ans. 1 of same chapter.*

For clinical and histological features, refer to Ans. 4 of same chapter.

Radiological Features

- Odontogenic keratocyst is oval in shape and it extends to the body of mandible with mediolateral expansion.
- It is very small in size or it can exceed the diameter of 5 cm.
- Margins of the cyst are hyperostotic.
- Mostly odontogenic keratocyst is unilocular and have smooth borders while some of the cysts show irregular borders too.
- Radiolucency is seen in the cystic part which appears to be hazy if keratin is present in the cavity.
- Radiolucency is surrounded by thin sclerotic rim.
- In some of the cases, perforation of lingual and buccal cortical plates is seen.
- Displacement of inferior alveolar canal is seen downwards.

Q.22. Give classification of osteomyelitis. Discuss in detail clinical features, etiology, histopathology of odontogenic keratocyst. *(Mar 2013, 8 Marks)*

Ans.

Classification of Osteomyelitis

- *Acute osteomyelitis*
  - Acute suppurative osteomyelitis
  - Acute subperiosteal osteomyelitis
  - Acute periostitis
- *Chronic osteomyelitis:*
  A. *Nonspecific type:*
     - Chronic intramedullary osteomyelitis
     - Chronic focal sclerosing osteomyelitis
     - Chronic diffuse sclerosing osteomyelitis
     - Chronic osteomyelitis with proliferative periostitis
     - Chronic subperiosteal osteomyelitis
     - Chronic periostitis
  B. *Specific type:*
     - Tuberculous osteomyelitis
     - Syphilitic osteomyelitis
     - Actinomycotic osteomyelitis
- Radiation-induced osteomyelitis
- Idiopathic osteomyelitis.

For clinical features and histopathology, refer to Ans. 4 of same chapter.

Etiology of Odontogenic Keratocyst

The cyst arises from:
- Dental lamina or its remnants.
- Primordium of developing tooth germ or enamel organ
- Basal cell layer of oral epithelium.

Q.23. Write short note on radicular cyst histopathology. *(Feb 2013, 8 Marks)*

Ans. *For details, refer to Ans. 5 of same chapter.*

Q.24. Write short note on OKC-etiology and histopathology. *(Nov 2014, 3 Marks)*

Ans. *For etiology of OKC, refer to Ans. 22 of same chapter.*

For histopathology of OKC, refer to Ans. 4 of same chapter.

Q.25. Write short note on Rushton bodies.
(Feb 2015, 5 Marks)

Ans. Rushton bodies are seen in the histological picture of radicular cyst or residual cyst.
- Rushton body is a hyaline body is found in great numbers in epithelium of radicular cyst or residual cyst.
- Rushton bodies are linear, straight or curved or of hair pain shaped.
- Rushton bodies measure up to 0.1 mm
- Rushton bodies appear amorphous in structure, eosinophilic in reaction and are brittle in nature.
- They are sometimes concentrically laminated and frequently fractured.

Origin

Related to origin of Rushton bodies two views were put forward, i.e.:
- Rushton bodies were of odontogenic epithelial origin and are probably a form of keratin. **—By Shear**
- Hyaline bodies has hematogenous origin and they were derived from thrombi in venules of connective tissue that had become varicose and strangled by the cuffs of epithelium which encircle it and these bodies reacted histochemically as hemoglobin. According to the authors who had given this view also suggested that thrombi shrinks centrifugally and undergo splitting or calcify.

Q.26. Discuss histology and reasons for recurrence of odontogenic keratocyst. *(May 2018, 3 Marks)*

Ans. *For histology of odontogenic keratocyst, refer to Ans. 4 of same chapter.*

For recurrence of odontogenic keratocyst, refer to Ans. 19 of same chapter.

6. BACTERIAL INFECTIONS OF ORAL CAVITY

Q.1. Write notes on oral manifestations of syphilis.

(Mar 2007, 2.5 Marks)

Ans. Oral manifestations of syphilis are given below:

Charac-teristic	Primary syphilis	Secondary syphilis	Tertiary syphilis
Site	Chancre occurs at the site on entry of *Treponema*. It occurs on lip, oral mucosa, lateral surface of tongue, soft palate, tonsillary region, pharyngeal region and gingiva	Mucus patches are present on tongue, buccal mucosa, pharyngeal region, tonsillar region. Split papules develop at commissure of lips	Gumma can occur anywhere in jaw but more frequent site is palate, mandible and tongue
Appearance	It has narrow copper-colored slightly raised borders with reddish-brown base in center	Mucus patches appear as slightly raised grayish white lesions surrounded by erythematous base. Split papules are cracked in middle giving "Split pea appearance"	Gumma manifests as solitary, deep punched out mucosal ulcer. Lesion is sharply demarcated and necrotic tissue at base of ulcer may slough leaving punched out defects
Symptom	Intraoral chancers are slightly painful due to secondary infection and are covered with grayish white film	Mucus patches are painless but some-times mild-to-moderately painful	In gumma, the breathing and swallowing difficulty may be encountered by the patients
Signs	White sloughy material is present	Snail track ulcers and raw bleeding surfaces are present	Perforation of palatal vault is present
Tongue	Tongue lesion may be commonly seen on lateral surface of anterior two-thirds or on dorsal surface and often there is enlargement of folate papilla	Tongue gets fissured	• Numerous small healed gumma in tongue results in series of nodules or sparse in deeper area of organ giving tongue an upholstered or tufted appearance

Contd...

Contd...

Charac-teristic	Primary syphilis	Secondary syphilis	Tertiary syphilis
			• Luetic glossitis: There is complete atrophy of papillary coating and firm fibrous texture is seen • Chronic superficial interstitial glossitis: Tongue can involve diffusely with gumma and appear, large, lobulated and irregular shaped
Lip	Extraoral lip chancre has more typical brown crusted appearance which can be multiple. Lower lip is mainly involved	Split papule is a raised papular lesion which develops at commissure of lip and whic fissure which separates upper lip portion from the lower lip portion	Lip is not commonly involved

Q.2. Describe oral manifestations of leprosy, tuberculosis and syphilis.

(Mar 1998, 16 Marks)

Ans.

Oral Manifestations of Leprosy

♦ In oral cavity, the disease produces tumor like lesions called "lepromas" which are found on lips, gingiva, tongue and hard palate.

♦ Oral lesion appears as yellowish soft or hard sessile growth which have tendency to breakdown and ulcerate.

♦ Ulceration, necrosis and perforation of palate.

♦ Fixation of palate with loss of uvula.

♦ Difficulty in swallowing and regurgitation.

♦ Cobble stone appearance of tongue with loss of taste sensation.

♦ Chronic gingivitis, periodontitis and candidiasis are present.

♦ Enamel hypoplasia of teeth, pinkish discoloration of teeth and tapering of teeth is present.

Oral Manifestations of Tuberculosis

♦ Tuberculous infection in oral cavity may produce nodules, vesicles, fissures, plaque, granulomas or verrucal papillary lesions.

- Tuberculous lesions of oral cavity are tuberculous ulcers, tuberculous gingivitis and tuberculosis of salivary gland.
- Tongue is most common location for the occurrence, besides this palate, gingiva, lips, buccal mucosa, alveolar ridge and vestibules may also be affected.
- **Tongue lesion:** Tuberculous lesion of tongue develops on the lateral borders and appears as single or multiple ulcers which are well defined, painful, firm and yellowish gray in color.
- **Lip lesions:** Lesions produce small, nontender, granulating ulcer at mucocutaneous junction.
- **Gingival lesions:** These lesions produce small granulating ulcers with concomitant gingival hyperplasia.
- **Tuberculous lesion of jaw bone:** Chronic osteomyelitis of maxilla and mandible may occur and infection reaches to bone via blood or root canal or extraction socket. Tuberculous osteomyelitis of jaw bone produces pain, swelling, sinus or fistula formation.

Oral Manifestations of Syphilis

Refer to Ans. 1 of same chapter.

Q.3. Write note on congenital syphilis. *(Mar 2000, 5 Marks)*

Or

Write short note on congenital syphilis.

(Dec 2015, 3 Marks) (Sep 2006, 5 Marks)
(June 2015, 5 Marks) (Apr 2017, 4 Marks)

Or

Write in brief on congenital syphilis.

(Sep 2018, 5 Marks)

Ans. *Congenital syphilis is a rare entity that occurs in children born of an infected mother.*

- This condition occurs due to transplacental infection with *T. palladium* during fetal development.
- Deciduous teeth are less frequently affected as compared to the permanent teeth.

Features of Congenital Syphilis

- Mulberry molars and screw driven shaped incisors occur due to involvement of developing tooth germs.
- Rhagades, i.e., fissuring and scaring at the corners of the mouth.
- Saddle nose or bull dog appearance is seen.
- There is mandible prognathism and increased inter dental spaces.
- Delayed eruption of teeth is present.
- Hypodontia and enamel hypoplasia is seen.
- *There is occurrence of Hutchinson's triad which consists of:*
  - Hypoplasia of incisors and molar teeth
  - 8th nerve deafness
  - Interstitial keratitis of eyes.

Treatment

High doses of penicillin are given.

Q.4. Write note on NOMA. *(Mar 2000, 5 Marks)*

Or

Write short answer on cancrum oris.

(Oct 2019, 3 Marks)

Ans. It is also called as gangrenous stomatitis.

It is rapidly spreading gangrene of oral and facial tissues occurring usually in debilitated or nutritionally deficient patients.

Predisposing Factors

- Occurs in undernourished persons.
- Debilitated from infections, such as diphtheria, measles, pneumonia, scarlet fever, TB and blood dyscrasias.
- Excessive mechanical injury.
- It is a specific infection by Vincent's organism.

Clinical Features

- It is seen chiefly in malnourished children.
- Common sites are areas of stagnation around the fixed bridge or crown.
- Commencement of gangrene is denoted by blackening of skin. Small ulcers of gingival mucosa spread rapidly and involves surrounding tissue of jaw, lips and cheeks by gangrenous necrosis.
- Odor is foul and patient have high temperature.
- Overlying skin is inflamed, edematous and finally necrotic.

Treatment

- Reconstructive surgery should be done along with palliative treatment.

Q.5. Describe histopathology of actinomycosis.

(Sep 2006, 5 Marks)

Or

Describe histologic features with diagram of actinomycosis *(Nov 2008, 5 Marks)*

Ans. Actinomycosis is a chronic granulomatous suppurative and fibrosing infection. It is caused by filamentous, gram-positive and anaerobic actinomycosis group of infections, i.e., *Actinomycosis israelii, Actinomycosis viscosus*, etc.

Histopathology

- Actinomycosis under microscope shows numerous abscesses whose centers are occupied by bacterial colonies.
- Bone tissue often exhibits extensive necrosis with multiple areas of granuloma formation.
- Bacterial colony consists of dense, eosinophilic masses of Gram-negative filaments.

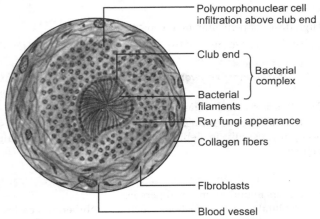

Fig. 73: Actinomycosis *(For color version, see Plate 13).*

- Periphery of each colony shows club-shaped swellings and produces a "Ray fungus" like appearance.
- Colonies are surrounded by polymorphonuclear neutrophils followed by lymphocytes, plasma cells and multinucleated giant cells.
- Colonies are surrounded by the fibrous tissue wall at outer margin.

Q.6. Write note on tuberculosis.

(Mar 2011, 5 Marks) (Feb 2013, 5 Marks)

Ans. Tuberculosis is a infectious granulomatous disease caused by *Mycobacterium tuberculosis*.

Pathogenesis

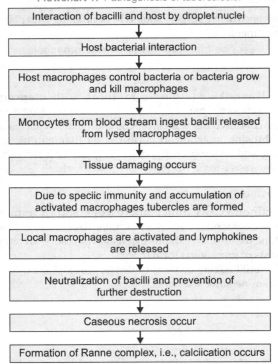

Flowchart 1: Pathogenesis of tuberculosis.

Interaction of bacilli and host by droplet nuclei

↓

Host bacterial interaction

↓

Host macrophages control bacteria or bacteria grow and kill macrophages

↓

Monocytes from blood stream ingest bacilli released from lysed macrophages

↓

Tissue damaging occurs

↓

Due to speciic immunity and accumulation of activated macrophages tubercles are formed

↓

Local macrophages are activated and lymphokines are released

↓

Neutralization of bacilli and prevention of further destruction

↓

Caseous necrosis occur

↓

Formation of Ranne complex, i.e., calciication occurs

Clinical Features

- Patient suffer from episodic fever and chills, easy fatigability and malaise.
- There is gradual loss of weight with persistent cough with or without hemoptysis.
- Choroid tubercles are seen in children.
- Lupus vulgaris may occur in children.

Oral Manifestation

- Tongue is the most common site involved followed by palate, lips, buccal mucosa, gingiva and frenula.
- There is presence of irregular, superficial or deep ulcer which is painful and will increase in size.
- There is presence of diffuse hyperemic, nodular or papillary proliferation of gingival tissues.
- Tuberculous osteomyelitis occurs in the later stages of disease.

Histological Features

There is formation of granuloma exhibiting, foci of caseous necrosis surrounded by epithelioid cells, lymphocyte and occasionally multinucleated giant cells.

- Epithelioid cells are morphologically altered macrophages and appear like epithelial cells.
- Multinucleated giant cells are of Langhans type.
- Area of caseous necrosis appears eosinophilic.
- Granuloma is surrounded by fibrous tissue and lymphocytes. At times dystrophic calcification is seen.

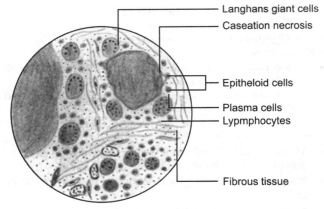

Fig. 74: Tuberculosis *(For color version, see Plate 13).*

Treatment

Multidrug therapy (MDT) is recommended.

Q.7. Write oral manifestations of tuberculosis.

(Dec 2010, 8 Marks)

Or

Write short note on oral manifestations of tuberculosis. *(Jan 2017, 5 Marks)*

Ans. Following are the oral manifestations of tuberculosis:

Tuberculous infection in oral cavity may produce nodules, vesicles, fissures, plaque, granulomas or verrucal papillary lesions.

- Tuberculous lesions of oral cavity are tuberculous ulcers, tuberculous gingivitis and tuberculosis of salivary gland.
- Tongue is most common location for the occurrence, besides this palate, gingiva, lips, buccal mucosa, alveolar ridge and vestibules may also be affected.
- *Tongue lesion:* Tuberculous lesion of tongue develops on the lateral borders and appears as single or multiple ulcers which are well defined, painful and firm in consistency. Ulcers are deep and are painful. Margins of ulcer are undermined with no induration. Area surrounding the ulcer remains inflamed and edematous. Base of the ulcer is yellowish.
- *Lip lesions:* Lesions produce small, nontender, granulating ulcer at mucocutaneous junction.
- *Gingival lesions:* These lesions produce small granulating ulcers. Gingiva appear diffuse, hyperemic and nodular papillary proliferation is seen.
- *Tuberculous lesion of jaw bone:* Chronic Osteomyelitis of maxilla and mandible may occur and infection reaches to bone via blood or root canal or extraction socket. Tuberculous osteomyelitis of jaw bone produces pain, swelling, sinus or fistula formation. As jaw bone is involved patient complains of swelling and difficulty in eating.
- Miliary lesion of oral mucosa in military tuberculosis is a small gray colored tubercle which breakdown and ulcerate.
- Periapical tissue can also be involved by the tubercle. Tooth socket is filled with tuberculous granulation tissue and has small pink and red elevations.

Q.8. Write short note on actinomycosis.

(Feb 2015, 5 Marks) (Dec 2009, 5 Marks)
(Mar 2006, 5 Marks) (Aug 2012, 5 Marks)

Or

Write short essay on actinomycosis.

(Jan 2012, 5 Marks)

Ans. It is a chronic granulomatous suppurative disease which is caused by anaerobic or microaerophilic gram-positive non-acid fast branched filamentous bacteria.

- The most common organism is *Actinomyces israelii, A. naeslundii, A. viscosus, A. odontolyticus* and *A. propionica.*

Classification of Actinomycosis Based on Location

- **Cervicofacial:** When there is involvement of face and cervical area
- **Abdominal:** When there is involvement of abdomen
- **Pulmonary:** When there is involvement of pleural cavity.
- **Cutaneous:** When there is involvement of skin
- **Central:** When there is involvement of bone
- **Periphery:** When there is involvement of soft tissue.

Pathogenesis

Disease originates when there is disruption of mucosal barrier which leads to invasion of bacteria. There is occurrence of initial acute inflammation which is followed by chronic indolent phase. Lesions appear as single or multiple indurations.

Clinical Features

Cervicofacial Actinomycosis

- Its occurrence is more common in males.
- Disease may remain localized to soft tissues or spread to involve salivary glands, bone or skin of face and neck. Most commonly involve area is submandibular region.
- Presence of trismus is there before formation of pus.
- The disease is characterized by presence of palpable mass which is indurated and is painless. Skin surrounding the lesion has wooden indurated area of fibrosis.

Abdominal Actinomycosis

- It is more severe form of disease.
- Patient complains of fever with chills and vomiting.
- There is involvement of liver and spleen.
- On palpation abdominal mass is felt which is the sign in diagnosis of disease.

Pulmonary Actinomycosis

- Patient complains of fever with chills, cough and presence of pain in pleural cavity.
- Empyema is present and there is formation of sinus.

Histopathology

Refer to Ans. 5 of same chapter.

Treatment

Patient should be kept on high antibiotic therapy, such as penicillin, cephalosporin, clindamycin, etc.

Q.9. Write short essay on pyogenic granuloma.

(Jan 2012, 5 Marks)

Or

Write short note on pyogenic granuloma.

(Apr 2015, 3 Marks) (Apr 2017, 5 Marks)

Or

Write short answer on pyogenic granuloma.

(Apr 2019, 3 Marks)

Ans. Pyogenic granuloma is considered as an exaggerated conditioned response to minor trauma.

Pyogenic granuloma is a misnomer since condition is not associated with pus formation.

Etiology

- It is caused by microorganisms, such as streptococci and staphylococci.
- If there is minor trauma to the tissue it provides the pathway for the nonspecific microorganisms which can cause pyogenic granuloma.
- Hormonal imbalance can lead to pyogenic granuloma.
- Sulfhydryl molecule is the agent which lead to pyogenic granuloma.

Clinical Features

- It occurs at the age of 10 to 40 years.
- Female predilection is present.
- Most affected sits are lip, gingiva, tongue, palate, vestibule. Lesion is more common in maxillary anterior region.
- Lesion is elevated, pedunculated or sessile mass with a smooth, lobulated or warty surface which is ulcerated.
- On manipulation the ulcer bleeds.
- Lesion is pink to red to purple in color depending on age of the lesion. It is usually painless and is soft in consistency.
- Size of the lesion ranges from 1 mm to centimeters.

Histopathology

- Overlying epithelium is thin and atrophic. At times, it is hyperplastic too.
- Surface of the epithelium is usually ulcerated and is replaced by thick fibrinopurulent membrane.
- Underlying connective tissue has number of endothelial lined vascular spaces engorged with RBCs and extreme proliferation of fibroblasts and budding endothelial cells.
- There is presence of moderate infiltration of PMN leukocytes, lymphocytes and plasma cells.
- Areas of hemorrhage and hemosiderin pigmentation is seen in connective tissue stroma.

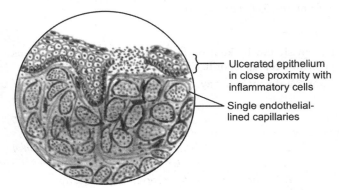

Ulcerated epithelium in close proximity with inflammatory cells

Single endothelial-lined capillaries

Fig. 75: Pyogenic granuloma (For color version, see Plate 13).

Treatment

Surgical excision of the lesion is done.

Q.10. Write short note on histopathology of pyogenic granuloma. *(Aug 2012, 5 Marks)*

Ans. For histopathology, refer to Ans. 9 of same chapter.

Q.11. Write short note on pathogenesis of tuberculosis. *(Jan 2016, 5 Marks)*

Ans. Following is the pathogenesis of tuberculosis:

Pathogenesis of Tuberculosis

- The interaction of the bacilli and the host begins when droplet nuclei from infectious patients are inhaled.
- The majority of the bacilli are trapped and exhaled by ciliary action and a fraction less than 10% enters alveoli.

- In the initial stage of the host-bacterial interaction, either host's macrophages control the multiplication of the bacteria or the bacteria grow and kill the macrophages.
- Non-activated monocytes attracted from blood stream to the site by various chemotactic factors ingest the bacilli released from the lysed macrophages.
- Initial stages are asymptomatic; about 2–4 weeks after infection tissue damaging and macrophage activating responses develop.
- With the development of specific immunity and accumulation of a large number of activated macrophages at the site of primary lesion, granulomatous reaction or tubercles are formed.
- The hard tubercle consists of epithelioid cells, Langhans giant cells, plasma cells, and fibroblasts. These lesions develop when host resistance is high.
- Due to cell-mediated immunity in the majority of individuals, local macrophages are activated and lymphokines are released, which neutralize the bacilli and prevent further tissue destruction.
- The central part of the lesion contains caseous, soft, and cheesy necrotic material (caseous necrosis). This necrotic material may undergo calcification at a later stage called Ranne complex, in the lung parenchyma and hilar lymph nodes in few cases.
- Caseous necrotic material under goes liquefaction and discharges into the lungs leading to the formation of a cavity. Spontaneous healing of the cavity occurs either by fibrosis or collapse.
- Calcification of the cavities may occur in which bacteria persist.
- In early stages, the spread of infection is mainly by macrophages to lymph nodes, other tissues, and organs. However, in children with poor immunity hematogenous spread results in fatal miliary TB or tuberculous meningitis.

For flowchart of pathogenesis of tuberculosis, refer to Ans. 6 of same chapter.

Q.12. Enumerate bacterial lesion involving oral cavity. Describe clinical features, investigations, histopathology and management of tuberculosis. *(Jan 2018, 10 Marks)*

Ans.

Bacterial Lesions Involving Oral Cavity

- Syphilis
- Non-venereal treponematoses
- Gonorrhea
- Streptococcal tonsillitis and pharyngitis
- Leprosy
- Tuberculosis
- Actinomycosis
- Noma
- Scarlet fever
- Diphtheria
- Cat scratch disease

♦ Tularemia
♦ Tetanus
♦ Rhinoscleroma
♦ Botryomycosis
♦ Melioidosis
♦ Granuloma Inguinale
♦ Lymphogranuloma venereum
♦ Myiasis.

For clinical features and histopathology, refer to Ans. 6 of same chapter.

Investigations

♦ *Serology:* In this ELISA technique is used which helpful in diagnosis of tuberculosis in children. PCR technique is more specific and sensitive serological test than ELISA, but PCR is less used due to its high cost.
♦ *Chest X-ray:* Presence of multiple nodular infiltrations or ill defined opacities in one of upper lobes is characteristic for pulmonary tuberculosis. An area of translucency in radiopacities is indicative of cavitation. Presence of cavity is indicative of an active lesion. In some of the patients, multiple thick-walled cavities can be seen. At the time of fibrosis, trachea and mediastinum shift to same side. Fibrosis can also cause calcification.
♦ *Pathological tests:*
  • *Blood examination:* Peripheral blood examination shows monocytosis, i.e., 8 to 12%
  • ESR is elevated.
  • *Tuberculin test:* It is a test to recognize prior tubercular infection, and is done by injecting one unit of purified protein derivative (PPD) on the forearm and readings taken after 48 hours. Induration of more than 15 mm indicates a positive test. The younger is the patient, greater is significance of positive test. A negative test does not always exclude tubercular infection since it may be negative in patients of blood malignancies, malnourishment and those on immunosuppressive therapy. Tuberculin test is nonspecific and only indicates prior infection. Its sensitivity wanes with age.

Management

Chemotherapy.

Drugs for Primary Chemotherapy (First Line Antitubercular Drugs)

Drug	Daily dose (Adult)	Thrice weekly dose
Rifampicin	>50 kg 600 mg <50 kg 450 mg	(10 mg/kg) (10 mg/kg)
Isoniazid	200–300 mg (in miliary TB 10 mg/kg)	(5 mg/kg) (10 mg/kg)
Pyrazinamide	>50 kg 2 g (25 mg/kg max 2 g) <50 kg 1.5 g	(35 mg/kg, max 3 g)
Ethambutol	25 mg/kg in initial phase,	(30 mg/kg) 15 mg/kg in continuation phase

Under DOTs following treatment regimen is used

Indication		Intensive phase		Continuation phase	
		Drugs	Duration	Drug	Duration
Category I	New sputum smear positive New sputum smear negative New extra-pulmonary tuberculosis	Isoniazid rifampicin, pyrazinamide and ethambutol	Thrice weekly for 2 months	Isoniazid and rifampicin	Thrice weekly for 4 months
Category II	Sputum smear positive Sputum smear-positive failure Sputum smear-positive treatment after default	Isoniazid rifampicin, pyrazinamide, ethambutol and streptomycin	Thrice weekly for 2 months followed by		
		Isoniazid rifampicin, pyrazinamide and, ethambutol	For 1 months	Isoniazid rifampicin and pyrazinamide	5 months

Second line anti-tuberculous Drugs

Drug	Dose
Streptomycin	20–40 mg/kg/day od im
Kanamycin	15–30 mg/kg/day od im
Amikacin	15–22.5 mg/kg/day od im
Capreomycin	15–30 mg/kg/day od im
Ofloxacin	15–20 mg/kg/day bd orally
levofloxacin	7.5–10 mg/kg/day od orally
Moxifloxacin	7.5–10 mg/kg/day orally
Ethionamide	15–20 mg/kg/day bd orally
Prothionamide	15–20 mg/kg/day bd orally
Cycloserine*	10–20 mg/kg/day od or bd orally
PAS'	150 mg/kg/day bd or tds orally

*Cycloserine and 'PAS are bacteriostatic others are bactericidal.

Treatment Regimen under RNTCP for MDR-TB (Multi-drug resistant TB) and XDR-TB (Extensively drug resistant TB)

♦ *For MDR-TB:*
  • *Six drugs in intensive phase for 6–9 months:* Kanamycin, levofloxacin, ethionamide, cycloserine, pyrazinamide and ethambutol.
  • *Four drugs in continuation phase for 18 months:* Levofloxacin, ethionamide, cycloserine and ethambutol.
  • Reserve drug is p-aminosalicylic acid.
♦ *For XDR-TB:*
  • Seven drugs in intensive phase for 6–12 months: Capreomycin, p-aminosalicylic acid, moxifloxacin, high dose isoniazid, clofazimine, linezolid, Amoxicillin and clavulanic acid.

- *Six drugs in continuation phase for 18 months:* p-aminosalicylic acid, moxifloxacin, high dose Isoniazid, clofazimine, linezolid, amoxicillin and clavulanic acid.
- *Reserve drugs:* Clarithromycin, thiacetazone
- *Corticosteroids:* They are to be given in the severe cases to enable them to survive till antitubercular drugs become effective. Oral prednisolone is given in doses of 20 mg orally for 6 to 8 weeks. Steroids produce euphoria and increase appetite in the patients.
- *Surgery:* Surgical resection of infected lobe is feasible.
- *Symptomatic treatment:*
  - *Cough:* If it is irritative, linctus codeine is given. Smoking should be stopped
  - *Laryngitis:* Rest is given to the voice. If pain is present anesthetic powders, spray and lozenges are given.

Q.13. **Enumerate bacterial lesions with oral manifestations. Describe syphilis in detail.** *(Sep 2018, 5 Marks)*

Ans.

Enumeration of Bacterial Lesions with Oral Manifestations

Name of the bacterial lesion	Oral Manifestations
Syphilis	*For details refer to Ans. 1 of same chapter*
Leprosy	*For details refer to Ans. 2 of same chapter*
Tuberculosis	*For details refer to Ans. 7 of same chapter*
Actinomycosis	• It enters tissue via oral mucus membrane and may either remain localized to adjacent soft tissue or spread to salivary gland, bone or skin of face and neck. • Trismus can also occur before formation of the pus. • It leads to swelling and induration of tissue. It can develop into single or multiple abscess which discharge on skin surface liberating pus consisting of sulfur granules. • There is also presence of non-healing tooth socket, exuberant granular tissue and periosteal thickening of alveolus. • Skin present over the abscess is purple red. • Presence of sinus is there, via which abscess is drained. Now abscesses are formed which can perforate via skin surface. • There is also disfigurement of face. Infection of maxilla and mandible is present. • Formation of periapical granuloma is also noted. • If lesion occurs on tongue, it is a painful nodule which ulcerates. If case becomes chronic tongue also becomes fixed.
Scarlet fever	• Main oral manifestation is stomatitis scarlatina. • Mucosa over the palate appears to be congested. Ulceration can also occur on the palate. • At face mainly the temporal region and cheeks become flushed and red, pale area of circumoral pallor is also seen around the mouth.

Contd...

Contd...

Name of the bacterial lesion	Oral Manifestations
	• Tongue consists of white coating and fungiform papillae become edematous and hyperemic projecting above the surface of tongue as small red knobs known as strawberry tongue. • As coating of the tongue get lost, tip of the tongue and its lateral margins along with organ become deep red, glistening and smooth except for swollen hyperemic papilla. Now in this state tongue is also known as raspberry tongue. • Presence of hypoplasia of teeth is seen in permanent teeth
Diphtheria	• There is formation of patchy "diphtheritic membrane" which start on the tonsils and enlarges becoming confluent over the surface. This is thick and gray in color. • The membrane tends to adhere and leave raw bleeding surface on removal. • There is also presence of temporary paralysis of soft palate at 3rd and 5th week of disease.
NOMA	• Areas of stagnation are seen around fixed bridge or crown. • Small ulcers of gingival mucosa spread rapidly and involve surrounding tissue of jaws, lips and cheek by gangrenous necrosis. • Lesion has foul odor. • In the jaw, large masses may be sloughed out leaving the jaws exposed.
Tularemia	• It is seen commonly on soft palate, tongue, gingiva and at the angle of mouth. • There is presence of ulcer which is shallow with white fibrinous pseudomembrane formation. • Generalized stomatitis is present.
Tetanus	• Presence of rigidity of muscle of mastication. • Rigidity of facial muscles may occur, producing typical risus sardonicus. Here corners of mouth are drawn back with protruded lip, wrinkling of forehead is not possible. • Patient complaints of difficulty in chewing and swallowing, in edentulous cases patient is unable to insert denture. • As there is increase in the spasm of muscle of mastication, jaw become locked and trismus occur
Lymphogranu-loma venereum	• It occurs because of orogenital contact or anti-inoculation. • Tongue is the most common site involved. • Appearance of lesion is small, slightly painful superficial ulceration with non-indurated borders appear on lip. • In chronic cases, a zone of cicatricial refraction, dark red area along with loss of superficial epithelium or opaque lichenoid grayish papules.

Contd...

Contd...

Name of the bacterial lesion	Oral Manifestations
	• Tongue can also get enlarged along with areas of scarring and grooves over its dorsal surface. • There is also presence of dysphagia, red soft palate and small granulomatous lesions accompanied by regional lymphadenopathy.
Gonorrhea	Pharyngeal gonorrhea is a condition which occurs in homosexuals and heterosexuals, pregnant women which practice oral sex. Patient also has sore throat and pharyngitis. In gonococcal stomatitis, there is multiple painful, round elevated gray white eroded spots, with/without the pseudomembrane formation. There is development of acute gingivitis around extraction site in patients who practice fellation repeatedly for days after dental extraction. Gingiva becomes erythematous, with/without necrosis. Painful acute ulcerations develop on lips which limits its motion. Tongue may present red, dry ulcerations or become glazed and swollen with painful erosion with same lesion in buccal mucosa and palate. *Gonococcus* involving articulating joint. There is presence of difficulty in jaw movement due to pain and swelling of both TMJs.

Syphilis in Detail

Syphilis is also known as Lues.

Syphilis is caused by *Treponema pallidum* which is a spirochete, it is characterized by gram-positive, motile, microaerophilic microorganism.

Mode of Transmission

♦ Sexual contact with infectious person.
♦ Person, such as dentist who working on an infected patient in contagious stage.
♦ Transplacental transmission, i.e., from mother to fetus in utero.
♦ Due to infected blood transfusion.
♦ Break in the skin which comes in contact with infectious lesion.

Stages of Development

Syphilis is mainly classified as:
1. Acquired syphilis: It manifest in three stages:
   a. Primary
   b. Secondary
   c. Tertiary
2. Congenital syphilis

Clinical Features

Primary Syphilis

♦ This start as painless papule which can be single or multiple, with 5 mm to several centimeters in size and later on causes ulcer.

♦ Primary lesion occurs after 3 weeks at site of transmission after initial exposure. Primary lesion is known as chancre.
♦ Chancre is a painless ulcer which show dark pink color along with erythematous margin, punched out base, raised indurated roller edges with button like consistency and non-bleeding.
♦ Lesion is seen on genital organs and other extra-genital organ, such as fingers, lips, tongue, palate, gingiva, tonsil and oropharynx.
♦ Enlargement and non-tenderness on regional lymph node is seen.
♦ Lesion heals under 4 to 6 weeks and lymphadenopathy can persist for months.

Secondary Syphilis

♦ It is seen during 4 to 10 weeks after appearance of primary lesion.
♦ At this stage, spirochetes multiply and spread to entire body, it can also involve palm, sole and oral mucosa.
♦ There is also presence of malaise, headache, sore throat, headache, weight loss, fever, painless lymphadenopathy and musculoskeletal pain.
♦ Mucocutaneous lesions are present as macular, pustular, papular, papulosquamous and annular.
♦ Macule is a round, discrete, nonpruritic, symmetric, reddish brown in color. It is 5 mm or small in diameter and distributed on trunk and proximal extremities.
♦ There are also focal painless region which are smooth, silvery gray erosion with erythematous margin. Lesions undergo necrosis with slough and are referred to as mucous patches. It is visible on palate, tongue, buccal mucosa and tonsils. As mucus patches get coalesce they give rise to snail track ulcer.
♦ Split papule is double papule which occur at skin fold and commissure of lip which.
♦ Condyloma lata is usually a painless, papillary lesion which commonly develops at warm and moist sites, e.g., uvula, scrotum, inner thigh and axilla.
♦ Alopecia is present which is characterized by patchy loss of hair over the scalp and face including eyebrows.
♦ Leus maligna is present which is characterized by fever, headache and muscle pain which is followed by necrotic ulceration which involves both face and scalp.
♦ There is presence of generalized painless lymphadenopathy.
♦ Lesion heals in 3 to 12 weeks, but exacerbation may occur during month or several years.
♦ After secondary syphilis, patient enters the period free of lesions as well as symptoms which is known as latent stage of syphilis. It last from 1 to 30 years. Now tertiary syphilis develops.

Tertiary Syphilis

♦ It usually manifest as gumma, cardiovascular syphilis, neurosyphilis and as ocular lesions.
♦ Gumma is considered to be the scattered active foci of granulomatous inflammation over skin, oral mucosa, upper respiratory tract, stomach, liver and larynx. Gumma appears as indurated nodular or ulcerative lesion that leads

to extensive tissue destruction and its size varies from millimeters to centimeters.

♦ Cardiovascular syphilis is rare and appear after 20 or more years of the infection. Most common is aortitis, aortic aneurysm, aortic valvulitis with regurgitation and stenosis of coronary ostia.

♦ In neurosyphilis, there is tabes dorsalis, general paresis, psychosis, dementia and death.

♦ Ocular lesions are chorioretinitis, iritis and Argyll–Robertson pupil.

Congenital Syphilis

For details, refer to Ans. 3 of same chapter.

Oral Manifestation of Syphilis

For details, refer to Ans. 1 of same chapter.

Histopathology

♦ Both primary and secondary syphilis show same features except the surface epithelium which is ulcerated in primary syphilis and can be ulcerated or hyperplastic in secondary syphilis.

♦ Underlying lamina propria show increase in the number of vascular channels and an intense chronic inflammatory reaction is present. Inflammatory infiltrate consists of lymphocytes and plasma cells and often shows perivascular infiltration of inflammatory cells.

♦ In secondary syphilis, ulceration is not present and surface epithelium often shows hyperplasia with significant spongiosis and exocytosis.

♦ Oral tertiary syphilitic lesion exhibits the surface ulceration with peripheral pseudoepitheliomatous hyperplasia. Inflammatory infiltrate show granulomatous inflammation with collection of histiocytes and multinucleated giant cells.

♦ Silver impregnation technique, such as Warthin–Starry or steiner stains on the immunoperoxidase reactions are directed against the organisms show scattered corkscrew, such as spirochaetal organisms inside the surface epithelium.

Laboratory Diagnosis

♦ Demonstration of *T. pallidum* via dark field examination

♦ Non-specific and not highly sensitive serologic screening tests:
   1. VDRL test
   2. Rapid plasma regain test (RPR)

♦ Specific tests
   Treponemal tests
   1. Using killed *T. pallidum*
      – Fluorescent treponemal antibody-absorption (FTA-ABS) test
      – *T. pallidum* agglutination (TPA) test
      – *T. pallidum* immune adherence (TPIA) test
   2. Using *T. pallidum* extract
      – *Treponema pallidum* hemagglutination assay (TPHA)
      – Microtiter hemagglutination —*T. pallidum* (MHA-TP) test

   – *Treponema pallidum* particle agglutination (TP-PA)
   – Western blot
   – Enzyme immunoassay (EIA)
   3. Using live *T. pallidum*: *Treponema pallidum* immobilization (TPI) test

Treatment

♦ Single dose of parenteral long acting benzathine penicillin G is given.

♦ For latent or tertiary syphilis, intramuscular penicillin should be given weekly for 3 weeks.

Q.14. Write short answer on Hutchinson's teeth.
(Oct 2019, 3 Marks)

Ans. Hutchinson's teeth are seen in syphilis as syphilitic hypoplasia.

Teeth involved as Hutchinson's teeth are maxillary and mandibular permanent incisors.

Hutchinson incisors exhibit crowns which are like straight edge screw driver shaped with greatest circumference present in the middle one-third of crown and a constricted incisal edge. Both mesial and the distal surfaces of crown are tapering as well as converging towards the incisal edge of tooth, rather than towards the cervix. Additionally, incisal edge shows central hypoplastic notch. Main reason of notching is absence of central tubercle or calcification center.

Hutchinson's teeth can show barrel shaped outline.

7. VIRAL INFECTIONS OF ORAL CAVITY

Q.1. Write short note on clinical features of AIDS.
(Sep 2004, 5 Marks)

Ans. AIDS is predominantly lethal type of viral infection caused by the HIV and is characterized by the depletion of T4 lymphocytes in the body.

Clinical staging of AIDS is done by WHO in 1990 and is revised on 2007. So based on the clinical staging following are the clinical features of AIDS.

In Primary HIV Infection

♦ Patient is asymptomatic

♦ There is presence of acute retroviral syndrome, i.e., presence of sore throat, fever, maculopapular rash, headache, myalgia, arthralgia, photophobia.

Clinical Stage I

♦ Patient remains asymptomatic

♦ Presence of generalized lymphadenopathy

Clinical Stage II

♦ Presence of unexplained weight loss, i.e., less than 10% of body weight.

♦ Presence of recurrent respiratory infections

- Herpes zoster or shingles
- Presence of minor mucocutaneous diseases, i.e., aphthous ulcers, pruritic eruptions, etc.

Clinical Stage III

- Presence of severe weight loss, i.e., greater than 10% of body weight.
- Presence of diarrhea more than a month.
- Presence of pyrexia of unknown origin for more than one month.
- Presence of oral candidiasis which is persistant
- Pulmonary tuberculosis since last two years
- Multiple bacterial infections
- Presence of acute necrotizing ulcerative gingivitis and acute necrotizing ulcerative periodontitis.

Clinical stage IV

- There is presence of HIV wasting syndrome
- Pneumocystis pneumonia.
- Presence of herpes simplex infection for more than a month.
- Candidiasis extends to esophagus.
- Presence of extrapulmonary tuberculosis
- Kaposi's sarcoma
- HIV encephalopathy.

Q.2. Classify viral lesions of oral cavity. Describe in detail herpes simplex. *(Feb 2006, 6.5 Marks)*

Or

Write short note on herpes simplex.

(Sep 2007, 3 Marks)

Or

Write short note on herpes simplex viral infection.

(Nov 2008, 5 Marks)

Ans.

Classifications of Viral Lesions in Oral Cavity

The classification depends on the presence of the major viruses.

I. RNA Virus

- Orthomyxovirus, i.e., influenza
- Paramyxovirus, i.e., measles and mumps
- Rhabdovirus, i.e., rabies
- Arena virus, i.e., Lassa fever
- Calicivirus, i.e., upper respiratory tract infection
- Coronavirus
- Bunyavirus
- Picornavirus
- Reovirus
- Togavirus
- Retrovirus

II. DNA Virus

- *Herpes virus:*
  - Herpes simplex
  - Herpes zoster
  - Epstein-Barr virus

- *Poxvirus*
  - Smallpox
  - Monkeypox
  - Adenovirus, i.e., pharyngoconjunctival fever
  - Parvovirus
  - Iridovirus
  - Papovavirus, i.e., papillomas.

Primary Herpes Simplex Infection

It is also known as acute herpetic gingivostomatitis or infectious stomatitis or herpes labialis.

Pathogenesis

As the herpes virus enters in sensory autonomic nerve endings and remain latent in ganglia. Replication of virus occurs and it spread to the mucosal as well as skin surfaces by centrifugal distribution of virions through peripheral nerves.

Etiology

- It occurs during close personal contact, i.e., by sexual contact or kissing.
- Primary infection of newborn is caused by vaginal secretion during birth.
- Dentist may experience primary lesion of finger from contact with the lesion of mouth and saliva of patient who are asymptomatic carrier of HSV also known as herpetic whitlow.
- In cadence varies according to socioeconomic group.

Clinical Features

- It is seen in children as well as young adults.
- Incubation period of virus lies from 5–7 days.
- Patient complains of irritability, fever, headache, nausea, vomiting and pain in oral cavity.
- Cervical and submandibular lymph nodes are enlarged.

Oral Manifestations

- In oral cavity hard palate, tongue and gingiva are commonly involved.
- Oral symptoms are flattening of mucosa, followed by vesicle formation over keratinized mucosa.
- The vesicle consists of clear fluid and rupture to leave multiple, small and shallow painful ulcers these are followed by diffuse, large, whitish ulcers which are surrounded by red ring of inflammation.
- Ulcer is about 2 to 5 mm in diameter. Base of the ulcer is coated with grayish white or yellowish membrane.
- Excoriation of lip is seen with hemorrhage.
- Speech of patient become painful and difficult.
- Generalized acute marginal gingivitis is present. Gingiva become edematous as well as swollen.
- Small ulcers are seen over gingiva.
- Inflammation is present over posterior part of pharynx and patient feels difficulty in swallowing.
- Patient also suffers from myalgia or muscle soreness and difficulty in mastication.

Histopathology

- Infected cells are swollen have pale eosinophilic cytoplasm and large vesicular nuclei known as ballooning degeneration.
- Acantholysis is seen and acantholytic cells are known as Tzanck cells.
- Some of the cells contain intranuclear inclusion bodies known as Lipschutz bodies.
- Lipschutz bodies are eosinophilic, ovoid, homogenous structures in the nucleus which displaces nucleolus and nuclear chromatin peripherally.
- Multinucleated epithelial cells are formed when fusion occur between adjacent cells.
- Intercellular edema is present which leads to the development of intraepithelial vesicle.
- Underlying connective tissue stroma shows chronic inflammatory infiltrate.

Treatment

- Symptomatic treatment is done.
- Patient should be kept on antiviral therapy.

Recurrent or Secondary Herpes Simplex Infection

It is of two types:
1. Recurrent herpes labialis.
2. Recurrent Intraoral herpes.

Pathogenesis

As primary infection is over, virus can no longer recover from the ganglion and viral DNA is seen in ganglionic cells. Humoral and cell mediated immunity is responsible for the recurrence of the disease.

Etiology/Trigger Factors

- Any surgery which involves trigeminal ganglion leads to recurrent herpes.
- Low immunity leads to recurrent herpes.
- Trauma as in exodontias can precipitate recurrent herpes.
- Upper respiratory infection can lead to recurrent herpes.
- Other factors which lead to recurrent herpes are fatigue, pregnancy, fever, menstruation, etc.

Clinical Features

- Recurrent herpes occur at varying intervals.
- Patient complains of tingling and burning sensation, feeling of toughness and soreness before development of vesicle.
- Edema is seen at the site of lesion and is followed by development of multiple clusters of vesicles.

Oral Manifestations

- In recurrent herpes labialis grayish or whitish vesicles are seen which rupture and leave small red ulcers. There is presence of very slight erythematous halo over the lip which is covered by brown-colored crustation. Size of crust is 1 to 4 mm in diameter.
- In intraoral type vesicles are seen which rupture and leave small red ulcers with very slight erythematous halo.

Treatment

- Trigger factors should be suppressed or removed.
- Antiviral therapy should be given.

Q.3. Describe etiology, histopathology and clinical features of acute herpetic gingivostomatitis.

(Mar 2000, 15 Marks)

Or

Write short note on primary herpetic gingivostomatitis. *(Sep 2005, 5 Marks)*

Ans. *For etiology, histopathology and clinical features, refer to Ans. 2 of same chapter.*

Q.4. Write short answer on herpes zoster.

(Apr 2019, 3 Marks)

Or

Write short note on herpes zoster.

(Jan 2018, 5 Marks) (Feb 2019, 5 Marks)

Ans. It is also called as shingles or zona.

It is an acute infectious viral disease of extremely painful and incapacitating nature, characterized by inflammation of dorsal root ganglion.

Clinical Features

- It affects males and females with same frequency.
- There is prodromal period of 2 to 4 days in which shooting pain, paresthesia, burning and tenderness appears along the course of affected nerve.
- It may be found on buccal mucosa, tongue, uvula, pharynx and larynx.
- Trigeminal herpes zoster occur during tooth formation causes pulpal necrosis and internal root resorption.
- First branch of trigeminal is most commonly affected.

Oral Manifestations

- Herpes zoster may involve the face by infection of trigeminal nerve, mainly first branch.
- There is usually involvement of skin and oral mucosa supplied by trigeminal nerve.
- Lesions of the oral mucosa are extremely painful vesicles which may be found on the buccal mucosa, tongue, pharynx, larynx and uvula.
- This vesicle generally ruptures and leaves the area of erosion.
- Erosive ulcers heal up in a few days without scar formation.
- In herpes zoster, neuralgic pain in oral cavity stimulates tooth ache.
- Pain may persist long after the lesion heals up and the condition is known as postherpetic neuralgia.

Histopathology

- Herpes zoster is histologically characterized by swelling of infected epithelial cell cytoplasm due to intercellular edema (Ballooning degeneration).
- Margination of nuclear chromatin and formation of intra nuclear inclusion bodies.

- Reticular degeneration of epithelial cells along with the presence of multiple multinucleated giant cells.

Treatment

Antiviral drugs, such as acyclovir is given along with antibiotics to prevent secondary infection.

Q.5. Write short note on aphthous ulcers.
(Apr 2015, 3 Marks) (Apr 2007, 5 Marks)
Or
Write note on aphthous stomatitis.
(Feb 2013, 5 Marks)
Or
Write short note on aphthous stomatitis.
(June 2015, 5 Marks)
Or
Write short answer on aphthous ulcer.
(Apr 2019, 3 Marks)
Or
Write in brief aphthous ulcers.
(Sep 2018, 5 Marks)
Or
Write short answer on aphthous stomatitis.
(Sep 2018, 3 Marks)
Or
Write short note on recurrent aphthous stomatitis.
(Feb 2019, 5 Marks)

Ans. Aphthous ulcer or aphthous stomatitis is a common disease characterized by painful, recurrent, solitary or multiple ulcerations of oral mucosa with no other signs of any other disease.

Etiology

- **Bacterial infection:** Alfa hemolytic *Streptococcus* and *S. sanguis* has implicated as causative agent of disease.
- **Immunological abnormalities:** IgG and IgM binding of epithelial cells of spinous layer of oral mucosa is seen in patients suffering from recurrent aphthous ulcer.
- Iron deficiency or folic acid deficiency.
- Hematological deficiencies, serum iron or vitamin B12 deficiency.
- **Allergic factors:** Patients may have history of asthma, hay fever and food or drug allergy.

Clinical Features

- It occurs between second and third decades of life and females are more commonly infected.
- Clinically aphthous ulcer occur in three types, i.e.:
  1. *Minor aphthous ulcer:*
     - It is a single lesion or in cluster of 1 to 5 lesions.
     - Ulcers are painful, shallow, round or elliptical in shape and measure 0.5 cm in diameter.
     - They develop over lips, soft palate, anterior fauces, floor of mouth and ventral surface of tongue.

- Lesion is usually surrounded by an erythematous and is covered by yellowish, fibrous membrane.
  2. *Major aphthous ulcer:*
     - They are large and much painful lesions and measure 1 to 5 cm in diameter.
     - They are most severe and often makes patient ill.
     - Only one and two lesions develops at the time and mostly seen over lips, soft palate and fauces.
     - Lesions heal slowly and leaves scars, which result in decreased mobility of uvula and tongue.
  3. *Herpetic ulcer:*
     - They are multiple, small, shallow ulcers around 100 in number.
     - Lesions are painful than would be suspected by their size.
     - They are found on any intraoral mucosal surface.
     - They are present continuously for 1 to 3 years, with relatively short remissions.

Histopathology

- Fibrinopurulent membrane covers the ulcerated area.
- Intense inflammatory cell infiltrate is present in connective tissue beneath the ulcer with considerable necrosis of tissue near the surface of lesion.
- Neutrophils are predominant below the ulcer.
- Epithelial proliferation along the margins of lesion.
- Cells are present with elongated nuclei containing linear bar of chromatin with radiating process of chromatin extending towards nuclear membrane known as Anitschkow cells.

Treatment

Topical and systemic administration of steroids is beneficial.

Q.6. Enumerate ulcerative lesions of oral cavity. Describe etiology, histopathology and clinical features of aphthous stomatitis. *(Feb 1999, 15 Marks)*
Or
Enumerate ulcerative lesions of oral cavity, describe histopathology and clinical features of aphthous stomatitis. *(Dec 2009, 15 Marks)*
Or
Describe etiology, histopathology and clinical features of acute aphthous stomatitis. *(Mar 2001, 15 Marks)*

Ans.

Classification of Ulcerative Lesions

I. Microbial Origin

- **Bacterial:**
  - Streptococcal
  - Tuberculosis
  - Syphilis
  - Scarlet fever
  - Diphtheria
  - Typhoid
  - Noma

♦ **Fungal:**
- Histoplasmosis
- Blastomycosis
- Paracoccidioidomycosis
- Coccidioidomycosis
- *Cryptococcus*
- Zygomycosis
- Aspergillosis

♦ **Viral:**
- Herpes
- HIV
- Poxvirus

♦ **Protozoal:**
- *Entamoeba histolytica*
- Leishmaniasis
- Toxoplasmosis.

II. Physical Origin

♦ Cheek bite (Morsicatio Buccarum)
♦ Traumatic
♦ Thermal
♦ Electrical
♦ Osteoradionecrosis
♦ Anesthetic.

III. Chemical Origin

♦ Phenol
♦ Silver nitrate
♦ Hydrogen peroxide
♦ Aspirin.

IV. Immunological

♦ Behcet's syndrome
♦ Reiter's syndrome
♦ Erythema multiforme
♦ Erosive lichen planus (Secondary ulcer)
♦ Lupus erythematosus
♦ Sarcoidosis
♦ Cyclic neutropenia
♦ Ulcerative colitis
♦ HIV
♦ Pemphigus
♦ Epidermolysis bullosa

V. Metabolic Ulcers

♦ Diabetes
♦ Uremia
♦ Neutropenia
♦ Sickle cell anemia
♦ Agranulocytosis
♦ Crohn's disease.

VI. Nonspecific Ulcers

♦ HIV ulcers
♦ Graft Vs host reaction
♦ Necrotizing sialometaplasia
♦ Reynaud's phenomenon
♦ Bacterial angiomatosis

VII. Neoplastic

♦ Squamous cell carcinoma

For etiology, histopathology and clinical features of aphthous stomatitis, refer to Ans. 5 of same chapter.

Q.7. Write short note on mumps. *(Mar 2001, 5 Marks)*

Ans. It is an acute contagious viral infection, characterized by unilateral or bilateral swelling of salivary glands, but also affects testis, meninges, pancreas, heart and mammary glands.

Etiology

♦ It is caused by paramyxovirus.
♦ It spreads from human reservoir by air-borne infection of infected saliva and possibly urine.

Clinical Features

♦ It is seen between age of 5 to 15 years.
♦ It is most common in boys.
♦ It is preceded by onset of headache, chills, moderate fever, vomiting and pain below ear which lasts for one week.
♦ Parotid gland is most common site.
♦ Elongation of parotid gland causes elevation of ear lobule and produces pain on mastication especially while eating sore food.
♦ Papilla on opening of parotid duct is puffy and reddened.

Histopathology

♦ Microscopic section of diseased tissue reveals presence of degenerative changes in ductal epithelium of salivary gland.
♦ Interstitial infiltration of lymphocyte and mononuclear cells in glandular lobes and in few acinar atrophy occur.

Treatment

Only symptomatic treatment is done.

Q.8. Discuss in detail about clinical features, histopathology and laboratory investigations of oral herpes simplex infection. *(Jun 2010, 15 Marks)*

Ans. *For clinical features and histopathology, refer to Ans. 2 of same chapter.*

Laboratory Investigations

♦ **Tzanck smear:** It is a rapid, sensitive and inexpensive diagnostic method. Smears are prepared from the lesions, from the base of vesicles and is stained with 1% solution of toluidine blue for 15 seconds. Smear shows multinucleated giant cells with faceted nuclei and ground glass chromatin, i.e., Tzanck cells.
♦ In giemsa stained smears Type A inclusion bodies are seen.
♦ Electron microscopy show virus particle.
♦ Fluorescent antibody techniques show herpes virus antigen in smears and sections.
♦ ELISA is a serological test which helps in the detection of rise in titer of antibodies. It helps in detection in primary infection.
♦ **Virus Isolation:** The isolation of herpes virus can be done and can be identified by various systems.

Q.9. Enumerate viral lesions occurring in oral cavity. Discuss oral manifestation of herpes simplex infection. *(Aug 2012, 15 Marks)*

Ans. *For enumeration of viral lesions and oral manifestations of herpes simplex infection, refer to Ans. 2 of same chapter.*

Q.10. Describe in brief oral manifestations of AIDS.
(June 2015, 5 Marks) (Apr 2008, 10 Marks)

Or

Write short answer on oral manifestations of HIV diseases. *(May 2018, 3 Marks)*

Or

Write short note on oral manifestations of AIDS.
(Sep 2018, 5 Marks)

Or

Write short answer on most commonly associated oral manifestations of HIV infection.
(Feb 2019, 3 Marks)

Ans. Following are the oral manifestations of AIDS:

Classification of Oral Manifestations by EC-Clearing house

Group 1: Strongly associated with HIV infection
- *Candidiasis:* Erythematous, pseudomembranous, angular cheilitis
- Hairy leukoplakia
- Kaposi's sarcoma
- Non-Hodgkin's lymphoma
- *Periodontal diseases:* Linear gingival erythema, necrotizing gingivitis, necrotizing periodontitis

Group 2: Less commonly associated with HIV infection
- *Bacterial infections: Mycobacterium avium*—intracellular, *Mycobacterium tuberculosis*
- Melanotic hyperpigmentation
- Necrotizing ulcerative stomatitis
- *Salivary gland disease:* Dry mouth, unilateral or bilateral swelling of major salivary glands.
- Thrombocytopenia purpura
- Oral ulcerations NOS (not otherwise specified)
- *Viral infections:* Herpes simplex, human papilloma virus, varicella-zoster

Group 3: Seen in HIV infection
- *Bacterial infections: Actinomyces israelii, Escherichia coli, Klebsiella,* pneumonia.
- Cat-scratch disease (Bartonella henselae).
- Epithelioid (bacillary) angiomatosis (*Bartonella henselae*)
- *Drug reactions:* Ulcerative, erythema multiforme, lichenoid, toxic epidermolysis.
- *Fungal infections other than candidiasis: Cryptococcus neoformans, Geotrichum candidum, Histoplasma capsulatum, Mucoraceae* (Mucormycosis/Zygomycosis), *Aspergillus flavus.*
- *Neurologic disturbances:* Facial palsy, trigeminal neuralgia
- Recurrent aphthous stomatitis.
- *Viral infections: Cytomegalovirus,* Molluscum contagiosum.

Description of Oral Manifestations

- Candidiasis is the most common oral manifestation of HIV infection. All the three types, i.e., erythematous, pseudomembranous and hyperplastic forms are seen. Erythematous candidiasis is seen when the CD4 count drops below 400 cells/mm^3 and pseudomembranous develop when CD4 count drop below 200 cells/mm^3.
- *Hairy leukoplakia:* Presence of soft painless plaque on the lateral border of tongue with corrugated surface.
- *Kaposi's sarcoma:* Single or multiple bluish swellings are seen with or without ulceration over gingiva and palate.
- *Angular cheilitis:* Linear fissures or linear ulcers are seen at the angle of mouth.
- *Linear gingival erythema:* It is fiery red band along the gingival margin and attached gingiva with profuse bleeding.
- *Necrotizing ulcerative gingivitis:* Destruction of interdental papillae is seen.
- *Necrotizing ulcerative periodontitis:* There is advanced necrotic destruction of periodontium, rapid bone loss, loss of periodontal ligament and sequestration.
- *Oral ulcerations:* Single or multiple major recurrent aphthous ulcers are seen with white pseudomembrane surrounding the erythematous halo.
- *Non-Hodgkin's lymphoma:* It is the malignancy of HIV infected individuals. It occurs in extranodal locations and CNS is the common site. Intraosseous involvement is also seen.
- *Mycobacterial infection:* Mycobacterial infection in form of tuberculosis is seen. When present tongue is affected most commonly. Affected areas show common ulcerations.
- *Herpes simplex virus:* Recurrent or secondary herpes simplex infection is seen in the patients. Herpes simplex lesions increase when CD4 cell count drops below 50 cells/mm^3.
- *Herpes zoster:* It is common in HIV infected individuals. Orally, involvement is severe and leads to sequestration of bone as well as loss of teeth.
- *Histoplasmosis:* It is the fungal infection caused by histoplasma capsulatum. Sign and symptoms of disease are fever, weight loss, splenomegaly and pulmonary infiltrate.
- *Molluscum contagiosum:* It is caused by poxvirus. Lesions are small, waxy, dome-shaped papules which demonstrate central depressed crater.

Q.11. Write short note on herpes stomatitis.
(June 2014, 5 Marks)

Ans. This is a contagious viral infection, which produces ulceration and inflammation of mouth and gums.

It is a contagious viral illness caused by herpes simplex virus (HSV-1).

This condition is probably a child's first exposure to the herpes virus.

Clinical Features

- Occur in children of 2 to 4 years.
- Irritability and refusal of food due to difficulty in swallowing.

- High fever
- Vesicles on the tongue, buccal mucosa, gums and skin around the mouth. The ulcers are very painful.
- Mucosa becomes red, swollen and bleeds easily.
- Vesicles breakdown to form ulcers.
- Secondary bacterial infection may occur with enlarged lymph nodes and difficulty in swallowing.
- It is self-limiting and lasts between 7 to 10 days.

Prevention

Approximately 80% of the population carry the HSV which makes it difficult to prevent children contacting the virus. Parents should avoid kissing their children when they have a cold sore. Also avoid sharing glasses, food and utensils.

Complication

A secondary herpes infection of the eye may occur, i.e., herpetic keratoconjunctivitis.

Treatment

- Acyclovir, which fights the virus causing the infection.
- A mostly liquid diet of cool/cold nonacidic drinks.
- Numbing medicine (viscous lidocaine) applied to the mouth if there is severe pain.

8. FUNGAL INFECTIONS OF ORAL CAVITY

Q.1. Enumerate fungal lesions of oral cavity. Describe clinical features, histopathology and investigation of oral candidiasis. *(Dec 2010, 18 Marks)*

Or

Describe in brief moniliasis. *(May/June 2009, 5 Marks)*

Or

Write short note on candidiasis.

(Jan 2016, 5 Marks) (Feb 2019, 5 Marks)

Or

Write short note on oral candidiasis.

(Mar 2001, 5 Marks)

Ans.

Fungal Lesion of Oral Cavity

Fungal lesions affecting oral tissues are:
- Candidiasis
- Coccidioidomycosis
- Histoplasmosis
- Blastomycosis
- Paracoccidioidomycosis
- Sporotrichosis
- Chromomycosis and phaeomycotic abscess
- Aspergillosis
- Cryptococcosis
- Zygomycosis

- Mycetoma.
  - Candidiasis is the disease caused by the fungus called as *Candida albicans*.
  - Oral involvement is probably most common manifestation.

Etiology

- Hormonal disturbances
- Local or systemic steroid therapy
- Xerostomia
- Poor oral hygiene
- Denture wearing
- Heavy smoking
- Prolong antibiotic therapy.
- Nutritional deficiency, e.g., vitamin A and vitamin B6.

Clinical Features

- Common sites are roof of mouth, retromolar area and mucobuccal fold.
- It is more common in women.
- Prodromal symptom is rapid onset of bad taste. Spicy food causes discomfort.
- There is presence of inflammation, erythema and painful eroded areas may be associated with this disease.
- White patches of candidiasis are easily wiped out with wet gauge which leaves erythematous area or atrophic area.
- Deeper invasion by the organism leaves an ulcerative lesion upon removal of patch.

1. **Acute Pseudomembranous Candidiasis**
   - Common sites are roof of mouth, retromolar area and mucobuccal fold.
   - It is more common in women.
   - Prodromal symptom is rapid onset of bad taste. Spicy food causes discomfort.
   - There is presence of inflammation, erythema and painful eroded areas may be associated with this disease.
   - White patches of candidiasis are easily wiped out with wet gauge which leaves erythematous or atrophic area.
   - Deeper invasion by the organism leaves an ulcerative lesion upon removal of patch.

2. **Acute Atrophic Candidiasis**
   - It can be seen anywhere in the oral cavity but most commonly site involved are tongue as well as the tissue underlying prosthesis.
   - It appears as an erythematous area.
   - Patient complains of burning sensation in lesional area along with vague pain.

3. **Chronic Hyperplastic Candidiasis**
   - Male predilection is seen.
   - Most common in heavy smokers.
   - Oral sites involved are tongue, cheek and lips.
   - There is presence of firm and white leathery plaques.
   - Lesion cannot be rubbed with the lateral pressure. Lesion is whitish or creamy whitish in color. Borders of the lesion are vague.

Histopathology

♦ Epithelium show increase thickness of parakeratin at lesional area in conjunction with elongation of rete ridges.

♦ Small collection of neutrophils, i.e., microabscess is seen in parakeratin layer and superficial spinous layer.

♦ Hyphae or mycelia and yeast cells are seen in parakeratin layer of epithelium.

♦ There is presence of chronic inflammatory infiltrate cells, such as lymphocytes and plasma cells immediately subjacent to infected epithelium.

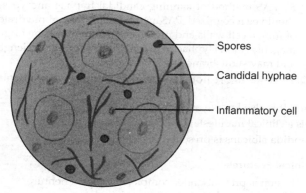

Fig. 76: Candida albicans *(For color version, see Plate 13).*

Treatment

♦ Topical and systemic administration of nystatin is done.

♦ In immunosuppressed patients systemic administration of amphotericin B and fluconazole is given.

♦ Improvement of oral hygiene is essential.

For investigations, refer to Ans. 4 of same chapter.

Q.2. Write short note on acute pseudomembranous candidiasis. *(Sep 2011, 3 Marks)*

Or

Write short note on oral thrush. *(July 2016, 3 Marks)*

Ans. It is commonly known as "oral thrush".

♦ Acute pseudomembranous candidiasis appears as a smooth, thick, creamy-white or allow, soft and friable plaque on the oral mucosa.

♦ Plaque can be easily wiped off by gentle scraping, which leaves an erythematous, raw, bleeding surface in the underlying area.

♦ Lesions may occur at any mucosal site and vary in size ranging from small areas to confluent plaques.

♦ Plaque consists of fungal organisms, keratotic debris, inflammatory cells, desquamated epithelial cells and fibrin, etc.

♦ Oral thrush commonly occurs among children, debilitated elderly persons and AIDS patients.

Histopathology

♦ Hyperplastic epithelium with superficial necrotic and desquamating parakeratinized layer.

♦ Hyperplastic epithelium is infiltrated by candidal hyphae and yeast cells along with PMNs.

♦ Often there is separation between the superficial pseudomembrane and the deeper layers of epithelium.

♦ Candidal hyphae often appear as a weakly basophilic thread like structure.

♦ Lamina propria is infiltrated by chronic inflammatory cells, i.e., lymphocytes and plasma cells.

Treatment

♦ Anti-fungal drugs, i.e., nystatin, amphotericin-B should be given.

♦ Proper oral hygiene should be maintained.

Q.3. Write short note on burning mouth syndrome. *(Dec 2010, 4 Marks)*

Ans.

♦ Burning mouth syndrome (BMS) is a painful, frustrating condition often described as a scalding sensation in the tongue, lips, palate, or throughout the mouth. Although BMS can affect anyone, it occurs most commonly in middle-aged or older women.

♦ BMS often occurs with a range of medical and dental conditions, from nutritional deficiencies and menopause to dry mouth and allergies. But their connection is unclear, and the exact cause of burning mouth syndrome cannot always be identified with certainty.

Signs and Symptoms

Moderate to severe burning in the mouth is the main symptom of BMS and can persist for months or years. For many people, the burning sensation begins in late morning, builds to a peak by evening, and often subsides at night. Some feel constant pain; for others, pain comes and goes. Anxiety and depression are common in people with burning mouth syndrome and may result from their chronic pain.

Other symptoms of burning mouth syndrome include:

♦ Tingling or numbness on the tip of the tongue or in the mouth

♦ Bitter or metallic changes in taste

♦ Dry or sore mouth.

Causes

There are a number of possible causes of burning mouth syndrome, including:

♦ Damage to nerves that control pain and taste

♦ Hormonal changes

♦ Dry mouth, which can be caused by many medicines and disorders, such as Sjögren's syndrome or diabetes

♦ Nutritional deficiencies

♦ Oral candidiasis, a fungal infection in the mouth

♦ Acid reflux

♦ Poorly-fitting dentures or allergies to denture materials

♦ Anxiety and depression.

Diagnosis

A review of your medical history, a thorough oral examination, and a general medical examination may help identify the source of your burning mouth. Tests may include:

- Blood work to look for infection, nutritional deficiencies, and disorders associated with BMS, such as diabetes or thyroid problems
- Oral swab to check for oral candidiasis
- Allergy testing for denture materials, certain foods, or other substances that may be causing your symptoms.

Treatment

- Treatment should be tailored to your individual needs. Depending on the cause of your BMS symptoms, possible treatments may include: Adjusting or replacing irritating dentures
- Treating existing disorders, such as diabetes, Sjögren's syndrome, or a thyroid problem to improve burning mouth symptoms.
- Recommending supplements for nutritional deficiencies
- Switching medicine, where possible, if a drug you are taking is causing your burning mouth.
- *Prescribing medications to:*
  - Relieve dry mouth
  - Treat oral candidiasis
  - Help control pain from nerve damage
  - Relieve anxiety and depression.

When no underlying cause can be found, treatment is aimed at the symptoms to try to reduce the pain associated with burning mouth syndrome.

Q.4. Give classification of candidiasis and enumerate its laboratory tests. *(Sep 2011, 5 Marks)*

Ans.

Classification of Candidiasis by Axell Et Al 1997

- Primary oral candidiasis:
  - *Acute form:*
    - Pseudomembranous candidiasis
    - Erythematous candidiasis
  - *Chronic form:*
    - Hyperplastic candidiasis
    - Erythematous candidiasis
    - Pseudomembranous candidiasis
  - *Candida associated lesion:*
    - Denture stomatitis
    - Angular stomatitis
    - Median rhomboid glossitis
  - *Keratinized primary lesion super-infected with candida:*
    - Leukoplakia
    - Lichen planus
    - Lupus erythematosus
- *Secondary candidiasis:*
  - Candidal endocrinopathy syndrome

Laboratory Test for Candidiasis

- Fragments of plaque material are smeared on a microscopic slide, macerated with 20% potassium hydroxide and examined for typical hyphae.

- Gram-stained smears from lesions or exudates show budding gram-positive cells.
- Sample can also be cultured on Sabouraud's broth and ordinary bacteriological culture. Colonies appear as creamy white, smooth and with yeasty odor.
- *Candida albicans* alone forms chlamydospores on cornmeal agar culture at 20°C.
- A rapid method of identifying *Candida albicans* is based on its ability to form germ tubes within 2 hours when incubated in human serum at 37°C.
- By PAS method of staining candidal hyphae and yeasts should be recognized. PAS method stains the carbohydrates of fungal cell walls and organisms are identified by bright magenta color. Hyphae are 2 μm in diameter, vary in length and may show branching.

Q.5. Write short note on chronic atrophic candidiasis. *(June 2014, 5 Marks)*

Ans. It is also known as denture-induced stomatitis.

It is a clinical manifestation of erythematous candidiasis.

Candida albicans is present in the lesion.

Clinical Features

- Lesion is present under complete or partial denture.
- Most commonly seen in females in palate.
- Patient complains of soreness and dryness of mouth.
- Lesion shows patchy distribution and is associated with speckled curd like white lesion.
- Tissue of palate becomes bright red, edematous and granular.
- Redness of mucosa is limited till the area covered by denture.

Investigations

Refer to Ans. 4 of same chapter.

Treatment

Clotrimazole and nystatin ointments are applied after meal and at bed time 3 to 4 times.

Q.6. Classify candidiasis. Describe in detail etiology, pathogenesis, clinical features, histopathology and treatment of acute pseudomembranous candidiasis. *(Dec 2015, 8 Marks)*

Ans. *For classification of candidiasis, refer to Ans. 4 of same chapter.*

For etiology, refer to Ans. 1 of same chapter.

For clinical features of acute pseudomembranous candidiasis, refer to Ans. 1 of same chapter.

For histopathology and treatment of acute pseudomembranous candidiasis, refer to Ans. 2 of same chapter.

Pathogenesis of Acute Pseudomembranous Candidiasis

Overgrowth of yeast occurs on oral mucosa causing desquamation of epithelial cells. This overgrowth also leads to accumulation of bacteria, keratin, necrotic tissue and debris and form a pseudomembrane which can closely adhere to mucosa.

9. DISEASES OF PERIODONTIUM

Q.1. Write note on acute necrotizing ulcerative gingivitis.

(Mar 2003, 5 Marks)

Or

Write short note on acute necrotizing ulcerative gingivitis. *(Mar 2007, 2.5 Marks) (Sep 2011, 3 Marks)*

(Mar 2016, 3 Marks)

Or

Write short note on ANUG.

(Nov 2014, 3 Marks) (June 2014, 5 Marks)

(Apr 2015, 3 Marks) (Feb 2019, 5 Marks)

Ans. It is an endogenous oral infection which is characterized by the necrosis of gingiva.

It is also called as Trench mouth, Vincent's infection, acute ulceromembranous gingivitis and acute ulcerative gingivitis.

Etiology

It is caused by the fusiform bacilli and spirochete.

Predisposing Factors

Systemic Predisposing Factors

♦ *Malnutrition:* This may lead to acute necrotizing ulcerative gingivitis
♦ *Nutritional deficiency:* Deficiency of Vitamin C, Vitamin B1, Vitamin B2 leads to the exaggeration of pathologic changes caused by fusospirochetal bacteria.
♦ *Psychosomatic conditions:* Disease is associated with the stress and with increment in adrenocortical secretion.
♦ Diseases, such as leukemia, syphilis, AIDS and gastrointestinal disturbances also leads to ANUG.

Localized Predisposing Factors

♦ Marginal gingivitis
♦ Poor oral hygiene
♦ Faulty dental restorations
♦ Deep periodontal pockets
♦ Tobacco smoke

Clinical Features

♦ Acute necrotizing ulcerative gingivitis usually occurs among young and middle aged adults, between the ages of 16 and 30 years and males suffer more often than females.
♦ Stressed professionals like army recruits tend to suffer more from the disease.
♦ Moreover, young children suffering from malnutrition are also prone to the disease.
♦ Initially the gingiva becomes red, edematous, hemorrhagic and painful.
♦ Later, on, a sharply demarcated "punched- out" crater-like erosion of the interdental papillae occurs.
♦ Gingiva is often covered by a gray "pseudomembrane" with accumulation of necrotic tissue debris.

♦ Patient have pronounced spontaneous bleeding tendency, exquisite pain and an extremely unpleasant fetid odor in the mouth.
♦ Patients often develop headache, fever, malaise and lymphadenopathy of the affected area.
♦ Often there is difficulty in taking food due to increased salivation and a metallic taste in the mouth.
♦ When the necrotizing process leads to the development of periodontitis with loss of epithelial attachment the condition is called necrotizing ulcerative periodontitis.
♦ When the necrotizing process of ANUG extends further through the oral mucosa and reaches to the extraoral skin surface, the condition is called 'noma' or cancrum oris.

Histopathology

♦ It involves both stratified squamous epithelium and underlying connective tissue.
♦ Surface epithelium is destroyed and is replaced by pseudo-membranous meshwork of fibrin, necrotic epithelial cells, polymorphonuclear neutrophils and various microorganisms.
♦ Underlying connective tissue is hyperemic with numerous engorged capillaries and dense infiltration of polymorphonuclear neutrophils.
♦ Numerous plasma cells may appear in periphery of infiltrate.

Treatment

♦ Conservative treatment is employed, i.e., superficial cleaning of oral cavity by chlorhexidine, diluted hydrogen peroxide or warm salt water. This is followed by scaling and polishing. Topical anesthetics are used to produce pain during procedure.
♦ Use of antibiotics is coupled with local treatment.

Q.2. Write short note on etiology of gingivitis.

(Sep 2005, 5 Marks)

Ans. Gingivitis is the inflammation of gingiva and occurs in acute, subacute and chronic form.

Etiology

♦ **Local Factors**
  • *Microorganisms:* Plaque associated with gingivitis is complex and heterogeneous. *Actinomyces* group of organisms are dominant in supragingival plaque.
  • *Calculus:* Supragingival or subgingival or both causes irritation of contacting gingival tissue. Irritation is produced by the mechanical friction resulting form hard, rough surface of calculus.
  • *Food impaction:* Impaction of food and accumulation of debris on teeth due to oral negligence results in gingivitis.
  • Faulty and irritating restorations or appliance may act as irritant to gingival tissue and induce gingivitis.
  • *Mouth breathing:* It leads to drying of oral mucus membrane which results in gingival irritation with accompanying irritation.

- **Systemic factors**
  - *Nutritional disturbances:* The nutritional imbalance if frequently manifested leads to changes in gingiva.
  - *Pregnancy:* During pregnancy gingiva undergoes changes causing pregnancy gingivitis.
  - Diabetes mellitus
  - *Hormonal changes:* Puberty and menstruation may result in gingival inflammation.

Q.3. Describe in detail necrotizing ulcerative gingivitis.
(Sep 2011, 8 Marks)

Ans. It is an endogenous oral infection characterized by necrosis of gingiva. It is also called as trench mouth.

Etiopathogenesis

Proliferation of anaerobic fusiform bacteria and spirochetes results in ANUG. Infection mostly occurs in presence of pschycological stress. Stress related corticosteroid hormones are thought to alter T4/T8 lymphocyte ratios and may cause the decreased neutrophilic chemotaxis and phagocytic response seen in patients with ANUG. Stress related epinephrine may result in localized ischemia which predisposes gingiva to ANUG.

Following are the predisposing factors for acute necrotizing ulcerative gingivitis:

- Systemic predisposing factors
- Local predisposing factors

Systemic Predisposing Factors

- *Malnutrition:* This may lead to acute necrotizing ulcerative gingivitis
- *Nutritional deficiency:* Deficiency of Vitamin C, Vitamin B1, Vitamin B2 leads to the exaggeration of pathologic changes caused by fusospirochetal bacteria.
- *Psychosomatic conditions:* Disease is associated with the stress and with increment in adrenocortical secretion.
- Diseases like leukemia, syphilis, AIDS and gastrointestinal disturbances also leads to ANUG.

Localized Predisposing Factors

- Marginal gingivitis
- Poor oral hygiene
- Faulty dental restorations
- Deep periodontal pockets
- Tobacco smoke

Clinical Features

- Acute necrotizing ulcerative gingivitis usually occurs among young and middle-aged adults, between the ages of 16 and 30 years and males suffer more often than females.
- Stressed professionals like army recruits tend to suffer more from the disease.
- Moreover, young children suffering from malnutrition are also prone to the disease.
- Initially the gingiva becomes red, edematous, hemorrhagic and painful.

- Later, on, a sharply demarcated "punched- out" crater-like erosion of the interdental papillae occurs.
- Gingiva is often covered by a gray "pseudomembrane" with accumulation of necrotic tissue debris.
- Patient have pronounced spontaneous bleeding tendency, exquisite pain and an extremely unpleasant fetid odor in the mouth.
- Patients often develop headache, fever, malaise and lymphadenopathy of the affected area.
- Often there is difficulty in taking food due to increased salivation and a metallic taste in the mouth.
- When the necrotizing process leads to the development of periodontitis with loss of epithelial attachment the condition is called necrotizing ulcerative periodontitis.
- When the necrotizing process of ANUG extends further through the oral mucosa and reaches to the extraoral skin surface, the condition is called 'noma' or cancrum oris.

Investigations

Investigations are associated with testing of fusiform bacilli and spirochetes:

- Spirochetes and fusiform bacilli are demonstrated in stained smears of exudates from the lesion on microscopic examination. The spirochete *T. pallidum* is visible on dark ground microscopy.
- Direct fluorescent antibody test is done for detection of spirochete *T. pallidum*
- Enzyme immunoassays are also done to detect for spirochetes present in ANUG.
- Antibody tests, i.e., detection of specific IgM antibody is helpful in detection of *Treponema*.

Differential Diagnosis

- *Benign mucous pemphigoid:* In this as compared to ANUG, it is seen in elderly people and no necrosis is evident.
- *Pemphigoid lichen planus:* It does not show any acute course, no foul breadth is observed.
- *Pemphigus:* It present a very regular histology. Seen in older people.
- *Syphilitic gingivitis:* Lesion is seen on gingiva and it does not get spread to adjacent gingiva.
- *Streptococcal gingivostomatitis:* Diffuse erythema is seen on posterior parts of oral mucosal lining and no necrosis is evident.
- *Gingivostomatitis by candida:* Covering of white membrane is seen which can be removed by scrapping. On laboratory investigation, the membrane reveals of candida.

Complications

Patient affected by ANUG develop systemic complications, such as:

- Pulse rate get increased
- High fever
- Loss of appetite
- Generalized lassitude.

Treatment

- The involved areas are isolated with cotton rolls and dried. A topical anesthetic is applied and after 2 to 3 minutes, areas are gently swabbed with a cotton pellet to remove pseudomembrane. After the area is cleaned with warm water, superficial calculus is removed.
- Patient is told to rinse the mouth every 2 hours with glassful of an equal mixture of warm water and 3% hydrogen peroxide. Twice daily rinsing with 0.12% chlorhexidine are effective.
- Penicillin V 250 or 500 mg, 6 hourly or erythromycin 250 or 500 mg, 6 hourly are given.
- Scaling is performed, if sensitivity permits. After disease process is diminished, complete gingival curettage and root planing is done.
- Supportive treatment consists of copious fluid consumption and administration of nutritional supplements.

Q.4. Describe in detail the clinical features, etiology and histopathology of necrotizing ulcerative gingivitis.

(May/Jun 2009, 15 Marks)

Ans. *For clinical features, refer to Ans. 3 of same chapter.*

Etiology

- It is caused by fusiform bacilli and by a spirochete known as *Borrelia vincentii*.
- Mainly precipitating factors are there which lead to necrotizing ulcerative gingivitis.

For precipitating factors in detail, refer to Ans. 3 of same chapter.

Histopathology

- Affected gingiva show inflammation, ulceration and necrosis.
- Gingival stratified squamous epithelium is replaced by thick fibrinopurulent pseudomembrane.
- Pseudomembrane shows PMNs and necrotic debris.
- In unaffected areas of gingiva keratinization is absent.
- Underlying connective tissue show hyperemia and acute inflammatory cells, i.e., PMNs.

Q.5. Classify gingival hyperplasia. Describe clinical features and histopathology of idiopathic gingival hyperplasia.   *(Dec 2009, 15 Marks)*

Ans.

Classification of Gingival Hyperplasia

On basis of etiological factors and pathologic changes
- Inflammatory enlargement
  - Chronic
  - Acute
- Drug-induced enlargement
- Enlargement associated with systemic disease
  - Conditional enlargement
    - Pregnancy
    - Puberty
    - Vitamin C deficiency
    - Plasma cell gingivitis
    - Nonspecific conditioned enlargement (Pyogenic granuloma)
- Systemic diseases causing gingival enlargement
  - Leukemia
  - Granulomatous disease (e.g., Wegener's Granulomatosis, sarcoidosis)
- Neoplastic enlargement
  - Benign tumors
  - Malignant tumors
- False enlargement

Using the criteria of location and distribution gingival enlargement is designated as follows:
- *Localized:* Gingival enlargement limited to one or more teeth.
- *Generalized:* Involving the gingiva throughout the mouth.
- *Marginal:* Confined to marginal gingiva.
- *Papillary:* Confined to interdental papilla.
- *Diffuse:* Involving the marginal and attached papillae.
- *Discrete:* Isolated sessile or pedunculated tumor like enlargement.

On basis of degree of gingival enlargement

Grade 0: No sign of gingival enlargement.

Grade I: Enlargement confirmed to interdental papilla

Grade II: Enlargement involves papilla and marginal gingiva.

Grade III: Enlargement covers three quarters or more of the crown.

Idiopathic Gingival Hyperplasia

- Idiopathic gingival enlargement is a rare condition of undetermined cause.
- It is also known as gingivomatosis or elephantiasis gingivae or idiopathic fibromatosis or hereditary gingival hyperplasia or congenital fibromatosis.

Clinical Features

- Enlargement affects attached gingiva, gingival margin and interdental gingiva.
- Facial and lingual surfaces of mandible and maxilla are affected.
- Involvement may be limited to one jaw.
- Enlarged gingiva is pink, firm and leathery in consistency and has minutely pebbled surface.
- In severe cases, teeth are completely covered by enlarged gingiva.

Histopathology

- Epithelium is hyperplastic with elongation of rete ridges.
- Mild hyperkeratosis is also seen.
- Underlying connective tissue stroma consists of dense bundles of collagen and numerous fibroblasts.
- At times presence of chronic inflammatory infiltrate is seen.

Q.6. Write short note on gingival fibromatosis.

(Feb 2014, 3 Marks)

Ans. It is also known as hereditary gingival fibromatosis or elephantiasis gingivae.

Gingival fibromatosis is the condition characterized by the diffuse gingival enlargement and it also covers major parts of total tooth surfaces.

It is the slowly progressive gingival enlargement caused by collagenous overgrowth of gingival fibrous connective tissue.

It may be familial or idiopathic.

Clinical Features

♦ Gingival enlargement starts before age of 20 years and it is correlated with eruption of deciduous and permanent teeth.
♦ It occurs as diffuse or nodular growth of gingiva over maxillary or mandibular arch. Maxilla is affected more frequently.
♦ Surface of gingiva is pebbled.
♦ Gingiva is pink or pale in color.
♦ Consistency of gingiva is firm and leathery.
♦ Gingiva is nontender and does not bleed.
♦ Gingival swelling leads to spacing between the teeth.
♦ Extension of gingiva is so severe that it can cover the crown of the erupted tooth.

Histology

♦ Surface epithelium exhibits long, thin rete ridges that extend deep into underlying fibrous connective tissue.
♦ Connective tissue is dense hypocellular and hypovascular.
♦ Collagen fibers are present in form of bundles which are interspersed with fibroblasts.
♦ Inflammation is mild to absent.
♦ At times scattered islands of odontogenic epithelium, foci of dystrophic calcification or areas of osseous metaplasia may be seen.

Treatment

Gingivectomy should be done.

Q.7. Write short note on gingival enlargement.

(Feb 2019, 5 Marks) (June 2015, 5 Marks)

Or

Write short note on gingival hyperplasia.

(Jan 2017, 5 Marks)

Ans. Gingival enlargement is the increase in size of gingiva.

For classification of gingival enlargement, refer to Ans. 5 of same chapter.

Gingival Hyperplasia Associated with Vitamin C Deficiency

Vitamin C deficiency leads to scurvy and the disease has following manifestations:

♦ Gingiva becomes tender, edematous and swollen.
♦ Frequent bleeding is present from gingiva.
♦ Crest of the interdental papillae appear reddish or purple in color.
♦ Ulceration and necrosis of gingiva occur.
♦ Foul smell is present from the mouth.

Gingival Hyperplasia Associated with Leukemia

♦ Gingiva becomes soft, edematous and swollen.
♦ Gingiva is painful and has purplish and has glossy appearance.
♦ Surrounding mucosa is pale and petechiae is seen.
♦ Ulceration and severe hemorrhage occur on gingiva.

Gingival Hyperplasia Associated with Endocrine Imbalance

Hormonal imbalance mostly increases the proliferative potential of gingival tissue in response to irritation caused by plaque, bacteria and local irritants. Following manifestations develop clinically:

♦ Gingiva becomes red, edematous and swollen.
♦ Frequent bleeding is present.
♦ At times localized tumor growth develops on gingiva during pregnancy.
♦ Gingiva becomes soft, edematous and swollen.

Gingival Hyperplasia Associated with Dilantin Sodium Therapy

It causes gingival hyperplasia as its side effect. Manifestations associated are:

♦ Presence of painless enlargement of interdental papilla.
♦ Swelling is rough, lobulated and has a pebbled surface.
♦ Gingiva is normal in color and increased stippling is present.
♦ Gingiva is firm and tender and there is no tendency to bleed.
♦ As drug therapy is stopped gingival growth ceases.

Idiopathic Gingival Enlargement

For idiopathic gingival enlargement, refer to Ans. 5 of same chapter.

Q.8. Classify gingival enlargement. Give a detailed account of enlargement caused by drugs.

(Jan 2018, 10 Marks)

Ans. *For classification of gingival enlargement, refer to Ans. 5 of same chapter.*

Gingival Enlargement Caused by Drugs

♦ Drug-related gingival enlargement is an abnormal growth of gingival tissue which is secondary to the use of systemic medication.
♦ Drug related gingival enlargement is a misnomer because neither the epithelium and nor the cells inside the connective tissue undergo hyperplasia or hypertrophy. Increase in the size of gingiva is because of increased amount of extracellular matrix mainly collagen.
♦ Strong association of drug induced gingival enlargement is related to three drugs, i.e., cyclosporine, phenytoin and nifedipine. All the drugs causing gingival enlargement lead to calcium dysregulation which disrupt normal collagen phagocytosis and remodeling process.
♦ Prevalence related to use of phenytoin is 50% while cyclosporine and nifedipine produce changes in 25%.

- Degree of drug-induced gingival enlargement is related significantly to patient's susceptibility and level of oral hygiene.
- Degree of drug-induced gingival hyperplasia is higher in smokers.
- Dilantin sodium was the first drug reported to cause gingival enlargement.

Clinical Features

- Phenytoin is commonly given in young patients so it induces a problem in people younger than 25 years of age. Patients taking calcium channel blockers are of middle age and cyclosporine has a broad age range.
- As any of the drug is used for 1 to 3 months enlargement occur in interdental papillae and spread to the tooth surface. Anterior and facial segments are more frequently involved areas. Enlargement is painless.
- In extensive cases of hyperplasia gingiva cover almost complete crown surface.
- If there is extension of gingiva lingually and occlusally this can interfere with speech and mastication.
- Edentulous areas are usually not affected, but hyperplasia is seen under poorly maintained dentures as well as around the implants.
- Non-gingival soft tissue growths which look like pyogenic granulomas are seen in allogenic bone marrow transplant recipients who are taking cyclosporine for graft versus host disease.
- Enlarged gingiva is normal in color and is firm, it has smooth, stippled or granular surface.
- If inflammation occurs affected gingiva is dark red and edematous, surface become friable, bleeds easily and occasionally ulcerated.

Histopathology

- Gingival overgrowth caused by phenytoin shows redundant tissue of normal composition.
- Gingival overgrowth caused by cyclosporine shows increase amount of collagen per unit volume with normal density of fibroblast.
- Overlying surface epithelium show elongation of rete ridges with long extension in underlying lamina propria.
- Patients with secondary inflammation show increased vascularity and increased chronic inflammatory cell infiltrate composed of lymphocytes and plasma cells.

Treatment

- Discontinue the offending medication which leads to regression in size of gingiva.
- If drug substitution can be done than cyclosporine is replaced with tacrolimus; phenytoin with carbamazepine, lamotrigine, gabapentin, etc., and nifedipine with atenolol.
- Professional cleaning, frequent re-evaluation and home plaque control is done.
- Systemic or topical folic acid is beneficial in some cases.
- Cyclosporine induced gingival hyperplasia resolve after short course of metronidazole or azithromycin.

- When objectionable alterations are present and all other interventions fail, gingivectomy is the treatment of choice.

10. DENTAL CARIES

Q.1. Describe in brief etiology of dental caries. *(Sep 2008, 3 Marks)*

Ans. Following is the etiology of dental caries:

Host factors	Components
Tooth	• Composition • Morphologic characteristics • Position
Saliva	• Composition • pH • Quantity • Viscosity • Anti-bacterial factors
Diet	• Physical factors • Local factors
Systemic conditions	

Tooth

Composition

- Structure and composition of the teeth influence initiation and rate of progression of dental caries.
- Surface enamel is more resistant to caries as compared to subsurface enamel. Surface enamel consists of more quantity of fluoride, zinc, lead and iron. Concentration of carbonate, magnesium and sodium is lower in surface layer. Level of carbon dioxide is also lower in the surface layer which causes dissolution of surface layer by acids in lower rate and it consists of less organic and water content.
- Age changes in enamel, such as decrease in the density and permeability and increase in nitrogen and fluoride content causes teeth to become more caries resistant.

Morphologic Characteristic

- Deep and narrow occlusal fissures or buccal and lingual pits lead to development of dental caries.
- As age increases attrition of teeth occur and this leads to less accumulation of food in fissures, and there is less occurrence of caries.

Position

Malaligned tooth or rotated tooth has more chances of predisposition of caries as it tends to accumulate more food debris, cariogenic plaque and bacteria. In all these teeth cleaning cannot be done.

Saliva

Composition

- *Inorganic components of saliva:* In normal aspect saliva is supersaturated with calcium and phosphate ions. This causes prevention of dissolution of enamel and also precipitates apatite crystals in surface of enamel of carious lesion which helps in partial repair of tooth damaged by dental caries. During caries saliva is unsaturated with calcium and phosphate ions which lead to dissolution of enamel. Fluoride has also got excellent role in reduction of the dental caries.

♦ *Organic components of saliva:* High concentration of ammonia retards plaque formation and neutralizes acid. Urea increases the neutralizing power of saliva. Enzyme salivary amylase leads to the degradation of starch and makes it more soluble in this way starch is washed away from tooth surface.

pH

♦ Critical pH is the pH at which saliva appears to be saturated with the calcium and phosphorus ions. Value of critical pH is 5.5, below the critical pH inorganic portion of tooth starts dissolving. As there is increase in concentration of hydrogen ion in cariogenic plaque, this leads to the loss of more phosphate ions from the tooth.

♦ Buffering property of saliva leads to diffusion of bicarbonate ions in dental plaque and neutralizes the acid during caries process.

Quantity

♦ Quantity of saliva is inversely proportional to dental caries activity.

♦ More is the salivary flow less is the caries index.

♦ Hyposalivation occurs due to the conditions like diabetes mellitus, uremia and usage of anti-sialogogues.

Viscosity

If saliva is thick mucinous there is presence of high caries incidence.

Anti-bacterial Factors

♦ Saliva consists of many anti-bacterial products, such as lysozyme, salivary peroxidase and immunoglobulins.

♦ Lysozyme under the presence of sodium lauryl sulfate can lyse cariogenic streptococci.

♦ Salivary peroxidase inactivates bacterial enzymes of glycolytic pathway and inhibits their growth. This is more effective against lactobacillus bacteria.

♦ IgA immunoglobulin inhibits *S. mutans* in saliva.

Diet

Physical Factors

♦ Raw unrefined food consists of roughage which cleans the teeth but presence of soil and sand leads to attrition of occlusal and proximal surfaces of teeth and reduces dental caries.

♦ Soft and refined foods stick to the teeth and causes increased accumulation of debris which causes increased risk of dental caries.

Local Factors

♦ Carbohydrates, i.e., starch, sucrose, lactose, glucose, fructose or maltose play important role in process of dental caries. Synthesis of extracellular polysaccharides, glucans and levan helps in adherence of bacteria to teeth.

♦ In lipids medium chain fatty acids and their salts have anti-bacterial properties at low pH.

♦ Deficiency of vitamin A and D can lead to enamel hypoplasia which can lead to dental caries in affected teeth.

Systemic Conditions

♦ *Hereditary:* There is possibility of dental caries which leads to the inheritance of tooth form or structure which predisposes to dental caries.

♦ *Pregnancy:* In later stages of pregnancy because of lack of oral hygiene there is increased risk of dental caries.

Q.2. Describe the theories of etiology of dental caries.
(Mar 2003, 15 Marks)

Or

Define dental caries and theories associated with dental caries. *(Sep 2009, 8 Marks)*

Ans. "Dental caries is an irreversible progressive microbial disease of the calcified tissues of the teeth, characterized by the demineralization of the inorganic portion and distortion of the organic substances of the tooth, which often leads to cavitation".

♦ Etiology of dental caries is a very complex process, which is often explained with the help of some theories.
  • Acidogenic theory
  • Proteolytic theory
  • Proteolytic chelation theory
  • Sucrose chelation theory
  • Autoimmune theory.

Acidogenic Theory

♦ This theory is also known as Miller's chemicoparasitic theory.

♦ It proposes that acid formed due to the fermentation of dietary carbohydrates by oral bacteria leads to progressive decalcification of the tooth. Structures with subsequent degeneration of the organic matrix.

♦ Acidogenic theory states that the process of dental caries involves two stages.
  1. **Initial stage:** Production of organic acid occurs as a result of fermentation of the carbohydrates by the Plaque bacteria.
  2. **Later stage:** Acid causes decalcification of enamel followed by dentin and thereby causes total destruction of these two along with dissolution of their softened residues. Final result is cavity formation.

♦ According to Miller there are four important factors, which can influence the process of tooth destruction in dental caries.
  1. Dietary carbohydrates
  2. Microorganisms
  3. Acids
  4. Dental plaque.

Role of Carbohydrates

♦ Fermentable dietary carbohydrates play an important role in the causation of caries, e.g., glucose, fructose and sucrose.

♦ Among them sucrose is more potent.

♦ These sugars are easily and rapidly fermented by cariogenic bacteria in the oral cavity to produce acid at or near the tooth surface and causes dissolution of the hydroxyapatite crystal of the enamel followed by the dentin.

♦ Risk of caries incidence increases greatly if the dietary sugar is sticky in nature which remains adheres to the tooth surface for long time after taking the meal.

♦ Following the ingestion of these sugars the pH of the Plaque falls to 4.5 to 5 within 1 to 3 minutes and neutralization occurs after 10 to 30 minutes.

♦ Glucose, sucrose and fructose, etc., are rapidly defused into the plaque due to their low molecular weight.

Role of Microorganisms

♦ A large number of microorganisms play individual role in dental caries production and among them the most important one is *Streptococcus mutans*.
  • It readily ferments the dietary carbohydrate to produce acid, which causes tooth destruction.
  • It synthesizes dextran from sucrose, which helps in adhering the plaque bacteria as well as the acid on to the tooth surface.
  • *S. mutans* has the ability to adhere and to grow on hard and smooth surface of the teeth.

♦ Actinomycosis group, e.g., *Actinomycosis israelii*, *Actinomycosis viscosus*, etc., are the important organisms to cause root caries.

♦ *Lactobacillus acidophilus* is important organism for the progress of dental caries.

Role of Acids

♦ During the process of caries formation, a large variety of acids are produced in the oral cavity due to the bacterial fermentation of dietary carbohydrate.

♦ These acids are lactic acid, aspartic acid, acetic acid, butyric acid, glutamic acid.

♦ They can cause demineralization of enamel and dentin and causes the tooth decay.

Role of Bacterial Plaque

♦ Plaque is a thin, transparent film produced on tooth surface and it consists of microorganisms suspended in salivary mucin, also contain desquamated epithelial cells, leukocytes and food debris, etc.

♦ The dental plaque helps in initiation of dental caries by:
  • It harbors the cariogenic bacteria on the tooth surface.
  • It holds the acids on the tooth surface for long duration.
  • It protects the acids from getting neutralized by buffering action of saliva.

Proteolytic Theory

According to this theory, the proteolytic enzymes liberated by cariogenic bacteria causes destruction of organic matrix of enamel, as a result of which the inorganic crystals of the enamel become detached from one another and finally the whole structure collapse, leading to a cavity formation.

This theory cannot explain the role of sucrose, pH, fluoride, etc., in dental caries.

Proteolysis-chelation Theory

♦ According to this theory during caries, first of all proteolytic breakdown of the organic portion of the enamel matrix takes place.

♦ Following this a chelating agent is formed by the combination of the proteolytic breakdown products, acquired pellicle and food debris, etc.

♦ Chelating agent (negatively charged) release the calcium ion (positively charged) from enamel and dentin, this process is called as chelation and eventually results in tooth decay.

Sucrose Chelation Theory

♦ This theory propose that if there is very high concentration of sucrose in the mouth, there can be formation of complex substances like calcium saccharide and calcium complexing intermediaries.

♦ These complexes causes release of calcium and phosphorus ions from the enamel and thereby results in tooth decay.

Autoimmune Theory

This theory suggests that few odontoblast cells at some specific sites, within the pulp of few specific teeth are damaged by autoimmune mechanisms.

Current Concept of Caries Etiology

♦ Dental caries is a multifactorial disease in which there is interplay of three primary factors—the host, microflora and the substrate. In addition a fourth factor, i.e., time.

♦ Caries formation requires a host, a cariogenic flora and a suitable substrate that must be present for a sufficient length of time.

Q.3. Define dental caries describe histopathology of caries in enamel and dentin. *(Dec 2009, 15 Marks)*

Or

Describe in brief histopathology of dental caries.
(June 2010, 5 Marks)

Ans. "Dental caries is an irreversible progressive microbial disease of the calcified tissues of the teeth, characterized by the demineralization of the inorganic portion and distortion of the organic substances of the tooth, which often leads to cavitation".

Histopathological Features of Caries in Enamel

Early Enamel Caries

♦ There will be loss of inter prismatic or interrod substances with increase in prominence of these enamel rods.

♦ Dark line often appears at right angles of the enamel rods, suggesting segments.

♦ Accentuation of the incremental striae of retzius often occurs.

Advanced Enamel Caries

♦ It presents several zones in the tissues, out of which four zones are clearly visible, starting from the inner advancing front of the lesion the zones are:

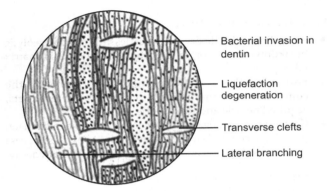

Fig. 77: Dentinal caries H and E (DS)
(For color version, see Plate 14).

Zone I: Translucent Zone

♦ It is the deepest zone lies at the advancing front of the enamel lesion.
♦ This zone is more porous than normal enamel.
♦ Pores are larger than the normal enamel.
♦ Pore volume is 1%.
♦ This zone appears structureless.
♦ This zone contains more fluoride than normal enamel.

Zone II: Dark Zone

♦ Dark zone is located just superficial to the translucent zone and its dark appearance is due to the excessive demineralization of the enamel.
♦ Zone is narrower in rapidly advancing caries and it is wider in slowly advancing lesion.
♦ Zone contains 2 to 4% pore volume.
♦ Pores are larger than normal but smaller than those of translucent zone.
♦ This zone reveals some degree of remineralization of carious lesion.

Zone III: Body of Leison

♦ Zone is situated between the dark zone and the surface layer of enamel.
♦ It represents the area of greatest demineralization.
♦ Pore volume is 5 to 25%.
♦ This zone contains appetite crystals larger than those of the normal enamel.
♦ Large crystals results from the reprecipitation of minerals dissolved from the deeper zone.

Zone IV: Surface Zone

♦ Surface zone when examined by the polarizing light appears relatively unaffected, it may be due to the surface remineralization by the salivary mineral ions.

Histological Features of Caries in Dentin/Dentinal Caries

Dentinal caries histologically presents five zones in the tissue, which are:

Zone I: Normal Dentin

♦ This zone represents the inner most layer of the carious dentin, here the dentinal tubules appears normal.
♦ There is evidence of fatty degeneration of the Tome's process.
♦ No crystals in the lumen of the tubules.
♦ No bacteria in the tubules.
♦ Inter tubular dentin has normal cross banded collagen and normal dense appetite crystals.

Zone II: Sub-transparent Dentin

♦ This is the zone of dentinal sclerosis and is characterized by the deposition of very fine crystal structures within the dentinal tubules.
♦ Superficial layer shows area of demineralization and damage of the odontoblastic processes.
♦ No bacteria in the tubules.
♦ Dentin is capable of remineralization.

Zone III: Transparent Dentin

♦ This zone appears transparent and this is because of decalcification of dentin.
♦ It is softer than normal dentin.
♦ No bacteria in tubules.
♦ Cross banded inter tubular collagen is still intact.
♦ This zone is capable of self-repair and remineralization.

Zone IV: Turbid Dentin

♦ This zone is marked by widening and distortion of dentinal tubules, which are packed with microorganisms.
♦ There is very little amount of minerals in dentin, denaturation of collagen fibers also takes place.
♦ Zone cannot undergo self-repair or remineralization.
♦ This zone must be removed before restoration.

Zone V: Infected Dentin

♦ This is the outermost zone of the carious dentin.
♦ It is characterized by complete destruction of dentinal tubules.
♦ In this zone, the area of decomposition of dentin, which occur along the direction of dentinal tubules are called "Liquefaction foci of Miller", which occur perpendicular to dentinal tubules are called "Transverse clefts".
♦ In the process, the entire dentinal structures become destroyed and cavitation begins from dentinoenamel junction.

Q.4. Describe the histopathology of caries in dentin.

(Feb 2002, 8 Marks)

Or

Describe histopathology of dentinal caries.

(Mar 2006, 5 Marks)

Or

Write short note on histopathology of dentinal caries.

(Jan 2017, 5 Marks)

Ans. *Refer to Ans. 3 of same chapter.*

Q.5. Describe dental caries and describe chemical and histopathological characteristics of caries in enamel.

(Sep 2004, 15 Marks)

Ans. "Dental caries is an irreversible progressive microbial disease of the calcified tissues of the teeth, characterized by the demineralization of the inorganic portion and distortion of the organic substances of the tooth, which often leads to cavitation".

Chemical Characteristics

Refer to acidogenic theory in, Ans. 2 of same chapter

For histopathological characteristics, refer to Ans. 3 of same chapter.

Q.6. Write short note on dentinal caries.

(Dec 2010, 3 Marks)

Or

Write note on dentinal caries. *(March 2007, 2.5 Marks)*

Ans. Caries of the dentin begins with the natural spread of process along the DEJ and the rapid involvement of the great number of dentinal tubules, each of which act as a tract leading to dentinal pulp along which the microorganisms may travel at a variable rate of spread.

Also refer to Ans. 3 of same chapter.

Q.7. Write short essay on caries activity test.

(Jan 2012, 5 Marks)

Or

Write short note on caries activity test.

(Dec 2015, 5 Marks)

Ans. A number of caries activity test have been evolved which are as follows:

Snyder Test

♦ This test measures the ability of salivary microorganisms to produce organic acids from carbohydrate metabolism.
♦ Glucose agar media containing an indicator dye, i.e., Bromocresol green is useful.
♦ The indicator dye changes from green to yellow in range of Ph between 5.4 to 3.8
♦ Paraffin stimulated saliva is added into the medium, change of the medium from green to yellow is indicative of degree of caries activity.

Salivary Reductase Test

♦ It measures the activity of Reductase enzyme present in salivary bacteria.
♦ Paraffin stimulated saliva is collected in the plastic container and an indicator dye "Diazoresorcinol" is added to it which colors the saliva blue.
♦ The reductase enzyme liberated by the cariogenic bacteria causes color changes in the medium from blue to other colors, which indicates the caries "conductiveness" of the patients.

Microbiological Test

♦ Microbiological test helps to measure the number of *Streptococcus mutans* and *Lactobacillus acidophilus*.
♦ Two samples of paraffin stimulated saliva is collected and diluted 10 times and each is cultivated in two different special media.
♦ Rogosa's SL agar medium for *Lactobacillus*.
♦ Mit's Salivarius agar medium for *S. mutans*.
♦ After incubation the numbers of colonies that develop in two separate media are counted and then are multiplied by 10 to estimate the number of bacteria in 1 mL of saliva.
♦ *Result:* If count is more than 10, 00,000 S. *mutans* and more than 1,00,000 *L. acidophilus*, than the caries susceptibility of individual is very high.

Alban's Test

It is the modification of synder test. It uses less agar, i.e., 5 mL per tube. The saliva is drooled directly into the tubes and the tubes are incubated for 4 days at 37°C. The color change is noted from bluish green to yellow and the depth to which the change has occurred is noted.

Strip Test for *S. Mutans* Level in Saliva

Saliva/plaque samples are obtained by using tongue blades and toothpicks (after air drying the tooth for plaque samples) and are transferred to the *S. Mutans* strip which is incubated in M.S.B. agar (Mitis Salivarius Bacitracin agar). The number of *S. Mutans* colonies are used to estimate the caries activity and more than 105 colonies per mL of saliva is indicative of high caries activity.

Buffer Capacity Test

10 mL of stimulated saliva is collected at least one after eating and stored under paraffin oil to prevent the loss of volatile bicarbonate ions, 4 mL of this is measured in beaker. After correcting the pH meter to room temperature the pH of the saliva is adjusted to 7.0 by addition of acid or base. The level of lactic acid in the graduated cylinder is then again recorded. Lactic acid is then added to the sample until a pH of 6.0 is reached. The amount of lactic acid needed to reduce pH from 7.0 to 6.0 is the measure of the buffer capacity.

Fosdick Calcium Dissolution Test

25 mL of gum stimulated saliva is collected. Part of this is analyzed for calcium content. The rest is placed in an 8 inch sterile test tube with about 0.1 g of powdered human enamel. The tube is sealed and shaken for four hours at body temperature after which it is again analyzed for calcium content. If paraffin is used, a concentration of about 5% glucose is added. The amount of enamel dissolution increases as the caries activity increases.

Dewar Test

This test is similar to the Fosdick calcium dissolution test except that the final pH after four hours is measured instead of the calcium dissolved.

Swab Test

The swab test involves sampling of the oral flora by swabbing buccal tooth surfaces and placing it in the Snyder media. This is incubated for 48 hours and the pH changes are read and correlated with the caries activity.

Interpretation

pH 4.1 and less than 4.1—Marked caries activity

pH 4.2–4.6—Active

pH 4.5–4.6—Slightly active

pH greater than 4.6—Caries active.

Q.8. Define dental caries. Enumerate the theories associated with dental caries. Explain different measures in preventing and controlling dental caries.

(Mar 2000, 15 Marks)

Ans. "Dental caries is an irreversible progressive microbial disease of the calcified tissues of the teeth, characterized by the demineralization of the inorganic portion and distortion of the organic substances of the tooth, which often leads to cavitation".

For theories, refer to Ans. 1 of same chapter.

Preventive and Controlling Methods of Caries

♦ Chemical measures
♦ Nutritive measures
♦ Mechanical measures

Chemical Measures

♦ Substances which alter the tooth surfaces or tooth structures.
  • **Fluorine:**
    – It has cariostatic activity
    – Fluorine makes the teeth more resistant to acid attack into oral cavity.
    – It decreases microbial acid production and enhance the remineralization of underlying enamel.
    – It is given in the form of:
      » Communal water fluoridation
      » Fluoride containing dentifrices
      » Fluoride mouth rinses
      » Dietary fluoride supplement.
  • **Bis biguanides:** Chlorhexidine and alexidine. They are antiplaque agents
  • Silver nitrate
  • Zinc chloride and ferrocyanide
♦ Substance which interfere with carbohydrate degradation through enzymatic alteration:
  • Vitamin K: It prevents acid formation in mixture of glucose into saliva.
  • Sarcoside.
♦ Substance which interfere with bacteria growth and metabolism:
  • Urea and ammonium compounds
  • Chlorophyll
  • Nitrofurans
  • Penicillin.

Nutritive Measures

♦ Groups of patients whose diet is high in fat, low in carbohydrate and practically free from sugar have low caries activity.
♦ Phosphates diet causes significant reduction in indication of caries.

Mechanical Measures

♦ **Tooth brushing:** Tooth brushing reduces the number of oral microorganisms. If the teeth are brushed after each meal.
♦ **Mouth rinsing:** The use of mouthwash looses the food debris from the teeth and prevents the caries.
♦ **Dental floss:** It removes plaque from an area of gingiva to contact area on proximal surfaces of teeth, an area impossible to reach with the toothbrush.
♦ **Detergent foods:** Fibrous foods prevent lodging of food in the pit and fissures of the teeth and in addition acts as detergent.
♦ **Pit and fissure sealants:** The pits and fissure of occlusal surface are most difficult areas on teeth to keep clean, so pits and fissure sealants are generally used.

Q.9. Write short note on contributing factors in dental caries. *(Sep 2005, 5 Marks)*

Ans. The following are the contributing factors in the dental caries.

♦ **Dietary factors:** Carbohydrates with types like monosaccharides, disaccharidase or polysaccharides and the amount consumed and whether it is between the meals.
♦ **Microorganisms:** Acidogenic *Streptococcus mutans* and *Actinomycosis viscosus*.
♦ **Systemic factors:** Hereditary, pregnancy and lactation factors have been suggested as etiological factors for dental caries.
♦ **Host factors:** Poor oral hygiene and improper brushing technique may lead to dental caries.
♦ **Immunological factors:** The functional role of circulating antibodies as protective agents against tooth decay has been demonstrated in nonhuman primates.

Q.10. Write notes on nursing bottle syndrome.

(Feb 2006, 2.5 Marks)

Ans. It is also called as nursing caries or baby bottle syndrome and bottle mouth syndrome.

This is a type of rampant caries affecting deciduous dentition.

Etiology

It occurs due to prolong use of:

♦ A nursing bottle containing milk or milk like formula, fruit juice or sweetened water.
♦ Breastfeeding
♦ Sugar or honey sweetened pacifiers.

Clinical Features

♦ The disease presents clinically as widespread carious destruction of deciduous tooth maxillary the fourth maxillary anterior followed by 1st molar and then the cuspid if the habit is prolonged.

♦ It has been emphasized that it is the absence of caries in mandibular incisors which distinguishes this disease from ordinary rampant caries.

♦ The carious process in affected teeth may be so severe that only root stumps remain

♦ The mandibular incisors usually escape because they are covered and protected by the tongue.

Q.11. **Write note on microbial plaque.**
(Mar 2000, 5 Marks) (Sep 2002, 6 Marks)

Ans. Microbial plaque is also called as dental plaque or bacterial plaque.

♦ It was demonstrated first time by William in 1897.

♦ Microbial plaque is the soft, non-mineralized bacterial deposit which forms on teeth and dental prosthesis that are not adequately cleaned. It is composed of 80% water and 20% solids.

♦ Bacterial and salivary proteins comprise one half of dry weight of plaque. Plaque has high concentration of protein, carbohydrates and lipids. Inorganic components of plaque are calcium and phosphate.

♦ It forms on the tooth surfaces which are not properly cleaned.

♦ Dental pellicle which is a glycoprotein and is derived from the saliva is adsorbed over the tooth surfaces and serve as nutrient for plaque microorganism.

♦ Plaque is classified into two types based on its anatomical location, i.e., supragingival plaque and subgingival plaque.

♦ Supragingival plaque play important role in origin of dental caries while subgingival plaque is responsible for the causation of periodontal diseases.

Q.12. **Describe the histopathology of enamel caries.**
(May/June 2009, 5 Marks) (Sep 2006, 5 Marks)

Or

Write short note on histopathology of enamel caries.
(Apr 2017, 4 Marks) (Jan 2018, 4 Marks)

Ans. *Refer to Ans. 3 of same chapter.*

Q.13. **Define and classify and write in detail on etiopathogenesis on dental caries.** *(Apr 2007, 15 Marks)*

Ans. "Dental caries is an irreversible progressive microbial disease of the calcified tissues of the teeth, characterized by the demineralization of the inorganic portion and distortion of the organic substances of the tooth, which often leads to cavitation".

Classification of Dental Caries

♦ **Based on location of the lesion**
  • Pit and fissure caries
    – Occlusal
    – Buccal or lingual pit
  • Smooth surface caries
    – Proximal
    – Buccal or lingual surface
  • Root caries

♦ **Based on tissue involved**
  • Enamel caries
  • Dentinal caries
♦ Cementum caries **Based on virginity of the lesion**
  • Primary caries
  • Secondary caries
♦ **Based on progression of lesion**
  • Progressive caries
    – Rapidly progressive like nursing caries and radiation caries
    – Slowly progressing
  • Arrested caries:

For etiopathogenesis, refer to Miller's chemico-parasitic theory in Ans. 2 of same chapter.

Q.14. **Draw diagram of histopathology of pit and fissure caries and dentinal caries.** *(Sep 2007, 5 Marks)*

Ans. Pit and fissure caries:
For dentinal caries, refer to Ans. 3 of same chapter.

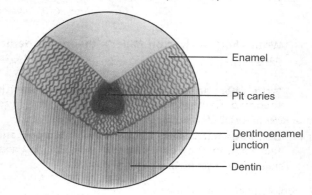

Fig. 78: Pit and fissure caries (GS) *(For color version, see Plate 14).*

Q.15. **Write short note on *Streptococcus mutans* in dental caries.** *(Jan 2012, 5 Marks)*

Ans. It was first isolated by Clarke in 1924 and is termed as *Streptococcus mutans*.

♦ It is a catalyse negative gram-positive cocci forming short to medium chains.

♦ *S. mutans* synthesizes insoluble polysaccharides from sucrose and is homofermentative.

♦ Most important substrate for involvement of *S. mutans* in caries process is disaccharide sucrose.

♦ *S. mutans* produces acid from fermentation of sucrose, glucose, lactose, mannitol, etc., This leads to demineralization of tooth structure and finally caries.

♦ *S. mutans* can survive at pH as low as 4.2 and can demineralize the tooth causing dental caries.

♦ *S. mutans* synthesizes dextran which helps in adhering plaque bacteria to tooth surface which leads to more decay.

♦ *S. mutans* adhere to acquired pellicle and helps in plaque formation which finally cause caries.

♦ *S. mutans* has ability to adhere on hard and smooth surfaces of tooth structure.

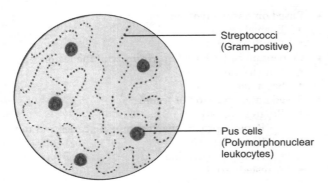

Fig. 79: *Streptococcus mutans (For color version, see Plate 14).*

Q.16. Write notes on Miller's acidogenic theory.

(Apr 2008, 5 Marks)

Or

Write in brief on Miller's acidogenic theory.

(Feb 2013, 8 Marks)

Or

Write short answer on Miller's theory for dental caries.

(Apr 2019, 3 Marks)

Or

Write short answer on Miller's chemicoparasitic theory for dental caries.   *(Oct 2019, 3 Marks)*

Ans. *Refer to Ans. 2 of same chapter.*

Q.17. Define dental caries. Describe microbiology and factors promoting dental caries. *(Nov 2008, 15 Marks)*

Ans. *For definition, refer to Ans. 2 of same chapter.*

Microbiology of Dental Caries

♦ In the pathogenesis of dental caries an important role play cariogenic bacteria, i.e., oral streptococci, especially of group mutans and lactic acid bacteria (*Lactobacillus* spp.).

♦ It is believed that bacteria of the species *Streptococcus mutans* is the main factor that initiates caries and very important factor of enamel decay.

♦ The bacteria of the genus *Lactobacillus* are important in further caries development, especially in the dentin.

♦ *Streptococcus mutans* and lactobacilli are characterized by the ability to grow in an acid environment and the property of rapid metabolism of sugars supplied in the diet to organic acids, including lactic acid.

♦ The microbial community from dentinal lesions is diverse and contains many facultatively and obligately anaerobic bacteria belonging to the genera *Actinomyces, Bifidobacterium, Eubacterium, Lactobacillus, Parvimonas and Rothia.*

♦ Streptococci are recovered less frequently. Caries can also be caused by other bacteria, including members of the mitis, anginosus and salivarius groups of streptococci, *Propionibacterium, Enterococcus faecalis* and *Scardovia*.

Streptococcus Mutans

Streptococcus mutans are the most cariogenic pathogens as they are highly acidogenic, producing short-chain acids which dissolve hard tissues of teeth. They metabolize sucrose to synthesize insoluble extracellular polysaccharides, which enhance their adherence to the tooth surface and encourage biofilm formation. The reactions are catalyzed by three isozymes of glycosyltransferases. The most important mutans streptococci isolated from tooth caries samples are *S. mutans* and *S. sobrinus*. *S. mutans* is more cariogenic than *S. sobrinus* because specific cell-surface proteins, which aid in its primary attachment to the tooth. *S. sobrinus* lacks such proteins.

S. mutans is able to metabolize a number of sugars and glycosides, such as glucose, fructose, sucrose, lactose, galactose, mannose, etc., In the presence of extracellular glucose and sucrose, *S. mutans* synthesizes intracellular glycogen-like polysaccharides (IPSs). *S. mutans* produces also mutacins (bacteriocins), what is considered to be an important factor in the colonization and establishment of *S. mutans* in the dental biofilm.

Streptococcus Sobrinus

S. sobrinus has been implicated in caries development particularly in instances where caries development appears to be independent of *S. mutans*. It is interesting that *S. sobrinus* displays higher acid production and acid tolerance compared to *S. mutans*.

Lactobacilli

Among the *Lactobacillus* rods in the oral cavity occur: *L. acidophilus, L. casei, L. fermentum, L. delbrueckii, L. plantarum, L. jensenii, L. brevis, L. salivarius* and *L. gasseri*. Lactobacilli are divided into two main groups: homofermentative which in the fermentation process of glucose produce mainly lactic acid, e.g., *Lactobacillus casei, Lactobacillus acidophilus,* heterofermentative which in addition to lactic acid produce acetate, ethanol and carbon dioxide, e.g., *Lactobacillus fermentum*.

Lactobacilli are isolated from deep caries lesions but rarely just before the development of dental caries and in the early tooth decay. It is believed that they are pioneering microorganisms in the caries progress, especially in dentin.

Veillonella

It is a gram-negative cocci which is commonly found in plaque. It utilizes lactic acid by converting it to propionic acid and other weak acids.

Factors Promoting Dental Caries

Tooth Factors

♦ Tooth factors, such as composition of tooth, structure of enamel, morphologic characteristics of tooth, position of tooth are the caries promoting factors.

♦ In composition of tooth surface enamel is more resistant to caries than subsurface enamel. This is because surface enamel is highly mineralized.

♦ Presence of deep, narrow occlusal fissures, buccal and lingual pits leads to the development of dental caries.

♦ Teeth which are malaligned, out of position, rotated or otherwise not normally situated are difficult to clean and favor accumulation of food and debris which lead to dental caries.

Salivary Factors

♦ Salivary factors, such as composition of saliva, pH, quantity, viscosity and antibacterial factors in saliva play role in promotion of dental caries.

♦ When salivary flow rate is normal it leads to cleaning of bacteria from tooth surface and reduces the chances of dental caries while in xerostomia incidence of caries is high.

♦ As viscosity of saliva is increased deposition of plaque increases because thick saliva does not produce proper cleaning action. If viscosity of saliva is decreased normal contents of mineral is less and saliva does not produce anticaries functions.

♦ As the buffering action of saliva is decreased acid demineralization of tooth by dental caries become high this is because low concentration of salivary bicarbonate does not cause neutralization of acids which is produced by cariogenic bacteria.

• Salivary enzymes, such as amylase leads to breakdown of starch (which is a residual carbohydrate) from tooth surface which is washed easily from mouth. As if levels of salivary amylase are too low this will lead to dental caries.

• Certain antibacterial agents are found in saliva, such as lysozyme, thiocyanate, etc., These agents leads to the destruction of cariogenic bacteria by anti-bacterial action and reduces caries incidence. As if deficiency of such agents is present this will lead to the promotion of dental caries.

• Salivary immunoglobulins, such as IgA and IgG inhibit *S. mutans* by facilitating destruction process through phagocytosis and lead to decrease in dental caries. If salivary immunoglobulin levels are decreased this leads to the increase in dental caries.

Diet Factors

♦ Diet factors, such as physical nature, carbohydrates, vitamins and fluoride content play important role.

♦ More and more intake of soft and sticky food increases possibility of dental caries.

♦ Foods rich in carbohydrates lead to the dental caries.

♦ Physical nature of diet is important as soft refined foods cling to the teeth and are not removed because of lack of roughage. This collection of debris is due to reduction in mastication because of softness of diet. This leads to dental caries.

♦ Fluoride ions limit rate of carbohydrate metabolism by cariogenic bacteria and reduce acid attacks on tooth. Lagging of fluoride in diet leads to the increase incidence of dental caries.

Dental Plaque

♦ Dental plaque is the soft, non-mineralized bacterial deposit which forms on teeth and dental prosthesis that are not adequately cleaned.

♦ Plaque harbors cariogenic bacteria on tooth surface.

♦ Rapid production of high amount of acids in plaque occur through fermentation of carbohydrates by cariogenic bacteria.

♦ Plaque hold the acids on tooth surfaces for longer duration.

♦ Increased thickness of plaque does not allow salivary buffers to enter into neutralize the acids produced by the cariogenic bacteria.

Q.18. **Define dental caries. Discuss in detail about theories and histopathology of dental caries. Add a note on caries activity tests.** *(Aug 2012, 10 Marks)*

Ans. *For definition and theories of dental caries, refer to Ans. 1 of same chapter.*

For histopathology of dental caries, refer to Ans. 3 of same chapter.

For caries activity test, refer to Ans. 9 of same chapter.

Q.19. **What is dental caries. Enumerate different theories of etiology of caries. Describe in detail Miller's chemico-parasitic theory.** *(Feb 2014, 8 Marks)*

Ans. *Refer to Ans. 2 of same chapter.*

Q.20. **Write short note on zones of dentinal caries.**
(Jun 2014, 5 Marks)

Ans. *Refer to Ans. 3 of same chapter.*

Q.21. **Write short note on sequel of dental caries.**
(Dec 2012, 3 Marks)

Ans. Following is the sequel of dental caries

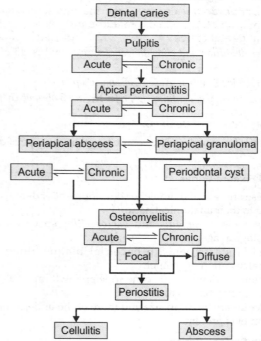

Flowchart 2: Sequel of dental caries.

Q.22. **Write short answer on role of carbohydrates in dental caries.** *(May 2018, 3 Marks)*

Ans. Fermentable dietary carbohydrates play an important role in the causation of caries, e.g., glucose, fructose and sucrose. Among them sucrose is more potent.

♦ Cariogenic carbohydrates are dietary in origin, as uncontaminated human saliva has negligible amount of carbohydrates regardless of blood sugar level.

♦ Salivary carbohydrates get bound to proteins as well as other compounds. They are not readily available for microbial degradation.

♦ Cariogenicity of dietary carbohydrates varies along with frequency of ingestion, physical form and the chemical composition, route of administration and presence of other food constituents.

♦ Sticky solid carbohydrates are more cariogenic as compared to their liquid form.

♦ Carbohydrates which get readily cleared from oral cavity via saliva and swallowing is less conducive to caries than to those which get slowly cleared.

♦ Polysaccharide gets less easily fermented by plaque bacteria as compared to monosaccharides and disaccharides. Organisms of plaque release less acid from sugar alcohols, sorbitol, xylitol, mannitol. This implies that all these carbohydrates are non-cariogenic.

♦ Carbohydrates which are fed through stomach tube or intravenously do not contribute to decay as they are unavailable for microbial breakdown.

♦ Food consisting of high fat, carbohydrate, protein or salt decreases oral retentiveness of carbohydrates.

♦ Refined pure carbohydrates are more carious as compared to crude carbohydrates which is complexed with other food elements which are capable of reducing enamel solubility or possessing antibacterial properties.

Q.23. Define dental caries. Describe etiopathogenesis, microbiology, clinical features and histopathology of dental caries. *(Sep 2018, 10 Marks)*

Ans. *For definition and etiopathogenesis, refer to Ans. 13 of same chapter.*

For microbiology, refer to Ans. 17 of same chapter.

For histopathology of dental caries, refer to Ans. 3 of same chapter.

Clinical Features of Dental Caries

Clinical features of dental caries are based on the type of dental caries:

Pit and Fissure Caries

♦ These areas are favorable for development of dental caries due to their anatomical nature.

♦ *S. mutans, S. sanguis* and *Lactobacillus* species are the etiological agents.

♦ Lesion starts beneath bacterial plaque along with decalcification of enamel.

♦ Lesion is triangular or cone in shape with apex at outer surface and base is towards DEJ.

♦ Cavities are larger in size and more of the undermining of enamel is present.

Smooth Surface Caries

♦ Most earliest sign is the presence of smooth, chalky white area of decalcification.

♦ Lesion here is of cone shaped with apex towards DEJ and base is towards the surface of tooth.

Cervical Caries

♦ It occurs as chalky, crescent shaped are of decalcification at gingival margin of labial and buccal surfaces which forms the cavity.

♦ Cavities are usually saucer shaped and are wider.

♦ It is due to poor oral hygiene.

Root Caries

♦ It is the caries of cementum and the underlying dentin and occurs at age of 40 to 50 years because of recession of gingival margin.

♦ Lesion appears shallow and saucer shaped, ill-defined area which is discolored and soft.

♦ Lesion starts CEJ and spreads laterally rather than in depth.

Acute Caries

♦ Caries progress rapidly and lead to the involvement of pulp quickly.

♦ It is seen in both children and adolescent.

♦ Depth of cavity is more in spite of small opening inside enamel.

♦ Wide undermining of enamel is present; soft and pale dentin is present.

♦ It is very painful since pulp is soon exposed and infected.

♦ Secondary dentin is present which is very less or is absent.

Chronic Caries

♦ There is slow progression of dental caries and there is more of secondary dentin formation.

♦ Wide cavity is present along with stained enamel and more destruction because of secondary enamel caries.

♦ It is less painful due to blockage of dentinal tubules and other pulp reactions to lesion.

♦ It occurs in patients more than 30 years of age.

Arrested Caries

♦ It is an area of remineralization of carious lesion because of change in pH.

♦ It is seen as discolored region which is more resistant to caries attack.

♦ Cavity becomes self-cleansing and with no stagnation caries is arrested.

♦ Formation of secondary dentin is below the cavity.

♦ It is seen on the occlusal surface as brown stained polished smooth area, i.e., eburnated dentin which is hard as well as shiny.

Primary Caries

It is the caries which occur for first time on any surface of a tooth.

Recurrent Caries

This is the caries which recur near the margin of restoration due to leaky margin of the restoration.

Q.24. Write short answer on enamel caries.

(Sep 2018, 3 Marks)

Ans. Enamel caries is believed to be preceded by formation of dental plaque.

Depending on the site of involvement, enamel caries is of two types, i.e., smooth surface caries and pit and fissure caries.

Depending on the degree of advancement, enamel caries is of two types, i.e., early caries or advanced caries.

Smooth Surface Caries

Early Enamel Caries

♦ Here, earliest macroscopic evidence of incipient caries is appearance of an area of decalcification beneath dental plaque which resembles smooth chalky white area mainly at cervical margin of interdental facet which is also known as white spot.

♦ Intact surface lesions can appear brown in color and this is known as brown spot, this depends on the degree of exogenous materials absorbed the porous region.

♦ Loss of interprismatic or interrod substances causes prominence of enamel rods.

♦ Smooth surface caries mainly of proximal surface consists of distinctive shape, i.e., it forms a triangular or cone-shaped lesion with apex towards the junction and base towards the surface of tooth.

Advanced Enamel Caries

It microscopically present four zones which start from inner advancing front of the lesion, i.e.:

1. Translucent zone
2. Dark zone
3. Body of the lesion
4. Surface zone

For details, refer to Ans. 3 of same chapter.

Pit and Fissure Enamel Caries

♦ Process of dental caries is same in pit and fissures as seen in smooth surface caries. Main variation is in anatomical and histological structure.

♦ Occlusal fissures consists of deep invagination of enamel which are broad or funnel shaped, constricted hour glass, various multiple invaginations with Y shaped divisions or are irregularly shaped.

♦ These pit and fissures leads to food stagnation along with bacterial decomposition at base.

♦ Often carious lesion start at both sides of the fissure wall and visual changes, i.e., chalkiness or yellow, brown or black discoloration can be seen.

♦ Enamel at bottom of pit and fissure can be very thin, so that early dentin involvement frequently occurs. Some of the pit and fissures are shallow and have relatively thick layer of enamel covering the base.

♦ In both types of pit and fissures, enamel rods flare laterally at bottom of pit and fissures. Caries follow the direction of enamel rods and form either triangular or cone shaped lesion with apex at outer surface and base towards DEJ. Due to its shape, more of the dentinal tubules are involved as lesion reaches DEJ.

Ultrastructural Changes in Enamel Caries

♦ In enamel caries first alteration seen is the scattered destruction of individual apatite crystals, both within enamel prisms and at their border.

♦ Later on there is demineralization occurs both from periphery and center of rods leading to increased intercrystalline gap.

♦ Sometimes, there is remineralization and there will be change in structure of crystals because of combined effect of demineralization and remineralization.

11. DISEASES OF THE PULP AND PERIAPICAL TISSUES

Q.1. Describe the etiology, histopathology and clinical features of acute pulpitis.
(Sep 2008, 16 Marks) (Dec 2010, 8 Marks)

Or

Describe etiology, histopathology, clinical features and sequelae of acute pulpitis. *(Sep 2002, 16 Marks)*

Ans. Acute pulpitis is an irreversible condition characterized by acute, intense inflammatory reaction in pulp tissue.

Etiology

♦ Pulp exposure due to faulty cavity preparation.

♦ Caries progressing beyond the dentinal barriers and reaching the pulp.

♦ Chemical irritation to pulp.

♦ Cracked tooth syndrome.

♦ Metallic restoration in a tooth without proper thermal insulation.

♦ Blow to tooth with subsequent damage to pulp.

♦ Recurrent caries around the pre-existing restoration.

♦ Galvanic current produced due to dissimilar metallic restoration may transmitted to pulp and causing pulpitis.

Histopathology

♦ Severe edema in the pulp with vasodilatation.

♦ Moderate to dense infiltration of polymorphonuclear leukocytes.

♦ Focal of complete destruction of odontoblast cells at pulp dentin border.

♦ Many microabscess formations in pulp characterized by the area of liquefaction degeneration in pulp being surrounded by dense band of neutrophils and micro-organisms.

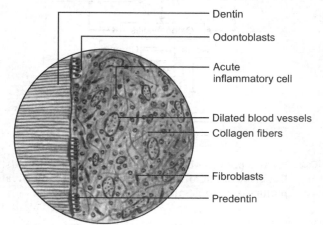

Fig. 80: Acute pulpitis *(For color version, see Plate 14).*

♦ There may be complete liquefaction and necrosis of pulp with total destruction of odontoblastic cell layer. This is known as acute suppurative pulpitis.

♦ Death of pulp is due to tissue dehydration. This is known as "dry gangrene of pulp".

Clinical Features

♦ Tooth is sensitive to cold and hot stimuli.

♦ Application of hot or cold stimuli causes an increase in intensity to pain and such pain persists for longer duration even after the stimuli is removed.

♦ Intensity of pain increases during the sleep and occurs due to increase in local blood pressure in head and neck region.

♦ As entrance of pulp is not wide, acute pulpitis helps in spread of inflammation throughout pulp with subsequent necrosis.

♦ Acute pulpitis is often associated with microabscess formation in pulp along with liquefaction degeneration.

♦ Pain subsides when drainage is established or when pulp undergo complete necrosis.

♦ Tooth is nontender to percussion unless the pulpal inflammation has spread beyond the root apex into periapical region.

♦ When intrapulpal pressure becomes very high during acute inflammation it cause collapse of apical blood vessels. This is known as "pulp strangulation".

Sequelae of Acute Pulpitis

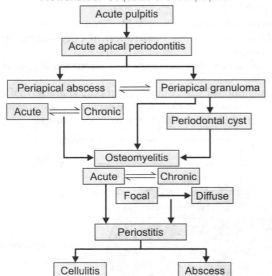

Flowchart 3: Sequelae of acute pulpitis.

Q.2. What is pulpitis? Explain different causes of pulpitis. Describe clinical features and histopathological picture of chronic open hyperplastic pulpitis.

(Mar 2000, 15 Marks)

Ans. Pulpitis refers to the inflammation of dental pulp within the tooth.

Causes of Pulpitis

♦ **Reversible pulpitis:** It is caused by an agent capable of injuring the pulp, such as trauma, disturbed occlusal relationship and thermal shock.

♦ **Irreversible pulpitis:** It is caused by the bacterial involvement of pulp through caries, chemical or thermal or mechanical injury.
  • *Acute pulpitis: Refer to Ans. 1 of same chapter*
  • *Chronic pulpitis: Refer to Ans. 3 of same chapter.*

Chronic Open Hyperplastic Pulpitis

♦ It is also known as chronic hyperplastic pulpitis or pulp polyp or pulpitis aperta.

♦ It is a productive pulpal inflammation due to an extensive carious exposure of young pulp. It is characterized by development of granulation tissue covered by epithelium and resulting from long standing low grade infection.

Clinical Features

♦ Pulp polyp appears as small, pinkish, red lobulated mass, which protrudes from pulp chamber and fills up the carious cavity.

♦ Condition is seen in young adults and children. It commonly develops in deciduous molar and first permanent molars.

♦ Affected tooth has a large open carious cavity, which is present for long duration.

♦ Lesion bleeds profusely on provocation.

♦ Involved tooth is painless and is sensitive to thermal stimuli.

Histopathology

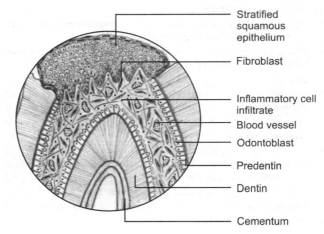

Fig. 81: Pulp polyp/chronic hyperplastic pulpitis
(For color version, see Plate 14).

♦ Hyperplastic pulp tissue lesion presents the feature of granulation tissue mass, consisting of numerous proliferating fibroblasts and young blood capillaries.

- Inflammatory cell infiltration by lymphocytes, plasma cells and sometimes polymorphonuclear neutrophils in tissue are common.
- Stratified squamous epithelium is present on the surface of hyperplastic pulpitis which resembles oral epithelium.
- Epithelium surface show well-formed rete peg formation.
- Epithelial cells on surface are believed to be desquamated epithelial cells which came either from buccal mucosa or from salivary gland ducts.

Q.3. Write short note on pulpitis. *(Mar 2003, 5 Marks)*

Ans. *Refer to Ans. 1 and Ans. 2 of same chapter.*

Chronic Pulpitis

It is a condition characterized by the low grade fever often persistent inflammatory reaction in pulpal tissue with little or no constitutional symptoms.

Etiology

Refer to Ans. 1 of same chapter.

Clinical Features

- The tooth with chronic pulpitis may remain asymptomatic for long time.
- There may be an intermittent dull and throbbing pain in the tooth.
- Tooth is less sensitive to hot and cold stimuli.
- Tooth responds to a higher level of current when electric pulp tester is used.
- Exposed pulp tissue may be manipulated by small instrument but bleeding can occur.

Histopathology

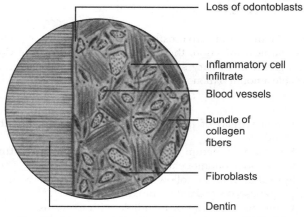

Fig. 82: Chronic pulpitis *(For color version, see Plate 15).*

- Chronic inflammatory response in the pulp is characterized by cellular infiltration by the lymphocytes, plasma cells and macrophages.
- Prolong chronic inflammation may encourage fibroblastic activity in pulp with formation of collagen bundle and in some cases leads to internal resorption of the tooth.

- Blood capillaries are prominent and few microorganisms are found in the pulpal tissue.
- Persisting chronic pulpitis may cause diffuse or solitary areas of calcification in the pulp.

Treatment

- Extraction of tooth
- Root canal therapy

Q.4. Write short note on pulp polyp.
(Mar 2013, 3 Marks) (Dec 2009, 5 Marks)
(Apr 2007, 5 Marks) (Sep 2007, 2.5 Marks)
(Aug 2011, 10 Marks) (June 2014, 5 Marks)
(Nov 2014, 5 Marks)

Or

Write short note on chronic hyperplastic pulpitis.
(Mar 2011, 3 Marks)

Or

Write short answer on pulp polyp.
(Mar 2018, 3 Marks)

Ans. *Refer to Ans. 2 of same chapter.*

Treatment

- Elimination of polypoid tissue, following the extirpation of the pulp.
- After removing hyperplastic pulp tissue bleeding can be stopped by pressure.
- Extraction of tooth or root canal treatment.

Q.5. Describe etiology, histopathology and clinical feature of periapical granuloma. *(Sep 1999, 15 Marks)*

Ans. It is also called as chronic apical periodontitis.

Periapical granuloma is a localized mass of granulation tissue around the root apex of nonvital tooth which develop in relation to infection and inflammation.

Etiology

- Extension of pulpal inflammation
- Occlusal trauma
- Orthodontic tooth movements with excessive uncontrolled force
- Acute trauma due to blows on tooth.
- Spread of periodontal infection in root apex.
- Perforation of root apex into endodontic therapy.

Clinical Features

- Tooth involves produce sensitivity to percussion which occurs due to edema, hyperemia and inflammation of apical periodontal ligament.
- Mild pain and discomfort in tooth during chewing solid foods.
- Involved tooth is slightly elongated from the socket.
- Periapical granuloma may be asymptomatic in many cases.
- Tooth may be vital or partially vital in initial stages of development of lesion but in fully developed periapical granuloma the affected tooth is nonvital.

Histopathology

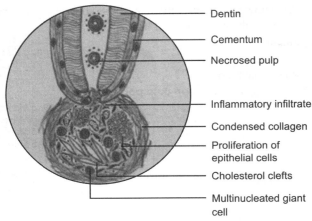

Dentin

Cementum

Necrosed pulp

Inflammatory infiltrate

Condensed collagen

Proliferation of epithelial cells

Cholesterol clefts

Multinucleated giant cell

Fig. 83: Periapical granuloma *(For color version, see Plate 15).*

♦ Lesion appears as granulation tissue mass consisting of proliferating fibroblasts, endothelial cells and numerous immature blood capillaries.
♦ Chronic inflammatory cells, i.e., macrophages, lymphocytes and plasma cells are present in the lesion.
♦ There is presence of epithelial islands, cholesterol clefts and foam cells.
♦ Plasma cells often produce immunoglobulin there is also present of T lymphocytes in the lesion.
♦ Epithelial rest cell of Malassez, proliferate in response to chronic inflammation and these proliferating cells undergo cystification.
♦ Bony tissue at the periphery of lesion is lined by the osteoclast cells with area of bone resorption.
♦ Few bacterias are present in the lesions which are not affected by the cellular immune mechanism.
♦ Occasionally Russell bodies are also found.
♦ Resorption of cementum and dentin often occurs as a result of chronic inflammation. In some areas along root, cementoblastic activity predominates leading to hypercementosis.

Q.6. Write notes on periapical granuloma.

(Sep 1999, 5 Marks)

Ans. *Refer to Ans. 5 of same chapter.*

Treatment

Extraction of involved tooth or under certain conditions root canal therapy with apical curettage.

Q.7. Describe etiology, histopathology and clinical features of acute alveolar abscess.

(Mar 1998, 15 Marks)

Ans. It is also known as dentoalveolar abscess.

It is defined as acute suppurative infection in periapical region of tooth.

Etiology

♦ Extension of pulpal infection in periapical tissue.
♦ Fracture of tooth with pulp exposure.
♦ Accidental perforation of apical foramen during root canal treatment

♦ Extension of periodontal infection in periapical tissues.
♦ Anachoretic infection of periapical tissues.

Clinical Features

♦ It is common odontogenic infection and constitutes 2% of apical radiolucencies.
♦ Due to acute abscess there is pain in the affected tooth.
♦ Localized swelling and an erythematous change in overlying mucosa is present.
♦ Affected area of jaw may be tendered during palpitation.
♦ Pain aggravates during percussion and when pressure is applied with the opposing tooth.
♦ Application of heat intensifies pain, whereas application of cold relieves pain temporarily.
♦ Pus discharging sinus often develops on alveolar mucosa over the affected root apex and sometimes on skin overlying the jaw bone.
♦ Infection from acute periapical abscess often spread to facial spaces, leading to space infections.

Histopathology

♦ Lesion appears as zone of liquefaction necrosis, which is made up of proteinaceous exudates, necrotic tissue and large number of dead neutrophils
♦ Adjacent tissue surrounding the bone has many dilated blood vessels and infiltration with the neutrophils.
♦ Inflammatory changes are observed in the PDL and adjoining bone marrow.
♦ Bony trabeculae in periapical region may show empty lacunae, which results from death of osteocytes.

Q.8. Describe etiology, histopathology and clinical features and complications of acute suppurative osteomyelitis in adult patient mandible.

(Mar 2000, 15 Marks)

Ans. Acute suppurative osteomyelitis is serious sequelae of periapical infection, there is diffuse spread of infection throughout medullary spaces with subsequent necrosis of variable amount of bone.

Etiology

♦ Direct spread of infection from dental pulp into the mandible.
♦ Spread of infection in the mandible from presenting suppurative odontogenic infections.
♦ Spread of infection following removable of tooth without proper asepsis and antibiotic coverage.
♦ Compound fracture of mandible with exposure of bone outside the mucosa.
♦ Post-radiation secondary infection.
♦ Infection to the preexisting bony lesions, e.g., Paget's disease of bone and fibrous dysplasia.

Clinical Features

♦ It occurs after the 50 years of age and males are more commonly affected.
♦ Mandibular lesions are diffuse in nature.
♦ Acute suppurative osteomyelitis of mandible in young adult causes severe pain, diffuse and enlarged swelling of mandible.

- There is loosening and soreness of the regional teeth with difficulty in food intake.
- Multiple intraoral and extraoral pus discharging sinuses often develops and moreover discharge of pus is seen from gingival crevice of the affected teeth.
- Paresthesia of lip is common.
- Patient is slightly febrile and general symptoms include fever, malaise, anorexia and vomiting.

Histopathology

- In acute suppurative osteomyelitis bone marrow undergoes liquefaction and purulent exudates occupy the marrow space.
- A large number of acute inflammatory cells infiltrations are present which shows PMNs with occasional presence of lymphocytes and plasma cells.
- Some areas of affected bone undergo necrosis with generation of osteoblast and osteocytes cells and therefore results in development of sequestrum (a piece of dead bone).
- When acute phase of infection subsides in new shell of bone called "involucrum" is formed over inflammatory focus.

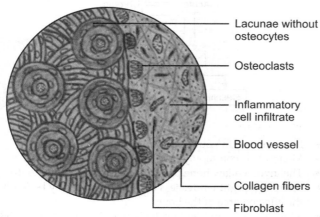

Fig. 84: Osteomyelitis *(For color version, see Plate 15).*

Complications

- Periostitis
- Cellulitis
- Abscess.

Q.9. Define and classify osteomyelitis. Describe in detail chronic osteomyelitis. *(Sep 2008, 8 Marks)*

Or

Write short note on chronic osteomyelitis.
(Jan 2017, 5 Marks) (June 2015, 5 Marks)

Or

Write short answer on chronic osteomyelitis.
(Sep 2018, 3 Marks)

Ans. Chronic osteomyelitis is the persistent abscess of the bone characterized by the complex inflammatory process including necrosis of mineralized and marrow tissues, suppuration, resorption, sclerosis and hyperplasia.

Osteomyelitis is defined as an inflammatory condition of bone that begins as an infection of medullary cavity and haversian systems of the cortex and extends to involve the periosteum of the affected area.

Classification of Osteomyelitis

- Acute osteomyelitis
  - Acute suppurative osteomyelitis
  - Acute subperiosteal osteomyelitis
  - Acute periostitis
- Chronic osteomyelitis
  - Non-specific type
    - Chronic intramedullary osteomyelitis
    - Chronic focal sclerosing osteomyelitis
    - Chronic diffuse sclerosing osteomyelitis
    - Chronic osteomyelitis with proliferative periostitis
    - Chronic subperiosteal osteomyelitis
    - Chronic periostitis
  - Specific type
    - Tuberculous osteomyelitis
    - Syphilitic osteomyelitis
    - Actinomycotic osteomyelitis
  - Radiation induced osteomyelitis
  - Idiopathic osteomyelitis

Pathogenesis

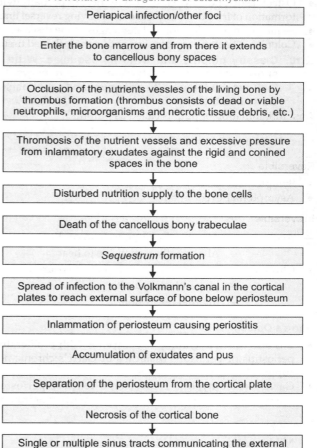

Flowchart 4: Pathogenesis of osteomyelisis.

| Periapical infection/other foci |
| Enter the bone marrow and from there it extends to cancellous bony spaces |
| Occlusion of the nutrients vessels of the living bone by thrombus formation (thrombus consists of dead or viable neutrophils, microorganisms and necrotic tissue debris, etc.) |
| Thrombosis of the nutrient vessels and excessive pressure from inlammatory exudates against the rigid and conined spaces in the bone |
| Disturbed nutrition supply to the bone cells |
| Death of the cancellous bony trabeculae |
| *Sequestrum* formation |
| Spread of infection to the Volkmann's canal in the cortical plates to reach external surface of bone below periosteum |
| Inlammation of periosteum causing periostitis |
| Accumulation of exudates and pus |
| Separation of the periosteum from the cortical plate |
| Necrosis of the cortical bone |
| Single or multiple sinus tracts communicating the external surface of the skin and mucous membrane |

Contd...

Contd...

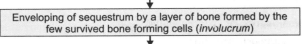

Enveloping of sequestrum by a layer of bone formed by the few survived bone forming cells (*involucrum*)

↓

Pus discharge from the involucrum can reach the skin through the sinus openings called cloacae

Clinical Features

- Molar area of mandible is more frequently affected.
- Pain is usually mild and insidious and is not related to the real severity of disease.
- Jaw swelling is common feature but mobility of teeth and sinus tract formation are rare.
- Anesthesia and paresthesia of lip is uncommon.
- Regional lymphadenopathy is common.
- There is thickened, woodened feeling of bone and slow increase in jaw size.

Histopathology

- Chronic inflammatory reaction of bone with accumulation of exudate and pus within medullary spaces.
- Lymphocytes, macrophages and plasma cells predominate among the inflammatory cells.
- Osteoblastic and osteoclastic cavity occurs partially with formation of irregular bony trabeculae having reversal lines.
- Sequestrum may develop in later stages of the disease.
- Colonies of bacteria are also seen within the inflamed tissue.

Q.10. Classify pulpitis and write its sequelae. Write in short etiology, clinical features, roentgenographic features, histology with treatment and prognosis of Garre's osteomyelitis. *(Feb 2006, 15 Marks)*

Ans. Inflammation of pulp is called as pulpitis.

Classification of Pulpitis

Reversible

- Symptomatic (acute)
- Asymptomatic (chronic).

Irreversible

- Acute — Abnormally responsive to cold
  — Abnormally responsive to heat
- Chronic — Asymptomatic with pulp exposure
  — Hyperplastic pulpitis
  — Internal resorption.

Garre's Osteomyelitis

- It is also called as chronic osteomyelitis with proliferative periostitis or periostitis ossificans or Garre's chronic non suppurative sclerosing osteitis.
- Garre's osteomyelitis represents a reactive periosteal osteogenesis in response to low grade infection or trauma.

Etiology

- Mild infection
- Chronic periapical abscess

- Infected periapical cyst
- Mechanical irritation in the jaw from dentures
- Chronic trauma in the jaw bone.

Sequelae of Pulpitis

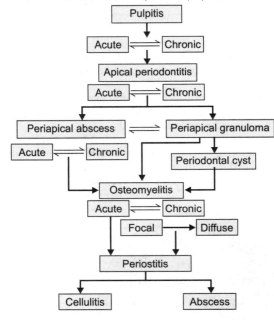

Flowchart 5: Sequelae of pulpitis.

Clinical Features

- It is common in young children and adults.
- Mandible is commonly involved in the posterior part.
- The involved jaw bone presents a carious nonvital tooth.
- There is a slight tenderness or a vague pain may be felt in the affected area of the bone.
- Slight pyrexia and leukocytosis may be present but ESR is normal.

Roentgenographic Features

- There is presence of a shadow of thin convex shell of bone over cortex.
- As the infection proceeds cortex become thick and laminated with alternating radiolucent and radiopaque layers. This is also known as onion skin appearance.
- Cancellous bone adjacent to the lesion can be normal, become sclerotic or it can show some areas of osteolytic changes.
- In the new bone osteolytic radiolucencies, i.e., small sequestra are seen.

Histology

- There is presence of newly formed bone consisting of multiple osteoids and primitive bony tissue in sub periosteal region.
- Osteoblastic as well as osteoclastic activities are observed in central part of the bone.

◆ Marrow space contains fibrous tissues showing patchy areas of chronic inflammatory cell infiltration.

◆ Trabeculae are oriented perpendicular to the cortex with trabeculae arranged, parallel to each other shows "retiform pattern".

◆ Connective tissue between the bony trabeculae shows a diffuse or patchy sprinkling of lymphocytes and plasma cells.

Treatment and Prognosis

◆ Elimination of causative agent

◆ Extraction of carious infected tooth and antibiotic therapy

◆ Prognosis is good so no any additional surgical intervention is required.

Q.11. **Describe pathogenesis, histopathology and clinical picture of osteomyelitis.** *(Mar 2003, 15 Marks)*

Ans. Osteomyelitis is defined as the inflammation of bone and bone marrow along with the surrounding periosteum.

◆ *Pathogenesis: Refer to Ans. 9 of same chapter.*

◆ *Histopathology: Refer to Ans. 8 and Ans. 9 of same chapter*

◆ *Clinical Features: Refer to Ans. 8 and 9 of same chapter.*

For pathogenesis of osteomyelitis, refer to Ans. 9 of same chapter.

For clinical features and histopathology of acute osteomyelitis, refer to Ans. 8 of same chapter.

For clinical features and histopathology of chronic osteomyelitis, refer to Ans. 9 of same chapter.

Q.12. **Write short note on Garrey's osteomyelitis.**
(Sep 2004, 5 Marks) (Aug 2011, 5 Marks)
(Mar 2013, 3 Marks)

Or

Give descriptive note on Garrey's osteomyelitis.
(Mar 2006, 5 Marks)

Ans. *Refer to Ans. 10 of same chapter.*

Q.13. **Define osteomyelitis and give an account of acute suppurative osteomyelitis in detail.**
(Mar 2007, 6.5 Marks)

Ans. Osteomyelitis is defined as the inflammation of bone and bone marrow along with the surrounding periosteum.

For acute suppurative osteomyelitis, refer to Ans. 8 of same chapter.

Q.14. **Draw well-labeled histopathological diagram of chronic hyperplastic pulpitis.** *(Dec 2007, 3 Marks)*

Ans. *Refer to Ans. 2 of same chapter.*

Q.15. **Classify pulpitis. Describe etiology, clinical features and sequelae of acute pulpitis.** *(Sep 2009, 7 Marks)*

Ans. *For classification of pulpitis, refer to Ans. 10 of same chapter.*

For etiology, clinical features and sequelae of acute pulpitis, refer to Ans. 1 of same chapter.

Q.16. **Write short note on osteomyelitis.** *(Feb 2013, 5 Marks)*

Ans. *For definition, classification and pathogenesis, refer to Ans. 9 of same chapter.*

For clinical features and histopathology of acute osteomyelitis, refer to Ans. 8 of same chapter.

For clinical features and histopathology of acute osteomyelitis, refer to Ans. 9 of same chapter.

Q.17. **Describe in brief etiology of pulpitis.**
(Apr 2008, 5 Marks)

Ans. Following is the etiology of pulpitis

◆ Dental caries which extend beyond the dentinal barrier and reaches pulp lead to pulpitis.

◆ During cavity preparation if pulp exposure occurs this will lead to pulpitis.

◆ When blow to the tooth occur which lead to damage of pulp.

◆ If cavity preparation is done without using the water spray this lead to the excessive heat production to tooth which lead to pulpitis.

◆ Chemical irritation to pulp

◆ Cracked tooth syndrome

◆ If metallic restoration is given in the tooth without providing proper thermal insulation this will lead to pulpitis.

Q.18. **Write short note on periapical abscess.**
(Dec 2009, 5 Marks)

Ans. Periapical abscess is an acute or chronic suppurative process of dental periapical region.

It is also known as dentoalveolar abscess or alveolar abscess.

Acute exacerbation of chronic periapical lesion is called as phoenix abscess.

Types of Periapical Abscess

◆ *Acute:* It is associated with severe pain in tooth.

◆ *Chronic:* It is long standing and symptoms are of low grade.

Clinical Features

Acute Periapical Abscess

◆ Patient complains of severe pain which is of throbbing variety.

◆ There is also presence of swelling in the associated area.

◆ Mucosa surrounding the swelling becomes tough and inflamed.

◆ Slight fever is present.

◆ Regional lymphadenitis is present.

◆ Patient feels sensitivity with the affected tooth.

◆ Tooth is tender to palpation and is mobile.

Chronic Periapical Abscess

◆ Pain is present from a longer time. Nature of pain is dull.

◆ Sinus formation is seen either intraorally and extraorally.

◆ At opening of sinus mass of inflamed granulation tissue is present known as parulis.

◆ Lymphadenopathy is present.

Histopathology

◆ Area of suppuration consists of central area of disintegrating PMN leukocytes surrounded by lymphocytes, cellular debris, necrotic material and the bacterial colonies.

◆ Dilated blood vessels are seen in PDL and adjacent marrow spaces of bone.

◆ Inflammatory cell infiltrate is seen in marrow spaces.

◆ In chronic periapical abscess chronic inflammatory infiltrate consist of lymphocytes, plasma cells, macrophages.

Treatment

Drainage of abscess is done followed by opening of root canal or extraction of tooth.

Q.19. Describe etiopathogenesis of periapical granuloma.

(Feb 2013, 8 Marks)

Ans.

Etiopathogenesis of Periapical Granuloma

♦ Periapical granuloma is caused as a response to prolonged irritation from infected root canals which leads to the extension of chronic apical periodontitis in PDL.

♦ Since pulp is infected it presents the release of inflammatory mediators, such as prostaglandins, kinins and endotoxins. Elevated levels of IgG are seen in pulpoperiapical lesion.

♦ Inflammation as well as increase in the vascular pressure leads to abscess formation and resorption of bone in affected area which is replaced by the granulation tissue.

Q.20. Classify osteomyelitis. Write in detail the clinical, radiological and histopathological features of Garre's osteomyelitis. *(Apr 2015, 8 Marks)*

Ans. *For classification of osteomyelitis, refer to Ans. 9 of same chapter.*

For clinical, radiological and histopathological features of Garre's osteomyelitis, refer to Ans. 10 of same chapter.

Q.21. Write short note on phoenix abscess.

(Jan 2017, 5 Marks)

Ans. Acute exacerbation of chronic periapical lesion is called as phoenix abscess.

Phoenix abscess is also known as recrudescent abscess.

Phoenix abscess is also defined as an acute inflammatory reaction superimposed on existing chronic lesion, such as cyst or granuloma.

Etiology

Chronic periradicular lesions, such as granulomas are in state of equilibrium during which they can be completely asymptomatic. But, sometimes, influx of necrotic products from diseased pulp or bacteria and their toxins can cause the dormant lesion to react and this leads to initiation of acute inflammatory response. Lowered body defenses and mechanical irritation during root canal treatment also trigger an acute inflammatory response.

Clinical features

♦ First symptom is that, there is tenderness on percussion. Tooth is slightly extruded from socket and is mobile.

♦ Patient can or cannot have swelling. Swelling, if present is localized and if left untreated may become diffuse (cellulitis), leading to asymmetry of the patients face. In case of upper canines, it may even extend to the eyelids.

♦ Patient can be present with fever, malaise and lymphadenopathy.

♦ Tissue at the surface of swelling appears taut and inflamed; pus starts to form beneath it.

♦ As the liquefaction continues, tissue ruptures due to the pressure to form a sinus tract which opens on the labial/buccal mucosa. This process is the beginning of chronic alveolar abscess.

Histopathology

There is presence of areas of liquefaction necrosis with disintegrated polymorphonuclear leukocytes and cellular debris surrounded by macrophages. lymphocytes, plasma cells in periradicular tissues.

Treatment

♦ Establishment of drainage is done.

♦ As symptoms subsides root canal therapy should be done.

Q.22. Classify diseases of pulp. Discuss pulp polyp.

(Apr 2019, 5 Marks)

Ans.

Classification of Diseases of Pulp

Grossman's Clinical Classification

1. Inflammatory diseases of dental pulp
   a. Reversible pulpitis
   b. Irreversible pulpitis
      i. Symptomatic irreversible pulpitis (acute irreversible pulpitis)
      ii. Asymptomatic irreversible pulpitis (chronic irreversible pulpitis)
      iii. Chronic hyperplastic pulpitis
      iv. Internal resorption
2. Pulp degeneration
   a. Calcific degeneration (radiographic diagnosis)
   b. Atrophic degeneration (histopathologic diagnosis)
   c. Fibrous degeneration
3. Pulp necrosis.

Ingle's Classification

1. Inflammatory changes
   A. Hyperactive pulpalgia
      a. Hypersensitivity
      b. Hyperemia
         i. Acute: Decrease flow of blood
         ii. Chronic: Decreased drainage of venous blood
2. Acute pulpalgia
   A. Incipient
   B. Moderate
   C. Advanced
3. Chronic pulpalgia
   A. Hyperplastic pulpitis
   B. Necrosis of pulp
4. Degenerative changes
   A. Atrophic changes
   B. Calcific pulposis

Histologic Classification by Seltzer and Bende

1. Inflammatory change
   a. Intact pulp with scattered chronic inflammatory cells
   b. Acute pulpitis
   c. Chronic total pulpitis with partial necrosis
   d. Chronic partial pulpitis
   e. Pulp necrosis
2. Degenerative changes
   a. Atrophic pulp
   b. Dystrophic mineralization

For details of pulp polyp, refer to Ans. 2 and Ans. 4 of same chapter.

III   INJURIES AND REPAIR

12. SPREAD OF ORAL INFECTION

Q.1. Write note on cellulitis. *(Apr 2007, 10 Marks)*

Or

Write short note on cellulitis. *(Apr 2017, 4 Marks)*

Ans. It is also known as phlegmon.

Cellulitis is defined as an acute edematous purulent inflammatory process which spreads diffusely through different tissue spaces or facial planes.

Clinical Features

♦ There is wide spread swelling, redness and pain without definite localization.
♦ Soft tissue swelling is firm and browny.
♦ When cellulitis involves the superficial tissue spaces, the overlying skin appears purplish.
♦ Fever, chills leukocytosis are often present which make the patient slight ill.
♦ Regional lymphadenopathy often develops.
♦ Some lesions resolve completely however in other cases pus discharging intraoral or extraoral sinuses may develop.
♦ If maxillary tooth is involved there may be redness of eye.

Histopathology

♦ There is collection of large amount of fibrin and serum fluid as well as tissue.
♦ Acute inflammatory cell infiltration by PMNs and occasionally lymphocytes.
♦ Formation of sinus tracts over skin or mucosal surfaces.
♦ Pus may develop in the later stages of the disease.

Treatment

♦ Bacteriological examination of exudates or pus.
♦ Drainage of pus is carried out.
♦ Antibiotic therapy.
♦ Elimination of primary source of inflammation.

Q.2. Write short note on Ludwig's angina.

(Sep 2018, 5 Marks)
(Sep 2006, 6 Marks) (Mar 2001, 5 Marks)
(Jan 2016, 5 Marks) (Feb 2013, 5 Marks)

Or

Describe in brief Ludwig's angina. *(Apr 2008, 10 Marks)*

Ans. Ludwig's angina is an acute toxic cellulitis begin in submandibular space and secondarily involving sublingual and submental spaces as well.

Etiology

♦ Dentoalveolar abscess in relation to mandibular 2nd or 3rd molar.
♦ Deep periodontal abscess or pocket.
♦ Pericoronal infection in relation to mandibular 3rd molar.
♦ Osteomyelitis.
♦ Injection of contaminated needle.
♦ *Traumatic injuries:* Fracture of mandible if infected or contaminated.
♦ Deep laceration or penetrating injury.

Rare Causes

♦ Sublingual sialadenitis
♦ Submandibular sialadenitis.
♦ Purulent tonsillitis.

Bacteriology

♦ Main microorganism is streptococci
♦ Others are staphylococci, gram-negative (*E. coli* and *Pseudomonas*), anaerobes, bacteroids and *peptostreptococcus*.

Clinical Features

♦ It produces a board like swelling of floor of mouth and consequent elevation of tongue.
♦ The swelling is firm, painful and diffuse showing no evidence of localization.
♦ There is difficulty in eating, swallowing and breathing.
♦ Patient has high fever, rapid pulse and fast respiration.
♦ Moderate leukocytosis is present.
♦ The swelling may spread to the neck with development of edema glottis.

Laboratory Findings

♦ Streptococci are invariably seen.
♦ Fusiform bacilli and spiral forms, various staphylococci, diphtheroids and other microorganisms are cultured.
♦ It is a nonspecific mixed infection.

Complication

♦ Asphyxia: Due to edema of glottis.
♦ Septicemia and cavernous sinus thrombosis.
♦ Mediastinitis.
♦ Meningitis
♦ Brain abscess.
♦ Death.

(The most common cause of death is as asphyxia).

Treatment

♦ Early diagnosis.
♦ Maintenance of patient airway.
♦ Intense and prolonged antibiotic therapy.
♦ Extraction of offending teeth.
♦ Surgical drainage of facial space.

Q.3. Write short note on focus of infection.

(Dec 2012, 3 Marks) (Mar 2013, 3 Marks)

Or

Write short note on focus of infection and focal infection. *(Feb 2019, 5 Marks) (July 2016, 5 Marks)*

Ans. Focus of infection refers to "the circumscribed area of tissue which is infected with exogenous pathogenic microorganisms and is located near mucous or cutaneous surface". **—Billings**

♦ As there is local or general infection which is caused by dissemination of microorganisms or toxic products from focus of infection this lead to focal infection.

♦ Foci may be primary or secondary. Primary foci usually are located in tissues communicating with a mucous or cutaneous surface.

♦ Secondary foci are the direct result of infections from other foci through contiguous tissues, or at a distance through the blood stream or lymph channels.

Mechanism of Focal Infection

Two of the accepted mechanisms are:

♦ Metastasis of microorganisms from an infected focus by hematogenous or lymphogenous spread.

♦ Toxins or toxic products may be carried through the blood or lymphatic channels from a focus to a distant site where they may incite a hypersensitive reaction in the tissues.

Oral Foci of Infection

Various infections of the oral cavity may act as sources of infection and may be responsible for spread of microbes to a distant site causing metastases. The potential foci in the oral cavity include:

♦ Infected periapical lesions, particularly the chronic lesions, such as the periapical abscess, granuloma and cyst.

♦ Teeth with infected root canals are the potential sources of dissemination of microbes as well as their toxins.

♦ Periodontal disease following tooth extraction or dental manipulation is also significant focus of infection; particularly the tooth extraction is an important cause of bacteremia.

Impedance of Oral Foci of Infection

Oral foci of infection either cause or aggravate many systemic diseases. Most frequently encountered systemic diseases are:

♦ *Arthritis:* Arthritis of the rheumatoid type and rheumatic fever type. Which are manifested because of the occurrence of streptococcal infection in mouth. The causal microbe (Group A streptococci) may not be cultured from the joints and blood, but the patients have a high titer of antibodies against these microbes. The presence of these antibodies suggests that tissue hypersensitivity reaction is the cause of inflammatory reactions that occur.

♦ *Subacute bacterial endocarditis (infective endocarditis):* Majority of these cases are related to oral infection and occur following tooth extraction. The close similarity between the causative agent of subacute bacterial endocarditis and the *Streptococcus* of *viridans* group in the oral cavity, in the dental pulp and periapical lesions, and frequent occurrence of transient streptococcal bacteremia following tooth extraction are the indication that oral foci are the cause of this disease.

♦ *Gastrointestinal diseases:* It has been reported that constant swallowing of streptococci from mouth may lead to a variety of gastrointestinal diseases. Gastric and duodenal ulcers are related to oral foci of infection.

♦ *Ocular diseases:* In many ocular diseases, such as iritis, cyclitis, choroiditis, uveitis, etc., microbes associated with the teeth, oral cavity, tonsils, sinuses, etc., have been considered as primary foci of infection.

♦ *Skin diseases:*, such as some form of eczema and possibly urticaria can be related to oral foci of infection.

♦ *Renal diseases:* Streptococci, particularly *S. haemolyticus* present in dental root canals or periapical or gingival areas appears to have some relation with certain type of renal diseases and may play a role in causing renal diseases.

Q.4. Describe in detail on diseases of maxillary sinus.
(June 2010, 10 Marks)

Ans. Following are the diseases of maxillary sinus:

Classification

♦ *Developmental:*
  • Crouzon's syndrome
  • Treacher Collins syndrome
  • Binder syndrome

♦ *Inflammatory:*
  • Maxillary sinusitis
  • Mucositis
  • Empyema

♦ *Cyst:*
  • Non-dental
    – Mucocele
    – Benign mucosal cyst of maxillary antrum
    – Surgical ciliated cyst
  • *Dental:*
    – Radicular cyst
    – Globulomaxillary cyst
    – Dentigerous cyst
    – Odontogenic keratocyst

♦ *Benign tumor:*
  • Osteoma
  • Ameloblastoma
  • Antral polyp
  • Antral papilloma

♦ *Malignant tumor:*
  • Squamous cell carcinoma
  • Metastatic carcinoma of maxillary sinus
  • Local malignant tumor invades maxillary sinus

♦ *Due to trauma:*
  • Fractured root
  • Sinus contusion
  • Blow out fracture
  • Isolated injury
  • Complex fracture
  • Oroantral fistula
  • Foreign bodies

♦ *Calcification:* Antrolith

♦ *Miscellaneous*
  • Fibrous dysplasia
  • Pseudotumor

Crouzon Syndrome

It is also known as craniofacial dysostosis.

Following are the features

♦ Frontal defect is present and cranium is brachycephalic.
♦ Maxilla and maxillary sinus remains hypoplastic.
♦ High arch palate is seen.
♦ Dental arch is V shaped
♦ Partial anodontia is present.

Treacher Collins Syndrome

It is also known as mandibulofacial dysostosis.

♦ Maxillary sinus and malar bones are underdeveloped.
♦ Cheek bones are underdeveloped.
♦ Facial cleft is present.
♦ Palate is high arched.
♦ Malformation of external ear is seen.

Binder Syndrome

♦ It leads to hypoplasia of middle third of face.
♦ Retrognathic maxilla
♦ Presence of maxillonasal dysplasia
♦ Hypoplastic maxillary and frontal sinus

Maxillary Sinusitis

♦ Inflammation of mucosa of maxillary sinus is known as maxillary sinusitis.
♦ It can be acute, subacute and chronic.

Etiology

♦ It is caused due to periapical infection of teeth.
♦ Due to oroantral fistula
♦ By deep pocket
♦ Due to trauma of facial bones.
♦ Due to overpreparation of root canal which leads to gutta-percha filling in sinus.
♦ If implant is placed too deep

Clinical Features

Acute

♦ Patient complains of pain in eyeball, cheek or frontal areas which is severe and is constant. Pain gets exaggerated by downward positioning of head.
♦ Nasal discharge is present which is watery in beginning of disease and later on becomes mucopurulent.
♦ There is presence of erythematous color and inflammation of mucosa of anterior nares.
♦ Presence of tenderness on palpation.

Subacute

♦ Symptoms are diminished.
♦ Presence of purulent discharge. Nasal voice is present.
♦ Patient is unable to sleep because of presence of cough.

Chronic

♦ Nasal obstruction and headache are the constant features.
♦ Low fever and tiredness is present.

Histopathology

♦ Maxillary sinus lining have acute inflammatory infiltrate.
♦ Edema of connective tissue is present.
♦ At times hemorrhage is also seen.

Treatment

♦ Removal of the cause.
♦ Antibiotics, analgesics and nasal decongestants should be given.

Mucositis

♦ Inflammation of mucosa of maxillary sinus is known as mucositis.
♦ It is caused by periodontal or periapical infection.
♦ Disease is asymptomatic.

Benign Mucosal Cyst of Maxillary Antrum

♦ Occurs during 2nd and 3rd decades of life.
♦ Male predilection is present.
♦ Localized dull pain is present over antrum.
♦ Yellow fluid discharge is seen from nose.
♦ Histology reveals presence of chronic inflammatory cells in connective tissue wall.

Postoperative Maxillary Cyst

♦ It occurs due to the entrapped epithelial lining of maxillary sinus in wound closure during Caldwell-Luc surgery.
♦ Occurs from 2nd to 7th decades of life.
♦ Pain and swelling is present over cheek or palate or face or alveolus.
♦ Pus discharge is present.
♦ Histopathology reveals presence of squamous metaplasia in pseudo-stratified columnar epithelium.
♦ Enucleation should be done.

Osteoma

♦ It occurs from 2nd to 4th decade of life.
♦ Male predilection is seen.
♦ Mainly asymptomatic but obstruct the ostium of sinus.
♦ It can expand to maxillary sinus and leads to swelling of hard palate.
♦ Surgical excision is done.

Antral Polyp

♦ Mucosa of the chronically inflamed sinus leads to the formation of irregular folds known as polyp.
♦ Seen in young adults.
♦ Pain in the nose and nasal obstruction is present.
♦ Saint's triad is present, i.e., asthma, nasal and antral polyp and aspirin sensitivity.
♦ Excision of polyp is done.

Squamous Cell Carcinoma

♦ Squamous cell carcinoma of maxillary sinus occurs from metaplastic epithelium of sinus lining.

♦ Occurs during 6th decade of life and male predilection is seen.
♦ Patient complains of pain over face, nasal obstruction and swelling.
♦ Ulceration is present over the hard palate.
♦ Both medial and lateral walls of the sinus are involved.
♦ Involvement of floor of the sinus leads to expansion of boney plates, swelling, mobility of teeth and severe pain.
♦ Histopathology reveals features of squamous cell carcinoma.
For details, refer to Ans. 23 of chapter Benign and Malignant Tumors of Oral Cavity.

Oroantral Fistula

♦ It is an epithelialized pathological communication between oral cavity and maxillary sinus.
♦ It is caused by trauma to sinus, malignancies and osteomyelitis
♦ There is presence of tenderness over the maxilla especially in infraorbital region.
♦ Mild edema to cheek in infraorbital soft tissue.
♦ Ear ache-referred pain from antrum.
♦ On nose-red, shiny and swollen, mucous membrane, around osteum.
♦ Presence of pus or mucopurulent discharge in middle meatus.
♦ Oropharynx—mucopurulent discharge.
♦ Impairment of sense of smell.
♦ Foul smelling of mucopurulent discharge.
♦ Mild tenderness over infraorbital region.
♦ Closure of opening is done by surgical methods.

Antrolith

♦ It is the calcified mass present in the maxillary sinus.
♦ It can occur at any age
♦ Lesion is asymptomatic and at times nasal discharge is present which is blood stained and nasal obstruction too is seen.
♦ Removal is done if lesion is symptomatic.

13. PHYSICAL AND CHEMICAL INJURIES OF THE ORAL CAVITY

Q.1. Write notes on osteoradionecrosis.

(Mar 2001, 5 Marks)

Or

Write short note on osteoradionecrosis.

(Sep 2007, 3 Marks) (Sep 2011, 3 Marks)

Ans. Osteoradionecrosis is a radiation induced pathologic process characterized by the chronic and painful infection and necrosis is accompanied by the late sequestration and sometimes permanent deformity.

This is one of the most serious complications of radiation to head and neck seen frequently today because of better treatment modalities and prevention.

Factors Leading to Osteoradionecrosis

♦ Irradiation of an area of previous surgery before adequate healing had taken place.
♦ Irradiation of lesion in close proximity to bone.
♦ Prolong oral hygiene and continued use of irritants.
♦ Poor patient's corporation in managing irradiated tissues.
♦ Surgery in irradiated area.
♦ Failure to prevent trauma to irradiated bony areas.

Clinical Features

♦ Osteoradionecrosis is the result of nonhealing dead bone.
♦ Mandible is affected more commonly than maxilla.

Histology

♦ There is destruction of osteocytes, absence of osteoblasts and lack of new bone or osteoid formation.
♦ Walls of regional blood vessels are thickened by fibrous connective tissue.
♦ Radiation causes proliferation of intima of blood vessels leading to thrombosis of arteries which results in nonvital bone.

Treatment

♦ Debridement of necrotic tissue should be done along with removal of sequestrum.
♦ Administration of intravenous antibiotic and hyperbaric oxygen therapy are essential
♦ Maintenance of oral hygiene is necessary.

Q.2. Write short note on lead poisoning.

(Aug 2012, 5 Marks)

Ans. Lead poisoning leads to plumbism.

Etiology

♦ *Paints consisting of lead:* Workers and children are most commonly affected.
♦ Illicit alcohol consisting of lead can cause lead poisoning.
♦ Gasolining consisting of lead.
♦ Lead from automobile smoke can lead to occupational exposure.

Clinical Features

♦ Due to lead poisoning there is axon degeneration and demyelination.
♦ In more severe cases, there is presence of encephalopathy, seizures, mental retardation and cerebral palsy.
♦ Patient often complains of nausea, vomiting and constipation.
♦ Due to lead poisoning bone deposition and resorption is disturbed.

Oral Manifestations

♦ There is presence of excessive salivation, metallic taste and dysphagia.
♦ Burtonian line is seen in cases of lead poisoning with poor oral hygiene. A gray black line is seen along marginal gingiva which is known as burtonian line.

♦ Characteristic signs are pale lips, Ashen colored face, muscle tone is poor.
♦ Bilateral parotid gland hypertrophy is evident.

Treatment

Chelating agents, such as EDTA should be given to treat the patient.

Q.3. Write short note on chemical injuries of oral cavity.
(Jan 2018, 5 Marks)

Ans. Oral cavity manifests serious reaction to the wide variety of drugs and chemicals.

♦ Tissue injury can be due to local response to a severe irritant or due to administration of systemic drugs.
♦ Aspirin, sodium perborate, hydrogen peroxide, gasoline, turpentine, rubbing alcohol and battery acid is the examples.
♦ Various patients many children under psychiatric care hold medication under their mouth rather swallowing them. Such medications are potentially caustic when held in mouth for long duration.
♦ Following are the materials in detail which lead to chemical injuries of oral cavity:

Chemical Injuries by Materials used Locally in Dentistry

Aspirin

♦ Aspirin tablets or powder are mainly used mistakenly in oral cavity by patients as local obtundent mainly for relief of toothache.
♦ Initially, there is burning sensation present in oral mucosa.
♦ Affected surface appear blanched as well as white in appearance.
♦ Epithelial separation and sloughing of epithelium along with frequent bleeding is seen.
♦ Healing take place under 1 to 2 weeks.

Endodontic Materials

♦ Some of endodontic materials lead to soft tissue damage causing deep spread of inflammation and necrosis.
♦ Paraformaldehyde is used to devitalize inflamed pulp. It can leak from pulp chamber in surrounding tissue and lead to necrosis of gingiva and bone.
♦ Sodium hypochlorite produces same effect as paraformaldehyde when it leaks in surrounding supporting tissue or injected beyond the apex.
♦ Sodium hypochlorite when come in contact with vital tissue it leads to hemolysis and ulceration.
♦ Microscopically sodium hypochlorite inhibits neutrophil migration and damage endothelial and fibroblast cells.

Hydrogen Peroxide

♦ This is a caustic agent.
♦ As it comes under the contact with tissues it lead to burning of tissues and release toxic free radicals, perhydroxyl ion or both.

♦ About 30 to 35% of hydrogen peroxide is used with heat for bleaching teeth. This thermocatalytic process damages the tooth by causing irritation to cementum and periodontal ligament which also causes cervical root resorption.

Phenol

♦ It is cavity sterilizing and cauterizing agent.
♦ This is used in treatment of aphthous ulcers.
♦ As extensive necrosis is seen from medicaments consisting of 0.5% phenol, this product should be used with atmost care.

Silver Nitrate

♦ It is useful for treatment of aphthous ulcers as chemical cautery leads to pain relief by destroying the nerve endings.
♦ Its over usage leads to the painful burn of oral cavity.

Histopathology of Locally Acting Agents Leading to Chemical Injuries

♦ White slough removed from mucosal chemical burns shows coagulative necrosis of epithelium. Outline of epithelial cells and nuclei is visible.
♦ Necrosis starts over the surface and moves basally.
♦ Underlying connective tissue consists of mixture of acute and chronic inflammatory cells.

Chemical Injuries by Materials used Systemically in Dentistry

Lead

♦ Lead poisoning or plumbism is an occupational hazard.
♦ Lead line or Burtonian line is a gray or blue black line of sulfide pigmentation present on gingiva.
♦ Ulcerative stomatitis is seen.
♦ Excessive salivation and metallic taste are commonly present.

Mercury

♦ Mercury poisoning occur when it is used therapeutically.
♦ In this tongue and salivary glands are swollen.
♦ Metallic taste in mouth is present.
♦ Salivary flow is increased.
♦ Ulcerations are present on gingiva, palate and tongue.
♦ Exfoliation of teeth is also present.
♦ Acrodynia occurs due to chronic mercury exposure in infants and children.

Silver

♦ Subepithelial deposition of silver in mucus membrane leads to diffuse grayish discoloration.
♦ A blue silver line occurs at gingival margin due to secondary deposition of metallic silver.
♦ Amalgam tattoo is the most common finding. In this particles enter via lacerations which occur during removal

of old amalgam restorations. It appears as raised blue, black or gray lesion.

Bismuth

◆ It is used by oral surgeons in surgical packs.
◆ Pigmentation of bismuth is seen in gingiva and buccal mucosa.
◆ Bismuth line, i.e., blue black line is present at marginal gingiva.

Tetracycline

◆ It lead to the discoloration of permanent or deciduous teeth due to deposition of tetracycline during prophylactic or therapeutic regimens in pregnant female or postpartum in infant.
◆ Affected teeth are yellowish or show brown gray discoloration.
◆ Dentine is more stained than enamel.

---

14. REGRESSIVE ALTERATIONS OF THE TEETH

Q.1. Write short note on abrasion. *(Sep 2002, 5 Marks)*

Or

Give descriptive note on abrasion. *(Mar 2006, 5 Marks)*

Ans. Abrasion is a pathological wearing of dental tissues by friction with the foreign substances independent of occlusion.

Etiology

◆ Tooth brush abrasion
◆ Habitual abrasion, e.g., pipe smokers, tooth pick and dental floss causes abrasion on proximal surfaces of teeth.
◆ Occupation abrasion, e.g., hair dressers, carpenters and shoemakers.
◆ Abrasion by prosthetic appliances
◆ Ritual abrasions.

Clinical Features

◆ In abrasion of tooth, the type and severity of surface will depend upon the duration and type of faulty habit adapted by the person.
◆ Toothbrush abrasion commonly occurs in cervical region of labial surface of incisors, canines and premolars.
◆ Maxillary teeth are more commonly affected than the mandibular teeth.
◆ The produces a 'V" shaped or wedge-shaped groove on the tooth with sharp angles and highly polished dentin surface.
◆ Toothbrush abrasion may cause gingival recession.
◆ Occupational abrasion often produces a small, deep, well-polished ditch on an incisal edge of teeth.
◆ Sever abrasion may cause opening of dentinal tubules and hence the patient experiences sensitivity in affected teeth due to hot and cold substances.

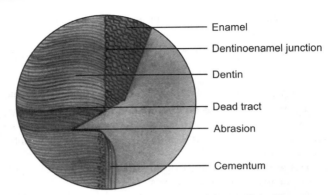

Fig. 85: Abrasion *(For color version, see Plate 15).*

Treatment

◆ Adaptance of normal brushing habits prevents abrasion.
◆ Restorative treatment helps to keep the tooth surface intact and prevents further tooth wear.

Q.2. Write short note on sclerotic dentin.

(Sep 2005, 5 Marks)

Ans. It is also known as transparent dentin.

◆ Dentinal sclerosis is the condition characterized by calcification of dentinal tubules of the tooth.
◆ It is the regressive alteration in the tooth surface.

Etiology

◆ Injury to dentin by caries
◆ Aging process
◆ Abrasion or erosion of the tooth.
◆ Sclerotic dentin is found under the slowly progressing caries
◆ It reduces the permeability of dentin and prolongs pulp vitality.
◆ Dentinal sclerosis presents a translucent zone in the teeth which is seen in the tooth by the transmitted light.
◆ Sclerosis often decreases the conductivity of the tubules.

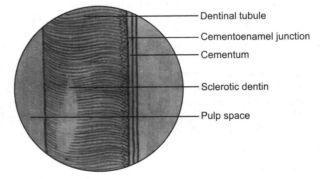

Fig. 86: Sclerotic dentin *(For color version, see Plate 15).*

Q.3. Describe regressive changes in pulp.

(Mar 2001, 15 Marks)

Or

Write short note on age changes in pulp.

(Dec 2012, 3 Marks)

Ans. Regressive changes of pulp mean aging of pulp.

Cell Changes

♦ Cells are characterized by decrease in size and number of cytoplasmic organelles.
♦ Pulpal fibrocytes or fibroblasts have abundant rough surface, cytoplasmic reticulum, Golgi bodies and numerous mitochondria with well-developed cristae.

Fibroblasts in aging pulp exhibit less perinuclear cytoplasm and long thin cytoplasmic processes.

Fibrosis

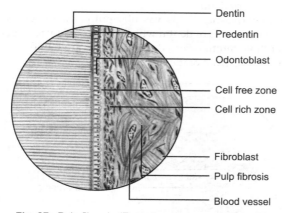

Fig. 87: Pulp fibrosis *(For color version, see Plate 16).*

♦ In aging pulp accumulation of diffuse fibrillar components and bundles of collagen fibers appears.
♦ Fiber bundles appear arranged longitudinally in bundles in radicular pulp and more diffuse arrangement on coronal area.
♦ Increase in fiber in pulp organ is generalized throughout the organ.
♦ Vascular changes occur in aging pulp organ.
♦ Atherosclerotic plaque may appear in pulpal vessels.
♦ Calcifications in the wall of blood vessels are found more often in region near the apical foramen.
♦ Outer diameter of vessel walls becomes greater, as collagen fibers increase in the medial and adventitial layer.

Pulp Stones/Denticles

♦ Pulp stones and denticles are nodular calcified masses appearing on coronal portions of the pulp organs.
♦ They are asymptomatic unless they impinge nerves on blood vessels.
♦ Pulp stones are classified according to their structures as true and false denticles.
♦ They are also classified as free, attached and embedded depending on the relation to dentin.
♦ Pulp stones may eventually fill substantial part of pulp chamber.

Pathogenesis of True Pulp Stone

♦ Development of true denticles is caused by inclusion of remnants of epithelial root sheath within pulp. These epithelial remnants induce cells of pulp to differentiate into odontoblasts which form dentin masses known as true pulp stone.

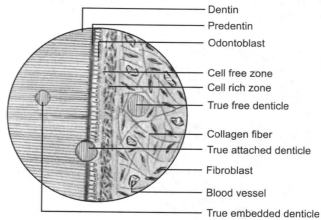

Fig. 88: True pulp stones *(For color version, see Plate 16).*

Pathogenesis of False Pulp Stone

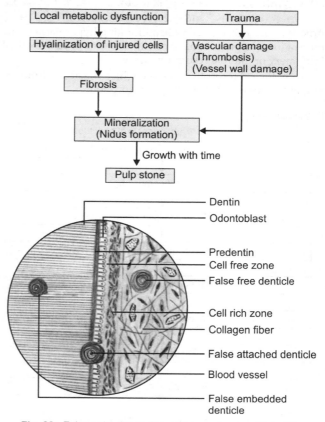

Fig. 89: False pulp stones *(For color version, see Plate 16).*

Diffuse Calcification

- They appear as irregular calcific deposit in pulp tissue following collagenous fibrous bundles in blood vessels.
- They persists as fine calcified spicules and sometimes develop into larger masses.
- Diffuse calcifications are found in root canal.
- Diffuse calcifications may surround the blood vessels.
- Diffuse calcification is also termed as "calcific degeneration."

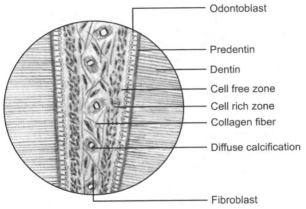

Fig. 90: Diffuse calcification *(For color version, see Plate 16).*

Q.4. Write short note on pink tooth. *(Feb 2002, 5 Marks)*
(Sep 2006, 5 Marks) (Mar 2016, 3 Marks)

Ans. It is also called as chronic perforating hyperplasia of the pulp or internal granuloma or odontoclastoma or pink tooth of Mummery or internal resorption of teeth.

Pathological resorption of tooth which is starting from the pulpal surface is called as internal resorption.

Pathogenesis

Flowchart 6: Pathogenesis of pink tooth.

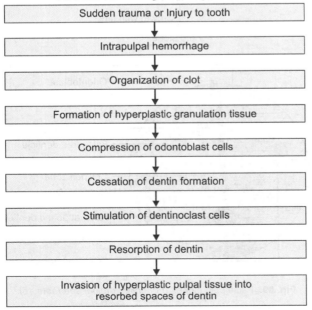

Clinical Features

- Internal resorption may involve either the crown portion of the tooth or the root portion.
- Any tooth may be involved and usually only a single tooth is affected.
- Pink appearance of tooth occur in advanced stage when the coronal dentin is involved.
- When internal resorption affects the root of the tooth no color change is found
- Affected tooth remains vital unless there is pulp necrosis due to fracture of tooth or due to its perforation.

Histopathology

- Multiple irregular or smooth areas of resorption in pulpal surfaces of dentin.
- A hyperplastic, highly vascular pulp tissue is projecting into the spaces of dentin which are created by resorption.
- Multiple multinucleated dentinoclasts are found near the resorpting front of the dentin.

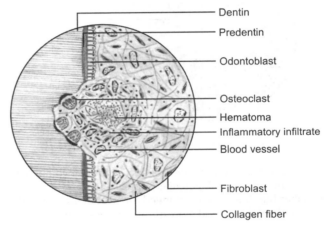

Fig. 91: Internal resorption of teeth or pink tooth *(For color version, see Plate 16).*

Treatment

- Extirpation (complete removal of part) of pulp tissue and conventional endodontic therapy
- When the tooth is perforated extraction is only the treatment.

Q.5. Describe in brief hypercementosis.
(Aug 2011, 5 Marks)

Ans. Hypercementosis is also known as cementum hyperplasia.

It increases the thickness of cementum on root surfaces of the tooth due to excessive cementogenesis and is called as hypercementosis.

Etiology

- Periapical inflammation
- Mechanical stimulation
- Functionless or unerupted tooth
- Paget's disease of bone
- Tooth repair.

Clinical Features

- Involved teeth are completely asymptomatic.
- There is no increase or decrease in tooth sensitivity, no sensitivity to percussion unless periapical inflammation is present.
- When the tooth with hypercementosis is extracted the roots appear larger in diameter than normal and present rounded apices.

Histological Features

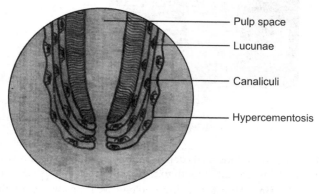

Fig. 92: Hypercementosis *(For color version, see Plate 17).*

- There is excessive amount of cellular cementum found deposited directly over the layer of acellular cementum.
- Area involved may be the entire root and the apical region.
- Cementum is arranged in the concentric layers around the root.
- Cementum shows numerous resting lines indicated by deeply staining hematoxyphilic line parallel to root surface.

Roentgenographic Features

Radiograph shows excessive cemental thickening with typical bulbous appearance of roots.

Treatment

No treatment is indicated for teeth exhibiting hypercementosis since the condition is itself innocuous.

Q.6. Write short note on attrition. *(Apr 2007, 5 Marks)*

Or

Write short answer on attrition. *(Sep 2018, 3 Marks)*

Ans. Attrition is a constant form of retrogressive change in teeth, characterized by the wear of tooth structure or restoration as a result of tooth to tooth contact during mastication.

Types

- *Physiological attrition:* Tooth loss is proportionate to age of individual.
- *Pathological attrition:* It occurs due to certain abnormalities in occlusion, chewing pattern or due to some structural defects.

Causes

- Abnormal occlusion, e.g., crowding of teeth or malposed teeth.

- Abnormal chewing habit, e.g., bruxism
- Structural defects in teeth, e.g., amelogenesis imperfecta, dentinogenesis imperfecta.

Clinical Features

- Attrition of tooth is manifested by formation of well-polished facet on tip of cusps, incisal edges and on proximal contact area of teeth.
- In advanced cases, attrition may lead to severe reduction in cuspal height with complete wearing of enamel and flattening of occlusal surface.
- When dentin is exposed it becomes discolored brown.
- Attrition in proximal surface of teeth causes transformation of proximal contact point to relatively bordered contact areas.
- Exposure of dentinal tubules in severe cases of attrition leads to hypersensitivity.
- Attrition may also lead to pulp exposure.

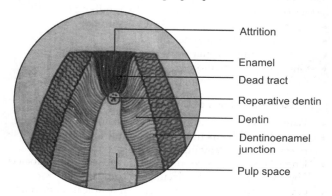

Fig. 93: Attrition *(For color version, see Plate 17).*

Treatment

- Correction of developmental abnormalities.
- Correction of parafunctional chewing habits.
- Protection of tooth by metal or metal ceramic crowns where structural defects are present.

Q.7. Write short note on attrition, abrasion, abfraction and erosion. *(Jan 2012, 5 Marks) (July 2016, 5 Marks)*

Ans. For attrition, refer to Ans. 6 of same chapter.

For abrasion, refer to Ans. 1 of same chapter.

Abfraction

Abfraction is the loss of tooth surface at the cervical areas of teeth caused by the tensile and compressive forces during tooth flexure.

Clinical Features

- Affects buccal/labial cervical areas of teeth.
- Deep, narrow V-shaped notch.
- Commonly affect single teeth with excursive interferences or eccentric occlusal loads

Erosion

It is defined as progressive loss of hard dental tissue by chemical process not involving bacterial action.

Clinical Features

♦ Broad concavities are present on tooth with smooth surface enamel.
♦ There is presence of cupping of occlusal surfaces with dentin exposure.
♦ Presence of increased incisal translucency
♦ Wearing away of nonoccluding surfaces.
♦ Amalgam restorations in erosive teeth get raised.
♦ Hypersensitivity is seen with the affected tooth.
♦ Pulp exposure is seen in deciduous teeth.

Q.8. Enumerate the diseases of cementum and describe the regressive alterations of cementum.

(Nov 2008, 15 Marks)

Ans.

Enumeration of Diseases of Cementum

Based on clinical radiographic and histological features boney lesions of cementum were classified by Pindborg et al (1971).

♦ Periapical cemental dysplasia (Cementoma)
♦ Benign cementoblastoma
♦ Cementifying fibroma
♦ Gigantiform cementoma
♦ Cemento-osseous dysplasia

Regressive Alterations of Cementum

♦ With aging, surface of cementum become more irregular.
♦ As thickness of cementum increases due to hypercementosis permeability of cementum decreases.
♦ Under light microscope only the surface layer of cementocytes appear viable. All other lacunae become empty.
♦ Greater amount of cementum appear in apical zone, middle third of the root and furcation areas.
♦ With age as a result of functional influences on teeth the location and shape of apical foramina undergo changes.
♦ Due to aging cementum can resorb or deposit creating reversal lines.
♦ **Hypercementosis:** *Refer to Ans. 5 of same chapter.*
♦ **Cementicles:** Calcifying spherical bodies composed of cementum either lying free within PDL, attached to cementum or within it. They are mostly 0.5 mm in size. They usually are ovoid or round with similar appearance to denticles and are classified as free, attached or embedded. Cementicles are a response to either local trauma or hyperactivity and appears in increasing numbers in an aging person. Found in 35% of human roots.

Pathogenesis or Formation of Cementicles

Flowchart 7: Pathogenesis or formation of cementicles.

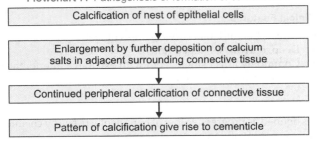

```
Calcification of nest of epithelial cells
                    ↓
Enlargement by further deposition of calcium
salts in adjacent surrounding connective tissue
                    ↓
Continued peripheral calcification of connective tissue
                    ↓
Pattern of calcification give rise to cementicle
```

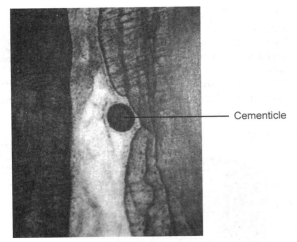

Fig. 94: Cementicle.

Q.9. Define attrition, abrasion and erosion.

(Feb 2019, 3 Marks) (Feb 2014, 3 Marks)

Ans. Attrition: Attrition is defined as physiologic wearing away of a tooth as a result of tooth to tooth contact as in mastication.

Abrasion: Abrasion is the pathologic wearing away of tooth substance through some abnormal mechanical process.

Erosion: Erosion is defined as irreversible loss of dental hard tissue by a chemical process that does not involve bacteria.

Q.10. Write short note on abfraction. *(June 2015, 5 Marks)*
(Jan 2017, 5 Marks) (Jan 2018, 5 Marks)

Ans. Abfraction is defined as the loss of tooth surface at the cervical areas of teeth caused by tensile and compressive forces during tooth flexure.

Pathogenesis

When occlusal forces are applied eccentrically to a tooth the tensile stress is concentrated at cervical fulcrum which causes flexure that leads to disruption in the chemical bonds of enamel crystals in cervical areas. Once damaged, cracked enamel can be lost or more easily removed by erosion or abrasion.

Etiology

♦ *Static forces:* These forces are produced during swallowing, clenching and tongue thrusting.
♦ *Cyclic forces:* These forces are produced at the time of chewing.
♦ People with open bite or deep class I cavity are prone for abfraction.

Clinical Features

♦ It can occur at any age.
♦ It affects buccal or labial cervical third or gingival third area of teeth.
♦ Most commonly affected teeth are facial surfaces of bicuspids and molars.
♦ There is presence of a narrow V-shaped notch.

- Single tooth is affected most commonly with excessive interferences or eccentric occlusal loads.
- Tooth becomes hypersensitive and there is wearing of occlusal surface.
- Since lateral forces damage the cervical area of tooth, repeated restoration failures are appreciated.

Treatment

- Etiological agent should be removed.
- Progression of the problem is stopped by bite guard.
- Areas of V-shaped notching should be restored by tooth colored restorative material.

Q.11. Write short note on erosion. *(Jan 2016, 5 Marks)*
Ans. Erosion is defined as progressive loss of hard dental tissue by chemical process not involving bacterial action.

Etiology

Dissolution of mineralized part of tooth occurs due to intrinsic causes and extrinsic causes.

Extrinsic causes are acidic beverages and citrus fruits.

Intrinsic causes are gastroesophageal reflux and vomiting

Extrinsic Causes

- It consists of acidic foods or due to iatrogenic exposure.
- Extrinsic causes consist of acidic beverages and foods, dietary acids, medication, environmental acids, sport drink, fruit juices, etc.
- Erosion is commonly seen in professional swimmers and occupational wine tasters.

Intrinsic Causes

- Gastric acids which regurgitate in esophagus and mouth because of acid reflux or due to excessive vomiting.
- Anorexia bulimia can also cause erosion of teeth, mostly the palatal surfaces of maxillary anterior teeth are involved.

Clinical Features

- Broad concavities are present on tooth with smooth surface enamel.
- There is presence of cupping of occlusal surfaces with dentin exposure.
- Presence of increased incisal translucency
- Wearing away of non-occluding surfaces.
- Amalgam restorations in erosive teeth get raised.
- Hypersensitivity is seen with the affected tooth.
- Pulp exposure is seen in deciduous teeth.

Treatment

- Proper etiology should be ruled out.
- Cases of acid reflux should be sent to physician for proper treatment.
- In cases with hyposalivation chewing gums are used to enhance the salivary flow.

Q.12. Write short note on pulp stones. (Mar 2016, 3 Marks)
Ans. Pulp stones are nodular calcified masses appearing on coronal portions of the pulp organs.

- They are asymptomatic unless they impinge nerves on blood vessels.
- Pulp stones are classified according to their structures as true and false denticles.
- They are also classified as free, attached and embedded depending on the relation to dentin.
- Pulp stones develop around central nidus of pulp tissue
- Pulp stones may eventually fill substantial part of pulp chamber.
- Pulp stones may arise as a part of age-related changes or local pathologic changes.

Pathogenesis of True Pulp Stone

- Development of true denticles is caused by inclusion of remnants of epithelial root sheath within pulp. These epithelial remnants induce cells of pulp to differentiate into odontoblasts which form dentin masses known as true pulp stone.

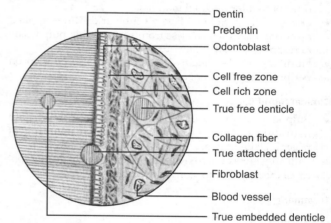

Fig. 95: True pulp stones *(For color version, see Plate 16).*

Pathogenesis of False Pulp Stone

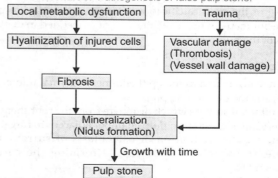

Flowchart 8: Pathogenesis of false pulp stone.

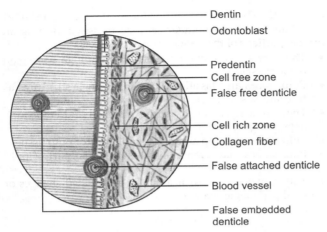

Fig. 96: False pulp stones *(For color version, see Plate 16).*

Labels (top to bottom): Dentin, Odontoblast, Predentin, Cell free zone, False free denticle, Cell rich zone, Collagen fiber, False attached denticle, Blood vessel, False embedded denticle

Histopathology

♦ Pulp stones show central amorphous mass of irregular calcification which is surrounded by concentric lamellar rings of regular calcified material.

♦ Occasionally peripheral layer of tubular dentin is applied by odontoblasts which arise from surrounding pulp tissue in response to pulp stone present.

♦ Fibrillar irregular calcified material can also be seen on periphery of pulp stone.

Clinical Significance

♦ Pulp stones are cause of pain, varying from mild pulp neuralgia to severe excruciating pain resembling of trigeminal neuralgia.

♦ Difficulty is encountered in extirpating the pulp during root canal therapy if pulp stones are present.

Treatment

No treatment is required.

Q.13. Write short note on pulp calcification.

(Apr 2017, 4 Marks)

Ans. Pulp calcifications are of three types, i.e., denticles, pulp stones and diffuse calcifications.

All of the pulp calcifications start as free bodies in pulp tissue but many of them get attached or embedded in dentinal walls of the pulp.

Denticles

♦ They occur due to the epithelio-mesenchymal interaction inside the developing pulp.

♦ Epithelial strands which originate from the root sheath or cervical extensions in pulp chamber adjacent to furcation, induce differentiation of osteoblasts of surrounding mesenchyme of dental papilla forming the core of denticle.

♦ Odontoblasts deposit tubular dentin as they migrate away from central epithelium and produce thimble-shaped structures which surround the epithelium.

♦ Denticles are formed at the time of root development and occur in root canal and pulp chamber adjacent to furcation areas of multirooted teeth.

♦ Most of the denticles remain attach or embedded in dentin.

Histopathology

♦ Denticles consist of tubular dentin which surround central nest of epithelium. As time progresses this central epithelium degenerates and tubules undergo sclerosis making their detection difficult.

♦ Mainly denticles are free or embedded but those remain free in pulp at times develop outer layers of irregular fibrillar calcification or lamellated layers of calcification.

Pulp Stones

♦ Pulp stones are nodular calcified masses appearing on coronal portions of the pulp organs.

♦ They are asymptomatic unless they impinge nerves on blood vessels.

♦ Pulp stones are classified according to their structures as true and false denticles.

♦ They are also classified as free, attached and embedded depending on the relation to dentin.

♦ Pulp stones develop around central nidus of pulp tissue

♦ Pulp stones may eventually fill substantial part of pulp chamber.

♦ Pulp stones may arise as a part of age related changes or local pathologic changes.

Histopathology

♦ Pulp stones show central amorphous mass of irregular calcification which is surrounded by concentric lamellar rings of regular calcified material.

♦ Occasionally peripheral layer of tubular dentin is applied by odontoblasts which arise from surrounding pulp tissue in response to pulp stone present.

♦ Fibrillar irregular calcified material can also be seen on periphery of pulp stone.

Diffuse Calcifications

♦ Diffuse calcification is also termed as "calcific degeneration."

♦ They are areas of fine, fibrillar, irregular calcification which are parallel to vasculature.

♦ They persist as fine calcified spicules and sometimes develop into larger masses.

♦ Diffuse calcifications are found in pulp chamber or root canal.

♦ Diffuse calcifications may surround the blood vessels.

Histopathology

♦ Its pattern is amorphous, unorganized linear strands or columns paralleling blood vessels and nerves of pulp.

Clinical Significance of Pulp Calcifications

♦ Pulp stones are cause of pain, varying from mild pulp neuralgia to severe excruciating pain resembling of trigeminal neuralgia.

- Difficulty is encountered in extirpating the pulp during root canal therapy if pulp stones are present.
- Pulp calcifications can also interfere with formation of root causing early periodontal destruction and tooth loss.
- Prominent pulp calcifications are associated with some diseases, such as dentin dysplasia, pulp dysplasia, Calcinosis universalis and Ehlers Danlos syndrome.

Treatment of Pulp Calcifications

No treatment is required.

Q.14. Discuss attrition and abrasion.   *(May 2018, 3 Marks)*

Ans. *For attrition in detail, refer to Ans. 6 of same chapter.*
For abrasion in detail, refer to Ans. 1 of same chapter.

Q.15. Write short answer on tooth reimplantation.
     (Feb 2019, 3 Marks)

Ans. Tooth reimplantation almost invariably results in severe resorption of root.

- Tooth substance regardless of whether root canal is filled or not should be considered as nonvital tissue, except in case of transplanting developing teeth where vascular supply to the tooth can be reestablished and vitality is maintained.
- An implanted tooth is analogous to a bone graft which act as temporary scaffold and is ultimately resorbed and get replaced.
- Root of the tooth is resorbed and is replaced by the bone leading to ankylosis.
- If root of the tooth does not completely resorbed, ensuing ankylosis may result in the functional tooth.
- Many of the reimplanted teeth, undergo complete resorption of root and get exfoliated.
- In reimplanted avulsed teeth, extensive external resorption of root is extremely common without rapid and appropriate intervention. If tooth remain outside the socket without being placed in proper storage medium, then PDL cells undergo necrosis. Without vital PDL cells, surrounding bone will view the tooth as foreign object and initiate resorption and replacement by the bone.

15. HEALING OF ORAL WOUNDS

Q.1. Enumerate various factors which promotes the healing process. Describe the healing of an extraction socket.   *(Sep 2004, 15 Marks)*

Ans. Healing is defined as restoration to a normal, mental or physical condition especially of an inflammation and wound.

Factors which Promotes the Healing Process

- **Localization of wound:**
  Wounds in the area in which there is good vascular bed heal helps in rapid healing of wound.
- **Physical factors:**
  - Mild traumatic injury favors the healing process.
  - Local temperature in the area of wound influences the rate of healing by its effect on local circulation and cell multiplication.
- **Circulating factors:**
  Good blood supply of wound tissues promotes healing process.
- **Nutritional factors:**
  - Presence of protein enhances the speed of wound healing.
  - Presence of vitamin C accelerates the rate of wound healing process.
  - Vitamin A and D accelerates the wound healing.
  - Vitamin B complex promotes wound healing.
- **Age of patient:**
  Wounds in younger patients heal rapidly due to increased circulatory insufficiency and presence of protein synthesis.
- **Infection:**
  A wound which is exposed to mild physical irritation or expose to bacteria heals quickly.

Healing Process of an Extracted Socket

Immediate reaction following an extraction:

After the removal of a tooth, blood which fills in the socket coagulates, red blood cells get entrapped in the fibrin meshwork and the ends of blood vessels in periodontal ligament are sealed off.

Healing in First Week

- There is proliferation of fibroblasts from connective tissue and these fibroblasts grow into a clot.
- There is endothelial proliferation which shows capillary growth.
- During, this period blood clot begins to undergo organization by ingrowth of fibroblasts and occasionally by small capillaries from residual periodontal ligament.
- Crest of alveolar bone shows beginning of osteoclastic activity.

Second Week Wound Healing

- During this period, remnants of PDL gradually undergo degeneration.
- Wall of bony socket appears slightly frayed.
- Margins of alveolar socket exhibits prominent osteoclastic resorption and fragments of necrotic bone are seen in the process of resorption or sequestration.

Third Week Wound Healing

- The clot is completely organized by maturation of granulation tissue.
- New uncalcified bone is formed around the periphery of wound from the socket wall.
- Original cortical bone of alveolar socket undergoes remodeling.
- Crest of alveolar bone is rounded off by osteoclastic resorption.

Fourth Week Wound Healing

- There is continuous deposition, remodeling and resorption of the bone filling in alveolar socket.

♦ Due to absorption of alveolar crest bone filling of the socket does not extend beyond the alveolar crest.

Q.2. Describe the healing of an extraction socket wound and complications of wound healing.

(Mar 1997, 15 Marks)

Ans. *For healing of extraction socket, refer to Ans. 1 of same chapter.*

Complications of Wound Healing

♦ **Infection:** Wounds may provide a portal entry to microsomal infections which delay the healing process.

♦ **Keloid and hypertrophic scar formation:** Keloids are the overgrowth scar tissues with no tendency for resolution. They occur in wounds which heal without any complication. Hypertrophic scars occur in wounds where healing is delayed.

♦ **Pigmentory changes:** These are common in healing of wounds on skin and appear as hypopigmented or hyperpigmented areas, e.g., lichen planus and lichenoid reactions.

♦ **Cicatrization:** It refers to late reduction in the size of the scar in contrast to immediate wound contraction. It is complication due to burns of skin.

♦ **Implantation cyst:** Epithelial cells may slide or get entrapped later in the wound and later may proliferate to form implantation cyst.

♦ **Healing after pulpal diseases:** It depends upon the degree of infection, inflammation, amount of the pulpal tissue involved and age of the patient.

♦ **Healing after periapical diseases:** It may result in the formation of fibrosis in the involved area.

Q.3. Write short note on dry socket.

(Nov 2014, 3 Marks) (Sep 2005, 5 Marks)
(Apr 2007, 5 Marks) (June 2014, 5 Marks)
(Dec 2010, 3 Marks) (July 2016, 5 Marks)

Or

Write note on dry socket.   *(Feb 2006, 2.5 Marks)*

Or

Write short answer on dry socket.   *(May 2018, 3 Marks)*

Or

Write in brief on dry socket.   *(Sep 2018, 5 Marks)*

Ans. It is also known as "Alveolitis Sicca Dolorosa" or alveolalgia or postoperative osteitis or localized acute alveolar osteomyelitis or alveolar osteitis.

♦ Dry socket is the common complication in healing of the extraction wound.

♦ It commonly occurs in the mandibular or molar areas.

♦ Dry socket is a very painful condition and the patient often has a foul breath.

♦ Clinical examination reveals a socket devoid of clot and bony walls of socket are bare and visible.

♦ Histological section of socket bone reveals formation of necrotic bone containing empty lacunae.

♦ There is balance inflammatory reaction in surrounding bone.

♦ Zinc oxide eugenol pack is given in the socket for palliative reaction.

Q.4. Describe the healing of fracture wound and complication in healing of the fracture.

(Mar 1998, 15 Marks)

Ans.

Healing of Fracture Wound

1. **Immediate effect of a fracture**
   • After fracture haversian vessels of bone are torn at the fracture site so the vessels periosteum and marrow cavity cross the fracture line.
   • There is considerable extravasation of blood in fractured area but at the same time, there is lack of circulation and loss of blood supply.
   • Due to disruption of blood supply and tearing of blood vessels there is death of bone marrow adjacent to fracture line.
   • Blood clot which forms plays an important role in healing of fracture through replacement by granulation tissue and its subsequent replacement of bone.

2. **Callus formation**
   • It is the structure which unites the fracture end of bone and consists of fibrous tissue, cartilage and bone.
   • There are two types of callus:
     1. External callus: It consists of new tissue which forms around the outside of two fragments of bone.
     2. Internal callus: It consists of new tissue arising from the marrow cavity.
   • Periosteum is an important structure in callus formation and ultimate healing of the fracture.
   • Cells of the periosteum torn at the fracture line usually die but peripheral to the area there is a flurry cellular activity within hours of injury.
   • The fibrous layer of periosteum is inert and lifted away from the surface of bone by proliferation of cell in osteogenic layer of periosteum which assumes features of osteoblasts which, in turn, begins the formation of small amount of new bone at some distance from the fracture site.
   • There is continuous proliferation of osteogenic cells forming collar of callus over the surface of fracture.
   • New bone which begins to form an external callus consists of irregular trabeculae.
   • This differentiation of cells into osteoblast and subsequent formation of bone occurs in deepest part of callus collar.
   • In rapidly growing area of collar, osteogenic layer differentiates into chondroblasts rather than osteoblast and forms cartilage.
   • The cartilage fuses with bone and begins to calcify by endochondral bone formation. The calcified cartilage is gradually resorbed and replaced by the bone.
   • Shortly after the fracture endosteum proliferates within the week to form new bone which unites and establish the continuity of bone.
   • After this bone external and internal callus remodel to form indistinguishable bone.

Complications

♦ Delayed union and non-union of the fragments of bones are the complication of the healing process. They result when the calluses of osteogenic tissue over each of two fragments fail to meet and fuse.
♦ Local infection and presence of foreign bodies
♦ Fibrous union in fracture arises usually as a result of lack of immobilization of damaged bone.
♦ Lack of calcification of newly formed bone in the callus may occur.

Q.5. Write about healing of oral tissues.

(Mar 2007, 3 Marks)

Ans. *For healing of extraction socket of oral cavity, refer to Ans. 1 of same chapter.*

Q.6. Write note on biopsy.

(Dec 2010, 8 Marks) (Sep 2002, 6 Marks)

(Sep 2011, 3 Marks)

Or

Write short note on biopsy.　　*(Sep 2018, 5 Marks)*

(Dec 2015, 3 Marks) (July 2016, 3 Marks)

Or

Write short answer on biopsy.

(Feb 2019, 3 Marks) (Sep 2018, 5 Marks)

Ans. Biopsy is the removal of tissue from the living organism for the purpose of microscopic examination and diagnosis.

Types of Biopsy

♦ *Excisional biopsy:* If a lesion is totally excised for histological evaluation, it is called as excisional biopsy.
♦ *Incisional biopsy:* When only a small section of tissue is removed from the lesion for the purpose of histological evaluation, it is called incisional biopsy.
♦ *Fine needle aspiration cytology (FNAC):* It is done by aspirating tissue material inside a lesion which is later on diagnosed microscopically after preparing a smear.
♦ *Frozen section biopsy:* It is performed in order to get an immediate histological report of a lesion. The tissue is obtained from the lesion and is kept in deep freeze and then frozen tissue is sectioned and stained to get a prompt diagnosis.
♦ *Punch biopsy:* A small cylindrical punch is applied to the lesion through full thickness of skin and a plug of tissue is removed.

Biopsy Procedure

♦ Area of wound from where the biopsy is taken and cleaned first.
♦ Area is anesthetized.
♦ Most representative site of wound is identified.
♦ A section of tissue from the identified site of wound is removed.
♦ Tissue is cleaned and put into 10% formalin solution for fixation.
♦ Biopsy site is sutured after achieving hemostasis.
♦ Biopsy specimen is sent to the histopathologist for diagnosis after labeling it properly.

Also refer to Ans. 8 of same chapter.

Q.7. Write note on exfoliative cytology.

(June 2015, 5 Marks) (Jan 2012, 5 Marks)

(Mar 2006, 5 Marks) (Aug 2012, 5 Marks)

Or

Write in brief about exfoliative cytology.

(Jan 2012, 5 Marks)

Or

Write short answer on exfoliative cytology.

(Sep, 2018, 3 Marks)

Ans. Exfoliative cytology is the microscopic study of cells obtained from the surface of an organ or lesion after suitable staining.

Procedure of Exfoliative Cytology

♦ Surface of lesion is cleaned by removing all debris and mucins.
♦ Gentle scrapping is done on the surface of lesion with metal cement spatula or a moistened tongue blade for several times.
♦ Thus material present on the surface of lesion are adhered or collected at the border of instrument.
♦ The collected material is then evenly spread over a microscopic slide and is immediately fixed with 95% of alcohol.
♦ The slide is then air dried and is stained by a special stain called as PAP stain (Papanicolaou stain).

Findings in Exfoliative Cytology

Class I (Normal): It indicates that only normal cells are present in the smear.

Class II (Atypical): It indicates the presence of minor cellular atypia.

Class III (Intermediate): This is an in between cytology that separates cancer from non-cancer diagnosis, the cells which display wider atypia are suggestive of cancer.

Biopsy is recommended for further diagnosis.

Class IV (Suggestive cancer): It indicates that in the lesion there is presence of few cells with malignant characteristic. Biopsy is mandatory.

Class V (Positive of cancer): The cells exhibit definite features of malignancy. Biopsy is mandatory.

Indication of Exfoliative Cytology

The exfoliative cytology is establishing in diagnosis of following oral lesion:

♦ Herpes simplex and herpes zoster
♦ Pemphigus vulgaris
♦ Pemphigoid
♦ Squamous cell carcinoma
♦ Aphthous ulcer.

Q.8. Define biopsy. Enumerate indications and contraindications of biopsy.　*(Sep 2011, 3 Marks)*

Ans. Biopsy is the removal of tissue from the living organism for the purpose of microscopic examination and diagnosis.

Indications

♦ Lesions that cannot be diagnosed by clinical and radiological examination.
♦ Lesions which does not respond to treatment
♦ For confirmation of precancerous conditions and lesions
♦ Lesions which exhibit rapid growth, paresthesia or loss of function.

Contraindications

♦ Acute inflammatory condition, such as cellulitis
♦ Normal anatomical variations, such as linea alba
♦ Patients with bleeding disorders, such as hemophilia
♦ Vascular lesions, such as hemangioma
♦ Patients who are on anticoagulant therapy.

Q.9. Write about healing of oral cavity injuries.

(Mar 2011, 5 Marks) (Sep 2011, 5 Marks)

Ans. When the cut surfaces of the oral cavity injuries be approximated or closely sutured, the wound heals up by primary intention. The process occurs in the following way:

Healing by Primary Intention

♦ In healing by primary intension wound edges are approximated by surgical sutures.
♦ In the initial phase, there will be formation of blood clot, which helps to hold the parts of the wound together.
♦ The tissue becomes edematous and an inflammatory process starts, with the infiltration of polymorphonuclear neutrophils (PMN) and lymphocytes into the area.
♦ The tissue debris collected in the wound are cleared either by the process of phagocytosis or by their lysis with the help of proteolytic enzymes, liberated by the inflammatory cells.
♦ Once the tissue debris are cleared, granulation tissue forms that replaces the blood clot in the wound, and it usually consists of young blood capillaries, proliferating fibroblasts, PMN and other leukocytes.
♦ The epithelium at the edge of the wound starts to proliferate and gradually it covers the entire wound surface.
♦ Finally, the healing process is complete with progressive increase in the amount of dense collagen bundles and decrease in the number of inflammatory cells in the area.

Healing by Secondary Intention

♦ When the opposing margins of the wound cannot be approximated together by suturing, the wound fills in from the base with the formation of a larger amount of granulation tissue, such type of healing of the open wound is known as healing by "secondary intention" or "secondary healing".
♦ Secondary healing occurs essentially by the same process as seen in the primary healing, the only difference is that a more severe inflammatory reaction and an exuberant fibroblastic and endothelial cell proliferation occur in the later.
♦ In secondary healing, once the blood clot is removed, the granulation tissue fills up the entire area and the epithelium begins to grow over it, until the wound surface is completely epithelized.

♦ Later on, the inflammatory exudates disappear slowly and the fibroblasts produce large amounts of collagen.
♦ Most of the healing processes occurring due to secondary intention, result in scar formation at the healing site. However, in the oral cavity these are rare.

Q.10. Enumerate the different techniques for biopsy taking. Describe in detail exfoliative cytology.

(Feb 2013, 16 Marks)

Ans.

Enumeration of Different Techniques for Biopsy Taking

♦ Excisional biopsy
♦ Incisional biopsy
♦ Intraosseous biopsy
♦ Punch biopsy
♦ Frozen section biopsy
♦ Oral brush biopsy or Oral CDX test
♦ Fine needle aspiration cytology

For details of exfoliative cytology, refer to Ans. 7 of same chapter.

Q.11. Write short note on factors affecting healing of wound. *(Jan 2016, 5 Marks)*

Ans. Following are the factors affecting wound healing:

♦ **Localization of wound**
Wounds in the area in which there is good vascular bed heal helps in rapid healing of wound.
♦ **Physical factors**
  • Mild traumatic injury favors the healing process.
  • Local temperature in the area of wound influences the rate of healing by its effect on local circulation and cell multiplication.
♦ **Circulating factors**
Good blood supply of wound tissues promotes healing process.
♦ **Nutritional factors**
  • Presence of protein enhances the speed of wound healing.
  • Presence of vitamin C accelerates the rate of wound healing process.
  • Vitamin A and D accelerates the wound healing.
  • Vitamin B complex promotes wound healing.
♦ **Age of patient**
Wounds in younger patients heal rapidly due to increased circulatory insufficiency and presence of protein synthesis.
♦ **Infection**
A wound which is exposed to mild physical irritation or expose to bacteria heals quickly.
♦ **Radiation**
Low dosages of ionizing radiation stimulate the healing while large doses suppress the healing. UV radiation facilitates the healing.
♦ **Hormonal factors**
Adrenocorticotropic hormone and cortisone interfere with the healing process. Patients receiving these hormones the growth of granulation tissue is inhibited due to inhibition of fibroblast proliferation, angiogenesis and decreasing of inflammatory reaction. Diabetes mellitus is the most common disease in which healing is hindered after surgical procedures.

IV   DISTURBANCE OF THE METABOLISM

16. ORAL ASPECTS OF METABOLIC DISEASES

Q.1. Write short note on pathologic calcification.

(Feb 2006, 6 Marks)

Ans. Pathologic calcification is abnormal deposition of the calcium in various tumors and organs of the body.

They are of three types:

1. Dystrophic calcification
2. Metastatic calcification
3. Calcinosis

Dystrophic Calcification

- It is a type of pathologic calcification in which calcium salts are deposited in the dead or degenerating tissue of the body.
- It is not associated with increased level of serum calcium and is related to change in local environment.
- This is the most frequent type of pathological calcification found in wide variety of tissues.
- In oral cavity dystrophic calcification is found in gingiva, tongue, cheek and pulp.
- One of the most common intraoral dystrophic calcification found in the pulp of the teeth, i.e., "Pulp Stone."

Metastatic Calcification

- Abnormal deposition of calcium in the tissue due to increase in amount of serum calcium.
- It occurs particularly in diseases like hyperparathyroidism which depletes the bone calcium and causes high level of blood calcium.
- Metastatic calcification also occurs in hypervitaminosis D. In this type of calcification, deposit of calcium occurs in kidney, lung, gastric mucosa and media of blood vessels.

Calcinosis

- Abnormal deposition of calcium under the skin is also known as calcinosis.
- There are two forms of calcinosis:
  1. *Calcinosis circumscripta:* It is circumscribed form.
  2. *Calcinosis universalis:* It is generalized form and is associated with scleroderma and dermatomyositis.

Q.2. Write short note on scurvy.   *(Sep 2006, 5 Marks)*
(Sep 2007, 2.5 Marks) (Sep 2008, 3 Marks)
(Dec 2009, 5 Marks) (Dec 2010, 8 Marks)

Ans. Scurvy is prolonged deficiency of vitamin C and is characterized by:

- Microvessels having least muscular support.
- Defective synthesis of osteoids.
- Impaired wound healing.

Clinical Features

- Lassitude, anorexia, painful limbs and enlargement of costochondral junction.
- Hair follicle rises above the skin and there is perifollicular hemorrhage.
- Hemorrhage may occur in the joint in the nerve sheath under the nails or conjunctiva.
- Scorbutic child usually assumes the frog like position.

Oral Manifestations

- It occurs chiefly in gingival and periodontal region.
- Interdental and marginal gingiva is bright red, swollen, smooth, shiny surface producing scurvy bud.
- There is presence of typical fetid breath of the patient with fusospirochetal stomatitis.
- In severe cases, hemorrhage and swelling of periodontal ligament membrane occurs followed by loss of bone and loosening of teeth which are exfoliated.

Histopathology

For details, refer to Ans. 5 of same chapter.

Treatment

Vitamin C 250 mg TDS daily is given.

Q.3. Write short note on hyperpituitarism.

(Sep 2004, 5 Marks)

Ans. It results from hyperfunction of anterior lobe of pituitary gland, most significantly if increases production of growth hormone.

Types

1. *Gigantism:* If the increase occur before the epiphysis of long bones are closed, gigantism results.
2. *Acromegaly:* If the increase occur later in the life after epiphysis, closure results in acromegaly.

Oral Manifestations of Hyperpituitarism

- Teeth in gigantism are proportional to size of jaw and the rest of the body and the root may be longer than the normal.
- Mandibular condylar growth is very important, overgrowth of mandible leads to prognathism.
- Mandible may be of extraordinary proportions creating a major discrepancy between the upper and lower jaw and class III malocclusion.
- The palatal vault is flattened and tongue increases in the size and causes crenation on its lateral border.
- In edentulous patients, enlargement of alveolus may prevent the comfortable fit of complete denture.
- The lip becomes thick and Negroid.

Treatment

- Transsphenoidal surgery should be done.
- Octreotide lowers the growth hormone.
- Dopamine antagonists are used.

Q.4. Write short note on vitamins.   *(Feb 2013, 5 Marks)*

Ans. Each vitamin is typically used in multiple reactions, and, therefore, most have multiple functions.

Vitamin generic descriptor name	Vitamin chemical names(s)	Solubility	Recommended dietary allowances	Deficiency disease	Overdose disease	Food sources
Vitamin A	Retinol	Fat	900 mg	Night-blindness, hyperkeratosis and keratomalacia	Hypervitaminosis A	Orange, ripe yellow fruits, leafy vegetables, carrots, pumpkin, squash, spinach, liver, soy milk, milk
Vitamin B1	Thiamine	Water	1.2 mg	Beriberi, Wernicke-Korsakoff syndrome	Drowsiness or muscle relaxation with large doses	Pork oatmeal, brown rice, vegetables, potatoes, liver, eggs
Vitamin B12	Cyanocobalamin, hydroxy-cobalamin methylcobalamin	Water	2.4 µg	Megaloblastic anemia	Acne-like rash	Meat and other animal products
Vitamin B2	Riboflavin	Water	1.3 mg	Ariboflavinosis		Dairy products, bananas, popcorn, green beans, asparagus
Vitamin B3	Niacin, niacinamide	Water	16.0 mg	Pellagra	Liver damage	Meat, fish, eggs, many vegetables, mushrooms tree nuts
Vitamin B5	Pantothenic acid	Water	5.0 mg	Paresthesia	Diarrhea; possibly nausea and heartburn	Meat, broccoli, avocados
Vitamin B6	Pyridoxine, pyridoxamine, pyridoxal	Water	1.3–1.7 mg	Anemia peripheral neuropathy	Impairment of proprioception, nerve damage (doses >100 mg/day)	Meat, vegetables, tree nuts, bananas
Vitamin B7	Biotin	Water	30.0 µg	Dermatitis, enteritis		Raw egg yolk, liver, peanuts, certain vegetables
Vitamin B9	Folic acid, folinic acid	Water	400 µg	Megaloblast and deficiency during pregnancy is associated with birth defects, such as neural tube defects	May mask symptoms of vitamin B12 deficiency; other effects	Leafy vegetables, pasta, bread cereal, liver
Vitamin C	Ascorbic acid	Water	90.0 mg	Scurvy	Vitamin C megadosage	Many fruits and vegetables, liver
Vitamin D	Cholecalciferol	Fat	10 µg	Rickets and Osteomalacia	Hypervitaminosis D	Fish, eggs, liver, mushrooms
Vitamin E	Tocopherols, tocotrienols	Fat	15.0 mg	Deficiency is very rare; mild hemolytic anemia in newborn infants	Increased congestive heart failure seen in one large randomized study.	Many fruits and vegetables, nuts and seeds
Vitamin K	Phylloquinone, menaquinones	Fat	120 µg	Bleeding diathesis	Increases coagulation in patients taking warfarin egg yolks	Leafy green vegetables, such as spinach, liver

Q.5. Describe histologic features with diagram of scurvy.
(Nov 2008, 5 Marks)

Ans. Following are the histologic features of scurvy:

♦ In scurvy osteoblasts fail to form osteoid on spicules of calcified cartilage matrix.

♦ Cartilage cells of epiphyseal plate proliferate normally and salts are deposited in matrix between column of cartilage cells.

♦ A wide zone of calcified but non-ossified matrix known as scorbutic lattice develop in metaphysis.

♦ As scorbutic lattice increases in width more fragile zone develops which leads to complete fracture of spicules with separation and deformity of cartilage shaft junction. Fracture of calcified matrix material lead to the classic picture of scurvy known as Trummerfeld zone.

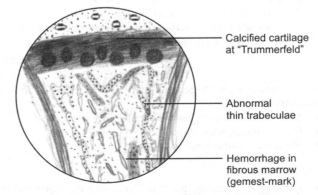

— Calcified cartilage at "Trummerfeld"

— Abnormal thin trabeculae

— Hemorrhage in fibrous marrow (gemest-mark)

Fig. 97: Scurvy *(For color version, see Plate 17).*

◆ Area beneath Trummerfeld zone is free of hematopoietic cells and is formed of connective tissue cells known as Gemest-mark.

Q.6. Write short note on hyperparathyroidism.

(Dec 2010, 8 Marks) (Jan 2018, 4 Marks)

Ans. Hyperparathyroidism is an endocrine disorder in which there is secretion of excess of circulating parathyroid hormone.

◆ Excess of parathyroid hormone stimulate osteoclast and mobilize calcium from bone which causes hypercalcemia.

Types of Hyperparathyroidism

◆ *Primary hyperparathyroidism:* In this excess secretion of parathyroid hormone is present because of parathyroid adenomas.

◆ *Secondary hyperparathyroidism:* It occurs when parathyroid continuously produced in response to low levels of serum calcium. This is related to chronic renal diseases. Kidney utilizes vitamin D which is important for calcium absorption from gut. So in patient with chronic renal disease active form of vitamin D is not produced and there is less calcium absorption from gut which results in low serum calcium levels.

◆ *Tertiary hyperparathyroidism:* As secondary hyperparathyroidism remains for longer time it is known as tertiary hyperparathyroidism.

Clinical Features

◆ It occurs mainly from 3rd to 6th decade of life.
◆ Female predilection is seen with male to female ratio of 1:3
◆ Patient has classic triad of kidney stones, resorption of bone and duodenal ulcers.
◆ Patient usually complains of back pain and blood in urination.
◆ Patient also suffers from emotional unstability.
◆ Presence of gastrointestinal problems is present, i.e., nausea, vomiting, anorexia.
◆ In severe cases, there is presence of headache, bone pain, pathological fractures and comma.

Oral Lesions

◆ A tumor like swelling is present either intraorally or extra-orally which is known as Brown's tumor.
◆ Mandible is affected more commonly.
◆ Presence of jaw bone fractures is present.
◆ There is presence of drifting, loosening and exfoliation of the teeth.
◆ Fetid odor or halitosis is present.
◆ Malocclusion is present because of drifting and spacing of the teeth.

Histopathology

◆ There is presence of osteoclastic resorption of multiple boney trabeculae and there is also formation of new bone by osteoblast cells.
◆ Areas of excessive hemorrhage and hemosiderin pigmentation are present.

◆ Multiple multinucleated osteoclast type of giant cells are often seen in tumor.
◆ At places bone marrow is replaced by fibrous connective tissue.
◆ As disease progresses osteoclastomas develop which are characterized by masses of fibroblasts growing in loose syncytium.

Treatment

◆ Administration of vitamin D and dietary phosphate supplements.
◆ Parathyroidectomy should be done if patient does not respond to the medicinal treatment.

Q.7. Write short essay on oral lesions of hyperparathyroidism. *(Jan 2012, 5 Marks)*

Ans. *Refer to Ans. 6 of same chapter.*

Q.8. Write short answer on oral manifestations of diabetes mellitus. *(Oct 2019, 3 Marks)*

Ans.

Oral Manifestations of Diabetes Mellitus

◆ Effect on periodontium: Patient having diabetes is prone to have periodontal disease as compared to normal persons. Directly, diabetes mellitus does not cause periodontal disease but it alters the response of periodontal lesion toward local irritants which leads to bone loss and it also decreases post-surgical healing of periodontal lesion.
◆ Periodontitis: A diabetic has fulminating periodontitis along with periodonal abscess formation. This causes mobility of teeth. Presence of severe and rapid bone resorption is also seen. Children with Type I diabetes mellitus have more destruction around first molars and incisors.
◆ Median rhomboid glossitis: Abnormal blood sugar levels can cause median rhomboid glossitis. There is impairment of blood supply to dorsum of tongue because of arteriosclerotic changes in blood vessels which supply the area.
◆ Oral candidiasis: This is the fungal infection caused by candida albicans which occurs because of encouragement of local multiplication of fungus because of impaired glucose level and immune mechanism.
◆ Localized osteitis: Dry socket in diabetes show delayed healing.
◆ Burning mouth: It is associated with many of unexplained oral symptoms, such as burning sensation, Atypical paresis, dysesthesia and dysgeusia.
◆ Trigeminal nerve involvement: It is recognized as polymorphic condition which is manifested as polyneuropathy, based on assumption that trigeminal nerve can be involved.
◆ Presence of xerostomia and increased caries activity.
◆ Presence of delayed healing of oral wounds.
◆ Diabetic sialadenosis: In diabetics, there is presence of diffuse, non – tender bilateral enlargement of parotid gland.
◆ Other features: Presence of angular cheilosis, altered taste sensation, lichen planus, pyogenic granuloma and diffuse enlargement of parotid gland.

V   DISEASES OF SPECIFIC SYSTEM

17. DISEASES OF BONE AND JOINTS

Q.1. Write short note on cleidocranial dysplasia.
(June 2014, 5 Marks)

Ans. It is also called as cleidocraniodysostosis or "Marie and Santon disease."

Etiology

♦ It appears as true dominant Mendelian characteristic.
♦ It is transmitted as an autosomal dominant trait with complete penetrance and variable expressivity.

Oral Manifestation

♦ Maxilla and paranasal air sinuses are underdeveloped resulting in maxillary micrognathia.
♦ Maxilla is underdeveloped in relation to mandible.
♦ There is prolonged retention of primary dentition.
♦ There is complete absence of cementum.
♦ Disorganization of developing permanent dentition.
♦ There is presence of supernumerary teeth usually in anterior region.
♦ High narrow arched palate and cleft palate is common.
♦ Roots of teeth are often short and thinner than the normal.
♦ The crown may be pitted as a result of enamel hypoplasia.

Clinical Features

♦ There is complete absence of clavicle.
♦ It primarily affects skull, clavicle and dentition.

Treatment

♦ Not specific
♦ Dental care should be taken.

Q.2. Write note on osteogenesis imperfecta.
(Feb 2015, 5 Marks)

Ans. It is also called brittle bone or lobstein disease or fragilitas ossium or osteopsathyrosis.

This is an autosomal dominant condition affecting bone formation.

It presents a hereditary autosomal dominant trait.

Types

♦ Congenital type
♦ Lobstein type.

Clinical Features

♦ It usually occur in infants.
♦ There is extreme fragility or porosities of bone with proneness of fracture.
♦ There is occurrence of pale blue sclera which is thin and pigmented choroids shows through and produces blue color.

♦ There is deafness due to osteosclerosis, laxity of ligaments and peculiar shape of skull.
♦ Increase tendency for capillary bleeding.

Oral Manifestations

♦ Osteogenic imperfecta is associated with dentinogenesis imperfecta.
♦ There is hypoplasia of teeth.
♦ Deciduous teeth are poorly calcified and semi-translucent or waxy.
♦ Teeth appear as faintly dirty pink, half normal size, with globular crown and relative short roots, in proportion to other dimensions.

Histopathological Features

♦ Osteoblastic activity appears as retarded and imperfect.
♦ Failure of fetus to be transformed with mature collagen.
♦ The trabeculae of cancellous bone are delicate and often show fracture.

Treatment

No known treatment.

Q.3. Enumerate fibro-osseous lesion. Describe in detail monostotic fibrous dysplasia. *(Sep 2005, 14 Marks)*

Ans. In fibrous dysplasia, normal bone is replaced by the benign fibrous tissue showing varying amount of mineralization.

Classification of Fibro-osseous Lesions

♦ *Developmental:*
  • Solitary bone cyst
  • Gigantiform cementoma
  • Cherubism
♦ *Reactive/Reparative:*
  • Aneurysmal bone cyst
  • Central giant cell granuloma
  • Garre's osteomyelitis
  • Osseous dysplasia
    – Florid osseous dysplasia
    – Cemental osseous dysplasia
    – Focal osseous dysplasia or sclerosing osteomyelitis
  • Osseous keloid
  • Traumatic periostitis
♦ *Neoplasms:*
  • Benign cementoblastoma
  • Ossifying fibroma
    – Conventional
    – Juvenile trabecular
    – Juvenile psammomatoid
  • Osteoma
  • Osteoid osteoma
  • Osteoblastoma

♦ *Endocrinal/Metabolic:* Brown tumor of hyperparathyroidism
♦ *Idiopathic:*
  • Fibrous dysplasia
  • Paget's disease.

Monostotic Fibrous Dysplasia

Monostotic fibrous dysplasia is a condition in which single bone is involved and is replaced by abnormal fibrous connective tissue which undergoes osseous metaplasia and the bone is transformed into dense lamellar bone.

Clinical Features

♦ It involves only one bone and pigmented skin lesions are present.
♦ The sites which affected are maxilla, mandible, ribs and femur.
♦ It occurs in children younger than 10 years and both the sexes are equally affected.

Oral Manifestations

♦ Maxilla is more commonly affected than the mandible and most of the changes occur in posterior region. The most common area involved is premolar area.
♦ There is presence of unilateral facial swelling which is slow growing with intact overlying mucosa.
♦ Swelling is painless but patient may feel discomfort.
♦ There is presence of enlarging deformities of alveolar process mainly buccal and labial cortical plates.
♦ In mandible, there is protrusion of inferior border of mandible.
♦ Teeth present in the affected area are malaligned and tipped or displaced.
♦ Supernumerary teeth are often impacted and affect the eruption of the teeth.

Histopathology

♦ Lesion is essentially a fibrous bone made up of proliferating fibroblasts in compact stroma of inter lacing collagen fibers.
♦ Irregular trabeculae of bone are scattered throughout the lesion.
♦ Some of the trabeculae are C-shaped and described as Chinese character shaped.
♦ There is permanent maturation arrest in woven bone stage.

Treatment

♦ Surgical removal of lesion
♦ Osseous countering is necessary for characterizing deformity for aesthetic or pre esthetic purposes.

Q.4. Write short note on monostotic fibrous dysplasia.
(Sep 2004, 5 Marks)

Ans. *Refer to Ans. 3 of same chapter.*

Q.5. Write note on fibrous dysplasia. *(Feb 2002, 6 Marks)*
Or
Write short note on fibrous dysplasia.
(Jan 2016, 5 Marks) (Nov 2014, 3 Marks)
(Feb 2019, 5 Marks) (Dec 2009, 5 Marks)

Or
Write short answer on histology of fibrous dysplasia.
(Feb 2019, 3 Marks)

Ans. Fibrous dysplasia is an idiopathic condition in which an area of normal bone is gradually replaced by abnormal fibrous connective tissue which then again undergoes osseous metaplasia and eventually the bone is transformed into dense lamellar bone.

Types of Fibrous Dysplasia

♦ *Monostotic fibrous dysplasia:* Only one of the bone is involved.
♦ *Polyostotic fibrous dysplasia:* More than one bone is involved.
  • *Jaffe's type:* Variable number of bones are involved accompanied by pigmented lesion of skin or cafe-au-lait spots.
  • *Albright syndrome:* It is a severe form of fibrous dysplasia involving all the bones in the body, accompanied by pigmented lesions of the skin and endocrine disturbances of various types.

Clinical Features

♦ It is seen during the first and second decades of life.
♦ Disease is more common among the females
♦ Polyostotic fibrous dysplasia commonly involve skull, facial bone, clavicle, pelvic bone, etc., and monostotic fibrous dysplasia involve maxilla and mandible.
♦ Monostotic form of disease can never be transformed into polyostotic form.
  For more clinical features and oral manifestations, refer to Ans. 3 of same chapter.

Histopathology

♦ Fibrous dysplasia reveals presence of highly cellular, proliferating well vascularized fibrillar connective tissue which replaces the normal bone.
♦ Within fibrous tissue the fibroblasts cells are arranged in "Whorled pattern".
♦ Trabeculae represent the Chinese letter pattern.
♦ Osteoblastic and osteoclastic activity may be present in relation to some trabeculae of bone.

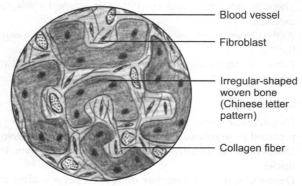

Fig. 98: Fibrous dysplasia *(For color version, see Plate 17).*

Treatment

Surgical removal of lesion.

Q.6. Write note on Paget's disease of bone.

(Sep 2006, 5 Marks) (Apr 2007, 10 Marks)

Or

Write notes on histopathology of Paget's disease.

(Feb 2006, 2.5 Marks)

Or

Write in detail on Paget's disease.

(Apr 2008, 10 Marks) (Feb 2006, 2.5 Marks)

Or

Write short note on Paget's disease.

(Apr 2015, 3 Marks) (June 2015, 5 Marks)

Ans. Paget's disease is a relatively uncommon bony disorder which is characterized by the excessive uncoordinated phases of resorption and deposition of osseous tissue in single or multiple bones.

It is also known as "Osteitis Deformans."

Etiology

- Inflammatory
- Circulatory disturbance
- Genetic and environmental factors
- *Others:* Vasculitis, trauma, hormonal balance and degenerative neurological disorders.

Clinical Features

- It occurs during 5th, 6th and 7th decades of life.
- Males are more commonly affected.
- It is prone to occur in axial skeleton especially in skull, femur, sacrum and pelvis.
- Most of the patient complain initially of the deep and aching bone pain with bilaterally symmetrical swelling of bone.
- Enlargement of skull, bowing of legs and curvature of spine are commonly seen.

Oral Manifestations

- Maxilla is more commonly involved than the mandible.
- There is movement and migration of affected teeth and malocclusion.
- As the disease progresses, the mouth remains open exposing the teeth.
- Extraction site heals slowly and incidence of osteomyelitis is higher.

Histopathology

- Osteoclastic bone resorption occurs and the bone is replaced by highly vascularized cellular connective tissue.
- Osteoclasts are usually larger and may contain over 100 nuclei.
- Deposition of new lamellar or woven bone within the connective tissue by osteoblast cells occur and fatty hemopoietic bone marrow is replaced by the fibrous stroma.

- Newly formed bone may again resorbed by osteoclast causing loss of normal architecture of bone.
- Chronic inflammatory cells and dilated blood capillaries are present within the bone.
- Bone resorption and deposition results in irregular fragments of bone formation characterized by prominent basophilic reversal and resting lines, and they produce mosaic pattern in bone.

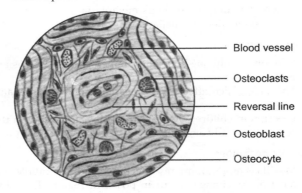

Fig. 99: Paget's disease of bone *(For color version, see Plate 17).*

Treatment

- Bisphosphonate therapy should be given.
- Calcitonin is administered.
- Surgical correction for bone deformities, fractures and severe degenerative arthritis

Q.7. Write short note on cementoma. *(Mar 2003, 5 Marks)*

Ans. It is a true neoplasm of functional cementoblasts which forms large masses of cementum like tissue or tooth root.

Recent Concept

Cementoma these days is known as periapical cemento-osseous dysplasia, this is because cementoma is an unorganized productivity of bone, PDL membrane cementum complex.

Clinical Features

- It occurs most frequently under the age of 25 years.
- Mandible is affected more commonly than maxilla.
- Mandibular first molar is most commonly affected tooth.
- It produces a slow enlarging bony hard swelling of jaw which causes expansion of jaw and displacement of regional teeth.
- Expansion of buccal and lingual cortical plates.
- Low-grade intermittent pain is present which felt more when area is palpated.
- A dull sound is produced when tooth is percussed.

Histopathology

- It presents a large mass of amorphous cemental tissue which shows the presence of multiple reversal line.
- Intervening connective tissue stroma contains many cementoblasts and cementoblasts cells.
- PDL adjacent to normal cementum becomes integrated with capsule and separate the neoplasm from surrounding bone.

♦ Multinucleated cells are present in the large number in central area and are associated with active resorption.
♦ Root of the involved tooth extends up to the center of lesion and neoplastic cemental tissue is continuous with normal cemental layer.

Treatment

Surgical excision is done.

Q.8. Give classification of bone disorders of face and jaw. Write shortly about the clinical features and histopathology of fibrous dysplasia.

(Mar 2007, 8 Marks)

Ans. Bone disorders of face and jaw:
1. **Developmental defects of bone formation of face and jaw:**
   • Agnathia
   • Micrognathia
   • Macrognathia
   • Facial hemiatrophy
   • Facial hemihypertrophy
   • Cleft palate.
2. **Benign and malignant lesions of bone:**
   • Osteoma
   • Osteosarcoma
   • Ewing's sarcoma.
3. **Fibro-osseous lesions**
   • Fibrous dysplasia of bone
   • Ossifying fibroma
   • Cementifying fibroma
   • Paget's disease of bone
   • Cherubism
   • Osteogenesis imperfecta
   • Cleidocranial dysplasia
   • Hurler's syndrome
   • Garre's osteomyelitis
   • Jaw lesions in hyperparathyroidism
   • Aneurysmal bone cyst.

For clinical features and histopathology of fibrous dysplasia, refer to Ans. 5 of same chapter.

Q.9. Classify fibro-osseous lesions of jaw. Give histopathology of Paget's disease. *(Sep 2008, 5 Marks)*

Or

Classify fibro-osseous lesions of jaw. Write about clinical features, histopathology of Paget's disease.

(Mar 2011, 6 Marks)

Ans. *Refer to Ans. 3 and 6 of same chapter.*

Q.10. Write short note on cherubism.

(Jan 2012, 5 Marks) (Dec 2009, 5 Marks)

Or

Describe in brief cherubism *(Jan 2010, 5 Marks)*

Or

Write short essay on cherubism. *(Jan 2012, 5 Marks)*

Or

Write short answer on cherubism. *(Sep 2018, 3 Marks)*

Ans. Cherubism is an autosomal dominant fibro-osseous lesion of the jaw which involves more than one quadrant that stabilizes after growth period leading to facial deformity and malocclusion.

Clinical Features

♦ Children of age 1 to 3 years are more commonly affected. Males are more commonly affected than females.
♦ Affected children are normal at birth but as soon the child's growth take place self-limited bone growth begins to slow down till patient reaches 5 years of age and stop at the age of 12–15 years.
♦ There is deforming mandibular and maxillary overgrowth with respiratory obstruction and impairment of vision and hearing.
♦ Enlargement of cervical lymph nodes contributes to patient's full faced appearance.
♦ A rim of sclera is may be beneath the iris, giving classic eye to heaven appearance.

Oral Manifestations

♦ Agenesis of 2nd and 3rd molars of mandible.
♦ Displacement of the teeth
♦ Premature exfoliation of primary teeth
♦ Delayed eruption of permanent teeth
♦ Transposition and rotation of teeth
♦ In severe cases tooth resorption occurs.

Histopathology

♦ Lesion presents a highly cellular and vascular connective tissue stroma, which is often arranged in a "whorled pattern".
♦ Numerous proliferating fibroblasts and variable numbers of multinucleated giant cells are also found within the stroma.
♦ Giant cells are relatively smaller in size and they often aggregate around the thin-walled blood capillaries.
♦ A hallmark of the disease is the presence of an "eosinophilic perivascular cuffing" of collagen fibers, which often surrounds the blood capillaries.
♦ Within the connective tissue extravasated blood and deposits of hemosiderin pigments are sometimes seen.
♦ Lymph nodes exhibit reactive hyperplasia, fibrosis and chronic inflammatory cell infiltration.

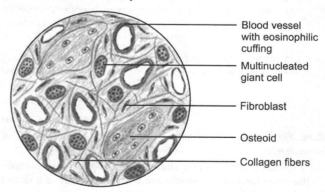

Fig. 100: Cherubism *(For color version, see Plate 18).*

Treatment

No treatment is required as cherubism is a self-limiting disease.

Q.11. Write short note on histopathology of Paget's disease and cherubism. *(Sep 2011, 3 Marks)*

Ans. *For histopathology of paget's disease, refer to Ans. 6 of same chapter.*

For histopathology of cherubism, refer to Ans. 12 of same chapter.

Q.12. Classify fibro-osseous lesions of oral cavity. Discuss clinical features, radiographic differential diagnosis and management of fibrous dysplasia.

(Nov 2008, 20 Marks)

Or

Classify fibro-osseous lesions of jaw. Discuss the clinical and histopathological features of fibrous dysplasia. *(Dec 2007, 8 Marks)*

Or

Classify fibro-osseous lesions of jaws. Describe in detail fibrous dysplasia. *(May/Jun 2009, 15 Marks)*

Or

Classify fibro-osseous lesions. Discuss in detail about the etiology, clinical, radiographic and histopathologic features of fibrous dysplasia.

(Aug 2012, 10 Marks)

Or

Enumerate fibro-osseous lesions of jaws and describe fibrous dysplasia in detail.

(Feb 2015, 10 Marks)

Or

Enumerate fibro-osseous lesions. Describe in detail the clinical radiological and histopathological features of fibrous dysplasia. *(Dec 2015, 8 Marks)*

Or

Classify fibro-osseous lesions affecting the jaws. Write in detail about the etiopathogenesis, clinical features, radiographic features of fibrous dysplasia. *(Apr 2017, 10 Marks)*

Or

Enumerate the fibro-osseous lesions involving orofacial region. Describe fibrous dysplasia in detail with diagram. *(Jan 2017, 10 Marks)*

Or

Classify fibro-osseous lesions. Write in detail about fibrous dysplasia. *(July 2016, 10 Marks)*

Or

Discuss fibrous dysplasia in detail.

(Apr 2019, 5 Marks)

Ans. *For classification of fibro-osseous lesions, refer to Ans. 3 of same chapter.*

Fibrous dysplasia is a skeletal developmental anomaly of the bone forming mesenchyme which manifest as a defect osteoblastic differentiation and maturation.

Etiology/Etiopathogenesis

- *Genetic:* Fibrous dysplasia is caused by postzygotic mutation in *GNAS1* gene which encodes a G-protein which stimulates production of cAMP. Mutation leads to excessive secretion of cAMP which leads to hyperfunction of endocrine organs, increase proliferation of melanocytes and affect differentiation of osteoblasts. If mutation occur in early preembryonic life polystotic fibrous dysplasia occur. If mutation occur in early postembryonic life monostotic fibrous dysplasia occur.
- *Developmental:* As the disease begins in early life, it was considered to be developmental.
- *Endocrine:* Some of the investigators thought that it occurs due to local endocrinal disorders.

Clinical Features

- **Monostotic Fibrous Dysplasia**
  - It involves only one bone and pigmented skin lesions are present.
  - The sites which affected are maxilla, mandible, ribs and femur.
  - It occurs in children younger than 10 years and both the sexes are equally affected.
  - Maxilla is more commonly affected than the mandible and most of the changes occur in posterior region. The most common area involved is premolar area.
  - There is presence of unilateral facial swelling which is slow growing with intact overlying mucosa.
  - Swelling is painless but patient may feel discomfort.
  - There is presence of enlarging deformities of alveolar process mainly buccal and labial cortical plates.
  - In mandible, there is protrusion of inferior border of mandible.
  - The teeth present in the affected area are malaligned and tipped or displaced.
  - Supernumerary teeth are often impacted and affected the eruption of teeth.
- **Polyostotic Fibrous Dysplasia**
  - It is seen during first and second decades of life.
  - Female predilection is seen with male to female ratio of 1:3.
  - Most common sites to be involved are skull, facial bones, clavicle, thighs, shoulder, chest and neck.
  - Café-au-lait spots are seen over the skin which are irregular in shape and are light brown melanotic spots.
  - Patient complains of recurrent bone pain.
  - There is expansion of jaws and asymmetry of facial bones which leads to enlargement and deformity.
  - Teeth eruption is not proper.

Radiographic Features

Lesions Representing Dominancy of Fibrous Tissue Or Osteolytic Stage of Fibrous Dysplasia

- Such lesions are generally radiolucent with ill-defined borders. Defect in bone is unilocular but at times bony septa presents a picture of multilocular activity.

♦ Margins of lesion are well defined.

♦ Loss of lamina dura is evident.

♦ Resorption of roots is evident.

Lesions presenting mixed radiolucent and radiopaque picture or mixed stage of fibrous dysplasia

♦ The lesion got both the fibrous and osseous tissue so, i.e., the lesion presents both mixed radiopaque and radiolucent picture.

♦ Newly formed bone represents multiple small opacities of poor density. As they increases in size they appear granular.

Mature Lesions with Radiopacity or Mature Stage of Fibrous Dysplasia

♦ In this stage, bone is prominent, i.e., they are referred to as mature lesions with radiopacity.

♦ Radiograph reveals orange peel appearance.

♦ In the affected area; teeth are bodily displaced and tilted.

♦ Bony expansion is seen on both distal and buccal aspect.

♦ As mandible get involved, vertical depth of bone is increased. Inferior border of mandible appears ribbon like cortex. In various cases, area over cortex is lost, there is a curved downward projection of inferior margins of mandible. This appearance is called as thumb print appearance.

♦ It also shows ground glass appearance.

Radiographic Differential Diagnosis

Osteolytic Stage of Fibrous Dysplasia

♦ *Central Giant cell granuloma:* Trabeculae in central giant cell granuloma are faint while in fibrous dysplasia internal calcifications are seen which are stippled and granular.

♦ *Traumatic bone cyst:* Cortical bulging as well as displacement of teeth is present in traumatic bone cyst while it is absent in fibrous dysplasia.

Mixed Stage of Fibrous Dysplasia

♦ *Osteosarcoma:* It presents its typical features as sunburst pattern and Codman's triangle while fibrous dysplasia show granular appearance.

♦ *Lymphoma of bone:* Lymphoma of bone appears irregular as well as bizarre in radiograph while fibrous dysplasia is smooth and has well contoured boney margins.

♦ *Cemento-ossifying fibroma:* Shape of cemento-ossifying fibroma is rounded while of fibrous dysplasia is rectangular. Margins in cemento-ossifying fibroma are sharply defined while in fibrous dysplasia they are indistinct.

Mature Stage of Fibrous Dysplasia

♦ *Paget's disease:* Ground glass appearance is present in both Paget's disease and fibrous dysplasia. But in Paget's disease complete effect is rarefaction.

Histopathology

Refer to Ans. 5 of same chapter.

Management

♦ Surgical removal of the lesion should be done.

♦ Osseous contouring is done to correct the deformities so that esthetics of patient should be improved.

Q.13. Describe in detail the serum investigations done in bone disorders and give detailed account of fibrous dysplasia. *(Dec 2012, 8 Marks)*

Ans. Serum investigations in bone disorders.

Following are the serum investigations done in bone disorders:

Serum Calcium

♦ In circulation, the calcium is present in three forms, namely—ionized calcium (48–50%) protein-bound fraction (40%) and rest as complex calcium.

♦ The estimated normal value of calcium is around 9 to 10.6 mg/dL and because of diurnal variation it reaches its peak value in mid-day and lowest in early morning. It is essential to correct serum calcium values to serum albumin levels as per formula.

Free Serum Calcium

♦ Serum calcium (mg/dL) + [4–serum albumin (g%) × 0.8]. It is advisable to avoid tourniquet while drawing blood for serum calcium estimation irrespective of fasting or non-fasting state.

Ionized Calcium

♦ It comprises 48 to 50% of total serum calcium, and is primarily responsible for physiological functions like muscle contraction, coagulation and bone mineralization. The normal value of ionized calcium is around 4.5 to 5.2 mg/dL in fasting state (1.12 to 1.3 micromoles/L) with maximum at 10:00 hours and minimum at 18:00 to 20:00 hours.

♦ Serum calcium decreases in osteomalacia, hypoparathyroidism, secondary hyperparathyroidism and increases in primary hyperparathyroidism.

Serum Phosphate

♦ Out of total phosphorus in plasma, Inorganic phosphate or phosphorus constitutes 1/3 fraction measurement of which is clinically useful for assessment of metabolic bone disorders.

♦ The normal range of inorganic phosphate is 2.5–4.5 mg/dL with higher values in elderly male and postmenopausal women. The inorganic phosphate is 20% protein bound and rest is free ionic form. The serum phosphorus level is higher in infants and children. Phosphate is essential to most biological systems. High levels are found in renal failure and hypoparathyroidism, while low levels are associated with primary hyperparathyroidism, hypophosphatemic rickets and osteomalacia.

Serum Magnesium

Magnesium is present mostly in ionized form (55%), protein bound (30%) and rest in complex form. The normal value of serum magnesium is 1.7 to 2.6 mg/dL. The hypomagnesemia is observed in hypoparathyroidism. Increase in serum magnesium level is seen in hemolysis. Severe and prolonged hypomagnesemia inhibits parathyroid hormone (PTH) release and induces resistance to PTH action on bones.

Serum 25-hydroxyvitamin D

Vitamin D status is best assessed using serum 25-(OH)D3, as 1,25(OH)D3 has a short half-life and does not accurately reflect true vitamin D status. Levels are only measured if disorders of vitamin D metabolism are suspected. Whilst rickets and osteomalacia occur with vitamin D deficiency. The deficiency is suspected at levels below <25 nmol/L (10 mg/mL) and insufficiency is suspected at <75 nmol/L (30 mg/mL).

Serum Alkaline Phosphatase

♦ The normal value in adults is 40–150 IU/L and in children 11–306 IU/L. The bone specific serum alkaline phosphatase (ALP) a marker of osteoblastic activity is raised in Paget's disease of bones, metastatic bone disease, osteomalacia, osteoporosis. However, it is important to exclude hepatobiliary disease where alkaline phosphatase level is also high, especially in patients with cholestasis.

♦ The bone specific alkaline phosphatase fraction has better predictive value in evaluating bone disorders.

For fibrous dysplasia in detail, refer to Ans. 12 of same chapter.

Q.14. Write oral manifestations of cherubism.

(Dec 2010, 8 Marks)

Ans. Following are the oral manifestations of cherubism:

♦ The most commonly affected site is angle of mandible bilaterally.

♦ Patient complains of problems in speech, mastication, deglutition and have restricted jaw movements.

♦ Presence of enlargement of mandible bilaterally which leads to the rounded appearance of the lower face. This is followed by bilateral enlargement of maxilla.

♦ Alveolar process become wide, this is because to occupy whole roof of mouth.

♦ Palate becomes narrow fissure like between alveolar process.

♦ Rapid expansion of mandible is seen at 7–8 years of age. After this age, lesion progresses very slowly till puberty. As puberty is over maxillary lesions regress. Mandibular lesions start regressing after 20 years of age before that lesion regresses slowly. Face of the patient becomes normal in 4th and 5th decades of life.

♦ Since the disease occur in childhood some of the primary teeth at time are absent. This leads to gapping between the erupted deciduous teeth.

♦ Premature loss of primary teeth too is seen.

♦ Permanent dentition is often defective with absence of numerous teeth and displacement and lack of eruption of those present.

♦ Malocclusion is also present.

Q.15. Write short note on trisomy 21. *(Aug 2012, 5 Marks)*

Or

Write short note on Down's syndrome.

(Jan 2018, 4 Marks)

Ans. It is also called as Down's syndrome or Mongolism

♦ It occurs due to excessive chromosomal material involving a part of chromosome 21 or complete chromosome 21.

♦ It is the form of a mental retardation which is associated with morphological features and many somatic abnormalities due to number of chromosomal aberrations.

♦ Trisomy 21 is one of the cytologic variants of Down's syndrome and occurs in 95% of patients with Down's syndrome.

♦ There is typical trisomy 21 with 47 chromosomes.

Clinical Features

♦ It occurs in children.

♦ Mental retardation is present.

♦ Head appears small, i.e brachycephaly.

♦ Flat facies are present with hypertelorism.

♦ Nasal bridge is depressed and there is presence of broad, short neck.

♦ Presence of narrow, upward and outward slanting of palpebral fissures.

♦ Ocular abnormalities are seen, such as strabismus, cataract and retinal detachment.

♦ Skeletal abnormalities, such as short stature, broad and short hands, feet as well as digits; dysplasia of pelvis; wide gap between first and second toes.

♦ Protuberant abdomen, hypogenitalism and delayed and incomplete puberty.

Oral Manifestations

♦ Macroglossia is present, scrotal tongue is seen.

♦ Maxilla is hypoplastic.

♦ Tooth eruption is delayed. Partial anodontia and enamel hypoplasia can also be seen.

♦ High-arched palate is present.

♦ Cleft lip or cleft palate can be seen.

♦ Juvenile periodontitis is present.

♦ There is fissuring and thickening of lips and angular cheilitis is present.

18. DISEASES OF BLOOD AND BLOOD FORMING ORGANS

Q.1. Write short note on pernicious anemia.

(June 2015, 5 Marks) (Sep 2004, 5 Marks)
(Feb 2013, 5 Marks)

Ans. Pernicious anemia is a type of a chronic progressive, megaloblastic anemia of adults and is caused by deficiency of intrinsic factors in stomach.

Etiology

♦ *Due to impaired absorption of vitamin B12:* This occurs due to the atrophy of gastric mucosa which results in lack of secretion of intrinsic factor.

♦ As autoimmune reaction to gastric parietal cells or intrinsic factor.

♦ Strict vegetarians suffer from vitamin B12 deficiency as it is present only in eggs, meat and milk.

♦ Malabsorption of vitamin B12 due to inadequate gastric production or defective functioning of intrinsic factor.

♦ Various other causes which lead to the deficiency of vitamin B12 are gastrectomy, celiac disease, Crohn's disease, alcoholism, prolong usage of drugs, i.e., proton pump inhibitors, colchicines.

Clinical Features

♦ Generalized weakness, palpitation, nausea, vomiting, anorexia, diarrhea and dyspnea.
♦ Patients have smooth, dry and yellow skin.
♦ Neurological manifestation includes tingling sensation in hand and feet, paresthesia of extremities due to peripheral nerve degeneration.
♦ Glossitis, glossodynia (painful tongue) and glossopyrosis (itching and burning tongue).
♦ Tongue appears beefy red in color.
♦ Sometimes loss of papilla produces a bald appearance of tongue.
♦ Sometimes hyperpigmentation occurs in mucosa.
♦ Inflammation and burning sensation surround entire oral mucosa.

Histopathology

♦ Oral epithelial cells become enlarged and show hyperchromatic nuclei with prominent nucleoli along with serrated nuclear membrane.
♦ Epithelium becomes atrophic.
♦ There is presence of subepithelial chronic inflammatory cell infiltration.

Laboratory Findings

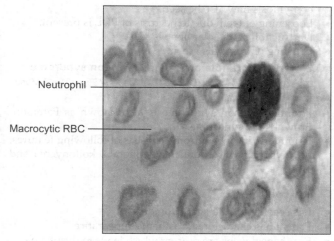

Fig. 101: Peripheral smear showing pernicious anemia
(For color version, see Plate 18).

Laboratory Diagnosis

♦ Macrocytosis is commonly seen.
♦ Red blood cell count is decreased, at times, it is 10 lakh/cubic mm of blood.
♦ Mild-to-moderate thrombocytopenia is also seen.
♦ MCV, MCH, MCHC concentration is normal
♦ Howell jolly bodies and Cabot rings are present.
♦ Neutrophils are hypersegmented.

♦ Buccal scrapings show nuclear abnormalities
♦ Schilling test show vitamin B12 deficiency.
♦ Serum lactate dehydrogenase is markedly increased while serum potassium, cholesterol and skeletal alkaline phosphatase are often decreased.
♦ Bone marrow is hypercellular and show trilineage differentiation. Erythroid precursors are large and oval. Nucleus is large and contains coarse motley chromatin clumps giving checkboard appearance.

Treatment

IM injection of vitamin B12 is given.

Q.2. Write notes on aplastic anemia. *(Mar 1997, 5 Marks)*

Ans. It is a rare disorder characterized by the peripheral blood pancytopenia (anemia, leukopenia and thrombocytopenia) associated with bone marrow suppression.

Etiology

♦ *Drug and chemicals:* Common drugs which can cause aplastic anemia are benzene derivatives, chloramphenicol, penicillin, sulfonamides and anticancer drugs.
♦ *Infections:* Patients with bacterial disease, such as tuberculosis and viral infections like hepatitis and infection mononucleosis can cause pancytopenia.
♦ *Radiation:* Long-term exposure to continuous radiation has lead to development of aplastic anemia.
♦ *Other causes:* Pregnancy and thymoma can cause aplastic anemia.

Clinical Features

♦ It is more common in young adults and elderly individuals.
♦ Marked pallor of skin and petechiae.
♦ Numbness and tingling of extremities.
♦ Generalized edema of body (anasarca).
♦ Fever and infections occur due to neutropenia.
♦ Spontaneous gingival bleeding and epistaxis.
♦ Multiple areas of ulceration in oral mucosa.

Treatment

Blood transfusion, splenectomy and bone marrow transplant.

Q.3. Write notes on sickle cell anemia.

(Aug/Sep 1998, 5 Marks)

Or

Write short note on sickle cell anemia.

(Mar 2007, 2.5 Marks) (Jan 2018, 4 Marks)

Ans. It is an autosomal dominant disorder.

In sickle cell anemia, the erythrocytes assume crescent shape and undergo lysis.

Clinical Features

♦ It is more common in females.
♦ Malaise, weakness and jaundice with yellow sclera.
♦ Pallor, loss of appetite and muscular rigidity.
♦ Fever, pain in abdomen and back in joints.
♦ Swelling in joints, hand and feet.

- There may be delayed eruption and hypoplasia of dentition.
- There is presence of mongoloid faces with high cheek bones and bimaxillary prognathism.

Radiographic Features

- Skull radiographs reveals multiple small spicules (small needle shaped body) across calvarium, which produces "Hair-on-end" appearance.
- IOPA reveals "Step ladder", such as trabeculae between contagious and posterior teeth.
- Increased osteoporosis and hyperplasia of bone marrow.

Treatment

No specific treatment.

Oxygen and blood transfusion in serious situation.

Q.4. Write notes on purpura. *(Mar 1996, 5 Marks)*

Ans. It is defined as purpulish discoloration of skin and mucous membrane due to subcutaneous and submucous extravasation of blood.

Clinical Features

- Purpura commonly occurs among adults below 40 years and females are more commonly affected.
- Sudden spontaneous occurrence of petechiae (small pin point hemorrhage under skin or mucosa), ecchymoses or hematomas in skin and mucous membrane.
- Bleeding spots on skin or mucosal surface which do not blanch on pressure.
- Women may have heavy menses or bleeding between periods.
- Spontaneous gingival bleeding is present.
- Bleeding into TMJ results in pain and trismus.

Treatment

- Steroid therapy and repeated blood transfusions.
- Splenectomy and immunosuppressive drug therapy is required.

Q.5. Write short note on hemophilia. *(Sep 2005, 5 Marks)*

Ans. Hemophilia is a potentially fatal inherited bleeding disorder characterized by the profuse hemorrhage due to deficiency of clotting factors.

Types

- Hemophilia A or classic hemophilia: In this factor VIII deficiency is present.
- Hemophilia B or Christmas disease: In this factor IX deficiency is present.
- von Willebrand's disease: In this factor VIII deficiency is present along with defective platelet function.

Clinical Features

- Disease is mostly characterized by the easy bruising and prolongs bleeding particularly often accidental, surgical and dental trauma.

- Spontaneous bleeding into subcutaneous tissue or internal organs leads to recurrent soft tissue hematoma formation.
- Gastric hemorrhage may occur in case of gastric ulcer.
- Joint problems occur due to degenerative changes in joint structures, osteoporosis and muscle atrophy.
- Severe hemorrhage from gingival tissue after dental extraction.
- Slight trauma may lead to hematoma formation in tongue, lips and palate.
- Hemophilic patient has high caries index and severe periodontal disease.

Treatment

- Immediate transfusion of factor VIII or IX concentrate is primary treatment.
- Patient need transfusion in every 12 hours until bleeding stops.
- Analgesic and corticosteroids reduce joint pain and swelling.
- In mild hemophilia, use of IV desmopressin is done.

Q.6. Write short note on oral manifestations of leukemia. *(Mar 2011, 5 Marks)*

Ans. Following are the oral manifestations of leukemia:

- Patient has got gingival hyperplasia which is the constant feature of leukemia.
- Gingiva become boggy, edematous and deep red and bleed easily.
- Gingival swelling is present due to leukemic infiltration.
- Purpuric lesions of oral mucosa analogous to cutaneous ecchymosis may also be seen.
- Loosening of teeth due to necrosis of PDL is present.
- Destruction of alveolar bone is seen.
- Crusting of lips is also seen.

Q.7. Write short note on Plummer-Vinson syndrome. *(Dec 2010, 8 Marks) (Sep 2011, 3 Marks)*

Ans.

- Plummer-Vinson syndrome is also known as Paterson-Brown-Kelly syndrome.
- Plummer-Vinson syndrome consists of following features, i.e., dysphagia, iron deficiency anemia, koilonychia and glossitis.

Clinical Features

- It is seen in middle-aged women.
- Patient has characteristic asthenic appearance.
- Esophageal webs are present which leads to dysphagia.
- Tongue is smooth and red.
- Angular cheilitis is also seen.
- Nails of the patient are spoon shaped.

Diagnosis

- Clinical diagnosis reveals all the above mentioned features.
- During blood examination picture of iron deficiency anemia is present.
- Biopsy reveals atrophy of epithelium, lamina propria as well as muscles.

Management

♦ Iron deficiency anemia should be corrected by giving hematinics to the patient.
♦ Esophageal dilatation should be done.

Q.8. Define and classify anemia. Describe iron deficiency anemia. *(Aug 2012, 15 Marks)*

Or

Write in detail on iron deficiency anemia.
(May/Jun 2009, 10 Marks)

Or

Write short note on iron deficiency anemia.
(Feb 2015, 5 Marks) (Apr 2017, 4 Marks)

Or

Define anemia. Describe iron deficiency anemia in detail. *(Jan 2017, 10 Marks)*

Or

What are the types of anemia? Describe iron deficiency anemia in detail. *(Sep 2018, 5 Marks)*

Ans. Anemia is defined as abnormal reduction in number of circulating RBCs, quantity of hemoglobin and the volume of packed red cells in a given unit of blood.

Classification of Anemia

Etiological classification of anemia (By **Lea and Febiger 1981**)
♦ Loss of blood
  • Acute posthemorrhagic anemia
  • Chronic posthemorrhagic anemia.
♦ Excessive destruction of red blood corpuscles
  • Extracorpuscular causes
    – Antibodies
    – Infections like malaria
    – Splenic sequestration and destruction
    – Associated diseases like lymphomas
    – Drugs, chemical and physical agents
    – Trauma to RBC.
  • Intracorpuscular hemolytic diseases
    – Hereditary
      » Disorders of glycolysis
      » Faulty synthesis or maintenance of reduced glutathione.
      » Qualitative or quantitative abnormalities in the synthesis of globulin
      » Abnormalities in RBC membrane
      » Erythropoietic porphyria
    – Acquired
      » Paroxysmal nocturnal hemoglobinuria
      » Lead poisoning.
♦ Impaired blood production resulting from deficiency of substances essential for erythropoiesis
  • Iron deficiency
  • Deficiency of various B vitamins: Vitamin B12 and folic acid (pernicious anemia and megaloblastic anemia); pyridoxine responsive anemia
  • Protein deficiency
  • Possibly ascorbic acid deficiency

♦ Inadequate production of mature erythrocytes
  • Deficiency of erythroblast
    – Atrophy of bone marrow: Aplastic anemia
      » Chemical or physical agents
      » Hereditary
      » Idiopathic.
    – Isolated erythroblastopenia
      » Thymoma
      » Chemical agents
      » Antibodies.
  • Infiltration of bone marrow
    – Leukemia, lymphomas
    – Multiple myeloma
    – Carcinoma, sarcoma
    – Myelofibrosis.
  • Endocrine abnormalities
    – Myxedema
    – Addison's disease
    – Pituitary insufficiency
    – Sometimes hyperthyroidism.
  • Chronic renal failure
  • Chronic inflammatory disease
    – Infectious
    – Noninfectious including granulomatous and collagen disease.
  • Cirrhosis of liver.

Morphological Classification of Anemia

Type of anemia	Description	Common causes
Macrocytic	Increased MCV, MCH and normal MCHC.	Lack of erythrocyte-maturating factors (intrinsic and extrinsic factors).
Normocytic	Reduction only in RBC number, Normal MCV, MCH MCHC.	Hemorrhage, hemolysis, lack of blood formation and dilution of blood with fluid.
Simple microcytic	Reduced MCV, MCH and normal MCHC.	Associated with infections and inflammatory diseases.
Hypochromic microcytic	Reduced MCV, MCH and MCHC.	Iron deficiency.

MCV = Mean corpuscular volume
MCH = Mean corpuscular hemoglobin
MCHC = Mean corpuscular hemoglobin concentration.

Iron Deficiency Anemia

Iron deficiency anemia results due to deficiency of iron in the body.

Etiology

♦ *Exogenous Cause:* It is due to dietary deficiency
♦ *Endogenous Cause:*
  • Absorption Defect as occurs in.
    – Histamine, i.e., fast achlorhydria.

– Gastric operations, i.e., total gastrectomy and partial gastrectomy.
- *Enterogeneous:*
  – Unusual hurry in the passage of chyme.
  – Abnormality in absorbing mucosa.
- *Transport defect*, i.e., atransferrinemia.
- *Loss in iron from body:*
  – Loss due to hemorrhage in peptic ulcer, hiatus hernia, Ca stomach, Ca colon and hookworm manifestation.
  – Excessive menstrual bleeding.
  – Excessive excretion.
- *Increased requirement of iron* in pregnancy and lactation.

Clinical Features

♦ Females are more commonly affected during 4th and 5th decades.
♦ Patient complains of lack of concentration, tiredness, headache, presence of tingling sensations over extremities.
♦ Nails of the patient become brittle and nail bed become spoon shaped which is also known as koilonychia.
♦ Patients feel difficulty in swallowing. This is also termed as dysphagia.
♦ Pigmentation can be seen over the dorsum of hand and metacarpophalangeal joint which is also known as knuckle pigmentation.
♦ Plummer-Vinson syndrome is associated with iron deficiency anemia and other features are dysphagia, koilonychia and glossitis.

Oral Manifestations

♦ Presence of pallor of oral mucosa as well as gingiva.
♦ Atrophy of oral mucosa is present. This is seen on tongue and buccal mucosa.
♦ Glossodynia, i.e., pain in the tongue and glossopyrosis, i.e., reddening of tongue is present.
♦ Atrophy of filliform and fungiform papillae is present giving tongue a bald or smooth or glistening appearance.
♦ Presence of cracking and fissuring is seen at corner of mouth suggestive of angular cheilitis.
♦ At times aphthous ulcers are also seen.

Laboratory Diagnosis

♦ Examination of peripheral blood picture shows:
  - *Chromicity:* Hypochromia of RBC
    – Central pallor increased
    – Anisochromia present
  - *Size:* Microcytic anisocytotic
  - *Shape:* Poikilocytosis often present, pear-shaped tailed variety of RBC, elliptical form common.
  - *Target cell:* Present
  - *Reticulocytes:* Present
  - *Osmotic fragility:* Slightly decreased
  - *ESR:* Seldom elevated
♦ RBC count is between 3,000,000 to 4,000,000 cells per cubic mm of blood.

♦ Presence of low serum iron and ferritin with an elevated total iron binding capacity.
♦ Hemoglobin level is at 4 mg/dL or below it.
♦ MCV, MCH and MCHC are decreased.

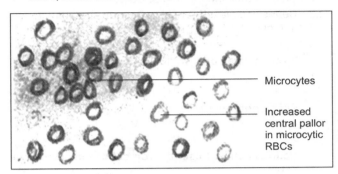

Fig. 102: Peripheral smear showing iron deficiency anemia
(For color version, see Plate 18).

Treatment

♦ Patient should be kept on oral iron therapy. Ferrous fumarate or ferrous sulfate should be given to the patient. 300 mg tablet should be given 3 to 4 times a day for six months duration.

Q.9. Describe in brief oral manifestations of anemia.
(Apr 2008, 5 Marks) (Jun 2010, 5 Marks)

Ans. *For oral manifestations, refer to Ans. 8 of same chapter.*

Q.10. Classify gingival hyperplasia and describe leukemia.
(Dec 2010, 18 Marks)

Ans.

Classification of Gingival Hyperplasia

On Basis of Etiological Factors and Pathologic Changes

♦ Inflammatory enlargement
  - Chronic
  - Acute
♦ Drug-induced enlargement
♦ Enlargement associated with systemic disease
  - Conditional enlargement
    – Pregnancy
    – Puberty
    – Vitamin C deficiency
    – Plasma cell gingivitis
    – Nonspecific conditioned enlargement (Pyogenic granuloma)
  - Systemic diseases causing gingival enlargement
    – Leukemia
    – Granulomatous disease (e.g., Wegener's granulomatosis, sarcoidosis)
♦ Neoplastic enlargement
  - Benign tumors
  - Malignant tumors.
♦ False enlargement.

Using the criteria of location and distribution gingival enlargement is designated as follows:

- *Localized:* Gingival enlargement limited to one or more teeth.
- *Generalized:* Involving the gingiva throughout the mouth.
- *Marginal:* Confined to marginal gingiva.
- *Papillary:* Confined to interdental papilla.
- *Diffuse:* Involving the marginal and attached papillae.
- *Discrete:* Isolated sessile or pedunculated tumor like enlargement.

On Basis of Degree of Gingival Enlargement

Grade 0: No sign of gingival enlargement.

Grade I: Enlargement confirmed to interdental papilla.

Grade II: Enlargement involves papilla and marginal gingiva.

Grade III: Enlargement covers three quarters or more of the crown.

Leukemia

Leukemia is a disease which is characterized by overproduction of WBCs which are present in circulating blood in an immature form.

Types of Leukemia

- Acute
- Chronic

Etiology

- Chromosomal abnormality: Presence of an abnormal chromosome, e.g., Philadelphia chromosome.
- Exposure to high doses of radiation therapy.
- Exposure to certain chemicals, e.g., phenylbutazone and benzene.
- Myeloproliferative disorders, such as polycythemia vera.
- Congenital or genetic abnormalities.
- Presence of primary immune deficiency
- Infection with human leukocyte virus.

Acute Leukemia

Classification of Acute Leukemia (FAB Classification)

1. **Acute myeloblastic leukemia (AMD)**
   - *M0:* Minimally differentiated: Myeloblasts lack definite cytologic and cytochemical features but have myeloid lineage antigens.
   - *M1:* AML without maturation: Myeloblasts predominate with distant nucleoli, few granules or Auer rods are present.
   - *M2:* AML with maturation: Myeloblasts with promyelocytes predominate and Auer rods may be present.
   - *M3:* Acute promyelocytic leukemia: Hypergranular promyelocytes often with multiple Auer rods are seen.
   - *M4:* Acute myelomonocytic leukemia: Mature cells of both myeloid and monocytic series in peripheral blood; myeloid cells resemble M2
   - *M5:* Acute monocytic leukemia: Promonocytes or undifferentiated blast.
   - *M6:* Acute erythroleukemia: Erythroblast predominate; myeloblasts and promyelocytes also increased
   - *M7:* Acute megakaryocytic leukemia: Pleomorphic undifferentiated blast cells predominate and react with anti-platelet antibodies.

2. **Acute lymphoblastic leukemia**
   - *L1:* Acute lymphoblastic (Seen in children): Homogeneous small lymphoblasts; scanty cytoplasm, regular round nuclei, inconspicuous nucleoli.
   - *L2:* Acute lymphoblastic (Seen in adults): Heterogeneous lymphoblasts; variable amount of cytoplasm, irregular or cleft nuclei, large nucleoli.
   - *L3:* Burkitt's type (Uncommon): Large homogenus lymphoblasts; nuclei are round to oval, prominent nucleoli, cytoplasmic vacuolation.

Clinical Features

Acute leukemias are more common in children and adults from 1st to 4th decades of life.

Clinical features are due to:

- **Bone marrow failure**
  - Anemia is seen leading to pallor, lethargy and dyspnea.
  - Pyrexia is present.
  - Bleeding manifestations are present, such as spontaneous bruises, petechiae, bleeding from gingiva.
  - Infections of multiple organs are present.
- **Organ infiltration**
  - Presence of pain and tenderness in bones.
  - Enlargement of tonsils is present.
  - Lymphadenopathy is seen.
  - Hepatomegaly and splenomegaly are common findings.
  - Chloroma or granulocytic sarcoma is a localized tumor mass occurring over the skin or orbit by local infiltration of tissues by leukemic cells.

Oral Manifestations

- Bleeding from gingiva is present. Gingiva becomes boggy, edematous and red in color.
- Presence of paresthesia of lower lip.
- Crustation over lips is seen.
- Mobility of permanent teeth is present.
- Oral mucosa appears pale with ulceration along with petechiae and ecchymosis.

Laboratory Findings

- *Anemia:* It is normochromic in type, moderate reticulocytes are seen, few nucleated red cells.
- *Thrombocytopenia:* Platelet count is below 50,000/µL of blood.
- *WBC count:* It ranges from sub-normal to markedly elevated. It is 1,00,000/µL of blood in advanced cases. Leukocytes in peripheral blood are blast cells.
- Bone marrow examination shows hypercellularity. Bone marrow is packed with leukemic blast cells. Erythropoietic cells are reduced. Megaloblastic features and ring sideroblasts are present.

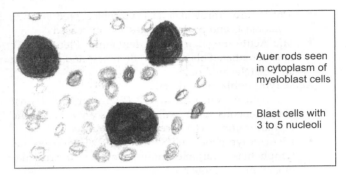

Fig. 103: Acute myeloid leukemia *(For color version, see Plate 18)*.

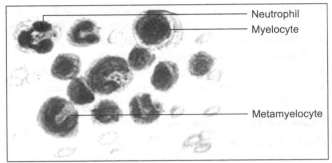

Fig. 105: Chronic myeloid leukemia
(For color version, see Plate 18).

Chronic Leukemia

These are hematologic malignancies in which predominant leukemic cells are initially well differentiated. They are of two types:

1. Chronic myeloid leukemia
2. Chronic lymphocytic leukemia

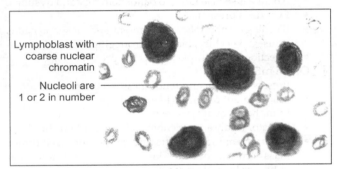

Fig. 104: Acute lymphoblastic leukemia
(For color version, see Plate 18).

Chronic Myeloid Leukemia

It consists of large leukemic cells and differentiated WBCs in bone marrow.

Clinical Features

♦ It occurs during 3rd and 4th decades of life.
♦ Splenomegaly is present.
♦ Patient complains of loss of weight, abdomen prominence.
♦ Presence of anemia leads to weakness, fatigue and dyspnea.
♦ Petechiae and ecchymosis is seen.

Laboratory Findings

♦ Anemia is normocytic and normochromic type.
♦ Marked leukocytosis is present, i.e., 2,00,000 cells/μL.
♦ There is increased proportion of basophils.
♦ Bone marrow shows hypercellularity with total or partial replacement of fat spaces by proliferating myeloid cells.

Chronic Lymphocytic Leukemia

It is the malignancy of mature B cells.

Clinical Features

♦ It occurs during 4th decade of life.
♦ Male predilection is seen.
♦ Features of anemia are seen, i.e., weakness, fatigue and dyspnea.
♦ Lymphadenopathy is commonly present.
♦ Hepatomegaly and splenomegaly is commonly seen.
♦ Hemorrhagic manifestations are common.

Oral Manifestations

♦ Gingival hypertrophy is present. Ulceration of gingiva with necrosis is present.
♦ Tongue is dark and swollen.
♦ Presence of mobility of teeth is seen.
♦ Necrosis of PDL is seen.
♦ Alveolar bone destruction is also present.

Laboratory Findings

♦ Anemia is mild-to-moderate and is normocytic normochromic type.
♦ Marked leukocytosis is present.
♦ Leukocytes are mature small lymphocytes.
♦ Platelet count is normal or moderately reduced.

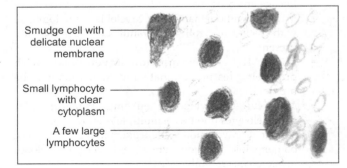

Fig. 106: Chronic lymphocytic leukemia
(For color version, see Plate 19).

Treatment

Chemotherapeutic drugs, radiation therapy and corticosteroids which leads to prolong remission and cures in some forms of disease.

Q.11. Define anemia. Give morphological classification of anemia. Describe in detail pernicious anemia.

(Apr 2015, 8 Marks)

Ans. *For definition of anemia and morphological classification of anemia, refer to Ans. 8 of same chapter.*

For pernicious anemia in detail, refer to Ans. 1 of same chapter.

Q.12. Write short note on erythroblastosis fetalis.

(July 2016, 5 Marks)

Ans. Erythroblastosis fetalis is a hemolytic anemia of newborn secondary to blood incompatibility mainly Rh factor between the mother and fetus.

Currently this disorder is uncommon due to use of anti-antigen gamma globulin at delivery in mothers with Rh negative blood.

Pathogenesis

It occurs due to the inheritance by the fetus of a blood factor from Rh positive father which act as foreign antigen to Rh negative mother.

Transplacental leak of RBCs from fetus to mother leads to immunization of mother and formation of antibodies which are transferred back to fetus transplacentally, this leads to fetal hemolysis.

Clinical Features

♦ Features depend on the severity of hemolysis, if it is severe child is stillborn or dead.
♦ Alive born child suffer from anemia with pallor, jaundice, compensatory erythropoiesis, i.e., medullary and extramedullary and edema.

Oral Manifestations

♦ Deposition of blood pigments in enamel and dentin of neonate which produces green, brown or blue hue.
♦ Enamel hypoplasia can also be present.
♦ A ring like defect is present at incisal edges of deciduous anterior teeth and middle portion of deciduous cuspid and first molar crown known as Rh hump.

Histopathology

Ground section of the affected teeth shows positive test for bilirubin.

Laboratory Findings

♦ RBC count at birth is from 1,000,000 cells/cu mm to normal level.
♦ Peripheral smear shows normoblasts or nucleated red cells.
♦ High bilirubin level.
♦ Direct Coombs test on cord blood is positive.

Treatment

No treatment is needed as the condition affects only deciduous teeth and not the permanent teeth.

Q.13. Write short note on megaloblastic anemia.

(Feb 2019, 5 Marks)

Ans. Megaloblastic anemia occurs due to deficiency of vitamin B12.

Term pernicious anemia is reserved for the patients with vitamin B12 deficiency due to lack of production of intrinsic factor in the stomach.

Clinical Features

♦ It is usually seen after the age of 30 years and increases in frequency with advancing age.
♦ It is characterized by the presence of triad of symptoms, such as generalized weakness, sore and painful tongue and numbness or tingling of the extremities.
♦ Other features are fatigability, headache, dizziness, nausea, vomiting, diarrhea, loss of appetite, shortness of breath, loss of weight, pallor and abdominal pain.
♦ Patient having severe anemia show yellow tinge of skin and sometimes sclera.
♦ Skin becomes smooth and dry.
♦ Nervous system involvement is present which include paresthetic sensation of extremities, difficulty in walking, general irritability, depression and drowsiness and loss of vibratory sensation.
♦ Psychiatric symptoms of memory loss, irritability, depression and dementia.

Oral Manifestations

♦ Glossitis is the more common symptom. Along with this glossodynia and glossopyrosis is seen.
♦ Presence of painful and burning lingual sensation.
♦ Small and shallow ulcers which resemble to aphthous ulcer are seen on the tongue.
♦ Gradual atrophy of papillae of tongue is seen which produces smooth or bald tongue, this is also known as Hunter's glossitis.
♦ Loss or distortion of taste is sometimes seen.

Histopathological Features

♦ It shows marked epithelial atrophy with loss of rete ridges, increased nuclear cytoplasmic ratio and prominent nucleoli. This pattern is misinterpreted as epithelial dysplasia at times, nuclei in pernicious anemia are pale staining and show peripheral chromatin clumping.
♦ Patchy diffuse chronic inflammatory infiltrate is noted in underlying connective tissue.

Laboratory Diagnosis

♦ Blood: Decrease in RBC count 1,000,000 or less per cubic millimeter.
  • Many of the cell exhibit macrocytosis.
  • Poikilocytosis or variation in shape is present.

- Leukocytes are remarkably reduced in number, increase in average size, increase in number of lobes to nucleus and anisopoikilocytosis.
- Mild to moderate thrombocytopenia is present.
♦ Serum: Elevation in indirect bilirubin.
- Serum lactate dehydrogenase is markedly increased.
- Serum potassium, cholesterol and alkaline phosphatase are often decreased.
♦ Bone marrow: Its biopsy and aspirate are hypercellular and show trilineage differentiation.
- Erythroid precursors are large and oval.
- Nucleus is large and has coarse motely chromatin clump which gives checkerboard appearance.
- Imbalanced growth of megakaryocytes is evidenced by hyperdiploidy of nucleus and presence of giant platelets in smear.
♦ Gastric secretion
- Most patients with anemia are achlorhydric, even with histamine stimulation.
- Intrinsic factor is either absent or markedly decreased.

Treatment

As diagnosis of megaloblastic anemia is made, monthly intramuscular injections of cyanocobalamin are given. Condition responds quickly to therapy with reports of clearing lesions within 5 days.

19. DISEASES OF SKIN

Q.1. Name the vesiculobullous lesions of oral cavity. Describe etiology, histopathology and clinical features of oral lichen planus. *(Dec 2010, 8 Marks)*

Or

Write short answer on clinical features and histology of lichen planus *(May 2018, 3 Marks)*

Or

Discuss clinical features and histopathology of lichen planus. *(Oct 2019, 3 Marks)*

Ans.

Vesiculobullous Lesions

Fitzpatrick Classification

♦ **According to anatomical plane:**
- Lntraepidermal blister granular layer
  - Pemphigus foliaceus
  - Frictional blisters
  - *Staphylococcus* scalded syndrome.
- Spinous layer
  - Eczematous dermatitis
  - Secondary to heat and cold
  - Herpes virus infection
  - Familial benign pemphigus

- Suprabasal
  - Pemphigus vulgaris
  - Pemphigus vegetans
  - Darier's disease
- Basal layer
  - Erythema multiforme
  - Toxic epidermal necrolysis
  - Lupus erythematosis
  - Lichen planus
  - Epidermolysis bullosa simplex
♦ **Dermal-epidermal junction zone:**
- Lamina lucida
  - Bullous pemphigoid
  - Cicatricial pemphigoid
  - Epidermolysis bullosa junctional
- Below basal lamina
  - Erythema multiforme
  - Epidermolysis bullosa dystrophica

Vesiculobullous Lesions

♦ **Primary blistering:**
- Pemphigus
- Bullous pemphigoid
- Cicatricial pemphigoid
- Epidermolysis bullosa acquisita.
♦ **Secondary blistering:**
- Contact
- Erythema mutltiforme
- Toxic epidermal necrolysis.
♦ **Infection:**
- Varicella zoster
- Herpes simplex
- Bullous impetigo.
♦ **Systemic disease:**
- Infection- cutaneous emboli
- Metabolic
  - Diabetic with bullae
  - Porphyria cutanea tarda.

Oral Lichen Planus

Lichen planus is also known as lichen ruber planus.

♦ It is a precancerous condition
♦ Lichen planus is a common mucocutaneous disease which arises due to an abnormal immunological reaction and the disease has some tendency to undergo malignant transformation.

Etiology

♦ *Immunology:*
- Due to cell mediated immune response
- Due to autoimmunity
- Immunodeficiency.
♦ *Genetic factors:* Lichen planus is reported in families, twins, husband and wife.

- *Infectious:* By spirochete.
- *Drugs and chemicals:* It is responsible for the lichenoid reaction.
- *Psychogenic factors:* Stress results, nervousness with emotional upset, overwork and some form of mental strain.
- *Habit:* Chewing of tobacco, betel nut and smoking.

Clinical Features

- It occurs among the middle aged and elderly people.
- There is slight predilection for the females.
- Lichen planus can involve several areas of oral cavity. *Oral lesion:* Mucosal surface of buccal mucosa, vestibule, tongue, lips, floor of mouth, palate and gingiva.
- Patient may report with burning sensation of oral mucosa.
- Oral lesion is characterized by radiating white and gray velvety thread like papules in linear, angular or retiform arrangement, tiny white elevated dots are present at the intersection of white lines known as "Wickhm's striae".

Histopathology

- Overlying surface epithelium exhibits hyperortho-keratinization or hyperparakeratinization or both.
- Acanthosis of spinal cell layer is present.
- Shortened and pointed rete pegs of epithelium which produces "Saw tooth" appearance.
- Intercellular edema in spinous cell layer is present.
- There is presence of necrosis or liquefaction degeneration of basal cell layer of epithelium.
- Few rounded or ovoid, amorphous eosinophilic bodies are present which are known as "Civatte bodies".
- These civatte bodies represent dead keratinocytes or other necrotic epithelial components which are transported to connective tissue for phagocytosis.
- Chronic inflammatory cell infiltration is present in juxtaepithelial lesion.

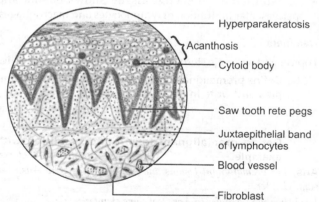

Fig. 107: Lichen planus *(For color version, see Plate 19).*

Q.2. Write short note on lichen planus.

(Apr 2007, 10 Marks)

Or

Write note on oral lichen planus. *(Mar 2006, 5 Marks)*

Or

Describe histopathology of lichen planus.

(Feb 2002, 5 Marks)

Or

Write in brief on lichen planus. *(June 2010, 5 Marks)*

Or

Write short note on oral lichen planus.

(Jan 2018, 5 Marks)

Or

Write short note on histopathology of oral lichen planus. *(July 2016, 5 Marks)*

Or

Write short note on histopathology of lichen planus.

(Sep 2018, 5 Marks)

Or

Write short answer on oral lichen planus.

(Sep 2018, 3 Marks)

Ans. *Refer to Ans. 1 of same chapter.*

Q.3. Enumerate vesiculobullous lesions and describe pemphigus. *(Sep 2002, 15 Marks)*

Or

Discuss in detail pemphigus vulgaris.

(Sep 2018, 10 Marks)

Ans. *For enumeration of vesiculobullous lesion, refer to Ans.1 of same chapter.*

Pemphigus

Pemphigus is a group of *vesiculobullous* lesion of skin and mucous membrane which is characterized by formation of intraepithelial vesicles or bulla causing separation of epithelium.

Clinical Features

- It occurs during 4th, 5th and 6th decades of life and is more prevalent among the females.
- Rapidly developing vesicle or bulla on several areas of skin and mucous membrane which contain clear fluid initially but later on there is formation of pus.
- Vesicle ruptures very soon and leaves painful, erythematous ulcers that bleed profusely.
- Gentle traction or oblique pressure on and affected area around the lesion causes stripping of the normal skin or mucous membrane which is known as "Nikolsky's Sign".
- Patient may die due to dehydration and septicemia.

Histopathology

- Formation of vesicle or bulla within the epithelium that result in supra basilar split.
- Following the suprabasilar split the basal cell layer remains attached to lamina propria and appears as row of "Tomb Stone".
- Loss of intracellular bridges and collection of edema fluid results in acantholysis within spinous cell layer which causes disruption of prickle cell layer.
- As result of acantholysis, clumps of large hyperchromatic epithelial cells lying free within the vesicular fluid, these

desquamated cells are round and smooth in appearance and are known as Tzanck cells.

♦ Small number of PMNs and lymphocytes may be found.

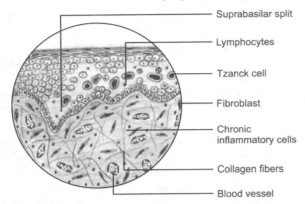

Fig. 108: Pemphigus *(For color version, see Plate 19).*

Treatment
♦ High dose of steroids
♦ Immunosuppressive agents
♦ Antibiotics to prevent secondary infection.
♦ Fluid and electrolyte balance must be strictly maintained.

Q.4. Write short answer on histology of pemphigus.
(Aug 2019, 3 Marks)

Or

Discuss about pemphigus. *(Sep 2005, 5 Marks)*

Or

Describe histopathology of pemphigus.
(Apr 2008, 5 Marks)

Ans. *Refer to Ans. 3 of same chapter.*

Q.5. Write short note on erythema multiforme.
(Feb 2006, 2.5 Marks) (Mar 2007, 2.5 Marks)
(Nov 2008, 5 Marks)

Ans. Erythema multiforme is an acute inflammatory dermatological disorder that involves skin, mucous membrane and sometimes internal organs.

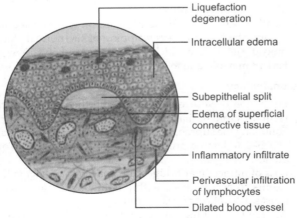

Fig. 109: Erythema multiforme *(For color version, see Plate 19).*

Etiology
♦ *Infection:* TB, herpes simplex.
♦ *Drug hypersensitivity:* Barbiturates, sulfonamides, salicylates.
♦ *Hyperimmune reaction:* Due to formation of antigen antibody complex against submucosal and derma blood vessels.

Types
♦ EM minor or erythema multiforme minor.
  It represents the localized eruption of skin with mild or no mucosal involvement.
♦ EM major or erythema multiforme major or Steven Johnson syndrome (SJS)
  It is more severe mucosal and skin disease and is potentially life-threatening disorder.

Clinical Features
♦ It occurs between the age of 15 to 40 years and males are more commonly affected.
♦ Rapidly developing erythematous macules, papules, vesicle or bulla appear symmetrically over hand and arm, legs and feet, face and neck.
♦ Classical dermal lesions of erythema multiforme which often appear on extremities are called "Bull's eye".
♦ Vesicles of mucosal surface are short lived and become eroded or ulcerated and bleed profusely.
♦ Patient also develops tracheobronchial ulceration and pneumonia.

Histopathology
♦ It usually consists of acanthosis, intercellular or intracellular edema and necrosis of epithelium.
♦ Vesicle may form within epithelium or at epithelial connective tissue junction.
♦ Subepithelial connective tissue shows edema and perivascular infiltration of lymphocytes and macrophages.

Treatment

Topical and systemic steroid therapy coupled with antibiotic.

Q.6. Define premalignant lesion and condition with examples and write in detail lichen planus.
(Sep 2006, 15 Marks)

Or

Define premalignant lesion and condition with example. *(Feb 2019, 3 Marks)*

Ans. *For premalignant lesions and conditions, refer to Ans. 7 of same chapter.*

For lichen planus, refer to Ans. 1 of same chapter.

Q.7. Define premalignancy. Enumerate the premalignant lesions and conditions. Describe in detail lichen planus. *(Dec 2007, 7 Marks)*

Ans. Premalignancy is an altered state of tissue which often has but not always has high potential to undergo malignant transformation.

Premalignant Lesion

Premalignant lesion is defined as "A morphologically altered tissue in which cancer is more likely to occur than its apparently normal counterparts". For example:

♦ Leukoplakia
♦ Erythroplakia
♦ Mucosal changes associated with smoking habits
♦ Carcinoma in situ
♦ Bowen disease
♦ Actinic keratosis, actinic cheilitis and actinic elastosis.

Premalignant Condition

Premalignant condition is defined as "A generalized state or condition associated with significantly increased risk for cancer development". For example:

♦ Syphilis
♦ OSMF
♦ Oral lichen planus
♦ Sideropenic dysplasia
♦ Dyskeratosis congenita
♦ Lupus erythematosus.

For lichen planus in detail, refer to Ans. 1 of same chapter.

Q.8. Write short note on oral manifestations of hereditary ectodermal dysplasia. *(Sep 2009, 3 Marks)*

Ans. Ectodermal dysplasia is a hereditary disorder characterized by defective formation of ectodermal structures, i.e., teeth, nail, sweat glands, sebaceous glands and hair follicles.

Oral Manifestations

♦ Anodontia and oligodontia
♦ Frequent malformation of any teeth in both deciduous and permanent teeth. Incisors appear to be conical, tapered or pointed while molars look narrow.
♦ Salivary glands including intraoral accessory glands are sometimes hypoplastic in this disease which leads to xerostomia.
♦ Patient have pharyngitis with dysphagia and there is hoarseness of voice.
♦ Alveolar process does not develop in absence of teeth, there is a reduction from normal vertical dimension resulting in protuberant lips
♦ Palatal arch is high and at times patient exhibits cleft palate.

Q.9. Define vesicle and bulla. Describe in detail etiopathogenesis, clinical features, histopathology and investigations of pemphigus vulgaris.
(Sep 2011, 8 Marks)

Ans. Vesicle is defined as a superficial blister which is 5 mm or less in diameter and is usually filled with clear fluid.

Bulla is defined as a larger blister which is greater than 5 mm in diameter.

Pemphigus vulgaris is an autoimmune, intraepithelial blistering disease affecting the skin and mucous membrane and is mediated by circulating autoantibodies directed against keratinocyte cell surfaces.

Etiopathogenesis

Flowchart 9: Etiopathogenesis of hereditary ectodermal dysplasia.

```
┌─────────────────────────────────────────────────┐
│ Pemphigus antibody binds to keratinocyte cell    │
│ surface molecules desmoglein 1 and desmoglein 3  │
└─────────────────────────────────────────────────┘
                      ↓
┌─────────────────────────────────────────────────┐
│ Patients have circulating and tissue bound       │
│ antibodies of IgG1 and IgG4 subclass             │
└─────────────────────────────────────────────────┘
                      ↓
┌─────────────────────────────────────────────────┐
│ Pemphigus antibody fixes components of complement│
│ to surface of epidermal cells                    │
└─────────────────────────────────────────────────┘
                      ↓
┌─────────────────────────────────────────────────┐
│ Antibody binding may active complement with      │
│ release of inflammatory mediators and            │
│ recruitment of activated T cells                 │
└─────────────────────────────────────────────────┘
```

Protease Theory

According to protease theory deposition of autoantibody within the epithelium induces the proteolytic activity by activating tissue plasminogen. This inturn generate proteolytic enzyme called plasmin which destroy desmosomes.

For clinical features and histopathology, refer to Ans. 3 of same chapter.

Investigations

♦ Incisional/punch biopsy of the involved area should be done and is histopathologically examined.
♦ *Immunofluorescent testing:* Direct immunofluorescence testing is done to demonstrate the presence of immunoglobulins, predominantly IgG but sometimes in combination with C3, IgA and IgM, in the intercellular spaces or intercellular substance in either oral epithelium or clinically normal epithelium adjacent to lesion.
♦ *Indirect immunofluorescence:* This is accomplished basically by incubating normal animal or human mucosa with serum from the patient suspected of having the disease and adding the fluorescein-conjugated human antiglobulin. A positive reaction in the tissue indicates presence of circulating immunoglobulin antibodies.

Q.10. Write short note on pemphigus vulgaris.
(Jan 2016, 5 Marks) (Aug 2011, 10 Marks)

Ans. *For clinical features and histopathology, refer to Ans. 3 of same chapter.*

For etiopathogenesis and investigations, refer to Ans. 9 of same chapter.

Q.11. Enumerate the mucocutaneous lesions of oral cavity. Describe in detail pemphigus. *(Jan 2012, 10 Marks)*

Or

Enumerate mucocutaneous lesions. Describe in detail pemphigus. *(Mar 2016, 8 Marks)*

Ans.

Mucocutaneous Lesions of Oral Cavity

Genodermatosis

♦ Darier's disease
♦ White sponge nevus

- Hereditary benign intraepithelial dyskeratosis
- Peutz-Jeghers syndrome
- Pachyonychia congenita
- Dyskeratosis congenita
- Pseudoxanthoma elasticum

Non-infective Disease

- Vesicular
  - Bullous pemphigoid
  - Benign mucous membrane pemphigoid
  - Pemphigus
  - Erythema multiforme
  - Lichen planus
  - Epidermolysis bullosa
- Non-vesicular
  - Geographic tongue
  - Lichen planus
- Collagen disorders
  - Wegener's granulomatosis
  - Midline lethal granuloma
  - Polyarteritis nodosa
  - Scleroderma
  - Lupus erythematosus
  - Vasculitis
- Degenerative disorder
  - OSMF
  - Amyloidosis
  - Solar elastosis
- Pigmentation
  - Anemia
  - Albert syndrome
  - Addison's disease
  - Racial pigmentation
  - Endocrinopathy

For pemphigus in detail, refer to Ans. 3 and Ans. 9 of same chapter.

Q.12. Write short note on Steven-Johnson syndrome.
(Mar 2011, 3 Marks)

Ans. Steven-Johnson syndrome is a severe bullous form of erythema multiforme with widespread involvement typically including skin, oral cavity, eyes and genitalia.

- **Skin lesions:** The cutaneous lesions in this mucocutaneous ocular disease are those of erythema multiforme although they are commonly hemorrhagic and are often vesicular or bullous.
- **Oral mucous membrane lesions:** Lesions are extremely painful and severe. Mucosal vesicles or bullae occur which rupture and leave surfaces covered with white or yellow exudates. Erosions of pharynx are common. Lips may exhibit ulceration with bloody crusting and are painful.
- **Eye lesions:** It consist of photophobia, conjunctivitis, corneal ulceration and panophthalmitis. Blindness may result.
- **Genital lesions:** There is nonspecific urethritis, balanitis, vaginal ulcers.

Q.13. Write notes on discoid lupus erythematosus.
(Apr 2008, 5 Marks)

Ans. Discoid lupus erythematosus remain confined to the mucosa and skin.

Etiology

- Genetic susceptibility
- *Autoimmune:* Patient develops antibodies to their own cells.
- *Endocrine:* Common in pregnant ladies.

Clinical Features

- It is seen during 3rd and 4th decades of life.
- Female predilection is present with ratio of 5:1.
- Lesion appears as circumscribed slightly elevated white patch surrounded by erythematous halo.
- Skin lesions are slightly elevated. They are purple or red macules and are covered by gray or yellow scales.
- As removal of scale is done it result in carpet track extension.
- There is presence of butterfly shaped distribution over malar region at bridge of nose.

Oral Manifestations

- Tongue, buccal mucosa, vermilion border of lip are most common involved oral sites.
- Patient complains of burning and tenderness in the involved area.
- Lesion begin as erythematous area with induration and white spots. At times pain is felt in ulcerated area with crusting and bleeding. Scale formation is absent.
- Fine white striae are seen radiating from the margins.
- Lips show erythematous area which is surrounded by keratotic border.

Histopathology

- It is characterized by hyperkeratosis with keratotic plugging.
- There is presence of atrophy of rete pegs.
- Presence of liquefaction degeneration of basal layer of cells.
- Perivascular infiltration of lymphocytes is present and their collection at about dermal appendages.
- Basophilic degeneration of collagen and elastic fibers is present.
- Hyalinization is also seen.
- Edema and fibrinoid change is present beneath the epithelium.

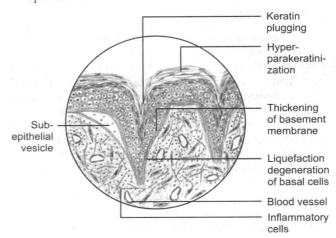

Fig. 110: Lupus erythematosus *(For color version, see Plate 19).*

Treatment

Corticosteroids along with immunosuppressant drugs is the choice.

Q.14. Describe in brief Tzanck cells.

(May/June 2009, 5 Marks)

Ans. Tzanck cell is a term given to a free floating epithelial cell in any intraepithelial vesicle.

Tzanck cells are seen in mainly two diseases, i.e.
1. Pemphigus vulgaris
2. Herpes simplex infection

Tzanck Cells in Pemphigus Vulgaris

Pemphigus consists of vesicle or bulla formation in spinous layer of epithelium just above basal cell layer which leads to suprabasilar split. Prevesicular edema weaken intercellular junctions and intercellular bridges between epithelial cells break and the epithelial cells fell apart which is known as acantholysis, due to this clumps of epithelial cells found free on the vesicular space. These loose cells are characterized by degenerative changes, such as hyperchromatic staining and swelling of nuclei, cells become round in shape, these cells are known as tzanck cells.

Tzanck Cells in Herpes Simplex Infection

Herpes simplex virus mainly affects the epithelial cells. Infected epithelial cells undergo ballooning degeneration and show following features, such as acantholysis, nuclear clearing and enlargement of nucleus. These acantholytic epithelial cells are known as tzanck cells.

Q.15. Write in detail on genodermatosis.

(May/June 2009, 10 Marks)

Ans. Genodermatoses are genetically determined skin conditions.
♦ Some of the genodermatosis are characterized particularly by alteration in normal keratinization process and are known as genokeratosis.

Following are the genodermatosis:
♦ Darier's disease
♦ White sponge nevus
♦ Hereditary benign intraepithelial dyskeratosis
♦ Peutz-Jeghers syndrome
♦ Pachyonychia congenita
♦ Pseudoxanthoma elasticum
♦ Porokeratosis
♦ Warty dyskeratoma.

Darier's Disease

It is also known as keratosis follicularis.

Clinical Features

♦ It occurs during childhood or in adults.
♦ Initially there is presence of papules over the skin which is red in color later on they become purple brown or gray in color.
♦ Changes in nails are also seen, such as splintering, longitudinal streaking and fissuring.
♦ White papule occurs in oral cavity over hard and soft palate, tongue and gingiva. It is rough on palpation.

Histopathology

♦ Histopathology reveals hyperkeratosis, papillomatosis, acanthosis and benign dyskeratosis.
♦ Benign dyskeratosis show typical cells, i.e., corps ronds and grains
♦ *Corps ronds:* These cells are larger than normal squamous cells and have round homogeneous basophilic nucleus with dark eosinophilic cytoplasm and distinct cell membrane. They are seen in granular layer and superficial spinous cell layer.
♦ *Grains:* Small, elongated, parakeratotic cells present in keratin layer.

White Sponge Nevus

It is also known as Cannon's disease.

Clinical Features

♦ It occurs most commonly at birth and its intensity increases till puberty.
♦ It is seen on buccal mucosa, gingiva and palate.
♦ It appears as thick, corrugated, soft textured, white opalescent line.
♦ White or keratotic area could be removed by rubbing and normal looking epithelium is seen.

Histopathology

♦ Histopathologically epithelium shows hyperparakeratosis and acanthosis.
♦ Cells of spinous layer show intracellular edema.
♦ Parakeratin plugging is seen which is projecting deep in spinous cell layer.

Hereditary Benign Intraepithelial Dyskeratosis

It is also known as Witkop-Von Sallmann syndrome.

Clinical Features

♦ It occurs commonly in children.
♦ Most commonly it involves eyes. In oral cavity it is seen in floor of mouth, buccal mucosa, tongue and palate.
♦ It appears as spongy, white macerated area.

Histopathology

♦ Histologically thick epithelium is seen with hydropic degeneration.
♦ Dyskeratotic cells are seen, i.e., round, eosinophilic, waxy appearing cells are seen.

Peutz-Jeghers Syndrome

It is also known as hereditary intestinal polyposis syndrome.

Features

♦ In it, there is pigmentation of face and oral cavity.
♦ Adenocarcinoma can occur in gastric, duodenum and colon.

Histopathology

Histologically acanthosis of epithelium is seen with elongation of rete ridges.

Pachyonychia Congenita

It is also known as Jadassohn-Lewandowsky syndrome.

Clinical Features

♦ It occur in neonates.
♦ It is seen on nails, palms, hands and feet.
♦ There is thickening of nail present, thickening increase toward free border of nail bed and get filled with yellow keratotic debris which lead to the projection of nail upward at free border.
♦ Hairs are sparse and corneal dyskeratosis is seen.
♦ Bullae are seen over the feet.

Histopathology

Histopathology of skin and mucous membrane showing acanthosis, parakeratosis and hyperkeratosis.

Pseudoxanthoma Elasticum

It leads to the degeneration of elastic fibers and make them susceptible for calcium.

Clinical Features

♦ It occurs at age of 13 years.
♦ Yellow papules are seen over the skin near neck, mouth, axilla.
♦ Skin surrounding the mouth give hound dog appearance.
♦ Lower lip is affected inside oral cavity.

Porokeratosis

It is also known as Mibelli's disease.

Clinical Features

♦ This disease occurs in childhood.
♦ Male predilection is present.
♦ It is seen commonly in face, neck, extremities and genitalia.
♦ Lesion appear as crateriform keratotic papule which later on form elevated plaque.
♦ Plaque from it margins is surrounded by raised border of epidermis.
♦ Nails of patient get thick and ridged.
♦ In oral cavity lesion is seen in upper lip and palate.

Histopathology

♦ Histologically elevated horny margin of the lesion show hyperkeratosis and acanthosis with deep groove filled with parakeratin and absence of underlying granular layer. This forms cornoid lamella.
♦ Central portion of the lesion show epithelial atrophy.

Warty Dyskeratoma

It is also known as isolated Darier's disease.

Clinical Features

♦ The disease occur in older age.
♦ Male predilection is present.
♦ Lesions are seen on scalp, neck, face and over the upper part of chest.
♦ Lesion present as elevated nodule which is umblicated.
♦ Borders of lesion are raised.
♦ Color of lesion is not specific and it varies from brown or yellow to black or gray.
♦ Orally lesion occurs very rarely and if present it can be seen as whitish area with central depression over it.

Histopathology

♦ Histopathologically intraoral lesions show central orthokeratin or parakeratin core below which epithelium show suprabasilar separation which result in cleft like space having acantholytic and dyskeratotic cells.
♦ Connective tissue papillae have single layer of basal cells.
♦ Underlying connective tissue show nonspecific chronic inflammatory infiltrate.

Q.16. Write in brief on ectodermal dysplasia.
(Dec 2010, 5 Marks) (Jan 2012, 5 Marks)

Ans. Term ectodermal dysplasia is a group of inherited diseases in which two or more ectodermal structures fails to develop.

♦ Disease can be autosomal dominant or autosomal recessive or it can be X-linked too.
♦ Most common ectodermal dysplasia is hereditary hypohidrotic ectodermal dysplasia.

Clinical Features

♦ Male predominance is seen.
♦ Patient is characterized by hypotrichosis, hypohydrosis and at times anhydrosis.
♦ Patient has characteristic saddle nose.
♦ Fine and sparse hair are seen on eyebrows and eyelashes
♦ Periocular skin has fine wrinkles with hyperpigmentation.
♦ Frontal bossing is commonly present.
♦ Nails appear dystrophic and brittle.
♦ Skin of the patient remains dry and there is absence or partial presence of sweat glands. Due to this patient cannot perspire and his heat regulation is disturbed which lead to increased temperature of patient.

Oral Manifestations

Refer to Ans. 8 of same chapter.

Histopathology

Histopathology of Skin Reveals Following Features

♦ There is reduction in number of sweat glands, hair follicles and sebaceous glands.
♦ Epidermis is thin and flattened.
♦ Eccrine sweat glands are few or poorly developed.
♦ In oral histopathology salivary glands show ectasia of ducts and inflammatory changes.

Treatment

♦ Condition is genetic so it is non-curable.
♦ Prosthetic rehabilitation of patient should be done by complete dentures, RPDs or fixed dentures.
♦ Dental implants can also be considered.

Q.17. Write short note on CREST syndrome.
(Aug 2012, 5 Marks)

Ans. It is considered to be a mild variant of systemic sclerosis.
The term CREST is an acronym for:
C- Calcinosis Cutis
R- Raynaud's phenomenon

E- Esophageal dysfunction

S- Sclerodactyly

T- Telangiectasia.

Clinical Features

♦ Female predilection is present.

♦ It most commonly occurs during sixth or seventh decades of life.

♦ Signs of the disease develop from months to years.

♦ *Calcinosis cutis:* It is characterized by deposition of calcium beneath the skin in form of nodules which are 0.5 to 2 cm in size and are movable, multiple and are nontender.

♦ *Raynaud's phenomenon:* It is seen when patient's hand or feet are exposed to cold. Characteristic clinical sign is blanching of digits which appear whitish in color because of vasospasm. After few minutes extremity become blue in color because of venous stasis. As area get warm it gives dusky-red hue which indicates of return of hyperemic blood flow. With all this presence of throbbing pain is there.

♦ *Esophageal dysfunction:* It is present because of deposition of abnormal collagen in esophageal submucosa.

♦ *Sclerodactyly:* In this fingers get stiff, skin becomes smooth and shiny. Flexure of fingers occurs resulting in claw deformity.

♦ *Telangiectasia:* In this bleeding from superficial dilated vessels is seen.

Q.18. Classify mucocutaneous lesions and describe in detail etiology, clinical features and histopathological features of oral lichen planus. *(Dec 2012, 8 Marks)*

Ans. *For classification of mucocutaneous lesions, refer to Ans. 11 of same chapter.*

For etiology, clinical features and histopathological features of oral lichen planus, refer to Ans. 1 of same chapter.

Q.19. Write short note on direct and indirect immunofluorescence. *(Dec 2012, 3 Marks)*

Ans. Direct and indirect immunofluorescence are the techniques which are used to detect immune mediated or immunobullous diseases.

Direct Immunofluorescence

It is the diagnostic method which is used for detection of autoantibodies which are bound to patient's tissue.

Method

♦ Frozen section of patient's tissue is placed over a slide.

♦ Tissue is incubated with fluorescein-conjugated goat antihuman antibodies.

♦ Antibodies bind to the human immunoglobulin site.

♦ Excess of antibodies are washed with buffered normal saline.

♦ Section is viewed under ultraviolet microscope.

Indirect Immunofluorescence

It is the diagnostic method which is used for detection of antibodies which are present in blood.

Method

♦ Frozen section of monkey's esophagus is placed over a slide and is incubated with patient's serum.

♦ Excess serum is washed off.

♦ Apply fluorescent conjugated anti-human Ig antibodies.

♦ Wash off excess antibody.

♦ Section is viewed under ultraviolet microscope.

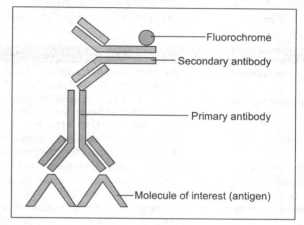

Fig. 111: Indirect immunofluorescence.

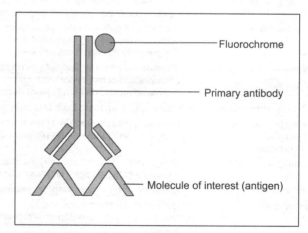

Fig. 112: Direct immunofluorescence.

Q.20. Describe etiopathogenesis of lichen planus. *(Feb 2013, 8 Marks)*

Ans.

Etiopathogenesis of Lichen Planus

♦ Oral lichen planus is a T cell mediated autoimmune disease in which cytotoxic CD8+ T cells trigger the apoptosis of oral epithelial cells. The CD8+ lesional T cells may recognize the antigen associated with major histocompatibility complex

(MHC) class I on keratinocytes. After antigen recognition and activation, CD8+ cytotoxic T cells may trigger keratinocyte apoptosis. Activated CD8+ T Cells may release cytokines that attract additional lymphocytes.

♦ As per the recent studies in psychoneuro-immunology pshycosomatic stress results in the autoimmunity reactions and this leads to lichen planus.

Q.21. What are vesiculobullous lesions. Describe in detail pemphigus. *(Nov 2014, 8 Marks)*

Ans. Vesicles are the superficial blisters which are 5 mm or less in diameter and are usually filled with clear fluid.

Bulla is a large blister which is greater than 5 mm in diameter.

The lesions which consist of vesicles or bullae are known as vesiculobullous lesions.

For classification of vesiculobullous lesions, refer to Ans. 1 of same chapter.

For pemphigus in detail, refer to Ans. 2 and Ans. 9 of same chapter.

Q.22. Enumerate dermal lesions with oral manifestation. Describe systemic lupus erythematosus in detail. *(June 2015, 10 Marks)*

Or

Enumerate the dermal diseases with oral manifestation. Describe the etiology, clinical and histopathological features of systemic lupus erythematosus in detail with diagram. Give its treatment plan. *(Jan 2017, 10 Marks)*

Ans. Enumeration of dermal lesions with oral manifestations

Dermal lesion	Oral manifestation
Ectodermal dysplasia	• Oligodontia or anodontia. • Presence of midfacial hypoplasia.
Oral lichen planus	• Presence of burning sensation in oral mucosa. • Presence of white and gray velvety thread-like papules in linear, angular and retiform arrangement. • Presence of Wickham's striae.
Psoriasis	• Lesions appear as plaques, silvery, scaly lesions with erythematous base. • Multiple popular eruptions are seen which can undergo ulceration.
Pityriasis rosea	• Lesions appear as erythematous macules with/without central area of grayish desquamation.
Erythema multiforme	• Lesions appear as bullae over the erythematous base and break in multiple major ulcers. • Lesions are larger, irregular, deep and bleed freely.
Pachyonychia congenita	• Presence of focal or generalized white opaque thickening of mucosa involving buccal mucosa, tongue and lips. • Angular cheilosis is commonly present. • Natal teeth are also present.
Keratosis follicularis	• Oral lesions appear as minute white papules which are rough on palpation. • Lesions occur commonly on gingiva, tongue, hard palate, soft palate, buccal mucosa and pharynx.
Incontinentia pigmenti	• Presence of delayed eruption of tooth. • Tooth crowns are peg or cone shaped. • Congenitally missing teeth are seen.
Dyskeratosis congenita	• Presence of mucosal leukoplakia on the buccal mucosa, tongue. • Stenosis and constriction occur due to dysphagia, dysuria, phimosis and epiphora. • Increased incidence of malignant neoplasms.
White sponge nevus	• Oral mucosa appears thick and corrugated with soft or spongy texture and a opalescent white hue.
Hereditary benign intraepithelial dyskeratosis	• Lesions are white, spongy and macerated associated with buccal mucosa, with/without folds. Lesions also appear as soft plaques with pin point elevation.
Acanthosis nigricans	• Tongue and lips are frequently involved. • Presence of hypertrophy of filiform papillae which produces a shaggy, papillomatous surface of dorsum of tongue.
Pemphigus	• Presence of ill defined, irregularly-shaped gingival, buccal or palatine erosions which are painful and slow to heal.
Pemphigoid	• Gingiva is commonly involved. • Vesicles or bullae develop on attached gingiva. As the vesicle rupture there is presence of raw bleeding surface. • There may be a formation of ulcer surrounded by zone of erythema.
Epidermolysis bullosa	• Bullae are present which are painful and when they rupture there is desquamation of epithelium. • Lesion heals with the formation of scar which results in obliteration of sulci and restriction of tongue.
Lupus erythematosus	• Intraoral lesion consists of central depressed red atrophic area which is surrounded by 2 to 3 mm elevated keratotic zone which merge in white lines.
Systemic sclerosis	• Presence of atrophy and induration of mucosal as well as muscular tissues. • Tongue become stiff and board like. • Gingiva become pale and firm. • Lips become thin, rigid and partially fixed. • Reduced opening of mouth. • Fixation of jaw.

Systemic Lupus Erythematosus

It is an autoimmune disease which is characterized by autoantibodies, immune complex formation as well as dysregulation of immune system which causes damage to any organ of body.

Etiology

Genetic predisposition: Higher incidence of auto-antibodies is seen in blood relations of patient.

Viral infection

Hormones, i.e., increase estrogen level in pregnancy.

Autoimmune: Antibodies are develops towards one's own body cells.

Pathogenesis

Antibodies are produced in reaction to exposure of normally unexposed self antigens. Dysregulation of immune system leads to excessive production of antibodies against DNA, ribosomes, other nuclear antigens, platelet, erythrocytes, leukocytes and various tissue specific antigens which causes tissue damage.

Clinical Features

♦ It occurs during 30 years of age in females and 40 years of age in males.
♦ Female predilection is seen. Female to male ratio is 2:1
♦ Most common sites affected are face, neck, upper arm, shoulders. Disease is characterized by repeated remission and exacerbations over these sites.
♦ Patient complaints of pain and fever in joints and muscles. Itching or burning sensation is also present along with the areas of hyperpigmentation. Symptoms aggravates under exposure to sunlight.
♦ The characteristic sign of the disease is presence of erythematous patches over the face which coalesce to form roughly symmetrical pattern over the cheeks and across the bridge of nose, this is known as butterfly distribution. In the kidney fibrinoid thickening of glomerular capillaries produces characteristic wire loops, this leads to renal insufficiency.
♦ In the heart, there is presence of typical endocarditis involving valves along with fibrinoid degeneration of epicardium and myocardium.

Oral Manifestations

♦ Buccal mucosa, lip and palate are most commonly affected.
♦ Patient complaints of presence of burning sensation in the mouth. Xerostomia is also seen.
♦ Lesions have very much similarity to lesions of discoid lupus except that they are hyperemic, edematous and extension of lesion is pronounced. Tendency for bleeding and petechiae is more as well as superficial ulcerations surrounded by red halo are also present.
♦ Intraoral lesion consists of central depressed red atrophic area which is surrounded by 2 to 3 mm elevated keratotic zone which merge in white lines.

Histopathology

♦ In systemic lupus erythematosus, areas of epithelial atrophy are present with absence of keratinization.
♦ There is presence of liquefactive degeneration of basal cell layer.
♦ There is presence of edema of subepithelial connective tissue with dilatation of vessels.
♦ In systemic lupus erythematosus degenerative areas and collagen disturbances are more prominent.
♦ Inflammatory features are less common.

For diagram, refer to Ans. 13 of same chapter.

Laboratory Findings

♦ LE cell inclusion phenomenon is used in which there is addition of blood serum from a person who is suspected to the buffy coat of normal blood. If patient is suffering from systemic lupus erythematosus, typical LE cells will appear. The test consists of rosette of neutrophils surrounding pale nuclear mass.
♦ There is also presence of anemia, leukopenia, thrombocytopenia and elevated ESR and serum gamma globulin level with positive Coombs test.
♦ Lupus band test is positive, i.e., there is deposition of IgG, IgM or complement component at epidermal-dermal junction or basement membrane zone of skin.

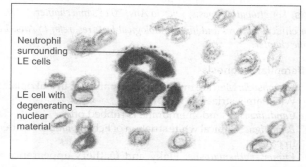

Neutrophil surrounding LE cells

LE cell with degenerating nuclear material

Fig. 113: LE cell inclusion phenomenon
(For color version, see Plate 19).

Treatment

♦ Exposure to sunlight should be avoided.
♦ Patient should be kept on systemic corticosteroid therapy.
♦ NSAIDs should also be given to combat the symptoms.

Q.23. Define genodermatosis and genokeratosis. Classify vesiculobullous lesions and describe in detail etiopathogenesis, clinical features and histopathology of pemphigus. *(Dec 2015, 8 Marks)*

Ans. Genodermatosis: Genodermatoses are genetically determined skin conditions.

Genokeratosis: Some of the genodermatoses are characterized particularly by alteration in normal keratinization process and they are referred to as genokeratosis.

For classification vesiculobullous lesions, refer to Ans. 1 of same chapter.

For etiopathogenesis of pemphigus, refer to Ans. 9 of same chapter.

For clinical features and histopathology of pemphigus, refer to Ans. 3 of same chapter.

Q.24. Describe pathogenesis, clinical manifestations and histopathological features of oral lichen planus.

(Jan 2016, 10 Marks)

Ans.

Pathogenesis

- Oral lichen planus is a T cell mediated autoimmune disease in which cytotoxic CD8+ T cells trigger the apoptosis of oral epithelial cells. The CD8+ lesional T cells may recognize the antigen associated with major histocompatibility complex (MHC) class I on keratinocytes. After antigen recognition and activation, CD8+ cytotoxic T cells may trigger keratinocyte apoptosis. Activated CD8+ T Cells may release cytokines that attract additional lymphocytes.
- As per the recent studies in pschyoneuro-immunology, pshycosomatic stress results in the autoimmunity reactions and this leads to lichen planus.

  For clinical manifestations and histopathological features of oral lichen planus, refer to Ans. 1 of same chapter.

Q.25. Write in detail etiopathogenesis, clinical features, histopathological features and differential diagnosis for oral lichen planus.   *(Feb 2019, 10 Marks)*

Ans. *For etiopathogenesis, refer to Ans. 20 of same chapter.*

For clinical features and histopathological features, refer to Ans. 1 of same chapter.

Differential Diagnosis

- *Leukoplakia:* Men are more commonly affected in leukoplakia. Wickham's striae are not present.
- *Candidiasis:* Pseudomembrane is rubbed off.
- *Pemphigus:* Clinical white striation of lichen planus is evident in cases.
- *Lupus erythematosus:* Flaky and feathery appearance of lupus lesion.
- *White sponge nevus:* It is seen at birth and puberty. Lichen planus is seen over age of 30 years.
- *Geographic tongue:* Presence of redness in the center with slightly raised margins which can change their shape.
- *Lichenoid drug reaction:* Systemic corticosteroids should be given for 2 weeks, if there is no improvement lichenoid reaction is the diagnosis.

Q.26. Write clinical, histological features and diagnosis of pemphigus vulgaris.   *(Feb 2019, 5 Marks)*

Ans. *For clinical features and histological features, refer to Ans. 3 of same chapter.*

Diagnosis

- *Clinical examination:* Patients having pemphigus vulgaris and active blistering, firm sliding pressure by the finger separates normal looking epithelium, this is Nikolsky's sign. Nikolsky's sign is positive in pemphigus vulgaris.
- *Biopsy:* On histopathological examination, there is presence of vesicle or bulla intraepithelially above the basal cell layer producing suprabasilar split. Disappearance of intercellular bridges leads to acantholysis due to which clump of epithelial cells are found lying free in vesicular space. These are known as Tzanck cells which are the diagnostic feature for the condition.
- *Tzanck smear:* In this, base of the blister is scrapped and is examined for the acantholytic cells. These acantholytic cells or Tzanck cells are free floating, round or ovoid in shape and their nucleus is enlarged, hyperchromatic and is centrally or eccentrically situated.
- *Compressed air test:* Compressed air stream is applied to oral mucous membrane of gingival tissues which can lead to shimmering of outer tissues followed by formation of bleb or blister.
- *Immunofluorescent testing:* Direct immunofluorescence testing is done to demonstrate the presence of immunoglobulins, predominantly IgG but sometimes in combination with C3, IgA and IgM, in the intercellular spaces or intercellular substance in either oral epithelium or clinically normal epithelium adjacent to lesion.
- *Indirect immunofluorescence:* This is accomplished basically by incubating normal animal or human mucosa with serum from the patient suspected of having the disease and adding the fluorescein-conjugated human antiglobulin. A positive reaction in the tissue indicates presence of circulating immunoglobulin antibodies.

20. DISEASES OF NERVES AND MUSCLES

Q.1. Write notes on Bell's palsy.   *(Sep 2008, 3 Marks)*
(Aug 2011, 5 Marks) (Dec 2010, 3 Marks)

Or

Write short note on Bell's Palsy.   *(Mar 2006, 5 Marks)*
(Nov 2014, 3 Marks)

Or

Write in brief on Bell's palsy.   *(June 2010, 5 Marks)*

Or

Write short essay on Bell's palsy.

(Jan 2012, 5 Marks)

Ans. Bell's palsy is an acute apparently isolated, lower motor neuron facial palsy.

Etiology

- Cold—It usually occurs after exposure to cold.
- Trauma—Extraction of teeth or injection of local anesthetic may damage to the nerve and subsequent paralysis.

♦ Surgical procedure—Such as removal of parotid gland tumor in which the facial nerve is sectioned can also cause facial paralysis.

♦ Tumors—Tumors of the cranial base, parapharyngeal space and infratemporal fossa cause 7th nerve palsy.

♦ Familial—Familial and hereditary occurrence is also reported in case of Bell's palsy.

♦ Facial canal and middle ear neoplasm.

♦ Herpes simplex—viral infection.

Clinical Features

♦ **Symptoms**
  - Sudden following exposure to chill or without any apparent precipitating causing maximum paralysis in 24 hours.
  - Post-auricular pain is common.
  - Spontaneous complaints of loss of sense of taste, hyperacusis (progressive loss of hearing and watering of the eye).
  - Sweating is less on the affected side.

♦ **Signs**
  - Forehead is not wrinkled and frowning is lost.
  - Eye of the affected side is not closed and on attempting closure eyeball turns upwards and outwards.
  - On showing teeth the lips do not separate on the affected side.
  - Cheeks puff out with the expiration because of buccinator paralysis and food collects between the teeth and paralyzed cheek.
  - Base of tongue is lowered.
  - Deafness may result.

Management

♦ *Local heat:* Infrared or moist heat over the face or parotid region or both if there is tenderness of nerve trunk.

♦ *Local treatment of muscles:* Patient should massage the facial muscles with bland oil for twice a day for 5 min.

♦ *Protection of eye:* It is done with dark glass or eye patch. Mild zinc boric solution is used to wash the eye to prevent conjunctivitis.

♦ *Corticosteroids:* Prednisolone 60 mg/day along with amoxicillin 250 mg 8 hourly help in reducing edema round about the nerve.

♦ Heavy doses of vitamin B12 1000 µg per day IM is given.

♦ *Galvanism:* It is given two weeks after the onset of paralysis three times in a week.

♦ *Surgery:* Plastic surgery is preferred.

Q.2. Write note on trigeminal neuralgia.

(Sep 2007, 2.5 Marks) (Jan 2012, 5 Marks)
(Feb 2013, 8 Marks)

Or

Write short note on trigeminal neuralgia.

(Dec 2009, 5 Marks) (Apr 2017, 5 Marks)

Ans. Trigeminal neuralgia is also called as Tic Douloureux.

A disorder characterized by the paroxysmal (occurring repeatedly without warning) attacks of neuralgic pain with affection of one or more division of trigeminal nerve. The pain involves the first and second divisions equally and rarely the first.

Clinical Features

♦ Pain is unilateral and is confined to one of the three divisions of nerve. Pain is sharp and onset is sudden. The pain is only of a few seconds.

♦ During attacks there is flushing of face, i.e., redness of the face.

♦ Dilatation of pupil is present.

♦ There is excessive lacrimation.

♦ After repeated attacks skin becomes shiny and hair in the area become gray.

♦ Sometimes secretion of nasal mucus and saliva may occur in the side of pain.

Etiology

Trigeminal neuralgia is spontaneous and following exposure to cold wind, blow on face, or chewing or eating, drinking hot or cold fluid and washing the face.

Management

♦ Elimination of all possible sources of infection.

♦ Drugs.
  - *Analgesics:* Potent analgesics must be used with caution because of danger of habituation.
  - *Carbamazepine:* 100–200 mg BD a day and increasing the dose to 600–800 mg per day.
  - *Phenytoin sodium:* 0.1 g TDS when carbamazepine is not tolerated.
  - *Vitamin B12:* 1000 µg IM daily for two weeks.

♦ Injection of alcohol: It is given in affected nerve, or gasserian ganglion. If more than one division is affected inject 10 minims of 90% alcohol after local anesthesia with 2 to 3 drops of procaine.

♦ Surgery: Selective or complete preganglionic selection of trigeminal root.

21. FORENSIC ODONTOLOGY

Q.1. Write short note on sex differences in tooth morphology and jaw anatomy. *(Sep 2011, 3 Marks)*

Ans.

Sex Differences in Tooth Morphology

♦ Amongst teeth, mandibular canines show greatest dimensional difference with larger teeth in males than in females.

♦ Mesiodistal width of mandibular canines was significantly greater in males than in females.

♦ Girls are more prone to caries as compared to boys because tooth erupt at an early age.

Sex Differences in Jaw Anatomy

♦ In males jaw bone is large, having broad ascending ramus while in females it is small, narrow ascending ramus.

♦ In males condyles of jaw bone are large while in females they are small.

♦ In males shape of chin is square while in females it is rounded/pointed.

♦ Gonial angle is less obtuse and flares in males while it is more obtuse and does not flare in females.

♦ Body height of jaw bone in males is high while it is low in females.

Q.2. Write short note on cheiloscopy. *(Feb 2013, 5 Marks)*

Or

Write short note on lip prints. *(Apr 2017, 4 Marks)*

Ans. External surface of the lip has many elevations and depressions forming a characteristic pattern called lip prints, examination of which is referred to as cheiloscopy.

♦ This is unique for individuals like the fingerprints.

♦ Lip prints can constitute material evidence left at a crime scene much like fingerprints.

♦ Lip prints provide direct link to the suspect.

♦ Use of lipstick was essential to leave behind color traces of lip prints.

Classification of Lip Prints

By Tsuchihashi

♦ Type I- Clear cut vertical grooves that run across entire lip

♦ Type I'- Similar to Type I but do not cover entire lip

♦ Type II- Branched grooves

♦ Type III- Intersected grooves

♦ Type IV- Reticular grooves

♦ Type V- Grooves that cannot be morphologically differentiated

♦ A combination of these grooves may be found on any given set of lips.

♦ To simplify recording lips are divided into quadrants similar to dentition, i.e., a horizontal line dividing the upper and lower lip and a vertical line dividing right and left sides. By noting the type of groove in each quadrant the individual's lip print pattern may be recorded.

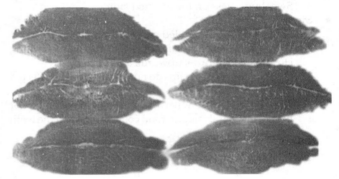

Type I: Complete straight grooves   Type I: Partial straight grooves

Type II: Branched grooves   Type II: Intersected grooves

Type III: Reticular grooves   Type III: Undifferentiated grooves

Fig. 114: Lip patterns *(For color version, see Plate 20).*

Q.3. Write short note on bite marks. *(Aug 2012, 5 Marks) (Apr 2015, 3 Marks) (Mar 2013, 3 Marks) (Feb 2015, 5 Marks) (June 2014, 5 Marks)*

Or

Write short answer on bite Marks.

(Sep 2018, 3 Marks)

Ans. Bite marks are defined as "A mark caused by the teeth either alone or in combination with other mouth parts".

—**MacDonald.**

Classification of Bite Marks

MacDonald's Classification

He had given an etiological classification

♦ *Tooth pressure marks:* Marks on tissue due to 'direct application of pressure by teeth'. Incisal and occlusal surfaces produce these marks.

♦ *Tongue pressure marks:* If sufficient amount of tissue is taken in mouth tongue presses the tissue against rigid areas, i.e., lingual surface of teeth as well as palatal rugae. Marks left over skin are called as suckling.

♦ *Tooth scrape marks:* They occur due to scraping of teeth over bitten material. They are caused by anterior teeth

Importance of Bite Marks

♦ They provide accurate identification since alignment of teeth is specific in each individual.
♦ Bite marks are contaminated by saliva and consist of amylin, ptyalin and blood group which help in determination of individual in criminal cases.

Bite Mark Collection

Collection of Bite Mark from Victim

Various methods are:

♦ **Case demographics:** All the information related to case is selected, such as name, age, address, etc.
♦ **Visual examination:** Visually examine the shape, size, color, contour, texture and other features of bite marks and document all of them.
♦ **Photography:** Photographs should be taken as quickly as possible. They provide permanent record of bite marks.
♦ **Impressions:** Impressions of bitten area is made by vinyl polysiloxane.
♦ **Saliva swab:** Saliva act as a source of DNA. It should be collected carefully and is preserved to match the DNA with suspect.

Collection of Bite Mark from Suspect

♦ Photographs of suspect's teeth should be taken.
♦ Impressions of maxillary and mandibular arch should be taken.
♦ Saliva swabs from buccal vestibule should be taken.

Bite Marks Analysis

It is done by:

♦ Metric analysis in conjunction with pattern association.
♦ *Direct method:* In which suspect's models are directly placed over bite mark.
♦ *Indirect method:* Incisal and occlusal edges of suspect's teeth are traced on clear acetate and superimposed on bite mark photographs.
♦ Adobe photoshop software.
♦ 3D/CAD supported photogrammetry.

Conclusion of Bite Marks Analysis

♦ *Definite biter:* Presence of reasonable medical certainty which indicate that bite mark is produced by suspect's dentition.
♦ *Probable biter:* There is some degree of specificity to suspect's teeth by sufficient number of matching points.
♦ *Possible biter:* Suspect's teeth could make the bite mark and there are no characteristic matches for certainty. Similarity of class characteristics is seen.
♦ *Not the biter:* Bite marks and suspect's dentition is not consistent.

Q.4. Write short note on dental DNA methods.

(Feb 2014, 3 Marks)

Ans. Following are the dental DNA methods:

♦ **Restriction fragment length polymorphism (RFLP) Typing:** It is used for analyzing the variable lengths of DNA fragments that result from digesting a DNA sample with a special kind of restriction enzyme called "restriction endonuclease" which sections DNA at a specific sequence pattern known as a restriction endonuclease recognition site. RFLP requires relatively large amounts of DNA. Hence, cannot be performed with the samples degraded by environmental factors and also takes longer time to get the results.

♦ **STRs typing:** These are described as short stretches of DNA that are repeated at various locations throughout the human genome and this technology is used to evaluate specific regions (loci) within nuclear DNA. Each person has some STRs that were inherited from father and some from mother, but however no person has STRs that are identical to those of either parent. The uniqueness of an individual's STRs provides the scientific marker of identity and hence is helpful in forensic identification and paternity testing. STR can be used for identification of bodies in the mass disasters and old skeletal remains.

♦ **Mitochondrial DNA (mtDNA) analysis:** Long intervals between the time of death and examination of tissues complicate the genetic identification with nuclear DNA and sometimes only bone and teeth may be available for analysis. Teeth provide an excellent source for high molecular weight mtDNA that offer several unique advantages for the identification of human remains. mtDNA is a powerful tool for forensic identification as it possesses high copy number, maternal inheritance, and high degree of sequence variability.

♦ **Y-chromosome analysis:** DNA-polymorphisms on the human Y chromosome are valuable tools for understanding human evolution, migration and for tracing relationships among males. Majority of the length of the human Y chromosome is inherited as a single block in linkage from father to male offspring as a haploid entity. Hence, Y chromosomal DNA variation has been mainly used for investigations on human evolution and for forensic purposes or paternity analysis.

♦ **X-chromosome STR:** Chromosome X specific STR is used in the identification and the genomic studies of various ethnic groups in the world. Since the size of X-chromosome STR alleles is small, generally including 100–350 nucleotides, it is relatively easy to be amplified and detected with high sensitivity. X-chromosome STR (X-STR) markers are a powerful complimentary system especially in deficiency paternity testing. Tooth-related jaw bone diseases can be divided in cysts and odontogenic tumors. Reactive bone diseases, fibro-osseous lesions, giant cell lesions, and bone tumors are taken together as the main second group.

Q.5. Write short note on forensic odontology.

(June 2015, 5 Marks) (Jan 2018, 5 Marks)

Ans. Forensic odontology is that branch of dentistry which in the interest of justice deals with the proper handling and examination of dental evidence and with the proper evaluation and presentation of dental findings. **Federation Dentaire Internationale (FDI)**

Scope of Forensic Odontology

♦ *Identification:* It helps in personal identification, i.e., individually or in mass disasters. This is done also through comparison of antemortem and postmortem dental information.

♦ *Age assessment:* This is done for assessing the age of person.

♦ *Record preparation:* Correct handling as well as examination of presentation of dental evidence in civil and criminal legal cases. These records make the foundation on which]

♦ *Identification of bite marks:* It is involved in identification of bite marks in criminal cases.

♦ *Child abuse:* For detection of child abuse or human abuse too.

♦ *Lip print:* For comparison and identification of suspect, lip prints are examined.

♦ *Legal aspect:* In cases with dental traumatology.

Parameters to be Compared in Forensic Dentistry

♦ Teeth

♦ Prosthetic appliances, i.e., bridges, partials, crowns, false teeth

♦ Shape, form (morphological) peculiarities

♦ Genetic anomalies

Q.6. Write short note on age estimation from radiographs.
(Feb 2019, 5 Marks)

Ans. Age estimation from radiographs is done by following methods:

1. Demirjian's method
2. Schour and Massler's method

Demirjian's method

♦ It is the method which assess the mandibular left side teeth.

♦ Development of the mandibular teeth as appeared on the radiographs was divided in 10 stages numbered from 0 to 9.

♦ Demirjian's and his colleagues provided different maturity scores for each tooth for each developmental stage.

♦ Considering the differences in dental development between girls and boys, authors provide separate maturity scores for both the sexes.

♦ Based on the developmental stage, each tooth is given an appropriate score.

♦ This method is most widely used technique for assessing age in children and adolescence probably due to detailed description and radiographic illustration of tooth developmental stages.

♦ The score assigned for each 8th teeth is added and total maturity score (S) is obtained.

Formula in Females:

$$Age = (0.0000615 \times S^3) - (0.0106 \times S^2) + (0.6997 \times S) - 9.3178$$

Formula in males:

$$Age = (0.000055 \times S^3) - (0.0095 \times S^2) + (0.6479 \times S) - 8.4583$$

Schour and Massler's Method

♦ They describe 20 chronological stages of tooth development starting from 5 months IU until 21 years of age.

♦ The chart is based on histological sections and permit direct comparison with radiographs.

♦ Dental development of males and females were combined and each stage include amount of age variation.

MULTIPLE CHOICE QUESTIONS

As per DCI and Examination Papers of Various Universities

1 Mark Each

1. Fordyce's granules actually are collection of:
   a. Salivary gland tissue
   b. Sweat gland
   c. Sebaceous gland
   d. Fatty tissue

2. In the lesion of median rhomboid glossitis, there is absence of:
   a. Filiform and foliate papillae
   b. Fungiform and filiform papillae
   c. Circumvallate and fungiform papillae
   d. Circumvallate papillae

3. Enzyme considered to be of special importance in establishment of *S. mutans* in dental plaque is:
   a. Glucosyltransferase
   b. Fructosyltransferase
   c. Dextranase
   d. Invertase

4. "Dead tracts" in ground section of teeth, are manifested as:
   a. White zone in transmitted light and black zone in reflected light.
   b. Black zone in transmitted light and white zone in reflected light.
   c. White zone in transmitted light and reflected light
   d. Black zone in transmitted light and reflected light.

5. Which of the following drugs may cause gingival enlargement:
   a. Nifedipine
   b. Cyclosporine
   c. Phenytoin sodium
   d. All of the above

6. Apoptosis of basal cell layer is a feature of:
   a. Psoriasis
   b. Pemphigus
   c. Lichen planus
   d. Erythema multiforme

7. White strawberry tongue is a feature of:
   a. Scarlet fever
   b. Syphilis
   c. Herpetic glossitis
   d. Pemphigus

8. Ramsay Hunt's syndrome is associated with:
   a. Herpes simplex
   b. Herpes zoster
   c. Mumps
   d. Measles

9. Most common cells affected in HIV patients are:
   a. CD 1 and 2
   b. CD 4 and 8
   c. CD 5 and 12
   d. CD 2 and 4

10. Hansen's disease is a:
    a. Syphilis
    b. Candidiasis
    c. Tuberculosis
    d. Leprosy

11. In xerostomia, the salivary pH is:
    a. Unaffected
    b. Low
    c. High
    d. Increased in morning and decreases in day

12. Organisms involved in cellulitis is:
    a. *S. mutants*
    b. *S. pyogenes*
    c. Pneumococci
    d. *Klebsiella*

13. Which is the following are a traid of the sign and symptoms of osteogenesis imperfecta:
    a. Blue sclera, sparse hair, anhydrosis
    b. Enlarged hand, feet, maxilla, mandible
    c. Blue sclera, brittle bones, opalescent dentin
    d. Blue sclera, arachnodactyly, brittle bone.

14. Starry sky appearance is seen in:
    a. Paget's disease
    b. Cherubism
    c. Garry's osteomyelitis
    d. Burkitt's lymphoma

15. Acanthosis is:
    a. Increase in mitotic division
    b. Increase in thickness of superficial layer
    c. Increase in thickness of spinous layer
    d. Disruption of basal lamina

Answers:
1. c. Sebaceous gland	2. b. Fungiform and...	3. c. Dextranase	4. b. Black zone in...
5. d. All of the above	6. c. Lichen planus	7. a. Scarlet fever	8. b. Herpes zoster
9. b. CD 4 and 8	10. d. Leprosy	11. b. Low	12. b. *S. pyogenes*
13. c. Blue sclera, brittle...	14. d. Burkitt's lymphoma	15. c. Increase in thickness...	

16. **Areca nut chewing is etiological factor in:**
    a. Leukoedema
    b. Oral submucous fibrosis
    c. Erythema multiforme
    d. Oral lichen planus

17. **Ameloblastoma most frequently occurs in:**
    a. Mandibular molar region
    b. Maxillary molar region
    c. Mandibular premolar region
    d. Maxillary premolar region

18. **One of them is not a true cyst:**
    a. Hemorrhagic cyst
    b. Median palatine
    c. Globulomaxillary
    d. Nasolabial

19. **Three stages in progression of acute odontogenic infection are:**
    a. Periapical osteitis, cellulitis, abscess
    b. Abscess, cellulitis, periapical osteitis
    c. Cellulitis, abscess, periapical osteitis
    d. Periapical osteitis, abscess, cellulitis

20. **Cyst with high recurrence rate:**
    a. Keratocyst
    b. Primordial
    c. Lateral Periodontal
    d. Radicular cyst

21. **An inability to absorb adequate amount of vitamin B12 from digestive tract may result in:**
    a. Thalassemia
    b. Pernicious anemia
    c. Aplastic anemia
    d. None of these

22. **Howell-Jolly bodies are seen in:**
    a. Malaria
    b. Pernicious anemia
    c. Iron deficiency anemia
    d. Leukemia

23. **On stretching, the cheeks lesion disappears in:**
    a. Leukoplakia
    b. Focal hyperkeratosis
    c. Leukoedema
    d. Typhoid

24. **The microscopic features of leukoedema consists of:**
    a. Increase in thickness of epithelium
    b. Intracellular edema of spinous or malpighian layer
    c. Broad rete ridges
    d. All of the above

25. **Greenspan syndrome is associated with:**
    a. Dyskeratosis congenita
    b. Psoriasis
    c. Leukoplakia
    d. Lichen planus

26. **Carpet track extensions are seen in:**
    a. Sarcoidosis
    b. Systemic sclerosis
    c. Discoid lupus erythematosus
    d. Erythema multiforme

27. **Serum alkaline phosphatase levels are seen in:**
    a. Osteoarthritis
    b. Dentinogenesis imperfecta
    c. Paget's disease
    d. Rheumatoid arthritis

28. **Strawberry tongue is associated with:**
    a. Syphilis
    b. Measles
    c. Scarlet fever
    d. Typhoid

29. **Which of the following cyst develops in place of tooth:**
    a. Primordial cyst
    b. Dentigerous cyst
    c. Keratocyst
    d. Radicular cyst

30. **Cyst having high recurrence rate is:**
    a. Dentigerous cyst
    b. Primordial cyst
    c. Odontogenic keratocyst
    d. Radicular cyst

31. **The most common form of actinomycosis is:**
    a. Cervicofacial
    b. Abdominal
    c. Pulmonary
    d. Any of the above

32. **Virus which may cause Burkitt's lymphoma is:**
    a. HSV Type-II
    b. Cytomegalovirus
    c. Epstein-Barr virus
    d. Varicella-Zoster virus

33. **Radiographic appearance of osteosarcoma is:**
    a. Sunray appearance
    b. Onion-peel appearance
    c. Honey comb appearance
    d. Ground glass appearance

16. b. Oral submucous...	17. a. Mandibular molar...	18. a. Hemorrhagic cyst	19. a. Periapical osteitis,...
20. a. Keratocyst	21. b. Pernicious anemia	22. b. Pernicious anemia	23. a. Leukoplakia
24. b. Intracellular edema...	25. d. Lichen planus	26. c. Discoid lupus...	27. c. Paget's disease
28. c. Scarlet fever	29. a. Primordial cyst	30. c. Odontogenic...	31. a. Cervicofacial
32. c. Epstein-Barr virus	33. a. Sunray appearance		

34. Presence of Bence-Jones protein in urine is characteristic of:
    a. Multiple myeloma
    b. Hodgkin's lymphoma
    c. Burkitt's lymphoma
    d. Hemangioma

35. A union of roots of adjacent teeth through the cementum is referred to as:
    a. Concrescence
    b. Fusion
    c. Gemination
    d. None of the above

36. Teeth that erupt in 30 days of birth are called as:
    a. Natal teeth
    b. Neonatal teeth
    c. Primary teeth
    d. Prenatal teeth

37. Talon's cusp is characteristic of which syndrome:
    a. Edward's syndrome
    b. Klinefelter's syndrome
    c. Rubinstein-Taybi syndrome
    d. Down's syndrome

38. Desquamative gingivitis may be seen in all of the following, *except*:
    a. Pemphigus vulgaris
    b. Recurrent aphthae
    c. Erythema multiforme
    d. Cicatricial pemphigoid

39. Organism in etiology of ANUG:
    a. Cocci and bacilli
    b. Bacilli and bacteriophage
    c. Spirochete and bacilli
    d. Bacteriophage and cocci

40. Areca nut chewing is an etiological factor in:
    a. Leukoedema
    b. Oral submucous fibrosis
    c. Erythema multiforme
    d. Lichen planus

41. Which of the following disease is characterized by fever, headache, sore throat and formation of pseudomembrane in pharynx:
    a. Scarlet fever
    b. Tuberculosis
    c. Cancrum oris
    d. Diphtheria

42. Tuberculosis of lymph nodes is known as:
    a. Lupus vulgaris
    b. Phthisis
    c. Scrofula
    d. Miliary tuberculosis

43. Ghost teeth is seen in which of the following:
    a. Dens in dente
    b. Regional odontodysplasia
    c. Dentin dysplasia
    d. None of the above

44. In Ramsay Hunt syndrome the crania nerve involved is:
    a. Trigeminal
    b. Facial
    c. Glossopharyngeal
    d. Oculomotor

45. Cherubism is associated with:
    a. Down's syndrome
    b. Edward syndrome
    c. Patau syndrome
    d. Noonan's syndrome

46. Which of the following is not a benign tumor of salivary glands:
    a. Pleomorphic adenoma
    b. Myoepithelioma
    c. Sialadenosis
    d. Cystadenoma

47. All of the following are true about pulp polyp, *except*:
    a. Excessive, exuberant proliferation of chronically inflamed dental pulp tissues
    b. Generally occur in children and young adults
    c. Lesion is tender
    d. Teeth most commonly involved are deciduous and permanent first molar

48. Squamous papilloma is associated with:
    a. EBV
    b. HIV
    c. HPV
    d. HSV

49. Basal cell nevus syndrome is associated with:
    a. Odontogenic keratocyst
    b. Dentigerous cyst
    c. Radicular cyst
    d. Nasopalatine cyst

50. Carcinoma usually metastasize by which route:
    a. Hematogenous spread
    b. Local spread
    c. Lymphatic spread
    d. Mechanical spread

34. a. Multiple myeloma   35. a. Concrescence   36. b. Natal teeth   37. c. Rubinstein-Taybi...
38. b. Recurrent aphthae   39. c. Spirochete and bacilli   40. b. Oral submucous...   41. d. Diphtheria
42. c. Scrofula   43. b. Regional...   44. b. Facial   45. d. Noonan's syndrome
46. c. Sialadenosis   47. c. Lesion is tender   48. c. HPV   49. a. Odontogenic keratocyst
50. c. Lymphatic spread

51. Neurofibroma is associated with:
    a. MEN syndrome
    b. Bechet syndrome
    c. Von-Recklinghausen's disease
    d. Cannon's disease

52. Malignant melanoma is a neoplasm of:
    a. Epidermal melanocytes
    b. Spinous cells
    c. Basal cells
    d. Keratin

53. Most common site for compound odontoma is:
    a. Anterior maxilla
    b. Posterior maxilla
    c. Anterior mandible
    d. Posterior mandible

54. Listed below are all methods to represent bite mark, *except*:
    a. Xeroradiography
    b. Transillumination
    c. Swab test
    d. Ultraviolet photography

55. Civatte bodies are also called as:
    a. Colloid bodies
    b. Cytoid bodies
    c. Hyaline bodies
    d. All of above

56. Which of the following is not type of oral lichen planus:
    a. Atrophic
    b. Hypertrophic
    c. Verrucous
    d. Erosion

57. Tzanck cells are characteristic of:
    a. Pemphigus
    b. Pemphigoid
    c. Lichen planus
    d. SLE

58. A fluid-filled elevated lesion of skin in called as:
    a. Papule
    b. Macule
    c. Vesicle
    d. Nodule

59. Gingiva is affected mainly by deficiency of vitamin:
    a. A
    b. B complex
    c. C
    d. D

60. Silver tattoo is deposition of amalgam in:
    a. Bone
    b. Dewtin
    c. Enamel
    d. Mucosa

61. Brown tumor is seen in:
    a. Hyperthyroidism
    b. Hyperparathyroidism
    c. Diabetes mellitus
    d. Acromegaly

62. Rodent ulcers are seen in:
    a. Basal cell carcinoma
    b. Gangrene
    c. Leprosy
    d. Syphilis

63. Most common supernumerary tooth is:
    a. Mesiodens
    b. Paramolar
    c. Peridens
    d. Lateral incisor

64. Most common microbial disease of oral cavity is:
    a. Candidiasis
    b. Dental caries
    c. Carcinoma
    d. Aphthous ulcer

65. Chronic hyperplastic pulpitis is also called as:
    a. Pulp polyp
    b. Acute pulpitis
    c. Chronic pulpitis
    d. Periapical abscess

66. Screening test is done to determine saliva from secretor is done with:
    a. Antigen-A
    b. Antigen-B
    c. Antigen-H
    d. Radioimmunoassay

67. All are types of acquired Nevi, *except*:
    a. Junctional nevi
    b. Compound nevi
    c. Blue nevi
    d. Garment nevi

68. Pregnancy tumor is histologically identical with:
    a. Aphthous ulcer
    b. Pyogenic granuloma
    c. Ameloblastoma
    d. Traumatic ulcer

---

51. c. Von-Reckling...	52. a. Epidermal...	53. a. Anterior maxilla	54. d. Ultraviolet photo...
55. d. All of above	56. c. Verrucous	57. a. Pemphigus	58. c. Vesicle
59. c. C	60. d. Mucosa	61. b. Hyperparathyroidism	62. a. Basal cell carcinoma
63. a. Mesiodens	64. b. Dental caries	65. a. Pulp polyp	66. d. Radioimmunoassay
67. d. Garment nevi	68. b. Pyogenic granuloma		

69. Most common site for compound odontoma is:
    a. Anterior maxilla
    b. Posterior maxilla
    c. Anterior mandible
    d. Posterior mandible

70. Which is not the odontogenic cyst:
    a. Lateral periodontal cyst
    b. Gorlin cyst
    c. Traumatic bone cyst
    d. Dentigerous cyst

71. 'Cafe aulait' spots are present in:
    a. Monostotic fibrous dysplasia
    b. Polyostotic fibrous dysplasia
    c. Paget's disease
    d. Cherubism

72. "Rathke's Pouch tumor" is another name for:
    a. Adamantinoma of lung bone
    b. Pituitary ameloblastoma
    c. Malignant ameloblastoma
    d. Ameloblastic carcinoma

73. Indentation of human premolar bite mark is:
    a. Oval in shape
    b. Spherical in shape
    c. Dual triangular or deep triangular in shape
    d. Square in shape

74. Type of ameloblastoma is most aggressive and high recurrence rate:
    a. Follicular
    b. Plexiform
    c. Granular
    d. Unicystic

75. Most common odontogenic cyst is:
    a. Dentigerous cyst
    b. Radicular cyst
    c. Keratocyst
    d. CEOC

76. Greenspan syndrome includes all, *except*:
    a. Lichen planus
    b. Diabetes mellitus
    c. Hypertension
    d. Pemphigus

77. A flat circumscribed discoloration of skin is called as:
    a. Macule
    b. Ulcer
    c. Papule
    d. Nodule

78. Bull's eye lesion of hand is seen in:
    a. Pemphigus
    b. Erythema multiforme
    c. Pemphigoid
    d. Lichen planus

79. Acanthosis is a feature of:
    a. Pemphigus
    b. Erythroplakia
    c. Leukoplakia
    d. OSMF

80. Blue sclera is seen:
    a. Marfan's syndrome
    b. Cherubism
    c. Osteogenesis imperfecta
    d. Vitamin C deficiency

81. Turner's tooth is associated with:
    a. Enamel hypoplasia
    b. Syphilis
    c. Multiple caries
    d. Cyst

82. Rushton bodies are seen in:
    a. Lichen planus
    b. SLE
    c. Radicular cyst
    d. Dental caries

83. 'Paul-Bunnell' test is positive in:
    a. Infectious mononucleosis
    b. Hodgkin's syndrome
    c. Leukemia
    d. Glandular fever

84. Fixative commonly used in histopathology techniques is:
    a. 10% formalin
    b. Dry heat
    c. 70% alcohol
    d. Saliva

85. Caféau lait spots are found in all, *except*:
    a. Peutz-Jeghers syndrome
    b. Cherubism
    c. Von-Recklinghausen's disease
    d. Fibrous dysplasia

86. Which condition will produce a negative pulp vitality test:
    a. Acute reversible pulpitis
    b. Apical periodontitis
    c. Chronic irreversible pulpitis
    d. Chronic hyperplastic pulpitis

---

69. a. Anterior maxilla   70. c. Traumatic bone cyst   71. b. Polyostotic fibrous...   72. b. Pituitary ameloblastoma

73. c. Dual triangular or...   74. a. Follicular   75. b. Radicular cyst   76. d. Pemphigus

77. a. Macule   78. b. Erythema multiforme   79. a. Pemphigus   80. c. Osteogenesis...

81. a. Enamel hypoplasia   82. c. Radicular cyst   83. a. Infectious...   84. a. 10% formalin

85. d. Fibrous dysplasia   86. b. Apical periodontitis

87. **Which is not a feature of Greenspan's syndrome:**
    a. Oral lichen planus
    b. Diabetes mellitus
    c. Leukoplakia
    d. Hypertension

88. **Which of the following cannot be used to investigate bite marks:**
    a. Photography
    b. Saliva swap
    c. Impression
    d. Bite detector

89. **Congenital absence of salivary gland duct is also known as:**
    a. Aberrancy
    b. Aplasia
    c. Atresia
    d. Xerostomia

90. **.......... is not a feature of Sjogren's syndrome:**
    a. Rheumatic arthritis
    b. Enlargement of salivary gland
    c. Xerostomia
    d. Keratoconjunctivitis

91. **Ghost cells are found in:**
    a. Calcifying epithelial odontogenic cyst
    b. Odontogenic cyst
    c. Residual cyst
    d. Paradental cyst

92. **Codman's triangle is a characteristic feature of:**
    a. Chondrosarcoma
    b. Ameloblastoma
    c. Osteosarcoma
    d. Ewing's sarcoma

93. **Reed-Sternberg cells are characteristic features of:**
    a. Non-Hodgkin's Lymphoma
    b. Burkitt's lymphoma
    c. Hodgkin's lymphoma
    d. Adenolymphoma

94. **Which of the following method is used to extract dental DNA:**
    a. Cryogenic method
    b. PCR
    c. Cheiloscopy
    d. DNA finger printing

95. **Which of the following deficiencies are associated with the disorders of hyperplasia of salivary glands and keratinization of salivary glands:**
    a. Vitamin A
    b. Vitamin B

    c. Vitamin C
    d. Vitamin K

96. **Talon's cusp is characteristics of which syndrome:**
    a. Edward syndrome
    b. Klinefelter syndrome
    c. Rubinstein-Taybi syndrome
    d. Down's syndrome

97. **Koilocytes are:**
    a. Cytomegalovirus altered epithelial cells
    b. Epstein-Barr virus altered cells
    c. Human papilloma virus altered cells
    d. RNA virus altered cells

98. **Denture sore mouth is caused by:**
    a. Actinomycosis
    b. Candida albicans
    c. Blastomycosis
    d. None of the above

99. **Hemophilia B is due to deficiency of:**
    a. Factor VII
    b. Factor IX
    c. Platelet
    d. Vitamin C

100. **Widely accepted theory of dental caries is:**
    a. Proteolytic theory
    b. Proteolytic chelation theory
    c. Acidogenic theory
    d. Autoimmune theory

101. **Number of zones seen in dental caries of dentin are:**
    a. One
    b. Two
    c. Four
    d. Five

102. **Lateral spread of caries is facilitated by:**
    a. Enamel spindles
    b. Dentinoenamel junction
    c. Enamel lamellae
    d. Striae of retzius

103. **All of the following may cause gingival enlargement, *except*:**
    a. Vitamin C deficiency
    b. Fibromatosis gingivae
    c. Monocytic leukemia
    d. Desquamative gingivitis

104. **Odontoma is:**
    a. Hamartoma
    b. Teratoma
    c. Choristoma
    d. None of the above

87. c. Leukoplakia	88. d. Bite detector	89. c. Atresia	90. b. Enlargement of...
91. a. Calcifying epithelial...	92. c. Osteosarcoma	93. c. Hodgkin's lymphoma	94. b. PCR
95. a. Vitamin A	96. c. Rubinstein-Taybi...	97. c. Human papilloma...	98. b. Candida albicans
99. b. Factor IX	100. c. Acidogenic theory	101. d. Five	102. b. Dentinoenamel...
103. d. Desquamative...	104. a. Hamartoma		

105. Self-healing carcinoma refers to:
    a. Verrucous xanthoma
    b. Keratoacanthoma
    c. Nevus
    d. Fibroma

106. A patient has filmy white opalescence bilaterally on buccal mucosa, the lesion fades on stretching. The most likely diagnosis is:
    a. White sponge nevus
    b. Leukoplakia
    c. Lichen planus
    d. Leukoedema

107. "Eye raised to heaven" look is clinical feature of:
    a. Marfan's syndrome
    b. Fibrous syndrome
    c. Albright's syndrome
    d. Cherubism

108. The most common gland involved in sialolithiasis is:
    a. Parotid gland
    b. Submandibular gland
    c. Sublingual gland
    d. Both (a) and (b)

109. Multiple OKC are found in the following syndrome:
    a. Gorlin-Goltz syndrome
    b. Ectodermal dysplasia
    c. Noonan's syndrome
    d. Down's syndrome

110. Radiographic finding in pindborg tumor is:
    a. Sunburst appearance
    b. Onion-Peel appearance
    c. Driven-Snow appearance
    d. Cherry-Blossom appearance

111. Rodent ulcer refers to:
    a. Squamous cell carcinoma
    b. Verrucous carcinoma
    c. Basal cell carcinoma
    d. Both a and b

112. Abtropfung effect is seen in:
    a. Junctional nevus
    b. Aphthous ulcer
    c. Erythema multiforme
    d. Pemphigus

113. Civatte bodies are seen in:
    a. Bowen's disease
    b. Leukoplakia
    c. Lichen planus
    d. OSMF

114. Racquet cell, strap cells and ribbon cells are typically seen in:
    a. Neuroblastoma
    b. Rhabdomyosarcoma
    c. Leiomyosarcoma
    d. Ewing's sarcoma

115. Van der Woude syndrome shows all, *except*:
    a. Bilateral lip pits
    b. Cleft lip
    c. Cleft palate
    d. Microdontia

116. Fordyce's granules are ectopic:
    a. Sebaceous glands
    b. Sweat glands
    c. Lacrimal glands
    d. Salivary glands

117. Hansen's disease is the another name of:
    a. Tuberculosis
    b. Leprosy
    c. Actinomycosis
    d. Diphtheria

118. In primary stage of syphilis the lesion is called as:
    a. Mucocutaneous patch
    b. Gumma
    c. Chancre
    d. Crust

119. Herpes virus infects all tissues, *except*:
    a. Skin
    b. Eyes
    c. CNS
    d. Salivary glands

120. Civatte bodies are seen in:
    a. Radicular cyst
    b. Lichen planus
    c. Pemphigus
    d. Pemphigoid

121. Iris lesions are seen in:
    a. Psoriasis
    b. Erythema multiforme
    c. Pemphigus
    d. Lupus erythematosus

122. Abrasion is wearing away of tooth due to:
    a. Mechanical forces
    b. Chemical
    c. Mastication
    d. None of the above

105. b. Keratoacanthoma	106. d. Leukoedema	107. d. Cherubism	108. b. Submandibular gland
109. a. Gorlin-Goltz...	110. c. Driven-Snow...	111. c. Basal cell carcinoma	112. a. Junctional nevus
113. c. Lichen planus	114. b. Rhabdomyosarcoma	115. d. Microdontia	116. a. Sebaceous glands
117. b. Leprosy	118. c. Chancre	119. d. Salivary glands	120. b. Lichen planus
121. b. Erythema...	122. a. Mechanical forces		

123. **Anitschkow cell is seen in:**
    a. Herpes infection
    b. Recurrent aphthous ulcers
    c. Tuberculosis
    d. None of the above

124. **Costen's syndrome has all, *except*:**
    a. Impairment of hearing
    b. Tinnitus
    c. Otalgia
    d. Blurring of vision

125. **Parakeratin plugging is seen in:**
    a. Verrucous carcinoma
    b. Liposarcoma
    c. Osteosarcoma
    d. Fibrosarcoma

126. **Jig saw puzzle or Mosaic pattern of bone is seen in:**
    a. Cherubism
    b. Paget's disease
    c. Fibrous dysplasia
    d. Achondroplasia

127. **Arcading pattern of rete pegs and Rushton bodies are seen in:**
    a. Radicular cyst
    b. Gorlin's cyst
    c. Paradental cyst
    d. Nasopalatine cyst

128. **Numbness in the palate, or area of looseness in palate are clinical features of:**
    a. Squamous cell carcinoma
    b. Necrotizing sialometaplasia
    c. Salivary duct carcinoma
    d. None of the above

129. **Duct like spaces lined by single cells and rosette pattern seen in:**
    a. AOT
    b. Ameloblastoma
    c. Odontogenic fibroma
    d. Odontogenic myxoma

130. **"Café au lait" spots are seen in:**
    a. Ganglioneuroma
    b. Fibroma
    c. Rhabdomyoma
    d. Neurofibroma

131. **Wickham's striae are seen in:**
    a. Leukoplakia
    b. Erythroplakia
    c. Lichen planus
    d. Both a and b

132. **Most common malignancy in AIDS:**
    a. Osteosarcoma
    b. Fibrosarcoma
    c. Ewing's sarcoma
    d. Kaposi's sarcoma

133. **Which of the following is an example of non-odontogenic cyst:**
    a. Eruption cyst
    b. Nasolabial cyst
    c. Primordial cyst
    d. Glandular odontogenic cyst

134. **Reed-Sternberg cells are characteristically seen in:**
    a. Thalassemia
    b. Glandular fever
    c. Hansen's disease
    d. Hodgkin's disease

135. **Cyst associated with root apex of a nonvital tooth is most likely to be:**
    a. Odontogenic keratocyst
    b. Dentigerous cyst
    c. Radicular cyst
    d. Glandular odontogenic cyst

136. **Microscopic appearance of "swiss cheese" pattern is seen in:**
    a. Pleomorphic adenoma
    b. Adenoid cystic carcinoma
    c. Mucoepidermoid carcinoma
    d. Acinic cell carcinoma

137. **Greatest demineralization is seen in the following zone of enamel caries:**
    a. Translucent zone
    b. Dark zone
    c. Body of the lesion
    d. Surface zone

138. **Mucous extravasation phenomenon most commonly occurs on:**
    a. Upper lip
    b. Lower lip
    c. Tongue
    d. Buccal mucosa

139. **Bleeding gums can be seen in patient with deficiency of:**
    a. Vitamin A
    b. Vitamin E
    c. Vitamin D
    d. Vitamin C

123. b. Recurrent aphthous... 124. b. Tinnitus
125. a. Verrucous carcinoma 126. b. Paget's disease
127. a. Radicular cyst   128. b. Necrotizing...
129. a. AOT   130. d. Neurofibroma
131. c. Lichen planus   132. d. Kaposi's sarcoma
133. b. Nasolabial cyst   134. d. Hodgkin's disease
135. c. Radicular cyst   136. b. Adenoid cystic...
137. c. Body of the lesion 138. b. Lower lip
139. d. Vitamin C

140. **Clinical finding of "pinkish discoloration" of tooth indicates:**
    a. Internal resorption
    b. External resorption
    c. Hypercementosis
    d. Tooth ankylosis

141. **"Parakeratin plugging" is the hallmark feature for:**
    a. Squamous cell carcinoma
    b. Basal cell carcinoma
    c. Malignant melanoma
    d. Verrucous carcinoma

142. **Most common tumor of parotid gland is:**
    a. Pleomorphic adenoma
    b. Adenoid cystic carcinoma
    c. Mucoepidermoid carcinoma
    d. Acinic cell carcinoma

143. **Punched out ulcers on interdental papillae are seen in:**
    a. ANUG
    b. Desquamative gingivitis
    c. Pericoronitis
    d. Crohn's disease

144. **Suprabasilar split in the epithelium is a feature of:**
    a. Lichen planus
    b. Pemphigus
    c. Erythema multiforme
    d. Pemphigoid

145. **Café-au-lait spots can be seen in:**
    a. McCune-Albright syndrome
    b. Neurilemmoma
    c. Neurofibromatosis
    d. Both a and c

146. **Multiple impacted supernumerary teeth are seen in the following:**
    a. Gardner syndrome
    b. Cowden's syndrome
    c. Klinefelter's syndrome
    d. Peutz–Jeghers syndrome

147. **Commonest opportunistic fungal disease of the oral cavity is:**
    a. Histoplasmosis
    b. Mucormycosis
    c. Candidiasis
    d. Blastomycosis

148. **Nikolsky's sign is positive in:**
    a. Lichen planus
    b. Pemphigus vulgaris
    c. Systemic sclerosis
    d. Lupus erythematosus

149. **Which of the following is not the feature of epithelial dysplasia:**
    a. Loss of basal cell polarity
    b. Nuclear and cellular pleomorphism
    c. Individual cell keratinization
    d. Koilocytic change

150. **Self-healing carcinoma is another name for:**
    a. Squamous papilloma
    b. Keratoacanthoma
    c. Verruca vulgaris
    d. Squamous cell carcinoma

151. **"Driven snow" appearance on radiograph is seen in:**
    a. Adenomatoid odontogenic tumor
    b. Ameloblastoma
    c. Calcifying epithelial odontogenic tumor
    d. Squamous odontogenic tumor

152. **Which of the following condition can cause difficulty in tooth extraction:**
    a. Microdontia
    b. Dilaceration
    c. Macrodontia
    d. Anodontia

153. **Malignant tumor of smooth muscle origin is:**
    a. Rhabdomyoma
    b. Rhabdomyosarcoma
    c. Leiomyoma
    d. Leiomyosarcoma

154. **Ghost cells are seen:**
    a. Odontogenic keratocyst
    b. Dentigerous cyst
    c. Radicular cyst
    d. Calcifying odontogenic cyst

155. **Which of the following shows "Driven snow appearance":**
    a. Ameloblastoma
    b. Pindborg tumor
    c. Squamous odontogenic tumor
    d. Fibrous dysplasia

156. **Syndrome associated with hemangioma:**
    a. Rubinstein-Taybi syndrome
    b. Noonan's syndrome
    c. Maffucci syndrome
    d. Grinspan syndrome

157. **Monroe's abscess is seen in:**
    a. White sponge nevus
    b. Acute apical periodontitis
    c. Cellulitis
    d. Psoriasis

.   140. a. Internal resorption   141. d. Verrucous carcinoma   142. a. Pleomorphic...   143. a. ANUG
    144. b. Pemphigus   145. d. Both a and c   146. a. Gardner syndrome   147. c. Candidiasis
    148. b. Pemphigus vulgaris   149. d. Koilocytic change   150. b. Keratoacanthoma   151. c. Calcifying epithelial...
    152. b. Dilaceration   153. d. Leiomyosarcoma   154. d. Calcifying...   155. b. Pindborg's tumor
    156. c. Maffucci syndrome   157. d. Psoriasis

158. Safety pin cells are present in:
    a. Thalassemia
    b. Pernicious anemia
    c. Aplastic anemia
    d. Polycythemia

159. Most common malignancy involving oral cavity:
    a. Carcinoma of tongue
    b. Squamous cell carcinoma
    c. Adenoid cystic carcinoma
    d. Ameloblastoma

160. Onion skin appearance radiography is seen in:
    a. Ewing's sarcoma
    b. Paget's disease
    c. Osteosarcoma
    d. Osteogenesis imperfecta

161. Which of these does not show presence of ghost cells:
    a. Odontoma
    b. Adenomatoid odontogenic tumor
    c. Ameloblastoma
    d. Calcifying odontogenic cyst

162. Monospot test is associated with:
    a. EBV
    b. HIV
    c. Hepatitis B
    d. Malaria

163. Lava flowing around boulders is the radiographic feature of:
    a. Dentin dysplasia
    b. Regional odontodysplasia
    c. Dentinogenesis imperfecta I
    d. Dentinogenesis imperfecta II

164. Etiological agent of Pink's disease is:
    a. Lead
    b. Bismuth
    c. Arsenic
    d. Mercury

165. Root surface caries is caused by:
    a. Streptococci
    b. Lactobacilli
    c. Actinomycetes
    d. *Prevotella*

166. Synonym of Warthin's tumor is:
    a. Cystadenoma papillary lymphomatosum
    b. Lymphoid papillary cystadenoma
    c. Papillary cystadenoma lymphomatosum
    d. Cyst papillary lymphomatosum

167. Most aggressive variant of adenoid cystic carcinoma:
    a. Cribriform type
    b. Solid type
    c. Tubular type
    d. Cystic type

168. Other name of Tic douloureux:
    a. Herpetic neuralgia
    b. Facial neuralgia
    c. Atypical facial neuralgia
    d. Trigeminal neuralgia

169. Which among this is a pseudocyst:
    a. Mucocele
    b. Dentigerous cyst
    c. OKC
    d. Globulomaxillary cyst

170. Which type of candidiasis is commonly associated with antibiotic usage:
    a. Atrophic
    b. Pseudomembranous
    c. Hyperplastic
    d. Erythematous

171. Causative organism of Kaposi sarcoma is:
    a. HPV
    b. HHV
    c. HSV
    d. EBV

172. Developmental anomaly associated with tongue are all, *except*:
    a. Macroglossia
    b. Ankyloglossia
    c. Microglossia
    d. Geographic tongue

173. Brown tumor is:
    a. Hypothyroidism
    b. Hyperthyroidism
    c. Hypoparathyroidism
    d. Hyperparathyroidism

174. Clark's and Breslow index is associated with:
    a. Basal cell carcinoma
    b. Squamous cell carcinoma
    c. Verrucous carcinoma
    d. Melanoma

175. Most common malignant salivary gland tumor in children is:
    a. Pleomorphic adenoma
    b. Mucoepidermoid carcinoma
    c. Adenoid cystic carcinoma
    d. All of the above

---

158. a. Thalassemia | 159. b. Squamous cell | 160. c. Osteosarcoma | 161. a. Odontoma
162. a. EBV | 163. a. Dentin dysplasia | 164. d. Mercury | 165. b. Lactobacilli
166. c. Papillary... | 167. b. Solid type | 168. d. Trigeminal neuralgia | 169. a. Mucocele
170. d. Erythematous | 171. b. HHV | 172. d. Geographic tongue | 173. d. Hyperparathyroidism
174. d. Melanoma | 175. b. Mucoepidermoid...

176. **In Down's syndrome cytogenetic investigations reveals chromosomal aberration in:**
    a. Chromosome 23
    b. Chromosome 21
    c. Chromosome 15
    d. Chromosome 27

177. **Herpetic infection of the fingers and hands is known as:**
    a. Koilonychia
    b. Herpetic paronychia
    c. Herpetic whitlow
    d. None of the above

178. **Which of the following is not a form of oral lichen planus:**
    a. Pustular
    b. Atrophic
    c. Erosive
    d. Reticular

179. **"Dry socket" is most frequently associated with:**
    a. Nutritional deficiencies
    b. Blood dyscrasias
    c. Traumatic extraction
    d. Bacteremia

180. **Most common site of occurrence of ameloblastoma is:**
    a. Maxillary anterior region
    b. Mandibular molar region
    c. Mandibular anterior region
    d. Maxillary molar region

181. **Acidogenic theory for dental caries is given by:**
    a. WD Miller
    b. GV Black
    c. Nickerson
    d. Churchill

182. **The odontoma which resembles anatomy of teeth are:**
    a. Composite odontoma
    b. Complex composite odontoma
    c. Compound composite odontoma
    d. Complex compound odontoma

183. **Which syphilitic lesion is most commonly seen by the dentist:**
    a. Chancre
    b. Mucous patches
    c. Gumma
    d. None of the above

184. **Pink tooth of Mummery is:**
    a. Internal resorption
    b. External resorption
    c. Mercury poisoning
    d. None of the above

185. **Bence Jones protein in urine is found in which disease:**
    a. Paget's disease
    b. Multiple myeloma
    c. Malignant melanoma
    d. Fibrous dysplasia

186. **Hunter's glossitis is seen in:**
    a. Aplastic anemia
    b. Iron deficiency anemia
    c. Sickle cell anemia
    d. Pernicious anemia

187. **Fixative/preservative generally used for biopsied specimen is:**
    a. Acetone 5%
    b. 10% Formalin
    c. 10% Alcohol
    d. 10% Normal saline

188. **Hemosiderin pigmentation in tissue is best seen in:**
    a. Masson's Trichrome stain
    b. Perl's Prussian blue stain
    c. Mallory stain
    d. PAS stain

189. **'Ghost teeth' is a characteristic radiographic feature of:**
    a. Bone dysplasia
    b. Regional odontodysplasia
    c. Osteogenesis imperfecta
    d. Dentinogenesis imperfecta

190. **Verocay bodies are histologically seen in:**
    a. Granular cell tumor
    b. Neurofibroma
    c. Schwannoma
    d. Rhabdomyoma

191. **Ludwig's angina involves space infection in:**
    a. Submandibular space
    b. Submental space
    c. Sublingual space
    d. All of the above

192. **Pin point hemorrhages on the skin are called as:**
    a. Petechiae
    b. Ecchymosis
    c. Papule
    d. Hematoma

---

176 b. Chromosome 21   177. c. Herpetic whitlow   178. a. Pustular   179. c. Traumatic extraction
180. b. Mandibular...   181. a. WD Miller   182. c. Compound...   183. b. Mucous patches
184. a. Internal resorption   185. b. Multiple myeloma   186. d. Pernicious anemia   187. b. 10% Formalin
188. b. Perl's Prussian...   189. b. Regional...   190. c. Schwannoma   191. d. All of the above
192. a. Petechiae

193. Which of the following oral cyst would be expected to have the highest rate of recurrence:
    a. Radicular
    b. Nasolabial
    c. Odontogenic keratocyst
    d. Eruption cyst

194. 'Branchless fruit laden tree' or 'Cherry blossom' appearance radiographically seen in:
    a. Adenoid cystic carcinoma
    b. Clear cell carcinoma
    c. Mucoepidermoid carcinoma
    d. Sjogren's syndrome

195. Herpetic whitlow is herpes infection of:
    a. Tongue
    b. Gingiva
    c. Fingers
    d. Eyes

196. Locally destructive inflammatory condition of salivary glands mimicking malignancy is:
    a. Necrotizing sialometaplasia
    b. Sjogren's syndrome
    c. Mikulicz disease
    d. None of the above

197. White lesion of oral cavity which disappears on stretching the mucosa is:
    a. Leukoplakia
    b. White spongy nevus
    c. Candidiasis
    d. Leukoedema

198. Joining of two tooth germs result in:
    a. Dilaceration
    b. Fusion
    c. Gemination
    d. Taurodontism

199. Multiple oral papilloma are the feature of:
    a. Cowden's syndrome
    b. Gorlin
    c. Goltz syndrome
    d. None of the above

200. "Verocay bodies" are seen in:
    a. Neurofibroma
    b. Schwannoma
    c. Traumatic fibroma
    d. PEN

201. Autoantibodies directed to desmoglein 1 and 3 leads to:
    a. Lichen planus
    b. Erythema multiforme
    c. Pemphigus
    d. Pemphigoid

202. Chinese letter pattern of bony trabeculae histologically seen in:
    a. Fibrous dysplasia
    b. Paget's disease
    c. Cherubism
    d. All of the above

203. Which of the following lesion does not show giant cell in histology:
    a. Tuberculosis
    b. Papilloma
    c. Cherubism
    d. Central giant cell granuloma

204. Most common minor salivary gland pathology is:
    a. Pleomorphic adenoma
    b. Sjogren's syndrome
    c. Sialadenosis
    d. Mucocele

205. Greatest degree of epithelial dysplasia is expected in:
    a. Homogeneous leukoplakia
    b. Erythroplakia
    c. OSMF
    d. Lichen planus

206. Which of the following does not have viral etiology:
    a. Herpes simplex
    b. Shingles
    c. Lupus vulgaris
    d. Chickenpox

207. "Target" or "Bull's eye" lesion is characteristic for:
    a. Lichen planus
    b. Erythema multiforme
    c. Pemphigus
    d. Pemphigoid

208. Most common site for leukoplakia is:
    a. Hard palate
    b. Tongue
    c. Lips
    d. Buccal mucosa

209. Histologically "starry sky" appearance is seen in:
    a. Burkitt's lymphoma
    b. Hodgkin's lymphoma
    c. Plasmacytoma
    d. Leukemia

193. c. Odontogenic...	194. d. Sjogren's syndrome	195. c. Fingers	196. a. Necrotizing...
197. d. Leukoedema	198. b. Fusion	199. d. None of the above	200. b. Schwannoma
201 c. Pemphigus	202. a. Fibrous dysplasia	203. c. Papilloma	204. a. Pleomorphic adenoma
205. b. Erythroplakia	206. c. Lupus vulgaris	207. b. Erythema...	208. d. Buccal mucosa
209. a. Burkitt's lymphoma			

210. **Lesion which shows spontaneous healing is:**
    a. Papilloma
    b. Leukoplakia
    c. Erythroplakia
    d. Keratoacanthoma

211. **Odontogenic cyst with highest rate of recurrence is:**
    a. Dentigerous cyst
    b. Odontogenic keratocyst
    c. Radicular cyst
    d. Eruption cyst

212. **Duct like pattern are seen in which of the following tumors:**
    a. Ameloblastoma
    b. Odontoma
    c. Adenomatoid odontogenic tumor
    d. Pindborg tumor

213. **Mandibular anterior teeth are spared in which caries:**
    a. Rampant caries
    b. Radiation caries
    c. Nursing bottle caries
    d. All of the above

214. **Zone of fatty degeneration is seen in:**
    a. Enamel caries
    b. Dentinal caries
    c. Cemental caries
    d. None of the above

215. **Tongue tie refers to:**
    a. Cleft tongue
    b. Fissured tongue
    c. Ankyloglossia
    d. Geographic tongue

216. **Loss of tooth structure due to non-bacterial chemical cause is:**
    a. Attrition
    b. Abrasion
    c. Erosion
    d. None of the above

217. **Reed–Sternberg cells are characteristic feature of:**
    a. Hodgkin's lymphoma
    b. Non-Hodgkin's lymphoma
    c. Plasmacytoma
    d. Burkitt's lymphoma

218. **Sulfur granules in the pus are seen in:**
    a. Actinomycosis
    b. Tuberculosis
    c. Leprosy
    d. ANUG

219. **Bell's palsy is paralysis of one of the following cranial nerves:**
    a. IX
    b. VII
    c. X
    d. IV

220. **Study of lip prints is known as:**
    a. Palatoscopy
    b. Rugoscopy
    c. Microscopy
    d. Cheiloscopy

221. **Following of ramus can be seen in:**
    a. Dentigerous cyst
    b. Odontogenic keratocyst
    c. Odontoma
    d. AOT

222. **Most common cause of oral candidiasis is:**
    a. *Candida albicans*
    b. *Candida glabrata*
    c. *Candida tropicalis*
    d. None of the above

223. **Loss of cohesion seen in epithelial dysplasia is a result of:**
    a. Acanthosis
    b. Acantholysis
    c. Atrophy
    d. Hypertrophy

224. **Prognosis is worst for which of the following histological type of adenoid cystic carcinoma:**
    a. Solid
    b. Cribriform
    c. Tubular
    d. All of the above

225. **Trauma can be the etiological factor in all of the following,** *except*:
    a. Oral mucocele
    b. Dilaceration
    c. Turner's hypoplasia
    d. Mulberry molar

226. **"Saw tooth rete ridges" can be seen in histopathology of:**
    a. Pemphigus
    b. Lichen planus
    c. Erythema multiforme
    d. SLE

210. d. Keratoacanthoma	211. b. Odontogenic...	212. c. Adenomatoid...	213. c. Nursing bottle caries
214. b. Dentinal caries	215. c. Ankyloglossia	216. c. Erosion	217. a. Hodgkin's lymphoma
218. a. Actinomycosis	219. b. VII	220. d. Cheiloscopy	221. a. Dentigerous cyst
222. a. *Candidia albicans*	223. b. Acantholysis	224. a. Solid	225. d. Mulberry molar
226. b. Lichen planus			

227. **Satellite cyst can be seen in:**
   a. Dentigerous cyst
   b. Radicular cyst
   c. Odontogenic keratocyst
   d. Eruption cyst

228. **Odontogenic tumor with predilection for anterior maxilla is:**
   a. Ameloblastoma
   b. Adenomatoid odontogenic tumor
   c. Pindborg's tumor
   d. Cementoblastoma

229. **Bilateral swelling of salivary gland can be seen in all, except:**
   a. Mumps
   b. Mickulicz's disease
   c. Sialosis
   d. Necrotizing sialometaplasia

230. **Tooth most frequently associated with microdontia is:**
   a. Mandibular central incisor
   b. Maxillary central incisor
   c. Maxillary lateral incisor
   d. Mandibular lateral incisor

231. **'Chinese letter pattern' is seen in histology of:**
   a. Fibrous dysplasia
   b. Cleidocranial dysplasia
   c. Achondroplasia
   d. Osteogenesis imperfecta

232. **Non-inflammatory, non-neoplastic swelling of salivary gland is:**
   a. Sialosis
   b. Sialolithiasis
   c. Sialorrhea
   d. Sialadenitis

233. **Lesion associated with HPV is:**
   a. Nevi
   b. Squamous papilloma
   c. Keratoacanthoma
   d. Mumps

227. c. Odontogenic...   228. b. Adenomatoid...   229. d. Necrotizing...   230. c. Maxillary lateral incisor
231. a. Fibrous dysplasia   232. a. Sialosis   233. b. Squamous...

FILL IN THE BLANKS

1 Mark Each

1. Complication of healing of extraction socket is called as ....
Ans. Dry socket

2. ANUG is caused by .... microorganism.
Ans. *P. intermedia, Borrelia* and *Treponema*

3. The other name of pindborg tumor is ....
Ans. Calcifying epithelial odontogenic tumor

4. Papilloma is caused by .... Virus.
Ans. HPV

5. "Pink tooth" is caused due to ....
Ans. Internal resorption

6. Dens in dente is called ....
Ans. Dens invaginatus

7. Syphilis is caused by ....
Ans. *Treponema pallidum*

8. Pseudocyst of jaws are ....
Ans. Solitary bone cyst and aneurysmal bone cyst

9. Kaposi's sarcoma is tumor of ....
Ans. Human herpes virus-8

10. Warthin's tumor is also called as ....
Ans. Papillary cystadenoma lymphomatosum

11. Bence-Jones protein is seen in ....
Ans. Plasmacytoma

12. Café au lait spots are seen in ....
Ans. Neurofibroma

13. "Liesgang's rings" are characteristic are features of ....
Ans. Calcifying epithelial odontogenic tumor

14. Phlegmon is also known as ....
Ans. Cellulitis

15. Hyaline or rushton bodies is seen in ....
Ans. Radicular cyst

16. Mulberry molars are seen in ....
Ans. Syphilis

17. Shell teeth is associated with ....
Ans. Dentinogenesis imperfecta- Type III

18. Virus implicated in squamous cell papilloma is ....
Ans. Human papilloma virus (HPV) 6 and 11

19. Self healing carcinoma is also known as ....
Ans. Keratoacanthoma

20. Abtropfung or dropping off effect is seen in ....
Ans. Junctional nevus and compound nevus

21. The chemical disintegration of enamel is referred to as ....
Ans. Erosion

22. Koplik's spots are an early intraoral manifestation of ....
Ans. Measles

23. Tumors of minor salivary glands are more frequently seen in ....
Ans. Palate

24. A fluid filled elevated lesion of skin is called as ....
Ans. Bulla

25. The most common sequel of pulpitis is ....
Ans. Periapical granuloma

26. Anitschkow cells are found in ....
Ans. Aphthous ulcers

27. Verocay bodies are the histologic feature of ....
Ans. Neurilemmoma

28. The term submerged tooth is used for ....
Ans. Deciduous molar

29. Reed-Sternberg cells are seen in ....
Ans. Hodgkin's lymphoma

30. Examination of lip prints is known as ....
Ans. Cheiloscopy

31. Cotton wool appearance radiographically is seen in ....
Ans. Paget's disease

32. Sunray appearance radiographically is seen in ....
Ans. Osteosarcoma

33. Wickham striae are characteristic features of ....
Ans. Lichen planus

34. Reed-Sternberg cells are seen in ....
Ans. Hodgkin's lymphoma

35. Codman's triangle is seen in ....
Ans. Osteosarcoma

36. Chicken wire pattern is seen in ....
Ans. Pemphigus vulgaris

37. Nikolsky's sign is a characteristic feature of ....
Ans. Pemphigus vulgaris

38. Hutchinson's triad is seen in ....
Ans. Syphilis

39. Ghost teeth appearance radiographically is seen in ....
Ans. Regional odontodysplasia

40. Parakeratin plugging is seen in ....
Ans. Verrucous carcinoma

41. **Swiss cheese pattern is seen in** ....
Ans. Cylindroma

42. **Screw driven-shaped incisors are seen in** ....
Ans. Syphilis

43. **Reed-Sternberg cells are feature of** ....
Ans. Hodgkin's lymphoma

44. **Grinspan syndrome is associated with** .... **mucocutaneous lesion**
Ans. Lichen planus

45. **Soap bubble appearance in X-ray is seen in** ....
Ans. Ameloblastoma, aneurysmal bone cyst, central hemangioma

46. **Ghost's teeth are seen in** ....
Ans. Regional odontodysplasia

47. **Chronic hyperplastic pulpitis is also called as** ....
Ans. Pulp polyp

48. **Most-accepted theory in etiopathogenesis of dental caries is** ....
Ans. Acidogenic theory

49. **Nikolsky's sign is a feature of** ....
Ans. Pemphigus vulgaris

50. **Keratin pearls are seen in** ....
Ans. Squamous cell carcinoma

51. **Syndrome associated with cherubism** ....
Ans. Noonan syndrome

52. **Monroe's abscess is seen in** ....
Ans. Psoriasis

53. **Shell teeth is also called as** ....
Ans. Brandywine type

54. **Virus infected cells are called as** ....
Ans. Koilocytes

55. **Candida grows in** .... **media.**
Ans. Sabouraud's broth

56. **Two lesion where we find keratin pearls** ....
Ans. Squamous cell carcinoma and pleomorphic adenoma

57. **Hair pin cells are seen in** ....
Ans. Radicular cyst

58. **Define neuralgia** ....
Ans. Neuralgia is defined as the pain along the pathway of nerve

59. **Other name of botryoid cyst** ....
Ans. Lateral periodontal cyst

60. **Subepithelial split is seen in** ....
Ans. Bullous pemphigoid

61. **HPV altered epithelial cells with perinuclear clear spaces and nuclear pyknosis found in squamous papilloma are** ....
Ans. Koilocytes

62. **Scattered macrophages with an abundant clear cytoplasm often containing phagocytic cellular debris, a characteristic histopathological pictures seen in African Jaw Lymphoma is** ....
Ans. Ans. Starry Sky appearance

63. **Characteristic malignant cells of Hodgkin's disease are large cells known as** ....
Ans. Reed-Sternberg cells

64. **Cells with elongated nuclei containing a linear bar of chromatin with radiating processes of chromatin with extension towards nuclear membrane found in aphthous stomatitis are called as** ....
Ans. Anitschkow cells

65. **Softened bone at the base of skull seen in Paget's disease is called as** ....
Ans. Platybasia

66. **Syndrome consisting of a triad of persistent or recurring lip or facial swelling, intermittent seventh (facial) nerve paralysis (Bell's palsy) and fissured tongue is** ....
Ans. Melkersson-Rosenthal syndrome

67. **Herpes simplex infection occurring in fingers due to autoinoculation is called as** ....
Ans. Herpetic Whitlow

68. **Degenerative cells showing swelling of the nuclei and hyperchromatic staining seen in pemphigus vulgaris is** ....
Ans. Tzanck cells

69. **Pronounced hyperextensibility in patients with Ehlers-Danlos syndrome give them appearance called as** ....
Ans. Rubber man

70. **Hunter's glossitis or Moeller's glossitis is characteristic feature of** ....
Ans. Deficiency of vitamin B12

71. **Ruston bodies are seen in** ....
Ans. Radicular cyst, dentigerous cyst and odontogenic keratocyst

72. **Most common carcinoma of skin on middle third of the face** ....
Ans. Basal cell carcinoma

73. **What is leukoedema?**
Ans. Leukoedema is the normal anatomic variant of the oral mucosa which has clinical appearance similar to potentially malignant white lesions

74. **What are natal teeth?**
Ans. Natal teeth are the teeth which are observed in oral cavity just after birth

75. **What is dilacerations?**
Ans. Dilaceration refers to an angulation or a sharp bend or a curve in the root and crown of the formed tooth.

76. Enumerate developmental disturbances in structure of teeth.
Ans. ◆ Amelogenesis imperfecta
    ◆ Dentinogenesis imperfecta
    ◆ Enamel hypoplasia
    ◆ Dentin dysplasia
    ◆ Regional odontodysplasia
    ◆ Dentin hypocalcification

77. Burtonian line is seen in...........................
Ans. Lead poisoning

78. Tuberculosis of lymph nodes is known as...................
Ans. Tuberculous lymphadenitis

79. Tzanck cells are characteristic features of....................
Ans. Pemphigus vulgaris and herpes simplex

80. Sarcoma metastasize through..............
Ans. Vascular system

81. Rootless teeth are seen in.................
Ans. Dentin dysplasia

82. Starry sky appearance is the histopathological feature in..........................
Ans. Burkitt's lymphoma

83. Papillary cystadenoma lymphomatosum is also known as...........................
Ans. Warthin's tumor

84. Raspberry tongue is seen in.................................
Ans. Scarlet fever

85. Hanson's disease is another name for.........................
Ans. Leprosy

86. ....cranial nerve involved in Bell's palsy.
Ans. Seventh

87. Radiographically hair on end appearance is seen in.......................
Ans. Thalassemia and sickle cell anemia

88. Bence Jones proteins are excreted in urine in...........................
Ans. Multiple myeloma

89. Leontiasis ossea is a feature of...........................
Ans. Paget's disease

90. Carpet track appearance is seen in...........................
Ans. Discoid lupus erythematosus

VIVA-VOCE QUESTIONS FOR PRACTICAL EXAMINATION

1. **Name the condition in which teeth get united by the cementum.**
Ans. Concrescence

2. **Name the condition in which in attempt for the division of a single tooth germ by an invagination which causes incomplete formation of two teeth.**
Ans. Gemination

3. **Name the condition in which there is sharp bent or curvature present in the root.**
Ans. Dilaceration

4. **What are the other names of geographic tongue?**
Ans. Wandering rash or erythema migrans

5. **Name the papillae affected in geographic tongue.**
Ans. Filiform papillae

6. **Name the condition characterized by heterotrophic collection of sebaceous glands at various sites in oral cavity.**
Ans. Fordyce's granules

7. **In hairy tongue which papillae of tongue get hypertrophied?**
Ans. Filiform papillae

8. **What is another name of dens evaginatus?**
Ans. Leong's premolar

9. **Which is the most common supernumerary teeth?**
Ans. Mesiodens

10. **Which is second most common supernumerary tooth?**
Ans. Distomolar

11. **By which structure predeciduous teeth are formed of?**
Ans. Hornified epithelial structures

12. **During which stage of tooth development, injury occur which result in enamel hypoplasia.**
Ans. Formative stage

13. **In which condition screw driven-shaped incisors and moon molars are seen?**
Ans. Syphilis

14. **Which condition consists of ghost teeth?**
Ans. Regional odontodysplasia

15. **Name the condition in which there is single tooth hypoplasia due to trauma or infection.**
Ans. Turner's hypoplasia

16. **Name the teeth which erupt prematurely in first thirty days of life.**
Ans. Neonatal teeth

17. **What does ankylosed deciduous tooth known as?**
Ans. Submerged teeth

18. **Name the condition in which there is presence of heart-shaped radiolucency and is bilateral, it is also lined by pseudostratified ciliated epithelium.**
Ans. Nasopalatine duct cyst

19. **What is the another name of klestadt cyst?**
Ans. Nasolabial cyst

20. **What is parulis?**
Ans. It is the inflammatory enlargement which is seen at the terminus of fistula or the sinus tract

21. **In which condition does Epstein pearls and Bohn's nodules are seen?**
Ans. Palatal cyst of neonate

22. **Name the cellular layer which proliferates in papilloma.**
Ans. Spinous cell layer

23. **Which is the most common benign soft tissue neoplasm of oral cavity?**
Ans. Fibroma

24. **Name the carcinoma which show no tendency for the metastasis.**
Ans. Basal cell carcinoma

25. **Name the route by which oral carcinoma metastatize.**
Ans. Lymphatic route

26. **Name the lymph nodes which commonly involved in metastasis of oral cancer.**
Ans. Submaxillary and cervical lymph nodes

27. **Name the disease which is known as self-healing carcinoma.**
Ans. Keratoacanthoma

28. **Name the nevus which is clinically benign but histologically malignant.**
Ans. Spindle cell nevus

29. **Which nevus show abtropfung or dropping off effect.**
Ans. Junctional nevus

30. **Which is the site of highest risk in leukoplakia?**
Ans. Floor of the mouth

31. **Which is the most common precancerous lesion and malignant precancerous lesion?**
Ans. Leukoplakia and erythroplakia

32. **Which is the most common malignancy in males and females?**
Ans. In males, it is lung cancer and in females it is breast cancer.

33. **Which is the most common malignancy in males and females in India?**

Ans. Oral cancer in males and breast cancer in females

34. **What is the hallmark of verrucous carcinoma?**

Ans. Parakeratin plugging

35. **What is the another name of lane tumor?**

Ans. Spindle cell carcinoma

36. **In which lesion epithelial melanocytes are distributed in pagetoid manner?**

Ans. Malignant melanoma

37. **Name the most common benign soft tissue tumor of oral cavity.**

Ans. Fibroma

38. **In which disease foam cells are evident?**

Ans. Verruciform xanthoma

39. **Which is the most common site for occurrence of lymphangioma?**

Ans. Tongue

40. **Which disease is known as Codman's tumor?**

Ans. Benign chondroblastoma

41. **In which disease Codman's triangle is seen?**

Ans. Osteosarcoma

42. **Which tumor show starry sky effect on cytoplasm?**

Ans. Burkitt's lymphoma

43. **In which disease Reed-Sternberg cell is seen?**

Ans. Hodgkin's lymphoma

44. **In which disease cartwheel or checker pattern histopathologic appearance is seen?**

Ans. Multiple myeloma

45. **In which disease Antoni A and Antoni B cells are seen?**

Ans. Neurilemmoma

46. **Name the salivary gland neoplasm in which predilection for men is seen?**

Ans. Warthin's tumor

47. **What is the histological similarity between Mikulicz disease and Sjogren's syndrome?**

Ans. Epimyoepithelial islands

48. **What is the another name of cylindroma.**

Ans. Adenoid cystic carcinoma

49. **Name the salivary gland neoplasm which spread along perineural spaces.**

Ans. Adenoid cystic carcinoma

50. **Which is the most common salivary gland neoplasm.**

Ans. Pleomorphic adenoma

51. **Which is the second most common salivary gland tumor?**

Ans. Warthin's tumor

52. **Name the most common malignant salivary gland neoplasm of children.**

Ans. Mucoepidermoid carcinoma

53. **Which is the most common etiology for necrotizing sialometaplasia?**

Ans. Ischemia

54. **Name the cyst consisting of Rushton bodies.**

Ans. Radicular cyst

55. **Which cyst consists of satellite cysts or daughter cysts?**

Ans. Odontogenic keratocyst

56. **What do you mean by satellite or daughter cyst?**

Ans. They represents the end of folds of lining epithelium of main cystic cavity which are cut in cross section

57. **Which tumor is known as pindborg tumor?**

Ans. Calcifying epithelial odontogenic tumor

58. **In which disease gastric acid decalcification of teeth is present?**

Ans. Anorexia nervosa

59. **What is the another name of pink tooth of Mummery?**

Ans. Internal resorption

60. **Which disease is known as Hansen's disease?**

Ans. Leprosy

61. **Where does pyogenic granuloma is seen commonly in oral cavity?**

Ans. Gingiva

62. **In which disease ballooning degeneration and Lipschutz's bodies are seen?**

Ans. Herpes

63. **Which disease is known as ray fungus?**

Ans. Actinomycosis

64. **Which disease is known as Lues?**

Ans. Syphilis

65. **What is hutchinson's triad?**

Ans. It is hypoplasia of incisor and molar teeth, eighth nerve deafness and interstitial glossitis

66. **Name the cells which are seen in cytologic margin of aphthous ulcer.**

Ans. Anitschkow cells

67. **Name the virus which causes hand, foot and mouth disease and herpangina.**

Ans. Coxsackie virus

68. **In which disease Koplik's spots are seen?**

Ans. Measles

69. **Which disease shows Henderson Peterson bodies?**

Ans. Molluscum contagiosum

70. **Name the syndrome with which herpes zoster is associated.**

Ans. James Ramsay Hunt syndrome

71. **Name the fungal lesion which closely mimics tuberculosis.**

Ans. Histoplasmosis

72. **Name the most common opportunistic infection of the world.**

Ans. Candidiasis

73. **Name the type of candidiasis which leads to pain.**

Ans. Acute atrophic form

74. **Who had given acidogenic theory.**

Ans. WD Miller

75. **Name the bacteria which cause dental caries.**

Ans. *S. mutans*

76. **Name the tooth which is least susceptible to dental caries.**

Ans. Mandibular central incisors

77. **Name the bacteria which leads to root caries.**

Ans. *A. viscosus*

78. **Name the condition in which bacteria circulating in blood leads to pulpal inflammation.**

Ans. Anachoretic pulpitis

79. **Which type of hypersensitivity is caused by periapical granuloma?**

Ans. Delayed hypersensitivity

80. **Name the cyst which develops in maxilla after Caldwell Luc operation.**

Ans. Surgical ciliated cyst of maxilla

81. **Name the disease in which pseudoepitheliomatous hyperplasia and plasma pooling is seen.**

Ans. Epulis fissuratum

82. **Name the mucocele which occurs in the floor of mouth.**

Ans. Ranula

83. **In which disease does test tube rete pegs are seen?**

Ans. Dilantin sodium induced gingival hyperplasia

84. **Name the compound which causes acrodynia or pink disease.**

Ans. Mercury

85. **Name the microorganism which leads to dry socket.**

Ans. *Treponema denticola*

86. **Deficiency of which ions causes tetany.**

Ans. Calcium and magnesium

87. **Which disease show punched out lesions of bone, exophthalmos and diabetes insipidus?**

Ans. Hand Schuller Christian Disease

88. **Deficiency of which vitamin shows Trummerfeld zone.**

Ans. Vitamin C

89. **Name the disease in which high predilection for osteomyelitis is seen after dental extraction.**

Ans. Osteomyelitis

90. **Name the most common complication of Paget's disease.**

Ans. It leads to pathologic fracture

91. **Which is the most common site for monostotic fibrous dysplasia?**

Ans. Ribs

92. **Name the most common cause for the ankylosis of temporomandibular joint.**

Ans. Trauma

93. **In which disease Hunter glossitis is seen?**

Ans. Pernicious anemia

94. **Name the constant feature of pernicious anemia.**

Ans. Achlorhydria

95. **Name the anemia in which there is lack of resistance to infection.**

Ans. Aplastic anemia

96. **Which type of leukemia is most common in children?**

Ans. Acute lymphocytic leukemia

97. **Which type of leukemia is most common in elders?**

Ans. Chronic lymphocytic leukemia

98. **Name the microorganisms causing ANUG.**

Ans. *Borrelia vincentii* and fusiform bacilli

99. **Name the disease in which saw tooth rete pegs with Civatte bodies are seen.**

Ans. Lichen planus

100. **Name the disease which show Auspitz sign, Monroe's abscess.**

Ans. Psoriasis

101. **What is Grinspan syndrome?**

Ans. Lichen planus + Diabetes mellitus + Vascular hypertension

102. **Corps rods and Grains are seen in which disease.**

Ans. Darier's disease.

103. **Name the sign in which there is loss of epithelium on normal rubbing.**

Ans. Nikolsky's sign

104. **Name the disease which show suprabasilar split and Tzanck Cells.**

Ans. Pemphigus

105. **Name the disease which shows histopathological appearance of rosettes of neutrophils which surrounds the lymphocytes.**

Ans. Systemic lupus erythematosus

106. **Name the disease which show hypermobility of TMJ and and increase tendency to form pulp stones.**

Ans. Ehlers-Danlos syndrome

107. **Name the neuralgia which show alarm clock headache with no trigger zone.**

Ans. Sphenopalatine neuralgia

108. **Name the condition in which there is shooting pain with trigger zone in tonsillar fossa.**

Ans. Glossopharyngeal neuralgia

109. **Name the condition in which there is severe pain which arise after sectioning of peripheral sensory nerve.**

Ans. Causalgia

110. **Name the disease in which there is sorrowful appearance of patient with histological appearance of lymphorrhage.**

Ans. Myasthenia gravis

111. **What is melasma?**

Ans. It is the condition in which there is pigmentary changes in associated with the pregnancy or taking the contraceptive pills.

112. **What do you mean by perimolysis?**

Ans. Perimolysis refers to the intrinsic dental erosion of teeth. This occurs in patients, in whom the gastric acid from stomach comes in contact with the teeth.

113. **What do you mean by ameloglyphics?**

Ans. These are tooth print patterns formed by enamel rods end at crown surface of tooth and are recorded by acetate peel technique.

114. **Name the solution which preserves the bite marks on apples presented at crime scene.**

Ans. Campden solution Or 5% acetic acid in 40% aqueous formaldehyde.

ADDITIONAL INFORMATION

Various Signs

Signs	Meaning	Seen in disease
Auspitz's sign	On removing the deep scales single or multiple tiny bleeding spots are seen	Psoriasis
Battle's sign	There is presence of ecchymosis in post-auricular region over mastoid process	In subcondylar fractures and fracture of base of skull
Chvostek's sign	While tapping at the angle of mandible, there is stimulation of facial nerve which leads to twitching of muscles of face over the same side	Tetany
Cluster of Jewel or Rosette sign or string of pearls	There is presence of new bullae over the old ones which show cluster of jewel appearance.	Chronic bullous disease of childhood
Crowe's sign	Presence of axillary freckling	Von Recklinghausen's neurofibromatosis
Dubois sign	Shortening of little finger	Congenital syphilis
Flag sign	Presence of horizontal alternating bands of discoloration over the hair shafts which correspond to the period of normal and abnormal hair growth	Kwashiorkor or ulcerative colitis
Forchheimer sign	Exanthem of red macules are seen over the soft palate	Rubella
Gorlin's sign	Patient touch the tip of nose with extended tongue	Ehlers-Danlos syndrome
Guiren's sign	Presence of ecchymosis near greater palatine foramen	Le Fort I fracture
Higoumenakis sign	Presence of irregular thickening of sternoclavicular portion of clavicle	Congenital syphilis
Hoagland's sign	Presence of early and transient bilateral upper lid edema	Infectious mononucleosis
Hutchinson's nose sign	Vesicles are seen over the tip of nose	Herpes zoster
Jellinek's sign	Pigmentation of eyelid which is occasionally seen	Hyperthyroidism
Nikolsky's sign	Epithelium become lost on rubbing and there is presence of raw or sensitive surface	Pemphigus, recessive form of epidermolysis bullosa
Raccoon sign	Present as periorbital ecchymosis due to subconjunctival hemorrhage	Basilar skull fracture
Shawl sign	Presence of confluent, symmetric, macular violaceous erythema over the shoulder and neck in posterior parts	Dermatomyositis
Tin tack or Carpet track sign	Horney track at the undersurface of scale removed from the lesion	Discoid lupus erythematosus
Trousseau's sign	Presence of carpal spasm after application of pressure on arm by inflating sphygmomanometer cuff	Hypoparathyroidism

Various Types of Cells and Their Associated Diseases

Various types of cells	Disease or pathology associated
Acantholytic cells	Pemphigus
Angulate body cells	Granular cell myoblastoma
Anitschkow cells	Sickle cell anemia, Aphthous ulcer, Iron deficiency anemia, Rheumatic heart disease
Arbiskov cells	Myeloblastoma
Benign dyskeratotic cells Or Corps, Ronds and Grains	Dyskeratosis follicularis
Centrocytes	Non-Hodgkin lymphoma (Follicular variety)
Downey cells	Infectious mononucleosis
Foam cells	Periapical granuloma

Gaucher cells	Gaucher's disease
Ghost cells	Craniopharyngioma, calcifying odontogenic cyst, ameloblastic fibroma and odontoma
Glycogen free clear cell	Mucoepidermoid carcinoma and acinic cell carcinoma
Glycogen rich clear cell	Gingival cyst of adult and lateral periodontal cyst
Hurler cell or Gargoyle cell	Hurler syndrome
Hyaline cell	Pleomorphic adenoma
Koilocytes	Papilloma
Lacunar cells	Hodgkin's lymphoma (Nodular variety)
LE cell	Systemic lupus erythematosus
Lepra cells	Lepromatous leprosy
Nevus cells	Pigmented mole
Pale cells	Odontogenic myxoma
Pericyte of Zimmerman	Glomus tumor
Popcorn cells	Hodgkin's lymphoma (Nodular variety)
Raquet or ribbon cells	Rhabdomyosarcoma
Reed–Sternberg cells	Hodgkin's lymphoma
Safety pin cells	Thalassemia
Touton type multinucleated giant cell	Fibrous histiocytoma
Tzanck cells	Herpes and pemphigus
Warthin Finkeldey giant cells	Measles

Various Spots Associated with Various Pathologies

Name of spots	Presentation of spot	Pathology
Bitot's spot	Present as white plaque in conjunctiva of children	Vitamin A deficiency
Café-au-lait spots	Presence of brown pigmentation on the skin	Fibrous dysplasia, neurofibromatosis, Peutz-Jeghers syndrome
Herald spot	Primary lesion of skin	Pityriasis rosea
Koplik spot	They are characterized as clustered, white lesions on the buccal mucosa opposite the lower 1st and 2nd molars	Measles
Pink spot	Color of tooth become pink	Internal resorption
Roth spot	Retinal hemorrhages with white or pale centers	Subacute bacterial endocarditis and typhoid fever
Sore spot	Presence of traumatic ulcers	Denture irritation

Various Inclusion Bodies Associated with Different Diseases

Inclusion body	Disease associated
Asteroid bodies	Sporotrichosis
Civatte or colloid or hyaline or cytoid bodies	Lichen planus
Cow dry Type A	Herpes simplex
Cow dry Type B	Poliomyelitis
Dohle bodies	Chédiak-Higashi syndrome
Fessas bodies	Thalassemia
Guarnieri bodies	Smallpox virus and Vaccinia virus
Heinz bodies	In G6PD deficiency individuals
Howell-Jolly body	Pernicious anemia
Lipschutz bodies	Primary herpetic stomatitis

Molluscum bodies or Henderson-Paterson inclusion	*Molluscum contagiosum*
Negri bodies	Rabies
Pappenheimer bodies	Sideroblastic anemia
Psammoma bodies	Papillary carcinoma of thyroid
Reilly bodies	Hurler syndrome
Rushton bodies	Inflamed dentigerous cyst, periapical cyst, gingival cyst of neonate
Russell bodies	Periapical granuloma, inflammatory conditions and multiple myeloma
Verocay bodies	Neurilemmoma

Various Specific Epithelial Rete Pegs Associated with Some Specific Diseases

Type of rete pegs	Disease associated
Absence of rete pegs	Oral submucous fibrosis
Saw tooth rete pegs	Lichen planus
Test tube rete pegs	Dilantin hyperplasia

Various Important Diagnostic Tests for Various Diseases

Diagnostic test	Disease
Dick test	Scarlet fever
Elisa and Western blot test	Acquired immunodeficiency syndrome (AIDS)
Figlu excretion test	Folic acid absorption
Freis test	Lymphogranuloma venereum
Gordons biological test	Hodgkin's lymphoma
VDRL and FTA ABS	Syphilis
Kveim test	Sarcoidosis
Mantoux test	Tuberculosis
Paul Bunnell test	Infectious mononucleosis
Prick skin or scratch skin test	For allergic skin reactions
Rose-Waller test	Rheumatoid arthritis
Schiller's test	Cervical carcinoma
Schilling's test	Vitamin B12 deficiency
Schimmer's test or Rose Bengal test	Sjögren's syndrome
Schick test	Diphtheria
Sweat test	Cystic fibrosis
Tzanck test	Pemphigus and Herpes simplex
Weil-felix test	Rickettsial manifestations

Incubation Periods of Various Diseases

Various diseases	Incubation periods
Chickenpox	2 to 3 weeks
Rubella	2 to 3 weeks
Mumps	2 to 3 weeks
Diphtheria	1 to 5 days
Typhoid	1 to 5 days
Cholera	1 to 5 days
Hepatitis A	2 to 7 weeks

Hepatitis B	7 to 23 weeks
Influenza	1 to 3 days
Measles	10 days
Tetanus	3 to 21 days

Characteristic Features of Tongue in Various Conditions

Appearance or changes in tongue	Condition
Atrophic glossitis	Iron deficiency anemia and pernicious anemia
Bald tongue of sandwith	Pellagra
Bifid tongue or cleft tongue	Orofacial digital syndrome
Black hairy tongue	Chronic antibiotic therapy
Cerebriform tongue	Pemphigus vegetans
Hunter's glossitis	Pernicious anemia
Luetic glossitis	Syphilis
Magenta colored tongue	Riboflavin deficiency
Migratory glossitis	Geographic tongue
Strawberry tongue	Scarlet fever
Tetanus	3 to 21 days

Various Theories of Dental Caries and Their Authors

Theory of dental caries	Author
Acidogenic theory or chemico-parasitic theory	Miller
Acidic theory	Robertson
Parasitic theory	Dubos
Proteolytic theory	Gottileb
Proteolysis chelation theory	Schartz and Martin
Sulfatase theory	Pincus
Sucrose chelation theory	Burch and Jackson

Important Terminologies with Their Meanings in Oral Pathology

Terminology	Meaning
Macule	It is the focal area of color change which is not elevated or depressed in relation to the surroundings
Papule	It is a solid and raised lesion which is less than 5 mm in diameter
Nodule	It is a solid and raised lesion which is more than 5 mm in diameter
Vesicle	It is a superficial blister which is 5 mm or less in diameter and is filled by the clear fluid
Bulla	It is a large blister which is more than 5 mm in diameter
Sessile	It is a tumor or the growth whose base is the widest part of lesion
Pedunculated	It is a tumor or the growth whose base is narrow and is widest part of lesion
Papillary	It is a tumor or growth having numerous projections
Verrucous	It is a tumor or growth having rough and warty surface
Pustule	It is a blister which is filled with purulent exudates
Ulcer	Ulcer is characterized by loss of epithelium along with underlying connective tissue
Erosion	It is characterized by the partial or total loss of surface epithelium
Fissure	It is a narrow slit like ulceration or groove

Plaque	It is a lesion which is slightly elevated and is flat on its surface
Petechiae	It is pinpoint area of hemorrhage
Ecchymosis	It is a non-elevated area of hemorrhage which is larger than petechiae

Various Skin Diseases and Their Fluorescent Appearance

Skin disease	Fluorescent appearance
Pemphigus	Granular intercellular space fluorescence
Lichen planus	Fluorescence is seen at basement membrane zone with multiple extension in lamina propria
Cicatricial pemphigoid	Presence of patchy linear pattern at basement membrane zone
Bullous pemphigoid	Presence of patchy linear pattern at basement membrane zone
Erythema multiforme	Presence of patchy linear pattern
Discoid lupus erythematosus	Presence of speckled or particulate pattern at basement membrane zone
Systemic lupus erythematosus	Fluorescence is seen at basement membrane zone with multiple extension in superficial lamina propria

Various Microorganisms and Their Associated Pathologies

Microorganism	Associated pathology
Streptococcus mutans	They causes initiation of smooth surface caries
Streptococcus sanguis	They causes dental caries and subacute bacterial endocarditis
Streptococcus salivarius	They causes subacute bacterial endocarditis
Streptococcus pyogenes	They leads to pharyngitis, Ludwig's angina, cellulitis
Staphylococci	They leads to skin infections, osteomyelitis, sialadenitis
Staphylococcus aureus	They lead to sialadenitis, toxic shock syndrome
Lactobacillus	They lead to the progression of dental caries
Actinomyces viscosus	They causes multiple abscess
Prevotella intermedia	It causes pregnancy gingivitis
Capnocytophaga	It causes puberty gingivitis
Porphyromonas gingivalis	It causes generalized juvenile periodontitis
A. Actinomycetemcomitans	It causes localized juvenile periodontitis
Clostridium tetani	Tetanus
Fusospirochete	Acute necrotizing ulcerative gingivitis
Treponema pallidum	Syphilis
Clostridium perfringens	Gas gangrene
Treponema denticola	Dry socket
TOGA virus	German measles
Human papilloma virus	Papilloma or wart
Paramyxovirus	Mumps and measles

Various Teeth Which are Associated with Specific Pathologies

Pathology	Teeth Associated
Natal teeth which is commonly seen	Deciduous mandibular central incisor
Most common ankylosed or submerged tooth	Deciduous mandibular second molar and permanent first and second molars
Most common permanent tooth which show variation in size and shape	Maxillary lateral incisor
Which tooth is affected commonly by dens evaginatus	Premolars

Teeth most commonly affected in concrescence	Permanent maxillary molars mainly the third molar
Teeth commonly affected by microdontia	Permanent maxillary lateral incisors and third molars
Teeth known as ghost teeth	Permanent maxillary and mandibular anterior teeth
Teeth which get impacted commonly	Third molars and maxillary canines
Teeth most commonly show supernumerary roots	Mandibular canine and the premolars
Name the permanent teeth which are most commonly missing	Third molars, permanent maxillary lateral incisor and permanent mandibular second molar
Name the deciduous teeth which are most commonly missing	Deciduous maxillary lateral incisor and deciduous mandibular lateral incisor
Which are the teeth which get commonly extracted for orthodontic purpose	Maxillary and mandibular first premolars
Name the tooth which most commonly shows variation in its eruption timing	Mandibular second premolar
Which tooth is known as taurodont or exhibit taurodontism	Deciduous or permanent molars
Name the tooth which is commonly affected by benign cementoblastoma and condensing osteitis	Permanent mandibular first molar
Name the tooth affected by pulp polyp	Deciduous molars and maxillary or mandibular permanent first molars
Name the teeth affected most commonly by nursing bottle caries	Deciduous maxillary incisors
Name the teeth which get prevented in nursing bottle caries	Deciduous mandibular incisors

Various Jaw Abnormalities and Their Association with the Diseases

Jaw abnormalities	Disease associated
Decrease in size of mandible or underdeveloped mandible	• Pierre Robinson syndrome • Treacher Collins syndrome
Decrease in size of maxilla or underdeveloped maxilla	• Cleidocranial dysostosis • Osteogenesis imperfect • Achondroplasia • Down syndrome
Decrease in size of both maxilla and mandible or underdeveloped maxilla and mandible	Hypopituitarism
Increase in size of maxilla	Monostotic fibrous dysplasia
Increase in size of mandible	Acromegaly
Increase in size of both maxilla and mandible	Paget's disease

Lesion/Condition	Radiological appearance
Acute osteomyelitis	Moth eaten radiolucency
Aneurysmal bone cyst	Honeycomb or soap bubble appearance
Apert's syndrome	Skull radiograph "Beaten metal" pattern
Calcifying epithelial odontogenic tumor	Driven snow appearance
Cemento-osseous dysplasia	Cotton wool radiopacities
Central hemangioma	Honey combed or sunburst or cotton wool appearance
Cherubism	Ground glass appearance; floating teeth syndrome
Chronic diffuse sclerosing osteomyelitis	Cotton wool appearance/mosaic pattern
Coronal dentin dysplasia	Thistle tube appearance
Crouzon syndrome	Skull radiograph "Beaten metal" pattern

Dentinogenesis imperfecta – 2	Shell teeth
Ewing' s sarcoma	Onion skin appearance; sunray appearance rarely
Fibrous dysplasia	Ground glass appearance; Rind sign
Garre's osteomyelitis	Onion peel appearance
Gaucher's disease	Erlenmeyer flask deformity of distal femur
Gigantiform cementoma	Cotton wool radio-opacities
Globulomaxillary cyst	Pear-shaped radiolucency between maxillary lateral incisor and canine
Gardner syndrome	Cotton wool radio-opacities
Hemangioma	Hair on end or crew cut appearance
Hyperparathyroidism	Partial loss of lamina dura; ground glass appearance of bone
Hypophosphatasemia	Metaphyses of long bone show spotty or streaky or irregular ossifications
Meningioma	Hair on end or crew cut appearance
Multiple myeloma	Punched out areas of radiolucency
Nasopalatine duct cyst	Heart-shaped radiolucency between roots of maxillary central incisors
Odontogenic myxoma	Honey comb/mottled appearance
Osteomalacia	Looser's zone pseudofracture line
Osteopetrosis	Vertebrae-Rugger-Jersey pattern; Ribs-Endo bone (Bone within bone) pattern; roots are not easily distinguishable from adjacent bone
Osteosarcoma	Intramedullary parts appears as cumulus cloud densities; sunray/sun burst pattern; widening of periodontal ligament; Codman's triangle (periosteum raised like tent)
Paget's disease	Osteoporosis circumscripta; cotton wool appearance; hypercementosis; loss of lamina dura
Plasmacytoma	Hair on end or crew cut appearance
Primary intraosseous carcinoma	Moth eaten radiolucency
Pseudohypoparathyroidism	Chevron pulp
Psoriatic arthritis	Pencil cup appearance; opera glass deformity in joints
Regional odontodysplasia	Ghost teeth
Rickets	Muller's line (Widened space @ the site of zone of preparatory calcification) Rachitic rosary—costochondral prominence
Scleroderma	Widening of lamina dura; bone resorption at angle, condyle or coronoid area
Scurvy and chronic vitamin C deficiency	Increased density @ end of long bones as white lines—"line of Frenkel"; Signet ring appearance of epiphyses; Zone of rarefaction around white lines—represents "Trummerfeld zone" Sclerotic ring around epiphyses—"Wimberger' line" Metaphyseal corner fracture—"Pelkan spur"
Severe iron deficiency in childhood	Hair on end or crew cut appearance
Sialadenosis (sialography)	Leafless tree
Sickle cell anemia	Hair on end or crew cut appearance
Sjögren's syndrome (sialography)	Branchless fruit laden tree or cherry blossom appearance
Synovial sarcoma	Spotty calcification; snow storm appearance
Synovial sarcoma	Snow storm appearance
Thalassemia	Rib within a rib appearance of rib; hair on end or crew cut appearance; salt and pepper effect; thin lamina dura

ABCDE Rule which Helps in Diagnosis of Malignant Melanoma

- Asymmetry in which one half does not match another half.
- Border irregularity
- Color irregularity
- Diameter more than 6 mm
- Elevated surface

Diseases which are Genetically Transmitted

Name of the Disease	Type of Inheritance
• Sickle cell anemia • Thalassemia • Chediak-Higashi syndrome • Agnathia	Autosomal recessive
Hemophilia	Sex linked recessive
Cleft lip and cleft palate	Polygenic and multifactorial
• Osteogenesis imperfecta • Amelogenesis imperfecta • Dentinogenesis imperfecta • Sickle cell trait • Von Willebrand's disease • White sponge nevus • Cherubism • Achondroplasia • Cleidocranial dysplasia • Apert syndrome • Color blindness	All are autosomal dominant
Van der Woude syndrome	Chromosome 1
Peutz-Jeghers syndrome	There is mutation of *STK11* gene which is located on Chromosome 19
Osteogenesis imperfecta	Chromosome 19
Marfan's syndrome	Chromosome 15
Cherubism	Chromosome 4

Various Diseases with some of the Similar Features

Keratin plugging	• Fordyce's granules • Verrucous carcinoma • Verrucous xanthoma • Keratoacanthoma • Discoid lupus erythematosis
Premature exfoliation of teeth	• Juvenile diabetes • Juvenile periodontitis • Papillon–Lefevre syndrome • Chediak–Higashi syndrome • Eosinophilic granuloma • Letterer–Siwe disease • Hand–Schuller Christian disease • Hypophosphatasia • Dentin dysplasia • Acrodynia • Cherubism
Intraepithelial bulla	• Herpes simplex • Herpes zoster • Chickenpox • Pemphigus • Familial benign pemphigus • Epidermolysis bullosa • As oral lesion in erythema multiforme
Subepithelial bulla	• Pemphigoid • Bullous pemphigoid • Bullous lichen planus • Epidermolysis bullosa • As skin lesion in erythema multiforme

Both intraepithelial and subepithelial bulla	• Erythema multiforme • Paraneoplastic pemphigus • Epidermolysis bullosa
Tzanck cells	• Pemphigus • Herpes
Multinucleated giant cells	• Tuberculosis • Cherubism • Herpes • Aneurysmal bone cyst • Hyperparathyroidism • Osteosarcoma • Osteoclastoma • Giant cell granuloma • Eosinophilic granuloma • Leprosy
Ghost cells	• Calcifying epithelial odontogenic cyst • Odontoma • Ameloblastic fibro-odontoma • Craniopharyngioma
Bence Jones protein	• Multiple myeloma • Leukemia • Polycythemia vera
Abnormal DEJ	• Ehlers–Danlos syndrome • Dentinogenesis imperfect
Nikolsky's sign	• Pemphigus • Familial benign pemphigus • Epidermolysis bullosa
Rushton bodies	• Periapical cyst • Dentigerous cyst • Neonatal cyst
Pseudoepitheliomatous hyperplasia	• Discoid lupus erythematous • Granular cell myoblastoma • Keratoacanthoma • Blastomycosis • Papillary hyperplasia • Necrotizing sialometaplasia
Café-au-lait pigmentation	• Polyostotic fibrous dysplasia • Peutz–Jegher's syndrome • Hypothyroidism • Neurofibroma
Russell bodies	• Multiple myeloma • Periapical granuloma
Juxtaepithelial hyalinization	• OSMF • Chondroectodermal dysplasia
Microcyst formation	• Neurilemmoma • Mucoepidermoid carcinoma • Acinic cell carcinoma • Squamous odontogenic tumor
Snake track ulcer	• Secondary syphilis • Pyostomatitis vegetans
True Koebner phenomenon	• Psoriasis • Vitiligo • Lichen planus

IMPORTANT CLASSIFICATIONS

Classification of Supernumerary Teeth
According to the Morphology
- **Conical:** This small peg-shaped conical tooth is supernumerary tooth.
- **Tuberculate:** This type of supernumerary tooth possesses more than one cusp or tubercle. It is of barrel shaped and may be invaginated.
- **Supplemental:** It refers to the duplication of the teeth in normal series. The most common tooth is permanent maxillary lateral incisor.
- **Odontome:** This represents the hamartomatous malformation.

According to Location
- **Mesiodens:** They are located between two upper central incisor.
- **Distomolars:** They are located on the distal aspect of regular molar teeth in dental arch.
- **Paramolar:** They are located either in buccal or lingual aspect of normal molars.
- **Extralateral incisors:** They are more common in maxillary arch.

Classification of Amelogenesis Imperfecta
Witkop, 1988 Four major categories-based primarily on phenotype (hypoplastic, hypomaturation, hypocalcified, hypomaturation-hypoplastic with taurodontism) subdivided into 15 subtypes by phenotype and secondarily by mode of inheritance.

Type I: Hypoplastic
Type IA: Hypoplastic, pitted autosomal dominant

Type IB: Hypoplastic, local autosomal dominant

Type IC: Hypoplastic, local autosomal recessive

Type ID: Hypoplastic, smooth autosomal dominant

Type IE: Hypoplastic, smooth X-linked dominant

Type IF: Hypoplastic, rough autosomal dominant

Type IG: Enamel agenesis, autosomal recessive

Type II: Hypomaturation
Type IIA: Hypomaturation, pigmented autosomal recessive

Type IIB: Hypomaturation, X-linked recessive

Type IIC: Hypomaturation, snow-capped teeth, X-linked

Type IID: Hypomaturation, snow-capped teeth, autosomal dominant?

Type II: Hypocalcified
Type IIIA: Autosomal dominant

Type IIIB: Autosomal recessive

Type IV: Hypomaturation-hypoplastic with taurodontism
Type IVA: Hypomaturation-hypoplastic with taurodontism, autosomal dominant

Type IVB: Hypoplastic-hypomaturation with taurodontism, autosomal dominant

Classification of White Lesions of Oral Cavity
- **Hereditary condition:**
  - Leukoedema
  - White sponge nevus
  - Hereditary benign intraepithelial dyskeratosis
  - Keratosis follicularis
  - Tylosis syndrome
- **Leukoplakia and malignancies:**
  - Chronic cheek biting
  - Friction or trauma-associated leukoplakia
  - Tobacco associated leukoplakia
  - Carcinoma in situ
  - Squamous cell carcinoma
  - Verrucous carcinoma.
- **Dermatosis:**
  - Lichen planus
  - Lupus erythematous.
- **Inflammation:**
  - Mucous patches of syphilis
  - Candidiasis
  - Koplik spots of measles.
- **Miscellaneous conditions:**
  - Oral submucous fibrosis
  - Papilloma
  - Lipoma
  - Hairy tongue
  - Geographic tongue
  - Fordyce's granules.

Classification of Hemangiomas by Watson and McCarthy
- Capillary hemangioma
- Cavernous hemangioma
- Angioblastic hemangioma
- Racemose hemangioma
- Diffuse systemic hemangioma
- Metastasizing hemangioma
- Port-Wine stain
- Hereditary hemorrhagic telangiectasia

Classification of Giant Cell Lesions of Oral Cavity
- According to the nature of different pathologic conditions
  - *infections*
    - Bacterial
    - Viral
    - Fungal
    - Protozoal
    - Parasitic
  - *Fibro-osseous lesions and osteodystrophies*
    - Immunologic
    - Idiopathic
    - Orofacial granulomatosis
    - Reaction to materials
    - Benign and malignant tumors